Oculofacial, Orbital, and Lacrimal Surgery

Acknowledgments

Throughout life, only by sharing knowledge can we understand what we do not know, which, thus continuously, pushes the envelope of learning further.

This compendium, containing 66 chapters covering much of the range of oculofacial plastic surgery, has required the immense time and support of numerous surgeons (oculofacial, plastic surgery, facial plastic surgery, otolaryngology, neurosurgery) and medical professionals from all over the world, all of whom are, first and foremost, generous souls who also happen to be dedicated physicians and teachers. Many of these internationally renowned experts have written their own books, which demonstrates the immense drive they feel to continuously give others the skills to become better providers for our patients. We wanted to let them freely format their own chapter, so that they could approach the topic and emphasize the highlights in a flow that would be similar to how they would teach you directly. I am truly humbled by the talent of all the authors.

I would like to recognize my coeditor, Adam, for his work in starting this vast endeavor, Springer for all their support, and Mr. Sushil Kumar Sharma (Project Coordinator) and their illustrator for their efforts through the publication process.

I would also like to thank my family, Jason and Hisa Schoephoester for their unwavering support, especially when this project required me to be apart from them for significant periods of time, and to my parents, Quang and Kim Nguyen, who brought me from Vietnam to give me amazing opportunities. Both Adam and I are also grateful for the critical foundations our preceptors have given us throughout our education.

We are all learning from the many past giants in our fields, and we will all move on as younger pioneers come forth. We should be proud of our vast accomplishments and help our field break new and exciting grounds together.

With respect,

Cat Nguyen Burkat, MD, FACS

This work was supported in part by an unrestricted grant from Research to Prevent Blindness, Inc. to the University of Wisconsin-Madison Department of Ophthalmology and Visual Sciences.

Contents

Contributors

Richard C. Allen, MD, PhD, FACS Section of Ophthalmology, Department of Head and Neck Surgery, The University of Texas MD Anderson Cancer Center, Houston, TX, USA

Shaloo Bageja, DNB, MBBS Senior Consultant, Ophthalmology, New Delhi, India

Francesco P. Bernardini, MD Oculoplastica Bernardini, Genova, Italy

Julie Jordan Brown Anaplastology, Medical Art Resources, Inc, Milwaukee, WI, USA

Kendall Burgett Indiana University School of Medicine, Fishers, IN, USA

Cat Nguyen Burkat, MD, FACS Department of Ophthalmology and Visual Sciences, University of Wisconsin-Madison, Madison, WI, USA

Alison B. Callahan, MD Tufts Medical Center, Ophthalmology, Boston, MA, USA

Ashley Campbell, MD Division of Oculoplastics, John Hopkins Wilmer Eye Institute, Baltimore, MD, USA

Ricardo L. Carrau, MD Department of Otolaryngology – Head and Neck Surgery, The Ohio State University Wexner Medical Center, Columbus, OH, USA

Scott R. Chaiet, MD, MBA, FACS Division of Otolaryngology – Head and Neck Surgery, Department of Surgery, University of Wisconsin-Madison, Madison, WI, USA

Christopher B. Chambers, MD Department of Ophthalmology/Plastic Surgery, University of Washington, Seattle, WA, USA

Valerie H. Chen, MD Department of Ophthalmology, Albany Medical College, Albany, NY, USA

Ophthalmic Plastic Surgery, Lions Eye Institute-Albany Medical Center, Slingerlands, NY, USA

Raymond I. Cho, MD, FACS Department of Ophthalmology and Visual Science, The Ohio State University Wexner Medical Center, Columbus, OH, USA

Adam J. Cohen, MD Eyelid & Facial Plastic and Reconstructive Surgery, Chicago and Glenview, IL, USA

Jordan R. Conger, MD Division of Oculofacial Plastic and Orbital Surgery, Gavin Herbert Eye Institute, Irvine, CA, USA

Department of Ophthalmology, University of California, Irvine, School of Medicine, Irvine, CA, USA

Ashley M. Crane, MD Division of Oculofacial Plastic and Reconstructive Surgery, Bascom Palmer Eye Institute, Department of Ophthalmology, University of Miami Miller School of Medicine, Miami, FL, USA

Sarah W. DeParis, MD Department of Oculoplastic Surgery, Wilmer Eye Institute/Johns Hopkins Hospital, Baltimore, MD, USA

Martin H. Devoto, MD Consultores Oftalmologicos, Ciudad de Buenos Aires, Argentina

Angela Maria Dolmetsch, MD Clínica de Oftalmología de Cali, Cali, Valle del Cauca, Colombia

Pontificia Universidad Javeriana, Cali, Valle del Cauca, Colombia

Jonathan J. Dutton, MD University of North Carolina, Durham, NC, USA

Moisés Enghelberg, MD Department of Ophthalmology, Larkin Community Hospital, South Miami, FL, USA

Benjamin P. Erickson, MD Division of Oculofacial Plastic and Reconstructive Surgery, Bascom Palmer Eye Institute, Department of Ophthalmology, University of Miami Miller School of Medicine, Miami, FL, USA

Joseph A. Eviatar, MD, FACS Facial Aesthetics, Omni Aesthetic MD, New York, NY, USA

Aaron Fay, MD Department of Ophthalmology, Harvard Medical School, Boston, MA, USA

John P. Fezza, MD Center for Sight, Sarasota, FL, USA

Jacinto García-Lorenzo Otorhinolaryngology Department, Hospital de Sant Pau, Barcelona, Spain

Alessandro Gennai, MD Oculoplastica Bernardini, Genova, Italy

Dan Georgescu, MD, PhD Oculofacial Institute, Fort Lauderdale, FL, USA

Shubhra Goel, MD Ophthalmic Facial Plastic and Cosmetic Surgery, Apollo Hospitals, Hyderabad, India

Juan-Ramon Gras-Cabrerizo Otorhinolaryngology Department, Hospital de Sant Pau, Barcelona, Spain

Gregory G. Grecco Indiana University School of Medicine, Indianapolis, IN, USA

Alexander Grigalunas, MD Departments of Ophthalmology and Neurology, Rush University Medical Center, Chicago, IL, USA

Seanna R. Grob, MD Division of Oculofacial Plastic and Orbital Surgery, Gavin Herbert Eye Institute, Irvine, CA, USA

Department of Ophthalmology, University of California, Irvine, School of Medicine, Irvine, CA, USA

A. K. Grover, MD, MNAMS, FRCS(GLAS), FIMSA Sir Ganga Ram Hospital, New Delhi, India

Andrew R. Harrison, MD Department of Ophthalmology, University of Minnesota, Minneapolis, MN, USA

Morris E. Hartstein, MD, FACS Department of Ophthalmology, Assaf Harofeh Medical Center, Tel Aviv University-Sackler School of Medicine, Tel Aviv, Israel

John T. Harvey, MD Division of Ophthalmology, McMaster University, Hamilton, ON, Canada

Sarah M. Jacobs, MD Department of Ophthalmology, University of Alabama at Birmingham, Birmingham, AL, USA

Miral Jhaveri, MD Rush University Medical Center, Chicago, IL, USA

James Johnston Ocularists Limited, Des Plaines, IL, USA

David R. Jordan, MD, FACS, FRCSC Department of Ophthalmology, University of Ottawa Eye Institute, Ottawa, ON, Canada

Naresh Joshi, MD, FRCOphth Oculoplastic and Craniofacial Service, Chelsea and Westminster Hospital, London, UK

William R. Katowitz, MD The Perelman School of Medicine at the University of Pennsylvania, Philadelphia, PA, USA

The Children's Hospital of Philadelphia, Philadelphia, PA, USA

Pelin Kaynak, MD Rufus Eye Microsurgical Center, Ophthalmic Plastic and Reconstructive Surgery Division, Istanbul, Turkey

Don O. Kikkawa, MD, FACS Division of Oculofacial Plastic and Reconstructive Surgery, UC San Diego Department of Ophthalmology, Shiley Eye Institute, La Jolla, CA, USA

Division of Plastic Surgery, UC San Diego Department of Plastic Surgery, La Jolla, CA, USA

Stephen R. Klapper, MD Department of Ophthalmology, Klapper Eyelid and Facial Plastic Surgery, Indiana University School of Medicine, Carmel, IN, USA

Christina Kong University of California, Irvine School of Medicine, Irvine, CA, USA

Qiang Kwong, MD, FRCOphth Oculoplastic and Craniofacial Service, Chelsea and Westminster Hospital, London, UK

Suzanne W. van Landingham, MD Department of Ophthalmology and Visual Sciences, University of Wisconsin-Madison, Madison, WI, USA

Paul D. Langer, MD Institute of Ophthalmology and Visual Science, Rutgers New Jersey Medical School, Newark, NJ, USA

Bradford W. Lee, MD, MSc Division of Oculofacial Plastic and Reconstructive Surgery, Bascom Palmer Eye Institute, Department of Ophthalmology, University of Miami Miller School of Medicine, Miami, FL, USA

Hui Bae Harold Lee, MD, FACS Department of Ophthalmology, St Vincent Hospital, Indianapolis, IN, USA

Iris Lee, MD Casey Eye Institute, Oregon Health & Science University, Portland, OR, USA

Emmy Y. Li, MPH, FRCS, FCOphthKH Department of Ophthalmology, Hong Kong Eye Hospital, Kowloon City, Hong Kong

Richard D. Lisman, MD, FACS Ophthalmology/Plastic Surgery, NYU School of Medicine, New York, NY, USA

Ophthalmology/Plastic Surgery, Manhattan Eye, Ear and Throat Hospital, New York, NY, USA

Christopher C. Lo, MD Oculoplastic and Orbital Surgery, UCLA Doheny and Stein Eye Institutes, Los Angeles, CA, USA

Daniele Lorenzano, MD Moorfields Eye Hospital, London, UK

Peter W. MacIntosh, MD Department of Ophthalmology, University of Illinois, Chicago, IL, USA

Nicholas Mahoney, MD Department of Ophthalmology, Johns Hopkins Hospital, Baltimore, MD, USA

Maureen Maloney-Schou Maloney's Custom Ocular Prosthetics Inc, Lake Oswego, OR, USA

Humbert Massegur Otorhinolaryngology Department, Hospital de Sant Pau, Barcelona, Spain

Medical School of Girona University, Girona, Spain

Dale R. Meyer, MD Ophthalmic Plastic Surgery, Lions Eye Institute-Albany Medical Center, Slingerlands, NY, USA

Ana Filipa Duarte, MD Department of Ophthalmology, Centro Hospitalar de Lisboa Central, Lisbon, Portugal

Department of Ophthalmology, Hospital Cuf Descobertas, Lisbon, Portugal

Meena Moorthy Carmel, IN, USA

Joshua M. Moran The Chicago Medical School at Rosalind Franklin University, North Chicago, IL, USA

Murali Nagarajan, MD Rush University Medical Center, Chicago, IL, USA

Akshay Gopinathan Nair, MBBS, DNB Ophthalmic Plastic Surgery and Ocular Oncology Services, Advanced Eye Hospital and Institute, Navi Mumbai, India

Ophthalmic Plastic Surgery and Ocular Oncology Services, Aditya Jyot Eye Hospital, Mumbai, India

John D. Ng, MD, FACS Departments of Ophthalmology and Otolaryngology/Head & Neck Surgery, Casey Eye Institute, Oregon Health & Science University, Portland, OR, USA

Daniel J. Oh, MD Illinois Eye and Ear Infirmary, University of Illinois at Chicago, Chicago, IL, USA

Jane Olver, MBBS, FRCOphth Oculoplastic and Lacrimal, Clinica London, London, UK

Rakesh M. Patel, MD Department of Ophthalmology, University of South Carolina and Prisma Health, Columbia, SC, USA

Alice Varanda Pereira, MD Plastic Reconstructive Surgery, Central Lisbon Hospital Center, Lisbon, Portugal

C. Blake Perry, MD Aesthetic Surgery Centre, Tacoma, WA, USA

Chau Pham, MD Department of Ophthalmology, University of Illinois, Chicago, IL, USA

Paul O. Phelps, MD Division of Ophthalmology, Department of Surgery, NorthShore University HealthSystem, Glenview, IL, USA

Ophthalmology and Visual Science, University of Chicago Medical Center, Chicago, IL, USA

Daniel L. Prevedello, MD Department of Neurological Surgery, The Ohio State University Wexner Medical Center, Columbus, OH, USA

Alkis J. Psaltis, MBBS(HONS), PhD, FRACS(ORL) Department of Otolaryngology Head and Neck Surgery, The Queen Elizabeth Hospital, Adelaide, South Australia

Department of Surgery, The University of Adelaide, Adelaide, South Australia

Allen M. Putterman, MD University of Illinois College of Medicine, Chicago, IL, USA

Vito Quatela, MD Quatela Center for Plastic Surgery, Rochester, NY, USA

Leon Rafailov, MD Institute of Ophthalmology and Visual Science, Rutgers New Jersey Medical School, Newark, NJ, USA

Geoffrey E. Rose, MBBS, DSc, MRCP, FRCS, FRCOphth Moorfields Eye Hospital, London, UK

Institute of Ophthalmology, London, UK

City University, London, UK

Katherine Rose, MD Division of Plastic and Reconstructive Surgery, University of Wisconsin-Madison, Madison, WI, USA

Preamjit Saonanon, MD Department of Ophthalmology, Faculty of Medicine, Chulalongkorn University, Bangkok, Thailand

Department of Ophthalmology, King Chulalongkorn Memorial Hospital, Thai Red Cross Society, Bangkok, Thailand

Amrita Sawhney, MBBS, DNB, MNAMS Associate Consultant, Ophthalmology, New Delhi, India

Richard Scawn, MD, FRCOphth Oculoplastic and Craniofacial Service, Chelsea and Westminster Hospital, London, UK

Katherine Schou Lake Oswego, OR, USA

Kevin R. Schou Maloney's Custom Ocular Prosthetics Inc, Lake Oswego, OR, USA

Robert Schwarcz, MD Ophthalmology, Division of Oculoplastic Surgery, Mount Sinai Hospital, ICAHN School of Medicine, New York, NY, USA

John Siebert, MD Division of Plastic and Reconstructive Surgery, University of Wisconsin-Madison, Madison, WI, USA

Pete Setabutr, MD Illinois Eye and Ear Infirmary, University of Illinois at Chicago, Chicago, IL, USA

Chirag M. Shah, MD Division of Oculofacial Plastic and Orbital Surgery, Gavin Herbert Eye Institute, Irvine, CA, USA

Department of Ophthalmology, University of California, Irvine, School of Medicine, Irvine, CA, USA

William E. Silver, MD Department of Otolaryngology, Head and Neck Surgery, Emory University, Atlanta, GA, USA

Atlanta Institute for Facial Aesthetic Surgery, Atlanta, GA, USA

Brent Skippen, MD Oculoplastica Bernardini, Genova, Italy

Danny J. Soares, MD Department of Otolaryngology, Head and Neck Surgery, University of Central Florida College of Medicine, Orlando, FL, USA

Mesos Plastic and Laser Surgery, Lady Lake, FL, USA

Eric A. Steele, MD Casey Eye Institute, Oregon Health & Science University, Portland, OR, USA

Krista Stewart, MD Department of Ophthalmology, University of Minnesota, Minneapolis, MN, USA

Michael C. Struck, MD University of Wisconsin School of Medicine and Public Health, Madison, WI, USA

Aimee J. Szewka, MD Departments of Ophthalmology and Neurology, Rush University Medical Center, Chicago, IL, USA

Jeremiah Tao, MD Division of Oculofacial Plastic and Orbital Surgery, Gavin Herbert Eye Institute, Irvine, CA, USA

Department of Ophthalmology, University of California, Irvine, School of Medicine, Irvine, CA, USA

Megan Spindel Thomas Anaplastology, Medical Art Resources, Inc, Milwaukee, WI, USA

Alexandre Bossi Todeschini, MD Department of Neurological Surgery, The Ohio State University Wexner Medical Center, Columbus, OH, USA

Ann Q. Tran, MD Department of Ophthalmology and Visual Sciences, University of Wisconsin-Madison, Madison, WI, USA

Kimberly D. Tran, MD Division of Oculofacial Plastic and Reconstructive Surgery, Bascom Palmer Eye Institute, Department of Ophthalmology, University of Miami Miller School of Medicine, Miami, FL, USA

Brian C. Tse, MD Division of Oculofacial Plastic and Reconstructive Surgery, Bascom Palmer Eye Institute, Department of Ophthalmology, University of Miami Miller School of Medicine, Miami, FL, USA

Roger E. Turbin, MD Institute of Ophthalmology and Visual Science, Rutgers New Jersey Medical School, Newark, NJ, USA

Kyle VanKoevering, MD Department of Otolaryngology – Head and Neck Surgery, The Ohio State University Wexner Medical Center, Columbus, OH, USA

Catherine Weng, MD Quatela Center for Plastic Surgery, Rochester, NY, USA

Edward J. Wladis, MD Department of Ophthalmology, Albany Medical Center, Albany, NY, USA

Ophthalmic Plastic Surgery, Lions Eye Institute, Slingerlands, NY, USA

Michael T. Yen, MD Cullen Eye Institute, Baylor College of Medicine, Houston, TX, USA

Alkek Eye Center, Baylor College of Medicine, Houston, TX, USA

List of Figures

List of Tables

Part I

Eyelid

Evaluation of the Oculofacial Patient

1

Dan Georgescu and Cat Nguyen Burkat

Evaluation of the Oculofacial Patient

Acquiring a thorough history and examination is key to the successful treatment of any patient presenting with oculofacial problems or concerns. Most patients presenting with functional concerns expect to look better after surgery, and all patients presenting with cosmetic concerns expect their face to function at least as good after as it did before surgery. In fact, most patients are bothered more by the cosmetic and social consequences of their disease than by the functional ones. As the fine line between "functional" and "cosmetic" is becoming more and more blurry, and especially in view of today's reimbursement changes, we need to perform a more holistic evaluation of our patients and take into consideration both the functional and the cosmetic aspects. In the end, there is no purely functional reconstructive or purely cosmetic surgery; rather, they are a fusion of both philosophies and approaches.

History

Successful diagnosis and treatment can be achieved only with good understanding of the problem that prompted the patient's visit. Not infrequently, the oculofacial surgeon finds out that his initial diagnosis is not the reason why the patient presented in the first place. This is particularly common with cosmetic patients who may focus on small blemishes and miss the more global changes. A thorough history taking should include:

D. Georgescu (✉)
Oculofacial Institute, Fort Lauderdale, FL, USA

C. N. Burkat
Department of Ophthalmology and Visual Sciences, University of Wisconsin-Madison, Madison, WI, USA
e-mail: cburkat@wisc.edu

Chief Complaint

A chief complaint should be elicited from every single patient. It is the reason why the patient came to see you, and it has to be addressed in order to achieve a satisfactory result. Imagine a 40-year-old male comes to see you for a droopy eyelid, and upon examination you conclude that he also has significant dermatochalasis, in addition to the minimal ptosis (less than 2 mm). The surgery you perform corrects the dermatochalasis with a spectacular result but not the ptosis, because you considered it unnecessary. In this situation, the patient will almost always be unhappy with the result because the reason for his visit was not addressed, despite the fact that the overall rejuvenation effect is remarkable.

History of Present Problem

This is as important in oculofacial plastic surgery as in any other medical speciality. Ophthalmology in general is very "visual," which makes history taking of somewhat lesser importance when compared to the eye exam. However, orbital and lacrimal pathology are difficult to diagnose with the naked eye or the slit lamp, so history can be very useful in formulating the diagnosis until the proper ancillary tests are obtained. For example, in a patient presenting with a bulging eye, rapidly progressive proptosis, pain with eye movements, and fever, this is likely due to acute orbital infection or inflammation, whereas slow progressive proptosis that is painless is likely due to thyroid orbitopathy or a benign orbital mass. It is important to remember that the most common cause of unilateral or bilateral proptosis is still thyroid eye disease. The history can also be important for the correct diagnosis of blepharoptosis. A slowly progressive unilateral blepharoptosis that does not fluctuate diurnally in a contact lens user is most likely aponeurotic in nature. In contrast, a highly variable ptosis that worsens in hot weather, associated with transient diplopia or swallowing problems, should be evaluated for myasthenia gravis.

A. J. Cohen, C. N. Burkat (eds.), *Oculofacial, Orbital, and Lacrimal Surgery*, https://doi.org/10.1007/978-3-030-14092-2_1

Ophthalmic History

The past ophthalmic history can be equally important for diagnosis making and for choosing the optimal therapeutic strategy. For example, intermittent but recurring tearing in a patient with a history of recurrent "herpes in the eye" may suggest canalicular obstruction. This is confirmed by examination, and the patient was treated successfully with a dacryocystorhinostomy (DCR) and canaliculoplasty. One year later, the patient returns for upper blepharoplasty and endoscopic forehead lifting. Knowing the past ocular history of recurrent HSV corneal infections, you perform a rather conservative blepharoplasty and maximize the browlift instead in order to prevent immediate and long-term corneal complications.

General Medical History

A thorough medical and surgical history should be obtained from all oculofacial patients even if the diagnosis is straightforward and the treatment plan already chosen. Imagine you have a female patient presenting with ptosis and dermatochalasis who has normal eye surface on examination but has been experiencing dry eyes and dry mouth and skin for the past few months despite drinking lots of fluids and not taking any medications. With further questioning you find out that she has not been feeling well for a couple of years and that she has had gastrointestinal problems and muscle aches intermittently. If this patient has subclinical or early Sjögren's syndrome, both ptosis and dermatochalasis correction can decompensate her dry eye syndrome. Therefore, anti-SSA antibodies (Ro/La) and a rheumatology consult should be obtained. The past medical history is important because many oculofacial, orbital, and lacrimal pathologies are associated with systemic disease. Classic examples are the association of Graves' disease with both orbitopathy and myasthenia gravis. Sinusitis and allergies are associated with acquired nasolacrimal duct obstruction and myasthenia gravis with ptosis. It is critical to elicit any history of bleeding problems prior to orbital, eyelid, or lacrimal surgery since hemorrhage around the eyes can be devastating. Hematoma formation outside the orbit in a cosmetic patient can be equally devastating if it leads to skin necrosis or scarring.

General Surgical History

This is important for both reconstructive and cosmetic patients. Cosmetic patients should be asked about prior surgeries and in particular about complications and overall experience. Patients who are dissatisfied with prior interventions and speak poorly of their other doctors are likely to be unhappy again and require special preoperative counseling. Any prior surgical complications, particularly hemorrhage, infections, wound dehiscence, or poor healing, should be noted and investigated. Any blood dyscrasia or immune deficiency can adversely affect the outcome and, in the worst case, the vision itself. Poor wound healing can be related to heavy smoking, nutritional deficiencies or malnutrition, or poorly controlled diabetes or rheumatologic disorders and need to be addressed before any oculofacial procedure or reconstruction.

Psychiatric History

This is particularly important with patients with cosmetic concerns. If numerous areas of dissatisfaction or unrealistic expectations are elicited, the surgeon should be on high alert for somatoform disease (body dysmorphic syndrome and dysmorphophobia), anxiety disorders, major depression, or bipolar disease. The patients should be asked whether they have ever seen or been advised to see a psychiatrist or psychologist and if they ever have mood changes. Patients who are overly concerned with minor or nonexistent aesthetic blemishes and/or have unrealistic expectations regarding the surgical outcome should raise suspicions for dysmorphophobia. These patients have the tendency to repeat themselves and ask the same questions multiple times. This is more frequently seen in young people in their late 20s to early 30s. An additional second opinion or referring the patient to another surgeon or therapist can be considered, as these patients tend to be extremely unhappy and highly litigious.

Allergies

All medical and environmental allergies should be noted. In addition, the patients should be asked to describe the allergy since many patients mistake adverse reactions (e.g., palpitations from lidocaine with adrenaline) for true allergies (e.g., anaphylactic shock following iodine-based contrast media intravenous infusion). The route of drug administration is also important. A patient with true allergy to intravenous iodine-based contrast media is not necessarily allergic to Betadine scrub solution. Environmental allergies are also important in the pathogenesis and prognosis of certain lacrimal diseases. For example, nasal allergies and chronic sinus disease are very common causes of acquired nasolacrimal duct obstruction, and the long-term outcome of dacryocystorhinostomy (DCR) surgery depends on proper allergy control.

Medications

A complete list of medications and over-the-counter vitamin supplements should be recorded. Some medications can be the cause of periocular disease, whereas others may adversely affect the treatment outcome. For example, prostaglandin drops routinely used for glaucoma are now known to be responsible for certain lacrimal, eyelid, and orbital manifestations. In addition, medications that can lead to intra- or postoperative complications should be recorded. This includes not only antiaggregants, anti-inflammatories, and anticoagulants but also many vitamins (e.g., C, E) and supplements (e.g., ginseng, *Ginkgo biloba*, garlic).

Antiaggregants, such as aspirin and Plavix, all vitamins, and all supplements should be stopped 2 weeks prior to surgery, whereas anti-inflammatory medications, such as ibuprofen and diclofenac, can be stopped only 5 days prior. However, these medications should never be stopped without the prior approval of the primary care physician or treating cardiologist. In certain situations, low-risk surgery can still be performed if the patient is unable to discontinue these drugs but only after proper counseling and documentation regarding bleeding risks and prolonged recovery time are discussed.

A particular situation in which good communication between the surgeon and the primary care physician or cardiologist is critical is in regard to perioperative anticoagulant bridging. If the patient is bridged with enoxaparin (Lovenox), or similar medication, this must be stopped 24 hours prior to surgery. In addition, the patient should *not* restart the enoxaparin after surgery. Rather, the patient should resume the normal anticoagulant dose the night of surgery and allow it to build back up to therapeutic level. Bleeding from enoxaparin (Lovenox) can be severe and extremely difficult to control, can occur as far out as 10–12 days after surgery, and can be vision threatening (such as after lower blepharoplasty or orbital surgery) or life threatening (after DCR).

Motivation for Treatment

The factors that motivate a patient to have surgery can be internal or external and should be carefully identified. The internal factors pertain to the patient's desire to feel or look better. These desires can be realistic or unrealistic, but they are organic. External factors, however, can relate to personal relationships, marriage, social pressures, or pecuniary factors. Some people believe that changing the way they look will improve an important relationship or elevate professional status, which is usually not the case. A study of cosmetic patients demonstrated that patients with internal motivations were more likely to be happy with the results of surgery than those driven by external factors. Consequently, the goals of surgery as agreed upon by the patient and surgeon should always be organic and realistic to achieve. Patients with external motivations should be properly and extensively counseled prior to proceeding with surgery.

Examination

Visual Acuity

Vision should always be checked first by the technician before the rest of the oculofacial exam and especially prior to performing any periocular surgery. This is essential for comparison if a patient complains of vision changes after surgery. For certain pathologies, such as thyroid eye disease, visual acuity should be carefully assessed in conjunction with color vision testing and red desaturation that may suggest optic neuropathy.

Pupils

Pupillary reaction should be documented in the preoperative examination for all functional and cosmetic cases, in the event of visual complaints arising after surgery. This is particularly important if a bleeding complication occurs. Size, symmetry, reaction to light and dark, and any relative afferent defect should be measured. Routine examination of the pupils is also mandatory with orbital pathology as it helps monitor disease evolution and thus guides medical or surgical treatment.

Motility

Many orbital diseases can affect eye movements; therefore, motility testing can be helpful in distinguishing between paralytic and restrictive disease. It is also useful for monitoring the evolution of orbital inflammation or infection. In the setting of facial trauma, altered ocular motility should raise the suspicion of muscle entrapment in an orbital fracture, although can also be secondary to muscle contusion and swelling. Extraocular muscle entrapment tends to be more common in children rather than in adults. New-onset diplopia following lower eyelid blepharoplasty may be a result of injury to the inferior oblique muscle during fat manipulation.

Ocular Surface

It is important to note that blepharoplasty surgery can exacerbate or result in ocular surface problems after surgery, and the surgeon should be comfortable managing the condition or referring the patient to an appropriate ophthalmologist. Occasionally, eyelid surgery can trigger meibomian gland dysfunction, leading to tear film instability and hyperosmolarity. This in turn leads to apoptosis and ocular surface inflammation with goblet cell loss and cytokine release that further increases tear film instability. Virtually any periocular disease or surgery can precipitate this vicious cycle and negatively impact both the patient's vision and comfort. The following factors should be explored preoperatively:

Tear Film

The tear film quality and breakup time (TBUT) should be measured. An unstable or scarce tear film will likely become worse immediately after surgery due to temporary loss of normal eyelid function from swelling. The need for frequent artificial tear use should be discussed with the patient before surgery as many may not find it acceptable and consider it very cumbersome. In some cases, the dry eye syndrome may not completely resolve despite appropriate management. In contrast, a high tear film suggests either a lacrimal excretory problem or reflex hypersecretion due to dryness or ocular surface irritation.

Eyelid Function

The role of the eyelids is to protect the eyes, so any alteration in eyelid position (ectropion, entropion, retraction) and function (lagophthalmos) can affect the ocular surface. This can subsequently lead to discomfort and vision changes. Meibomian gland secretion is dependent on tight eyelid closure. Patients with impaired blinking, as commonly occurs in facial paralysis or immediately after eyelid surgery, suffer from rapid tear film evaporation and high tear film osmolarity as the lipid layer (produced by the meibomian glands) is inadequate and the eyes are not protected by the eyelids. Eyelid malfunction can affect not only tear film production but also tear distribution and evaporation. Proper eyelid functioning is also important for tear drainage as the lacrimal pump depends on proper blinking and requires tight eyelid closure to create negative pressure in the lacrimal sac to draw tears down. Lax eyelids can also lead to tearing in the absence of tear drainage obstruction or eyelid malposition, as the lacrimal pump is not able to adequately create positive pressure to force the tears into the puncta.

Corneal Sensation

An absent or diminished corneal sensation can alter the ability to protect the eyes and lead to neurotrophic ulcers. Cranial nerve V sensation needs to be evaluated prior to upper eyelid ptosis or blepharoplasty surgery, as eyelid elevation can decompensate the ocular surface, even if the margin-reflex height appears appropriate. A gentle wiping of the corneal surface with a cotton tip applicator, or tissue, can indicate decreased corneal sensation. If corneal sensation is significantly affected, and/or neurotrophic ulcers are present, oculofacial surgery should proceed only with extreme caution. In combination with facial nerve paralysis or weakness (VIIth nerve), a partial lateral or complete tarsorrhaphy is typically indicated.

Trichiasis

In patients complaining of eye irritation, foreign body sensation, grittiness, or tearing, the presence of abnormally directed eyelashes should be carefully evaluated for. Trichiatic eyelashes are normal eyelashes growing from the eyelash follicles but are misdirected posteriorly toward the ocular surface. They are usually an acquired sequela of eyelid margin inflammation, although rarely, congenital trichiasis may occur. It differs from entropion, in which the eyelid margin itself (not just the eyelashes) is rotated back toward the globe. Distichiasis refers to abnormal lashes that originate from the meibomian gland orifices of the posterior lamella, rather than the eyelash follicles, and can be congenital or acquired in etiology.

Basic Tear Secretion Testing

The Schirmer test can identify those patients at risk for dry eyes after oculofacial surgery and should be considered before any ptosis surgery or blepharoplasty especially if the past ocular and medical history are suggestive of dry eyes or Sjögren's syndrome. Schirmer strips are placed in between the globe and the lower eyelid after a drop of topical anesthetic has been instilled in the eyes. Normal values are more than 15 mm of wetting at 5 min. In patients with Sjögren's syndrome, the amount of wetting of the strip is typically less than 5 mm. Burkat and Lucarelli also described that the tear lake meniscus, measured using the small narrowed beam of the slit lamp, is 0.2 mm in height, on average [1]. Greater heights of the tear lake meniscus suggest hypersecretion of tears or lacrimal excretory outflow obstruction, and a lower or nonexistent tear film will be highly indicative of dry eye syndrome.

General Facial Assessment

Before focusing on the areas of interest, it is always important to look at the overall face as any surgery should be considered in a continuum with the rest of the face, and careful evaluation for asymmetry or pathognomonic signs is critical. Any orbitofacial asymmetry or globe dystopia should alert the physician to the presence of an orbital process (Fig. 1.1).

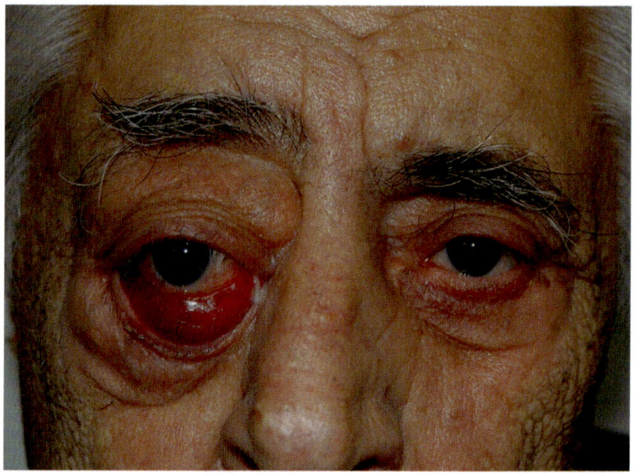

Fig. 1.1 A 68-year-old male patient presenting with rapidly progressive right eye proptosis and inferior dystopia from a superior orbital mass

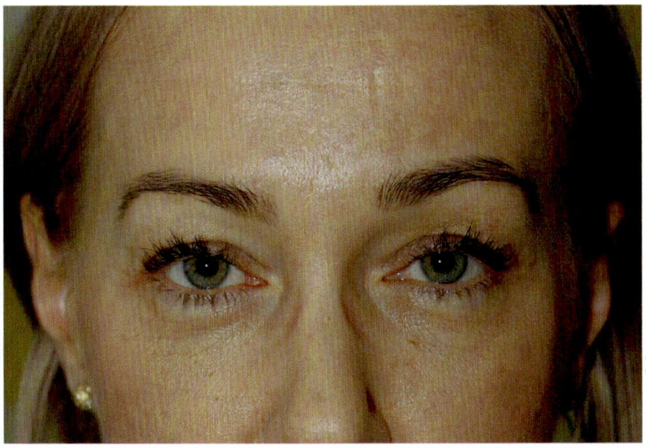

Fig. 1.2 A 50-year-old woman presenting for excess skin on the right upper eyelid. Examination shows significant eyebrow asymmetry to be the actual cause of her eyelid asymmetry

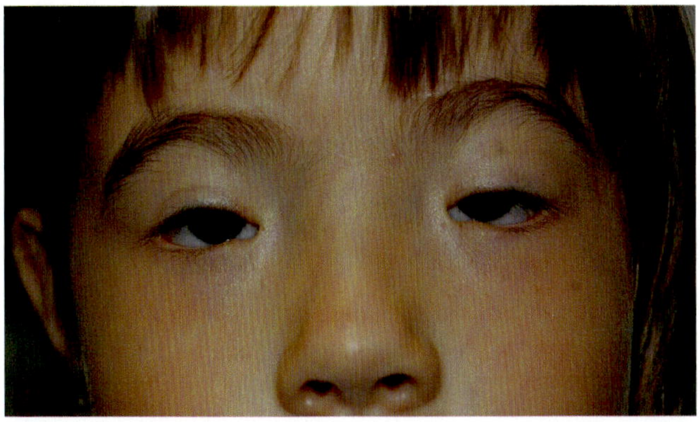

Fig. 1.3 A 4-year-old girl with congenital telecanthus, ptosis, and epicanthus inversus from blepharophimosis syndrome

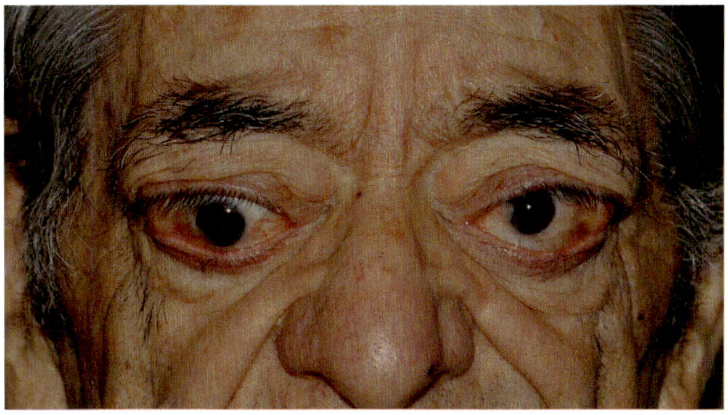

Fig. 1.4 A 74-year-old male presenting in the active phase of Graves' orbitopathy with bilateral compressive optic neuropathy

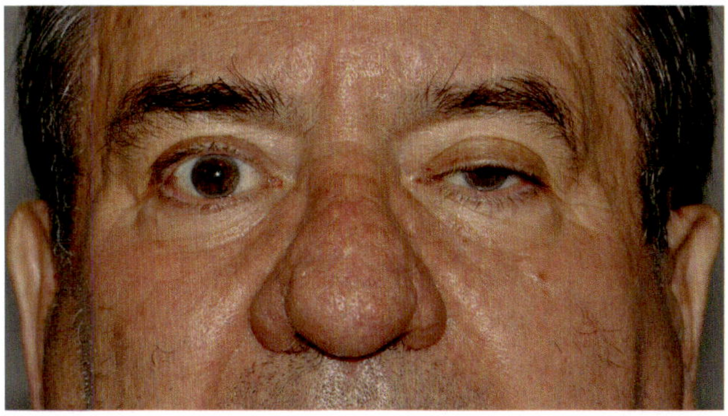

Fig. 1.5 A 63-year-old male presenting for left upper eyelid ptosis also has rhinophyma and dry eyes from rosacea. The increased margin-to-crease distance on the left side suggests levator disinsertion

Asymmetry should be documented and photographed and the patient informed of its presence prior to surgery (Fig. 1.2). It is very common for patients to be unaware of preexisting oculofacial asymmetry until after the surgery, at which point they attribute it to a faulty procedure. It is important to counsel the patient that natural facial asymmetry is difficult to treat and that surgery usually achieves only a partial and temporary improvement [2–4].

Telecanthus is present when the intercanthal distance is longer than half the interpupillary distance. This is commonly seen in blepharophimosis syndrome (Fig. 1.3) and with naso-orbito-ethmoidal (NOE) fractures if the medial canthal tendon or its attachment to the medial orbital wall is disrupted. Signs of localized or generalized facial inflammation should be noted. Periocular inflammation and eyelid edema are commonly seen in Graves' orbitopathy (Fig. 1.4) but are also present in many types of eyelid, orbital, or lacrimal infections. Orbital tumors and inflammation can also lead to asymmetrical periocular changes. Rosacea is a general skin condition that is most prominent on sun-exposed areas such as the face (Fig. 1.5) and can be a risk factor for dry eye symptoms or ocular irritation after eyelid surgery.

Eyebrows and Forehead

Eyebrow ptosis is a common finding in patients presenting for excess upper eyelid skin and tends to be underdiagnosed (Fig. 1.6). Patients rarely complain of droopy eyebrows; therefore, proper evaluation of eyebrow position is critical for obtaining optimal functional and cosmetic results after blepharoplasty. Male eyebrows are generally situated at the supraorbital rim, while female eyebrows rest higher above the rim. Individual variations exist; however, thus reviewing old photographs of the patient can better ascertain whether a low-sitting eyebrow is normal for that individual. Eyebrow ptosis is usually the result of brow fat pad (BFP, also known as the retroorbicularis oculi fat (ROOF)) and forehead deflation which make the eyelid skin slide down with gravity. These changes can also be appreciated from old photographs, particularly from a lateral or oblique view in which the three-dimensional deflation is seen. The shape and arch of the eyebrows (ascending, flat, or

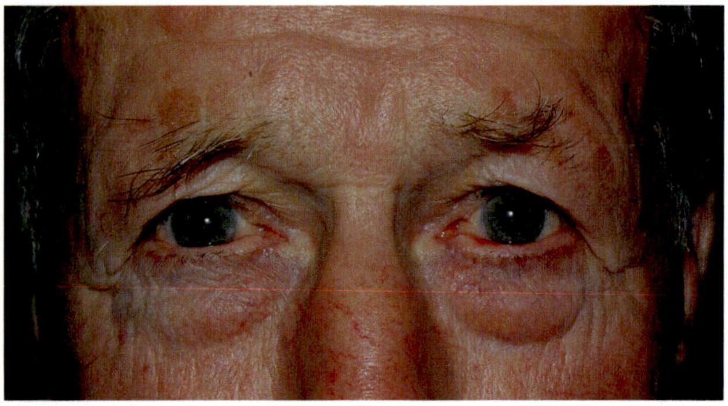

Fig. 1.6 A 71-year-old man with severe eyebrow ptosis presents for excess skin on the upper eyelids

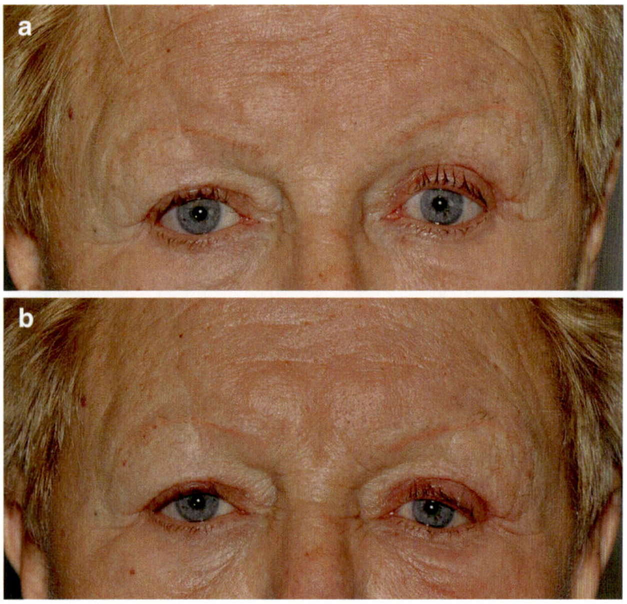

Fig. 1.7 (a) A 75-year-old female complains of the left eyebrow being higher after bilateral ptosis surgery. (b) Four units of botulinum toxin injected above the left eyebrow was sufficient for reversing this habit she had had since prior to surgery

descending) should also be noted since they can be influenced by the type of procedure performed.

Preoperative eyebrow asymmetry should be thoroughly discussed with the patient as this is very difficult to correct. Asymmetry may be secondary to underlying frontal bone/orbital rim differences or frontalis muscle preference in which one frontalis muscle is habitually elevated more prominently. These factors will likely result in persistent eyebrow asymmetry after surgery. In contrast, if the higher eyebrow is a compensatory mechanism due to visual axis blockage on that side, the patient may often unlearn the eyebrow lifting habit postoperatively. In those in whom the compensatory habit is difficult to reverse, forced relaxation of the frontalis muscle can be achieved with one or two injections of botulinum toxin injections above the eyebrow (Fig. 1.7).

Eyebrow ptosis that descends below the supraorbital rim and is severe enough to produce significant visual field loss may be covered by insurance. The amount of eyebrow ptosis can be objectively measured by manually lifting the ptotic eyebrow to the desired position while measuring the distance of movement with a ruler held up to the eyebrow [5].

Glabellar rhytids, which are the result of corrugator supercilii, depressor supercilii, and procerus muscle contractions, are a common cosmetic complaint and can be improved with botulinum toxin or surgery to selectively weaken or excise these muscles. Low medial eyebrows also suggest corrugator and depressor muscle hyperactivity and can be moderatively improved with botulinum toxin. When treated properly with botulinum toxin, the eyebrows can relax to a higher and slightly more lateral position (Fig. 1.8). Significant medial eyebrow ptosis is best corrected with cosmetic forehead lifting procedures and release of arcus marginalis attachments. Soft tissue fillers in the glabella should be approached very cautiously due to the risks of vascular emboli and skin necrosis [6].

In some patients, eyebrow ptosis may not be initially apparent due to frontalis muscle hyperactivity which raises the eyebrows. This manifests as prominent forehead horizontal rhytids. Botulinum toxin treatment of the forehead creases can therefore unmask an underlying eyebrow ptosis or lead

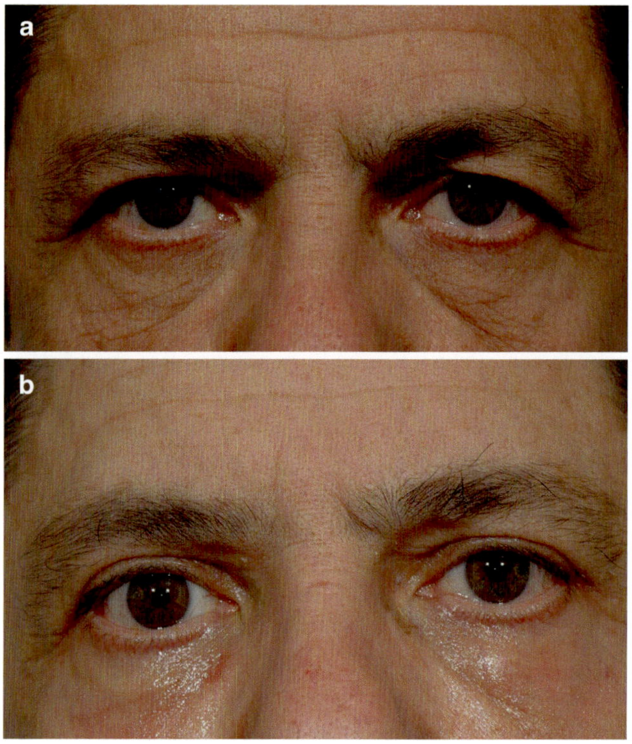

Fig. 1.8 (a) This male patient complains of excess upper eyelid skin and prominent vertical glabellar lines with expression (shown here in the relaxed state). (b) Improved overall eyebrow position is seen after upper blepharoplasty with corrugator muscle removal

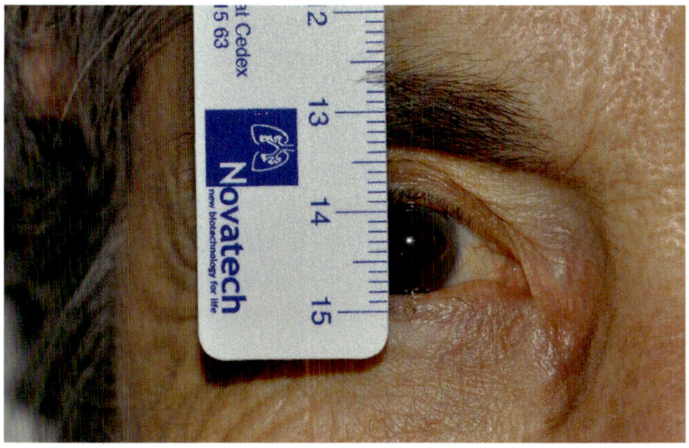

Fig. 1.9 Measurement of MRD1, PF, and MRD2 using a ruler and small light

to significant eyebrow/eyelid ptosis if doses are too aggressive, resulting in an unhappy patient.

Upper Eyelids

The upper eyelids are important for both vision and social interaction. Pathology that disturbs eyelid function can have a dramatic impact on the patient's quality of life. A patient complaining of droopy eyelids can have eyelid ptosis, dermatochalasis, eyebrow ptosis, or a combination. The following measurements should be performed routinely to formulate the correct diagnosis and treatment plan:

- *MRD1* (margin-reflex distance 1) is the distance from the upper eyelid margin to the pupillary light reflex with the patient looking in primary gaze and can be positive or negative. Normal values are considered 4–4.5 mm in Caucasians (Fig. 1.9), which correlate to the eyelid margin resting just below the superior limbus. Values less than 4 mm are consistent with ptosis, whereas values greater than 4.5 mm suggest upper eyelid retraction, such as seen in thyroid eye disease. If the eyelid margin is situated below the light reflex, the distance necessary to raise the eyelid until the light reflex becomes visible in the central pupil is marked in negative millimeters. Starting from the normal MRD1 measurements, the degree of ptosis can be quantified as mild (<2 mm), moderate (3–4 mm), and severe (>4 mm). If the eyelid margin and eyelash lash are not visible at all due to skin hooding over the margin, then the redundant skin should be gently elevated to assess if occult levator ptosis is also present or if the actual MRD1 is normal under the excess skin.
- *PF* (palpebral fissure height) is the vertical distance between the upper and the lower eyelid margins in straight primary gaze and usually measures 9.5–10.5 mm (Fig. 1.9).

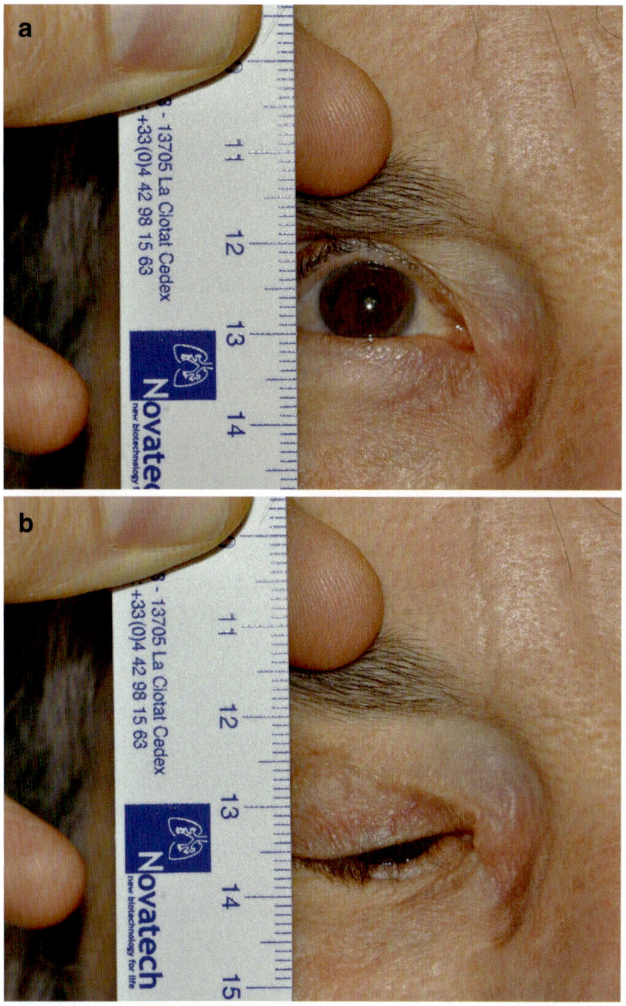

Fig. 1.10 LF measurement. (**a**) The eyebrow is firmly stabilized with the patient looking up "at the ceiling," and the position of the eyelid margin is red on the ruler. (**b**) The patient is asked to look down "to the floor" and the new value is red. The difference between the two values is the LF

- *LF* (levator function) is the maximal excursion of the upper eyelid measured when looking downgaze to extreme upgaze or from upgaze to downgaze (Fig. 1.10). It is important to firmly stabilize the eyebrow during this test as frontalis muscle contraction will elevate the eyebrow and secondarily the eyelid, resulting in falsely elevated levator measurements. Normal LF values are 12–15 mm. Good levator function is measured to be 8–15 mm, 5–7 mm fair, and <4 mm to be poor levator function.
- *MCD* (margin to crease distance) is the distance between the upper eyelid margin and the eyelid crease. A high MCD in the presence of eyelid ptosis suggests levator disinsertion, the most common type of acquired ptosis (Fig. 1.5). This distance is also important during blepha-

roplasty to accurately mark incisions in the eyelid crease and varies widely with race and gender. In Asian eyelids, the MCD is much lower at 4–5 mm due to the low insertion of the orbital septum onto the levator aponeurosis. In some patients of Asian descent, the crease is absent completely, or multiple creases may be present.

Proper upper eyelid measurements are important both for making the correct diagnosis and for treatment planning.

Blepharoptosis should be evaluated with the patient sitting up and looking straight ahead with a relaxed forehead. The photographs should be taken ideally without flash with the patient focusing at a point straight ahead, as the eyelids will appear higher if looking upward or appear lower if gazing slightly downward. The Hering phenomenon should be tested whenever a unilateral or asymmetric ptosis is present. This is tested by either mechanically raising the ptotic eyelid or by placing one drop of 2.5% phenylephrine solution in the ptotic eye while observing for a drop in height of the contralateral upper eyelid (Fig. 1.11). According to Hering's law, equal innervation is distributed to both levator muscles; thus when the brain is trying to raise the droopier eyelid, the contralateral "normal" eyelid also receives equal innervation to elevate. If only the ptotic eyelid is corrected, the apparently normal contralateral eyelid will then droop postoperatively as the innervation to elevate the eyelid is lost. Recognizing a Hering's phenomenon preoperatively can avoid patient dissatisfaction, as both levator repairs can then be performed simultaneously.

Distinguishing acquired from congenital ptosis in an older patient who believes, but is not sure, that the droopy eyelid was present since birth is tested in downgaze. In congenital ptosis, the droopy eyelid becomes higher than the contralateral upper eyelid in downgaze due to tethering by the fibrosed dystrophic levator muscle (Fig. 1.12). This is referred to as eyelid lag and is characteristic of congenital ptosis. If myasthenia gravis is suspected, an ice test can be useful in the office. Ice application to the ptotic eyelid for 3–5 minutes (the recommended 5 minutes is extremely painful and rarely necessary) leads to a transient improvement in eyelid position due to a decreased amount of anti-acetylcholine receptor antibodies available to block the neuromuscular junction. Unfortunately, the ice test has high sensitivity but very low specificity and should be confirmed with single-fiber EMG. Another easily performed test is to ask the patient to look up for approximately 30 seconds. In myasthenia gravis, eyelid fatigue occurs faster and ptosis manifests. Jaw-winking should be tested in all children with congenital ptosis as parents may not mention the abnormal facial movements as these tend to be less bothersome to them than the ptosis. Children with jaw-winking congenital ptosis often do not require surgery as they learn to elevate the ptotic eyelid themselves with certain jaw movements. As mentioned previously, a good Bell's phenomenon and intact corneal sensitivity should be present in patients undergoing blepharoptosis correction to ensure proper corneal protection after surgery.

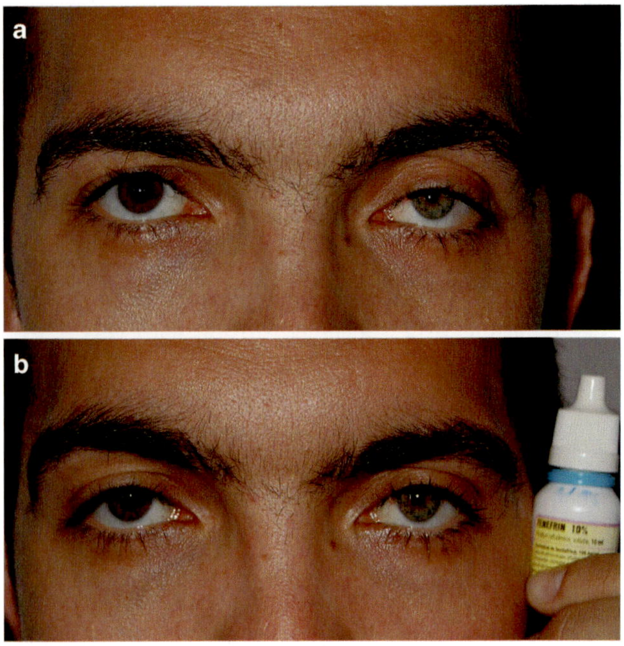

Fig. 1.11 Hering's law of equal innervation. (a) Left upper eyelid ptosis and apparent normal position of the right upper eyelid. (**b**) Drooping of the right upper eyelid occurs after 2.5% phenylephrine instillation in the left eye

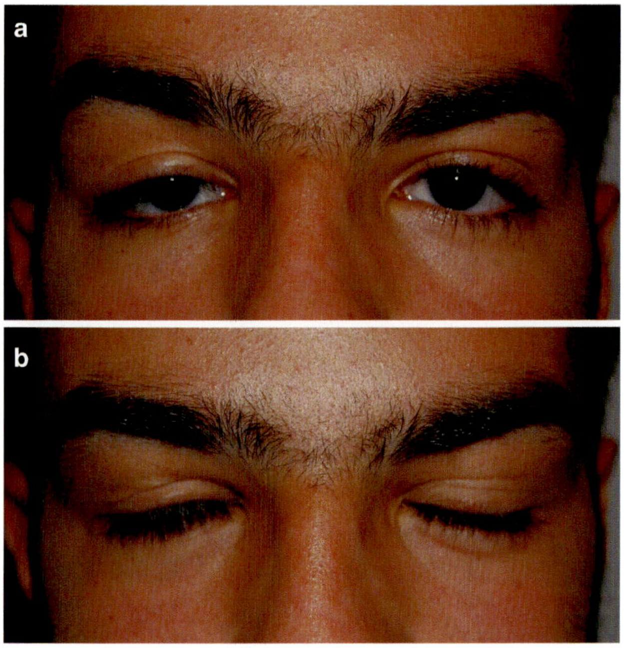

Fig. 1.12 (**a**) Right congenital blepharoptosis. (**b**) Lid lag in downgaze on the affected side is due to fibrosis of the dystrophic levator muscle

Dermatochalasis should be evaluated in relation to eyebrow position and upper eyelid/brow deflation. The skin does not grow or lengthen with age. Apparent excess skin in the eyelids is similar to the sagging that develops in the rest of the aging face due to volume deflation. Dermatochalasis is due partly to loss of the preaponeurotic fat pad, as well as to loss of brow fat pad volume resulting in downslanting lateral eyebrows. These aging changes are further exacerbated by atrophy of the superior orbital rim and the periorbital muscles. In addition, the medial fat pad deflates less than the central fat pad and contributes to the aged appearance. When prominent, the medial fat can be debulked or transposed to fill in the hollowness of the central sulcus. Lacrimal gland prolapse is not uncommon even in young cosmetic patients and should be noted to avoid mistaking it for orbital fat and inadvertently excising part of the gland. Intraoperatively, the prolapsed gland should be repositioned under the lateral superior orbital rim to avoid a persistent lateral eyelid bulge after surgery. Symmetry of the upper eyelid creases is critical after blepharoplasty surgery as patients will always complain if the postoperative creases are asymmetric, even if the creases were asymmetric before surgery. Preexisting asymmetric or multiple creases, such as seen in Asian eyelids, can also be corrected at the time of blepharoplasty or ptosis surgery.

Floppy eyelid syndrome should be considered every time a patient complains of red, irritated eyes in the morning, whether or not he or she has a diagnosis of sleep apnea. The test is very simple and involves distracting the upper eyelid up and outward with the thumb (Fig. 1.13). If the eyelid easily everts to the point where the tarsus flips outward, the patient has floppy eyelid syndrome and should be referred for sleep studies. Although the disease is partly reversible with medical treatment, surgery is almost always necessary to alleviate symptoms. Horizontal tightening and/or wedge resection techniques to improve the floppy eyelid must be performed prior to ptosis surgery as the tarsal plate will be displaced laterally.

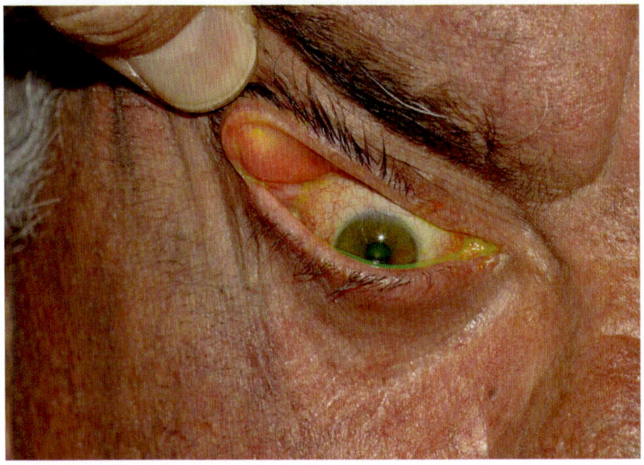

Fig. 1.13 Significant upper eyelid eversion seen in floppy eyelid syndrome

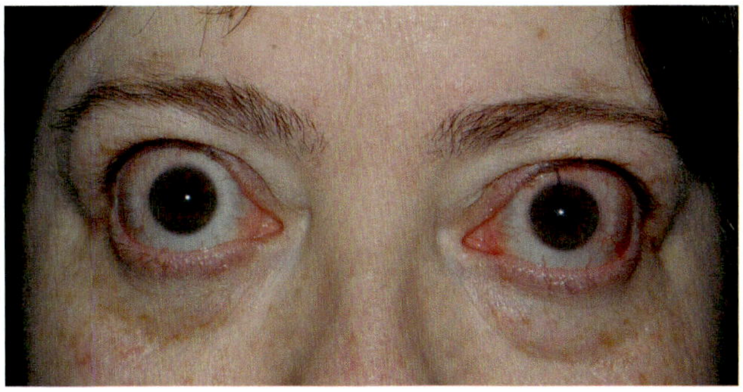

Fig. 1.14 Bilateral upper and lower eyelid retraction are commonly seen in Graves' orbitopathy

Upper eyelid retraction is commonly seen with thyroid eye disease but can also be present in other conditions, such as after filtering glaucoma blebs, strabismus surgery, or trauma (Fig. 1.14). An MRD1 greater that 4.5 mm is suggestive of upper eyelid retraction, although symmetry, history, old photographs, and associated ocular findings are useful in establishing the correct diagnosis.

Lower Eyelids

Similar to the upper eyelids, the lower eyelids provide ocular protection and contribute to the lacrimal pump mechanism. They contain the lower tear ducts which drain 60% or more of the tears. The most useful measurements are:

- *MRD2* (margin-reflex distance 2) is the distance between the corneal light reflex and the lower eyelid margin and normally measures less than 5.5 mm (Fig. 1.9). This correlates to the lower eyelid margin resting at the inferior limbus, or 0.5–1.0 mm below the limbus, on average. Higher measurements, in the absence of ectropion, suggest lower eyelid retraction.
- *Snapback test* is a simple measure of horizontal laxity. The normal lower eyelid should immediately snap back in contact with the globe when pulled down with a finger. If the eyelid stays away from the globe until the patient blinks, or the snapback is slower than normal, horizontal eyelid laxity is present (Fig. 1.15).
- *Eyelid distraction* is another test for horizontal laxity. If the lower eyelid can be pulled anteriorly away from the globe more than 6 mm, horizontal laxity is present (Fig. 1.16). Medial canthal laxity can be evaluated by pulling the eyelid laterally and observing the displacement of the punctum (Fig. 1.17). Different surgeons may describe slightly different measurements for the test, but

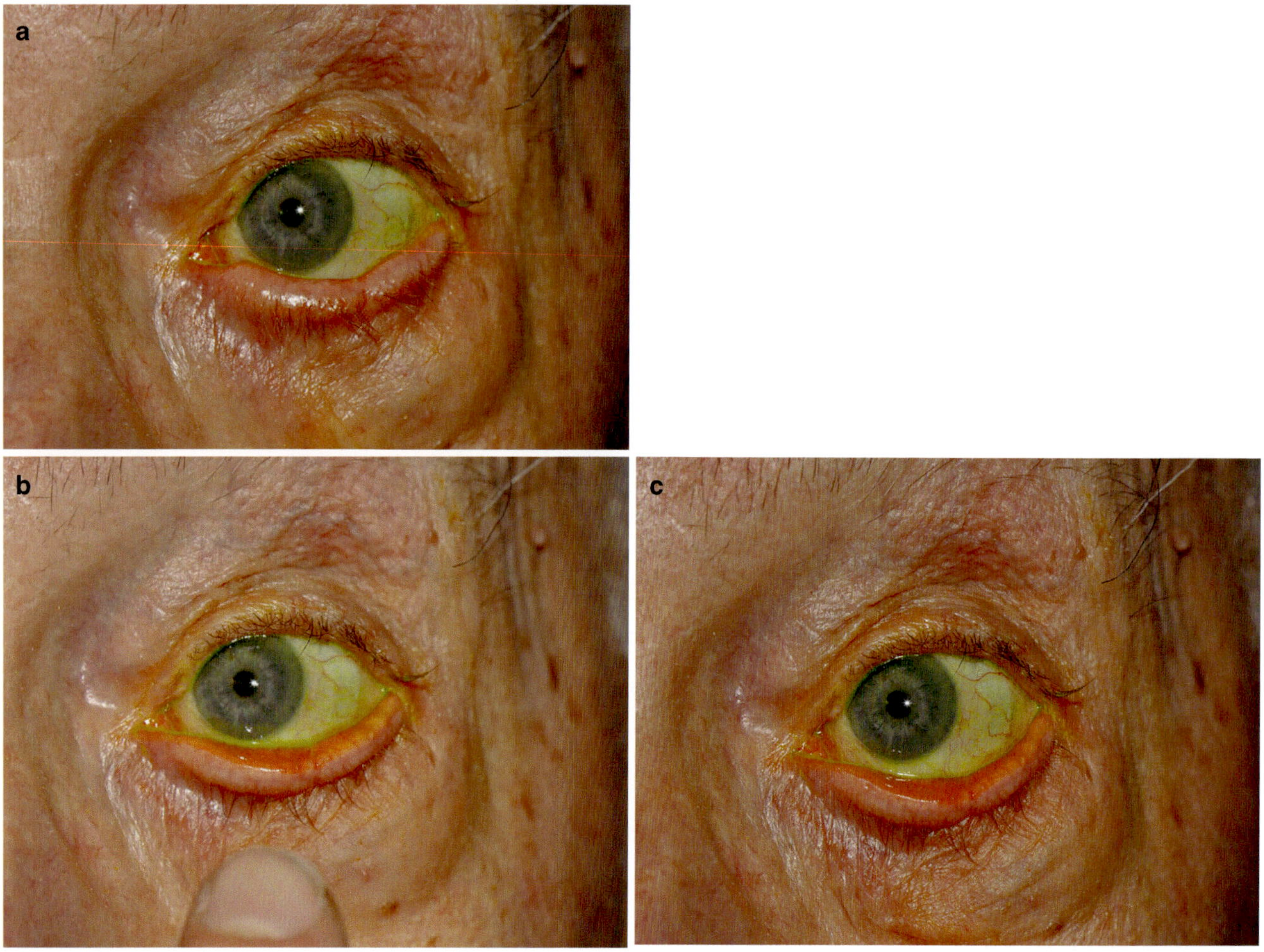

Fig. 1.15 Snapback test. (**a**) Left lower eyelid slightly everted in normal position. (**b**) Immediately after the eyelid is pulled down with a finger. (**c**) Five seconds after the eyelid was pulled down and before the patient blinked again

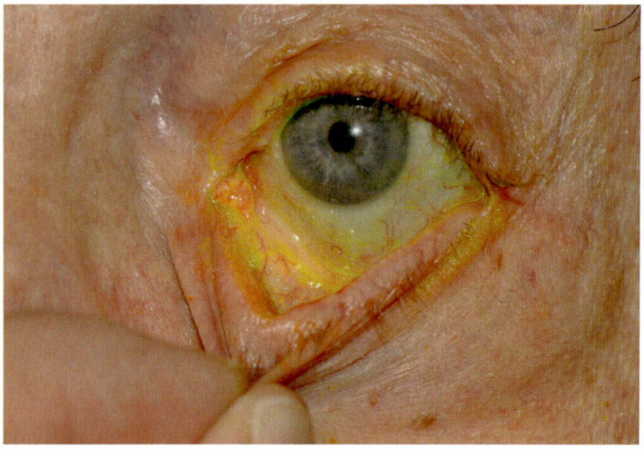

Fig. 1.16 Eyelid distraction test. A lax lower eyelid can be pulled away from the globe more than 6 mm

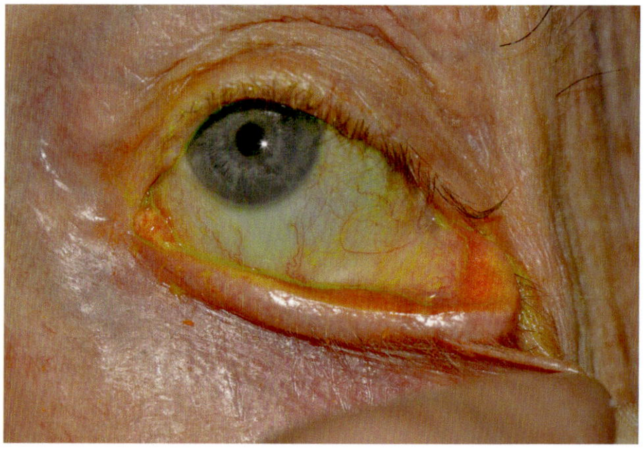

Fig. 1.17 Lateral distraction test for medial canthal tendon (MCT) laxity. When the MCT is lax, the lower punctum can be displaced more than 5–6 mm

in general, if the medial punctum can be easily lateralized to the medial limbus or pupil level, medial canthal tendon laxity should be addressed.

- *Vertical laxity* can be evaluated with the patient looking downward. If the lower eyelid fails to follow the globe, the lower eyelid retractors are either lax or dehisced from the inferior tarsus. This may also lead to the inward or outward turning of the eyelid margin. In addition, the lower fornix may be deeper than normal because the disinserted retractors pull down on the fornix, which could lead to excessive mucous trapping on the eye. This is similar to the deep upper eyelid crease in aponeurotic ptosis.

Lower eyelid ectropion is the outward turning of the lower eyelid (Fig. 1.18). It can be diffuse, medial or lateral, and usually associated with dry eyes or tearing. The dry eye symptoms are due to decreased corneal protection and decreased tear film which can be evaluated at the slit lamp (superficial punctate keratopathy and TBUT). Tearing is both reflex, from dryness, and secondary to eversion of the lacrimal punctum. In addition, the lacrimal pump does not function properly when the eyelids are lax. The ectropion can be involutional (horizontal laxity and/or laxity of the lower eyelid retractors), mechanical (mass effect usually tumor), or cicatricial (anterior lamella deficiency). Cicatricial ectropion is present if the eyelid does not regain normal apposition to the globe with manual horizontal tightening at the lateral canthus. This is in contrast to involutional ectropion where lateral distraction at the canthus corrects the eyelid malposition [7].

Lower eyelid entropion is the inward turning of the lower eyelid margin and is typically either involutional (horizontal laxity and laxity of the lower eyelid retractors) or cicatricial (scarring of the posterior lamella) in nature. The precise etiology should be determined prior to surgery, as cicatricial entropion secondary to undiagnosed ocular cicatricial pemphigoid, Stevens-Johnson syndrome, topical glaucoma medications, or ocular burns or trauma will all require further evaluation and medical optimization prior to considering surgery. On exam, cicatricial entropion is present if the eyelid does not remain in the straight upward position after manual repositioning, and often posterior conjunctival or forniceal linear scars or symblepharon can be seen. In contrast, simple digital eversion of the margin temporarily corrects an involutional entropion until the patient blinks or squeezes the eyes (Fig. 1.19).

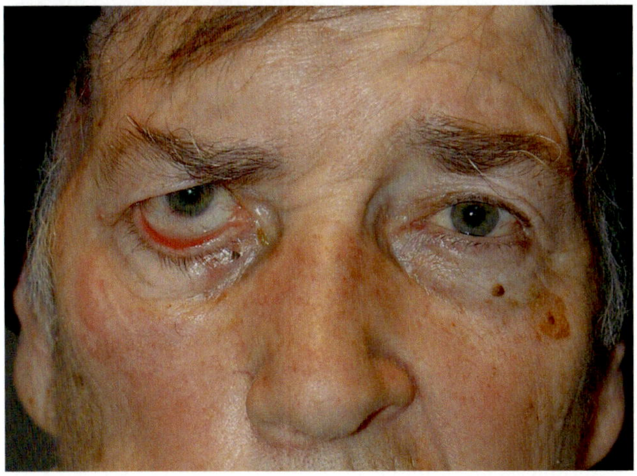

Fig. 1.18 Paralytic lower ectropion in a 75-year-old woman after resection of an acoustic neuroma

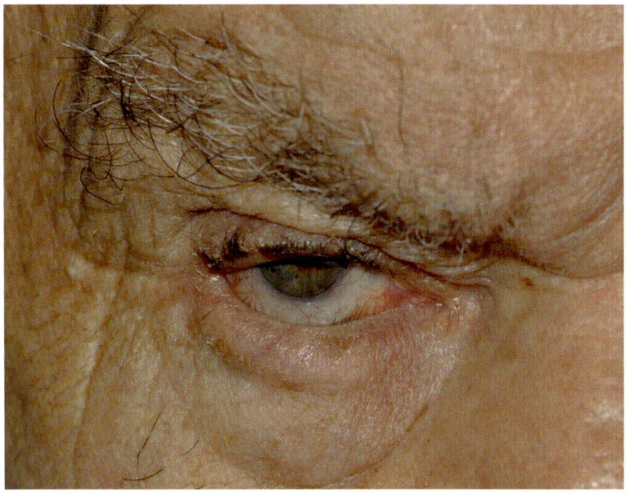

Fig. 1.19 Lower entropion: the entire eyelid margin is rolled in toward the ocular surface

Lower eyelid retraction is defined as MRD2 greater than 5.5 with a normal eyelid margin apposition to the ocular surface. A greater scleral show is seen below the inferior limbus, and there is typically no entropion or ectropion. The globe may be proptotic and thus should be measured by exophthalmometry. Eyelid retraction is often due to scarring or retraction in the middle or posterior lamella and is commonly seen in Graves' orbitopathy or after strabismus surgery and posterior approach eyelid surgery or trauma, such as following transconjunctival lower blepharoplasty or orbital floor fracture repair (Fig. 1.14). It is not usually associated with horizontal laxity.

Lower eyelid dermatochalasis with or without fat prolapse should be evaluated when a patient desires rejuvenation for "fat bags" or deep hollow circles under the eyes. Orbital fat may herniate anteriorly in the lower eyelids due to gravity and weakening of the orbital septum, which manifest as unsightly mounds above the inferior orbital rim (or tear trough). The tear trough, also referred to as the nasojugal groove, is the medial third of the inferior periorbital hollow and is situated at the junction of the thin eyelid skin with the thicker naso-malar skin (Fig. 1.20). The skin here can be more pigmented than the

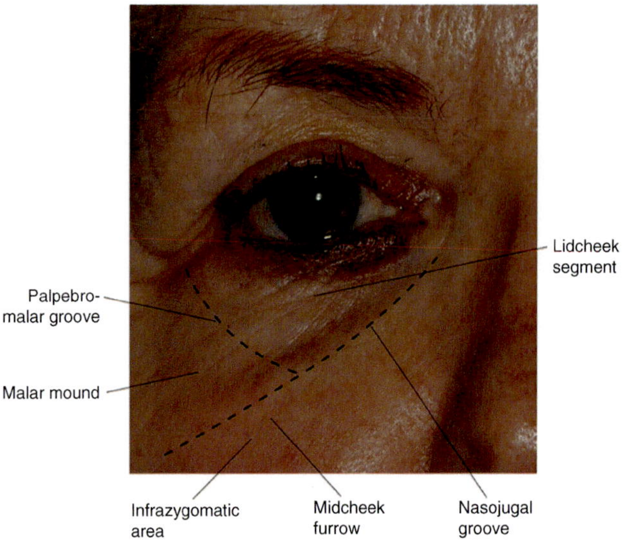

Fig. 1.20 Lower eyelid hollowing

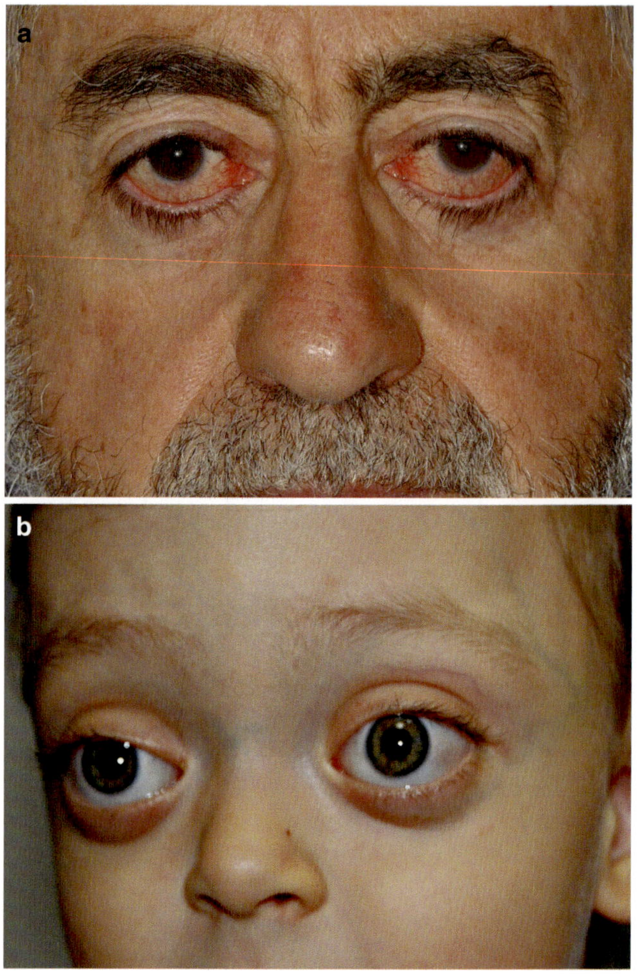

Fig. 1.21 Negative vector orbit. (**a**) Severe scleral show and exposure keratopathy in an adult patient. (**b**) Malar hypoplasia with lower eyelid retraction in a 4-year-old boy with Crouzon syndrome

adjacent eyelid, nasal, and cheek skin and may sometimes be so thin that the deep vessels are visible and project a bluish appearance to the eyelid. The skin at the bottom of the groove and the lower edge of the orbicularis oculi muscle are tethered down to the inferior orbital rim by the orbital retaining ligament or orbitomalar ligament. The groove becomes more prominent with age due to a combination of orbital fat herniation above and malar volume loss below the groove. Treatment differs widely according to whether the patient demonstrates skin excess versus fat prolapse, hollowing, dark shadows, facial ptosis, or a combination of these factors. Skin pigmentation in the nasojugal groove can be treated with intradermal injections of autologous fat cells. A mild to moderate nasojugal groove in a younger patient can be treated with hyaluronic acid injections in the office. Superficial pigmentation contributing to the shadowing can often be minimized with intense pulsed light therapy. A deep nasojugal groove extending laterally in the presence of fat herniation above and malar atrophy below is best treated with preperiosteal or subperiosteal transconjunctival fat repositioning. Occasionally, excess fat and skin may need to be removed, but the orbicularis oculi muscle should always be minimally manipulated, as this is a common cause of postoperative lower eyelid retraction or ectropion.

Midface

The midface is anatomically and functionally related to the lower eyelid, so conditions affecting the midface can also impact on the lower eyelids, both functionally and aesthetically. Volume deficiency in the midface, either congenital (malar hypoplasia) or acquired (involutional deflation), can decrease lower eyelid support, thus leading to retraction or ectropion. An example is facial paralysis where the loss of muscle tone in the face leads to midfacial ptosis and subsequent downward pull on the atonic lower eyelid. This also leads to recurrence of paralytic and mechanical ectropion over time that will require repeated lateral canthal surgeries. Malar hypoplasia is a common cause of the negative vector orbit. This occurs when the globe projects anterior to the lower eyelid margin and the malar eminence (Fig. 1.21). Patients with proptosis are more likely to have negative vector orbits and therefore develop lower eyelid retraction or ectropion than patients with deep-set eyes. Malar deflation due to aging is one reason why lower eyelid retraction after lower skin-muscle blepharoplasty occurs sometimes many years after the original surgery. In such cases, effective treatment of lower eyelid retraction after excessive skin-muscle lower blepharoplasty can be malar augmentation with fat, hyaluronic acid, or malar implants. Another consequence of malar deflation with normal aging is the deepening of the nasojugal and palpebro-malar grooves. Therefore, treatment of the dark hollow circles under the eyes typically involves a form of replacement of the lost malar volume. Festoons or malar mounds are a common but extremely difficult finding to treat, as surgery is usually ineffective or only partially beneficial. Although not completely understood, festoons seem to be due to alterations in the lower eyelid orbicularis muscle function leading to malar edema. Whereas steroid injections and various surgical techniques can provide some improvement, the results are usually transient only; therefore, proper documentation and preoperative counseling are critical. Nasolabial folds are another consequence of malar descent with aging due to midfacial volume loss, and there is a direct correlation between the depth of the nasolabial fold and the midcheek furrow. Patients should be counseled that proper treatment of the nasolabial fold involves malar volume augmentation in conjunction with nasolabial fold filling.

Lower Face

Age-related changes in the lower face are similar to those occurring in the rest of the face. Jowling and neck bands result from the same general process of facial deflation. Although volume loss is a major component in facial aging, the decreased tonus of facial muscles and ligament laxity also play a role. This is seen in facial paralysis where the loss of muscle tone leads to sagging of the entire hemiface, similar in many ways to the age-related changes. The lower face should be inspected carefully for jowls, neck bands, skin laxity, and double-chin deformity. Individual patients manifest varying degrees of soft tissue and bony volume loss versus tissue descent that should be addressed prior to surgery to adequately meet the patient's expectations. Retrognathia may require chin implants or fillers to improve the facial balance and overall results.

Lacrimal System

A complete history of tearing or epiphora should include the nature of the tearing, exacerbating or alleviating factors, chronicity, discharge, bloody tears, or pain. Emphasis should be placed on eliciting any history of environmental allergies, sinusitis, eyelid or facial trauma, nasal or sinus surgery, ocular viral infections (HSV, adenovirus), or punctal plugs. A thorough lacrimal system evaluation performed in the office is often sufficient for determining the correct diagnosis in the majority of patients.

Tear Film and Adnexa

Examination of the tear lake quality and quantity should be done at the slit lamp and compared between the two sides before touching the eyelids. A higher tear film in the watering eye suggests impairment of the draining system versus secondary hypersecretion from ocular irritation, whereas a lower tear film suggests dry eyes. Mucoid reflux on compression of the lacrimal sac suggests nasolacrimal duct obstruction. All four lacrimal puncta should be examined for stenosis and/or punctal ectropion. If both upper and lower puncta are completely closed, the cause of tearing could be simply punctal stenosis or a combination of punctal stenosis and downstream blockage which cannot be evaluated until punctal dilation or punctoplasty is performed [4, 8].

Dye Disappearance Test

This is a physiologic test of tear drainage, performed by measuring the tear meniscus 5 minutes after one drop of fluorescein is instilled in both eyes. A higher tear film on one side compared to the contralateral side suggests decreased outflow and thus blockage at any level from the canaliculi to the nasolacrimal duct. Blockage can be partial or complete. With nasolacrimal duct obstruction, reflux of dye with compression of the sac will also be seen. Degree and location of stenosis or obstruction are best assessed tactilely using a 0 or 00 Bowman probe passed through each canaliculus into the lacrimal sac.

Lacrimal Irrigation Test

Lacrimal irrigation is not a physiologic test but helps in differentiating partial from complete stenosis. At the same time, the canaliculi can be carefully probed with the Bowman probe or irrigation cannula to assess for stenosis or grittiness which would suggest occult canaliculoliths. When irrigating the canaliculus, reflux from the same punctum suggests canalicular stenosis. In contrast, reflux through the opposite canaliculus suggests common canalicular stenosis. In nasolacrimal duct obstruction, partial drainage into the nasopharynx combined with reflux from either canaliculus would distinguish partial duct stenosis from complete duct obstruction, in which only reflux would occur in the absence of nasal drainage.

Pay particular attention to the sensitivity of the canaliculi upon irrigation as this could indicate canalicular inflammation with partial obstruction. This is commonly seen in allergic conjunctivitis and after viral infections. Any ocular signs of allergies and prior HSV or adenoviral infections are useful in formulating the correct diagnosis. Canaliculitis caused most commonly by *Actinomyces israelii* presents as painful erythematous swelling of the punctum and medial eyelid margin between the punctum and the canthal angle. Compression of the medial eyelid over the canaliculus is typically tender and can result in extrusion of purulence or fine yellow-white canaliculoliths through the punctum. Probing and irrigation in the presence of active canaliculitis is contraindicated, as the risks of iatrogenic canalicular trauma and false passages are greater due to the inflamed mucosa. Canaliculitis is definitively treated with canaliculotomy and curettage of canalicular stones, with or without canalicular intubation.

Nasal Endoscopy

Office or intraoperative endoscopy is useful whether an external or an internal dacryocystorhinostomy technique is used, as it can assess for septal deviation, polyps, or other nasal pathology that could potentially alter the success rate of dacryocystorhinostomy (DCR). Endoscopy can be helpful in the diagnosis of certain pathologies such as Wegener's granulomatosis (granulomatosis with polyangiitis), sinusitis, or trauma. It can also be used to assess the patency and function of the DCR ostium in patients who continue to complain of epiphora following surgery.

Imaging

A maxillofacial CT is useful if trauma or mass lesions are suspected to contribute to altered nasolacrimal duct anatomy. CT is also useful when an acute dacryocystitis may have progressed to orbital cellulitis or abscess. Other imaging studies such as dacryocystography, dacryoscintigraphy, and lacrimal endoscopy are more cost-intensive, require additional instruments, and often do not contribute significant additional information.

Lacrimal Gland

The lacrimal gland can be evaluated by simply everting the lateral third of the upper eyelid with a finger at the slit lamp. Biomicroscopy can reveal inflammation (dacryoadenitis), cysts (dacryops), or even stones. Palpation of the lacrimal gland through the skin should also be performed if a lacrimal gland mass is suspected.

Orbit

The orbit is often more challenging for physicians to evaluate as there is often a need for additional tests, such as ultrasound, CT, and MRI. However, many orbital pathologies can be diagnosed with high accuracy based on a careful history and physical examination.

External Evaluation

Any external signs of inflammation, edema, asymmetry, or globe proptosis should be noted. Graves' orbitopathy is the most common cause of both unilateral and bilateral proptosis and can be associated with periorbital inflammatory signs. However, periorbital inflammation, erythema, and edema can also be seen in preseptal cellulitis, orbital cellulitis, or idiopathic orbital inflammation. Ocular or orbital dystopia (the uneven position of the eyes or orbits) can be appreciated directly on exam or from old photographs and can be suggestive of a mass effect (Fig. 1.1). The location of the orbital mass can be inferred from the direction of globe displacement as the lesion is normally situated on the opposite side from the direction of displacement. For example, inferomedial displacement of the globe would be seen with most lacrimal gland tumors or axial anterior proptosis seen with intraconal masses, such as a cavernous hemangioma. Blepharoptosis is commonly seen with acute infectious or noninfectious orbital inflammation, whereas upper eyelid retraction is usually seen in Graves' orbitopathy. This should also be distinguished from pseudoretraction seen with severe proptosis or from pseudoretraction compensating for a contralateral eyelid ptosis. Chemosis can be seen with allergies, outflow obstruction, and orbital congestion, following ocular, eyelid, or orbital surgery or secondary to corneal exposure from proptosis or lagophthalmos, among many other etiologies. Engorged and dilated bulbar conjunctival vessels warrant evaluation for a more severe form of congestion, such as direct (carotid-cavernous) or indirect (dural) arteriovenous fistulas.

Asymmetric fullness or bulging of the temple region, especially in conjunction with pulsatile movement, is highly suggestive of a sphenoid wing dysplasia or mass.

Palpation

Palpation is very useful for evaluating eyelid and orbital masses. Pain induced with minor pressure is suggestive of inflammation or infection. Resistance to retropulsion is frequently seen in Graves' orbitopathy and with intraconal space-occupying masses. The mass is best palpated if located in the anterior orbit or lacrimal gland fossa, and its consistency should be noted, as well as if the mass is freely mobile or adherent to underlying tissues or bone. A rubbery or fluctuant mass can suggest a vascular (lymphangioma, varix) or cystic (dermoid) lesion, whereas a firm, hard mass is more suggestive of a primary or metastatic malignant lesion, osteoma, or similar solid lesion.

Auscultation

Auscultation over closed eyes is indicated if a patient presents with acute proptosis and engorged bulbar conjunctival vessels. The presence of a bruit is suggestive of a high-flow fistula such as a carotid-cavernous fistula.

Extraocular Muscle Motility

Impaired ocular motility can assess for muscle restriction or paralysis. Restriction is suggestive of an infiltrative process such as thyroid eye disease or neoplastic disease or entrapped muscle or fibrous septa in an orbital fracture. Extraocular muscle paralysis is more frequently seen with myositis and orbital apex lesions. Saccadic velocity analysis is a simple method of distinguishing between the two in the office. With the patient looking suddenly (saccadic movement) from primary gaze to the direction of EOM limitation, a high velocity saccade that stops abruptly suggests muscle restriction, whereas a slow saccade (10 x slower) suggests paralysis. In children, however, this test may be difficult to perform in the office, thus necessitating forced duction testing performed in the OR under general anesthesia.

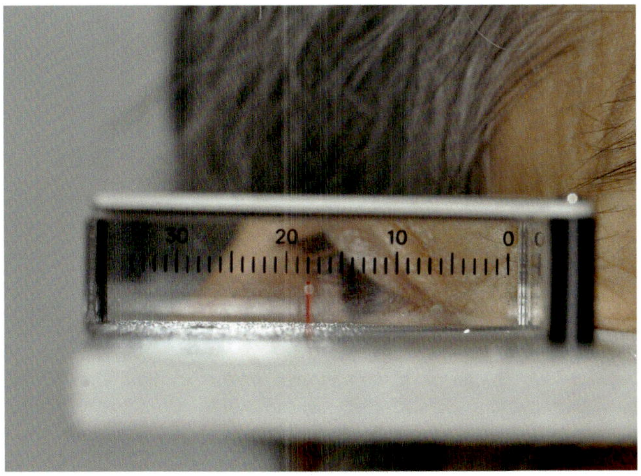

Fig. 1.22 Hertel exophthalmometry

Exophthalmometry

Exophthalmometry is an objective way of measuring proptosis as long as the interpupillary distance (IPD) is the same each time, the same instrument is used, and the repeat measurements are taken by the same person (Fig. 1.22). Most Hertel exophthalmometers commercially available today are single mirror, as the more precise double-mirror Zeiss model is no longer available. Exophthalmometry can be measured at rest (static) or after certain maneuvers (dynamic). If a venous malformation is suspected, Valsalva maneuvers, such as asking the patient to bend forward with the head down, can lead to increased orbital pressure and engorgement of the venous malformation with transient increase in proptosis. In contrast, lymphangiomas do not increase in size with Valsalva maneuvers but may enlarge during viral infections due to the presence of lymphoid tissue. Rarely, these enlarged lymphangiomas can bleed spontaneously or in response to trauma, forming "chocolate cysts" of varying ages as seen on imaging.

Differential Intraocular Pressure

Intraocular pressure measurements are useful for assessing orbital pressure and the tightness of the extraocular muscles. Increased intraocular pressure correlates in general with increased orbital pressure from various causes. In a patient with Graves' orbitopathy with a tight inferior rectus muscle, the intraocular pressure can increase in upgaze more than 10 mm Hg, suggesting that close monitoring for the development of compressive optic neuropathy is indicated.

Imaging

Imaging should always be used judiciously and guided appropriately by the findings of the clinical examination. A computed tomography (CT) scan with or without contrast is typically the most useful as it allows for high-quality detail of both bones and soft tissues (Fig. 1.23). It is the imaging study indicated if an intraocular or orbital foreign body is suspected and the most useful study in trauma for optimal evaluation of orbital and facial fractures. Two millimeter coronal and axial sections without contrast are usually sufficient. CT is also critical for preoperative planning in orbital fracture repair, orbital decompression, and orbitotomy for biopsy/excision of masses. The thickness of the sphenoid trigone can help determine if lateral orbital wall decompression is the adequate decompression technique. Similarly, the depth of the ethmoidal recess has to be evaluated before medial wall decompression is performed to avoid an inadvertent CSF leak. A low or extremely downward slanting ethmoidal roof, the fovea ethmoidalis, should also be noted prior to medial decompression or dacryocystorhinostomy. Magnetic resonance imaging (MRI) is slightly more superior in the evaluation of soft tissues; therefore, an MRI is ordered first or after a CT scan to better define the nature of orbital lesions and their relationship to surrounding vital structures. Vascular lesions are best evaluated with magnetic resonance angiography (MRA) (Fig. 1.24). In all instances, communication of the preliminary clinical diagnosis to the radiologist is critical for choosing the optimal study. Orbital ultrasound can be an inexpensive modality for lacrimal and orbital lesions without the risks of radiation, but requires the expertise of a specially trained technician or ophthalmologist, and provides less anatomic detail overall.

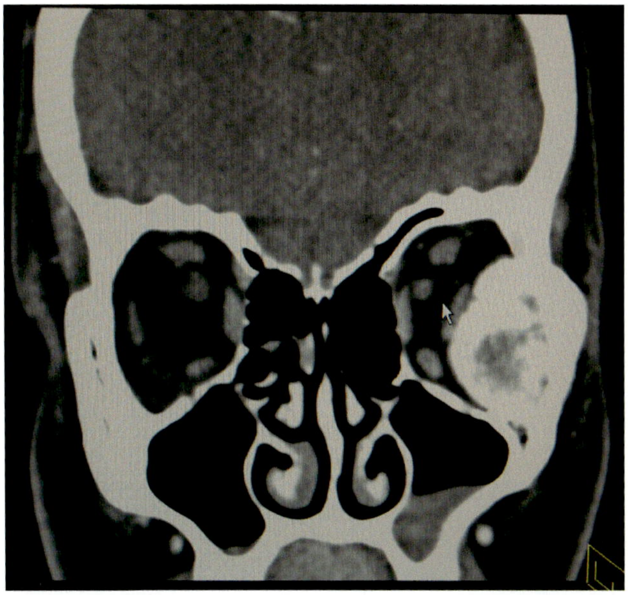

Fig. 1.23 Coronal section of orbital CT scan showing a left orbital lesion originating in the bone of the lateral orbital rim

Skin

The skin is the most superficial layer of the face and can bear many signs of aging or disease. A lesion suspicious for skin malignancy should be evaluated at the

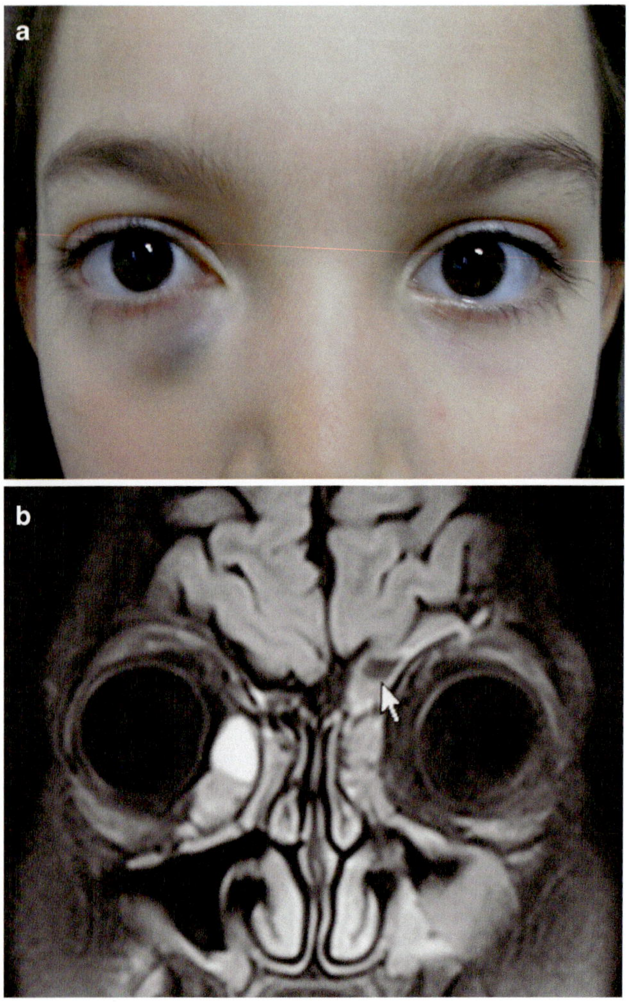

Fig. 1.24 Orbital vascular malformation in a child complaining of pain and double vision. (**a**) The lesion producing a bluish discoloration of the skin is palpable through the right lower eyelid. (**b**) Coronal MRI sections showing a large cystic space filled with contrast in the inferomedial right orbit, compressing the globe. The fluid level indicates the presence of a clot, which is seen in a low-flow lesion

slit lamp whenever possible, and biopsied for pathology, rather than treated with liquid nitrogen. Unusual xanthelasma lesions associated with orbital changes require imaging and biopsy to rule out orbital xanthogranuloma (Fig. 1.25). Xanthelasmas, if multiple and presenting in a young patient, should also be evaluated for lipid disorders. Facial pigmentation should always be documented before cosmetic surgery, chemical peels, or laser treatments, to avoid confusion for postinflammatory hyperpigmentation. Facial wrinkles and textural changes due to chronic sun exposure and aging should be discussed with the patient before surgery, as adjunctive chemical peels and laser skin resurfacing can improve the overall results dramatically.

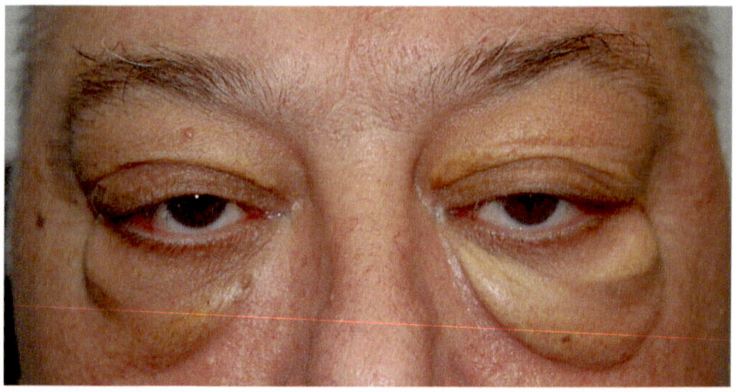

Fig. 1.25 A 58-year-old patient referred for xanthelasma. The unusual presentation and associated proptosis and orbital symptoms warranted further evaluation for orbital xanthogranuloma. This was confirmed with an orbital biopsy

Visual Field Testing

Visual fields, taped and untaped, have become mandatory before functional ptosis or upper blepharoplasty surgery. Generally, a 30% decrease in superior visual field is required by most insurance companies, but there are variabilities among states and different individual carriers. Currently, only Humphrey and Goldmann automated perimetry fields are accepted. Visual fields are also necessary in the setting of optic nerve or orbital pathology, or if monitoring for compressive optic neuropathy in thyroid eye disease, and should be obtained using the same machine and protocol each time to best follow evolution over time.

Photography

Photographs should be obtained before surgery, and after surgery as needed, as they can serve as medical documentation. They can also be helpful preoperatively to explain the pathology and the treatment plan to the patient. Requesting old photographs from the patient can frequently help in understanding how the pathological process or facial aging has affected his or her appearance. Comparison of preoperative and postoperative photographs also demonstrates to the patient the improvement obtained with surgery. It is surprising how often patients forget how they used to look or instead focus on minor concerns. When presented with the preoperative pictures, this helps put things in better perspective for the patient. In addition, certain anatomic features such as facial asymmetries that are present before surgery tend to persist after surgery. Clinical photographs can also be useful in preparation for surgery when reviewing the patient chart. At a minimum, full-face and periocular frontal, lateral, and oblique 45° angle photographs should be obtained (Fig. 1.26). The photographs should be taken using the same camera and light conditions each time.

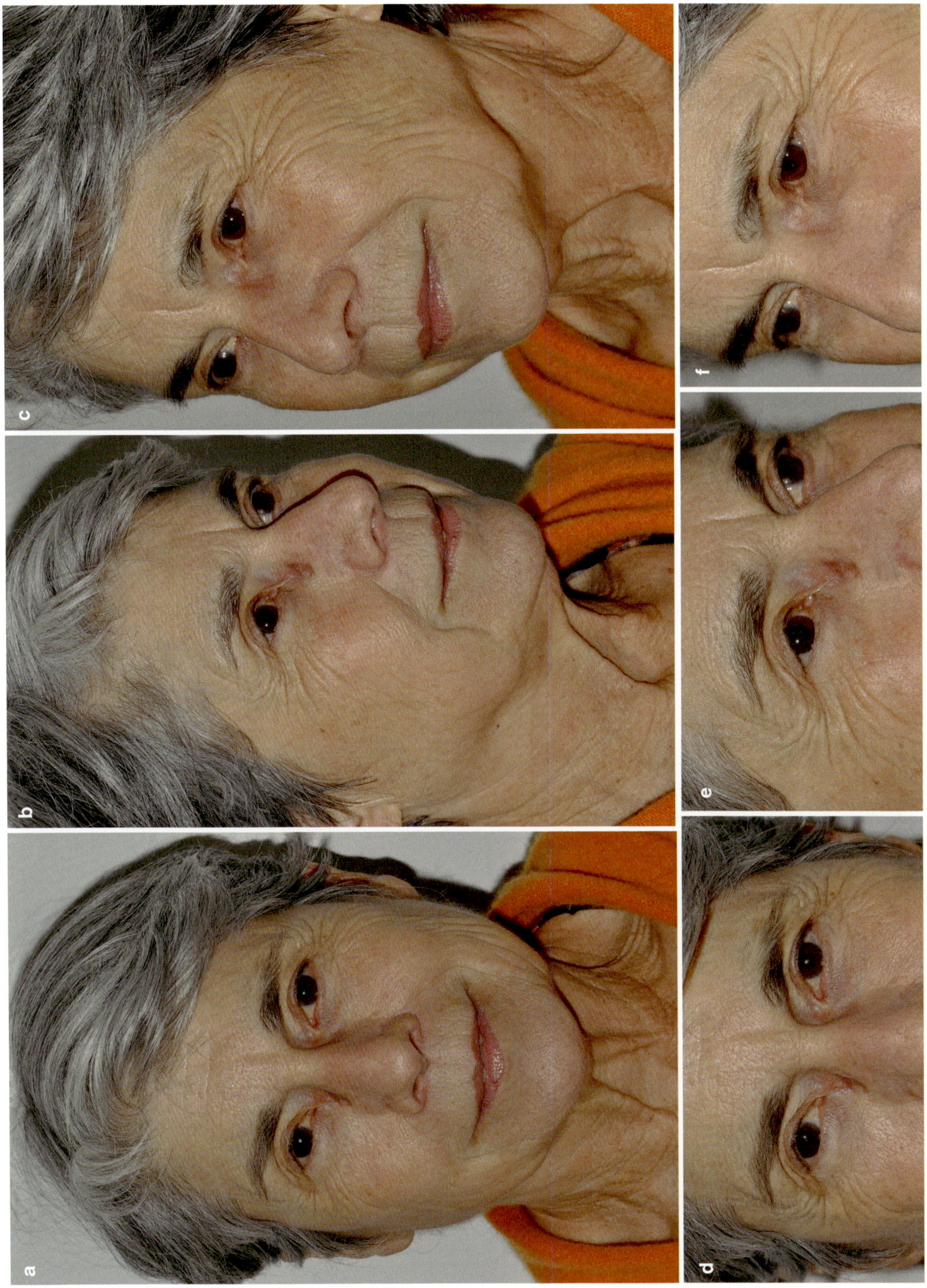

Fig. 1.26 Standard photographic documentation: (**a**) full-face frontal; (**b**, **c**) full-face 45° angle; (**d**) eyes frontal; (**e**, **f**) eyes at 45° angle

Consultation

After a thorough history taking and examination, sufficient face-to-face time between the surgeon and patient is mandatory to discuss the findings and treatment plan. The patient must be able to leave with all questions adequately addressed and feel that the surgeon is understanding of their personal concerns or anxieties. It is particularly important to discuss with the cosmetic patient what can be realistically achieved with the treatment proposed. The goal should always be to under-promise and over-deliver. Many patients are also not aware of their individual facial asymmetry or negative vector orbit that can influence the final result, which should be discussed with the patient using their photographs. The informed consent should be covered in detail with the patient, including all the risks, benefits, and alternatives of the procedures proposed. Preoperative instructions should be given to the patient and the patient aware of the importance of stopping the antiaggregants 2 weeks prior and anticoagulants 5 days prior to the procedure. Permission from the general practitioner or the treating cardiologist should always be requested before stopping these medications. Payment information or insurance preauthorization should be done by the office manager or a surgery scheduling person. Patients who have additional concerns and questions may require subsequent visits to adequately discuss their concerns in person again.

References

1. Burkat CN, Lucarelli MJ. Tear meniscus level as an indicator of nasolacrimal obstruction. Ophthalmology. 2005;112(2):344–8.
2. Fagien S. Putterman's cosmetic oculoplastic surgery. Philadelphia: WB Saunders; 2008.
3. Mauriello JA. Techniques of cosmetic eyelid surgery: a case study approach. Philadelphia: Lippincot Williams & Wilkins; 2004.
4. Tyers AG, Collin JRO. Colour atlas of ophthalmic plastic surgery. Philadelphia: Butterworth-Heinemann; 2002.
5. Georgescu D, Anderson RL, McCann JD. Brow ptosis correction: a comparison of five techniques. Facial Plast Surg. 2010;26(3):186–92. https://doi.org/10.1055/s-0030-1254328. Epub 2010 Jun 3.
6. Georgescu D, Jones Y, McCann JD, Anderson RL. Skin necrosis after calcium hydroxylapatite injection into the glabellar and nasolabial folds. Ophthal Plast Reconstr Surg. 2009;25(6):498–9.
7. Georgescu D, Anderson RL, McCann JD. Lateral canthal resuspension sine canthotomy. Ophthal Plast Reconstr Surg. 2011;27(5):371–5.
8. Jones YJ, Georgescu D, McCann JD, Anderson RL. Snip conjunctivoplasty for postoperative conjunctival chemosis. Arch Facial Plast Surg. 2010;12(2):103–5.

Etiologies of Blepharoptosis

2

Alexander Grigalunas and Aimee J. Szewka

Introduction

Blepharoptosis, herein referred to as ptosis, is a common complaint of patients presenting for medical evaluation and can be a presenting sign for a myriad of diseases. Strong examination skills and familiarity with all possible causes of ptosis are essential for proper diagnosis and workup of these findings. While many causes of ptosis are benign and age-related, several potentially life-threatening causes of ptosis need to be considered, which will be the focus of this chapter. This chapter will first address acquired ptosis, with its indicated evaluations and treatments, followed by a discussion of congenital ptosis.

Neurogenic Causes of Acquired Ptosis

Acute third nerve (CN III) palsy may herald a medical emergency, the most concerning being unstable cerebral aneurysm. Pathology inducing a CN III palsy can occur at any point along the course of the nerve. Determining the cause of third nerve palsy requires working knowledge of the anatomy and course of the nerve. CN III originates in the midbrain and courses anteriorly near the medial longitudinal fasciculus (MLF), red nucleus, and substantia nigra. It exits in the interpeduncular cistern, coursing through the subarachnoid space superior to the superior cerebellar artery and inferior to the posterior cerebral artery. CN III then enters the cavernous sinus along the lateral wall superiorly, near the internal carotid artery. Parasympathetic fibers are located superficially on CN III. The ophthalmic division of CN V joins CN III within the cavernous sinus. CN III then enters the orbit through the superior orbital fissure, dividing into a superior and inferior branch. The superior branch courses medial to the optic nerve and supplies the superior rectus and levator palpebrae superioris muscles. The inferior branch, carrying the parasympathetic fibers, eventually supplies the medial rectus, inferior rectus, and inferior oblique muscles.

The most dangerous causes of CN III palsy are cerebral aneurysm, subarachnoid hemorrhage, ischemic or hemorrhagic stroke of the brain stem, space-occupying lesion, cavernous sinus thrombosis, giant cell arteritis, or infectious etiologies, such as meningitis or mucormycosis. Other causes include autoimmune disorders (e.g., sarcoidosis, myasthenia gravis, multiple sclerosis), inflammation, trauma, and microvascular ischemia. Pupil-sparing CN III palsy is thought to be caused by microvascular ischemia in up to 70% of cases [1], and these tend to resolve fully without treatment over the course of 3 months [2].

CN III palsies have classically been categorized as pupil-involving (complete) and pupil-sparing (incomplete). In a study of 1400 referred outpatients with CN III palsy, 33% had complete involvement [3]. Involvement of the pupil suggests an external source of disease, in particular compression, as the parasympathetic fibers course on the outer layer of CN III. Signs of a complete, pupil-involving third nerve palsy include ipsilateral ptosis, mydriasis, and a depressed and abducted eye at rest. These findings can vary based on involvement of the CN III, but any amount of pupil abnormality should be considered pupil-involving. With any pupil-involving CN III palsy or partial CN III palsy without pupil involvement, an emergent MRI with contrast and an MRA (or CT/CTA) are indicated to look for masses, stroke, carotid dissection, aneurysms, and other abnormalities. Complete CN III involvement without pupil involvement is unlikely to be caused by external compression and is typically microvascular in etiology. However, any worsening of symptoms or signs on follow-up would warrant emergent imaging [4].

All patients with CN III palsy should have basic blood work consisting of a complete blood count, sedimentation rate, C-reactive protein, lipid profile, and hemoglobin A1C if diabetic status is unknown. Noninvasive neurovascular

A. Grigalunas · A. J. Szewka (✉)
Departments of Ophthalmology and Neurology, Rush University Medical Center, Chicago, IL, USA
e-mail: Aimee_J_Szewka@rush.edu

A. J. Cohen, C. N. Burkat (eds.), *Oculofacial, Orbital, and Lacrimal Surgery*, https://doi.org/10.1007/978-3-030-14092-2_2

imaging (MR angiogram or CT angiogram) should be considered in any patient without a complete pupil-sparing CN III palsy. Obtained imaging should ideally be reviewed with a neuroradiologist to avoid missing aneurysms and other critical causes [5]. Any underlying disease should be treated appropriately. Upon stabilization, ptosis and strabismus secondary to CN III palsy may be corrected surgically. Typically, strabismus should be addressed first, as muscle surgery may alter the position of the eyelid.

Lesions of the brain stem can cause bilateral ptosis. It is important to note that a *lesion of the oculomotor nucleus* presents with distinctively different signs than a lesion of the CN III nerve or fascicle. Unilateral *oculomotor nucleus* lesion causes ipsilateral adduction and depression weakness with a bilateral upgaze palsy and bilateral ptosis. The oculomotor nucleus is composed of individual nuclei for the medial rectus, inferior rectus, superior rectus, and inferior oblique. All of these nuclei control the muscle on the ipsilateral side except for the superior rectus, which controls the contralateral superior rectus muscle. There is one nucleus (central caudal subnucleus) that supplies bilateral levator palpebrae superioris muscles. Lesion of this nucleus causes *midbrain ptosis*. Lesions of the oculomotor nucleus are rare and almost always associated with other neurologic findings. Possible etiologies include ischemia, demyelination, infiltration, compression, and toxic/metabolic etiologies.

Horner's syndrome (HS), or Horner syndrome, is a syndrome of sympathetic autonomic dysfunction characterized by ipsilateral miosis causing anisocoria that is greater in the dark than in the light, mild ptosis secondary to impaired Müller's muscle function, and, less often, anhidrosis of the upper face. The underlying cause of an HS may be found anywhere along the sympathetic pathway from the hypothalamus to the eye. HS may be caused by an idiopathic condition in up to 40% [6] but may also be secondary to an emergent condition. The differential diagnosis for HS is broad, including brain stem stroke, brain tumor, demyelinating disease, arteriovenous malformations, Pancoast tumor of the lung, thyroid cancer, carotid dissection, carotid aneurysm, cavernous sinus thrombosis, and cluster headache. Therefore, prompt diagnosis and proper workup of a HS may be life-saving.

The sympathetic chain consists of a three-neuron pathway. The central neuron originates in the hypothalamus and courses inferiorly through the brain stem and spinal cord to the level of C8-T2 where it synapses with the second-order neuron in the ciliospinal center of Budge. The second-order neuron exits the spinal cord and traverses superiorly over the apex of the lung via the cervical sympathetic chain and brachial plexus. It then synapses with the third-order neuron at the superior cervical ganglion, which is located near the bifurcation of the common carotid artery. The third-order neuron runs with the internal carotid artery to the level of the cavernous sinus where it joins the first division of the trigeminal nerve (CN V1), and enters the orbit through the superior orbital fissure. Departing from CN V1, the third-order neuron travels through the ciliary ganglion to the iris dilator and Müller's muscle. Norepinephrine is released from the presynaptic terminal to innervate the iris dilator.

Eyedrop testing may aid in the diagnosis and localization of HS. Cocaine, which inhibits the reuptake of norepinephrine, may be used to diagnose HS. Sixty minutes after instillation of cocaine eyedrops, the normal pupil will dilate, while the Horner's pupil will remain miotic, increasing the anisocoria. Apraclonidine, a direct alpha-adrenergic agonist with weak alpha-1 and strong alpha-2 activity, has been shown to be non-inferior to cocaine testing in diagnosing HS [7] and may be used to diagnose HS. The denervated pupil dilator from HS will exhibit hypersensitivity, causing an upregulation of alpha-1 receptors. Forty to 60 minutes after instillation of 0.5% apraclonidine eyedrops in both eyes, the Horner's pupil will dilate, while the normal pupil will exhibit mild constriction, thereby exhibiting reversal of anisocoria. Hydroxyamphetamine causes a release of stored norepinephrine and may help localize an HS to a central (first- or second-order neuron) or peripheral (third-order neuron) cause. When damage occurs proximal to the third-order neuron, it maintains a store of presynaptic norepinephrine. Therefore, the Horner's pupil will dilate upon instillation of hydroxyamphetamine eyedrops. The normal pupil will also dilate, but the anisocoria will be reduced and, in some cases, reversed. However, if the third-order neuron is damaged, there will be no norepinephrine to release. Therefore, the Horner's pupil will stay miotic, while the normal pupil will dilate, thus increasing anisocoria. Of note, pharmacologic testing of pupils should only be done with one agent at a time and should be separated by 48 hours to allow a proper washout period.

Once HS is diagnosed, finding the underlying cause is of utmost importance. Urgent imaging of the complete sympathetic pathway should be pursued. This includes MRI or CT scan of the head, neck and upper chest, including the apex of the lung. Vascular imaging, such as MRA or CTA of the neck, should be obtained to evaluate for carotid dissection or other vascular abnormalities. Table 2.1 provides a concise summary of this information.

Ptosis may be corrected in Horner's syndrome after diagnosis and treatment of the underlying cause and stabilization of the lid height for several months. Interestingly, Müller's muscle resection may be done with good results [8]. Success has also been found using the Fasanella-Servat procedure [9] as well as anterior tarsectomy [10].

Apraxia of lid opening (ALO) is a rare entity where patients have difficulty opening their eyes. It is in the differential for ptosis but likely represents a dystonic phenomenon [11]. Once the patient's eyes are open, strength is relatively normal, but opening the eyes may take significant time or

Table 2.1 Summary of Horner's syndrome localization

	First-order neuron	Second-order neuron	Third-order neuron
Associated symptoms	Neurologic symptoms (ataxia, numbness, weakness)	Cough, chest pain	Neck pain, headaches
Hydroxyamphetamine response	Pupil dilates	Pupil dilates	No response
Structures involved	Hypothalamus, brain stem, cervical spinal cord	Brachial plexus, apex of the lung, subclavian artery injury	Internal and external carotid arteries, cavernous sinus
Imaging study	MRI brain and cervical spine	Chest radiograph, CT of the chest	MR angiogram of the head and neck
Possible causes	Ischemia, tumor, demyelination	Pancoast tumor, infiltrative malignancy	Carotid dissection, aneurysm, neck tumor, post procedural

even sensory "tricks" such as touching the eyelids. Often the forehead frontalis contractions will be prominent to try to lift the eyelids and will precede the slow opening of the eyelids. The entity can be isolated or with concurrent benign essential blepharospasm and may be associated with Parkinson's disease or Parkinsonism syndromes such as progressive supranuclear palsy. Treatment with levodopa may be helpful [12], but it can also be treated with botulinum toxin injections [13]. Surgical intervention may be necessary if injections fail.

Neuromuscular Junction Causes of Ptosis

Myasthenia gravis (MG) is a disease of the neuromuscular junction that causes painless unilateral or bilateral ptosis. Autoantibodies are formed that interfere with the functioning of acetylcholine receptors (AChR) on the muscle membraines, impeding proper muscle contraction in response to the nerve's signal. MG can present at any age, with weakness of the extraocular muscles as the presenting sign in 50–85% of cases [14, 15]. Eyelid position becomes more ptotic with use and may be accompanied by diplopia that does not follow a specific cranial nerve or specific muscle pattern. Ptosis may also be unilateral and sudden and sometimes alternate sides. MG may generalize and progress quickly to affect muscles involved in respiration; therefore, patients with MG should be informed to go directly to an emergency room if they experience any shortness of breath or difficulty breathing.

Examination of patients with MG may reveal orbicularis oculi muscle fatigability, which can be measured by having the patient continuously close their eyes with maximal force while the examiner attempts to open them for 1 minute. Progressive decrease in closure strength may be noted. Upper eyelid fatigability can also be elicited by having the patient look up for an extended period of time (up to 2 minutes) and watching for the upper eyelid to slowly drift down. The presence of a Cogan's lid twitch, a flick overshooting of the eyelid when the eyes saccade from downgaze to primary gaze, can be strongly suggestive of neuromuscular junction dysfunction. Strength evaluation of other muscle groups, including facial, neck, and appendicular muscles, is indicated to evaluate for generalized symptoms. If other muscle groups are weak, the patient requires more urgent evaluation by a neurologist.

Once clinically suspicious of MG, confirmatory tests should be performed. The ice pack test, where an ice pack is placed over closed eyelids at rest, is easily done in clinic. This is a particularly helpful test in the setting of atypical ptosis. As ice cools the tissue, acetylcholinesterase activity is diminished, thereby increasing acetylcholine at the neuromuscular junction and resulting in a transient improvement in ptosis and diplopia [16]. Recent studies place the sensitivity at 92% and specificity at 79%, with a negative predicative value of 94%, emphasizing the test's usefulness in ptosis suspected to be from MG [17]. However, icing the eyelids for more than 5 minutes has also been shown to cause more false-negative results. Edrophonium, a fast-acting acetylcholinesterase inhibitor, can be given intravenously to assess for muscular improvement, but due to potential adverse effects of bradycardia, bronchospasm, and syncope, its use is limited to situations where cardiac monitoring and access to atropine are available.

Serology is typically ordered to assess for AChR antibodies; and in the appropriate clinical setting, positive results are highly specific for MG [18]. AChR antibodies are found in 85% of patients with systemic MG and 50% of ocular MG. There are three types AChR antibodies typically tested: binding, modulating, and blocking. When AChR antibodies are not present, anti-muscle-specific kinase antibodies (anti-MuSK) are positive in 39–49% of patients with generalized MG [19]. However, these are not often positive in patients with isolated ocular MG. Electromyography (EMG) may be helpful in the diagnosis of myasthenia gravis, with repetitive nerve stimulation testing being most helpful in the case of generalized MG. Further EMG maneuvers, particularly single-fiber EMG, may be necessary to confirm the diagnosis, especially with isolated ocular MG [20].

Coexisting thymoma occurs in approximately 21% of patients with MG [21]. A CT of the chest without contrast should be done as part of the routine workup of the patients to assess for thymoma and thymic hyperplasia. As 5–10% of patients with MG have coexisting thyroid disease, patients should also undergo serologic testing for thyroid abnormalities [22].

Patients with ocular MG who eventually progress to develop systemic MG usually do so within the first 2 years following diagnosis [23]. All patients with myasthenia should be referred to a neurologist for further classification and disease monitoring/management. Treatment consists of systemic therapy with cholinesterase inhibitors (pyridostigmine) and/or immunosuppressive agents (prednisone, azathioprine). Plasmapheresis and intravenous immunoglobulin therapy are used primarily to treat myasthenic crises. Thymectomy is indicated when thymic hyperplasia or thymoma is present. Surgical management of MG-induced ptosis may be considered once the disease has been stable for over 6 months to 1 year.

Myogenic causes of ptosis include *myotonic dystrophy (DM1 and DM2)*, an autosomal dominant trinucleotide repeat disease that presents with myotonia and muscle atrophy. Type 1 DM (DM1) maps to a CTG repeat sequence on chromosome 19, while type 2 DM (DM2) shows a CCTG repeat on chromosome 3. Disease incidence ranges from 1 in 8000 in the general population to 1 in 1830 in the Finnish population [24].

Manifestations of DM1 consist of distal muscle weakness, grip myotonia, slurred speech, gonadal atrophy, respiratory muscle weakness, hearing deficits, and cardiac arrhythmia [25]. DM2 consists of proximal muscle weakness but with far less gonadal atrophy, cardiac arrhythmia, respiratory weakness, and ptosis [26]. Classic ocular findings of myotonic dystrophy consist of reduced visual acuity, ptosis, ophthalmoplegia, low intraocular pressure, subcapsular "Christmas-tree" cataract, and peripheral pigmentary retinopathy. Diagnosis of myotonic dystrophy consists of increased creatine kinase levels and hypogammaglobulinemia. EMG is helpful and can demonstrate a unique pattern of myotonic discharges. Genetic testing for the nucleotide repeats is available and diagnostic. An electrocardiogram should be ordered for all patients suspected of having myotonic dystrophy, as cardiac conduction defects are common. As there is currently no treatment of the underlying cause of muscle dysfunction from myotonic dystrophy, patients should receive symptomatic treatment. Based on clinical findings, ptosis may be managed by levator advancement or frontalis sling. Surgery must be carefully selected, as eyebrow weakness may be present, thus rendering a frontalis sling ineffective.

Chronic progressive external ophthalmoplegia (CPEO) is an inherited mitochondrial disease typically passed maternally, less often in an autosomal dominant or autosomal recessive fashion and, rarely, through non-inherited somatic mutations. The disease consists of progressive ptosis and ophthalmoplegia. Exercise intolerance, hearing loss, ataxia, hypogonadism, and other skeletal muscle myopathy may occur. Kearns-Sayre syndrome is a specific subtype consisting of CPEO with heart block and pigmentary retinopathy. Diagnosis is based on clinical findings in addition to muscle biopsy, which shows groupings of enlarged mitochondria, called "ragged-red fibers." An EKG is essential to assess for cardiac abnormalities. Currently, there is no proven treatment for CPEO. A small study of eight patients suggested that the use of coenzyme Q10 improves markers of cellular energy dysfunction with little symptomatic benefit [27]. Ptosis may be corrected by surgery [28]; however, long-term follow-up is required as patients may progressively lose their ability to close their eyelids and develop exposure keratopathy.

Oculopharyngeal muscular dystrophy (OPMD) is a muscular dystrophy that usually becomes symptomatic in the fifth or sixth decade of life and more common in women. It is inherited mainly in an autosomal dominant fashion but may also be autosomal recessive. Like DM, it is a product of trinucleotide repeat with most common mutation being a GCG repeat on chromosome 14. Prevalence ranges from 1 in 100,000 in the European population to 1 in 1000 in the French-Canadian population [29] and to 1 in 600 in the Bukharan Jewish population [30]. Symptoms of OPMD include ptosis, dysphagia, and proximal limb weakness that exhibits progressive skeletal muscle weakness and slowly worsening ophthalmoplegia. Diagnosis is based on symptomatology and confirmatory genetic testing for trinucleotide repeats. If suspicion is high and genetic testing reveals two normal alleles, a muscle biopsy may be performed. Although gene therapy treatments are being investigated [31], there is currently no treatment for OPMD. Ptosis from OPMD may be surgically corrected with good results.

Mechanical Causes of Ptosis

The most common cause of blepharoptosis is *aponeurotic or involutional ptosis*. Gradual stretching of the aponeurosis over time may lead to dehiscence or disinsertion of the levator aponeurosis from the tarsal plate. This results in decreased MRD1 despite normal levator function (greater than 10 mm of elevation). Typically, the upper eyelid crease will be located more superiorly than normal, indicating dehiscence or disinsertion with resulting slippage superiorly. Hering's law of equal innervation may mask bilateral ptosis. The apparently ptotic eyelid should be lifted, while the contralateral eyelid is observed for manifestation of any underlying ptosis. Depending on the amount of levator function and the amount of lift required to relieve the ptosis, levator advancement or Müller's muscle conjunctival resection may be appropriate for correction of involutional ptosis. Involutional ptosis is most often age-related, compared to ptosis secondary to blunt shearing trauma, frequent eyelid rubbing, stretching from eyelid speculum, or other causes that can attenuate the levator complex.

Direct trauma to the eyelid may induce ptosis. If tissue is present and identifiable, lacerations of the eyelid involving the levator muscle or Müller's muscle may undergo primary repair. An eyelid laceration that has fat prolapsing through the wound indicates violation of the orbital septum and thus warrants exploration of the levator complex. Blunt trauma to the eyelid may cause permanent ptosis through aponeurotic changes. Finally, ecchymosis and edema may cause mechanical ptosis, both of which usually resolve over time.

Post-cataract traumatic ptosis may occur in up to 7.3% of those undergoing cataract surgery [32]. The use of a rigid eyelid speculum as opposed to flexible wire speculum has been associated with damage to the levator aponeurosis [33]. Superior bridle suture placement during surgery is also associated with an increased risk of ptosis. When compared to a transconjunctival bridle suture, subconjunctival dissection and placement of a superior rectus bridle suture have been shown to significantly reduce the amount of postsurgical ptosis [34]. Ptosis as a surgical complication should be discussed with all patients undergoing ocular surgery that requires a superior bridle suture or eyelid speculum.

Rigid contact lens wearers are 20 times more likely to develop ptosis than non-contact lens wearers [35]. To a lesser degree than rigid contact lens wear, soft contact lens wear has also been associated with ptosis [36]. Ptosis occurring through involutional changes of the eyelid levator aponeurosis may be exacerbated by long-term microtrauma to, and stretching of, the levator aponeurosis from the contact lens during each blink. Removal of rigid contact lenses, which typically requires lateral pulling of the eyelid to blink the lens off, also contributes to stretching. Patients who are being prescribed contact lenses should be informed of the increased risk of ptosis.

A mass of the superior orbit or eyelid may induce a *mechanical ptosis* causing improper function of the levator muscle. Mechanical ptosis may be induced by any space-occupying mass of the eyelid and/or orbit (chalazion, neurofibroma, capillary hemangioma, dermoid cyst, epidermal cyst, hidrocystoma, pilomatrixoma, nevi, lipoma, xanthogranuloma, hemangiopericytoma, lacrimal gland cyst, varix, lymphangioma, meningoencephalocele, mucocele, metastasis, basal cell carcinoma, squamous cell carcinoma, rhabdomyosarcoma, papillae from vernal conjunctivitis). Amyloid deposition [37] and gouty tophi [38] have also been reported to induce ptosis. Hematomas, ecchymosis, and edema may also induce transient mechanical ptosis. Removal of the mass may be indicated to address ptosis. However, preoperative assessment, including a CT (if bony involvement is suspected) or MRI (to assess soft tissues), may be imperative, as some masses (e.g., meningoencephalocele) should not be operated on without a multispecialty approach.

Ocular cicatricial pemphigoid [39], Stevens-Johnson syndrome, alkali burns, trachoma, or surgical trauma may induce scarring that creates ptosis. Ptosis repair in these cases consists primarily of lysis of adhesions and eyelid reconstruction. Care must be taken to avoid exposure keratopathy in these cases, as the conjunctiva is usually abnormal.

Pseudoptosis

Some disease entities give the appearance of ptosis when the neuromuscular apparatus of the eyelid is normal. Cases of pseudoptosis are important to diagnose as surgery of the eyelid muscle apparatus will not correct the underlying issue.

Patients with *enophthalmos* often present with complaints that an eye appears smaller due to pseudoptosis. Common causes of enophthalmos are orbital floor/wall fractures, silent sinus syndrome, fat atrophy (e.g., aging, ocular prostaglandin use, linear scleroderma), and bony lytic lesions (e.g., scirrhous metastatic breast cancer). Contralateral exophthalmos with eyelid retraction can cause the appearance of pseudoptosis. Common causes of exophthalmos are thyroid eye disease, orbital tumor, orbital inflammation, retrobulbar hemorrhage, orbital cellulitis, and vascular fistulas. A difference between the two eyes of greater than 2–3 mm on Hertel exophthalmometry is typically considered abnormal, and enophthalmos or exophthalmos should be considered.

A congenitally smaller globe (*microphthalmia*) may appear ptotic, as will a contralaterally larger eye. Slit-lamp examination, corneal diameter, and axial length can be used to confirm microphthalmos, nanophthalmos, and buphthalmos.

Dermatochalasis occurs when excessive skin of the eyelid droops down past the eyelid margin. The "pinch test," where the examiner pinches the redundant skin of the upper eyelid with forceps, may be performed to mark the amount of excess to remove without inducing eyelid margin ectropion. In pure dermatochalasis, the eyelid margin is in a normal position and height near the superior limbus. Surgical treatment consists of blepharoplasty.

Brow ptosis occurs when the soft tissues of the eyebrow lay abnormally low below the superior orbital rim, typically occurring from involutional changes. When the eyebrows descend below the orbital rim, this causes the eyelid skin to also hang lower, thus exacerbating eyelid ptosis or pseudoptosis. Additionally, paralysis of the frontalis muscle from any cause or mass effect may induce brow ptosis. Surgical treatment consists of eyebrow or forehead lifts, as well as treatment of the underlying cause.

Blepharochalasis is a rare inflammatory disorder that is characterized as painless, episodic attacks of bilateral edema of the upper and/or lower eyelids generally resolving on its own over the course of a few days. Greater than 75% of patients with this disorder will develop aponeurotic ptosis after multiple episodes [40, 41]. Surgery should be deferred until no further episodes occur and findings are stable.

Congenital Ptosis

Congenital ptosis may result from a myogenic, neuropathic, or genetic cause and may have lasting implications on vision if severe enough to be amblyogenic. The eyelid may occlude the visual axis, inducing sensory deprivation, or may change the shape of the cornea by inducing astigmatism, thus leading to significant anisometropia. Additionally, congenital ptosis may be a manifestation of a more complex syndrome. Therefore, prompt assessment and treatment of congenital ptosis are essential.

Myogenic causes include *agenesis or dysgenesis of the levator palpebrae superioris muscle*. Clinically, the patient may show an absent eyelid crease or reduced eyelid crease. Additionally, levator function measurements will be reduced or absent. A myopathological analysis in congenital ptosis reported hypoplasia or aplasia of the levator palpebrae muscle in 16 of 20 pediatric patients that underwent palpebral resection with hypoplasia or agenesis of Müller's muscle in 3 of 20 of the same patients. Of note, if the levator palpebrae muscle was hypoplastic or absent, the Müller's muscle was normal, and if Müller's muscle was hypoplastic or absent, the levator muscle was normal [42]. In levator dysgenesis, the levator muscle may be highly fibrotic, causing a restrictive lagophthalmos. The eyelid may also demonstrate a characteristic "lid lag" in downgaze, such that the ptotic eyelid is higher than the contralateral normal eyelid when looking down, due to levator restriction.

Without additional symptoms or clinical signs, true levator dysgenesis requires no further workup. Treatment options are dependent on the amblyogenic potential of ptosis. If the eyelid is deemed to be non-amblyogenic, then observation is sufficient until the child is older. However, if patient has amblyogenic potential, then frontalis sling procedure may be indicated earlier. Fascia lata autograft is the gold standard, but should be carefully considered in children under 3 years of age as there may not be enough tissue to safely harvest and risk of scarring [43]. Many other options also exist to use in frontalis suspension surgery that do not require a secondary site, including sutures, silicone slings, expanded polytetrafluoroethylene (Gore-Tex), and fascia lata.

Congenital third nerve palsy is a neurogenic cause of ptosis typically associated with ipsilateral dysfunction of extraocular movement that correlates to the third cranial nerve. Pupil involvement, either mydriatic or miotic secondary to aberrant regeneration, may be present. Congenital CN III palsy frequently is associated with underlying neurologic disorders, but the most common cause is peripheral trauma [44]. Imaging (MRI) should be done to evaluate for potentially life-threatening causes and neurologic abnormalities such as septo-optic dysplasia [45]. Surgery is indicated if the ptosis is deemed to be amblyogenic.

Congenital Horner's syndrome is another neurogenic cause of congenital ptosis and presents with ptosis, miosis, and anhidrosis, often with associated iris heterochromia. Horner's syndrome results from a diminished, absent, or otherwise abnormal sympathetic chain. Ptosis arises from lack of innervation of Müller's muscle. Iris heterochromia develops secondary to the lack of proper melanocyte migration during embryogenesis. Miosis is secondary to reduced sympathetic tone to the iris dilator muscle, resulting in an imbalance where the constrictor muscle is unopposed. The incidence of congenital HS has been noted to be 1.42 per 100,000 patients [46].

The most common cause of congenital HS is birth trauma, particularly to the brachial plexus. More insidious causes of congenital HS include neuroblastoma and carotid artery pathology. Appropriate workup of a congenital ptosis includes MRI of the head, neck, and thorax to fully assess the sympathetic pathway. Other tests may include carotid ultrasound to evaluate for artery abnormalities and abdominal ultrasound to assess for neuroblastoma. Ptosis secondary to congenital HS may be managed conservatively, but a Müller's muscle conjunctival resection procedure (if less than 2 mm of elevation is needed) or a levator advancement (if more than 2 mm of elevation is required) may be necessary.

Marcus Gunn jaw-winking syndrome is an autosomal dominant condition with incomplete penetrance [47, 48] characterized by synkinetic innervation of the levator palpebrae upon activation of the external pterygoid muscle. It is best noted by elevation of the eyelid with movement of the jaw, although depression of the eyelid may occur as well. While the exact mechanism is unknown, it is thought that the connection between the trigeminal nerve and the oculomotor nerve occurs when motor fibers from CN V aberrantly reach the levator palpebrae superioris muscle. Fifty percent of cases of these patients develop strabismus and 20–50% develop amblyopia [49]. Surgical repair must be evaluated on a case-to-case basis [50], as it may be repaired with levator resection alone, strabismus surgery with levator resection, or a levator resection and concurrent frontalis sling procedure [51]. It is important to discuss with the patient and family that while the ptosis may be improved, the jaw-winking synkinesis will often persist.

Blepharophimosis syndrome (BPS) is a genetic cause of congenital ptosis causing blepharophimosis (horizontal shortening of the palpebral fissures), ptosis, epicanthus inversus, and telecanthus. High-arched eyebrows, low-set ears, short nasal philtrum, and a broad nasal bridge are other facial findings. It is typically an autosomal dominant syndrome of chromosome 3q23 (FOXL2 gene) [52]. However, up to 50% of cases are sporadic. The involvement of the FOXL2 gene in BPS type 1 also leads to infertility secondary to primary ovarian failure, while BPS type 2 is isolated to the eyelids

[53]. Surgery is considered if the ptosis is amblyogenic. Traditionally, telecanthus and epicanthal folds are corrected first, followed by ptosis surgery later, although some recent studies have demonstrated good results when performed together rather than staged. As levator function is usually poor, the ptosis surgery of choice for BPS is a frontalis sling.

Conclusion

The etiology of ptosis is most often benign. However, regardless of whether the ptosis is congenital or acquired, it can be a sign of a dangerous underlying issue and must be recognized and treated appropriately. With timely diagnosis and proper treatment, patients with ptosis may enjoy improved vision and cosmesis while avoiding morbidity and, in rare cases, mortality.

References

1. Rush JA, Younge BR. Paralysis of cranial nerves III, IV, and VI. Cause and prognosis in 1,000 cases. Arch Ophthalmol. 1981;99(1):76–9.
2. Keane JR, Ahmadi J. Most diabetic third nerve palsies are peripheral. Neurology. 1998;51(5):1510.
3. Keane JR. Third nerve palsy: analysis of 1400 personally-examined inpatients. Can J Neurol Sci. 2010;37(5):662–70.
4. Kung NH, Van Stavern GP. Isolated ocular motor nerve palsies. Semin Neurol. 2015;35(5):539–48.
5. Elmalem VI, Hudgins PA, Bruce BB, Newman NJ, Biousse V. Underdiagnosis of posterior communicating artery aneurysm in noninvasive brain vascular studies. J Neuroophthalmol. 2011;31(2):103–9.
6. Maloney WF, Younge BR, Moyer NJ. Evaluation of the causes and accuracy of pharmacologic localization in Horner's syndrome. Am J Ophthalmol. 1980;90(3):394–402.
7. Koc F, Kavuncu S, Kansu T, Acaroglu G, Firat E. The sensitivity and specificity of 0.5% apraclonidine in the diagnosis of oculosympathetic paresis. Br J Ophthalmol. 2005;89(11):1442–4.
8. Glatt HJ, Putterman AM, Fett DR. Muller's muscle-conjunctival resection procedure in the treatment of ptosis in Horner's syndrome. Ophthalmic Surg. 1990;21(2):93–6.
9. Pang NK, Newsom RW, Oestreicher JH, Chung HT, Harvey JT. Fasanella-Servat procedure: indications, efficacy, and complications. Can J Ophthalmol. 2008;43(1):84–8.
10. Baylis HI, Shorr N. Anterior tarsectomy reoperation for upper eyelid blepharoptosis or contour abnormalities. Am J Ophthalmol. 1977;84(1):67–71.
11. Zadikoff C, Lang AE. Apraxia in movement disorders. Brain. 2005;128(Pt 7):1480–97.
12. Lee KC, Finley R, Miller B. Apraxia of lid opening: dose-dependent response to carbidopa-levodopa. Pharmacotherapy. 2004;24(3):401–3.
13. Kanazawa M, Shimohata T, Sato M, Onodera O, Tanaka K, Nishizawa M. Botulinum toxin a injections improve apraxia of eyelid opening without overt blepharospasm associated with neurodegenerative diseases. Mov Disord. 2007;22(4):597–8.
14. Grob D, Arsura EL, Brunner NG, Namba T. The course of myasthenia gravis and therapies affecting outcome. Ann N Y Acad Sci. 1987;505:472–99.
15. Meriggioli MN, Sanders DB. Autoimmune myasthenia gravis: emerging clinical and biological heterogeneity. Lancet Neurol. 2009;8(5):475–90.
16. Sethi KD, Rivner MH, Swift TR. Ice pack test for myasthenia gravis. Neurology. 1987;37(8):1383–5.
17. Fakiri MO, Tavy DL, Hama-Amin AD, Wirtz PW. Accuracy of the ice test in the diagnosis of myasthenia gravis in patients with ptosis. Muscle Nerve. 2013;48(6):902–4.
18. Cromar A, Lozier BK, Haven TR, Hill HR. Detection of acetylcholine receptor blocking antibodies by flow cytometry. Am J Clin Pathol. 2016;145(1):81–5.
19. Guptill JT, Sanders DB, Evoli A. Anti-MuSK antibody myasthenia gravis: clinical findings and response to treatment in two large cohorts. Muscle Nerve. 2011;44(1):36–40.
20. Gwathmey KG, Burns TM. Myasthenia gravis. Semin Neurol. 2015;35(4):327–39.
21. Mao ZF, Mo XA, Qin C, Lai YR, Hackett ML. Incidence of thymoma in myasthenia gravis: a systematic review. J Clin Neurol. 2012;8(3):161–9.
22. Mao ZF, Yang LX, Mo XA, Qin C, Lai YR, He NY, et al. Frequency of autoimmune diseases in myasthenia gravis: a systematic review. Int J Neurosci. 2011;121(3):121–9.
23. Kupersmith MJ. Ocular myasthenia gravis: treatment successes and failures in patients with long-term follow-up. J Neurol. 2009;256(8):1314–20.
24. Suominen T, Bachinski LL, Auvinen S, Hackman P, Baggerly KA, Angelini C, et al. Population frequency of myotonic dystrophy: higher than expected frequency of myotonic dystrophy type 2 (DM2) mutation in Finland. Eur J Hum Genet. 2011;19(7):776–82.
25. Romeo V. Myotonic dystrophy type 1 or Steinert's disease. Adv Exp Med Biol. 2012;724:239–57.
26. Day JW, Ricker K, Jacobsen JF, Rasmussen LJ, Dick KA, Kress W, et al. Myotonic dystrophy type 2: molecular, diagnostic and clinical spectrum. Neurology. 2003;60(4):657–64.
27. Chen RS, Huang CC, Chu NS. Coenzyme Q10 treatment in mitochondrial encephalomyopathies. Short-term double-blind, crossover study. Eur Neurol. 1997;37(4):212–8.
28. Rajabi MT, Tabatabaie SZ, Rajabi MB, Abrishami Y, Hosseini SS, Oestreicher J. Management of myogenic ptosis in chronic progressive external ophthalmoplegia. Iran J Neurol. 2014;13(3):185–7.
29. De Braekeleer M. Hereditary disorders in Saguenay-Lac-St-Jean (Quebec, Canada). Hum Hered. 1991;41(3):141–6.
30. Blumen SC, Nisipeanu P, Sadeh M, Asherov A, Blumen N, Wirguin Y, et al. Epidemiology and inheritance of oculopharyngeal muscular dystrophy in Israel. Neuromuscul Disord. 1997;7(Suppl 1):S38–40.
31. Harish P, Malerba A, Dickson G, Bachtarzi H. Progress on gene therapy, cell therapy, and pharmacological strategies toward the treatment of oculopharyngeal muscular dystrophy. Hum Gene Ther. 2015;26(5):286–92.
32. Hosal BM, Tekeli O, Gursel E. Eyelid malpositions after cataract surgery. Eur J Ophthalmol. 1998;8(1):12–5.
33. Altieri M, Truscott E, Kingston AE, Bertagno R, Altieri G. Ptosis secondary to anterior segment surgery and its repair in a two-year follow-up study. Ophthalmologica. 2005;219(3):129–35.
34. Loeffler M, Solomon LD, Renaud M. Postcataract extraction ptosis: effect of the bridle suture. J Cataract Refract Surg. 1990;16(4):501–4.
35. Kitazawa T. Hard contact lens wear and the risk of acquired blepharoptosis: a case-control study. Eplasty. 2013;19(13):e30.
36. Bleyen I, Hiemstra CA, Devogelaere T, van den Bosch WA, Wubbels RJ, Paridaens DA. Not only hard contact lens wear but also soft contact lens wear may be associated with blepharoptosis. Can J Ophthalmol. 2011;46(4):333–6.
37. Mun KS, Pailoor J, Reddy SC. Primary localised deep cutaneous amyloidosis of the eyelid. Malays J Pathol. 2005;27(2):113–5.

38. Yang CC, Vagefi MR, Davis D, Mamalis N, Anderson RL, McCann J. Gouty tophus of the upper eyelid. Ophthal Plast Reconstr Surg. 2008;24(5):404–6.
39. Scuderi G, Mutolo MG, Lambiase A, Recupero SM. Surgical management of concomitant ptosis and cicatricial entropion in a patient with ocular cicatricial pemphigoid. Int J Ophthalmol Clin Res. 2015;2(3):32.
40. Koursh DM, Modjtahedi SP, Selva D, Leibovitch I. The blepharochalasis syndrome. Surv Ophthalmol. 2009;54(2):235–44.
41. Langley KE, Patrinely JR, Anderson RL, Thiese SM. Unilateral blepharochalasis. Ophthalmic Surg. 1987;18(8):594–8.
42. Sarnat HB, Flores-Sarnat L, Kherani F. Palpebral myopathology of congenital ptosis. Presented at the 57th annual meeting of the German Society for Neuropathology and Neuroanatomy. Erlangen, Germany; 2012.
43. Crawford JS. Repair of ptosis using frontalis muscle and fascia lata: a 20-year review. Ophthalmic Surg. 1977;8(4):31–40.
44. Hamed LM. Associated neurologic and ophthalmologic findings in congenital oculomotor nerve palsy. Ophthalmology. 1991;98(5):708–14.
45. Langmann A, Lindner S. Congenital third nerve palsy in septo-optic dysplasia. Br J Ophthalmol. 2004;88(7):969.
46. Smith SJ, Diehl N, Leavitt JA, Mohney BG. Incidence of pediatric Horner syndrome and the risk of neuroblastoma: a population-based study. Arch Ophthalmol. 2010;128(3):324–9.
47. Yamada K, Hunter DG, Andrews C, Engle EC. A novel KIF21A mutation in a patient with congenital fibrosis of the extraocular muscles and Marcus Gunn jaw-winking phenomenon. Arch Ophthalmol. 2005;123(9):1254–9.
48. Kirkham TH. Familial Marcus Gunn phenomenon. Br J Ophthalmol. 1969;53(4):282–3.
49. Demirci H, Frueh BR, Nelson CC. Marcus Gunn jaw-winking synkinesis: clinical features and management. Ophthalmology. 2010;117(7):1447–52.
50. Bowyer JD, Sullivan TJ. Management of Marcus Gunn jaw winking synkinesis. Ophthal Plast Reconstr Surg. 2004;20(2):92–8.
51. Ibrahim HA. Use of the levator muscle as a frontalis sling. Ophthal Plast Reconstr Surg. 2007;23(5):376–80.
52. Fukushima Y, Wakui K, Nishida T, Ueoka Y. Blepharophimosis sequence and de novo balanced autosomal translocation [46,XY,t(3;4)(q23;p15.2)]: possible assignment of the trait to 3q23. Am J Med Genet. 1991;40(4):485–7.
53. De Baere E, Dixon MJ, Small KW, Jabs EW, Leroy BP, Devriendt K, et al. Spectrum of FOXL2 gene mutations in blepharophimosis-ptosis-epicanthus inversus (BPES) families demonstrates a genotype – phenotype correlation. Hum Mol Genet. 2001;10(15):1591–600.

External Levator Advancement and Resection

3

Ann Q. Tran and Cat Nguyen Burkat

Introduction

Blepharoptosis occurs from congenitally or acquired mechanical, neurogenic, myogenic, or traumatic etiologies leading to drooping of the upper eyelid. Ptosis in elderly patients most commonly presents as dehiscence of the levator aponeurosis insertion and thinning of the aponeurotic fibers [1]. The aponeurotic repair of ptosis, originally described by Everbrush in 1883, grew in popularity in 1975 after Jones reported a new technique resecting a portion of the flaccid aponeurotic tissue [2]. The technique continued to be modified over time as the role of the disinsertion of the levator aponeurosis in involutional ptosis was more clearly understood [3].

The most common surgical approaches of symptomatic involutional levator aponeurotic blepharoptosis include anterior approaches with the levator aponeurosis advancement or resection, tarsoaponeurectomy, modified small-incision levator repair, and posterior approaches with a conjunctival Müller's muscle resection. The aim of these procedures targets reattaching the levator aponeurosis to the tarsal plate. This chapter aims to discuss the anterior surgical approaches for blepharoptosis including external levator advancement, levator resection, and small-incisional surgery.

Preoperative Evaluation

A careful history of trauma, duration of symptoms, progression, variation, and severity of ptosis should be documented to help assess the etiology of ptosis. Common complaints include decrease in peripheral vision, heaviness, forehead fatigability, or constant brow elevation and droopy eyelids. Prior ocular history should encompass previous eyelid or intraocular surgery, recurrent intravitreal injections, and surgical glaucoma history of trabeculectomy or glaucoma drainage implant device. Theoretical concern of placement of sutures through the palpebral conjunctiva or alteration of the eyelid margin could result in possible glaucoma drainage implant exposure, erosion, or bleb failure.

A thorough assessment and treatment of patients with dry eye complaints should be completed prior to surgery. All patients should be aware that dry eyes may occur or become more noticeable after surgery due to greater ocular surface exposure that may lead to increased tear film evaporation. Postoperatively, patients may benefit from a regimen of preservative-free artificial tears and eyelid hygiene. Patients with poor corneal integrity, lagophthalmos, or severe dry eyes despite medical management may experience worsening of symptoms after surgery and thus may wish to defer surgery or have a more conservative elevation. Punctal plugs or permanent punctal cautery before or after surgery can aid in patients with severe dry eye syndrome and corneal punctate keratopathy.

Clinical features to document include the location of the eyelid crease, presence of excess dermatochalasis or an epicanthal fold (Fig. 3.1), degree of ptosis, vertical palpebral fissure, marginal distance reflex, levator function, obstruction of pupil in downgaze (Fig. 3.2), fatigability, and Hering's law. Complete obstruction of the pupil in downgaze, or less than 1 mm of vertical palpebral fissure in reading position, typically qualifies as visually significant.

Levator function is measured with a ruler held to the eyelid margin while the patient looks down and then in extreme upgaze, measuring the distance of maximal levator excursion in millimeters. It is important to eliminate the use of the frontalis muscle with the examiner's hand to prevent the patient from using the forehead to elevate the eyelid (Fig. 3.3).

If unilateral or asymmetric ptosis is present and the ptotic eyelid manually lifted, the contralateral eyelid may become droopy, consistent with Hering's law of equal innervation. If the contralateral eyelid droops enough to approach the visual

A. Q. Tran · C. N. Burkat (✉)
Department of Ophthalmology and Visual Sciences, University of Wisconsin-Madison, Madison, WI, USA
e-mail: cburkat@wisc.edu

A. J. Cohen, C. N. Burkat (eds.), *Oculofacial, Orbital, and Lacrimal Surgery*, https://doi.org/10.1007/978-3-030-14092-2_3

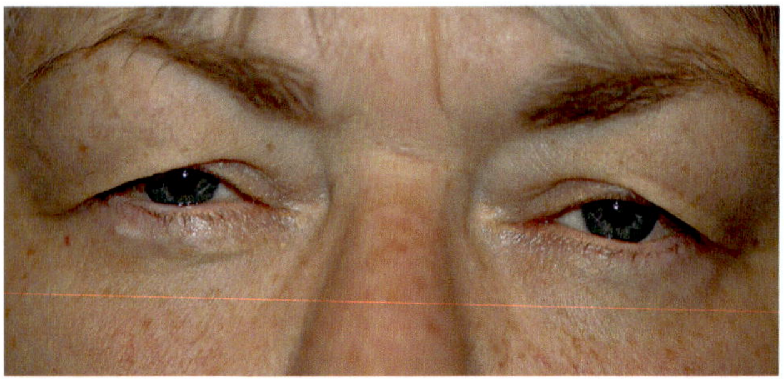

Fig. 3.1 Dermatochalasis hooding over the eyelid margin is also present in addition to involutional ptosis

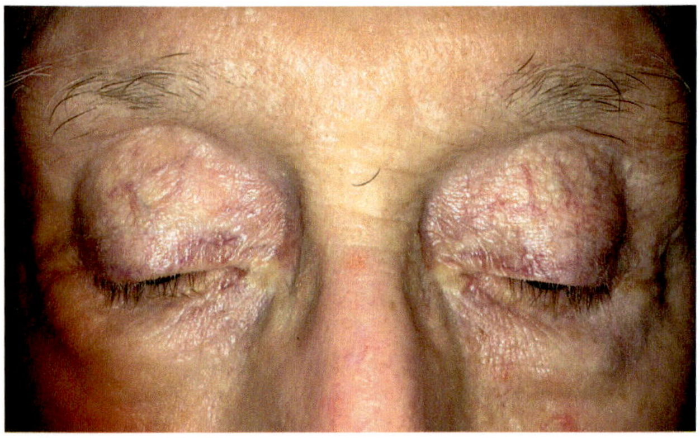

Fig. 3.2 In involutional ptosis (in contrast to congenital ptosis), the eyelids may block the pupil completely in downgaze or reading position

axis, this would suggest that bilateral ptosis surgery should be performed. Beard's classification of levator function has historically served as a surgical guideline for the degree of ptosis: with good levator function categorized as 8–16 mm of eyelid excursion, fair 5–7 mm, and poor being ≤4 mm of levator function [4]. For patients with fair to good levator function, aponeurotic advancement or repair serves as a good surgical option. Patients with mild to moderate ptosis (1–3 mm) that elevates after instillation of a drop of 2.5% or 10% phenylephrine on the ptotic side may be suitable for a posterior conjunctival Müller's muscle resection (CMMR). However, in instances where the ptosis is more severe or the patient has failed prior conjunctivomüllerectomy, additional elevation with an anterior levator approach may result in better outcomes and more subtle contour adjustments. Although some surgeons have performed repeat conjunctival Müller's muscle resection with reportedly good results, the algorithms and outcomes may be less predictable. Myogenic (such as in chronic progressive external ophthalmoplegia, myotonic dystrophy, myasthenia gravis, or oculopharyngeal dystrophy) or involutional ptosis with poor levator function will often require a more conservative approach to minimize postoperative complications of dry eye syndrome, lagophthalmos, or exposure keratopathy.

Eyebrow ptosis and eyebrow asymmetry must be corrected concurrently with levator repair as patients postoperatively may otherwise perceive asymmetry or lack of ptosis improvement despite elevation of the actual margin-reflex distance (Fig. 3.4). Patients with frontalis muscle preference,

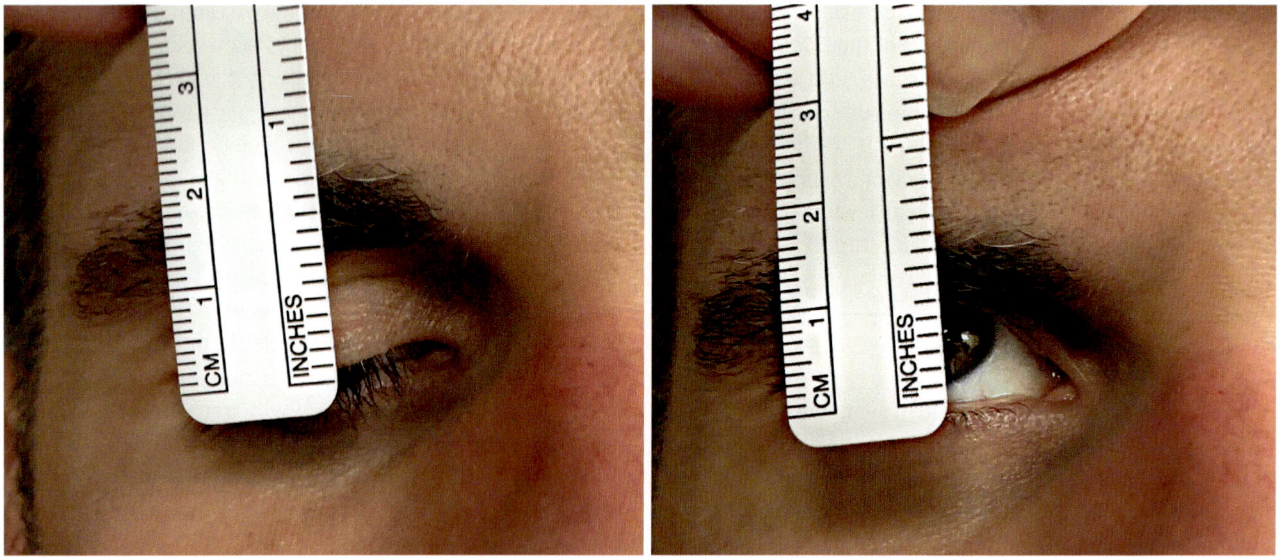

Fig. 3.3 Levator function, or levator excursion, is measured while holding the eyebrow steady to negate compensatory frontalis muscle elevation

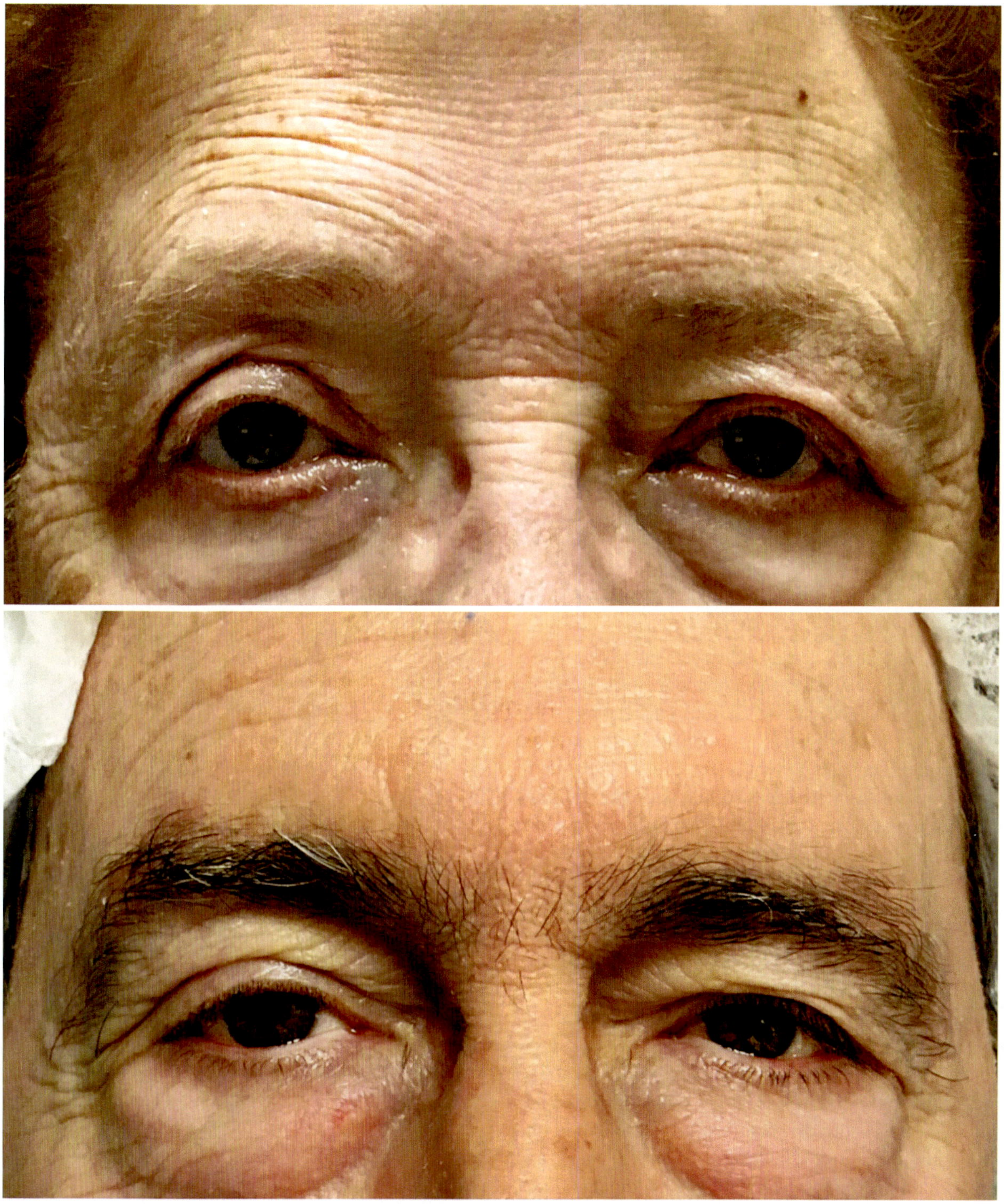

Fig. 3.4 Asymmetric frontalis preference is evident, as noted by the higher right eyebrow and increased horizontal rhytids on that side. This results in the appearance of greater pseudodermatochalasis or pseudoptosis on the contralateral side

raising one side of the forehead more prominently, may mask underlying eyebrow ptosis but may also feel that that side is more "open" after bilateral levator surgery. Excessive skin or dermatochalasis with concurrent ptosis should be assessed by taping up the excess skin or gently rolling the skin back with a cotton applicator to obtain accurate measurements of the upper eyelid crease position, vertical fissure height, and levator function.

For insurance authorization, clinical photographs and visual field defects showing substantial superior visual field constriction can aid in approval of surgical intervention and should be checked with the individual insurance prior to surgery. Conversations about patient expectations, postoperative care, and surgical risks that include bruising, bleeding, infection, asymmetry, need for additional surgery, recurrence, scarring, and loss of vision should also be thoroughly discussed.

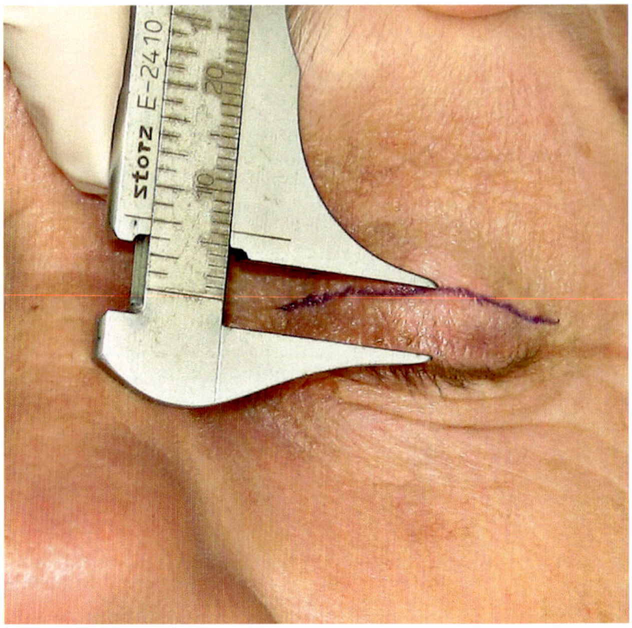

Fig. 3.5 Marking the eyelid crease incision

Surgical Techniques and Variations

External Levator Aponeurosis Advancement

The goal of the external levator advancement, also called a levator repair, is to reattach the levator aponeurosis to its anatomic position along the anterior surface of tarsal plate, without resection of levator tissue. The indications for external levator advancement are generally for ptosis with fair to good levator excursion of at least 6 mm. Contraindications for external levator advancement include ptosis with poor or absent levator function. External levator advancement has achieved excellent outcomes with postoperative satisfaction as high as 80–94% with reoperation rates in 8–10% of patients [5]. When compared to the posterior approach conjunctivomüllerectomy (CMMR), both groups have been shown to perform equally in effectiveness [6].

Although surgical variations exist, in general, the eyelid incision is marked prior to local anesthetic infiltration, as this could stretch the soft tissues or cause ecchymosis that affects the accuracy of the eyelid markings. The surgical incision line is typically marked within the natural eyelid crease at 8–12 mm above the eyelid margin for females, 7–9 mm for males, and 4–6 mm for Asian eyelids (Fig. 3.5). Local infiltration of lidocaine 2% with 1:100,000 epinephrine, with or without a longer acting agent such as marcaine, is injected along the incision line to provide hemostasis and analgesia. It is important to inject no more than 1–1.5 mL of anesthetic in each eyelid and to place the same volume between the two sides, as larger and asymmetric volumes can cause temporary paresis of the levator and Müller muscles and thus make the dynamic intraoperative adjustment of eyelid height unreliable.

The incision can be made with a #15 blade scalpel, CO_2 laser, and monopolar or radiofrequency cautery through the skin and orbicularis oculi. In patients in whom dry eyes or postoperative exposure may be a concern, or who have less levator function, the orbicularis muscle can be left intact without excision (if a skin blepharoplasty is concurrently performed) in order to facilitate eyelid closure (Fig. 3.6). Posterior to the preseptal orbicularis muscle lies the multilayered translucent orbital septum, and prolapse of the underlying preaponeurotic fat can be noted with gentle pressure on the globe. The orbital septum is then carefully opened to avoid injury to the underlying levator complex, and excessive preaponeurotic fat can be clamped with a curved hemostat and debulked or thermally shrunk with cautery. Gentle pushing with cotton-tipped applicators can also

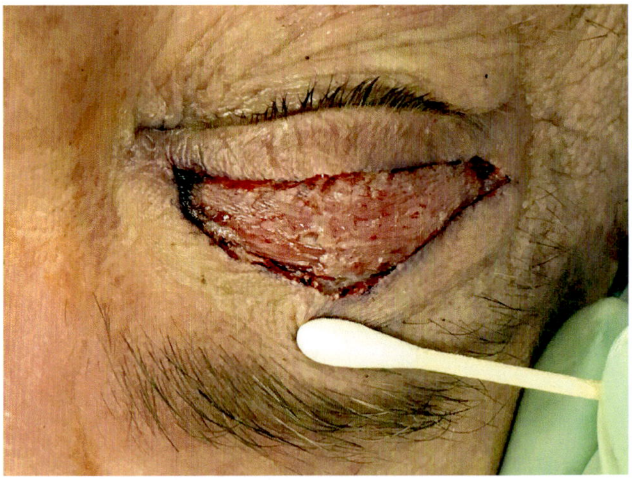

Fig. 3.6 Preseptal orbicularis muscle can be left intact after concurrent skin blepharoplasty, which may help minimize postoperative lagophthalmos as well as maintain volume

release the many fine septal attachments over the levator complex up toward Whitnall's ligament. Often the levator muscle itself may demonstrate significant rarefication or fatty infiltration of the normal muscle (Fig. 3.7). The anterior superior tarsal surface is also dissected clean, taking care to minimize pretarsal dissection along the inferior half of the tarsus that could lead to postoperative eyelash ptosis (Fig. 3.8). Next, 2–3 sutures through the levator aponeurosis and partial-thickness superior tarsus with 6-0 Prolene or 5-0 nylon suture are placed above the central pupil, or at the lateral and medial limbus, to create the desired eyelid height and contour (Fig. 3.9). Typically, the suture is passed starting from the musculoaponeurotic junction to behind the levator muscle (anterior to Müller's muscle), through the tarsus horizontally, and then back up behind the levator to exit several millimeters adjacent to the first pass. The suture is

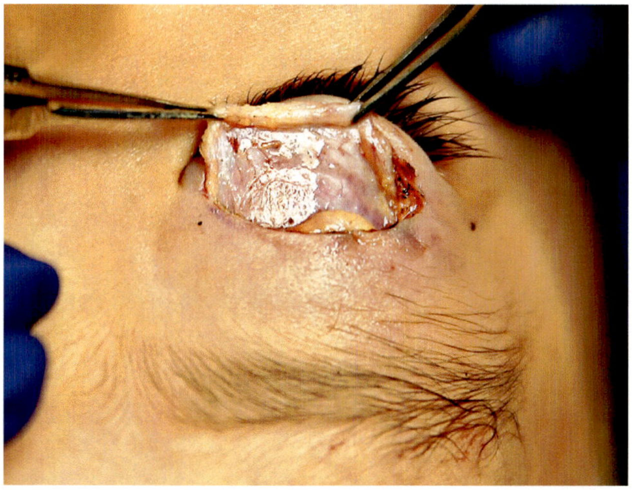

Fig. 3.7 The levator complex can demonstrate significant attenuation, or even fatty infiltration, of the muscle body and aponeurosis

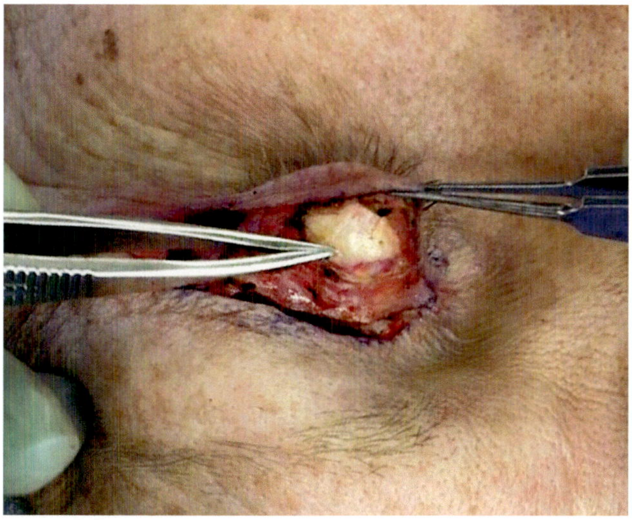

Fig. 3.8 The anterior superior portion of the tarsus is dissected in preparation for suture placement (surgeon view)

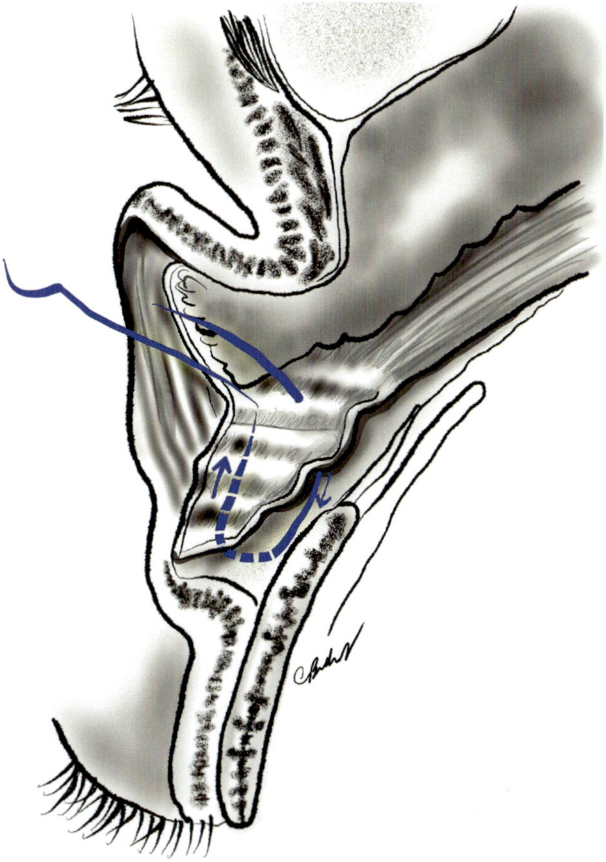

Fig. 3.9 Schematic of the levator advancement suture pass, starting from the musculoaponeurotic junction, behind the levator muscle, and through the tarsus horizontally

then cinched temporarily on the anterior surface of the levator aponeurosis. Note that placing the tarsal sutures too low in the tarsal plate may result in peaking of the eyelid margin, or eyelid margin ectropion off the globe surface. Therefore, the sutures should typically be passed in horizontal lamellar fashion through the upper one-third of the tarsus (Fig. 3.10). The eyelid should always be everted after each tarsal pass, to confirm that the suture is not exiting full-thickness, which would result in corneal abrasions (Fig. 3.11). Fine adjustments are made with the patient alert without sedation and sitting up to ensure adequate eyelid height and symmetry, as well as a natural curved contour without lateral retraction. Having the patient sitting up also allows for the natural forehead and eyebrow ptosis to manifest which affects the dynamics of the eyelid position. Eyelid closure should also demonstrate negligible lagophthalmos, or the sutures would need to be loosened. The sutures can be loosened to lower the medial or lateral margin, or tightened further to elevate the eyelid as desired, and then permanently tied without further cinching down the knot. The incision is closed with several interrupted eyelid crease reformation and orbicularis sutures with 6-0 polyglactin, followed by a running skin suture with 6-0 nylon or fast-absorbing plain gut suture.

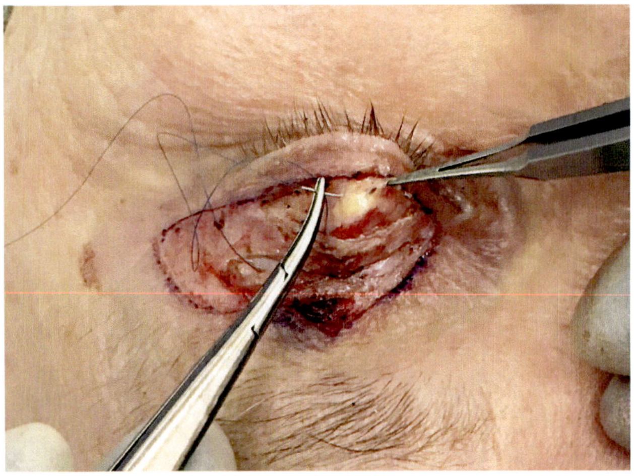

Fig. 3.10 The tarsal sutures are placed in the upper third of the tarsus, in a horizontal partial-thickness pass

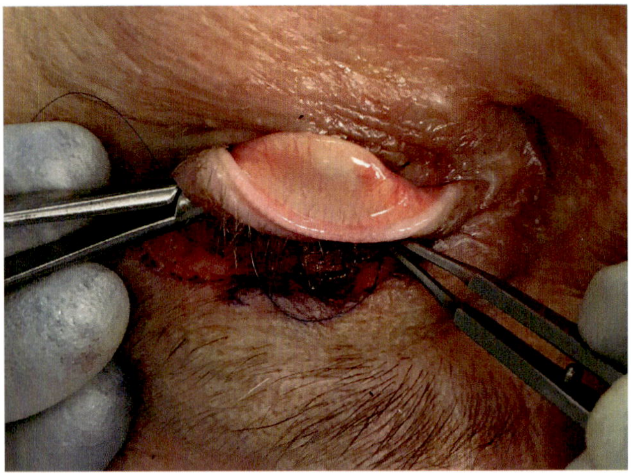

Fig. 3.11 The eyelid is everted to confirm lamellar tarsal bites, without exposure through the posterior tarsal conjunctiva

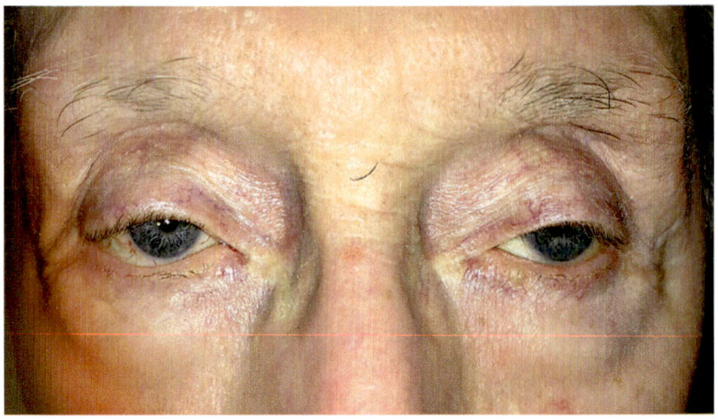

Fig. 3.12 Patient candidate for the small-incision levator technique due to deep sulci and lack of skin redundancy

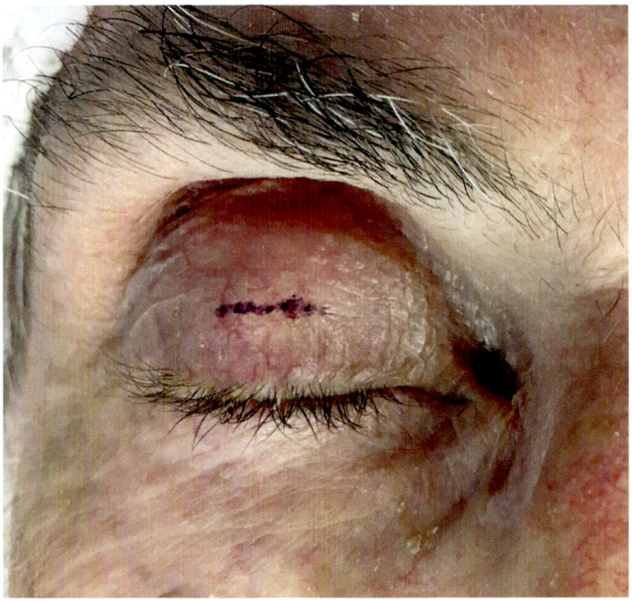

Fig. 3.13 Skin marking for the small-incision levator repair technique can be 7–12 mm in length

Small-Incision External Levator Repair

While a longer skin excision allows for complete visualization of the upper eyelid anatomy, the benefits of a smaller incision are to decrease the operative area, resulting in less scarring, ecchymosis, edema, incidence of hematoma, as well as less anesthetic and surgical time [7]. Indications and contraindications are similar to those for external levator advancement, with patients with ptosis of good to fair levator function having best outcomes. Initially popularized by Lucarelli and Lemke in 1999, their outcomes using small-incision external levator surgery demonstrated effective eyelid correction without significant postoperative complications [8]. When compared to the traditional full external levator approach, the small-incisional technique has been shown to produce similar results with shorter operating times [9]. This approach is also an ideal option for those who have had prior blepharoplasty, or do not need skin removal such as if deep superior sulci are present (Fig. 3.12), in reoperations, or for those concerned about lengthy scarring.

Using a cotton-tipped applicator to assess the eyelid elevation at multiple sites, a small 8 mm skin incision is marked in the eyelid crease at the location that achieves best eyelid contour, followed by 0.5–1.0 mL of local infiltrative anesthesia (Fig. 3.13). The surgical steps are the

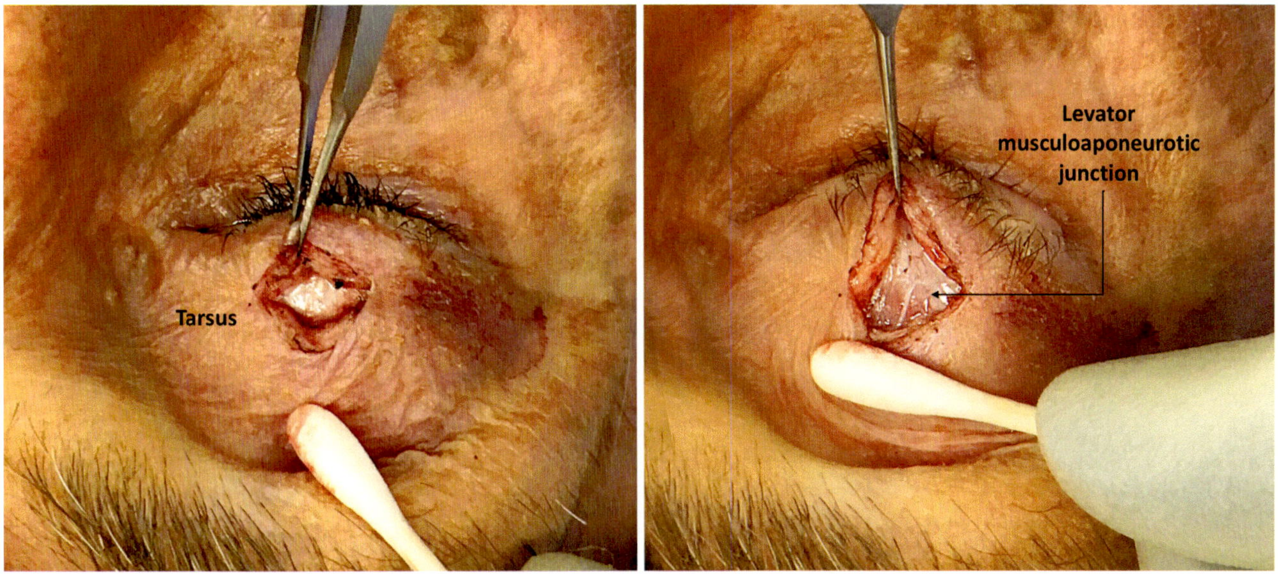

Fig. 3.14 Small-incision technique demonstrating the dissected superior tarsus and the levator muscle and aponeurosis junction

same, but overall the operative field is more confined, which may be more technically challenging for less experienced surgeons. With retraction of the skin edges, dissection down through the pretarsal orbicularis allows for exposure of the superior tarsus (Fig. 3.14). Some surgeons prefer to further release the levator complex from the underlying Müller muscle, although this is not required. Using a spatulated needle on a 6-0 Prolene suture or a 5-0 nylon suture, the suture is passed starting from the musculoaponeurotic junction under the levator muscle, horizontally through partial-thickness superior tarsus, followed by passing the needle superiorly in the plane between the levator and Müller's muscle to exit at the musculoaponeurotic junction and temporarily tied (Fig. 3.9). If the eyelid requires less elevation based on the preoperative margin-reflex distance, the suture can be placed lower than the musculoaponeurotic junction or higher on the tarsus to minimize the length of the hangback suture. Adjusting the suture tension with the patient in an upright position allows the eyebrows to rest in their natural position and more accurately reflect the eyelid height. An additional suture can be placed for contour if needed, even within the small incision. Once the eyelid height and contour are optimized, the suture can be clamped just under the knot with a needle driver to prevent the knot from cinching down further when tying down the suture permanently, which would thus inadvertently elevate the eyelid (Fig. 3.15). Eyelid crease reformation sutures are not required with this approach.

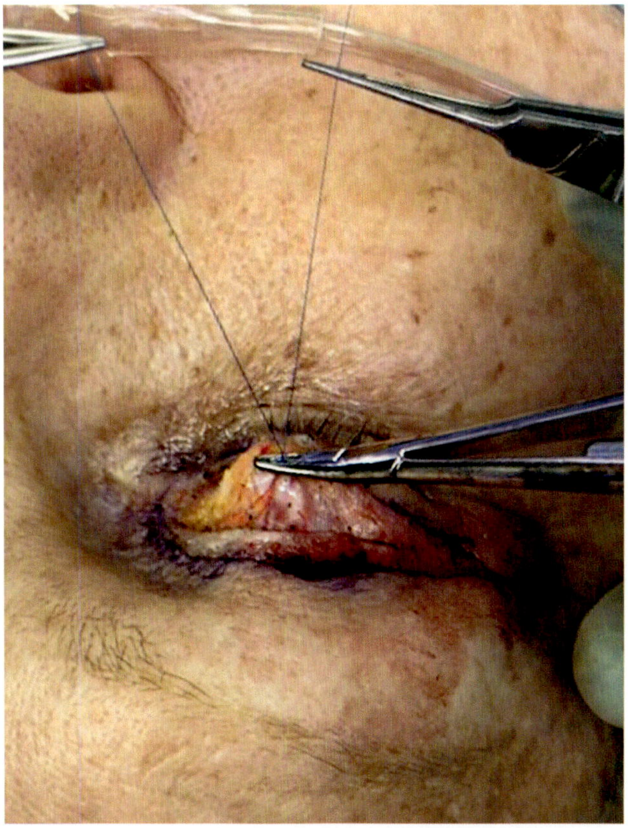

Fig. 3.15 Once the eyelid height and contour are optimized, the suture can be clamped just under the knot with a needle driver to prevent the knot from cinching down further when tying the suture permanently (surgeon view)

Levator Resection via External Approach

Indications for levator resection include patients with congenital, myogenic, or neurogenic severe ptosis with poor to fair levator function, often with structurally maldeveloped or abnormal levator muscles (Fig. 3.16). Levator resection surgery through the skin can result in greater eyelid elevation, as the levator aponeurosis and muscle are first resected and then further advanced to the tarsal surface [4]. Patients with good levator function should undergo levator advancement or posterior approach surgeries, and those with near-absent levator function require frontalis suspension surgery (frontalis sling). An external levator resection should also be used cautiously in Asian patients as an undesirable eyelid crease or double crease may be created.

The technique was initially described in 1953 by Johnson, with further modifications by Beard and others [9, 10]. Based on the degree of ptosis and measured levator function, many algorithms have been proposed to determine the amount of levator resection necessary (Table 3.1) [4, 11, 12]. Generally speaking, each quantitative technique serves as a guideline but each surgery requires individualization. In addition, it is often difficult to accurately measure levator function in children, which is reflected in the wide range of measurements seen in algorithms. This approach is primarily useful for congenital ptosis, often with fair or decreased levator function, as anterior levator resection can result in predictable eyelid elevation and clearance of the visual axis postoperatively [11, 13].

Table 3.1 Amount of resection for degree of ptosis and levator function in congenital cases

Levator function (LF)	Berke [11]	Beard [4]	Hendersen [12]	
Good (>8 mm)	3–4 mm resection/ mm ptosis	14–17 mm for 3 mm ptosis	>11 mm LF	6–11 mm LF
			Resection equal to amount of ptosis	Resection double to amount of ptosis
Fair (5–7 mm)	5–6 mm resection/ mm ptosis	18–22 mm for 3 mm ptosis	5–6 mm LF	<5 mm LF
			Resection double to amount of ptosis	Resection tripe to amount or ptosis
Poor (3–4 mm)	Maximal resection	Maximal resection possible secondary brow	Resection triple to amount or ptosis	
No function (<3 mm)	Not suitable for resection	Maximal levator resection and advancement of anterior tarsal face	Not suitable for resection	

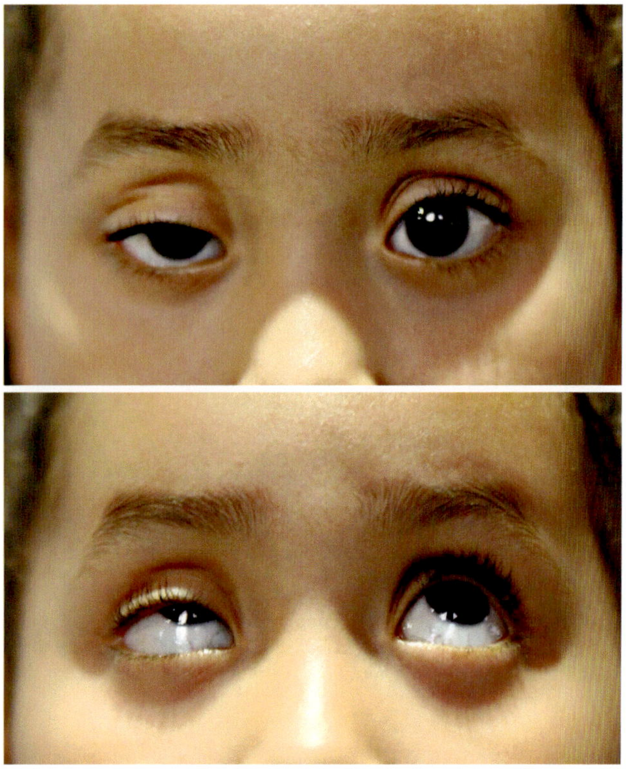

Fig. 3.16 Patient with right congenital ptosis and fair-poor levator function is a candidate for levator resection surgery

A major benefit of this technique in children, or adults with limited cooperation, is that the patient does not need to be awake during surgery for intraoperative suture adjustments. Contraindications would be the presence of a poor Bell's reflex or elevator palsy that would limit upgaze and thus risk corneal integrity after surgery. Using the charts to determine the amount of resection, the levator aponeurosis and most of the levator muscle are excised, with horizontal mattress sutures placed just above the incision line so that the residual muscle stump can be advanced to the superior tarsus. Maximal or supramaximal levator aponeurosis resection involves removal up to or above Whitnall's ligament, respectively, and is reserved for cases of severe ptosis with poor levator function [14]. External levator resection differs from an external levator advancement as the levator complex is actually excised, compared to imbricated, with reattachment to the superior tarsal plate.

When performing a levator resection, a traction suture at the gray line of the eyelid margin can provide inferior traction to facilitate dissection. The orbital septum is opened and the entire levator aponeurosis dissected horizontally off the tarsus. Dissection is continued superiorly toward the fornix in a plane behind the levator muscle or encompassing both the levator and Müller muscles depending on surgeon preference (Fig. 3.17). The medial and lateral horns of the levator aponeurosis are incised vertically and widely toward the fornix, taking care to avoid injury to the lacrimal gland and

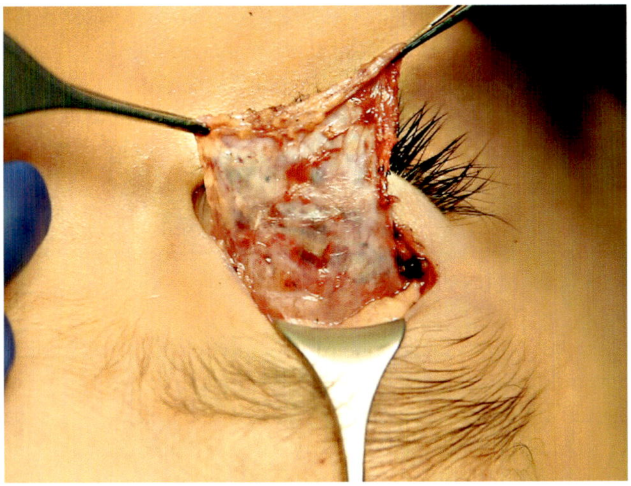

Fig. 3.17 Surgeon's view of superior dissection toward the fornix in a plane behind the dystrophic levator muscle or encompassing both the levator and Müller's muscles

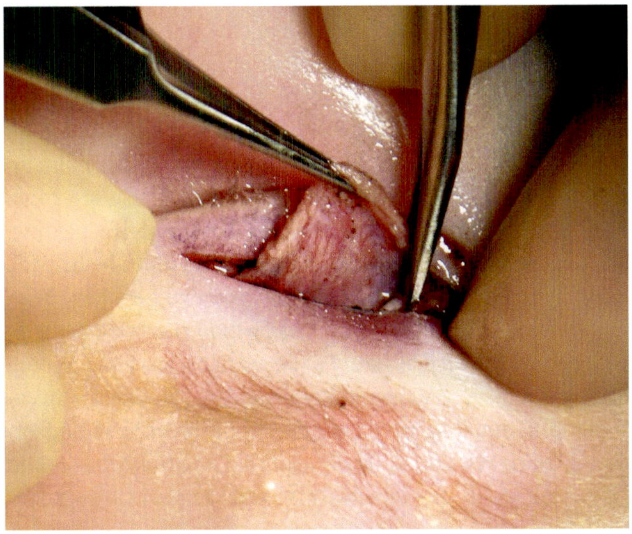

Fig. 3.18 The medial and lateral horns of the levator aponeurosis are incised vertically and widely toward the fornix, taking care to avoid narrowing the proximal muscle base (surgeon view)

avoid narrowing the proximal muscle base (Fig. 3.18). The elevated tissue is placed in a Berke ptosis clamp and the desired amount of tissue resection marked on the muscle with a surgical marker (Fig. 3.19). If more than 25–30 mm needs to be excised based on the severity of ptosis and decreased levator function, this may sometimes result in a resection that extends up to or past Whitnall's ligament (Fig. 3.20). Prior to transecting the muscle at the markings, it is useful to secure the remaining portion of levator with sutures, such as 6-0 Prolene mattress sutures, so that the proximal stump does not retract and become difficult to locate after cutting. These sutures pass horizontally through the anterior superior tarsus to advance the levator muscle and

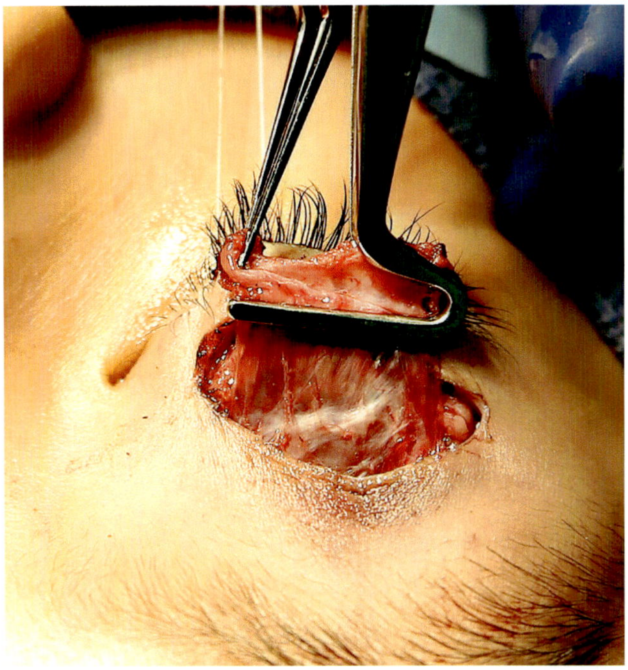

Fig. 3.19 The elevated levator tissue is placed in a Berke ptosis clamp and the desired amount of tissue resection measured on the muscle

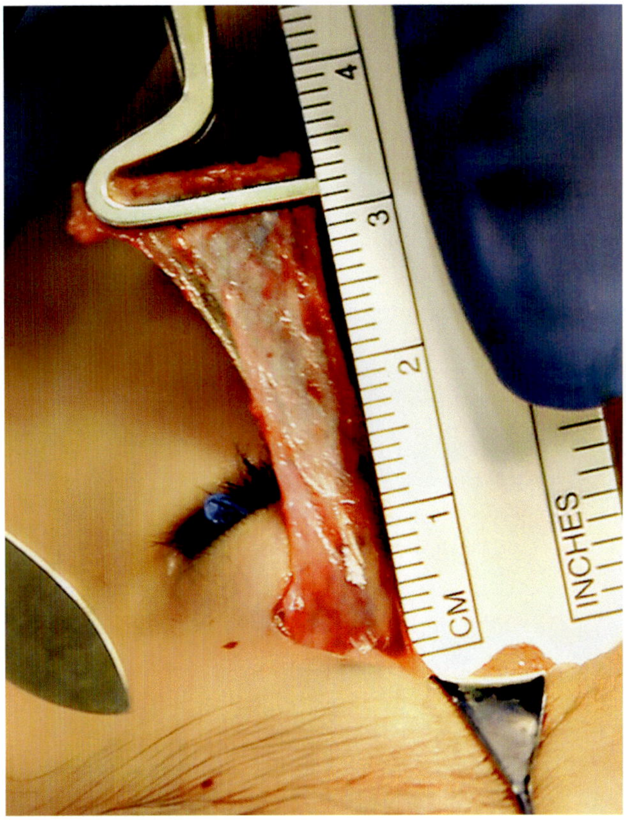

Fig. 3.20 The amount of levator resection can extend to or incorporate Whitnall's ligament if needed

elevate the eyelid. Alternatively, several 5-0 or 6-0 double-armed sutures (Prolene, nylon, chromic gut) can be first passed horizontally through the upper tarsus, and each of the suture arms passed upward behind the levator to exit at or just above the resection markings (Fig. 3.21). The double-armed sutures are tied as horizontal sutures to advance the levator muscle, followed by resection of the excess muscle (Fig. 3.22). Typically the desired eyelid margin height at the end of the procedure should rest at or above the superior limbus.

If the elevated eyelid creates a fold of skin over the margin that causes mechanical eyelash ptosis or entropion, then a thin strip of skin should be excised. The eyelid crease is reformed by suturing the orbicularis oculi muscle from the superior and inferior incision to the edge of the levator complex, followed by skin closure. Patients and families should be aware that postoperative lagophthalmos is not uncommon, but rather expected, following this technique, and therefore aggressive lubrication with tears and nighttime gel is often necessary.

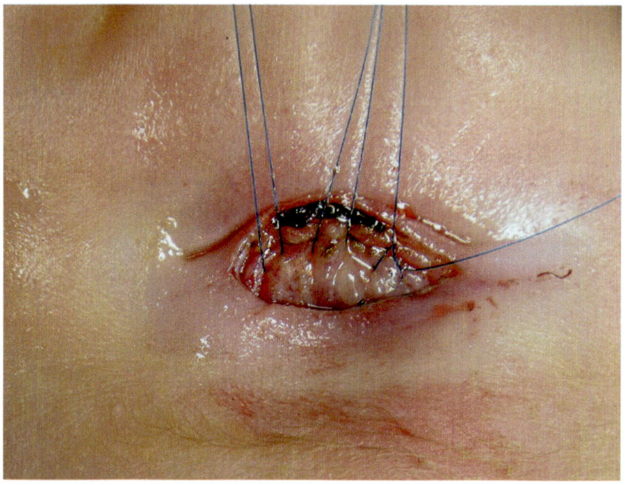

Fig. 3.21 Three Prolene mattress sutures are placed to secure the residual levator complex to the superior tarsus prior to excising the levator complex

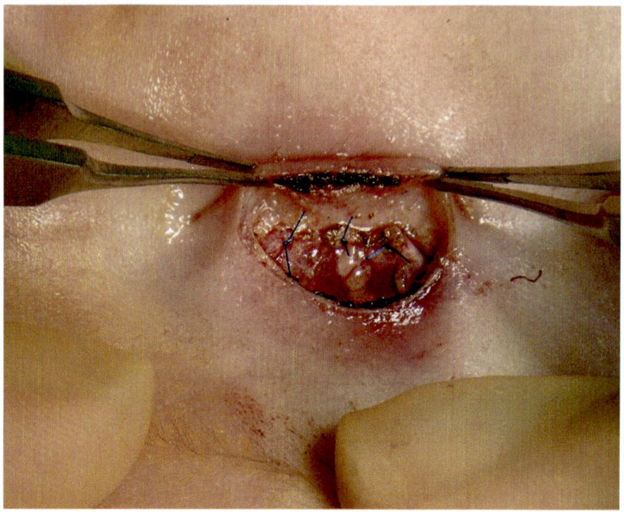

Fig. 3.22 After securing the residual levator complex to the superior tarsus, the Prolene sutures are tied and the levator complex resected

Postoperative Care

Cold wet compresses applied frequently for the first 48 hours and mild analgesics help control postoperative pain. Patients should be instructed to call for severe deep, aching pain or visual loss that may be an early manifestation of an orbital hemorrhage. Antibiotic ointment is applied on the sutures three times a day for 1 week, which may blur vision temporarily. Nonabsorbable skin sutures, if used, should be removed approximately 5–10 days after surgery. Artificial tears can be used for mild ocular irritation or dry eye symptoms. Exercise and heavy lifting or bending are also avoided for 1 week after surgery to minimize bleeding complications.

The most common risks of anterior approach levator surgery, besides edema and ecchymosis, include undercorrection, overcorrection, asymmetric eyelid creases, scarring, lagophthalmos and dry eyes, or suboptimal eyelid contour. Although noted immediately after surgery, these are often difficult to distinguish from normal postoperative healing, and thus observation for a month may sometimes be helpful. Reoperation rates for levator advancement surgery have been reported to occur in 8.7% of cases within the first operative year and up to twice as likely to occur in patients undergoing bilateral surgery versus unilateral surgery [5]. On rare occasion, a unilateral surgery may unmask a previously undiagnosed Hering's effect, such that the contralateral eyelid becomes ptotic postoperatively and requires secondary surgery.

In the first few weeks after surgery, if significant overcorrection or undercorrection is evident and edema is minimal, the incision can be opened in the office and the levator sutures adjusted as needed. Later reoperations, even up to 6 weeks postoperatively, have demonstrated similar adjustment outcomes; therefore, longer observation is reasonable to allow for more healing and spontaneous recovery [15].

Conclusion

Correction of eyelid blepharoptosis can be performed with various surgical techniques.

Anterior approaches with external levator advancement, small-incision levator repair, and levator resection all offer effective long-term outcomes with excellent eyelid height, contour, and function.

References

1. Anderson RL, Beard C. The levator aponeurosis. Attachments and their clinical significance. Arch Ophthalmol. 1977;95(8):1437–41.
2. Jones LT, Quickert MH, Wobig JL. The cure of ptosis by aponeurotic repair. Arch Ophthalmol. 1975;93:629–34.
3. Dortzbach RK, Sutula FC. Involutional blepharoptosis. A histopathological study. Arch Ophthalmol. 1980;98(11):2045–9.
4. Beard C. The surgical treatment of blepharoptosis: a quantitative approach. Trans Am Ophthalmol Soc. 1966;64:401–87.
5. McCulley T, Kersten RC, Kulwin DR, et al. Outcome and influencing factors of external levator palpebrae superioris aponeurosis advancement for blepharoptosis. Ophthal Plast Reconstr Surg. 2003;19:388–93.
6. Ben Simon GJ, Lee S, Schwarcz RM, et al. External levator advancement vs Müller's muscle-conjunctival resection for correction of upper eyelid involutional ptosis. Am J Ophthalmol. 2005;140(3):426–32.
7. Baroody M, Holds JB, Sakamoto DK, et al. Small incision transcutaneous levator aponeurotic repair for blepharoptosis. Ann Plast Surg. 2004;52(6):558–61.
8. Lucarelli MJ, Lemke BN. Small incision external levator repair: technique and early results. Am J Ophthalmol. 1999;127(6):637–44.
9. Frueh BR, Musch DC, McDonald HM. Efficacy and efficiency of a small-incision, minimal dissection procedure versus a traditional approach for correcting aponeurotic ptosis. Ophthalmology. 2004;111(12):2158–63.
10. Johnson CC. Blepharoptosis: a general consideration of surgical methods; with the results in 162 operations. Am J Ophthalmol. 1954;38(2):129–62.
11. Berke RN. Results of resection of the levator muscle through a skin incision in congenital ptosis. Arch Ophthalmol. 1959;61:177.
12. Henderson JW. Present status of blepharoptosis surgery. Postgrad Med. 1963;33:153–8.
13. Göncü T, Çakmak S, Akal A, et al. Improvement in levator function after anterior levator resection for the treatment of congenital ptosis. Ophthal Plast Reconstr Surg. 2015;31(3):197–201.
14. Mauriello JA, Wagner RS, Caputo AR, Natale B, Lister M. Treatment of congenital ptosis by maximal levator resection. Ophthalmology. 1986;93(4):466–9.
15. Shore JW, Bergin DJ, Garrett SN. Results of blepharoptosis surgery with early postoperative adjustment. Ophthalmology. 1990;97(11):1502–11.

4 Fasanella-Servat Procedure for Ptosis Correction

John T. Harvey

History

In 1959 Dr. Servat went to New Haven, Connecticut, for his ophthalmology residency at Yale University under the mentorship of Dr. Rocko M. Fasanella, the Chief of the Eye Service. On a busy surgical day in 1960, they operated on a child with ptosis who had Cooley anemia requiring multiple transfusions. Speed was essential. And on that day, the Fasanella-Servat procedure was created [1]. In 1961 [2], Fasanella and Servat described their procedure for correcting small amounts of ptosis in patients with normal levator function. The procedure, as they described it, involved everting the upper eyelid and infiltrating local anesthetic into the subconjunctival space above the tarsal plate, to then place 2 curved hemostats no more than 3 mm from the upper border of the tarsus. 5-0 chromic sutures in a horizontal mattress fashion were then passed above the two curved hemostats. The tissue enclosed within the hemostats was excised and two frost sutures were placed to prevent corneal abrasion. The procedure was described as the removal of tarsus, conjunctiva, Müller's muscle, and levator palpebrae superioris.

Mechanism of Action

Over the years, there have been a number of theories to explain how this procedure works. Fasanella and Servat proposed that it was the shortening of the levator, Müller's muscle, tarsus, and conjunctiva that caused the eyelid elevation [2]. However, Beard proposed that it was the shortening of the tarsus [3] and demonstrated in pathologic studies that excised tissues consisted of only conjunctiva, Müller's muscle, and tarsus – without levator muscle present [3]. Beard correctly noted that retraction of the aponeurosis prevented its inclusion in hemostats, and this was later confirmed by Putterman. Putterman concluded that resection and advancement of Müller's muscle was the basis for success in the Fasanella-Servat procedure [4]. He found that when an external levator resection was performed with a Putterman clamp in place, the levator aponeurosis was easily accessible and not trapped within the clamp [5]. Furthermore, Putterman pointed out that there is no associated eyelid elevation when tarsoconjunctival grafts are taken from the upper eyelid.

In 1989, Buckman et al. [6] performed a histopathologic study that showed that 87.5% of specimens displayed minimal or no smooth muscle, thus concluding that Müller's muscle resection had little, if any effect. However, it was further stated that no correlation was found between the amount of tarsus excised and the degree of eyelid elevation achieved. The mechanism of action of the Fasanella-Servat procedure has remained inconclusive.

Indications

The Fasanella-Servat procedure is best suited for no more than 3 mm of ptosis with levator function greater than 10 mm [2, 4, 7]. Ideally it is used for 1.5–2 mm of ptosis, with levator function of 13–15 mm. The procedure has been used for congenital, neurogenic, myogenic, traumatic, and bilateral ptosis, as well as for correction of eyelid contour abnormality from previous surgery or trauma. It is contraindicated in patients with significant posterior lamellar scarring or shortened tarsus (congenital, surgical, or traumatic). It is generally recommended that this procedure should not be repeated if unsuccessful on the first attempt as this could cause significant vertical shortening of the tarsus and eyelid instability. To our knowledge there have not been any studies that look specifically at complications after a Fasanella-Servat procedure in patients with corneal disease or following corneal surgery. However, it has been shown that in presumed high-risk patients

J. T. Harvey (✉)
Division of Ophthalmology, McMaster University, Hamilton, ON, Canada
e-mail: jtharvey@mcmaster.ca

A. J. Cohen, C. N. Burkat (eds.), *Oculofacial, Orbital, and Lacrimal Surgery*, https://doi.org/10.1007/978-3-030-14092-2_4

with glaucoma filtering blebs, Müller muscle-conjunctival resection can provide an effective and safe means for ptosis repair [8].

It has been previously suggested that the absence of eyelid elevation following instillation of phenylephrine demonstrates poor response of Müller's muscle to adrenergic stimulation, thus indicating that a tarsoconjunctivomullerectomy (Fasanella-Servat procedure) or an anterior approach (levator advancement surgery) may prove more beneficial than a pure conjunctivomullerectomy [5]. However, in 2007, Skibell showed that the Fasanella-Servat and Putterman procedures have equal outcomes, independent of adrenergic receptors [9].

Procedure

There have been multiple variations of the original procedure described by Dr. Fasanella and Dr. Servat. Beard modified the technique in 1969 using a running suture of catgut and externalizing the knot in the temporal crease [3]. In 1972, Putterman developed a clamp to supplant the use of curved hemostats for the Fasanella-Servat procedure [5]. The clamp was placed over the superior 3 mm of tarsus and Müller's muscle, and a double-armed 6-0 plain gut suture was placed in a running fashion above the clamp. This clamp is best known today for its use in the Müller's muscle-conjunctival resection procedure, also known as a conjunctivomullerectomy. In 1973, Crawford used a Desmarres retractor to evert the eyelid [10]. Bodian used a 5-0 running nylon suture that he externalized with bolsters to the eyelid [11]. In an effort to end the cut-and-sew technique, Fox excised all eyelid tissue above the hemostats and placed a running 5-0 plain gut suture across the inner eyelid [12]. Lauring in 1977 described a sutureless method in which two curved hemostats were placed on the everted eyelid for 1 minute [13]. Iris scissors were used to cut down the broad groove left by the clamps after the hemostats were removed. Others have also described a sutureless technique [14]. In 1983, Betharia et al. [15] used sutures instead of curved hemostats to isolate the eyelid tissue to be excised. Samimi and Dresner [16] described a modification of the technique and provided an algorithm for the amount of resection. Sohrab [17] compared the Fasanella-Servat procedure to small-incision external approach ptosis repair and found that the outcomes were comparable but the surgical time shorter for the Fasanella-Servat technique.

Since its inception in 1961, the Fasanella-Servat procedure has thus become more refined, as well as fluctuated in popularity. Beard and Putterman were responsible for two major advances in technique. Beard advocated a simplified suturing approach, and the Putterman clamp increased efficiency.

Surgical Technique

The patient is positioned in the usual fashion and prepped and draped in sterile technique fashion. Topical anesthetic drops are placed into the conjunctival sac, and the upper eyelid is infiltrated with local anesthetic.

If awake, the patient is instructed to "look down," which aids in everting the eyelid over a Desmarres retractor (Fig. 4.1). With toothed forceps, the tarsus is grasped at the medial and lateral "corners" (Fig. 4.2). The "corners" are an arbitrary location where the horizontal and vertical portions of the tarsus meet, if the tarsus was rectangular shaped. Grasping too narrow a portion of tarsus will give a peaked eyelid contour. The Putterman clamp is placed (Fig. 4.3). The placement of the clamp determines the amount of eyelid elevation that will occur. Small (1 mm), medium (2 mm), and large resections (3 mm) correspond to 1 clamp width, 2 clamp widths, or 3 clamp widths of resection. A double-armed

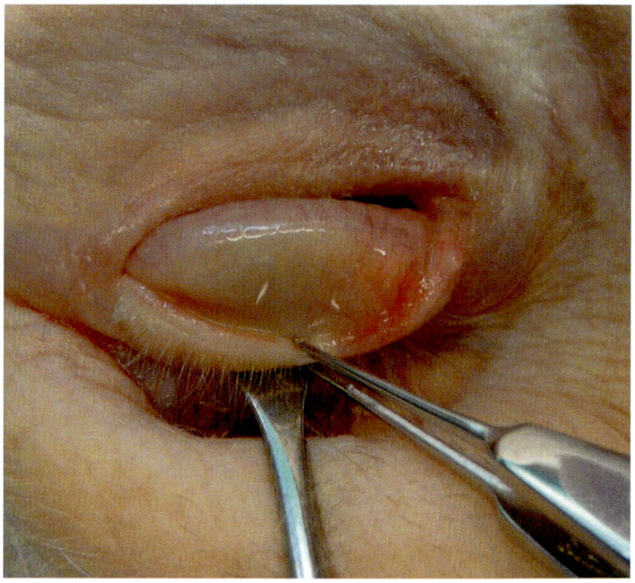

Fig. 4.1 The upper eyelid is everted over a Desmarres retractor

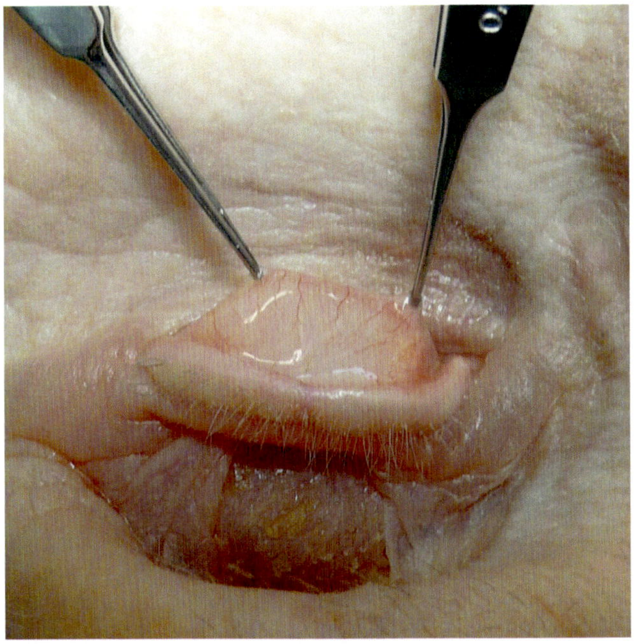

Fig. 4.2 The tarsus is grasped at the "corners" on both sides. The "corner" is the arbitrary location at the junction of the "horizontal" superior tarsal border and the "vertical" medial (or lateral) border

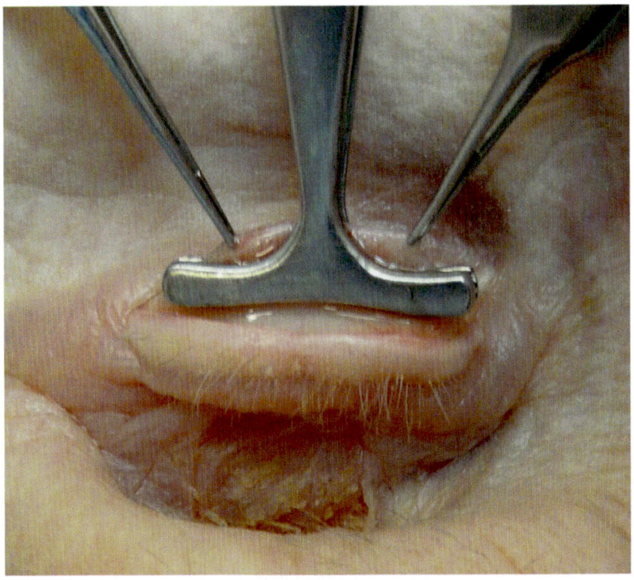

Fig. 4.3 The Putterman clamp is placed. The amount of tarsus included in the clamp will determine the amount of eyelid elevation

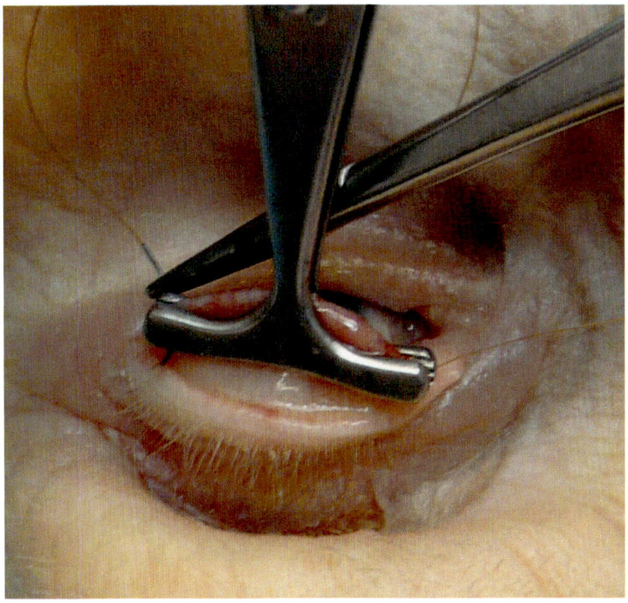

Fig. 4.4 A 5-0 chromic suture is placed "back and forth" below the clamp

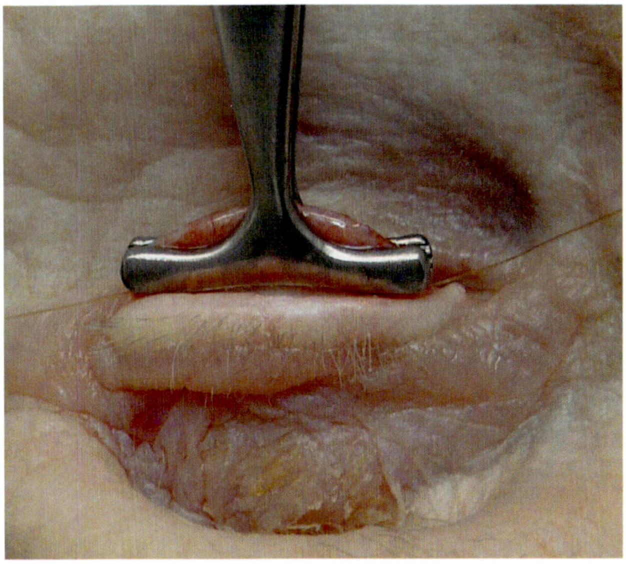

Fig. 4.5 The suture has been placed across the eyelid

absorbable suture is passed full-thickness "back and forth" in a serpentine manner below the edge of the clamp (Figs. 4.4 and 4.5). The clamp is removed and the "corners" are once again grasped (Fig. 4.6). The tarsus with attached conjunctiva and Müller's muscle is resected above the suture, taking care to avoid cutting too close to the suture (Figs. 4.7 and 4.8). The suture is tested to ensure that it has not been accidentally cut (Fig. 4.9). The lateral and medial arms of the suture are passed from the conjunctival side through to the skin side of the eyelid where they are then tied (Figs. 4.10, 4.11, and 4.12). Externalizing the sutures minimizes the risk of corneal abrasion from suture knots. Topical antibiotic ointment can be placed on the ocular surface.

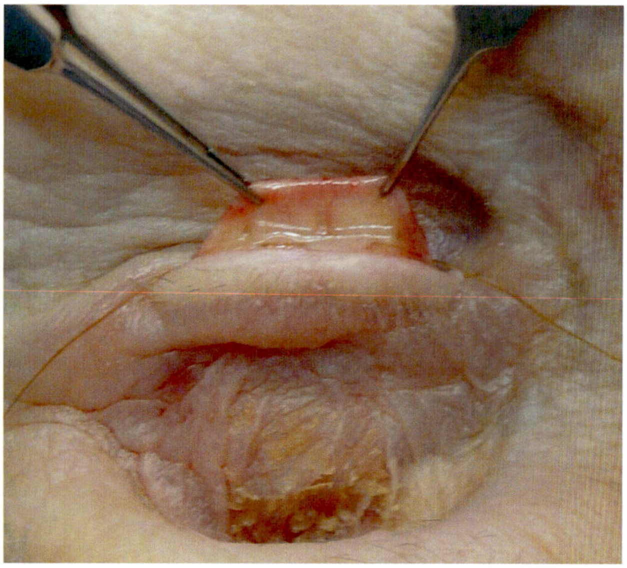

Fig. 4.6 The Putterman clamp is removed

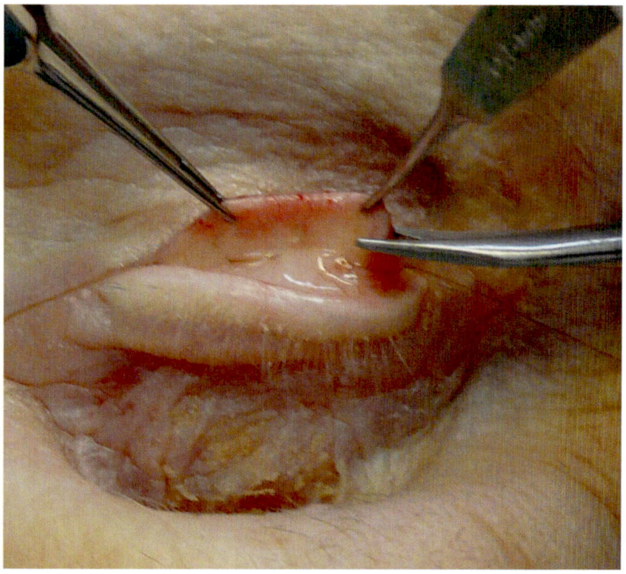

Fig. 4.7 The tarsus and adjacent conjunctiva/Müller's muscle are excised

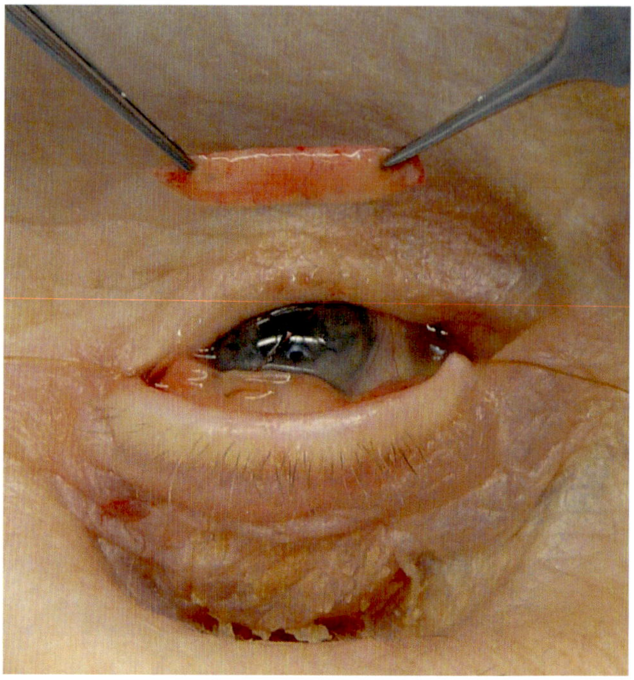

Fig. 4.8 The removed fragment of tarsus with reflected conjunctiva is shown. Bleeding is minimal from the cut edge due to the hemostatic effect of the clamp

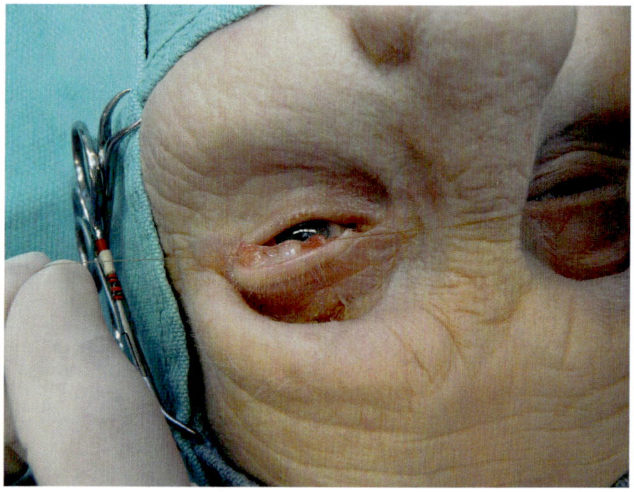

Fig. 4.9 The suture is pulled taut to ensure that it has not been inadvertently cut

Complications

Complications of the Fasanella-Servat procedure are most often undercorrection of the ptosis. Less common complications include overcorrection, contour abnormalities, duplicate eyelid creases, suture allergy, corneal abrasion, dry eye syndrome, hematoma, wound dehiscence, pyogenic granuloma, and bleeding [7, 18].

Undercorrection can be avoided by selecting patients with minimal ptosis and sufficient levator function. Eyelid peaking can be prevented by careful symmetric placement of the hemostat or Putterman clamp and precise suture placement in relation to the clamp. If some sutures are passed close to the clamp, and then others are placed several millimeters away from the clamp, this will result in an uneven resection and contour issues.

Patients should be aware of the potential for postoperative dermatochalasis and a double eyelid crease (Personal Communication, Dr. J. Oestreicher, University of Toronto, 2010). To prevent bleeding and hematoma formation, anticoagulants should be stopped preoperatively if possible. The

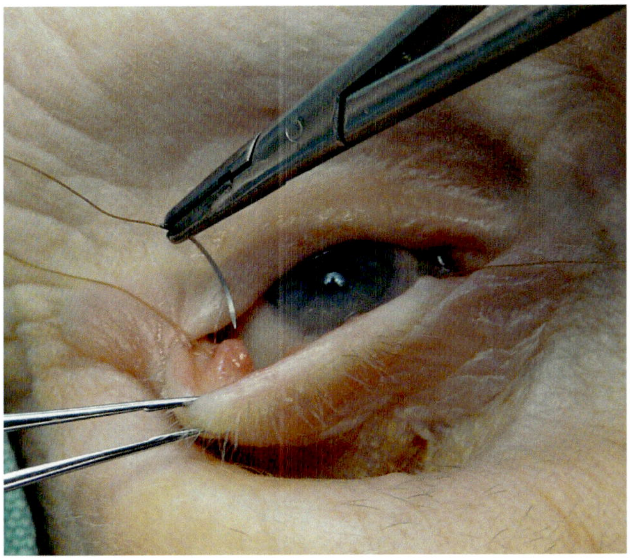

Fig. 4.10 The double-armed ends of the suture are passed from the medial and lateral ends of the conjunctival wound out to the skin surface of the eyelid

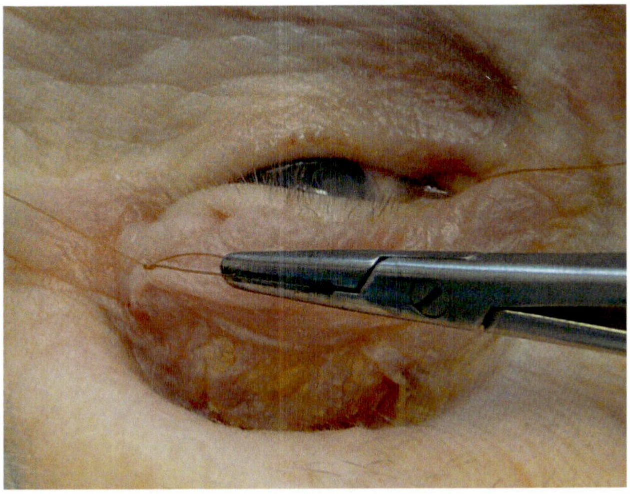

Fig. 4.11 The suture is passed through skin and knotted externally

insertion of a bandage contact lens can help avoid postoperative keratopathy.

In the event of significant contour and height abnormalities that are not believed to be secondary to normal edema, early postoperative adjustments can be considered. Beard [19] described using local anesthesia and "stretching" of the eyelid without suture removal. For overcorrection, downward eyelid massages can be effective [20, 21]. In 2009, Rosenburg [22] described an office procedure without anesthetic that caused minimal discomfort to the patient. At 6 days after surgery, when much of the edema had resolved but tissues were not yet densely fibrosed, gentle downward tugging was performed in the desired area of adjustment.

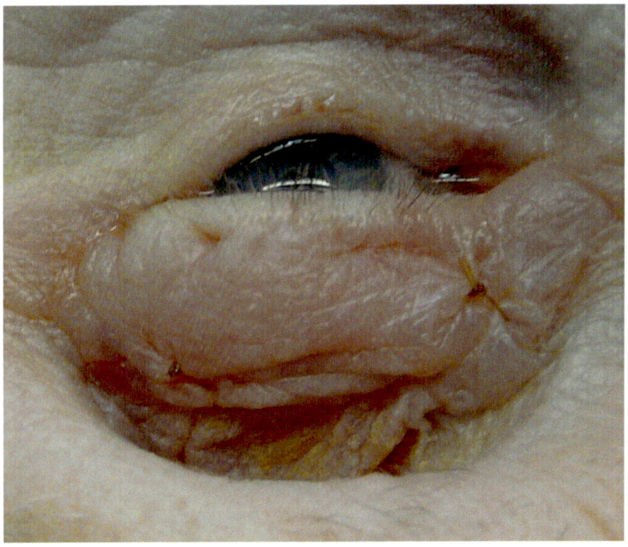

Fig. 4.12 Both the medial and lateral suture ends have been tied on the skin surface

Discussion

This long-standing procedure for ptosis correction has the advantage of high reliability in a patient that has met the appropriate preoperative criteria. Patients who have had prior posterior eyelid surgery, tarsal scarring, or short tarsal plates may be less optimal candidates as the stability of the eyelid tarsus may be at risk. The technique is minimally invasive and faster to perform than other levator approaches. The success rate of the Fasanella-Servat procedure has been reported to range from 28% [23] to 95% [14] for most types of ptosis, with very minimal complications.

In 2007, Pang [7] reported a success rate of 89.5% (137/153). The authors retrospectively reviewed 169 charts of 2 surgeons (JTH & JHO) from 1988 to 1996. Among subgroups, success was highest at 100% in Horner's syndrome (8/8) and post-levator surgery (11/11) and lowest in congenital ptosis at 76.4% (13/18). Seventy-five percent of failures were undercorrections. These results are summarized in Table 4.1.

The procedure is generally quick to perform, so that it can be done in frail patients relatively safely with local anesthetic in a treatment room. It has been advocated by some to be less likely to cause overcorrection or contour abnormalities than levator advancement surgery. In addition, the technique is easier to perform than external levator advancement for surgeons less comfortable with eyelid anatomy. The operation is very useful for small degrees of ptosis, and the likelihood of overcorrection is low. In cases where there is scarring in the eyelid skin crease from trauma or previous surgery, it avoids the scar by working posteriorly.

Table 4.1 Summarized results (Pang et al. [7])

Type of ptosis[a]	n	Success rate (%)	Preoperative ptosis (mean, in mm)	Amount excised (mean, in mm)	Levator function (mean, in mm)
Involutional	57	87.7	1.96	1.89	13.3
Post-intraocular surgery	53	92.4	2.33	2.10	12.5
Horner's syndrome	8	100	1.93	2.12	13.6
Congenital	17	76.4	1.56	1.91	10.5
Following previous surgery or contour abnormality	11	100	1.58	Variable	13.3
Myogenic/other	7	85.2	1.20	1.36	10.7
Total (or average)	153	89.5	1.76	1.88[a]	12.3

[a]Excludes cases of eyelid contour correction

Like any surgical procedure, proper patient selection is critical, and in the average oculoplastic practice, up to 75% of ptosis repairs can be done using this method. It can be combined with blepharoplasty, although this creates two separate incisions. Many surgeons therefore prefer external levator advancement in conjunction with blepharoplasty surgery.

Eyelid contour abnormalities can also be addressed by skewing the clamp to one side. In other words, if the medial portion of the eyelid is low but the lateral eyelid has good height, then the clamp can be placed on the medial half of the eyelid to elevate only the ptotic portion of the eyelid. This is especially valuable in revision surgeries.

In summary, this operation, with its refinements by other surgeons and demonstration of minimal complications, remains one of the mainstays of ptosis correction in modern oculoplastic surgery.

References

1. Fasanella RM, Shields MB. Obituaries – Javier Servat, MD. Arch Ophthalmol. 2002;120:104.
2. Fasanella RM, Servat J. Levator resection for minimal ptosis: another simplified operation. Arch Ophthalmol. 1961;65:493–6.
3. Beard C. Ptosis. 3rd ed. St. Louis: The C.V. Mosby Company; 1981. p. 232–66.
4. Putterman AM, Urist MJ. Müller's muscle-conjunctival resection ptosis procedure. Ophthalmic Surg. 1978;9(3):27–32.
5. Putterman AM. A clamp for strengthening Müller's muscle in the treatment of ptosis. Modification, theory, and clamp for the Fasanella-Servat ptosis operation. Arch Ophthalmol. 1972;87(6):665–7.
6. Buckman G, Jakobiec FA, Hyde K, et al. Success of the Fasanella-Servat operation independent of Müller's smooth muscle excision. Ophthalmology. 1989;96:413–8.
7. Pang NK, Newsom RW, Oestreicher JH, Chung HT, Harvey JT. Fasanella-Servat procedure: indications, efficacy, and complications. Can J Ophthalmol. 2008;43(1):84–8.
8. Georgescu D, Cole E, Epstein G, Fountain T, Migliori M, Nguyen Q, Mannor G, Weinberg D. Müller muscle-conjunctiva resection for blepharoptosis in patients with glaucoma filtering blebs. Ophthal Plast Reconstr Surg. 2007;23(4):285.
9. Skibell BC, Harvey JH, Oestreicher JH, Howarth D, Gibbs A, Wegrynowski T, Wing T, Deangelis DD. Adrenergic receptors in the ptotic human eyelid: correlation with phenylephrine testing and surgical success in ptosis repair. Ophthal Plast Reconstr Surg. 2007;23(5):367–71.
10. Crawford JS. Repair of blepharoptosis with a modification of the Fasanella-Servat operation. Can J Ophthalmol. 1973;8(1):19–23.
11. Bodian M. A revised Fasanella-Servat ptosis operation. Ann Ophthalmol. 1975;7(4):603–5.
12. Fox SA. A modified Fasanella-Servat procedure for ptosis. Arch Ophthalmol. 1975;93(8):639–40.
13. Lauring L. Blepharoptosis correction with the sutureless Fasanella-Servat operation. Arch Ophthalmol. 1977;95:671–4.
14. Gupta VP, Aggarwal R, Mathur SP. Blepharoptosis repair by modified sutureless Fasanella-Servat Operation (F.S.O.) – a large series of 50 cases. Indian J Ophthalmol. 1992;40:86–9.
15. Betharia SM. Transconjunctival levator resection: a modified simple technique. Ann Ophthalmol. 1988;20(6):234–8.
16. Samimi DB, Erb MH, Lane CJ, Dresener SC. The modified Fasanella-Servat procedure: description and quantified analysis. Ophthal Plast Reconstr Surg. 2013;29(1):30–4.
17. Sohrab MA, Lissner GS. Comparison of Fasanell-Servat and small incision techniques for involutional ptosis repair. Ophthal Plast Rescontr Surg. 2015. [Epub ahead of print] PMID 25719375.
18. Carroll RP. Preventable problems following the Fasanella-Servat procedure. Ophthalmic Surg. 1980;11:44–51.
19. Beard C. Blepharoptosis repair by modified Fasanella-Servat operation. Am J Ophthalmol. 1970;69(5):850–7.
20. Dortzbach RK, Kronish JW. Early revision in the office for adults after unsatisfactory blepharoptosis correction. Am J Ophthalmol. 1993;115:68–75.
21. Jordan DR, Anderson RL. A simple procedure for adjusting eyelid position after aponeurotic ptosis surgery. Arch Ophthalmol. 1987;105:1288–91.
22. Rosenberg C, Lelli GJ Jr, Lisman RD. Early postoperative adjustment of the Fasanella-Servat procedure: review of 102 consecutive cases. Ophthal Plast Reconstr Surg. 2009;25(1):19–22.
23. Sampath R, Saunders DC, Leatherbarrow B. The Fasanella-Servat procedure: a retrospective study. Eye. 1995;9(Pt 1):124–5.

Müller's Muscle-Conjunctival Resection (MMCR) for Management of Blepharoptosis: Posterior Approach

5

Joshua M. Moran and Adam J. Cohen

Background

Müller's muscle, otherwise known as the superior tarsal muscle, originates on the underside of the levator palpebrae superioris and inserts on the superior tarsal plate. It is sympathetically innervated and contributes to eyelid elevation. Paresis of the muscle will result in 2–3 mm of ptosis as can be seen in Horner's syndrome.

MMCR is a common technique used to correct blepharoptosis by clamping a portion of Müller's muscle and conjunctiva and excising it from the posterior aspect of the eyelid. The procedure was first described by Putterman and Urist in 1975 and has become well-known as a simple and reliable method of correcting phenylephrine test-positive cases of blepharoptosis with good levator function [1]. A variety of modifications to the procedure have been proposed since its introduction, a few of which will be discussed here.

The Phenylephrine Test

Typically, prerequisites for MMCR candidacy include good levator function and positive response to phenylephrine, an α-adrenergic agonist. Two drops of 2.5% phenylephrine are administered to the affected eye 1 minute apart, with the patient looking down during application to maximize delivery to Müller's muscle. Eyelid elevation is assessed after 5 minutes: the test is considered positive if blepharoptosis is corrected. Alternatively, 0.5% apraclonidine may be used [2].

Ten percent phenylephrine eye drops are frequently used during this procedure, though reported cardiovascular side effects have prompted some surgeons to use only 2.5% phenylephrine, especially in patients with known risk factors such as cerebral aneurysms, or coronary artery disease [7, 8]. Stavert et al. found that 10% phenylephrine drops caused transient but significant increases in heart rate and blood pressure, while 2.5% drops did not [9]. Lowering the concentration of phenylephrine may result in less elevation of the ptotic eyelid that was not found to be statistically significant and does change the absolute testing outcome [10].

Some studies have reported successful outcomes of MMCR with negative phenylephrine challenge [3, 4]; however, results are generally unsatisfactory if the patient has both poor levator function and a negative phenylephrine test [5]. MMCR may be used effectively in rare cases of patients with poor levator function but a positive response to phenylephrine [6].

Determining the Amount of Tissue to Resect

Preoperative eyelid position is easily assessed by measuring the margin-reflex distance 1 (MRD_1). This is the distance in millimeters between the eyelid margin and the corneal light reflex, seen when the physician holds a light source at pupil level directly in front of the patient [11].

A variety of algorithms have been proposed to determine how much Müller's muscle and conjunctiva should be resected. In their seminal work, Putterman and Urist proposed that 8.25 mm of conjunctiva (with underlying Müller's muscle) should be resected, ± 1 or 2 mm depending on whether phenylephrine administration over- or undercorrected the ptosis. Several linear relationships between tissue resection and ptosis correction have been proposed: Mercandetti et al. suggested a 3:1 ratio, Weinstein and Buerger described a 4:1 ratio, and Ayala et al. described an approximate 5:1 ratio [12–14].

Dresner found that the 4:1 linear relationship only extended to 8 mm of resection. For resections of 10 mm, he recommended 3 mm of resection and further stipulated that

J. M. Moran
The Chicago Medical School at Rosalind Franklin University, North Chicago, IL, USA

A. J. Cohen (✉)
Eyelid & Facial Plastic and Reconstructive Surgery, Chicago and Glenview, IL, USA
e-mail: acohen@theartofeyes.com

A. J. Cohen, C. N. Burkat (eds.), *Oculofacial, Orbital, and Lacrimal Surgery*, https://doi.org/10.1007/978-3-030-14092-2_5

this relationship is only sufficient in cases where the eyelid elevated 2 mm or greater in response to phenylephrine [15].

Perry et al. further modified the algorithm by incorporating tarsectomy into their MMCR procedure. They suggested that 9 mm of Müller's muscle and conjunctiva should be resected, plus an additional 1 mm of tarsal resection for each 1 mm of ptosis undercorrection after phenylephrine [16]. To avoid contour abnormalities, Samimi et al. set a limit of 5 mm of tarsal resection for a total possible elevation of 7 mm [17].

Patel et al. found that the postoperative amount of elevation did not significantly correlate with the amount of resection within the range of 8.0–9.5 mm. They attributed this variation to a general lack of consistency and precision when performing MMCR, factors which may vary depending on the surgeon [18].

Technique variation with MMCR is the likely factor for varying amounts of tissue resection and eyelid elevation within the literature. Surgeons are encouraged to examine individual publications and develop an algorithm that suits their own techniques and experience.

Surgical Technique

Anesthesia

Patient cooperation is not required in MMCR, and therefore general anesthesia, monitored anesthesia care (MAC), or local anesthetic may be used to equal effect. MAC carries the benefits of improved patient comfort and a decreased risk of patient movement during the procedure. This may be of greater importance if a frontal nerve block is performed, as the intraorbital injection does carry risk of damage to the globe and surrounding structures if the patient were to move.

With a frontal nerve block 25-gauge, 1½ inch sharp needle is passed just inferior to the mid-superior orbital rim parallel to the orbital roof. The needle is advanced to a depth of 1½ inch sliding the bevel of the needle along the orbital roof. One and one half to 2 milliliters (ml) of anesthetic solution is infiltrated, and gentle digital pressure is applied. Anesthetic selection varies based on surgeon preference with 2% lidocaine with epinephrine and/or 0.5–0.75% bupivacaine commonly used. Successful frontal nerve blocks result in complete ptosis.

A supraorbital nerve block carries less risk of inadvertent damage to surrounding structures. A short 27–30-gauge needle, with approximately 1 ml of local anesthetic, is injected just inside the superior orbital rim adjacent to the supraorbital notch.

With either technique subperiosteal infiltration is necessary for full anesthetic effect.

In cases where difficulty with clamp placement is anticipated, such as patients with prominent supraorbital ridges, deep sockets, and small upper eyelids without laxity, tumescent anesthesia may also be considered. In brief, a small amount of anesthetic is infiltrated in sub-Müller's muscle in the area of and massaged to aid dispersal. This markedly increases patient comfort, and the tumescent dissection plane allows Müller's muscle and conjunctiva to be more easily grasped by forceps and separated from the levator aponeurosis when applying the Putterman clamp.

If further anesthesia is required and tumescent anesthesia is not indicated, the lacrimal nerve may be blocked with an infiltration of local anesthetic just inside the superolateral orbital rim.

Technique

A Desmarres lid retractor is used to evert the eyelid and hold it in place. Optionally, a 4-0 silk suture may be passed through the eyelid margin to aid manipulation and is preferred by the author especially when using only local anesthesia and also facilitates accurate placement of the Putterman clamp (Fig. 5.1).

To determine their placement, a point cephalad to the superior tarsal border is demarcated using calipers and methylene blue. The distance from the tarsal border should be equal to one half of the predetermined resection amount if traction sutures are used and the full amount of planned resection without the use of traction sutures. If handheld cautery is used to demarcate, care should be taken to prevent welding of Müller's muscle to the levator aponeurosis as this could result in unintentional resection of the levator.

If traction sutures are used, two or three contiguous 6-0 silk traction sutures are passed through conjunctiva and Müller's muscle using long and relatively shallow needle pass. Alternatively, one double-armed silk suture may be used, one arm passing laterally and the other medially from

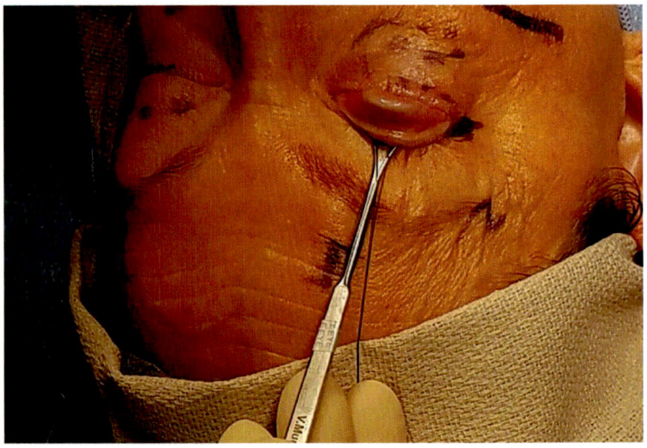

Fig. 5.1 Eyelid everted over Desmarres retractor with traction suture through eyelid margin

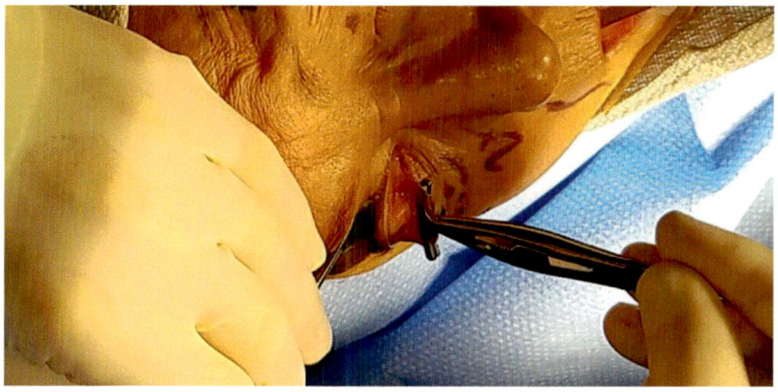

Fig. 5.2 Placement of clamp

a central bite. The medial and lateral passes should be equidistant and parallel to the initial central pass. The authors do not prefer this technique opting to perform the procedure without traction sutures.

Following gentle digital massage to displace the anesthetic, fine forceps may be used to gently grasp the conjunctiva and Müller's muscle and tent them upward, further freeing them from the levator followed by placement of the Putterman clamp (Ambler Surgical Corp, Exton, PA, USA) (Fig. 5.2).

The clamp should be centered with the tarsus to achieve optimal eyelid margin contour. This is especially important in older patients, who may display a lateral shift of the tarsal plate. Failure to do this may result in asymmetries such as nasal peaking or central flattening due to advancement of the levator muscle [19].

Following clamp application, a suture is placed approximately 1 mm below the clamp to plicate the conjunctiva. There are many techniques by which this may be performed. We prefer to use a 6-0 double-armed, plain gut suture on a G-3 needle (Ethicon, Inc. Skillman, NJ, USA) and suture lateral to medial in a horizontal mattress, running fashion. To excise the clamped tissue, a 15 blade is held at a 45° angle facing the clamp edge to avoid cutting any sutures (Fig. 5.3). The wound is closed in a medial to lateral continuous fashion to re-approximate the conjunctival edges. One needle is then trimmed and the suture externalized through the skin and tied once again to bury the knot and reduce corneal irritation.

Another technique begins similarly, passing a double armed 6-0 plain gut suture laterally to medially. Following tissue excision, the other arm of the suture is passed through conjunctiva and Müller's muscle, incorporating the superior border of the tarsus in a medial to lateral running fashion. The two arms of the suture are then passed toward each other at the lateral limit of the excision, retrieved from within the wound, and tied together with several throws. As the suture is tied, the edges of conjunctiva are approximated and the knot is buried [20].

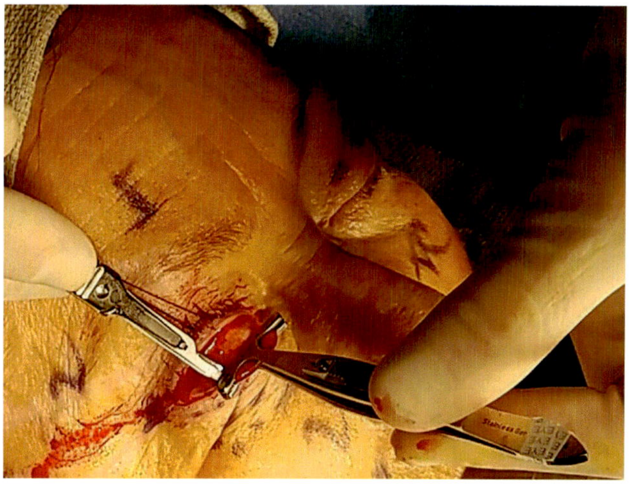

Fig. 5.3 Excision of tissue within clamp

Liao and Chuang, found that modification of this procedure to include tarsal resection can achieve additional eyelid elevation as well as a reduction in eyelid crease. This cosmetic outcome may be of particular concern for patients from Asian populations [21].

There have been several studies investigating the use of fibrin sealant for wound closure instead of sutures. The sealant was found to offer comparable cosmetic outcomes, with reduced need for revision surgeries and fewer postoperative complications [22–24].

Additional modifications have been developed to accommodate additional procedures and individual patient needs. To address asymmetric eyelid contour, if traction sutures are used, they pulled toward the corresponding side prior to clamping. If blepharoplasty is performed concomitantly, the surgeon should take care to externalize the suture through the tarsal skin to avoid severing the suture during blepharoplasty. Eyelid manipulation during MMCR may also cause blepharoplasty incision dehiscence, and so the surgeon may choose to leave the incision open until after MMCR is completed. The authors prefer to perform MMCR prior to blepharoplasty when performed during a single surgery.

Postoperative Care

At the end of the procedure, a combination antibiotic-steroid drop is used four times daily for 1 week. If the suture knot was not externalized, the surgeon may also consider applying a bandage contact lens to prevent keratoconjunctivitis. Follow-up intervals are based on surgeon comfort and intraoperative factors. It is safe to extend more than 1 week after surgery for patients without risk factors [25].

Additional Considerations

MMCR may cause or worsen dry eye symptoms due to the removal of goblet cells and glands of Wolfring. Some studies have found a transient increase in dry eye symptoms following unilateral MMCR, but note that scores were equal in both eyes within 2 months following the surgery [26, 27]. Rymer et al. did not find any difference in ocular surface scores or dry eye symptoms for MMCR with blepharoplasty when compared to blepharoplasty alone [28]. This supports the findings of studies by Uğurbaş et al. and by Putterman and Uris who evaluated tear formation and ocular surface conditions with a variety of tests.

Past history of glaucoma filtering procedures, corneal disease, or corneal surgery do not exclude patients from MMCR, though care should be taken when working near vulnerable thin walled filtering blebs [29, 30]. A negative phenylephrine test does not necessarily exclude the patient from MMCR. Patients with ptosis greater than 3 mm or with poor levator function are generally not considered for MMCR, except in rare cases with a positive phenylephrine test.

Recently, Saonanon and Sithanon conducted a randomized clinical trial which found MMCR to have significantly better cosmetic outcomes and lower revision rates than external levator advancement [31]. This supports similar findings in retrospective studies conducted by Simon et al. [32]. A study by Thomas et al. additionally found that MMCR had significantly lower risk of lid contour abnormalities and need for correction [33].

MMCR can be performed rapidly and easily and may be adapted to a variety of situations. It leaves no visible scar and can reliably yield excellent cosmetic outcomes. The utility of MMCR makes it a useful tool for any oculoplastic surgeon.

References

1. Putterman AM, Urist MJ. Müller muscle-conjunctiva resection. Technique for treatment of blepharoptosis. Arch Ophthalmol. 1975;93:619–23.
2. Yazici B, Beden U. Use of 0.5% apraclonidine solution in evaluation of blepharoptosis. Ophthal Plast Reconstr Surg. 2008;24:299–301.
3. Baldwin HC, Bhagey J, Khooshabeh R. Open sky Müller muscle-conjunctival resection in phenylephrine test-negative blepharoptosis patients. Ophthal Plast Reconstr Surg. 2005;21:276–80.
4. Georgescu D, Epstein G, Fountain T, Migliori M, Mannor G, Weinberg D. Müller muscle conjunctival resection for blepharoptosis in patients with poor to fair levator function. Ophthalmic Surg Lasers Imaging. 2009;40:597–9.
5. Maheshwari R, Maheshwari S. Muller's muscle resection for ptosis and relationship with levator and Muller's muscle function. Orbit. 2011;30:150–3.
6. Cohen AJ, Weinberg DA. Müller's muscle-conjunctival resection for blepharoptosis with poor levator function. Ophthalmic Surg Lasers. 2002;33:491–2.
7. Miller SA, Mieler WF. Systemic reaction to subconjunctival phenylephrine. Can J Ophthalmol. 1978;13:290–3.
8. Fraunfelder FW, Fraunfelder FT, Jensvold B. Adverse systemic effects from pledgets of topical ocular phenylephrine 10%. Am J Ophthalmol. 2002;134:624–5.
9. Stavert B, McGuinness MB, Harper CA, Guymer RH, Finger RP. Cardiovascular adverse effects of phenylephrine eyedrops: a systematic review and meta-analysis. JAMA Ophthalmol. 2015;133:647–52.
10. Glatt HJ, Fett DR, Putterman AM. Comparison of 2.5% and 10% phenylephrine in the elevation of upper eyelids with ptosis. Ophthalmic Surg. 1990;21:173–6.
11. Nemet AY. Accuracy of marginal reflex distance measurements in eyelid surgery. J Craniofac Surg. 2015;26:e569–71.
12. Mercandetti M, Putterman AM, Cohen ME, Mirante JP, Cohen AJ. Internal levator advancement by Müller's muscle-conjunctival resection: technique and review. Arch Facial Plast Surg. 2001;3:104–10.
13. Weinstein GS, Buerger GF. Modification of the Müller's muscle-conjunctival resection operation for blepharoptosis. Am J Ophthalmol. 1982;93:647–51.
14. Ayala E, Gálvez C, González-Candial M, Medel R. Predictability of conjunctival-Müellerectomy for blepharoptosis repair. Orbit. 2007;26:217–21.
15. Dresner SC. Further modifications of the Müller's muscle-conjunctival resection procedure for blepharoptosis. Ophthal Plast Reconstr Surg. 1991;7:114–22.
16. Perry JD, Kadakia A, Foster JA. A new algorithm for ptosis repair using conjunctival Müllerectomy with or without tarsectomy. Ophthal Plast Reconstr Surg. 2002;18:426–9.
17. Samimi DB, Erb MH, Lane CJ, Dresner SC. The modified fasanella-servat procedure: description and quantified analysis. Ophthal Plast Reconstr Surg. 2013;29:30–4.
18. Patel RM, Chuang AZ, Sartori J, Aakalu VK, Putterman AM, Setabutr P. The significance of minimal adjustments in the muller's muscle and conjunctiva resection procedure to achieve the phenylephrine result. Orbit. 2015;34:79–83.
19. Migliori ME. Avoiding lid contour abnormalities in Müller's muscle-conjunctival resection: recognizing the lateral shift. In: Pearls pitfalls cosmetic. Oculoplastic surgery. New York: Springer; 2015. p. 661–2.
20. Patel RM, Aakalu VK, Setabutr P, Putterman AM. Efficacy of Muller's muscle and conjunctiva resection with or without tarsectomy for the treatment of severe involutional blepharoptosis. Ophthal Plast Reconstr Surg. 2017;33:273–8.
21. Liao S-L, Chuang AY. Various modifications of Müller's muscle-conjunctival resection for ptosis repair. Arch Aesthet Plast Surg. 2015;21:31.
22. Kavanagh MC, Ohr MP, Czyz CN, Cahill KV, Perry JD, Holck DEE, Foster JA. Comparison of fibrin sealant versus suture for wound closure in Müller muscle-conjunctiva resection ptosis repair. Ophthal Plast Reconstr Surg. 2009;25:99.
23. Czyz CN, Rich NE, Foster JA, Kavanagh MC, Perry JD, Holck DEE. Comparison of postoperative eyelid position using fibrin sealant versus suture for wound closure in Müller's muscle-conjunctiva resection ptosis repair. Plast Reconstr Surg. 2011;128:423–30.
24. Foster JA, Holck DEE, Perry JD, Wulc AE, Burns JA, Cahill KV, Morgenstern KE. Fibrin sealant for Müller muscle-conjunctiva resection ptosis repair. Ophthal Plast Reconstr Surg. 2006;22:184–7.
25. Porteous AM, Haridas AS, Collin JRO, Verity DH. Upper lid ptosis surgery: what is the optimal interval for the postoperative review? A retrospective review of 300 cases. Eye. 2018;32:757–62.
26. Wee SW, Lee JK. Clinical outcomes of conjunctiva-Müller muscle resection: association with phenylephrine test-negative blepharoptosis and dry eye syndrome. J Craniofac Surg. 2014;25:898–901.
27. Dailey RA, Saulny SM, Sullivan SA. Müller muscle-conjunctival resection: effect on tear production. Ophthal Plast Reconstr Surg. 2002;18:421–5.

28. Rymer BL, Marinho DR, Cagliari C, Marafon SB, Procianoy F. Effects of Muller's muscle-conjunctival resection for ptosis on ocular surface scores and dry eye symptoms. Orbit. 2017; 36:1–5.
29. Michels KS, Vagefi MR, Steele E, Zwick OM, Torres JJ, Seiff SR, Dailey RA. Müller muscle-conjunctiva resection to correct ptosis in high-risk patients. Ophthal Plast Reconstr Surg. 2007;23:363–6.
30. Georgescu D, Cole E, Epstein G, Fountain T, Migliori M, Nguyen Q, Mannor G, Weinberg D. Müller muscle-conjunctiva resection for blepharoptosis in patients with glaucoma filtering blebs. Ophthal Plast Reconstr Surg. 2007;23:285–7.
31. Saonanon P, Sithanon S. External levator advancement versus Müller muscle-conjunctival resection for aponeurotic blepharoptosis: a randomized clinical trial. Plast Reconstr Surg. 2018;141:213e–9e.
32. Simon GJB, Lee S, Schwarcz RM, McCann JD, Goldberg RA. Müller's muscle–conjunctival resection for correction of upper eyelid ptosis: relationship between phenylephrine testing and the amount of tissue resected with final eyelid position. Arch Facial Plast Surg. 2007;9:413–7.
33. Thomas GN, Chan J, Sundar G, Amrith S. Outcomes of levator advancement and Müller muscle-conjunctiva resection for the repair of upper eyelid ptosis. Orbit. 2017;36:39–42.

Frontalis Sling

6

Paul O. Phelps and Dale R. Meyer

Introduction

The first reference that records an operation in which the eyelid margin was anchored to action of the frontalis muscle was described in a case of congenital ptosis [1]. Surgeons in those days used an incision in the brow to release a vertical band of fascial tissues from the forehead and then attach them near to the eyelid margin with catgut sutures. Since that time many different materials have been used, including autogenous fascia lata, [2] Supramid, [3] Gore-Tex, [4] silicone, [5] and others. All materials have specific advantages and disadvantages. However, the authors of this chapter have found silicone to be the material of choice because of its ease of readjustment and lack of complications sometimes seen with other materials. The surgical technique and type of needle used for performance of the frontalis sling vary by surgeon preference, and so we will explain in detail the operation for frontalis sling which has achieved excellent surgical outcomes in our hands.

Indications

Frontalis sling may be recommended for patients with moderate to severe ptosis (MRD1 of 2.0 mm or less) and poor levator function (4 mm or less). The procedure is generally performed bilaterally, but select patients with unilateral ptosis may be addressed with a unilateral frontalis sling, recognizing that the affected side cannot be made "normal" [6, 7].

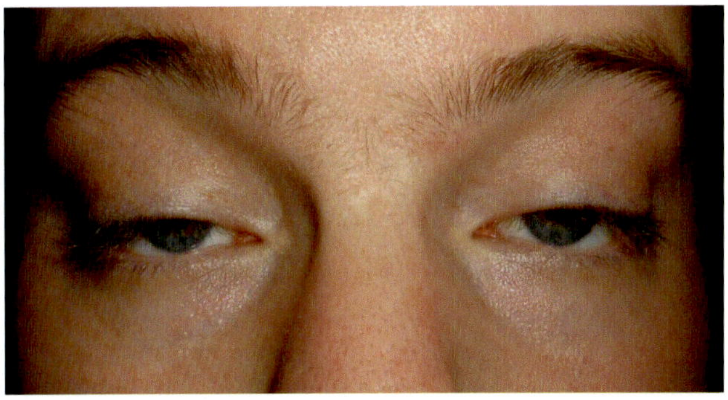

Fig 6.1 Preoperative photo of congenital ptosis patient demonstrates severe ptosis of both upper eyeids in primary gaze

The most common indication for frontalis sling is congenital ptosis (Fig. 6.1). These patients generally have poor levator function. If there is no evidence of amblyogenisis in these patients, it is appropriate to wait until 3–4 years old to perform surgery to allow the eyelid and facial tissues to develop. However, when the ptosis is amblyogenic, earlier intervention may be warranted. Other patients with moderate to severe acquired ptosis and poor levator function include patients with myasthenia gravis, progressive external ophthalmoplegia, and ptosis secondary to third nerve palsy.

Materials

As mentioned above, several materials have been recommended for frontalis slings. Silicone rods produced by Visitec have been useful in our hands. This material is ideal because it is easily inserted, adjusted, and removed (if necessary). Silicone also has good elasticity, which permits both good upper lid height and eye closure. Other materials have inherent advantages and disadvantages and include fascia lata, Supramid, and Gore-Tex. All of these procedures can

P. O. Phelps (✉)
Division of Ophthalmology, Department of Surgery, NorthShore University HealthSystem, Glenview, IL, USA

Ophthalmology and Visual Science, University of Chicago Medical Center, Chicago, IL, USA

D. R. Meyer
Ophthalmic Plastic Surgery, Lions Eye Institute-Albany Medical Center, Slingerlands, NY, USA
e-mail: meyerd@amc.edu

A. J. Cohen, C. N. Burkat (eds.), *Oculofacial, Orbital, and Lacrimal Surgery*, https://doi.org/10.1007/978-3-030-14092-2_6

have complications, including inclusion cysts, extrusion, over- or undercorrection, recurrent ptosis, exposure keratitis, chronic infection, granuloma formation, suture rupture, lid margin deformity, trichiasis, loss of apposition of the lid to the globe, and even frontalis muscle spasm.

Operative Procedure

The silicone rod material marketed by Visitec is particularly convenient in that the silicone rod material is directly attached to two stainless steel needles that can be used to pass the material through the tissue in any pattern desired by the surgeon. The material can be passed via either a transconjunctival or a transcutaneous approach. The authors use a transcutaneous approach with a single "pentagon" pattern as follows. In young children, the procedure is performed under general anesthesia. In cooperative older children and adults, the procedure can be performed under local anesthesia (with or without sedation).

The patient is placed in the supine position. Two skin incisions are marked, ~2–3 mm above the lash line in the upper lid approximating the medial and lateral corneal limbus. A 4-0 silk suture is placed at the upper lid margin for retraction. Two additional incisions are made in the superior brow cilia, slightly more medial and lateral to the previous eyelid incisions, down to the level of the periosteum. A forehead incision ~1.5 cm above the brow, also down to the periosteum, is placed midway between the two brow incisions. This incision may be placed in a forehead crease to hide a postoperative scar. A pocket is dissected with blunt Stevens tenotomy scissors (or a 15 blade scalpel) in the deeper aspect of the forehead incisions.

Some surgeons cut the silicone rod set in half; however, we leave the set intact and use both needles to pass the silicone rod material. Each needle is bent into a gentle curve. The needle is grasped with a large needle holder and passed from one eyelid incision to the other. This maneuver is generally performed with a corneal shield or a Jaeger lid plate beneath the lid to protect the globe. One needle is then passed from the medial eyelid incision to the medial brow incision, attempting to place the silicone rod posterior to the septum as it passes between the incisions. The second needle is then passed from the lateral eyelid incision to the lateral brow incision in a similar fashion (Fig. 6.2).

Each needle is then passed from the brow incisions to the central forehead incision. A silicone sleeve is used to secure the tubing. This silicone sleeve is cut at a total length of ~5 mm, and each end of the silicone rod material is passed through the sleeve. During insertion of the rod and sure of the incisions, care should be taken to avoid piercing or damaging the silicone rod material. The sleeve is "spread apart" with a device such as a Watzke spreader or a small mosquito clamp. The sleeve is then passed down the silicone rod into the forehead incision, while the tension on the silicone rods is adjusted to achieve the desired lid elevation.

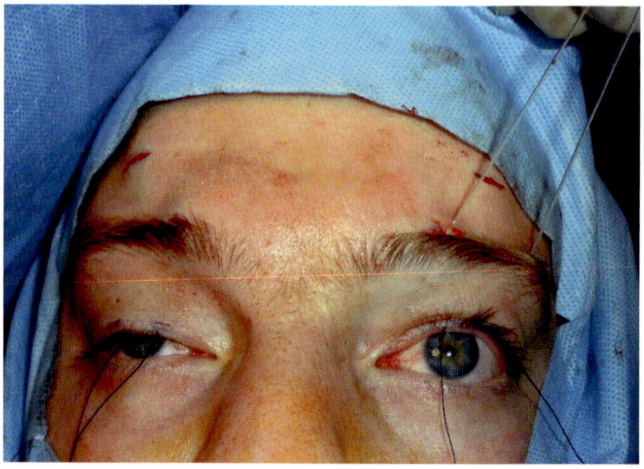

Fig. 6.2 Intraoperative photo demontrating the right upper eyelid after placment of frontalis sling, while on the left side the silicone sling is still being placed into position

The sleeve is then further secured by tying it to the rods with a 6-0 Vicryl suture, which is then tied to the frontalis muscle. The ends of the silicone rods are then cut (leaving ~1 cm "excess") and tucked deeply into the previously made pocket so that they lie flat on the periosteum. The brow incisions are closed with a 6-0 plain gut suture in a horizontal mattress fashion. The eyelid incisions do not require a suture. The incisions are irrigated before closure. Antibiotic ointment is placed on each incision in the eyelid. Light dressings may be applied to the brow incisions if desired.

The patient's eyelid position and closure are followed postoperatively, and vigorous topical eye lubrication is recommended in the early postoperative period and titrated as needed. The lid height can be adjusted as needed in the early period by opening the mid-forehead incision and adjusting the position of the silicone sleeve.

Follow-Up

Patients who have undergone frontalis sling are generally seen at 1 week and 1 month after surgery (Fig. 6.3). If there is a significant amount of asymmetry between the eyelid positions, they may be adjusted in the office or in the operating room by titration of the position of the sleeve and the silicone rods. Adjustment can be carried out soon after surgery if there is unsatisfactory eyelid position; otherwise, the patient is monitored on a more extended basis with adjustment if needed, again understanding the nature, risks, and limitations of surgery.

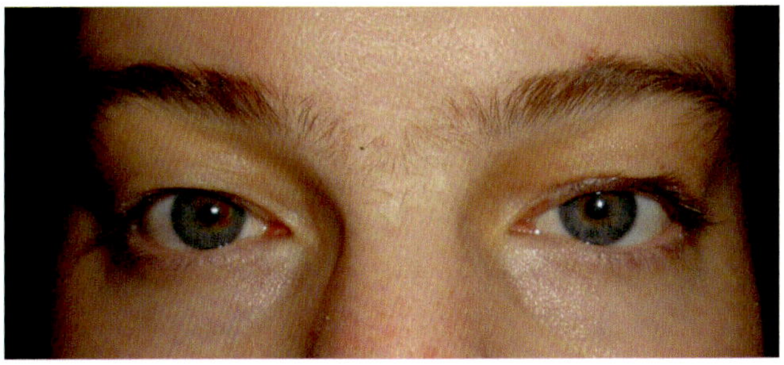

Fig. 6.3 Postoperative photo demonstrating good upper eyelid position in primary gaze

References

1. Fergus F. An easy operation for congenital ptosis. BMJ. 1901;1(2100):762.
2. Bartley GB. The enhanced frontalis sling for blepharoptosis repair. Am J Ophthalmol. 2002;134(5):782–4. https://doi.org/10.1016/S0002-9394(02)01630-6.
3. Wagner RS, Mauriello JA, Nelson LB, Calhoun JH, Flanagan JC, Harley RD. Treatment of congenital ptosis with frontalis suspension: a comparison of suspensory materials. Ophthalmology. 1984;91(3):245–8. https://doi.org/10.1016/S0161-6420(84)34298-1.
4. Steinkogler FJ, Kuchar A, Huber E, Arocker-Mettinger E. Gore-Tex soft-tissue patch frontalis suspension technique in congenital ptosis and in Blepharophimosis-ptosis syndrome. Plast Reconstr Surg. 1993;92(6):1057–60.
5. Carter SR, Meecham WJ, Seiff SR. Silicone frontalis slings for the correction of blepharoptosis: indications and efficacy. Ophthalmology. 1996;103(4):623–30. https://doi.org/10.1016/S0161-6420(96)30643-X.
6. Meyer DR. Congenital ptosis. In: Nerad JA, Daily R, Turgeon PW, editors. Focal points: clinical modules for ophthalmologists. American Academy of Ophthalmology. 2001;XIX(2).
7. Meyer DR. Surgery of ptosis. In: Wobig JL, Daily RA, editors. Oculofacial plastic surgery. New York: Thieme; 2004. p. 78–82.

Complications of Blepharoptosis Repair and Their Solutions

7

Rakesh M. Patel and Allen M. Putterman

When performed correctly, blepharoptosis correction can be one of the most rewarding procedures to the patient and to the surgeon. However, for the inexperienced surgeon and even the most experienced surgeon, it is a procedure fraught with potential for complications. Given that most ptosis surgeries are not technically difficult, complications are infrequently due to an intraoperative failure. Instead, the most common reason for complications is poor preoperative assessment of the patient. Without a thorough evaluation, an inappropriate surgical procedure may be selected for the patient such as performing a maximal levator resection when a frontalis sling was indicated or resecting only 6.5 mm of Müller's muscle in a mullerectomy when 9.5 mm resection would have been preferred.

The preoperative exam should include a detailed history to rule out conditions such as myasthenia gravis, third nerve palsy, or chronic progressive external ophthalmoplegia (CPEO) that may be the cause of ptosis [1]. In addition, meticulous eyelid measurements are necessary such as levator function and margin-reflex distance 1 (MRD-1) as well as performing a careful slit lamp exam looking for signs of dry eye [2]. The presence of a Bell's phenomenon should be checked as well as Schirmer's testing being performed in the dry eye patient.

The most commonly performed ptosis surgeries include external levator advancement (ELA) with or without levator resection, conjunctiva-Müller's muscle resection, Fasanella-Servat, or a frontalis sling operation [3]. The complications that can result from these surgeries include undercorrection, overcorrection, contralateral ptosis, suture keratopathy with corneal abrasion, eyelid contour irregularities, and dry eye due to exposure keratopathy among others. In addition, as implants are frequently used in frontalis sling surgery, implant rejection remains a potential complication. Various complications encountered with each ptosis procedure will be discussed.

Mullerectomy/Fasanella-Servat

Müller's muscle and conjunctiva resection (MMCR) is a posterior approach surgery that has gained significant popularity in the treatment of acquired involutional blepharoptosis [3]. It has shown great efficacy in the treatment of mild to moderate ptosis with good levator function that is responsive to phenylephrine testing. Fasanella-Servat (FS) is another method to perform posterior approach surgery. Although both techniques have high success rates, complications such as overcorrection, undercorrection, exposure or suture keratopathy, and development of contralateral ptosis may occur [4–7].

Undercorrection

An undercorrection from ptosis surgery is a frustrating complication for many surgeons, and its management can be challenging. It may be due to inappropriate procedure selection such as performing the MMCR or FS procedure on patients with poor or fair levator function. Insufficient resection of tissue during the procedure may also result in an undercorrection.

If the undercorrection is mild (<0.5–1.0 mm) in the early post-operative period, one may consider observation waiting for the post-operative edema to resolve as this may be contributing to the ptosis. However, if the undercorrection after surgery is more significant or the mild undercorrection does not resolve after the post-operative edema subsides, the patient will likely require a second ptosis surgery.

R. M. Patel
Department of Ophthalmology, University of South Carolina and Prisma Health, Columbia, SC, USA

A. M. Putterman (✉)
University of Illinois College of Medicine, Chicago, IL, USA
e-mail: drputterman@drputterman.com

A. J. Cohen, C. N. Burkat (eds.), *Oculofacial, Orbital, and Lacrimal Surgery*, https://doi.org/10.1007/978-3-030-14092-2_7

Surgical options to address the undercorrected ptosis include repeat MMCR/FS procedure or an external levator advancement presuming the patient has good levator function. One must ensure if a repeat MMCR procedure is performed, there is adequate conjunctiva remaining to prevent fornix shortening. If the FS procedure is repeated, there must be at least 4 mm of tarsus remaining to prevent an unstable upper eyelid. Repeat surgery is typically performed 3–6 months after the initial surgery to allow for adequate resolution of the tissue edema and for the eyelid to settle to a final MRD-1 so the appropriate amount of tissue to resect is determined.

For many surgeons, ELA is the preferred modality to manage undercorrected ptosis in a patient with good levator function. This method allows the surgeon to make intraoperative adjustments to better ensure the eyelid is of appropriate height before the conclusion of the case. If the undercorrection is a result of selecting the inappropriate procedure such as performing a MMCR/FS on a patient with poor or fair levator function, then one must perform a frontalis sling or levator resection, respectively, to address the undercorrected ptosis.

Overcorrection

Overcorrection occurs when the post-operative MRD-1 is higher than desired. It is a less frequently seen complication than undercorrection; however, it is often preferable to an undercorrection given it is frequently simpler to manage post-operatively than an undercorrection. In addition to poor cosmesis and eyelid asymmetry, overcorrection can lead to dry eyes and exposure keratopathy.

If an overcorrection is identified early and is mild (<1 mm overcorrection in MRD-1), the surgeon may have the patient initiate massage of the upper eyelid down. This may be done in a variety of ways; however, our preferred technique is to raise the brow with one hand and then apply firm and constant pressure on the eyelid at the level of the eyelid crease downward and inward. The patient is asked to perform this maneuver several times a day for about 30 seconds to 1 minute at a time [8]. Massage will stretch the internal wound in the upper eyelid decreasing the MRD-1 to a more acceptable level. Patients are frequently skeptical of the efficacy of massage, and therefore they must be strongly encouraged to perform this maneuver.

If a more severe overcorrection is identified at the first post-operative visit after the MMCR or FS procedure, the surgeon must give consideration to opening the wound. This is done by injecting the upper eyelid with a local anesthetic and placing a 4–0 silk traction suture through the upper eyelid. The eyelid is then everted over a Desmarres retractor. Topical tetracaine is placed on the wound and a small aliquot of local anesthetic is injected subconjunctivally adjacent to the wound. The suture from the MMCR or FS procedure is identified, cut, and removed. The Desmarres retractor is removed and the eyelid is reverted back to its normal anatomic position, and the 4-0 silk traction suture is taped down to the cheek placing the upper eyelid on stretch. This will leave the patient monocular and therefore the patient must be warned of this. The suture is removed the following day and the MRD-1 is reassessed. If eyelid height is satisfactory, then further treatment is not necessary. If MRD-1 still remains slightly overcorrected, massage therapy may be initiated again (Figs. 7.1, 7.2, and 7.3).

If severe overcorrection is identified several months after from the MMCR or FS procedure, the cicatrix in the upper eyelid is set in and therefore the aforemen-

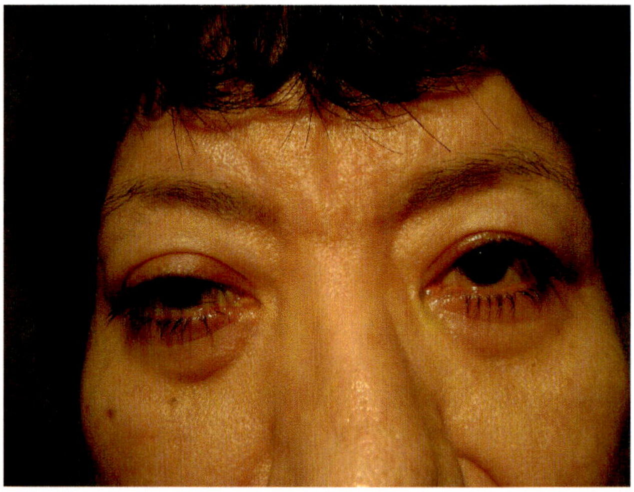

Fig. 7.1 Preoperative photograph of a patient with bilateral ptosis

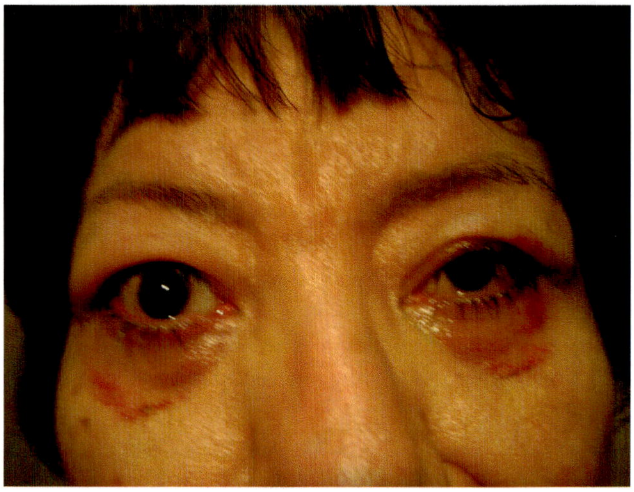

Fig. 7.2 After bilateral Müller's muscle and conjunctiva resection. Note the overcorrection on the right upper eyelid at post-operative day 6. The internal suture was removed and a tarsorrhaphy suture was placed on the upper eyelid and taped down to the cheek with tension

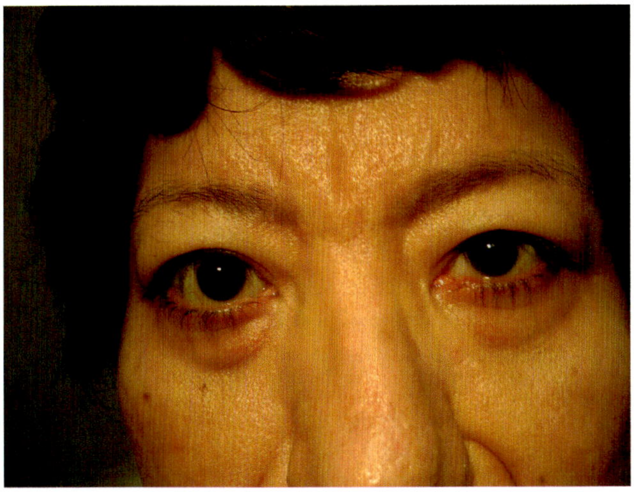

Fig. 7.3 Post-operative month 6. Note improved symmetry between the two eyelids

tioned techniques are unlikely to work. These patients will require a surgical correction of the eyelid retraction. A blepharotomy may be performed to address the retraction; however, the primary technique the authors prefer is internal Müller's muscle extirpation and levator recession [9, 10]. The technique involves injection of 1% lidocaine with 1:100,000 units of epinephrine both subcutaneously and subconjunctivally into the upper eyelid. The eyelid is everted over a Desmarres retractor, and the conjunctiva is incised at the superior tarsal border and separated from the Müller's muscle. The Müller's muscle is then dissected free from the underlying levator aponeurosis and then detached from the superior tarsal border for the temporal two-thirds of the eyelid. The patient is raised to a seated position and if the lid is in satisfactory position, this Müller's muscle is excised. If a nasal retraction does persist, then entire Müller's muscle may be released from the superior tarsal border and excised. If further lowering of the eyelid is necessary, this can be done by stripping the levator aponeurosis by using two toothed forceps to stretch the levator in the temporal eyelid until the eyelid is of desirable height. Of note, after a mullerectomy procedure, there may not be significant amount of Müller's muscle to resect, and therefore levator stripping and recession may have to be more aggressive. The conjunctiva is then closed to the superior tarsal border.

Suture Keratopathy/Corneal Abrasion

A known complication of internal ptosis repair is suture keratopathy or corneal abrasion of the eye. This is due to the internal suture rubbing on the cornea with each blink. This occurrence is more common when tarsus is resected such as in the Fasanella-Servat procedure due to the internal running suture being placed more inferiorly on the tarsus and therefore closer to the cornea. In addition, if the knot of the suture is not appropriately buried in the wound when tied, it can rub on the eye with each blink. This can be extremely painful for the patient. The surgeon should look for vertically oriented linear abrasions of the cornea with fluorescein staining in cobalt blue light to identify suture keratopathy.

Mild foreign body sensation after surgery is expected, and the patient is advised to lubricate with antibiotic ointment and artificial tears. However, if the patient is extremely uncomfortable or there is a corneal abrasion on exam, a soft bandage contact lens (BCTL) may be placed on the eye. In this case, the ointment is discontinued and the patient is started on prophylactic antibiotic drops such as ciprofloxacin while the contact lens is in place. The BCTL is removed once the corneal abrasion is healed and the internal suture is no longer irritating the cornea, typically about 1 week after surgery.

Contralateral Ptosis

If a unilateral internal ptosis repair is performed, the patient may develop ptosis in the contralateral eyelid. This is due to Hering's law where the innervation to the contralateral upper eyelid is relaxed upon raising the ipsilateral eyelid [11]. A careful preoperative exam can help assess for this potential complication by manually raising the ptotic eyelid to determine if the contralateral eyelid does indeed have an underlying ptosis. The phenylephrine test will also frequently identify contralateral eyelid ptosis after instillation of the drop in the more ptotic eye. It is strongly advised that the patient have bilateral surgery if bilateral ptosis is identified.

Nevertheless, even with the most careful preoperative evaluation to rule out bilateral ptosis, the patient may still develop contralateral ptosis after a unilateral MMCR/FS procedure. In such a case, the patient will require ptosis surgery on the contralateral eyelid.

External Levator Advancement

ELA has historically been the mainstay of blepharoptosis repair in the patient with good levator function. It allows for intraoperative adjustments to ensure the eyelid is satisfactory before the conclusion of the case. The procedure is not without complications that may include overcorrection, undercorrection, suture keratopathy, and contralateral ptosis similar to the MMCR/FS procedure. Another risk more specific to external levator advancement includes contour abnormalities of the upper eyelid.

Undercorrection

Similar to the MMCR/FS procedure, undercorrection is probably the most common complication after surgery. The etiologies of undercorrection include selection of the incorrect procedure or not advancing the levator aponeurosis adequately. For example, performing an ELA when the levator function is in fact poor or fair will certainly lead to an undercorrection.

The management of a ptosis undercorrection is similar to MMCR/FS procedure. If the undercorrection is mild (<0.5–1.0 mm) in the early post-operative period, the physician may observe the patient as the ptosis may resolve as the eyelid edema subsides. However, if a large undercorrection is identified in the early post-operative period, then one may consider early post-operative suture adjustment. This is preferably performed in the first few weeks after surgery once eyelid edema has improved but before significant scar tissue has formed [12]. The adjustment may be performed in the office under local anesthesia. The eyelid is infiltrated with 1% lidocaine with 1:100,000 epinephrine for no more than 1.5 ml to decrease the risk of levator paresis. The skin sutures are removed and the wound is opened. The previously placed sutures securing the levator to the tarsal plate are removed. New sutures can then be placed by advancing the levator aponeurosis further. The patient may be raised to a seated position to check for appropriate height of the eyelid. Once deemed satisfactory, the eyelid may then be closed in the usual fashion.

If the undercorrection is identified late after a few months, suture adjustment will not be possible at this point due to scarring. Therefore, it is advised to allow for adequate post-operative recovery from the initial eyelid surgery for up to 3–6 months. The patient must then be re-examined, checking for the amount of ptosis present and rechecking levator function to ensure the appropriate procedure was selected in the first place. If levator function is good, then a repeat external levator advancement may be performed. If levator function is fair or poor, then consideration must be given to alternative procedures such as an ELA with resection or frontalis sling.

Overcorrection

Overcorrection with eyelid retraction may also occur with the external levator advancement procedure. If a small overcorrection is present (<0.5–1.0 mm), massage may be instituted to the overcorrected eyelid as previously described. However, if the overcorrection is more significant or is not showing improvement with massage, early suture adjustment is advised. This is performed similar to early suture adjustment for undercorrection. After infiltrating the eyelid with local anesthetic and opening the wound, the sutures attaching the levator to the tarsus are cut in the area of the overcorrection. The levator aponeurosis may then be bluntly dissected away from the tarsus with cotton-tipped applicators. This maneuver alone frequently improves the eyelid retraction. If it does not, the other sutures from the levator to tarsus may need to be removed as well and further blunt dissection performed. Massage may also be instituted after revision to further improve the eyelid retraction. If the above maneuvers are unsuccessful, then a blepharotomy procedure or Müller's muscle extirpation with levator recession may be performed as previously described.

Contralateral Ptosis

Similar to when MMCR/FS procedure is performed unilaterally, performing an ELA unilaterally places the patient at risk of developing contralateral ptosis. As mentioned previously, this can be assessed for during the patient evaluation by manually raising the ptotic eyelid to see if the contralateral eyelid does descend to a ptotic level. In such a case, ptosis repair should be performed bilaterally or the patient will be unhappy. If contralateral ptosis does develop after unilateral surgery, the patient will require ptosis surgery on the opposite eyelid.

Suture Keratopathy

Corneal trauma from the suture rubbing on the eye is quite rare but a serious complication if it does occur. The etiology is often due to the suture that secures the levator to tarsus being passed full thickness through the tarsal plate leaving exposed suture on the palpebral conjunctiva. With every blink, the patient may feel the irritation from the suture and potentially cause a corneal abrasion. Similar to MMCR/FS, the surgeon should look for vertically oriented linear abrasions at the slit lamp.

If the suture utilized for the levator aponeurosis advancement was a resorbable suture such as polyglactin 910, one may first lubricate with ointment to see if that improves the symptomatology and the ocular surface. If it does not, a bandage contact lens may be placed to protect the eye from the suture. The patient should be placed on prophylactic topical antibiotic drops, and the BCTL may be removed once the suture resorbs. If this conservative approach is chosen, the surgeon should be aware that polyglactin 910 suture can take up to 2 months if not more to resorb so the patient may potentially require the BCTL for an extended period of time which is not ideal.

Many surgeons will choose to use a permanent suture for the ELA procedure such as polypropylene or polyester fiber among others. If these sutures are passed full thickness through the tarsal plate and is causing damage to the ocular surface, BCTL or ointment is only a temporizing measure since the sutures will not dissolve. Therefore, the surgeon must open up the wound, find and remove the offending suture, and place another suture in a lamellar fashion taking care to ensure the pass is not full thickness through the tarsus. The skin is then closed in the usual manner.

Another potential option in the management of suture keratopathy is everting the eyelid after instillation of topical anesthetic and cutting both ends of the exposed suture flush with the tarsus. This may allow enough of the suture to retract back into the eyelid leaving no exposed suture on the palpebral conjunctiva.

Contour

A known complication of external levator advancement procedures is an abnormal eyelid contour ranging from a residual segmental ptosis to a peaked eyelid. The management of eyelid contour abnormality depends on its severity. For example, if there is a mild segmental eyelid retraction, massage of the eyelid down in that focal area may help improve the contour to an acceptable level. If the segmental eyelid retraction is more severe, early post-operative suture adjustment to recess the levator is preferred using a technique similar to previously described for overcorrection.

If there is a residual segmental blepharoptosis after surgery, the wound may be opened releasing the levator-tarsus suture in the area of the blepharoptosis. The levator aponeurosis can then be further advanced and secured to the tarsus ensuring the ptosis has resolved with the patient in the seated position. An alternative option is the internal vertical shortening procedure [13]. This procedure is similar to the mullerectomy procedure with the difference being the tissue is resected focally only in the area of the blepharoptosis with 3–8 mm of tissue being resected depending on severity of the ptosis.

If a peaked eyelid is identified early, massage is unlikely to be successful. In this scenario, the etiology is likely the levator aponeurosis being advanced too far focally or orbital septum may have been incorporated into the closure. The wound should be opened and spread apart with cotton-tipped applicators. If the peak resolves with this maneuver, septum in the wound is the likely cause and the skin can simply be re-closed taking care to avoid septum. Otherwise, the aggressively advanced portion of the levator aponeurosis is identified and the suture removed in this area. Blunt dissection with cotton-tipped applicators is used to separate the levator aponeurosis from tarsus allowing the peak to resolve. If the eyelid height is satisfactory, no further sutures are needed from the levator to tarsus. If ptosis does recur, a new suture should be passed from levator to tarsus with the levator in a more recessed position to avoid a peaked eyelid. The skin is then closed in the usual manner.

If the eyelid peak is identified late, the management remains similar. However, given there will be significant scar tissue present, the surgeon needs to perform sharp dissection with scissors or cautery to recess the levator in the area of the peaked eyelid.

External Levator Resection

External levator resection (ELR) procedure has the same complications of ELA, and the management algorithm will be the same as for ELA with few slight variations discussed below.

Overcorrection

In a severe overcorrection, the levator will need to be recessed. However, there may not be enough levator muscle or aponeurosis available to position it on tarsus in a recessed manner due to the levator having been partially resected. Therefore the surgeon will need to use a hang-back suture in this circumstance to recess the levator an adequate amount or consider the use of a spacer graft such as decellularized porcine-derived membrane.

Undercorrection

In a significant undercorrection, the etiology may be due to the levator function being underestimated on preoperative exam leading to an insufficient resection of tissue. The options for correction include further advancement and resection of levator aponeurosis with consideration given to a Whitnall sling procedure or super-maximum levator resection with tarsectomy [14–16]. If a maximal levator resection had been performed or the levator function is quite poor, a frontalis sling is indicated for this patient.

Lagophthalmos

Although lagophthalmos is possible in an external levator advancement or MMCR/FS procedure, it is more common in an ELR procedure due to the shortening of the levator aponeurosis. Management will depend on severity of the lagophthalmos and the patient's symptoms. Without appropriate treatment, the patient is at risk of exposure keratopathy and its subsequent complications of corneal abrasion or corneal ulcer.

If lagophthalmos is mild and identified in the early post-operative period with mild exposure keratopathy, lubrication and ointment may suffice. A suture tarsorrhaphy may also be placed through the lower eyelid to minimize exposure. The lagophthalmos will typically improve over the first few weeks. However, if the lagophthalmos is more severe and there is upper eyelid retraction in primary gaze, massage may be instituted. If the eyelid retraction and lagophthalmos persists despite massage, the wound may then need to be opened and the sutures cut. This may be done in the office with infiltration of local anesthetic, opening the eyelid wound, and cutting the suture that secures the levator to the tarsus. More than one suture may need to be removed for optimal results. This is ideally performed within the first few weeks before significant scar tissue has formed. Fortunately, the suture removal rarely results in recurrent ptosis.

Frontalis Sling

Of the procedures mentioned thus far, frontalis sling may have the most complications due to its inherent nature of bypassing the eyelid retractors to achieve adequate eyelid height. The complications induced by frontalis sling procedures include overcorrection, undercorrection, abnormal eyelid contour, lash entropion, implant rejection, lagophthalmos, or having a palpable sling. Various materials are often utilized for frontalis slings including silicone, nylon suture, autogenous fascia lata, Supramid suture, and banked fascia lata among others. The management of the complications will depend partly on the material utilized for the ptosis repair [17].

Undercorrection

It is often advised to set the tension of the sling so the upper eyelid sits at the superior limbus during surgery. Yet it is not uncommon to see the eyelid descend to an undercorrected position either early after surgery or months later. Choice of sling material does influence the rate of undercorrection as autogenous fascia lata is the longest lasting and considered the gold standard while Supramid suture is believed to not last as long [17]. Silicone sling is another method to performing frontalis sling surgery, but this material is not immune to an undercorrection. If the undercorrection is small and not affecting the vision in the adult patient or not amblyogenic in a child, the patient may be observed although do not expect the eyelid position to improve. If the undercorrection is significant enough to affect peripheral vision in an adult or cause amblyopia in a child, surgical intervention is advised.

In a silicone sling undercorrection, the central forehead wound where both arms of the sling and the sleeve were placed may be opened and the sling retightened. For adults, this may be easily performed in the office. The ability to make such post-operative adjustments by opening a single wound gives the silicone sling an advantage over other materials.

With other materials aside from silicone, the management of undercorrection is more challenging. If a Supramid material or nylon suture was utilized and the ptosis is undercorrected, the suture needs to be tightened. As untying a suture is difficult, typically the suture is released and a new sling is placed. The same type of suture or Supramid material may be utilized in the repeat frontalis sling operation with the understanding the eyelid may descend rather quickly again. It may be advisable to utilize an alternative material such as silicone to give hopefully a longer-lasting result. The goal is to manage the ptosis with these materials until approximately age 3–4. By this time, there should be enough autogenous fascia lata to harvest for a frontalis sling providing a more long-lasting effect.

If fascia lata was utilized for the frontalis sling and undercorrection is identified quite early within days, attempts may be made to untie the sling and retie it in a tighter position. However, if the ptosis is identified late, then management is much more challenging as the fascia lata will have become integrated into the host tissue making untying it not feasible. If the ptosis is not visually significant in this situation, the patient may be observed; otherwise a new sling must be placed.

Overcorrection

Overcorrection is rare in frontalis sling surgery and even desired in the early post-operative period as the sling is expected to relax over time allowing the eyelid to descend. Due to this fact, a permanent overcorrection is quite rare. If mild overcorrection is identified early, lubrication with artificial tears and ointment is advised to prevent exposure keratopathy with the expectation the upper eyelid will ultimately descend. If the overcorrection is more severe, the patient is at risk of developing exposure keratopathy with a subsequent corneal abrasion. Aggressive lubrication and ointment may be instituted, a punctal plug may be placed, and/or a Frost suture tarsorrhaphy may be performed with the hope the upper eyelid will slowly descend over time. However, if the upper eyelid retraction does not improve over the first few weeks and the cornea is developing signs of severe exposure keratopathy, the sling itself needs to be addressed. Similar to undercorrection, the silicone sling may be easily loosened by opening a single forehead wound where the sling was set. If a Supramid material or nylon suture was utilized, the surgeon may attempt to untie the suture and retie it with less tension. Otherwise, a new sling will have to be passed. With fascia lata, if the overcorrection is identified early, the surgeon may be able to untie the knot of the fascia and retie it in a more relaxed position. However, if the overcorrection from fascia lata is identified late after months, the tissue is likely scarred into place by this point. The surgeon will likely have to release the material and potentially repeat the surgery.

Lagophthalmos/Exposure Keratopathy

Lagophthalmos is in fact expected when performing a frontalis sling operation. This is due to the inability of the sling to stretch upon eyelid closure. The post-operative lagophthalmos can be quite disturbing to the unwarned adult patient or to the parents of the child with congenital ptosis. Therefore, it is prudent for the surgeon to let the patient or the patient's family know that lagophthalmos will certainly occur after surgery and is not truly a complication. It will often improve over time as the sling relaxes but may not resolve completely. Therefore, aggressive lubrication early in the post-operative period to the ocular surface is strongly advised as a prophylactic measure to prevent exposure keratopathy.

Lagophthalmos is considered acceptable in the setting of an adequate MRD-1 and no signs of exposure keratopathy. However, if the patient does develop signs of exposure such as punctate epithelial erosions on slit lamp exam, lubrication is advised such as preservative-free artificial tears every 2 hours and an artificial tear ointment 4–8x/day. Punctal occlusion may also be considered to prolong the contact time of the tears to the ocular surface. Presuming the cornea does not deteriorate any further, the lubrication regimen may be maintained until the lagophthalmos improves at which point it may be slowly tapered off.

If the exposure keratopathy persists or is worsening despite aggressive lubrication, a suture tarsorrhaphy from the lower eyelid to the forehead may be placed. Various techniques are available in place of this tarsorrhaphy including a technique devised by the senior author which will be discussed in a subsequent section [18]. If this still does not resolve the exposure keratopathy or it recurs after release of the tarsorrhaphy, consideration must then be given to relaxing the sling. This will unfortunately decrease the MRD-1 but is necessary to prevent more serious complications such as a corneal ulcer. If a corneal ulcer does develop in the setting of significant lagophthalmos after frontalis sling surgery, the sling should be completely released and a consultation with a cornea specialist obtained for likely culture and administration of fortified topical antibiotics.

Contour Irregularities

Frontalis slings are known to cause eyelid contour abnormalities to the upper eyelid including a peaked eyelid. This can make an excellent lift of the eyelid appear suboptimal. The best method to manage this complication is to identify it on the operating room table and address it before the conclusion of the case. It almost certainly will not resolve with time. The etiology is due to one of the sutures securing the sling on the tarsal plate being too close to the lashes. Correction would involve release of the suture and reposition of the sling in a more superior location on the tarsal plate.

Segmental ptosis or segmental eyelid retraction of the upper eyelid may occur and is often related to the position of the sling on the tarsal plate or asymmetric tension of the arms of the sling. If segmental nasal or temporal ptosis is identified on the table, surgeon should attempt to tighten the arm of the sling controlling that portion of the eyelid. Similarly, if segmental eyelid retraction is noted, the arm of the sling should be loosened for that segment. If this does not adequately address the contour irregularity, the sling may need to be adjusted on the tarsal plate itself. For residual segmental ptosis, the sling may need to be advanced closer to the lid margin on the tarsal plate and/or the sling may need to be placed further nasally for nasal ptosis or further temporally for temporal ptosis on the tarsal plate. If segmental eyelid retraction is present, the sling will need to be positioned further away from the lid margin on the tarsal plate.

Eyelash Entropion

Entropion of the eyelashes after a frontalis sling procedure is frequently due to anterior lamella slippage relative to the posterior lamella. This may lead to trichiasis causing corneal keratopathy or frank corneal abrasion. The etiology is typically a lack of supratarsal fixation of the anterior lamella. This is another complication that is ideally identified and corrected at the time of the operation.

Various methods are available to achieve supratarsal fixation with eyelid crease formation [19]. One may pass an interrupted suture from the pretarsal orbicularis to the superior edge of the tarsal plate or the distal edge of the levator aponeurosis. Three to four sutures are typically passed in this manner. Whatever method is chosen, formation of an eyelid crease with supratarsal fixation will allow the anterior lamella to remain fixed in a taut manner preventing lash entropion.

Suture Keratopathy

The mechanism and management of suture keratopathy in the setting of a frontalis sling procedure is similar to ELA procedures. If a suture is passed full thickness through the tarsal plate when fixating the sling, the patient is at risk of the suture rubbing on the cornea. Since permanent sutures are used for frontalis slings, the suture needs to be removed and repassed in a partial-thickness lamellar fashion. The reader is noted that for the surgeon performing frontalis sling operations without tarsal fixation, this complication does not occur.

Other Implant-Specific Complications

Complications specific to the various implant materials utilized for frontalis sling surgery include implant extrusion, infection, granuloma, slippage, and implant breakage. Nylon or Supramid sutures are at risk for breakage and are known to have higher rates of ptosis recurrence. Silicone material carries the risk of implant rejection, extrusion, or granuloma formation (Fig. 7.4). The sling may require removal, and these patients may be an ideal candidate for autogenous fascia lata given its inherently lower risk of these complications. However autogenous fascia lata requires a second site surgery to harvest the tissue from the leg which carries the risk of muscle herniation or hematoma formation. Banked fascia lata has the theoretical risk of disease transmission and may undergo premature resorption leading to earlier recurrence of ptosis compared to autogenous fascia lata [17].

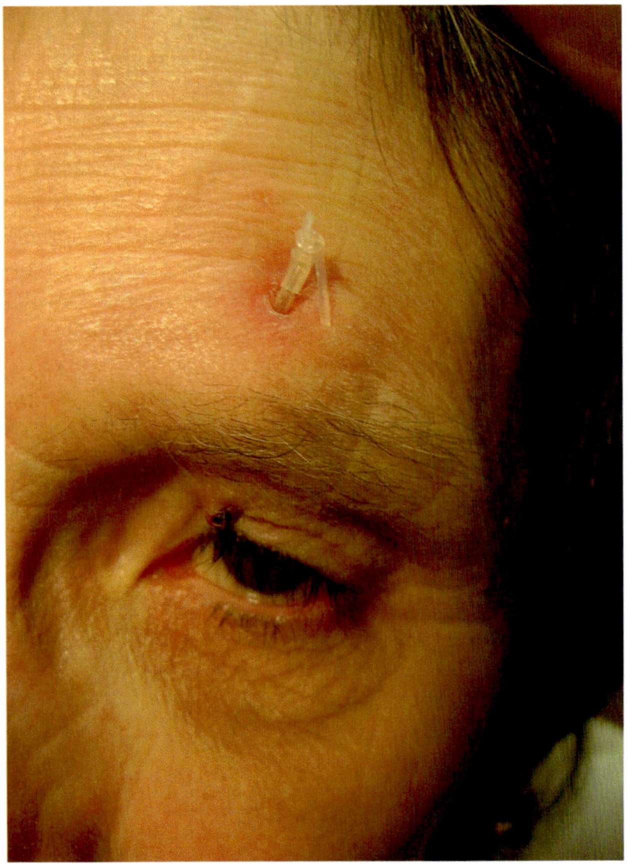

Fig. 7.4 Exposed frontalis silicone sling

Occasionally, the sling material is visible underneath the skin after a frontalis sling procedure, particularly in the upper eyelid. This is most commonly due to the sling being passed too superficial when it is passed from the eyelid to the brow. If the patient is not bothered by the appearance, this may be observed. Otherwise, the sling needs to be repassed in a retroseptal fashion to prevent visibility of the sling.

Special Considerations in Ptosis Surgery

Marcus Gunn Jaw-Winking Syndrome

In a patient with congenital ptosis undergoing frontalis sling operation, care must be taken to evaluate for Marcus Gunn jaw-winking syndrome preoperatively. This condition is due to cross innervation between cranial nerves III and V. With contralateral movement of the jaw, the ptotic eyelid elevates and is frequently noted by the parents when the child is feeding on a bottle. When performing a frontalis sling on these patients, the levator aponeurosis should be completely detached from the tarsal plate, dissected up to and past Whitnall's ligament, and the muscle along with the aponeurosis removed [20]. Without this step, the jaw-winking will persist post-operatively, and the patient and/or family will be unhappy.

Neurogenic/Myopathic Ptosis

In patients with neurogenic or myopathic ptosis such as myasthenia gravis, third nerve palsy, or CPEO among others, great care must be taken in performing ptosis surgery in these patients. These patients often have a poor Bell's phenomenon putting the cornea at great risk for exposure keratopathy with surgical elevation of the upper eyelid. A surgical result achieving a MRD-1 of 4 mm may be an excellent result in the standard ptosis patient yet may lead to devastating complications of corneal ulceration in the patient with a poor Bell's phenomenon.

Various options are available to minimize the risk of exposure keratopathy or corneal ulceration in these patients. For one, aggressive post-operative lubrication is a must for patients. The surgeon may consider undercorrecting the eyelid to decrease the vertical palpebral fissure and therefore decreasing the amount of corneal exposure. A punctal plug may also be placed to retain the tears on the ocular surface longer.

The senior author (AMP) utilizes a suture tarsorrhaphy system that is placed intraoperatively to manage these challenging patients, particularly for patients undergoing frontalis slings. Three double-armed 4-0 silk sutures are passed from the nasal, central, and temporal lower eyelid to the forehead and tied over cotton bolsters. A fourth suture is placed beneath the central lower eyelid suture and taped to the cheek. The sutures are removed gradually one by one over the ensuing 2 post-operative weeks, tapering off the ocular lubrication as well to allow for corneal adaptation to the increased exposure. If the corneal surface develops significant punctate epithelial erosions after sutures have been removed, the cheek suture may be taped to the forehead to bring the lower eyelid up and ocular lubrication increased. As the forehead and brow mobility begins to improve as the edema resolves, this allows for better closure of the eye at which point it is typically safe to remove the suture tarsorrhaphy completely and manage the patient with ocular lubrication [18].

An alternative method to correcting ptosis in these patients with poor levator function is performing a functional blepharoplasty of the upper eyelid. In this procedure, excess skin and orbicularis is excised from the upper eyelid utilizing the skin-pinch technique to determine the amount of tissue to resect. This creates a physiologic sling from the brow to the upper eyelid and therefore, upon raising the brow, the eyelid elevates to clear the visual axis. The patient may relax the brow when closing the eyes allowing for there to be minimal to no lagophthalmos, a significant advantage over traditional frontalis sling surgeries [21]. To determine if a patient is a candidate for such a procedure, the senior author has devised a blepharoplasty clamp [22]. This clamp may be placed on the excess upper eyelid skin in the office. If the patient notices an improvement in vision upon raising the eyebrows with the clamp in place, the patient will likely benefit from surgery.

Full-Thickness Ptosis Resection

In patients who have refractory ptosis despite multiple ptosis surgeries such as ELA with or without resection or MMCR procedure, a full-thickness ptosis resection may be beneficial. In this procedure, full-thickness eyelid is resected, typically 1 mm for every millimeter desired increase in the MRD-1. This surgery will also help improve asymmetric upper eyelid creases and folds [23].

The surgery is performed by making an eyelid crease incision on the ptotic eyelid and resecting full-thickness eyelid tissue either above or below this crease incision dependent on the crease position of the contralateral eyelid. If the crease is higher on the contralateral side, tissue is resected above the crease; conversely, if the crease is lower on the normal eyelid, tissue is resected below the crease incision of the ptotic eyelid. A double-armed 6-0 polyglactin 910 suture is passed from the superior tarsal border through the levator aponeurosis and tied over a knot releasing silk suture. Three of these sutures are placed. The patient is raised to a seated position to ensure the eyelid height is adequate. If not, more tissue may be resected and the sutures repassed. The polyglactin 910 sutures are then permanently tied off and left long. One arm of the needle is then passed through the superior skin edge, and the other arm is passed through the inferior skin edge and tied off to recreate the eyelid crease. The excess suture is cut and the skin is closed with surgeon's suture of choice.

Conclusion

Surgical correction of blepharoptosis can lead to an extremely satisfying result for the patient. Nevertheless, complications are inevitable for any surgeon performing this operation. Thorough knowledge of the various techniques discussed in this chapter will give the surgeon the confidence to overcome the complications that may result from blepharoptosis surgery.

References

1. Lim JM, Hou JH, Singa RM, et al. Relative incidence of blepharoptosis subtypes in an oculoplastics practice at a tertiary care center. Orbit. 2013;32:213–4.
2. Putterman AM. Margin reflex distance (MRD) 1, 2, and 3. Ophthal Plast Reconstr Surg. 2012;28:308–11.
3. Aakalu VK, Setabutr P. Current ptosis management: a national survey of ASOPRS members. Ophthal Plast Reconstr Surg. 2011;27:270–6.
4. Fasanella RM, Servat J. Levator resection for minimal ptosis: another simplified operation. Arch Ophthalmol. 1961;65: 493–6.
5. Pang NK, Newsom RW, Oestreicher JH, et al. Fasanella-Servat procedure: indications, efficacy, and complications. Can J Ophthalmol. 2008;43:84–8.
6. Putterman AM, Urist MJ. Muller muscle-conjunctiva resection: technique for treatment of blepharoptosis. Arch Ophthalmol. 1975;93:619–23.
7. Putterman AM, Fett DR. Muller's muscle in the treatment of upper eyelid ptosis: a ten-year study. Ophthalmic Surg. 1986;17: 354–60.
8. Putterman AM. Eyelid finger manipulation in the treatment of overcorrected blepharoptosis and postblepharoplasty ectropion-retraction. Plast Reconstr Surg. 2015;135:1073e–4e.
9. Putterman AM, Chalfin J. Muller's muscle excision and levator recession in retracted upper lid. Treatment of thyroid-related retraction. Arch Ophthalmol. 1979;97:1487–91.
10. Demirci H, Hassan AS, Reck SD, et al. Graded full-thickness anterior blepharotomy for correction of upper eyelid retraction not associated with thyroid eye disease. Ophthal Plast Reconstr Surg. 2007;23:39–45.
11. Carraway JH. The impact of Herring's law on blepharoplasty and ptosis surgery. Aesthet Surg J. 2004;24:275–6.

12. Tucker SM, Verhulst SJ. Stabilization of eyelid height after aponeurotic ptosis repair. Ophthalmology. 1999;106:517–22.
13. Gladstone GJ, Putterman AM. Internal vertical shortening for the correction of diffuse or segmental postoperative blepharoptosis. Am J Ophthalmol. 1985;99:429–36.
14. Epstein GA, Putterman AM. Super-maximum levator resection for severe unilateral congenital blepharoptosis. Ophthalmic Surg. 1984;15:971–9.
15. Pak J, Shields M, Putterman AM. Superior tarsectomy augments super-maximum levator resection in correction of severe blepharoptosis with poor levator function. Ophthalmology. 2006;113:1201–8.
16. Holds JB, McLeish WM, Anderson RL. Whitnall's sling with superior tarsectomy for the correction of severe unilateral blepharoptosis. Arch Ophthalmol. 1993;111:1285–91.
17. Takahashi Y, Leibovitch I, Kakizaki H. Frontalis suspension surgery in upper eyelid blepharoptosis. Open Ophthalmol J. 2010;4:91–7.
18. Putterman AM. Suture tarsorrhaphy system to control keratopathy after ptosis surgery. Ophthalmic Surg. 1980;11:577–80.
19. Yagci A, Egrilmez S. Comparison of cosmetic results in frontalis sling operations: the eyelid crease incision versus the supralash stab incision. J Pediatr Ophthalmol Strabismus. 2003;40:213–6.
20. Khwarg SI, Tarbet KJ, Dortzbach RK, Lucarelli MJ. Management of moderate-to-severe Marcus-gunn jaw-winking ptosis. Ophthalmology. 1999;106:1191–6.
21. Burnstine MA, Putterman AM. Upper blepharoplasty: a novel approach to improving progressive myopathic ptosis. Ophthalmology. 1999;106:2098–100.
22. Putterman AM. Functional ptosis blepharoplasty diagnostic clamp. Ophthal Plast Reconstr Surg. 2012;28:311–2.
23. Bassin RE, Putterman AM. Full-thickness eyelid resection in the treatment of secondary ptosis. Ophthal Plast Reconstr Surg. 2009;25:85–9.

Full-Thickness Blepharotomy

8

Ann Q. Tran and Cat Nguyen Burkat

Introduction

A blepharotomy is defined by any operation that transects through one or more layers of the eyelid lamella. The transconjunctival partial-thickness blepharotomy was first described in 1965 by Henderson for the relief of upper eyelid retraction by disinserting the levator and Müller's muscles [1, 2]. The rapid technique initially appeared to be useful in the management of mild upper eyelid retraction without atypical eyelid contour; however, many surgeons experienced unpredictability with this procedure. Subsequent surgical treatments were developed including Müller's muscle lengthening, excision or recession [2–4] using a posterior or anterior approach [5–8] in conjunction with adjustable and nonadjustable sutures [9], marginal myotomy [10], and placement of natural synthetic spacer grafts [11–13], none of which provided reliably consistent outcomes. Postoperative complications included dry eye, undercorrection, overcorrection, eyelid contour abnormalities, eyelid thickening, and eyelid crease elevation [14].

In the 1990s, Leo Koornneef described a full-thickness graded blepharotomy technique through the levator aponeurosis, Müller's muscle, and conjunctiva that was both effective and predictable in patients with mild to severe eyelid retraction. On June 10, 1999, Koornneef revealed his work at the University of Michigan (Ann Arbor). However, the results were not published due to his untimely death until 2003 when Elner and Frueh repeated the study [15, 16]. Since then, modifications of full-thickness blepharotomies and expansions of its uses outside of upper eyelid retraction have been reported. Currently, the full-thickness blepharotomy is a favored technique for eyelid retraction, given its predictable and satisfactory postoperative eyelid contour. The remaining portion of this chapter will investigate the indications, nonsurgical alternatives, techniques and pertinent variations to full-thickness blepharotomy, and its use in upper eyelid retraction. Variations of eyelid blepharotomy used in mild blepharoptosis will also be briefly discussed.

Indications

Upper Eyelid Retraction

Many studies report the use of full-thickness blepharotomy in the treatment of upper eyelid retraction in thyroid-associated orbitopathy or Graves ophthalmopathy (Fig. 8.1a, b), one of the most characteristic features and common symptoms of this autoimmune inflammatory disease [17]. Sympathetic overstimulation of Müller's muscle may initially be reversible, but most cases of upper eyelid become chronic and require treatment [18]. In chronic retraction,

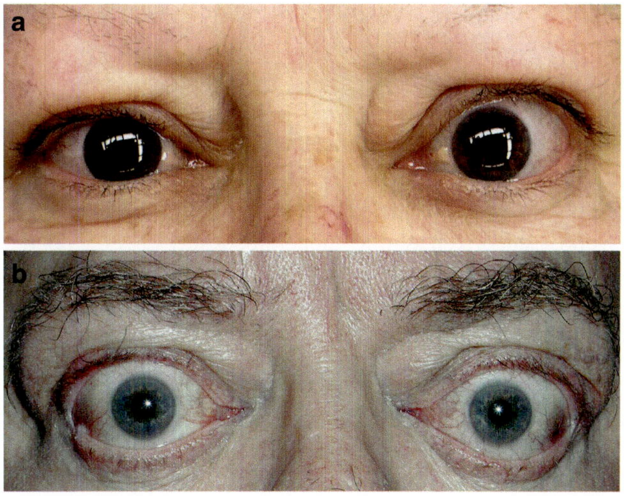

Fig. 8.1 Example of moderate unilateral (**a**) and bilateral (**b**) upper eyelid retraction secondary to thyroid eye disease

A. Q. Tran · C. N. Burkat (✉)
Department of Ophthalmology and Visual Sciences, University of Wisconsin-Madison, Madison, WI, USA
e-mail: cburkat@wisc.edu

A. J. Cohen, C. N. Burkat (eds.), *Oculofacial, Orbital, and Lacrimal Surgery*, https://doi.org/10.1007/978-3-030-14092-2_8

pathology demonstrates levator, conjunctival, and Müller muscle inflammation, fibrosis, atrophy, and fatty infiltration [19–20]. Upper eyelid retraction may lead to complications such as epiphora, foreign body sensation, punctate keratitis, corneal ulcers, and an exacerbation of proptotic appearance in patients [21]. Thus, to reduce corneal exposure and minimize the cosmetic disturbance, patients may require surgical correction.

The use of full-thickness blepharotomy has expanded outside of thyroid eye disease. In a study by Demirci et al., 21 eyelids of 18 patients underwent Koornneef's novel technique [22]. The demographics of the upper eyelid traction included cicatricial trauma, myectomy, graft-versus-host disease, upper eyelid blepharoplasty and idiopathic in 12 eyelids, overcorrected ptosis in 5 eyelids, and paralytic facial nerve palsy in 4 eyelids. Preoperative symptoms of discomfort, asymmetry, and epiphora improved in 94% and remained unaffected in 6%. Lagophthalmos resolved in 55% of patients, improved in 9% of patients, and remained unchanged in 36% patients. Preoperative SPK resolved in 1/3 of patients and improved in 2/3 of patients. No surgical or postoperative contour abnormality was noted after a 10-month follow-up period. One patient with cicatricial upper eyelid retraction had a slight contour abnormality with a lateral peak.

In children, upper eyelid retraction is most commonly idiopathic or secondary to congenital anomaly of oculomotor innervation, trauma, thyroid eye disease, hydrocephalus, dorsal midbrain syndrome, or other rare entities [23, 24]. A modified full-thickness anterior blepharotomy in a child with right upper eyelid retraction secondary to thyroid eye disease and ocular myasthenia gravis resulted in symptomatic improvement and cosmetically acceptable outcomes [25]. Marginal distance reflex improved from 8 mm to 4 mm on the right. The modified approach preserved a 5-mm bridge of intact conjunctiva centrally for optimal central margin curvature.

Mild Blepharoptosis and Congenital Ptosis

Blepharoptosis refers to a lower resting position of the upper eyelid, categorized as mild, moderate, or severe by the degree of drooping (typically 2 mm, 3 mm, and 4 mm, respectively) [26]. Congenital ptosis occurs from maldevelopment of the levator palpebrae superioris muscle within the first year of life, either unilateral or bilateral, associated in isolation or in combination of other conditions [27]. Acquired ptosis typically develops due to neurogenic, myogenic, mechanical, or aponeurogenic causes [28]. If the upper eyelid obscures the visual axis or creates a significant astigmatism, infants and children will benefit from early surgical repair to prevent the development of amblyopia. If visual development is not at risk, surgery may be deferred until age 3–4 years, in order to utilize an autogenous fascia lata [29, 30]. Ultimately, the proposed surgical procedure for congenital ptosis typically depends on the amount of levator function and degree of ptosis and can be quite controversial and challenging [31].

The classic blepharotomy technique used for ptosis correction is the Fasanella-Servat procedure and its modifications. In 1961, Fasanella and Servat introduced a fairly reliable and low technicality procedure with a maximum removal of 3 mm of the superior tarsus, conjunctiva, Müller muscle, and levator, performed through the posterior eyelid [32]. A subsequent retrospective review of 155 cases demonstrated a reoperation rate of 20% with an overall success rate of 71% [33]. More prominent dermatochalasis, duplicate eyelid creases, eyelid irregularities, hematoma, undercorrection, overcorrection, wound dehiscence, pyogenic granulomas, and bleeding are all reported complications of this procedure [34].

In 2008, Patel et al. studied a modified tarsal resection approach in 30 patients with congenital ptosis with follow-up ranging 6 weeks to 8 years. An en bloc resection of the tarsus, Müller muscle, and conjunctiva was performed in conjunction with a graded levator advancement [35]. The amount of en bloc resection predicted the amount of eyelid elevation, leading to 84% of patients having a good surgical outcome. In 2013, Dresner described a modified Fasanella-Servat tarsectomy procedure for patients with minimal blepharoptosis defined as less than 2.5 mm of ptosis, with good levator function, and negative phenylephrine test. He found results to be both reliable and with minimal complications [36].

Other Etiologies

Case reports have illustrated other eyelid irregularities where modified full-thickness blepharotomies may be used. A case report described an infracanalicular full-thickness transverse blepharotomy for medial entropion using rotational sutures. Eversion of the eyelid is achieved from the rotational sutures allowing a fibrous band to form at the site of full-thickness blepharotomy to prevent upward movement of the preseptal muscle. Unfortunately, this procedure does not correct for horizontal eyelid laxity and thus has not been widely expanded [37].

Nonsurgical Alternatives

While no studies have investigated the timing for when patients should undergo surgical repair of upper eyelid retraction secondary to thyroid eye disease, it is common practice that elective surgery for orbital decompression should be deferred until the patient is euthyroid with stable measurements for 6–9 months, unless urgent treatment for corneal ulceration or compressive optic neuropathy is indicated [38]. Conservative management of upper eyelid retraction and ptosis includes symptom control with artificial tears, lubricating ointment, eyelid taping, and topical and systemic steroids [39].

Local injection of neurotoxins to the upper lid may help weaken the Müller muscle function. The use of 5 units of onabotulinum toxin A (Botox) in 24 eyelids with thyroid eye disease resulted in a pharmacologic decrease in lid height by 3.81 mm in the fibrotic stage for 1 month and 3.05 mm during the congestive phase for 3 months [40]. Injection of abobotulinum toxin A (Dysport) using 25 units into the central superior tarsal border resulted in 3.24 mm reduction of lid height for 4 months or more [41]. Common complications included overcorrection with temporary ptosis lasting less than 1 month.

The use of soft tissue fillers may induce a relative mechanical ptosis to alleviate eyelid height asymmetry. The injection of hyaluronic acid fillers has been studied in eight patients with mild upper eyelid retraction from thyroid eye disease, surgery-induced asymmetry, Horner's syndrome, Bell's palsy, and involutional ptosis [42]. The average total volume injected was 0.2 mL bilaterally with statistically significant improvement in symmetry up to 8 months follow-up. No major complications occurred, and only one patient required repeat injection. Soft tissue fillers have since been applied to the lower eyelid as well for correction of lid retraction.

Another study reported that the subconjunctival injection of 0.5 mL triamcinolone acetonide (40 mg/mL) in 2-week intervals during the congestive phase of thyroid eye disease significantly improved eyelid height in 22 patients [43]. Patients in the fibrotic phase ($n = 8$) did not respond to the injection. Complications from injection, such as increased intraocular pressure and mild ptosis, occurred in two and one patients, respectively. This may serve as an alternative to neurotoxins during their decreased efficacy in the congestive phase.

Surgical Techniques and Variations

Upper Eyelid Retraction

Graded Full-Thickness Anterior Blepharotomy

The approach originally proposed by Koornneef and published by Elner et al. [15, 16] is performed through the upper eyelid crease incision following administration of local anesthesia (0.5% bupivacaine and 1% lidocaine with epinephrine 1,100,000). The levator aponeurosis inferior to the confluence with the orbital septum is carefully identified. Starting at the maximum point of eyelid retraction, a full-thickness blepharotomy is performed by incising through the levator aponeurosis, Müller's muscle, and conjunctiva superior to the tarsal plate (Fig. 8.2a). Care is taken to avoid the peripheral arcade at the superior tarsal border (Fig. 8.2b). Based on the preoperative lid height in primary gaze, the full-thickness blepharotomy is continued nasally and temporally if needed. Temporal flare is corrected by releasing the lateral horn of the levator aponeurosis, taking care to avoid injury to the lacrimal gland (Fig. 8.2c). A central bridge of intact tissue can help preserve eyelid curvature (Fig. 8.2d). The patient may be seated upright during surgery to assess the need for additional release or contour adjustment. A flattened eyelid contour can be adjusted by securing the levator aponeurosis to the tarsal plate using a 6-0 polyglactin mattress suture. Skin is closed with 6-0 nonabsorbable or absorbable suture.

This approach reported 93% resolved or improved symptoms in 32 patients [15, 16]. Statistically significant improvements were seen in upper eyelid position, lagophthalmos, and keratopathy (Fig. 8.3). Minimal eyelid irregularities <1 mm were noted in 7/50 eyes. Patients with mild retraction preoperatively demonstrated more symmetrical outcomes. Postoperative complications included ptosis, overcorrection, wound dehiscence, flattened contour, and full-thickness hole.

Modified Full-Thickness Blepharotomy

Hintschich and Haritoglou subsequently described a modification of this technique in a prospective interventional case series of 41 patients (60 eyelids) with thyroid eye disease [44]. Through a transcutaneous incision, all layers except the conjunctiva were divided. The conjunctiva was gradually transected starting at the temporal third of the eyelid until optimal lid height and contour were achieved, with more severe cases of retraction requiring conjunctival transection further medially. The central 3–4 mm bridge of the conjunctiva at the pupillary axis was left intact to maintain a natural postoperative eyelid contour and to avoid central ptosis or flattening. A nonabsorbable suture was used to reapproximate the levator aponeurosis to the tarsus if needed, and the skin was closed with a 6-0 running locking suture. The study reported success of 88% in achieving the desired eyelid height and contour with no complaints of postoperative dry eyes. Two lids required wound revision for superficial wound dehiscence, and six lids required reoperation for undercorrection or patient preference.

A similar technique was described by another group in 2013, in which the central 3–5 mm of the conjunctiva was also spared [45]. If overcorrection or a flattened contour occurred, a "hang-back" 6-0 polyglactin mattress suture between the levator aponeurosis and tarsal plate was placed, making sure intact conjunctiva was posterior to the suture. Over 75% of cases achieved symmetry within 1 mm of both

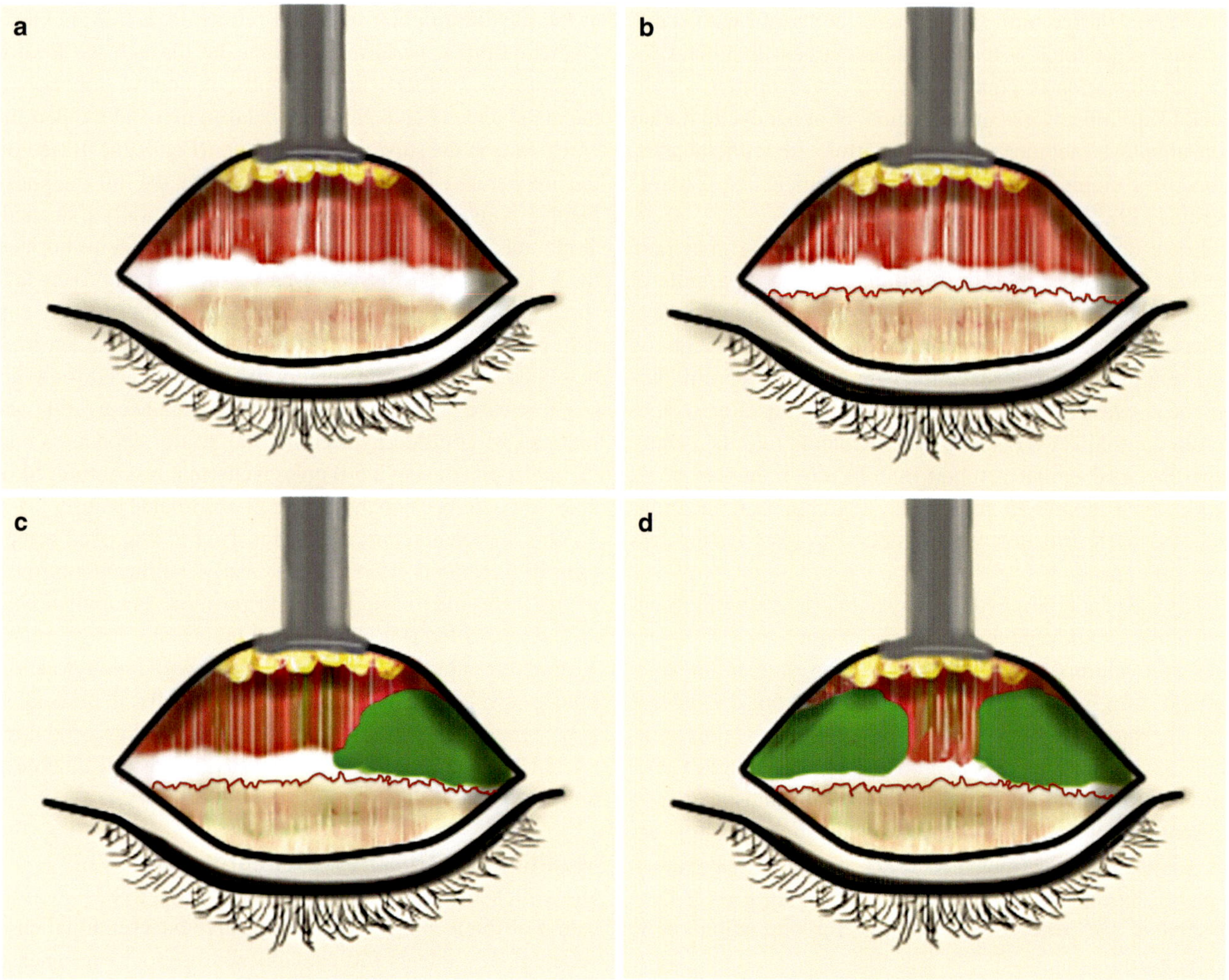

Fig. 8.2 Full-thickness blepharotomy technique, as popularized by Koornneef, through skin incision. (**a**) Exposure of levator muscle and aponeurosis; (**b**) incision should be placed above the peripheral vascular arcade along the superior tarsal border; (**c**) lateral full-thickness incision is first created, with release of the lateral horn if needed; (**d**) medial release may be performed, with a 4–5-mm bridge of intact tissue left centrally to maintain eyelid curvature. Underlying green corneal protector is visible

eyes. Eight cases required reoperation: six for undercorrection and two for overcorrection. One patient developed worsened retraction due to recurrent thyroid eye disease, and wound dehiscence occurred in two patients.

The modified technique preserving the central conjunctiva was also studied on 18 Asian patients (22 eyelids) with thyroid eye disease [46]. Due to anatomical eyelid differences in patients of Asian descent, the double eyelid fold was taken into account during the lid crease incision. An incision placed lower than the natural double fold prevented the formation of a high fold postoperatively. The procedure otherwise remained the same. Although sample size was small, almost 50% of patients complained of discomfort, and a quarter of patients described photophobia and epiphora. Lid margin height was improved postoperatively despite the severity of thyroid eye disease, with a mean reduction of 3 mm on average. After 6 months follow-up, patients reported a 90% satisfaction rate.

Congenital Ptosis

Modified Fasanella-Servat Procedure

For patients with minimal blepharoptosis <2.5 mm and a negative phenylephrine test, the modified Fasanella-Servat procedure was designed to minimize eyelid irregularities and suture keratopathy [36]. After local anesthetic, the eyelid is everted over a Desmarres retractor and the central tarsus along the pupillary axis marked to remove 2 mm of superior tarsus (Fig. 8.4). Two 4-0 silk sutures are placed medially and laterally for traction at the conjunctival-tarsal border. With the traction sutures elevated, a clamp is placed to enclose the tissues down to the tarsal marking. A 6-0 prolene

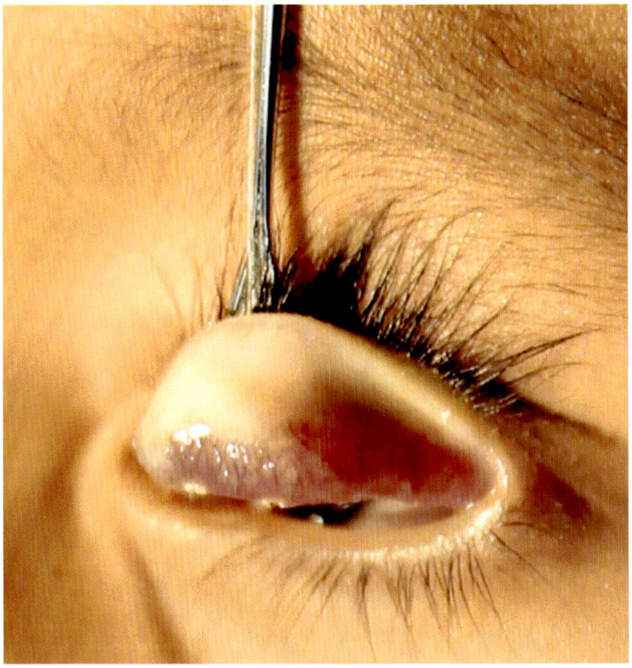

Fig. 8.3 Left upper eyelid everted over a Desmarres retractor to measure the tarsal resection in a Fasanella-Servat procedure

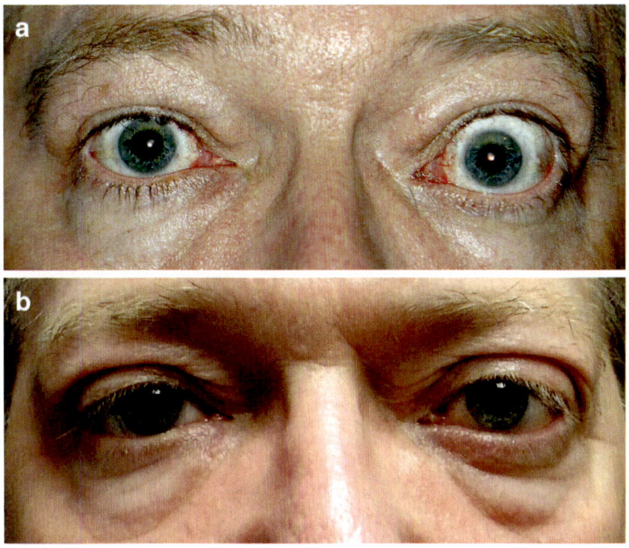

Fig. 8.4 (**a**) Preoperative photo of eyelid retraction, the left eye is worse than the right eye, from thyroid eye disease; (**b**) postoperative photo demonstrating improved margin-reflex distances and decreased lagophthalmos 4 weeks after surgery using the Koornneef blepharotomy approach

suture is passed through the skin 5 mm above the eyelid margin to exit conjunctiva just below the clamp and then passed in a serpentine fashion below the entire clamp. The enclosed conjunctival-tarsal tissue is then excised with a blade passed carefully along the clamp. The suture is tied loosely over the pretarsal skin and removed in 5–7 days.

Of 118 eyelids, 92% achieved symmetrical correction within 0.5 mm, with no incidence of overcorrection, tarsal buckling, instability, or corneal abrasion [36]. The tarsectomy ranged from 2 mm to 5 mm. There was no correlation or predictability between age, the resection amount, or levator function. Only one eyelid demonstrated contour irregularity. Complications such as overcorrection, tarsal buckling, or corneal abrasion did not occur.

Modified En Bloc Tarsal Resection

Patel et al. described a blepharotomy approach that combined an en bloc resection of the tarsus, Müller muscle, and conjunctiva, with a graded levator aponeurosis advancement for repair of congenital ptosis with good levator function (Fig. 8.5a, b) [35]. A blepharoplasty incision is made, with dissection carried down through the orbicularis muscle to the orbital septum. The levator aponeurosis is separated and reflected superiorly from the underlying Müller muscle (Fig. 8.6a). Using an algorithm to determine the amount of resection based on the amount of ptosis present (Table 8.1), the amount of conjunctiva and Müller muscle excised is approximately double the amount of tarsus removed (Fig. 8.6b, c). The tarsal portion to be resected is first incised horizontally and then vertically through the Müller muscle and conjunctiva, medially and laterally, to complete the en bloc resection (Fig. 8.6d). The edge of the remaining Müller muscle and conjunctiva is advanced to the new tarsal border

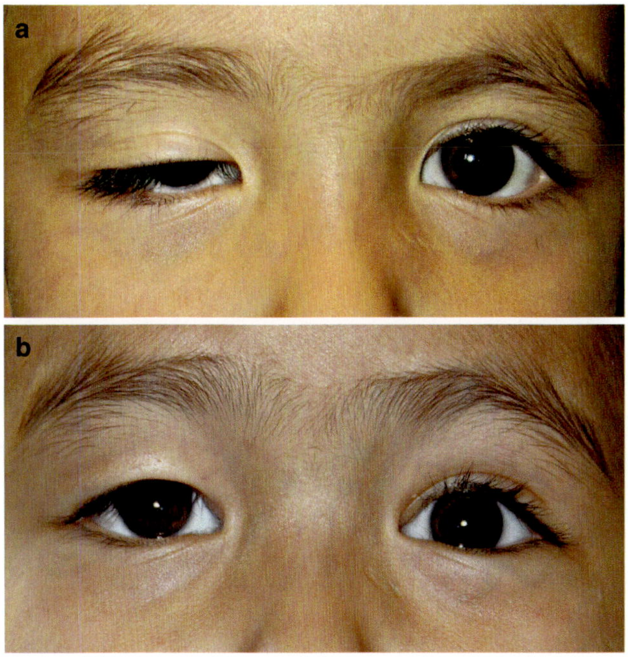

Fig. 8.5 (**a**) Preoperative photo of severe congenital ptosis of the right eye; (**b**) postoperative photo illustrating symmetric lid height at 5 weeks after surgery using an en bloc resection. Residual edema and skin fullness are still present

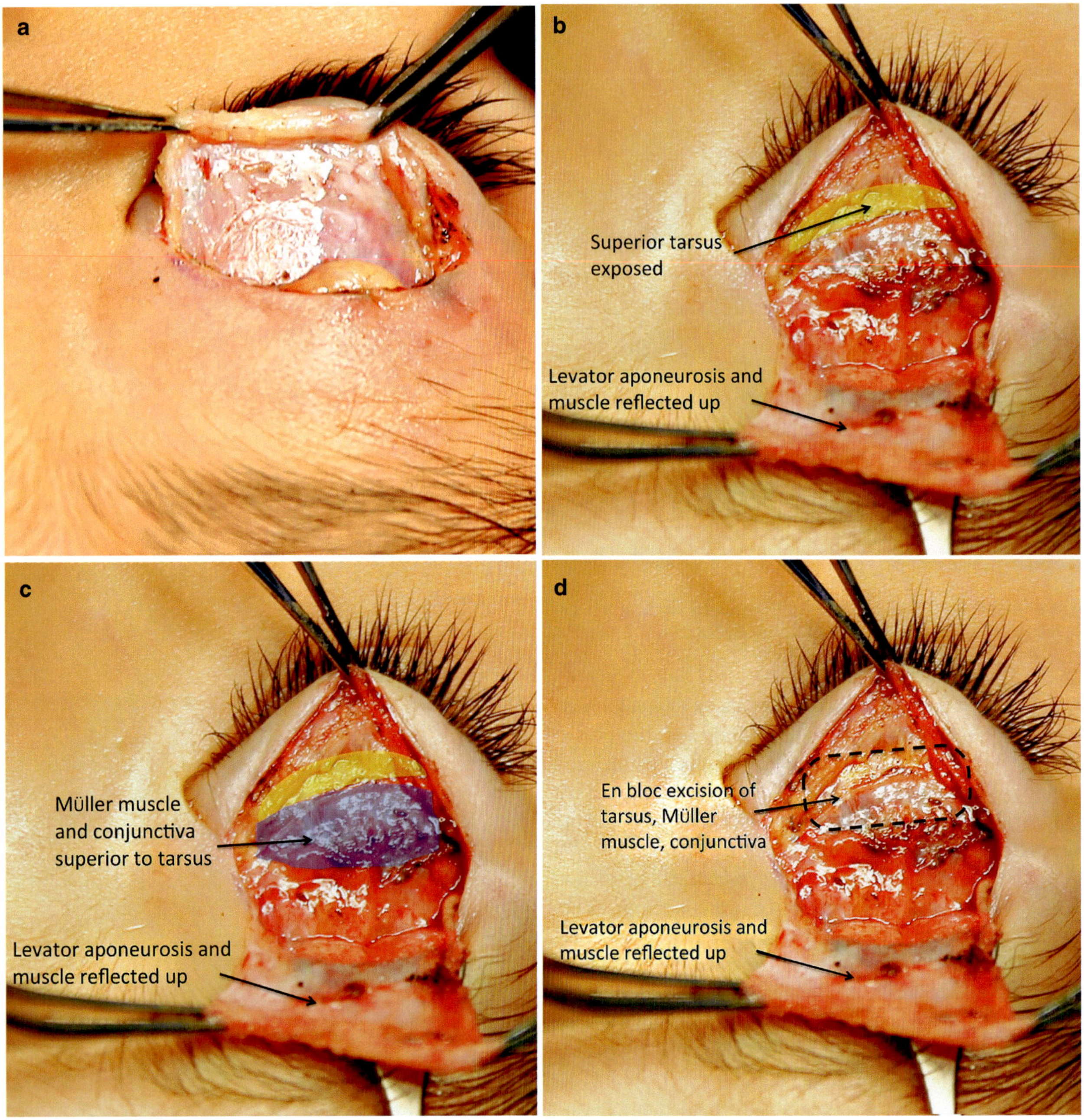

Fig. 8.6 Surgeon's view of the en bloc resection technique for congenital ptosis. (**a**) Levator aponeurosis dissected carefully off Müller's muscle; (**b**) levator complex reflected superiorly, demonstrating underlying Müller's muscle and the superior tarsus dissected for the amount of the tarsus to be resected (yellow highlight); (**c**) Müller's muscle and conjunctiva superior to the tarsus is measured for resection (blue highlight); (**d**) dotted line outlines the en bloc resection of the tarsus, Müller's muscle, and conjunctiva

Table 8.1 The severity of ptosis guides the amount of tarsus, Müller muscle, and conjunctival excision in the en bloc resection surgical approach [35]

Degree of ptosis	Amount of tarsal muscle resection	Amount of conjunctiva and Müller muscle resection
Mild (2 mm)	2–3 mm	4–6 mm
Moderate (3 mm)	3–4 mm	6–8 mm
Severe (≥4 mm)	4–5 mm	8–10 mm

using interrupted 7-0 chromic sutures. The levator aponeurosis is next advanced to the tarsus with 5-0 polyglactin sutures and adjusted for appropriate lid height and contour. Redundant aponeurosis can be excised followed by skin closure.

Eighty-four percent of patients with congenital ptosis with good levator function achieved a good surgical outcome. Preoperative and postoperative measurements of the eyelid height demonstrated a statistically significant difference. Only transient lagophthalmos that resolved after a few weeks of surgery and one suture abscess were recorded as complications.

Conclusion

In conclusion, full-thickness and partial-thickness blepharotomy techniques can be powerful procedures to correct eyelid height abnormalities, used successfully for correction of both eyelid retraction and ptosis. Subtle nuances such as eyelid crease incision placement, dissection plane, central conjunctival sparing, and understanding ethnic differences are all advanced considerations that will allow the surgeon to achieve optimal surgical results.

References

1. Henderson JW. Relief of eyelid retraction: a surgical procedure. Arch Ophthalmol. 1965;74:205–16.
2. Henderson JW. A surgical procedure for retraction of eyelids in endocrine exophthalmos (a moving picture). Trans Am Ophthalmol Soc. 1965;63:70–4.
3. Putterman AM, Fett DR. Mueller's muscle in the treatment of upper eyelid retraction: a 12 year study. Ophthalmic Surg. 1986;17(6):361–7.
4. Ceisler EJ, Bilyk JR, Rubin PA, et al. Results of Mullerotomy and levator aponeurosis transposition for the correction of upper eyelid retraction in Grave's disease. Ophthalmology. 1995;102(3): 483–92.
5. Haravey JT, Anderson RL. The aponeurotic approach to eyelid retraction. Ophthalmology. 1981;88(6):513–24.
6. Baylis HI, Cies WA, Kamin DF. Correction of upper eyelid retraction. Am J Ophthalmol. 1976;82(5):790–4.
7. Callahan A. Levator recession: with reattachment to the tarsus with collagen film. Arch Ophthalmol. 1965;73:800–2.
8. Putterman AM, Urist MH. A simplified levator palpebrae superioris muscle recession to treat overcorrected blepharoptosis. Am J Ophthalmol. 1974;77(3):358–66.
9. Tucker SM, Collin R. Repair of upper eyelid retraction: a comparison between adjustable and non-adjustable sutures. Br J Ophthalmol. 1995;79(7):658–60.
10. Grove AS. Eyelid retraction treated by levator marginal myotomy. Ophthalmology. 1980;87(10):1013–8.
11. Doxanas MT, Dryden RM. The use of sclera in the treatment of dysthyroid eyelid retraction. Ophthalmology. 1981;88(9): 887–94.
12. Downes RN, Jordan K. The surgical management of dysthyroid related eyelid retraction using Mersilene mesh. Eye (Lond). 1989;3:385–90.
13. Mourits MP, Koorneef L. Lid lengthening by sclera interposition for eyelid retraction in Graves' ophthalmopathy. Br J Ophthalmol. 1991;75(6):344–7.
14. George JL, Tercero ME, Angioi-Duprez K, et al. Risk of dry eye after mullerectomy via posterior conjunctival approach for thyroid related upper eyelid retraction. Orbit. 2002;21(1): 19–25.
15. Elner VM, Hassan AS, Frueh BR. Graded full-thickness anterior blepharotomy for upper eyelid retraction. Trans Am Ophthalmol Soc. 2003;101:67–75.
16. Elner VM, Hassan AS, Frueh BR. Graded full-thickness anterior blepharotomy for upper eyelid retraction. Arch Ophthalmol. 2004;122(1):55–60.
17. Bartley GB. The epidemiologic characteristic and clinical course of ophthalmopathy associated with autoimmune thyroid disease in Olmstead County, Minnesota. Trans Am Ophthalmol Soc. 1994;92:477–588.
18. Boulos PR, Hardy I. Thyroid-associated orbitopathy: a clinicopathologic and therapeutic review. Curr Opin Ophthalmol. 2004;15(5):389–400.
19. Grove AS. Upper eyelid retraction and Graves' disease. Ophthalmology. 1981;88(6):499–506.
20. Cockerham KP, Hidayat AA, Brown HG, et al. Clinic pathologic evaluation of the Mueller muscle in thyroid-associated orbitopathy. Ophthal Plast Reconstr Surg. 2002;18(1):11–7.
21. Chang EL, Rubin PA. Upper and lower eyelid retraction. Int Ophthalmol Clin. 2002;42(2):45–59.
22. Demirici H, Hassan AS, Reck SD, et al. Graded full-thickness anterior blepharotomy for correction eye disease. Ophthal Plast Reconstr Surg. 2007;23(1):39–45.
23. Stout A, Borchert M. Etiology of eyelid retraction in children: a retrospective study. J Pediatr Ophthalmol Strabismus. 1993;30(2):96–9.
24. Bartley GB. The differential diagnosis and classification of eyelid retraction. Trans Am Ophthalmol Soc. 1995;93:371–89.
25. Stewart KJ, Griepentrog GJ, Lucarelli MJ. Modified full-thickness anterior blepharotomy for upper eyelid retraction in children. J AAPOS. 2013;17(2):223–4.
26. Beard C. Ptosis. 2nd ed. St Louis: CV Mosby Co; 1976.
27. Sakol PJ, Mannor G, Massaro BM. Congenital and acquired blepharoptosis. Curr Opin Ophthalmol. 1999;10(5):335–9.
28. Frueh BR. The mechanistic classification of ptosis. Ophthalmology. 1980;87(10):1019–21.
29. Pescosolido N, Stefanucci A, Buomprisco G, et al. Amblyopia treatment strategies and new drug therapies. J Pediatr Ophthalmol Strabismus. 2014;51(2):78–86.
30. Harrad RA, Graham CM, Collin JR. Amblyopia and strabismus in congenital ptosis. Eye (Lond). 1988;2:625–7.
31. SooHoo JR, Davies BW, Allard FD, et al. Congenital ptosis. Surv Ophthalmol. 2014;59(5):483–92.
32. Fasanella RM, Servat J. Levator resection for minimal ptosis: another simplified operation. Arch Ophthalmol. 1961;65:493–6.
33. Berry-Brincat A, Willshaw H. Paediatric blepharoptosis: a 10-year review. Eye (Lond). 2009;23(7):1554–9.
34. Pang NK, Newsom RW, Oestreicher JH, et al. Fasanella-Servat procedure: indications, efficacy, and complications. Can J Ophthalmol. 2008;43(1):84–8.
35. Patel SM, Linberg JV, Sivak-Callcott JA, et al. Modified tarsal resection operation for congenital ptosis with fair levator function. Ophthal Plast Reconstr Surg. 2008;24(1):1–6.
36. Samimi DB, Erb MH, Lane CJ, et al. The modified Fasanella-Servat procedure. Ophthal Plast Reconstr Surg. 2013;29(1):30–4.
37. Kristan RW, Stasior OG. Infracanalicular full-thickness transverse blepharotomy for medial ectropion. Ophthal Plast Reconstr Surg. 1987;3(3):127–9.
38. Kacker A, Kazim M, Murphy M, Trokel S, et al. Balanced orbital decompression for severe Graves' orbitopathy: technique with treatment algorithm. Otolaryngol Head Neck Surg. 2003;128(2): 228–35.
39. Hamawy AH, Farkas JP, Fagien S, et al. Preventing and managing dry eyes after periorbital surgery: a retrospective review. Plast Reconstr Surg. 2009;123(1):353–9.
40. Costa PG, Saraiva FP, Pereira IC, et al. Comparative study of Botox injection treatment for upper eyelid retraction with 6-month follow-up in patients with thyroid eye disease in the congestive or fibrotic stage. Eye (Lond). 2009;23(4):767–73.

41. Salour H, Bagheri B, Aletaha M, et al. Transcutaneous dysport injection for treatment of upper eyelid retraction associated with thyroid eye disease. Orbit. 2010;29(2):114–8.
42. Mancini R, Khadavi NM, Goldberg RA. Nonsurgical management of upper eyelid margin asymmetry using hyaluronic acid gel filler. Ophthal Plast Reconstr Surg. 2011;27(1):1–3.
43. Lee JM, Lee H, Park M, et al. Subconjunctival injection of triamcinolone for the treatment of upper lid retraction associated with thyroid eye disease. J Craniofac Surg. 2012;23(6):1755–8.
44. Hintschich C, Haritoglou C. Full thickness eyelid transsection (blepharotomy) for upper eyelid lengthening in lid retraction associated with Graves' disease. Br J Ophthalmol. 2005;89(4):413–6.
45. Nimitwongsakul A, Zoumalan CI, Kazim M. Modified full-thickness blepharotomy for treatment of thyroid eye disease. Ophthal Plast Reconstr Surg. 2013;29(1):44–7.
46. Lee J, Lee H, Chang M, et al. Modified full thickness graded blepharotomy for upper eyelid retraction associated with thyroid eye disease in east Asians. Ann Plast Surg. 2016;77(6):592–6.

Congenital Eyelid Malpositions and Anomalies

9

Sarah M. Jacobs, Cat Nguyen Burkat, William R. Katowitz, and Christopher B. Chambers

Congenital Eyelid Malpositions and Anomalies

A variety of eyelid anomalies can be present at the time of birth, seen in isolation or in association with systemic syndromes. These anomalies can be broadly grouped as abnormalities of eyelid division, eyelid tissue defects (colobomas), congenital eyelid malpositions, and congenital eyelid lesions. Knowledge of basic embryology of the eyelid affords a better understanding of abnormalities, especially failures of eyelid development or palpebral fissure division such as cryptophthalmos and ankyloblepharon. Colobomatous eyelids must be considered from the standpoint of their potential for syndromic association. Congenital eyelid malpositions are often functionally and cosmetically significant, requiring effective management early in life. Finally, certain eyelid lesions may be apparent at birth or manifest in the weeks or months thereafter. Lesions with amblyogenic potential must be addressed in a more expeditious fashion if indicated.

S. M. Jacobs
Department of Ophthalmology, University of Alabama at Birmingham, Birmingham, AL, USA

C. N. Burkat
Department of Ophthalmology and Visual Sciences, University of Wisconsin-Madison, Madison, WI, USA
e-mail: cburkat@wisc.edu

W. R. Katowitz
The Perelman School of Medicine at the University of Pennsylvania, Philadelphia, PA, USA

The Children's Hospital of Philadelphia, Philadelphia, PA, USA

C. B. Chambers (✉)
Department of Ophthalmology/Plastic Surgery, University of Washington, Seattle, WA, USA
e-mail: cbc108@uw.edu

Normal Anatomic Variants

Certain normal anatomic variants of the eyelid may be seen which alter the slant of the palpebral fissure or the conformation of the skin at the medial canthus. While these variants do affect the appearance of the lid, its function is unaffected. Common normal variants include:

- *Epicanthus tarsalis*. A fold of skin and subcutaneous tissue originating from the upper lid is stretched across the medial canthus, terminating at the canthal angle. This anatomy is frequently seen in the upper eyelid of patients with Asian descent. It may also be seen in infants and young children, who often outgrow the clinical finding as the midfacial bones mature. It can also be seen in association with syndromes in which the nasal bridge is flat, such as fetal alcohol syndrome (FAS) and Trisomy 21 [1].
- *Epicanthus inversus*. In this variant, the prominent soft tissue fold arises from the lower lid, bridging the medial canthus and terminating on the upper lid. This may be seen independently, or as a part of the constellation of findings in blepharophimosis syndrome, which is discussed elsewhere (Fig. 9.1 Epicanthus Inversus).
- *Epicanthus palpebralis*. The fold is shared equally between the upper and lower lids, usually arising above the superior tarsus and extending to the skin overlying the inferior tarsus. The epicanthal fold decreases scleral show

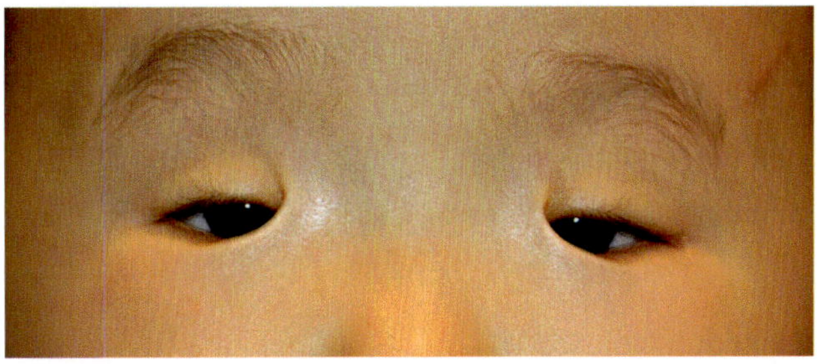

Fig. 9.1 Epicanthus inversus present on both medial lower eyelids

A. J. Cohen, C. N. Burkat (eds.), *Oculofacial, Orbital, and Lacrimal Surgery*, https://doi.org/10.1007/978-3-030-14092-2_9

nasally, which may result in a pseudoesotropic appearance and sometimes leads to an erroneous referral for strabismus evaluation.

- *Epicanthus supraciliaris*. The fold of skin and subcutaneous tissue arises near the head of the brow and extends toward the region overlying the lacrimal sac. This is the least common form of epicanthus but is seen as a strongly heritable trait in certain families.

While isolated epicanthus can be surgically addressed (e.g., by creating a new fold in the upper lid and performing a V-to-Y plasty at the medial canthus), the procedure is typically cosmetic rather than functional in nature and rarely applicable to the pediatric population [2].

Eyelid Embryology and Abnormalities of Eyelid Division

An understanding of the embryologic eyelid development gives insight into several eyelid anomalies, especially those related to abnormal eyelid division. By the third week of gestation, the embryonic plate has formed with ectoderm, mesoderm, and endodermal layers, and the neural tube has begun to close [3]. The forebrain, midbrain, and hindbrain head folds form at the anterior end of this plate. The optic pits form as depressions at the front of the forebrain on each side of the midline, and then the depressions deepen until they form spherical vesicles fully enclosed by surface ectoderm.

By the fifth week, five branchial arches have formed. The maxillary process of the first branchial arch gives rise to the lower eyelid and nasolacrimal duct structures. The upper eyelid forms from the paraxial mesoderm known as the frontonasal process, cephalad to the first arch [4].

During gestational weeks 8–10, adhesions form between the upper and lower lids, fusing them together [3]. In the subsequent weeks, all of the internal eyelid structures develop, including the tarsal plate, hair follicles, and the muscular complex encompassing the levator palpebrae superioris and superior rectus muscle.

The eyelids remain fused until the end of the fifth month of gestation, when the adhesions between the eyelids begin to break down due to traction exerted by the eyelid retractors, as well as eyelid margin keratinization and the effects of Meibomian gland secretions [4].

Failures of eyelid formation, fusion, or disjunction result in congenital eyelid abnormalities spanning a wide range of clinical severity.

Cryptophthalmos

In this rare, usually bilateral, condition, the eyelid folds fail to develop properly and are replaced by facial skin extending onto the ocular surface. Cryptophthalmos can be complete, incomplete, or abortive (Fig. 9.2 Amniotic banding with partial cryptophthalmos) [5].

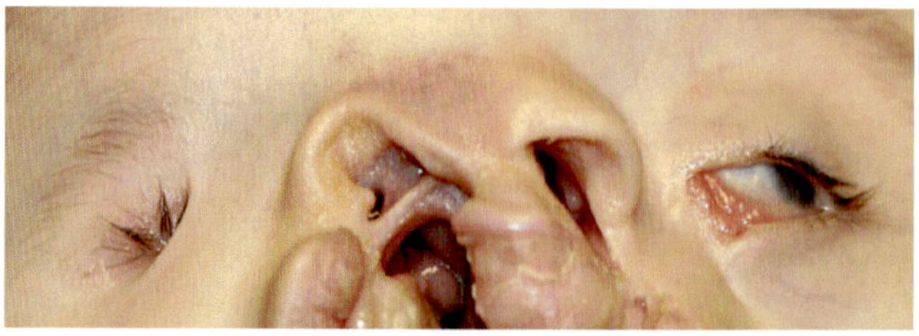

Fig. 9.2 Amniotic banding with partial symblepharon

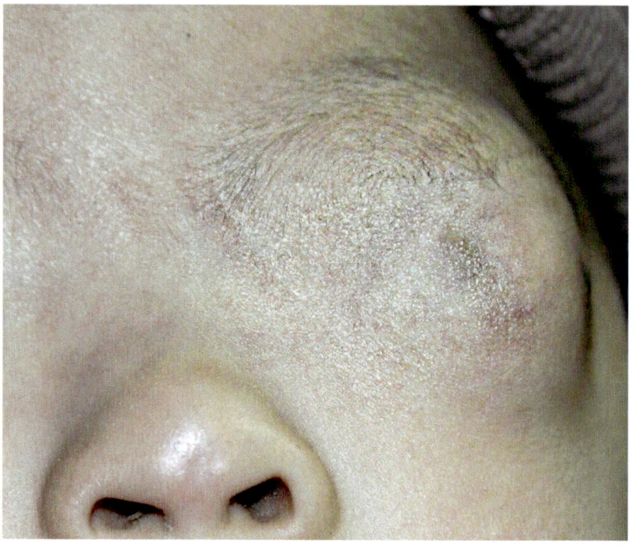

Fig. 9.3 Complete left eye cryptophthalmos, demonstrating lack of any eyelid margin opening or eyelid structures

- Complete: No upper or lower eyelid tissue forms. The exposed cornea undergoes metaplasia, and cutaneous epithelium grows across in a continuous plane from the forehead to the cheek, completely covering the eye with skin (Fig. 9.3 Complete cryptophthalmos, left).
- Incomplete: Rudimentary portions of the upper and lower eyelids form laterally, while the medial globe is covered by cutaneous epithelium that lacks normal eyelid structures.
- Abortive: The lower eyelid forms normally, but the upper eyelid fails to develop properly from the frontonasal process, with the forehead skin extending down to fuse with the superior cornea and conjunctiva. This condition is also known as congenital symblepharon.

Cryptophthalmos is typically sporadic, although autosomal dominant and recessive inheritance has been reported. In all three forms, the underlying globe often has significant abnormalities such as microphthalmia or anterior segment dysgenesis, resulting in a limited visual prognosis. It may also be associated with Fraser syndrome, the autosomal recessive constellation of cryptophthalmos, laryngeal stenosis, genital hypoplasia, and renal hypoplasia or agenesis [1].

Eyelid and orbital reconstruction in cryptophthalmos poses a challenge due to the lack of normal eyelid and lacrimal structures, as well as the decision-making involved in optimizing visual potential, postoperative exposure keratopathy, and cosmesis. Surgical steps must include dissection of corneal adhesions, mucous membrane grafting for forniceal reconstruction, and myocutaneous flaps or eyelid-sharing grafts for upper and lower eyelid reconstruction, typically in staged fashion [6].

Ablepharon or Microblepharon

The absence of eyelid tissue, with congenital shortening of the anterior lamella in particular, is described as ablepharon (total absence) or microblepharon (partial absence). These entities differ from cryptophthalmos in that there is no growth of cutaneous epithelium onto the ocular surface. Ablepharon is seen in several syndromes including Say-Barber, autosomal dominant ablepharon-macrostomia, and Neu-Laxova. Management depends on the degree of eyelid involvement present. Vertical stretching of the eyelid in order to surgically anchor it at the lateral orbital rim can protect the ocular surface from urgent exposure-related complications until more definitive eyelid reconstruction can be undertaken [7].

Ankyloblepharon

As described above, the upper and lower eyelids are fused together during gestational weeks 10–24 and then undergo disjunction. Failure of eyelid separation results in ankyloblepharon. The defect is usually isolated, with a well-formed eye and normal visual potential. The adhesions between the eyelids can be clamped with a hemostat and then separated with scissors (Fig. 9.4 Ankyloblepharon) [8].

Eyelid Tissue Defects

Unlike intraocular colobomas of the iris, lens, or retina, colobomatous soft tissue defects of the eyelid are not related to failure of embryologic fissure closure. Instead, these full-thickness soft tissue defects of the eyelid margin arise from abnormal development of the frontonasal process (upper eyelid) or first branchial arch (lower eyelid). In one 30-year case series, eyelid colobomas were found to be far more common in the upper eyelid (93%) and unilateral (76%), with approximately two-thirds of cases associated with additional ocular or craniofacial abnormalities [9]. Eyelid colobomas seen in association with facial clefting disorders are typically more severe.

Upper Eyelid Coloboma

The majority of upper eyelid colobomas occur as an isolated anomaly. However, approximately 20% of upper eyelid colobomas are associated with other systemic findings. One example is Goldenhar syndrome (oculo-auriculo-vertebral spectrum), a usually sporadic syndrome which can include eyelid coloboma, limbal dermoids, preauricular appendages, and microtia of the external ear, vertebral anomalies, and sometimes cardiac anomalies [10].

Lower Eyelid Coloboma

In contrast to upper eyelid coloboma, defects of the lower eyelid are more frequently associated with a facial clefting syndrome. Due to the shared embryologic origin of the lower eyelid and nasolacrimal duct structures from the first branchial arch, patients with inferior coloboma often have comorbid lacrimal system anomalies. Treacher-Collins is a well-described syndrome most commonly arising from a mutation in the TCOF1 gene, characterized by lower eyelid coloboma, zygomatic and mandibular hypoplasia, abnormalities of the external and inner ear structures, and sometimes cleft lip and/or cleft palate [11]. Treatment is tailored to each patient's individual needs, ideally by a multidisciplinary craniofacial team (Fig. 9.5 Lower eyelid coloboma in Treacher-Collins syndrome).

Strategies for Eyelid Coloboma Repair

Depending upon the size of the coloboma, successful repair can be accomplished with wedge excision and direct closure

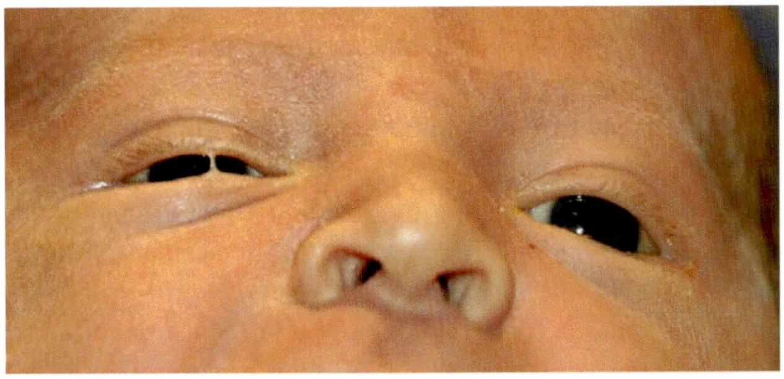

Fig. 9.4 Ankyloblepharon seen as a thin web of skin bridging the right upper and lower eyelids

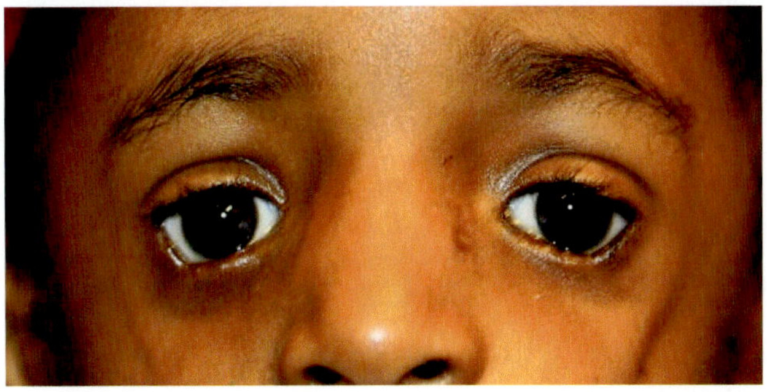

Fig. 9.5 Lower eyelid coloboma in Treacher-Collins syndrome

for smaller defects, versus lateral canthotomy/cantholysis, potentially with semicircular flap, allowing for adjacent tissue advancement into larger defects. Eyelid-sharing procedures such as Hughes or Cutler-Beard flaps are generally avoided in the pediatric population, due to the risk of amblyopia from obstruction of the visual axis.

Eyelid Malpositions

Congenital Eyelid Eversion

Complete eversion of the upper eyelids is occasionally seen in newborns and can be considered a form of acute ectropion (Fig. 9.6 Congenital eyelid eversion in a newborn with Trisomy 21). Classically, it occurs intermittently due to spasm of the orbicularis oculi muscle when the neonate cries and then spontaneously resolves when the muscle is relaxed. In some patients, especially those with a history of Trisomy 21, African origin, or inclusion conjunctivitis, the eversion is more persistent, leading to irritation and conjunctival chemosis. In such cases, initial treatment involved topical lubrication and short-term pressure patching. If necessary, full-thickness rotational sutures or a temporary tarsorrhaphy can be utilized to reposition the eyelids.

Congenital Ectropion

Outward rotation of the eyelid margin results in ectropion, which may lead to symptomatic exposure of the conjunctiva and cornea. Although it can be an isolated finding, most cases of congenital ectropion are associated with syndromes (e.g., Trisomy 21, blepharophimosis, or mandibulofacial dysostosis) or congenital skin disorders causing shortening of the anterior lamella of the eyelid (e.g., cutis laxa, lamellar ichthyosis, harlequin ichthyosis).

Mild ectropion may require no treatment; simple topical lubrication can be used on an as-needed basis in these cases. A more severe or symptomatic congenital ectropion can be treated with surgical tightening of the lateral canthal tendon.

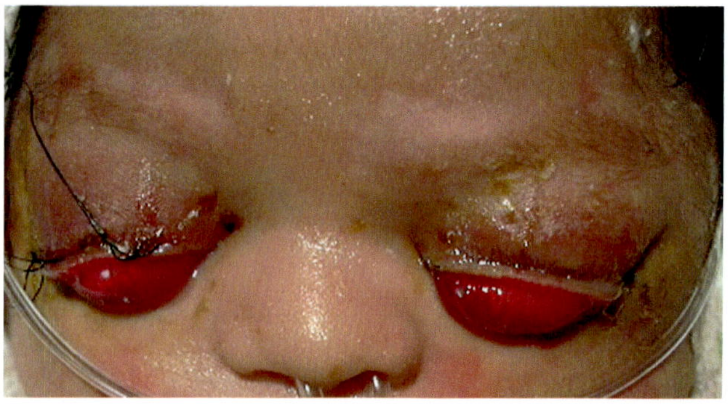

Fig. 9.6 Congenital upper eyelid eversion seen in a newborn with Trisomy 21

As with repair of cicatricial ectropion due to other causes, a full-thickness skin graft can be used to vertically lengthen the anterior lamella if necessary [12]. More recently, the usage of injectable hyaluronic acid fillers to support the lower eyelid in a properly rotated position has been proposed as a nonsurgical alternative, although requires repeated treatment and cost [13].

Congenital Entropion and Congenital Tarsal Kink

Inward rotation of the eyelid margin and tarsal plate results in congenital entropion, which is far more common in the lower eyelid but can also occur in the upper eyelid. Rarely, a horizontal flexure referred to as a "tarsal kink" can be present in the tarsus of the upper eyelid, causing misdirection of the eyelid margin toward the ocular surface. In other cases, microphthalmos, enophthalmos, or eyelid retractor dysgenesis can result in a lack of posterior support for the eyelid, allowing it to rotate inward. Shortening of the posterior lamella due to primary malformation or secondary cicatrization can also play a role. In many cases, the eyelashes on the entropic eyelid abrade the ocular surface.

A trial of lubrication can be considered in mild cases. However, surgical entropion repair is frequently indicated to protect the cornea from trichiasis-related infections and scarring. Horizontal tightening of the tarsal strip, debulking of the overriding orbicularis muscle, and/or reattachment of the lower eyelid retractors to the inferior tarsal border can be performed [12]. If present, a tarsal kink can be repaired with a full-thickness tarsotomy to allow for rotational repositioning of the tarsus and eyelid margin [14].

Epiblepharon

Unlike true entropion, epiblepharon involves inward rotation of the eyelashes *without* misdirection of the eyelid margin or tarsus. Override of the pretarsal orbicularis muscle creates a fold of skin that pushes the lashes toward the ocular surface. Epiblepharon is most common in Asian or Hispanic children, is usually asymptomatic, and typically diminishes as the facial bones mature. It occurs more frequently in the lower eyelid but upper eyelid involvement is possible, particularly in Trisomy 21.

Surgical correction is indicated for the rare cases in which eyelash misdirection results in significant keratitis despite a trial of lubricating ointment. Approaches include an infraciliary incision with excision of the excess fold of the skin and orbicularis, sometimes coupled with a medial epicanthoplasty [12, 15]. Excision of the skin and muscle may result in the formation of a new eyelid crease or changes to the existing crease, especially in upper eyelid epiblepharon surgery. Repair can also be complicated by postoperative ectropion, so care must be taken to avoid

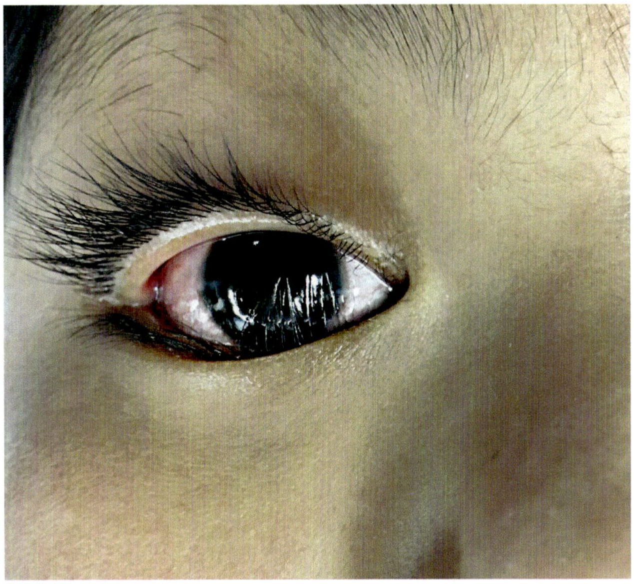

Fig. 9.7 Epiblepharon of lower eyelids causing eyelash rotation onto the ocular surface, exacerbated in downgaze

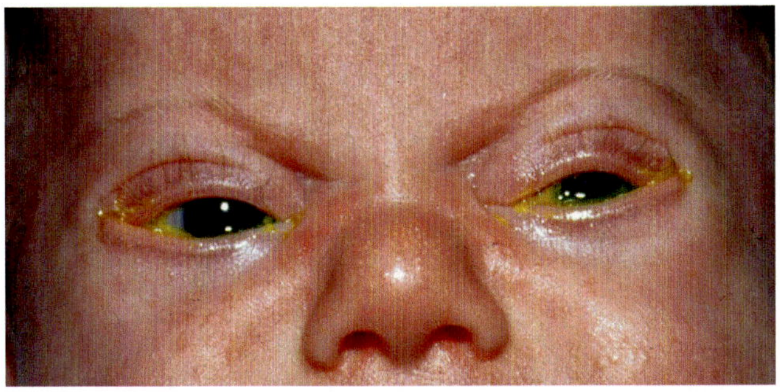

Fig. 9.8 Bilateral euryblepharon of the outer eyelids

over-shortening the anterior lamella (Fig. 9.7 Epiblepharon of lower eyelids).

Euryblepharon

This anomaly is characterized by enlargement of the palpebral fissure, usually due to horizontal lengthening and vertical shortening of the involved eyelids. It is especially notable laterally in the lower eyelid, with outward and downward displacement of the eyelid and lateral canthus. Euryblepharon may occur in isolation unilaterally or bilaterally or in conjunction with certain syndromes such as blepharophimosis syndrome, Down syndrome, blepharocheilodontic syndrome, and Kabuki syndrome [16]. Horizontal eyelid shortening surgery with lateral canthal repositioning can be utilized for reconstruction, sometimes along with a midface lift for further support of the lower eyelid and full-thickness skin grafts for vertical lengthening of the eyelid if necessary [16] (Fig. 9.8 Euryblepharon).

Blepharophimosis

Seen as an isolated defect or as part of a syndrome, blepharophimosis refers to palpebral fissures which are both horizontally and vertically shortened. Sporadic cases have a high correlation with fetal alcohol syndrome, with up to one-third of children with FAS demonstrating this finding [17]. The autosomal dominant blepharophimosis-ptosis-epicanthus inversus syndrome with telecanthus (BPES) has also been defined, with two clinical subtypes:

- BEPS I: Male transmission only, with ovarian failure in affected females resulting in infertility.
- BEPS II: Transmission through both sexes, without any associated infertility. Developmental motor delays due to hypotonia may be seen in the first years of life [5].

Some patients may also demonstrate other features, such as optic disk colobomas, strabismus, hypoplasia of the nasal bridge and the superior orbital rims, amblyopia, hypertelorism, and vertical eyelid deficiency causing euryblepharon or ectropion [16].

Although the majority of children with visually significant blepharophimosis adopt a chin-up head posture to optimize viewing through their restricted palpebral fissures, ptosis interfering with the visual axis poses a high risk for amblyopia. For this reason, surgical intervention is primarily directed toward ptosis repair. Poor or absent function of the levator palpebrae superioris muscle necessitates frontalis suspension. Some surgeons advocate coupling the ptosis surgery with repair of telecanthus and epicanthus inversus in a single operation [18]. Others recommend staging the procedures, addressing the telecanthus and epicanthus later if they have not sufficiently improved with maturation of the facial bones [16, 19]. Of note, medial canthoplasty may worsen blepharoptosis, which bears consideration when determining the staging order of operations (Fig. 9.9 Blepharophimosis syndrome).

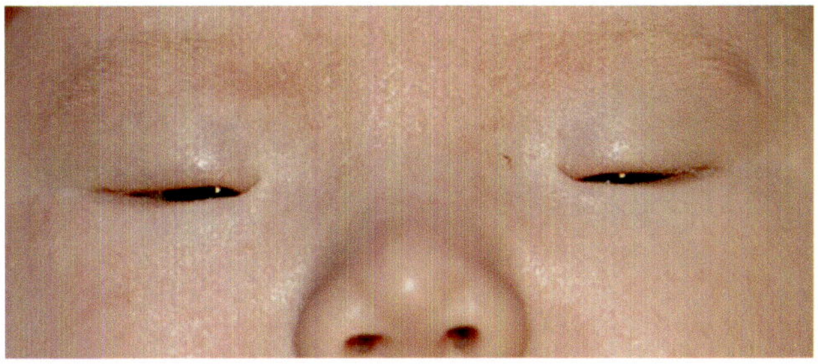

Fig. 9.9 Clinical appearance of blepharophimosis syndrome

References

1. Roy FH. Ocular syndromes and systemic diseases. 3rd ed. Philadelphia: Lippincott Williams & Wilkins; 2002.
2. Kwon B, Nguyen AH. Reconsideration of the epicanthus: evolution of the eyelid and the devolutional concept of Asian blepharoplasty. Semin Plast Surg. 2015;29(3):171–83.
3. Cook C, Ozanics V, Jakobiec F. Prenatal development of the eye and its adnexa. In: Tasman W, Jaeger E, editors. Foundations of clinical ophthalmology. Philadelphia: Lippincott-Raven; 1996. p. 1–18.
4. Bedrossian EH. Embryology and anatomy of the eyelid. In: Tasman W, Jaeger EA, editors. Duane's foundations of clinical ophthalmology. Philadelphia: Lippincott Williams & Wilkins; 2006.
5. Dollfus H, Verloes A. Developmental anomalies of the lids. In: Hoyt CS, Taylor D, editors. Pediatric ophthalmology and strabismus. Philadelphia: Elsevier Health Sciences; 2012. p. 147–64.
6. Saleh GM, Hussain B, Verity DH, Collin JR. A surgical strategy for the correction of Fraser syndrome cryptophthalmos. Ophthalmology. 2009;116(9):1707–12.
7. Jordan DR, Hwang IP, Pashby R. Microblepharon: A case report. Ophthalmic Surg Lasers. 2000;31(6):502–5.
8. Bordin G, Valerio E, Cutrone M. Ankyloblepharon filiforme adnatum in a newborn. AJP Rep. 2015;5(1):e12–3.
9. Smith HB, Verity DH, Collin JR. The incidence, embryology, and oculofacial abnormalities associated with eyelid colobomas. Eye (Lond). 2015;29(4):492–8.
10. Tasse C, Hohringer S, Fisher S, Ludecke HJ, Albrecht B, Horn D, et al. Oculo-auriculo-vertebral spectrum (OAVS): clinical evaluation and severity scoring of 53 patients and proposal for a new classification. Eur J Med Genet. 2005;48(4):397–411.
11. Katsanis SH, Jabs EW. Treacher Collins syndrome. In: Pagon RA, Adam MP, Ardinger HH, Wallace SE, Amamiva A, Bean LJH, et al., editors. GeneReviews. Seattle: University of Washington; 2004.
12. Nerad JA. Techniques in ophthalmic plastic surgery. Philadelphia: Saunders Elsevier; 2010.
13. Litwin AS, Kalantzis G, Drimtzias E, Hamada S, Chang B, Malhotra R. Nonsurgical treatment of congenital ichthyosis cicatricial ectropion and eyelid retraction using Restylane hyaluronic acid. Br J Dermatol. 2015;173(2):601–3.
14. Naik MN, Honavar SG, Bhaduri A, Linberg JV. Congenital horizontal tarsal kink: a single-center experience with 6 cases. Ophthalmology. 2007;114(8):1564–8.
15. Asamura S, Nakao H, Kakizaki H, Isogai N. Is it truly necessary to add epicanthoplasty for correction of the epiblepharon? J Craniofac Surg. 2013;24(4):1137–40.
16. Lewis C, Heher KL, Katowitz JA, Traboulsi EI. Malformations of the ocular adnexae. In: Traboulsi EI, editor. Genetic diseases of the eye. 2nd ed. London: Oxford University Press; 2012. p. 40–56.
17. Gummel K, Ygge J. Ophthalmologic findings in Russian children with fetal alcohol syndrome. Eur J Ophthalmol. 2013;23(6):823–30.
18. Sebastiá R, Herzog NG, Fallico E, Lessa S, Solari HP, Ventura MP. A one-stage correction of the blepharophimosis syndrome using a standard combination of surgical techniques. Aesthet Plast Surg. 2011;35(5):820–7.
19. Allen CE, Rubin PA. Blepharophimosis-ptosis-epicanthus inversus syndrome (BPES): clinical manifestation and treatment. Int Ophthalmol Clin. 2008;48(2):15–23.

Trichiasis, Distichiasis, and Eyelash Ptosis

10

Valerie H. Chen, Dale R. Meyer, and Edward J. Wladis

Normal Anatomy

Eyelashes develop from the ectoderm around 22–26 weeks of gestation. They are modified pilosebaceous units containing a hair follicle and sebaceous gland of Zeis. Unlike elsewhere in the body, cilia in the eyelid do not have an associated arrector pili muscle [1]. In the upper lid, the average follicular depth is 1.8 mm, and average follicular bulb width is 188 microns; in the lower lid, the average follicular depth is 1.0 mm, and average follicular bulb width is 132 microns [2]. Each cilium undergoes a three-stage cycle of anagen (growth), catagen (transition), and telogen (resting) that lasts a total of approximately 3 months [3].

The lash line emerges from the epidermis anterior to the mucocutaneous junction of the anterior lamella. It is composed of 100–150 longer cilia in 5–6 rows in the upper lid and 50–75 shorter cilia in 3–4 rows in the lower lid [3, 4]. These cilia are naturally oriented outward and curl upward in the upper lid and downward in the lower lid so as to avoid interlacing with each blink. Together, they function to protect the eye from airborne particles [5].

Trichiasis and Distichiasis

Introduction

Trichiasis refers to eyelashes in normal anatomic position that are misdirected posteriorly toward the ocular surface (see Fig. 10.1). This is in contrast to distichiasis where accessory eyelashes originate from an abnormal position at or near the Meibomian gland orifices (see Fig. 10.2). Both conditions can result in foreign body sensation (secondary to contact with the cornea and/or conjunctiva), pain, tearing, and photophobia. Untreated, these can lead to ocular and visual complications,

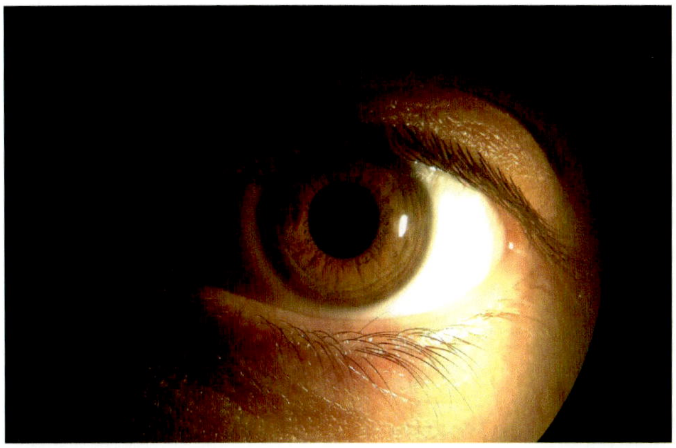

Fig. 10.1 Trichiasis in the central lower eyelid misdirected toward the ocular surface

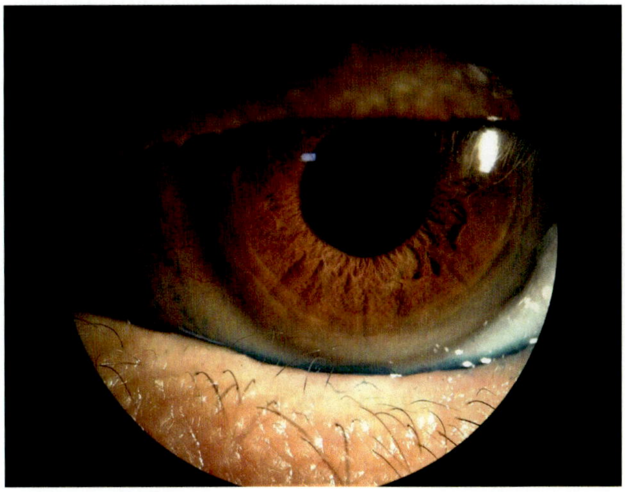

Fig. 10.2 Clinical photograph of lower eyelid distichiasis

V. H. Chen (✉) · E. J. Wladis
Department of Ophthalmology, Albany Medical College, Albany, NY, USA

Ophthalmic Plastic Surgery, Lions Eye Institute, Slingerlands, NY, USA
e-mail: wladise@amc.edu

D. R. Meyer
Ophthalmic Plastic Surgery, Lions Eye Institute-Albany Medical Center, Slingerlands, NY, USA
e-mail: meyerd@amc.edu

A. J. Cohen, C. N. Burkat (eds.), *Oculofacial, Orbital, and Lacrimal Surgery*, https://doi.org/10.1007/978-3-030-14092-2_10

Inflammatory: chronic blepharitis, Stevens-Johnson syndrome, ocular cicatricial pemphigoid

Infectious: trachoma, herpes simplex/zoster

Trauma: chemical or thermal burn, physical injury, previous lid margin surgery

Medications: topical prostaglandin

Fig. 10.3 Causes of trichiasis [5, 7, 9, 13–22]

including corneal abrasion and ulceration, corneal scarring and neovascularization, and ultimately blindness [6–11].

Pathogenesis

Several causes of trichiasis have been identified (see Fig. 10.3). Distichiasis can be either a congenital or acquired condition. Congenital distichiasis is most frequently inherited in an autosomal dominant fashion associated with systemic lymphedema due to abnormalities of the FOXC2 gene [12]. Acquired distichiasis results from certain inflammatory conditions similar to those seen in trichiasis. It is hypothesized that the inflammation causes dedifferentiation of the Meibomian gland into a complete pilosebaceous unit that possesses the hair follicle component [13].

Symptomatic Treatment

- Lubrication: Artificial tears, lubricating gel, eyelid hygiene to minimize blepharitis.
- Bandage contact lens: This may be indicated for more severe symptoms and keratopathy, until more definitive treatment can be performed.

Definitive Treatment

Lash treatment is aimed at removing the aberrant cilia and reducing the patient's symptoms and ocular sequelae. The number and distribution of pathologic lashes often dictate treatment selection.

- **Single or limited number of involved lashes**
  - *Mechanical epilation* can be done with forceps at the slit lamp or with magnifying loupes. Epilated lashes typically grow back within 4–6 weeks. It is important to remove the entire lash follicle as a broken lash can act as a "barb" and cause more irritation than mature lashes [5, 23]. Careful visual inspection can be utilized to ensure that the follicle has been removed in its entirety.
  - *Electrolysis or hyfrecation* directs a high-frequency electrical current through a probe or needle inserted into anesthetized skin along each hair follicle shaft until bubbles and a subtle whitening of the base of the lash are seen. The treated lash can then be freely removed, and the absence of resistance suggests adequate cauterization. Success rates have been reported as low as 50%; this may reach up to 100% with multiple treatments. Extensive or repeated treatments can cause lid notching or frank eyelid entropion due to tarsal scarring [5, 24, 25].
  - *Radiofrequency ablation* coagulates and destroys the cilia via a needle directed into the eyelash follicle. It is performed in a similar manner as electrolysis. Success rates have been reported to be 60–67% after a single treatment [7, 26]. A lower rate of recurrence may be seen with supplemental mitomycin C injection into the follicle following ablation [22].
    - *Settings*: 3.8 MHz, power setting 1.5–3
  - *Laser photoablation* uses selective photothermolysis to destroy the cilia. After topical or subcutaneous anesthesia is given, the laser beam is directed coaxially down the hair shaft, and repetitive applications are applied until a "white burn" crater is achieved, indicating that the hair follicle is destroyed and can be easily removed. Multiple lasers, including argon (514 nm) [7, 18, 27–31], ruby (694 nm) [32, 33], diode (810 nm) [33, 34], and Nd:YAG (1064 nm) [33], have been used. Success rates for argon laser have been reported to range from 39% to 90% [28–31]. This method is most useful for pigmented lashes and is generally well tolerated, although recurrence is not uncommon and there is a learning curve associated with use of the laser [5].
    - *Settings*: spot size 50–100 μ, duration 0.2–0.5 s, power 0.2–1.5 W, number 20–40 spots/aberrant lash
  - *Eyelash trephination* (e.g., lacrimal trephine, Sisler trephine) can be used to bore out individual lashes. The trephine is directed into the anesthetized lid margin, parallel to the aberrant lash follicle, to a depth of 2–3 mm. The instrument is then removed, and the cylindrical core of lid margin tissue containing the abnormal follicle is excised at the base with scissors [10].

While performing these techniques, it is helpful to recall that the average follicular depth is 1.8 mm in the upper lid and 1.0 mm in the lower lid. Thus, for a needle to completely contact 95% of all follicles, it must be inserted on average 2.4 mm into the upper lid and 1.4 mm into the lower lid. Further, laser spot size selection and diameter of treatment should fully encompass the follicular bulb width [2].

- **Focal or segmental lash involvement**
  - *Cryotherapy* is used to deliver a double freeze-thaw cycle (rapid freeze to −20 °C followed by a slow thaw) to the affected area(s) via a cryoprobe. Care is taken to avoid contact with the globe or a nonconducting shield can be used. While the success rates are higher (up to 90%) than those methods previously listed, there is also increased risk of complications (up to 26%), including lid swelling, lid margin distortion or notching, damage

to adjacent normal tissue and lashes, reactivation of herpes zoster, and skin depigmentation (especially in patients with increased skin pigmentation) [17, 35–37].
- *Full-thickness wedge resection* can remove a focal segment of aberrant lashes with excellent cosmesis [5, 23]. The lid segment containing the abnormal lashes is resected in a full-thickness pentagonal wedge manner. Reconstruction is then done with careful re-approximation of the lid margin in standard fashion; a lateral canthotomy and/or semicircular flap can be performed if there is insufficient laxity for direct closure.

– **Broad segments or diffuse lid involvement**
- *Eyelid splitting* techniques have many variations. All begin with making an incision anterior and parallel to the abnormal eyelashes (a large chalazion clamp may be helpful to stabilize the lid and aid in hemostasis). The incision is made approximately 3 mm in depth at the level of the gray line for full exposure of the hair follicle and bulb and sufficient lengthwise to encompass all aberrant lashes. Cryotherapy [6, 13], electrolysis [19], radiofrequency ablation [38], cautery [9], or direct excision [19, 39] can then be applied directly to the offending lash follicles. In trichiasis, some surgeons also advocate recessing the anterior lamella (e.g., chromic gut horizontal mattress sutures) [13]. The split lid margin can then be closed with a running suture or left to heal by secondary intention. Eyelid splitting allows for direct visualization of treatment to the hair follicle and is thought to minimize damage to the surrounding tissue (e.g., conjunctiva, lid margin). While this technique is effective, patients should be cautioned a cosmetically noticeable defect may be present during a healing process of several weeks.
- *Blepharotomy with tarsal rotation* was first described by Wies [40] in 1954 for senile or spastic entropion of the lower lid but has also found utility in the treatment of abnormal lashes in the setting of normal lid position. A full-thickness horizontal lid incision is made parallel to and approximately 3–4 mm from the lid margin. A double-armed horizontal mattress suture (e.g., 5–0 chromic gut) is placed partial thickness through proximal tarsus, threaded through the distal bridge of orbicularis muscle and skin adjacent to the lash line, and tied down (bolster optional) titrating tightness for the desired degree of lid eversion. Additional horizontal mattress sutures can be placed depending on the extent of lid involvement. The skin is then closed [21]. The World Health Organization currently recommends bilamellar tarsal rotation for trichiasis secondary to trachoma [11].

Antibiotic-steroid ointment can be applied to the lid for 1–2 weeks. Over-the-counter analgesia is often sufficient for pain control.

While there are many potentially beneficial treatments, recurrence is not uncommon, and additional treatment may be necessary. When occurring in conjunction with lid malposition, the latter may also warrant specific treatment.

Lash Ptosis

Introduction

Lash ptosis is the global declination of upper lid eyelashes (see Fig. 10.4). When severe, it can obscure vision and cause visual field defects. It is best identified and evaluated

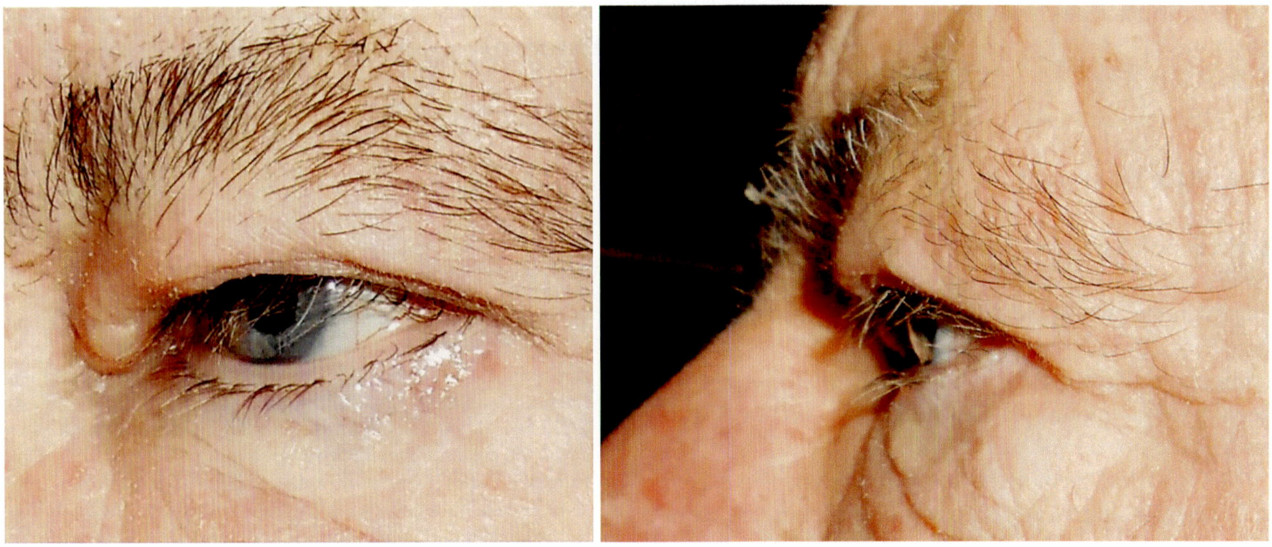

Fig. 10.4 Clinical photographs of eyelash ptosis in a patient with floppy eyelid syndrome

0	None (natural position of the lid; 0° to 30° above the horizontal)
1	Minimal (0° to 30° below the horizontal)
2	Moderate (31° to 45° below the horizontal)
3	Significant (more than 45° below the horizontal meridian)

Fig. 10.5 Lash ptosis rating scale

in primary gaze with the chin parallel to the floor. A four-point rating scale has been proposed by Malik et al. [41] (see Fig. 10.5).

It is most classically associated with floppy eyelid syndrome and recognition of this sign during routine eye examination can facilitate timely diagnosis of obstructive sleep apnea [42, 43]. Lash ptosis has also been associated with eyelid blepharoptosis, dermatochalasis, latanoprost use [44], facial palsy [45], long-standing ocular leprosy [46], failure to reform the eyelid crease during ptosis repair, and congenital lamellar ichthyosis [41]. Certain ethnicities, particularly Asian, have a higher natural prevalence of lash ptosis [47].

Pathogenesis

The eyelash bulb naturally lies in the space between the muscle of Riolan and the pretarsal orbicularis with possible extension posteriorly into the tarsus. Lash ptosis is thought to occur as a result of anatomic changes in these structures and/or their relationship to one another [43, 45]. Various studies have suggested deficiency of elastin in the tarsus and pretarsal orbicularis as well as excess skin laxity may contribute to insufficient lash support leading to lash ptosis [48, 49].

Symptomatic Treatment

- Eyelash curler

Definitive Treatment

Surgical intervention is typically directed at the underlying etiology, such as eyelid tightening procedures for floppy eyelid syndrome. While the full features and management of floppy eyelid syndrome is beyond the scope of this chapter, horizontal tightening as a primary surgical intervention has been shown to improve both eyelid and eyelash ptosis without any additional measures [43, 50, 51].

The following methods have also been discussed as general treatment options of lash ptosis or if further lash elevation is needed after addressing the underlying cause.

- *Anterior lamellar recession* can be done by splitting the eyelid (as described above) and suturing the skin and orbicularis further from the eyelid margin.
- *Lid crease formation sutures* were first described by Pang in 1961 based on his observations in the Far East for surgical creation of an upper lid fold [52]. This technique creates a full-thickness fibrous tract between the superior tarsal border and the skin. Horizontal mattress sutures (e.g., double-armed 5–0 chromic gut) are placed full thickness from the conjunctiva (1–2 mm superior to the tarsus) externally to the skin at the natural or desired lid crease, a few millimeters apart. The sutures are passed in a straight, through-and-through manner without rotating the needles. The double-armed suture is then tied down (bolster optional), titrating tightness for the desired degree of lash elevation. Eversion can be accentuated with displacing the skin exit of the suture closer to the lash line. Additional horizontal mattress sutures can be placed depending on the extent of lash involvement.
- *Lid eversion mattress sutures* are performed through an eyelid crease incision across the length of the eyelid. Dissection is carried out inferiorly over the tarsus to the level of the eyelash bed. Sutures are placed through the pretarsal orbicularis superior to the lash line and then passed partial thickness through the superior tarsus to evert the eyelashes. Overcorrection is desired as this will often settle lower in the postoperative period. High recurrences have been reported despite the use of absorbable and nonabsorbable sutures [41].

Antibiotic-steroid ointment can be used for 1–2 weeks. Over-the-counter analgesia is often sufficient for pain control.

Lash ptosis can be rather difficult to treat and may necessitate multiple and repeated treatments.

References

1. Paus R, Burgoa I, Platt CI, Griffiths T, Poblet E, Izeta A. Biology of the eyelash hair follicle: an enigma in plain sight. Br J Dermatol. 2016;174(4):741–52.
2. Elder MJ. Anatomy and physiology of eyelash follicles: relevance to lash ablation procedures. Ophthal Plast Reconstr Surg. 1997;13(1):21–5.
3. Thibaut S, De Becker E, Caisey L, et al. Human eyelash characterization. Br J Dermatol. 2010;162(2):304–10.
4. Montagna W, Ford DM. Histology and cytochemistry of human skin. 3. The eyelid. Arch Dermatol. 1969;100(3):328–35.
5. Kirkwood BJ, Kirkwood RA. Trichiasis: characteristics and management options. Insight. 2011;36(2):5–9.
6. O'Donnell BA, Collin JR. Distichiasis: management with cryotherapy to the posterior lamella. Br J Ophthalmol. 1993;77(5):289–92.
7. Salour H, Rafati N, Falahi MR, Aletaha M. A comparison of argon laser and radiofrequency in trichiasis treatment. Ophthal Plast Reconstr Surg. 2011;27(5):313–6.

8. Moosavi AH, Mollan SP, Berry-Brincat A, Abbott J, Sutton GA, Murray A. Simple surgery for severe trichiasis. Ophthal Plast Reconstr Surg. 2007;23(4):296–7.
9. Chi MJ, Park MS, Nam DH, Moon HS, Baek SH. Eyelid splitting with follicular extirpation using a monopolar cautery for the treatment of trichiasis and distichiasis. Graefes Arch Clin Exp Ophthalmol. 2007;245(5):637–40.
10. McCracken MS, Kikkawa DO, Vasani SN. Treatment of trichiasis and distichiasis by eyelash trephination. Ophthal Plast Reconstr Surg. 2006;22(5):349–51.
11. Merbs S, Resnikoff S, Bedri Kello A, Mariotti S, Greene G, West SK. Trichiasis surgery for trachoma. Geneva: WHO Publication; 2015.
12. Dellinger MT, Thome K, Bernas MJ, Erickson RP, Witte MH. Novel FOXC2 missense mutation identified in patient with lymphedema-distichiasis syndrome and review. Lymphology. 2008;41(3):98–102.
13. Anderson RL, Harvey JT. Lid splitting and posterior lamella cryosurgery for congenital and acquired distichiasis. Arch Ophthalmol. 1981;99(4):631–4.
14. Chiou AG, Florakis GJ, Kazim M. Management of conjunctival cicatrizing diseases and severe ocular surface dysfunction. Surv Ophthalmol. 1998;43(1):19–46.
15. Bearden W, Anderson R. Trichiasis associated with prostaglandin analog use. Ophthal Plast Reconstr Surg. 2004;20(4):320–2.
16. Mabey DC, Solomon AW, Foster A. Trachoma. Lancet (London, UK). 2003;362(9379):223–9.
17. Wood JR, Anderson RL. Complications of cryosurgery. Arch Ophthalmol. 1981;99(3):460–3.
18. Al-Bdour MD, Al-Till MI. Argon laser: a modality of treatment for trichiasis. Int J Biomed Sci. 2007;3(1):56–9.
19. Vaughn GL, Dortzbach RK, Sires BS, Lemke BN. Eyelid splitting with excision or microhyfrecation for distichiasis. Arch Ophthalmol. 1997;115(2):282–4.
20. Reacher MH, Munoz B, Alghassany A, Daar AS, Elbualy M, Taylor HR. A controlled trial of surgery for trachomatous trichiasis of the upper lid. Arch Ophthalmol. 1992;110(5):667–74.
21. Bleyen I, Dolman PJ. The Wies procedure for management of trichiasis or cicatricial entropion of either upper or lower eyelids. Br J Ophthalmol. 2009;93(12):1612–5.
22. Kim GN, Yoo WS, Kim SJ, et al. The effect of 0.02% mitomycin C injection into the hair follicle with radiofrequency ablation in trichiasis patients. Korean J Ophthalmol. 2014;28(1):12–8.
23. Ferreira IS, Bernardes TF, Bonfioli AA. Trichiasis. Semin Ophthalmol. 2010;25(3):66–71.
24. Sakarya Y, Sakarya R, Yildirim A. Electrolysis treatment of trichiasis by using ultra-fine needle. Eur J Ophthalmol. 2010;20(4):664–8.
25. Bartley GB, Bullock JD, Olsen TG, Lutz PD. An experimental study to compare methods of eyelash ablation. Ophthalmology. 1987;94(10):1286–9.
26. Kezirian GM. Treatment of localized trichiasis with radiosurgery. Ophthal Plast Reconstr Surg. 1993;9(4):260–6.
27. Yung CW, Massicotte SJ, Kuwabara T. Argon laser treatment of trichiasis: a clinical and histopathologic evaluation. Ophthal Plast Reconstr Surg. 1994;10(2):130–6.
28. Gossman MD, Yung R, Berlin AJ, Brightwell JR. Prospective evaluation of the argon laser in the treatment of trichiasis. Ophthalmic Surg. 1992;23(3):183–7.
29. Huneke JW. Argon laser treatment for trichiasis. Ophthal Plast Reconstr Surg. 1992;8(1):50–5.
30. Awan KJ. Argon laser treatment of trichiasis. Ophthalmic Surg. 1986;17(10):658–60.
31. Basar E, Ozdemir H, Ozkan S, Cicik E, Mirzatas C. Treatment of trichiasis with argon laser. Eur J Ophthalmol. 2000;10(4):273–5.
32. Moore J, De Silva SR, O'Hare K, Humphry RC. Ruby laser for the treatment of trichiasis. Lasers Med Sci. 2009;24(2):137–9.
33. Wanner M. Laser hair removal. Dermatol Ther. 2005;18(3):209–16.
34. Pham RT, Biesman BS, Silkiss RZ. Treatment of trichiasis using an 810-nm diode laser: an efficacy study. Ophthal Plast Reconstr Surg. 2006;22(6):445–7.
35. Zabriskie NA, Nordlund JJ, Nerad JA. Unusual skin depigmentation following eyelid cryosurgery. Ophthal Plast Reconstr Surg. 1996;12(4):296–8.
36. Sullivan JH. The use of cryotherapy for trichiasis. Trans Sect Ophthalmol Am Acad Ophthalmol Otolaryngol. 1977;83(4 Pt 1):708–12.
37. Johnson RL, Collin JR. Treatment of trichiasis with a lid cryoprobe. Br J Ophthalmol. 1985;69(4):267–70.
38. Rosner M, Bourla N, Rosen N. Eyelid splitting and extirpation of hair follicles using a radiosurgical technique for treatment of trichiasis. Ophthalmic Surg Lasers Imaging. 2004;35(2):116–22.
39. Wojno TH. Lid splitting with lash resection for cicatricial entropion and trichiasis. Ophthal Plast Reconstr Surg. 1992;8(4):287–9.
40. Wies FA. Surgical treatment of entropion. J Int Surg. 1954;21:758–60.
41. Malik KJ, Lee MS, Park DJ, Harrison AR. Lash ptosis in congenital and acquired blepharoptosis. Arch Ophthalmol. 2007;125(12):1613–5.
42. Culbertson WW, Ostler HB. The floppy eyelid syndrome. Am J Ophthalmol. 1981;92(4):568–75.
43. Langford JD, Linberg JV. A new physical finding in floppy eyelid syndrome. Ophthalmology. 1998;105(1):165–9.
44. Casson RJ, Selva D. Lash ptosis caused by latanoprost. Am J Ophthalmol. 2005;139(5):932–3.
45. Mulhern MG, Aduriz-Lorenzo PM, Rawluk D, Viani L, Eustace P, Logan P. Ocular complications of acoustic neuroma surgery. Br J Ophthalmol. 1999;83(12):1389–92.
46. Guimaraes FC, Cruz AA. Eyelid changes in long-standing leprosy. Ophthal Plast Reconstr Surg. 1998;14(4):239–43.
47. Lee TE, Lee JM, Lee H, Park M, Kim KH, Baek S. Lash ptosis and associated factors in Asians. Ann Plast Surg. 2010;65(4):407–10.
48. Netland PA, Sugrue SP, Albert DM, Shore JW. Histopathologic features of the floppy eyelid syndrome. Involvement of tarsal elastin. Ophthalmology. 1994;101(1):174–81.
49. Schlotzer-Schrehardt U, Stojkovic M, Hofmann-Rummelt C, Cursiefen C, Kruse FE, Holbach LM. The pathogenesis of floppy eyelid syndrome: involvement of matrix metalloproteinases in elastic fiber degradation. Ophthalmology. 2005;112(4):694–704.
50. Dutton JJ. Surgical management of floppy eyelid syndrome. Am J Ophthalmol. 1985;99(5):557–60.
51. Mills DM, Meyer DR, Harrison AR. Floppy eyelid syndrome: quantifying the effect of horizontal tightening on upper eyelid position. Ophthalmology. 2007;114(10):1932–6.
52. Pang HG. Surgical formation of upper lid fold. Arch Ophthalmol. 1961;65:783–4.

Entropion

11

Jonathan J. Dutton

Introduction

Entropion is a turning inward of the eyelid margin. Like ectropion, the causes are numerous, but unlike the latter, the results may be far more devastating to the ocular surface. Regardless of the specific etiology, in the presence of entropion, the mucocutaneous border of the eyelid margin and the eyelashes turns toward the globe resulting in conjunctival irritation and corneal abrasion. Corneal contact causes symptoms of foreign body sensation, secondary blepharospasm, reflex epiphora, ocular discharge, and superficial keratopathy and ultimately may lead to corneal stromal scarring. In some cases, distortion of eyelid tissues may include a true trichiasis. However, in most patients with entropion, the eyelashes are in a normal position relative to the lid margin, but the resulting corneal touch is secondary to the eyelid malposition.

Entropion is classified into a number of subtypes, each with its own specific anatomic characteristics. These include medial or lateral canthal tendon laxity, capsulopalpebral fascia redundancy or disinsertion, preseptal orbicularis muscle override, posterior lamellar contraction or scarring, and tarsal deformity. These must be determined during the initial examination and understood if appropriate long-term corrective procedures are to be undertaken. In most cases, the goal is to restore eyelid structures to a more normal anatomic relationship.

Other conditions can simulate entropion and cause similar symptoms. In most cases, however, these occur in the presence of an eyelid margin that is oriented in a normal anatomic position with respect to the ocular surface. Trichiasis is a condition frequently misdiagnosed as entropion. While there are numerous variations of this disorder, for the most part, this is an acquired anomaly where eyelashes originate from normally positioned follicles in the eyelid margin but are misdirected toward the cornea [1] (Fig. 11.1) While the lid is usually in a normal anatomic orientation in most cases, it also can be associated with entropion. Distichiasis is a distinct condition where aberrant eyelashes arise from metaplastic meibomian glands posterior to the normal eyelash follicles (Fig. 11.2). Because of their more posterior location on the mucosal tarsal border, they more commonly lie in contact with the ocular surface [2].

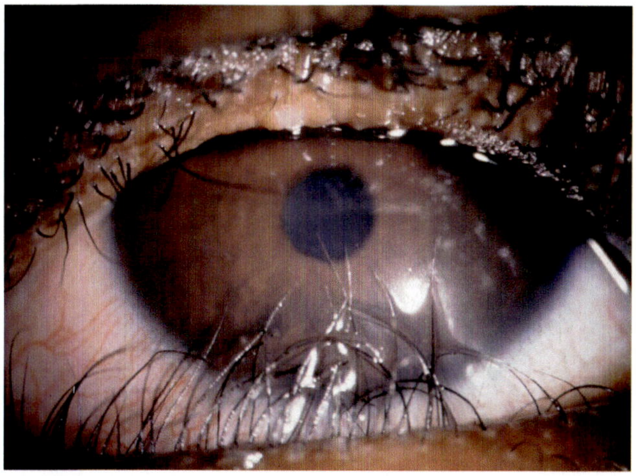

Fig. 11.1 Trichiasis of the right lower eyelid with lashes directed backward against the cornea

Relevant Anatomy

An understanding of eyelid anatomy and function is essential for evaluating the etiology of specific cases of entropion and for planning medical or surgical intervention. Externally the eyelids form the boundaries of the palpebral fissure and provide a vital interface between the lid and the corneal surface. The upper and lower eyelids join at the medial and lateral canthi and are suspended by canthal tendons to the periosteum along the medial and lateral orbital rims. The eyelid

J. J. Dutton (✉)
University of North Carolina, Durham, NC, USA
e-mail: Jonathan_dutton@med.unc.edu

A. J. Cohen, C. N. Burkat (eds.), *Oculofacial, Orbital, and Lacrimal Surgery*, https://doi.org/10.1007/978-3-030-14092-2_11

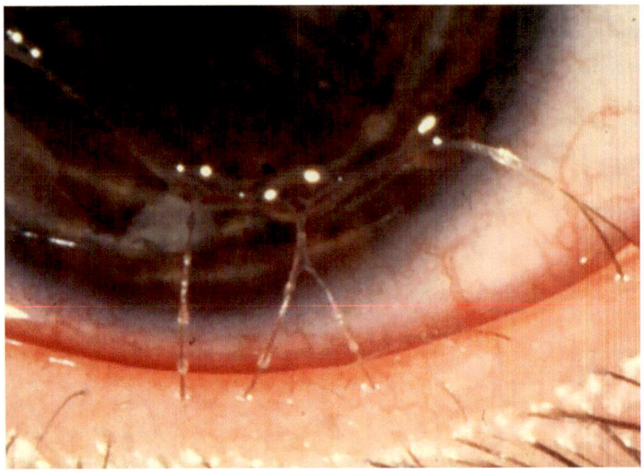

Fig. 11.2 Distichiasis of the right lower eyelid; aberrant lashes emerge along the meibomian gland orifices, posterior to the normal row of eyelashes

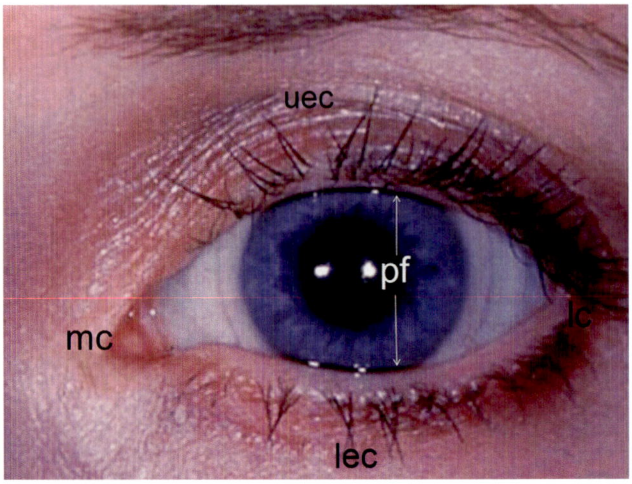

Fig. 11.4 Normal eyelids. *uec* upper eyelid crease, *mc* medial canthus, *lc* lateral canthus, *pf* palpebral fissure, *lec* lower eyelid crease

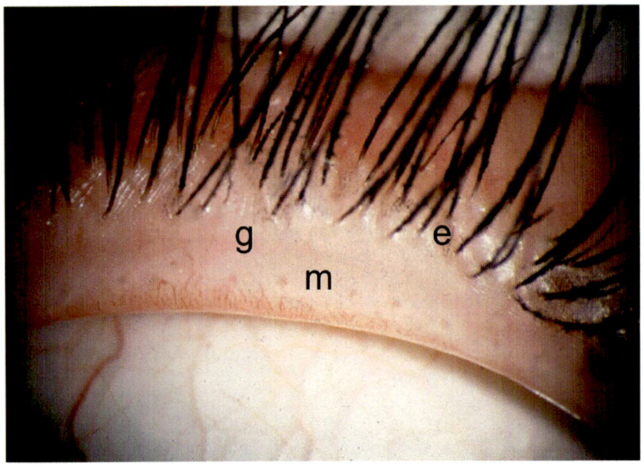

Fig. 11.3 Normal lower eyelid margin. *m* meibomian gland orifices, *e* eyelashes, *g* gray line

margins are covered posteriorly by conjunctiva, and anteriorly by the skin, separated horizontally by the gray line. The eyelashes emerge just anterior to the gray line, and the meibomian gland orifices open immediately behind it (Fig. 11.3). The eyelid crease is a horizontal fold in the skin. It is well developed in the upper lid but rather poorly defined in the lower lid (Fig. 11.4). Between the lid margin and the eyelid crease, anterior and posterior lamellae are joined together by fibrous attachments so that they move as a single anatomic unit. This is important for eyelid function since disruption or absence of this adhesion zone is a potential cause of mechanical entropion and epiblepharon where the anterior lamella rides over the tarsus.

The eyelid is a layered structure with anterior and posterior lamellae [3–6]. The anterior lamella consists of skin with its adnexal structures, and beneath it is the orbicularis muscle (Fig. 11.5). The posterior lamella is composed of the tarsal plate near the lid margins, and behind that is the conjunctiva against the eye. The eyelid muscles fall into two groups, the protractors that close the lid and the retractors that open the lid. The major protractor is the orbicularis oculi muscle that surrounds the eyelids in circular fashion. This muscle is divided arbitrarily into three portions: the orbital portion overlies the bony orbital rims, the preseptal portion overlies the orbital septum, and the pretarsal portion overlies the tarsal plates. It is innervated by branches of the facial nerve (CN.VII). Eyelashes are hairs that have their bulbs between the skin and orbicularis muscle along the lid margins. There are approximately 100 lashes in the upper lid and 50 in the lower lid.

The tarsal plates are dense fibrous structures that give rigidity and support to the eyelid margins, and maintain a contour that conforms to the ocular surface. They are about 1 mm in thickness. In the upper eyelid, the tarsus is typically 8–12 mm in height tapering medially and laterally, and in the lower lid, it is 3–4 mm in height (Fig. 11.6). Medially and laterally, the tarsal plates are fixed to the orbital rims by the medial and lateral canthal tendons. The tarsal plates contain meibomian holocrine sebaceous glands that provide the superficial lipid layer to the precorneal tear film. There are about 25 in the upper lid and 20 in the lower lid.

The palpebral conjunctiva is a mucous membrane that lines the posterior surface of the eyelids. It is continuous around the superior and inferior fornices with the bulbar conjunctiva covering the sclera and Tenon's capsule. Conjunctiva contains goblet cells that secrete mucin, as well as apocrine Moll glands and holocrine Zeis glands along the lid margin that open into the eyelash follicles. Several types of accessory lacrimal glands lie beneath the conjunctiva. Twenty to forty glands of Krause are mostly situated near the lateral superior fornix and discharge via long ducts into the fornix space. Glands of Wolfring are large and fewer in number

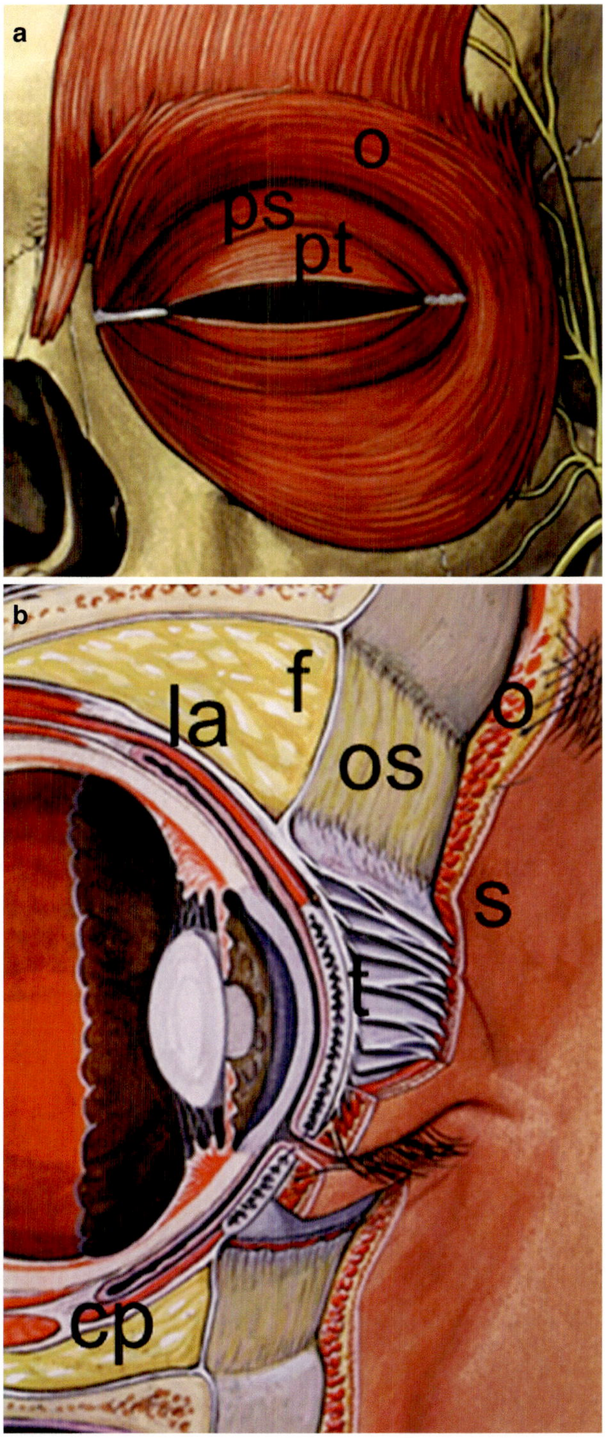

Fig. 11.5 Eyelid anatomy. (**a**) Orbicularis muscle. *o* orbital portion, *ps* preseptal portion, *pt* pretarsal portion. (**b**) Lamellar structure of the eyelids. *s* skin, *o* orbicularis muscle, *t* tarsus, *c* conjunctiva, *la* levator aponeurosis, *mm* Müllers muscle, *os* orbital septum, *cp* lower eyelid retractor, *f* preaponeurotic fat

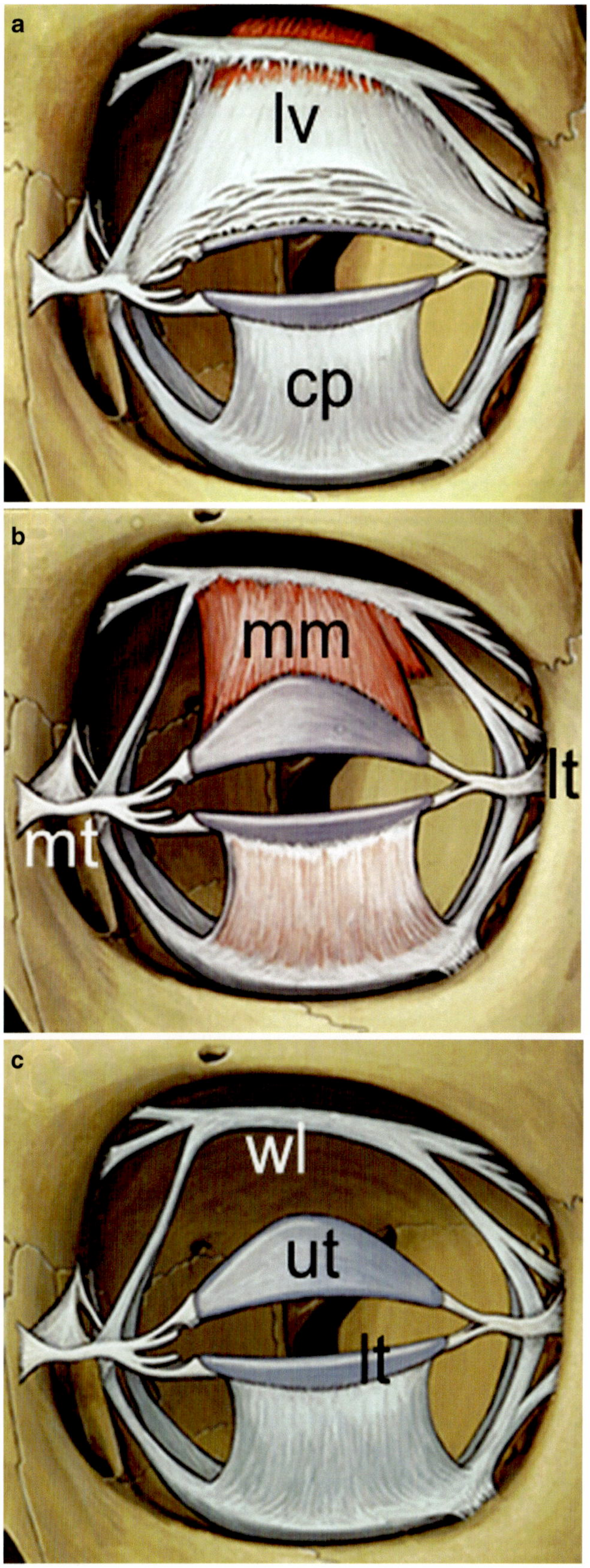

Fig. 11.6 Eyelid anatomy. (**a**) *lv* Levator aponeurosis, *cp* capsulopalpebral fascia. (**b**) *mm* Müllers muscle, *mt* medial canthal tendon, *lt* lateral canthal tendon. (**c**) *ut* upper lid tarsus, *lt* lower lid tarsus, *wl* Whitnall's ligament

located near the proximal tarsal border in both upper and lower eyelids.

In the upper lid, the levator muscle is the major eyelid retractor, although it is properly an orbital structure not an eyelid one (Fig. 11.6). Near the orbital rim, the muscle passes into its thin aponeurosis that fans downward between the posterior and anterior lamellae to insert near the lid margin onto the tarsus and interfascicular orbicularis muscle fibers. Between the levator aponeurosis and the conjunctiva is Müllers muscle, an accessory smooth muscle of eyelid retraction. In the lower lid, the capsulopalpebral fascial sheet extends from the inferior tarsus to Lockwood's ligament, a conjoined fascia around the inferior oblique and inferior rectus muscles. This not only retracts the lid on downgaze but also stabilizes the inferior tarsus. As such, it is a major factor in the etiology of some forms of entropion.

The canthal tendons join the tarsal plates to the orbital rims. Each consists of a superior and inferior crus from the tarsal plates that join into a common tendon that inserts onto the medial and lateral orbital rims [7]. Redundancy or disinsertion of these structures can result in eyelid laxity that is often associated with entropion or ectropion.

Clinical Features and Evaluation

Most patients with entropion present with symptoms of foreign body sensation, burning, tearing, and photophobia. The conjunctiva may be inflamed with mucoid or mucopurulent discharge. The cornea often shows areas of punctate keratopathy but in severe cases can even show areas of frank ulceration. The eyelid margin is turned inward to varying degrees. In mild cases, the lashes may only show ptosis, but in moderate cases, they are more typically in contact with the corneal epithelium. In severe cases, the eyelid may be so inverted that the skin will directly contact the cornea.

Clinical evaluation begins with a thorough medical and ocular history to uncover any conditions that might predispose to entropion. The onset and course of the ocular symptoms are recorded. A history of trauma or prior eyelid or ocular surgery may offer possible clues to etiology. A thorough ophthalmic examination is performed in all patients. Slit-lamp evaluation of the conjunctiva and corneal surface may reveal evidence of corneal abrasions. Blepharitis, trichiasis, or evidence of past or current infectious or inflammatory diseases is noted.

Eyelid examination should include all aspects of eyelid anatomy and suspensory structures, including the medial and lateral canthal tendons, the tarsal plates, the orbicularis muscle tone, and the integrity of the capsulopalpebral fascia. Horizontal laxity of the tarsus or canthal tendons is a predisposing factor in developing both ectropion and entropion. The lateral canthal tendon is more commonly associated with eyelid laxity than is the medial tendon. Laxity is evaluated with the eyelid distraction test. This is performed at the central eyelid by pulling the lid margin outward away from the cornea (Fig. 11.7). When released, a normal lid quickly snaps back into a normal position. With cicatricial entropion, the lid returns to a position turned toward the globe. In cases

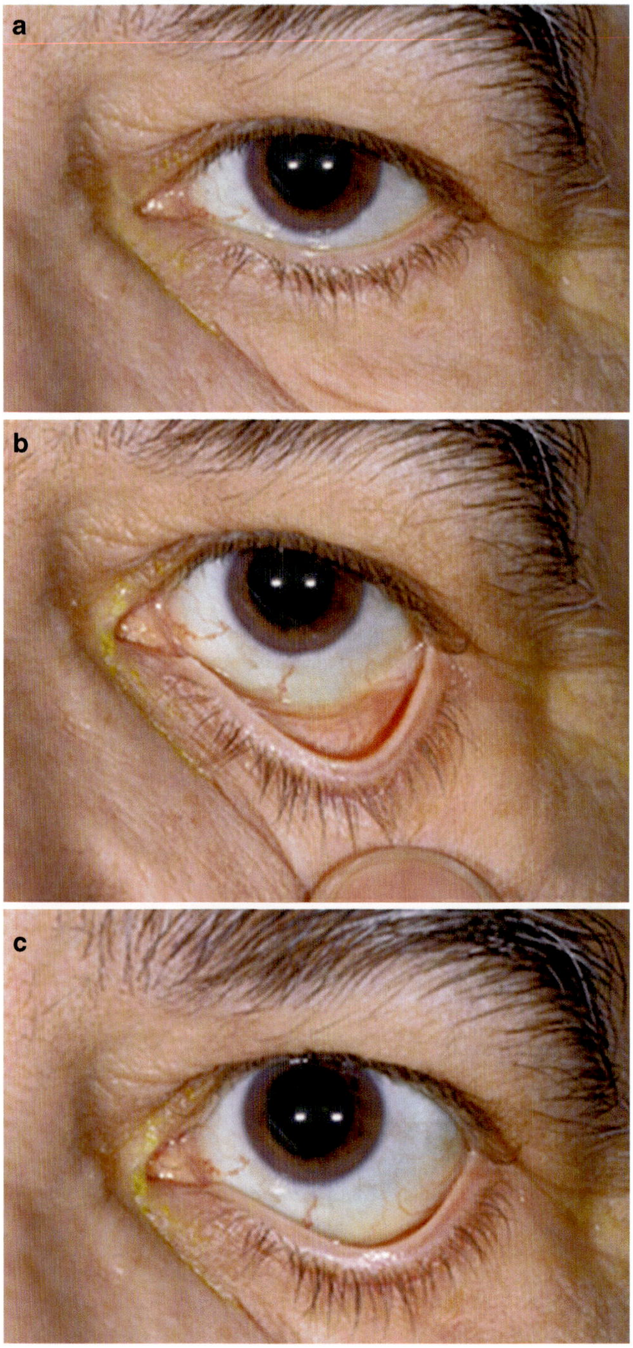

Fig. 11.7 Distraction test for eyelid laxity. (**a**) Lower eyelid showing signs of horizontal laxity. (**b**) The lower eyelid is manually pulled away from the cornea. (**c**) When released the eyelid slowly drifts back to its original position or may remain away from the globe until the next blink

of involutional entropion associated with eyelid laxity, the lid usually drifts back toward the globe slowly and may not assume a normal position against the cornea until the next blink. When the lid is pulled outward, a distance of 6–8 mm or more between the eyelid and corneal surface is usually considered abnormal. However, Beigi et al. failed to show any significant difference in this measurement between the eyelid with entropion and the normal side in 80 tested patients [8].

In cases of intermittent entropion, the eyelid may appear normal on clinical examination, but the entropion can often be elicited by certain maneuvers. Asking the patient to close their eyelids forcefully will usually elicit internal rotation of the margin when the lid is predisposed to entropion. If this test is negative, the "TIE test," as described by Faria-E-Sousa [9], may uncover the entropion. In this test with the eye in downgaze, the lid margin is pinched, and the skin is rolled up over the lid margin. The skin is spread medially and laterally with the finger and then released. With a predisposition to entropion, the lid assumes a stable inward rotation.

Evaluation of the canthal tendons is done by manually stretching the lid horizontally toward the medial or lateral canthus. Redundancy or less likely dehiscence of the canthal tendons is suggested if the lid moves more than about 5 mm. The canthal tendons normally measure about 8–10 mm in length, so that a lax stretched tendon can palpate on examination in many cases.

The capsulopalpebral fascia between the inferior oblique and inferior rectus conjoined fascial complex, and the tarsus serves as the major retractor of the lower eyelid. Laxity or frank disinsertion of this structure is a major cause of involutional entropion. Palpation just beneath the tarsus during vertical gaze shifts may reveal the disinserted edge of the capsulopalpebral fascia. In such cases, the conjunctival fornix may appear pink from the presence of orbicularis muscle instead of the retractor. Beigi et al. found increased forniceal fat prolapse in cases where the retractors were disinserted [8]. It may not be easy to demonstrate abnormalities of this structure, but the eyelid may lie at a higher resting position in primary gaze, and manual passive vertical distraction may be increased [10].

The conjunctiva and posterior tarsus are examined to evaluate for any scars, symblephara, or cicatricial contractions (Fig. 11.8). The fornix depth may offer some useful information. With retractor disinsertion, the fornix depth may be increased, but with cicatricial conditions, it can be decreased. Khan et al., in a study on 240 Asian subjects, noted mean lower and upper fornix depths as 10.9 mm and 15.8 mm, respectively [11]. They also found that the depths in females were on average about 0.5 mm less than in males and that the fornices become slightly shallower with age by about 1 mm in the lower lid and 2 mm in the upper lid. Clinical measurements of less than 13 mm in the upper lid and less than 9 mm in the lower lid should raise the suspicion of pathology.

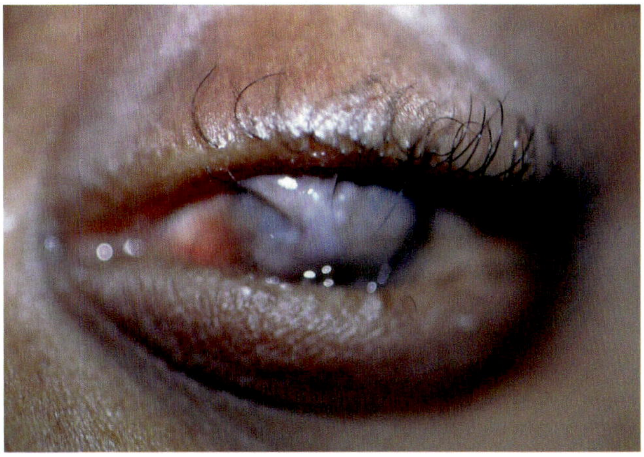

Fig. 11.8 Symblephara between the upper eyelid and cornea obliterating the superior conjunctival fornix in cicatricial pemphigoid

Kemp and Collin presented a grading system for cicatricial changes in the posterior lamella [12]. This system relied upon assessment of posterior lamellar scarring, position of meibomian gland orifices, conjunctivalization of the eyelid margin, position of the eyelashes, palpable assessment of tarsal plate morphology, and keratinization of the palpebral conjunctiva. They graded the entropion from mild to severe and correlated these to proposed surgical techniques.

Mobility of the preseptal orbicularis muscle with override onto the tarsus is seen in many cases of involutional and spastic entropion. Asking the patient forcibly to squeeze the eyelids closed may demonstrate such override with an increased fullness along the lid margin. The inferior border of the tarsus can sometime be seen as it rotates forward beneath the skin.

Classification of Entropion

Entropion is classified into several types based on specific anatomic abnormalities responsible for the malposition. While all have similar clinical characteristics and symptomatology, each has findings that allow the clinician to determine the anatomic pathology. Appropriate clinical evaluation is necessary to be able to undertake the most appropriate treatment.

The following types are discussed here:

- Congenital entropion
- Involutional entropion
- Cicatricial entropion
- Mechanical entropion
- Spastic entropion

Congenital Entropion

Primary congenital entropion of the upper eyelid is a very rare condition that can cause significant corneal damage and visual compromise in young children. It is associated with a variety of anatomic anomalies and syndromes including levator aponeurosis disinsertion [13], congenital facial nerve palsy [14], and Down syndrome [15]. Hiles and Wilder proposed that congenital upper eyelid entropion could be associated with multiple systemic abnormalities [16], and Zak observed cardiovascular, musculoskeletal, and central nervous system abnormalities in a child with congenital primary upper eyelid entropion [17]. In most cases the upper eyelid crease is absent. The skin and orbicularis muscle drape over the tarsus and eyelid margin. Repair is with reformation of the eyelid crease through a skin incision and fixation of the pretarsal orbicularis muscle to the levator aponeurosis (Fig. 11.9).

One type of congenital entropion occurs with deformity of the tarsal plate known as the tarsal kink syndrome. First described by Kettesy in 1948, this is a rare but severe form of entropion in which there is a fold or kink in the upper tarsal plate along its horizontal length [18]. The upper eyelid crease is typically absent on the affected side [19], and the eyelid margin is turned inward. In 50% of cases, the condition is bilateral [20].

The cause of tarsal kink syndrome is unknown. Suggested etiologies have been attributed to a primary tarsal defect [21], direct mechanical pressure on the tarsus in utero [22, 23], disinsertion of the levator aponeurosis [13], secondary blepharospasm from corneal abrasion, or overaction of the marginal fibers of the orbicularis muscle [20]. Lucci et al. reported a case associated with trisomy 13 [22]. Most patients present within the first 8 weeks of age, but when tarsal folding and symptoms are mild, recognition may be delayed for several years [19]. The condition is characterized clinically by entropion of the entire eyelid margin and absence of the upper eyelid crease. Corneal abrasion is typical [24], and corneal opacity or infiltrate at birth may be seen in 50–80% of cases [19]. Corneal ulceration occurs in 50% of patients and is typically sterile on culture. Amblyopia can be seen in up to 25% of cases [25], and secondary blepharospasm is common, making clinical examination difficult [20, 26].

Surgical correction will be needed in most cases of tarsal link syndrome. A variety of procedures have been described, all resulting in good outcomes. These include direct excision of the kink [21], excision with posterior lamellar scleral graft [27], lamellar tarsoplasty [28], eyelid everting sutures [29, 30], anterior lamellar repositioning [23, 31, 32], margin rotation [19], partial tarsotomy with levator repositioning [33], levator aponeurosis reattachment and crease reformation (13), and intermarginal suture tarsorrhaphy [25].

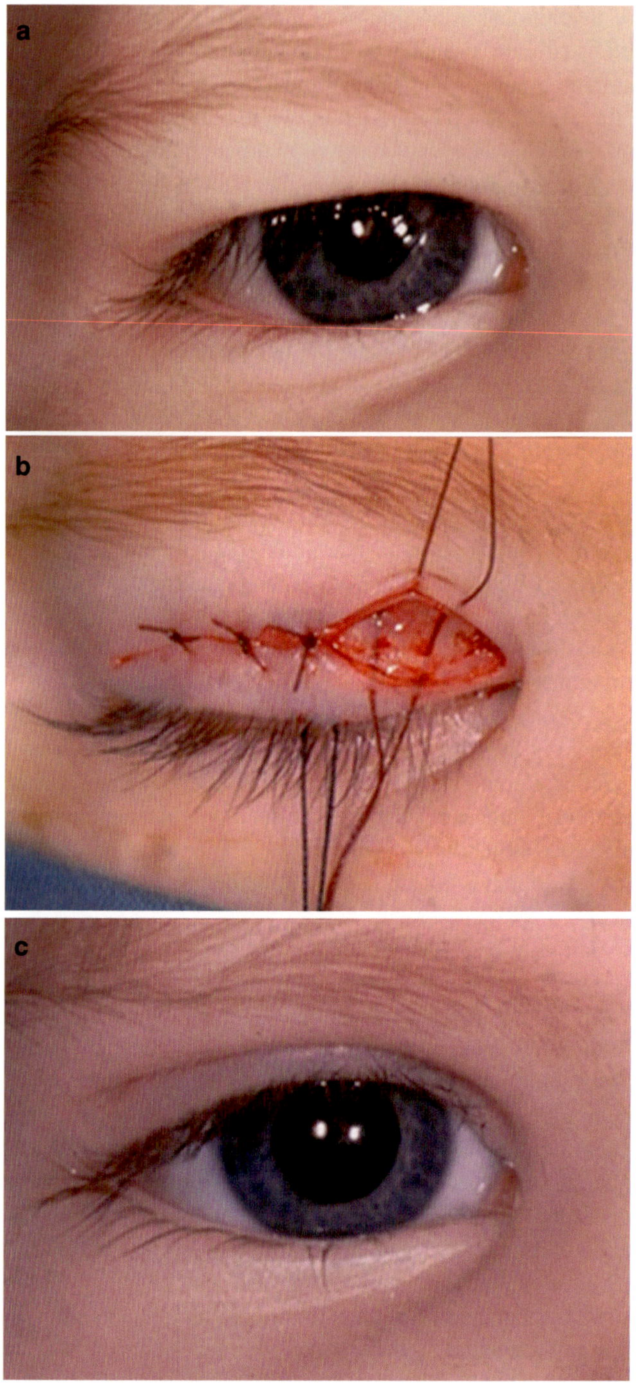

Fig. 11.9 (**a**) Congenital entropion of the upper eyelid with absence of the lid crease and overhang of the skin and orbicularis muscle onto the eyelid margin. (**b**) Skin incision, excision of a strip of muscle, and reformation of the eyelid crease. (**c**) Correction of the entropion with fixation of the anterior and posterior lamellae along the crease

Involutional Entropion

This is the most common form of entropion seen as an aging phenomenon in older individuals. The etiology is varied but usually involves one or more of several mechanisms. Probably the most important is vertical eyelid laxity from redundancy or disinsertion of the capsulopalpebral fascial eyelid retractor with consequent loss of tarsal fixation and resultant instability. This often is associated with a riding up of the preseptal orbicularis muscle onto the tarsus, mechanically inverting the margin toward the globe. Horizontal laxity is a confounding factor, most frequently resulting from stretching of the lateral canthal tendon, which is the weakest segment of lower eyelid support. However, it may also involve generalized laxity of the entire tarsal plate or the medial canthal tendon as well. Initially, the entropion may occur only intermittently, but as it progresses, the lid assumes a more permanent inward orientation.

Damasceno et al. evaluated more than 24,000 elderly patients including 565 with involutional entropion [34]. They reported an overall incidence for involutional entropion of 2.1%, greater in females and in Caucasians. They also noted a progressively increased prevalence with age, increasing from 0.9% in the seventh decade to 7.6% in the ninth decade and above. These authors identified potential risk factors including retractor laxity, canthal tendon laxity, chronic blepharitis, conjunctivitis, and dry eyes.

A less common etiology is a vertically narrow tarsal plate. In some cases, this alone may be sufficient to result in entropion. Bashour et al. measured the heights of upper and lower eyelid tarsal plates in various age groups [35]. Narrower plates were noted in older patients as an involutional phenomenon and especially in those individuals who develop entropion. They proposed an age-related atrophy of the tarsus that can predispose to entropion by allowing it to rotate on the axis along the canthal tendons. Awan et al. described a young patient with congenitally narrow lower lid tarsal plates of only 2.5 mm in width who developed recurrent entropion at age 15, presumably from increased orbicularis muscle tone and override [36]. After numerous failed attempts at repair, she was finally corrected with hard palate mucosal grafts to lengthen the tarsal height.

The clinical spectrum of involutional entropion may vary from a mild intermittent backward tilting of the marginal tarsus associated with only occasional corneal touch to severe 180° inversion of the eyelid with the lashes and skin in full contact with the globe (Figs. 11.10 and 11.11). The resulting ocular surface irritation is associated with conjunctival injection, reflex lacrimation and epiphora, and ocular discomfort from corneal touch. Corneal abrasion and even frank ulceration may evolve if the condition is not corrected. A secondary blepharospasm is frequently present which exacerbates the condition.

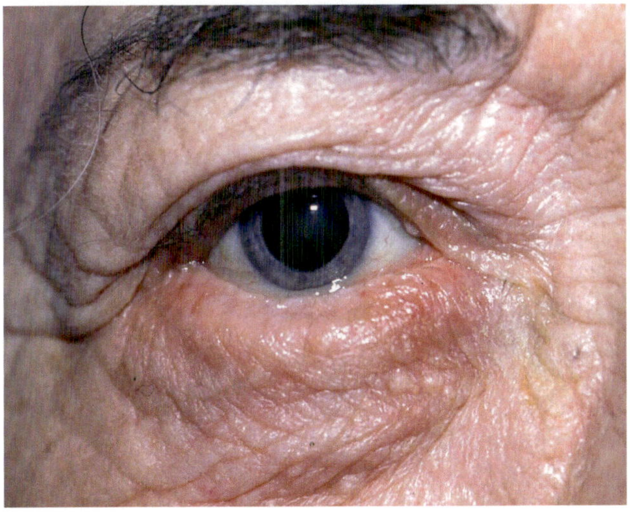

Fig. 11.10 Moderate lower eyelid involutional entropion with the lid margin turned against the corneal surface

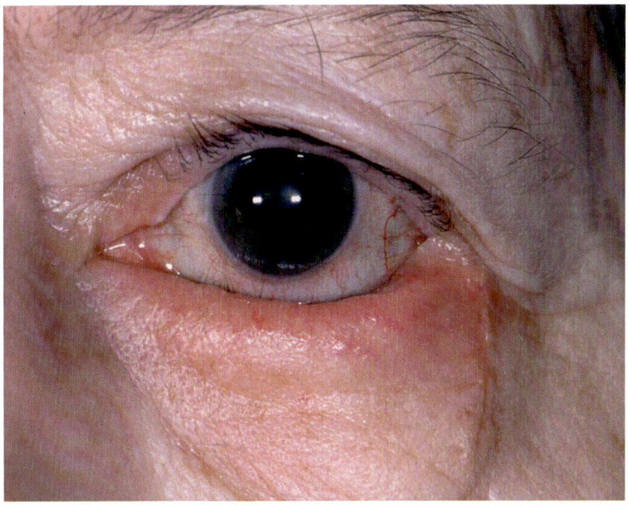

Fig. 11.11 Severe involutional entropion with the tarsus inverted 180°

Symptomatic medical management is offered to patients who may not be able to tolerate surgery or to those awaiting definitive surgical intervention. These include topical lubrication to help protect the cornea, taping the eyelid skin to the cheek or brow to evert the lid margin, or the temporary use of botulinum toxin to weaken the orbicularis muscle and prevent override onto tarsus that often is part of the etiologic mechanism.

The surgical correction of involutional entropion is directed at repair of the primary anatomic defects. In mild cases, shortening of the anterior lamella with laser ablation or cautery can correct the defect [37]. If horizontal eyelid laxity is a significant finding, repair may be achieved with simple horizontal eyelid shortening. This is achieved with a full-thickness wedge resection in the lateral third of the eyelid and primary layered closure [38, 39]. More commonly a lateral tarsal strip (LTS) canthal reconstruction is used, often combined with other procedures [40, 41] (Fig. 11.12). Olver et al. described a minimally invasive modification of the LTS procedure performed through a 1 cm lateral incision. The lateral canthal tendon is reconstructed through this opening along with a diagonal tightening of the orbital septum and capsulopalpebral fascia [42].

When horizontal eyelid laxity is minimal but retractor redundancy or frank disinsertion is the major factor, tightening or reattachment of the capsulopalpebral fascia alone will usually correct the entropion. A minimally invasive technique is the placement of full-thickness Quickert-Rathbun type sutures to tightening the retractors and of equal importance to fix the preseptal orbicularis muscle to the posterior lamella to prevent override [43, 44]. This procedure can also rotate the lid margin outward by placing the conjunctival suture insertions lower on the lid than the emerging skin sutures. Chromic or Vicryl sutures elicit an inflammatory reaction to form a cicatrix between the included tissues

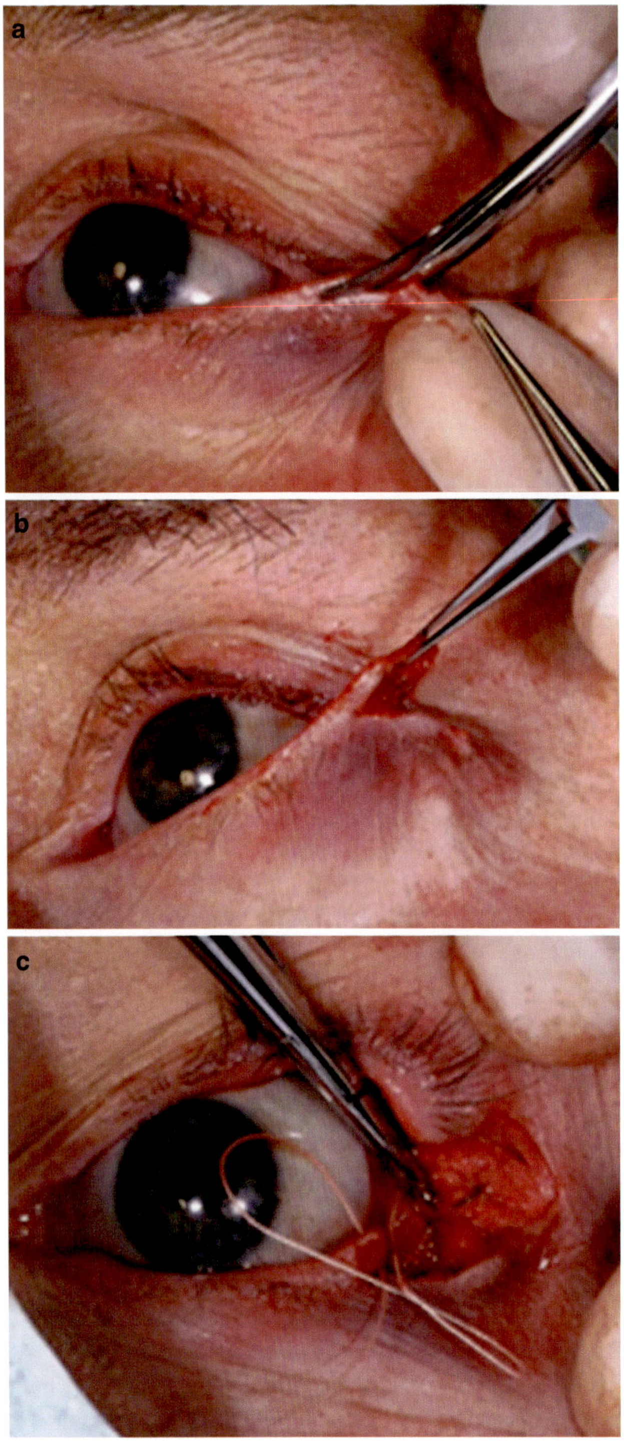

Fig. 11.12 Lateral tarsal strip procedure for horizontal eyelid tightening. (**a**) Lateral canthotomy along the lateral canthal tendon. (**b**) The lid is split along the gray line, and the tarsal strip is formed laterally. (**c**) The tarsal strip is sutured to periosteum along the inner surface of the lateral orbital rim

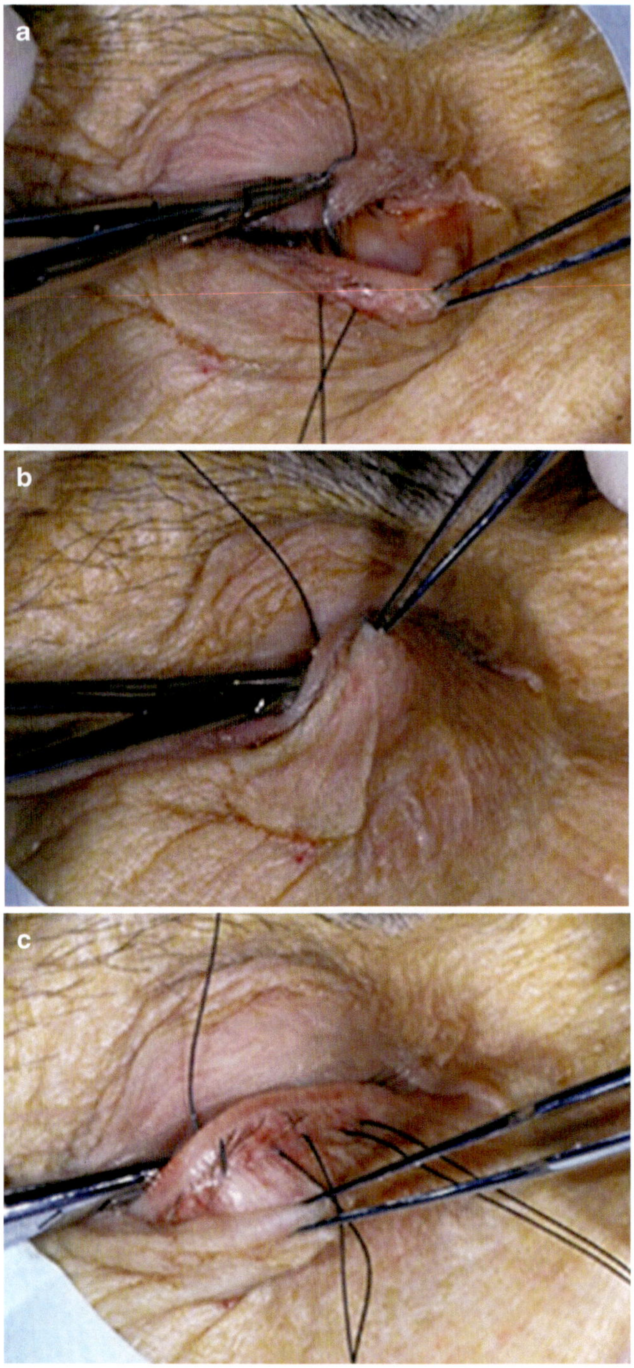

Fig. 11.13 Quickert-Rathbun sutures. (**a**) Three double-armed 6-0 chromic sutures are passed through the conjunctival surface below the tarsus. (**b**) As the needles pass through full-thickness eyelid, they are directed upward closer to the lid margin. (**c**) The needles emerge through the skin just below the lash line and are tied to evert the lid margin

(Fig. 11.13). The advantage of this operation is that it can be performed at the bedside of patients who are unable to undergo a more definitive surgery. However, results tend to be temporary because it does not permanently reattach the tucked retractors to the tarsal plate so that recurrence rates are as much as 50% at 2 years [45].

A more permanent approach to address lower lid retractor dysfunction is with direct open reattachment of the retractor to the tarsal plate. Several minor modifications have been

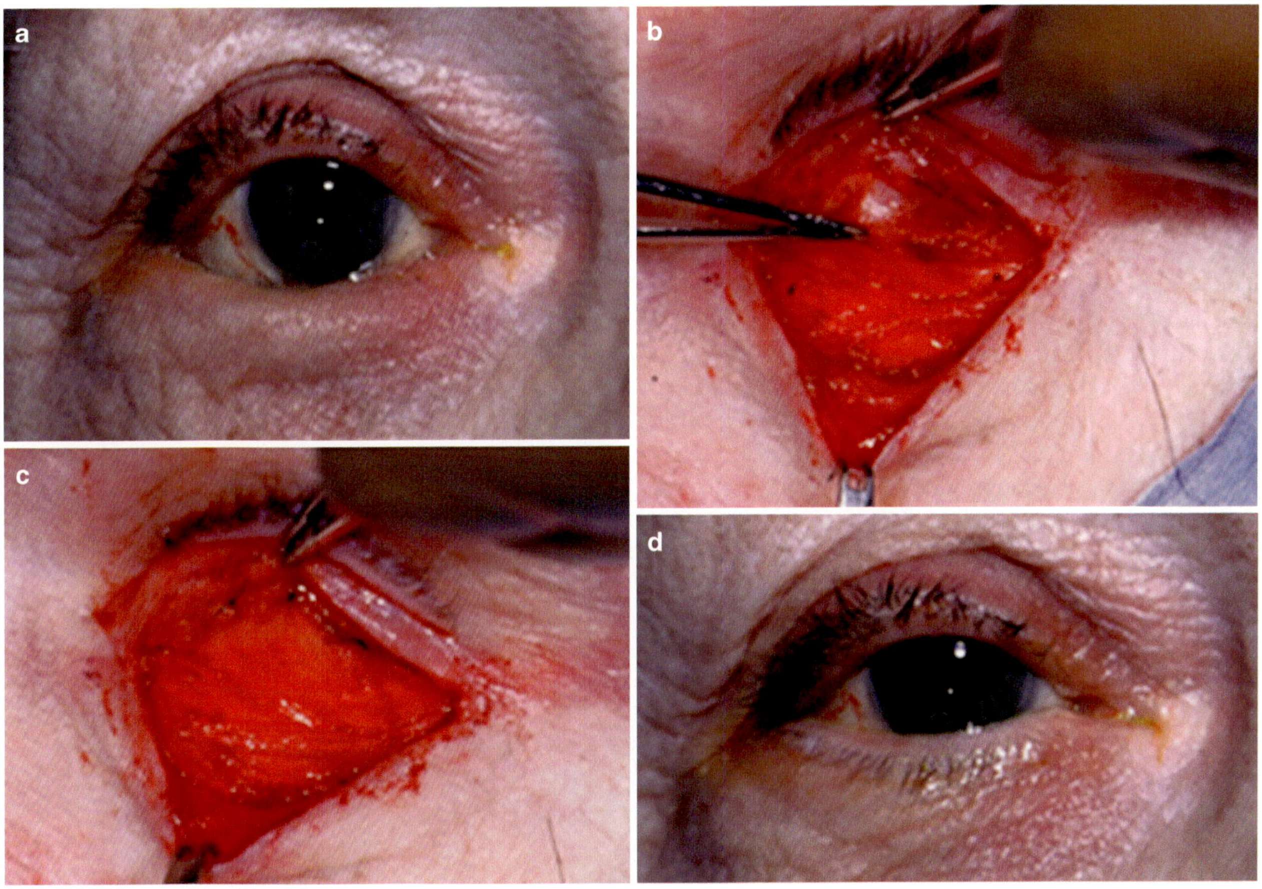

Fig. 11.14 Retractor reinsertion procedure. (**a**) Involutional entropion with outward rotation of the inferior tarsal border. (**b**) Exposure of the disinserted capsulopalpebral fascia. (**c**) The retractor is sutured to the inferior tarsal border. (**d**) Postoperative position of the lower eyelid

described using a variable number of sutures [46, 47], placed through transcutaneous or transconjunctival approach [48, 49]. The procedure involves exposure of the inferior tarsal edge with either shortening or reattachment of the capsulopalpebral fascia directly to the inferior tarsal border (Fig. 11.14). In my experience orbicularis muscle override is a very common associated finding. The eyelid crease is reformed by placing several 7-0 chromic sutures between the preseptal orbicularis and the retractor [3, 50].

In most cases of involutional entropion, some degree of both vertical and horizontal laxities is present simultaneously. This will require a combination of horizontal and vertical tightening [51–53]. In a recent report, Ding et al. introduced an orbicularis transposition procedure in which the pretarsal portion of the muscle is transposed downward to a preseptal positon [54]. This changes the pressure dynamics away from the eyelid margin to the tarsal base. The authors reported a high success rate with less than 5% recurrence.

When orbicularis muscle override is significant in involutional entropion, temporary improvement can be achieved with botulinum toxin into the preseptal orbicularis muscle [55, 56]. This is especially useful in symptomatic patients for whom surgery may not be indicated because of medical issues or for relief while awaiting definitive surgical repair.

Cicatricial Entropion

In cicatricial entropion, there is a shortening of the posterior tarsoconjunctival eyelid lamella relative to the anterior lid surface. The normally balanced anterior and posterior forces shift in favor of the posterior vector. These forces deform the tarsus so that the eyelid margin turns inward toward the globe, even in the absence of any significant horizontal or vertical eyelid laxity. The condition is seen with a variety of cicatricial diseases of the conjunctiva such as ocular cicatricial pemphigoid, Steven-Johnson syndrome, and linear IgA bullous dermatosis [57]. Conjunctival scarring, cicatrization, and symblepharon formation may also result from allergic blepharoconjunctivitis, erythema multiforme, chemical burns, traumatic injuries, and infectious processes such as trachoma and herpes zoster. A number of topical medications are also associated with cicatricial conjunctival contraction.

These include miotics, idoxuridine, timolol, pilocarpine, and dipivefrin (Propine) [58, 59]. Recently prostaglandin periorbitopathy has been recognized, with several patients developing cicatricial entropion [60].

The symptoms associated with cicatricial entropion are similar to those seen from other causes of entropion, with the frequent addition of severe dry eyes due to loss of conjunctival goblet cells and accessory lacrimal glands. If there is significant conjunctival or tarsal scarring and keratinization, significant keratitis, vascularization, and ulceration of the cornea may result.

Correction of cicatricial entropion is aimed at restoration of the eyelid margin to a more normal position. The choice of surgical procedure is dictated by the severity of the deformity, involvement of conjunctiva and/or tarsus, and coexistence of trichiasis or keratinization of the eyelid margin. The health of the patient and their ability to undergo a surgical procedure are also important. A large number of procedures are described, but they all fall into only four basic approaches depending upon the anatomic defect. These include margin rotation, recession of the anterior lamella (Fig. 11.15), lengthening of the posterior lamella, excisional procedures along the eyelid margin, or a combination of all three [61].

In mild cases not associated with appreciable tarsal deformity, removing the lash line alone may be enough to relieve symptoms. The lashes can be removed with cryotherapy or electroablation (Fig. 11.16), but the recurrence rate can be greater than 50% at 1 year [62]. Direct internal eyelash bulb excision is a more definitive method performed through an eyelid crease incision. Dissection is carried in the postorbicular plane to the lash bulbs that are then removed with fine scissors or bipolar cautery [63] (Fig. 11.17). The entire lash-bearing lid margin can also be excised by splitting the lid along the gray line and excising a strip of the anterior lamella containing skin along with the eyelash bulbs [64].

In cases of mild to moderate cicatricial entropion, eyelid margin rotation can be achieved with full-thickness Quickert-Rathbun type sutures [43, 44]. Recession of the anterior skin and muscle lamella may relieve symptoms by moving the lashes and skin away from the lid margin. This is achieved by splitting the lid along the gray line and recessing the skin and muscle [61, 65]. The lash-bearing margin may be resected at the same time [66]. Shortening of the skin lamella with cautery or laser resurfacing to apply gentle outward traction on the tarsus has also been reported to give good results [67, 68].

When the posterior lid surface is severely scarred or deficient, restoration of conjunctiva alone or conjunctiva plus tarsus is indicated. In cases of active cicatricial disease, such as ocular cicatricial pemphigoid, surgery should be delayed until adequate immunosuppression has been achieved. When the major pathology is conjunctival contraction without significant tarsal warping, grafting with oral mucous membrane [69] (Fig. 11.18) or amniotic membrane [70] (Fig. 11.19) can correct the length disparity. Where there is fixed tarsal deformity, a lid margin rotation can be performed using a horizontal blepharotomy with marginal rotation, as with the Wies procedure [71, 72]. Here a full-thickness horizontal tarsotomy incision is carried along the lid and repaired by suturing the anterior skin lamella of the marginal segment to the posterior lamella of the main lid segment. This will rotate the marginal bridge outward (Fig. 11.20). Several minor variations of this technique have been described [73]. The major problem of all of them is that it does not reappose similar

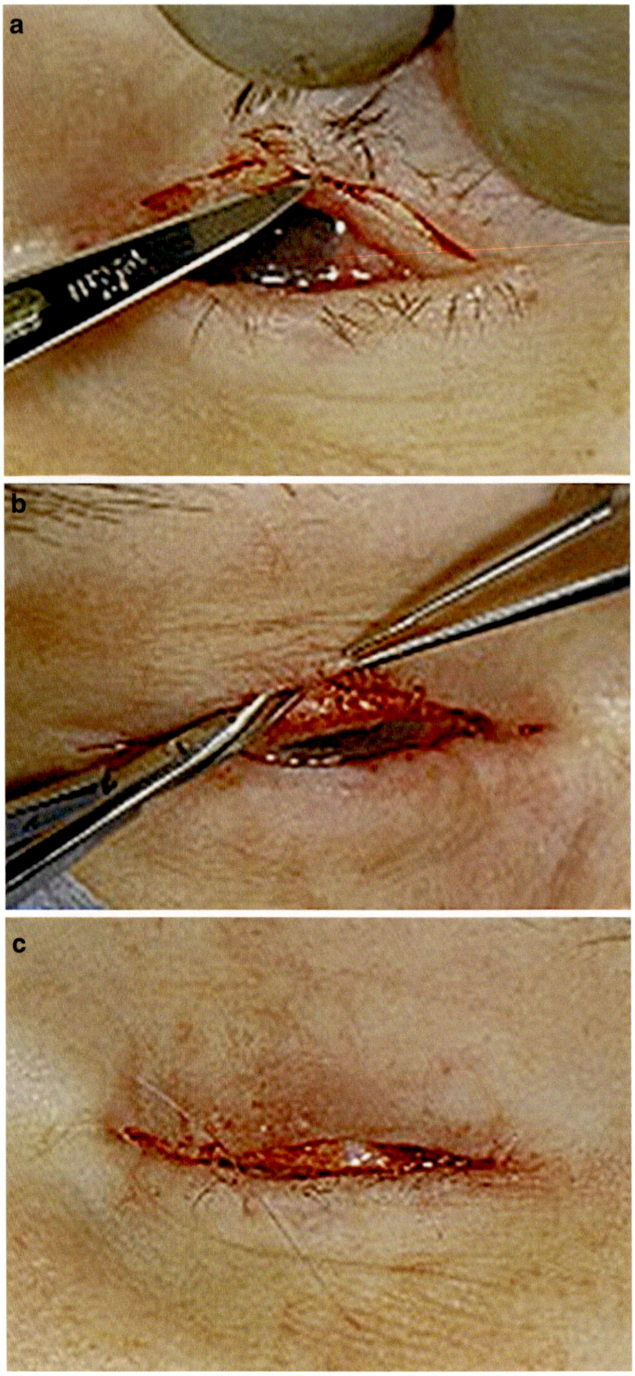

Fig. 11.15 Anterior lamellar recession. (**a**) The lid is split along the gray line to separate anterior and posterior lamellae. (**b**) The anterior lamella is separated upward for a distance of about 10 mm, and a strip of marginal skin and lashes is resected. (**c**) The skin is sutured to the tarsus several mm above the lid margin

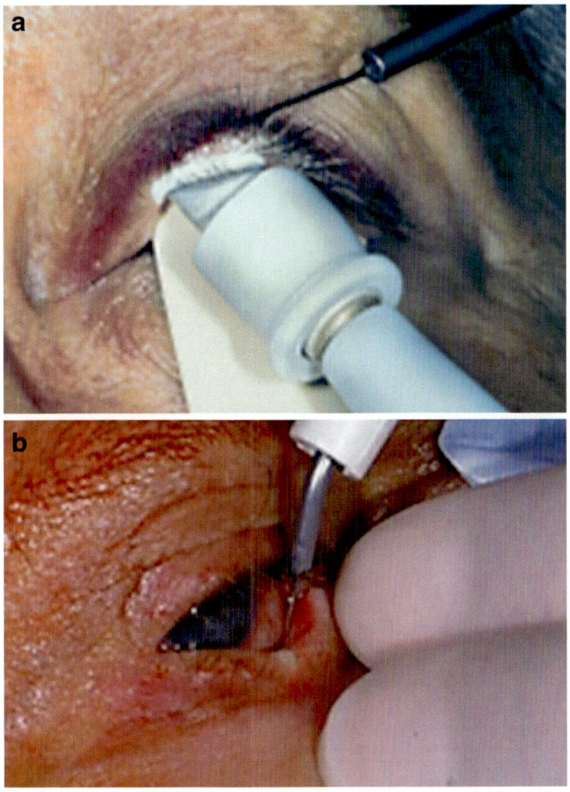

Fig. 11.16 Treatment of trichiatic or distichiatic eyelashes. (a) Cryosurgery of the lid margin. (b) Electrolysis of individual lashes

tissue layers and therefore is not anatomical. Consecutive ectropion is a significant complication requiring reconstruction for correction [74, 75], and recurrence rates as high as 30% have been reported [76]. Dutton et al. [77] described a

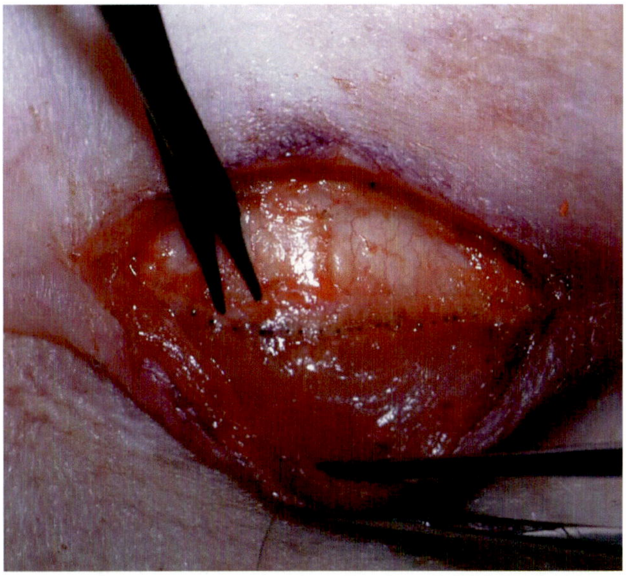

Fig. 11.17 Direct resection of eyelash bulbs. Through a lid crease incision, the anterior lamella is dissected from the tarsal surface to the lid margin, and lash bulbs are individually cauterized or excised

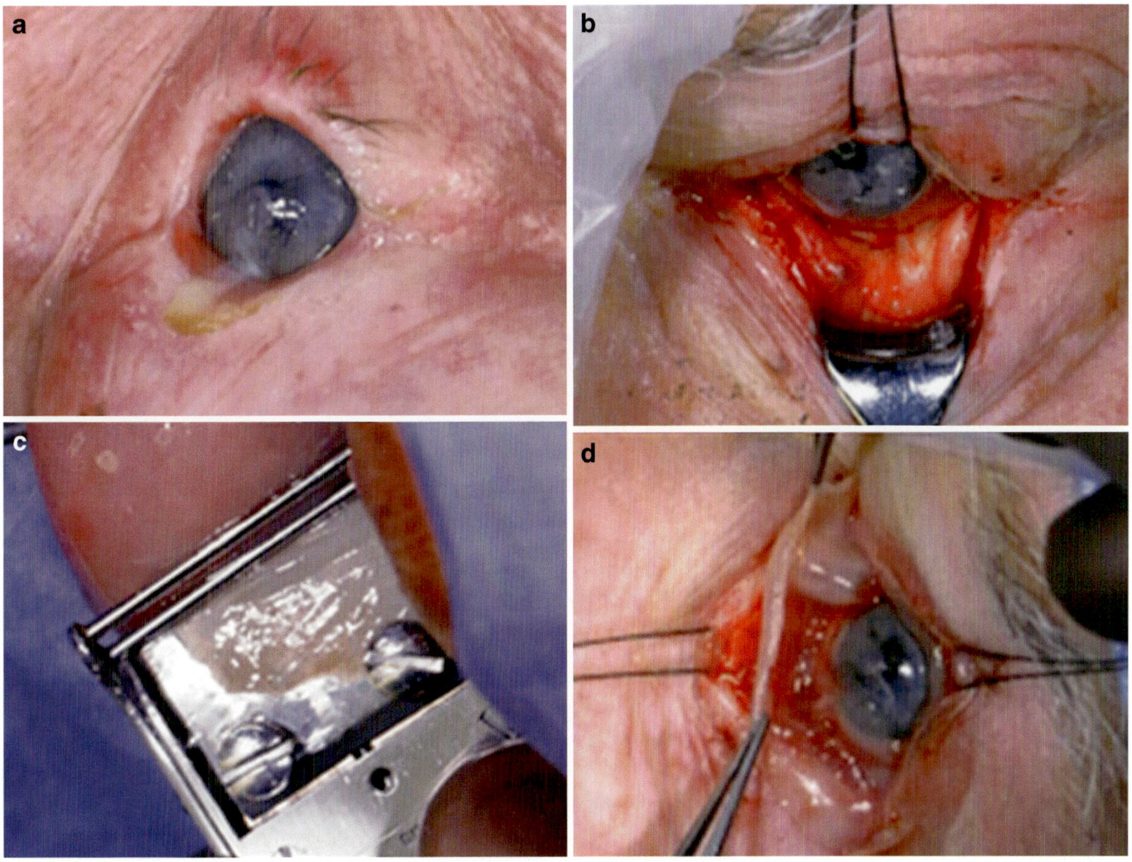

Fig. 11.18 Mucous membrane grafting. (a) Severe loss of conjunctiva from cicatricial disease. (b) The lids are separated from the globe to deepen the fornices. (c) Oral mucosa is harvested from the lower lip. (d) The mucosal graft is sutured to the eyelid and globe to reconstruct the fornices

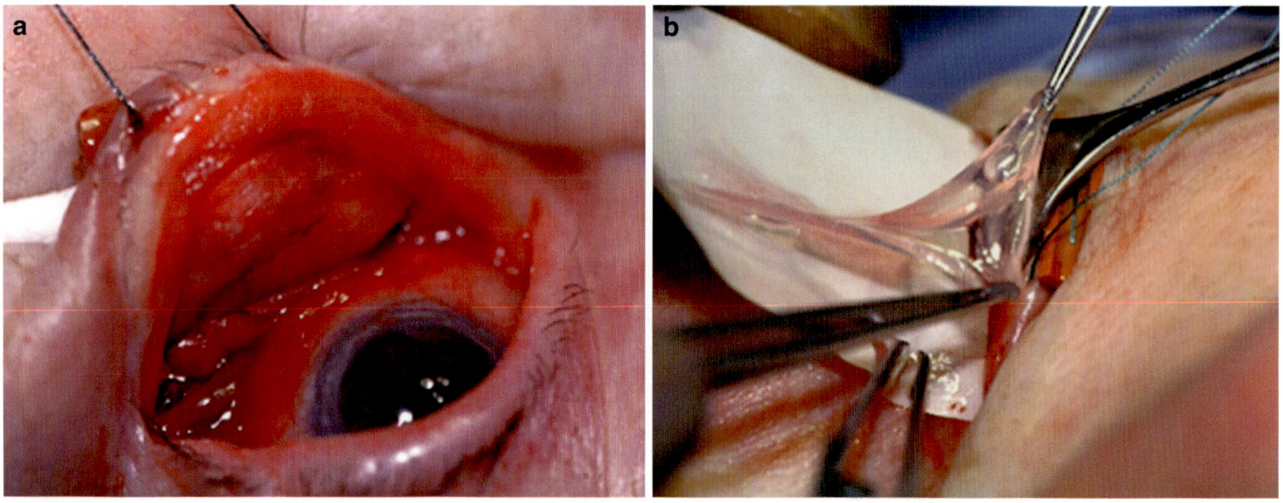

Fig. 11.19 Amniotic membrane resurfacing to reconstruct a shallow fornix. (**a**) The lid is separated from the globe to the desired depth of the fornix. (**b**) Amniotic membrane is sutured to line the exposed surfaces

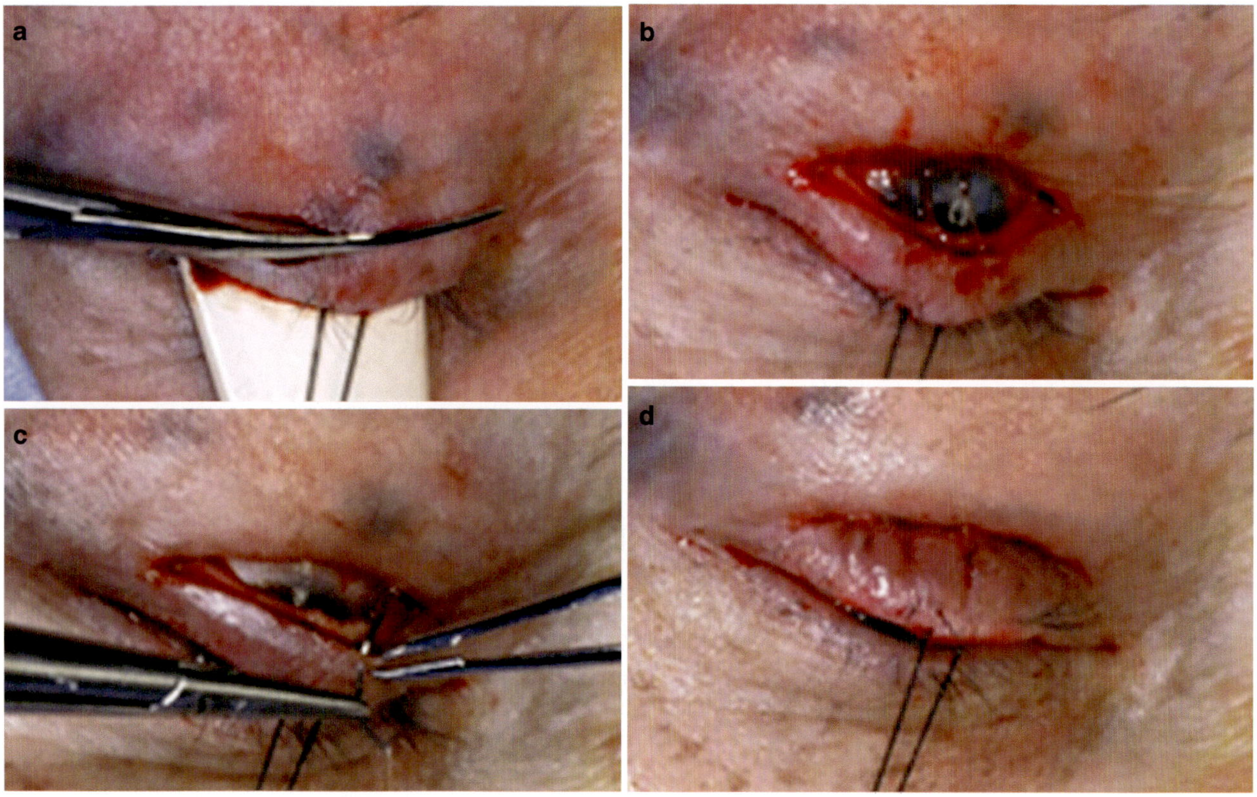

Fig. 11.20 Wies marginal rotation procedure. (**a**) A horizontal incision is started within the tarsus. (**b**) A full-thickness horizontal blepharotomy incision is cut across the upper tarsal plate. (**c**) The skin of the lower wound margin is sutured to the tarsus of the upper wound incision. (**d**) Postoperative position of the eyelid

more anatomic eyelid rotation procedure where a 90% thickness horizontal V-shaped groove is cut along the anterior tarsus. The edges of the V are closed with 6-0 Vicryl sutures that rotate the lid margin forward (Fig. 11.21).

When tarsus is permanently buckled inward and is the principle cause of the entropion, lengthening or reshaping the tarsus is necessary to restore the margin to proper alignment with the corneal surface. This is achieved with a variety of interpositional graft materials that are added to the tarsus. The tarsus can be lengthened with a free tarsoconjunctival graft from the upper or opposite eyelid [3, 78] (Fig. 11.22); hard palate mucosal graft [79, 80] (Fig. 11.23), nasal

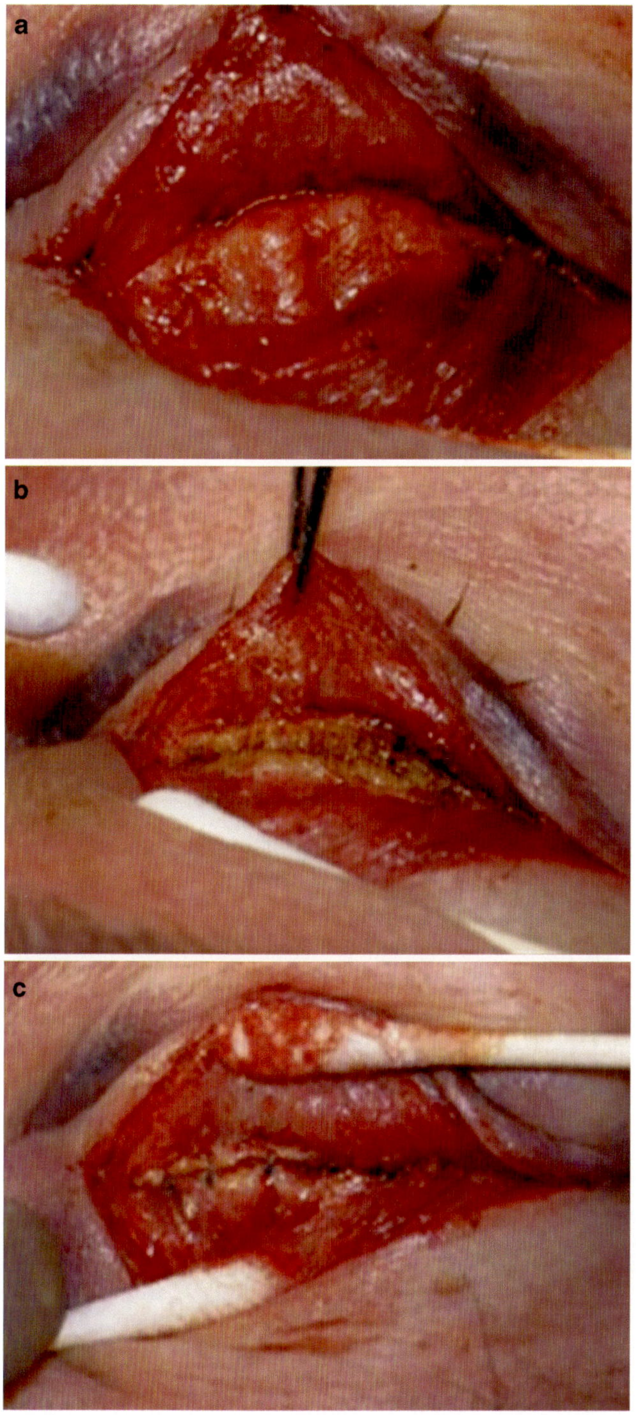

Fig. 11.21 V-groove marginal rotation procedure. (**a**) The anterior tarsal surface is exposed through a lid crease incision. (**b**) A 90% thickness horizontal V-shaped groove is cut across the tarsus. (**c**) Closure of the V edges with 6-0 Vicryl sutures rotates the lid margin outward

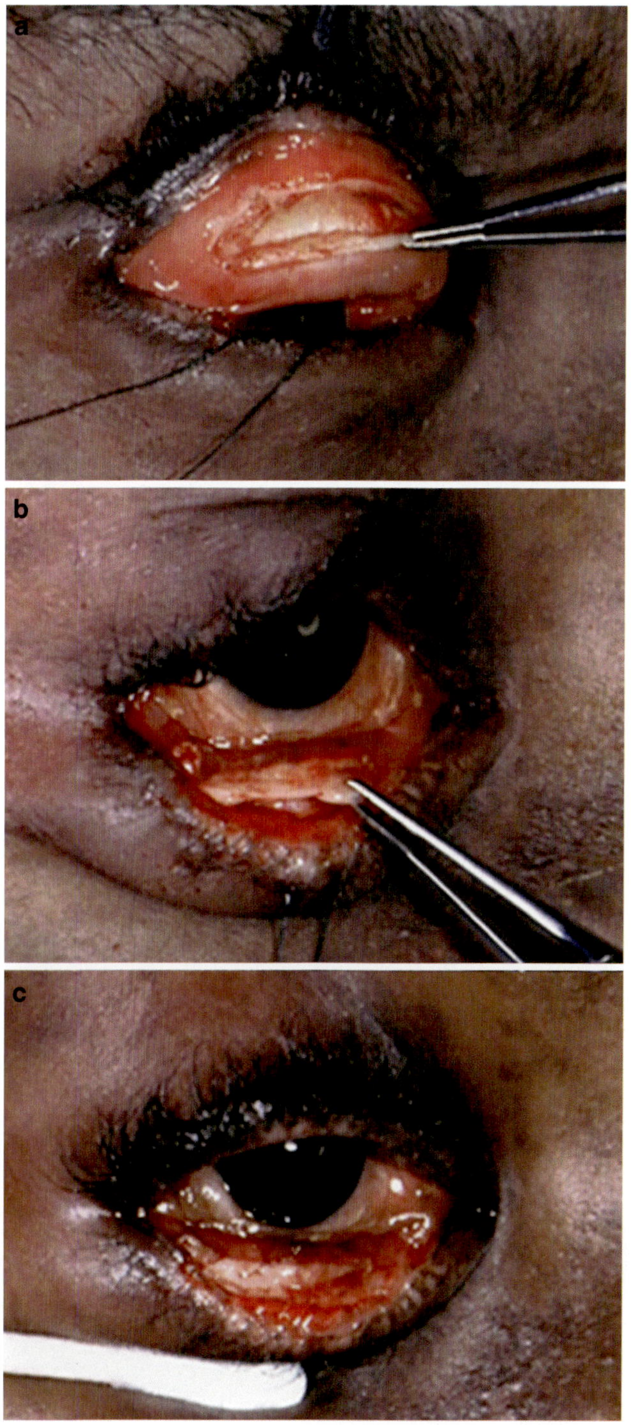

Fig. 11.22 Free tarsoconjunctival graft. (**a**) A block of tarsus and conjunctiva is harvested from the upper eyelid. (**b**) The lower eyelid retractors are separated from tarsus, and the graft is sutured between the tarsus and retractors. (**c**) The graft lengthens the posterior lamella rotating the lid margin outward

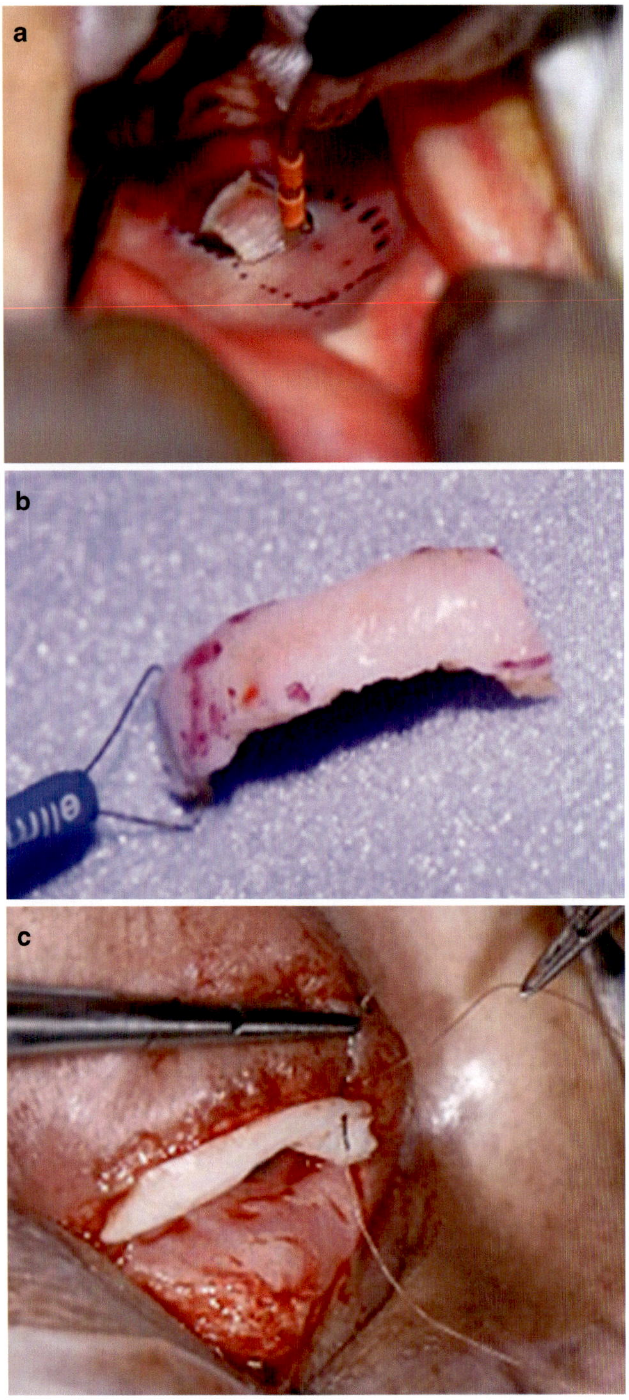

Fig. 11.23 Hard palate mucosal graft. (**a**) A rectangular graft measuring about 5 mm wide by 20–25 mm in length is cut from the hard palate with a radiofrequency wire tip or a scalpel. (**b**) The graft is inspected. (**c**) The graft is sutured into a horizontal space created in the tarsus with the mucosal side toward the cornea

cartilage-mucosal graft [81], scleral graft (Fig. 11.24), or alloplastic material such as acellular human dermis [82–84] may be necessary to achieve adequate lid margin elevation and rotation [78].

Mechanical Entropion

Mechanical entropion is not a category that is often included in the classification of entropion. However, there are several causes that do not easily fit into the usually categories. With these the eyelid anatomy, including the tarsus, canthal tendons, retractors, conjunctiva, and skin, is all normal. The lid margin becomes oriented backward against the globe by factors external to the normal eyelid structures. These include facial or brow involutional changes or inflammatory, infectious, or neoplastic diseases that affect eyelid suspension.

Mass lesions in the anterior eyelid lamella may physically rotate the lid margin inward. These include abscesses, tumors, lid edema, or excess eyelid fat (Fig. 11.25). Dermatochalasis with full upper eyelids or severe brow ptosis may induce a mechanical entropion along with blepharoptosis [85] (Fig. 11.26). This manifests as lateral upper lid entropion seen more common in Asian patients [86]. Mechanical entropion also occurs with excess upper eyelid skin associated with cutis laxa [87–89], eyelid laxity associated with progeria premature aging syndrome [90, 91], and with blepharochalasis [92]. Heydenrych et al. described a trauma case with CSF loculated in the superior orbit and upper eyelid causing a mechanical entropion [93]. Raina et al. reported a case of morbid obesity with full cheeks and lower lids presenting with entropion that could only be managed with extensive tissue and fat debulking [94]. Upper eyelid entropion can sometimes be seen with severe eyelid retraction in Graves' disease. Here the posterior lamella is mechanically pushed inward by the overhanging anterior skin and orbicularis muscle (Fig. 11.27). Lin reported several cases of eyelid retraction and mechanical entropion from aponidine treatment [95]. They suggested that this was more common in Asian patients due to the lower insertion of the orbital septum and more inferior position of the preaponeurotic fat pockets.

Floppy eyelid syndrome (FES) is a condition in which the eyelid, usually the upper, is lax and floppy, associated with papillary conjunctivitis. It occurs more commonly in obese individuals who preferentially sleep with the involved side against a pillow. The lid is horizontally elongated and easily everted especially during sleep. The excess eyelid bulk can cause a mechanical entropion (Fig. 11.28). When it occurs in the lower lid, it most commonly presents with ectropion but can occasionally cause a mechanical type of entropion [96]. FES is repaired with a horizontal shortening of the eyelid, usually with a 10–15 mm wedge resection.

Enophthalmos may be seen with loss of orbital fat, after orbital trauma, following orbital decompression surgery, or with an anophthalmic socket. When significant, the cornea will lay at the level of or posterior to the canthal tendon insertions so that the lid margin inverts toward the globe from purely mechanical relationships (Fig. 11.29). Kersten et al. [97] found no significant difference in exophthalmom-

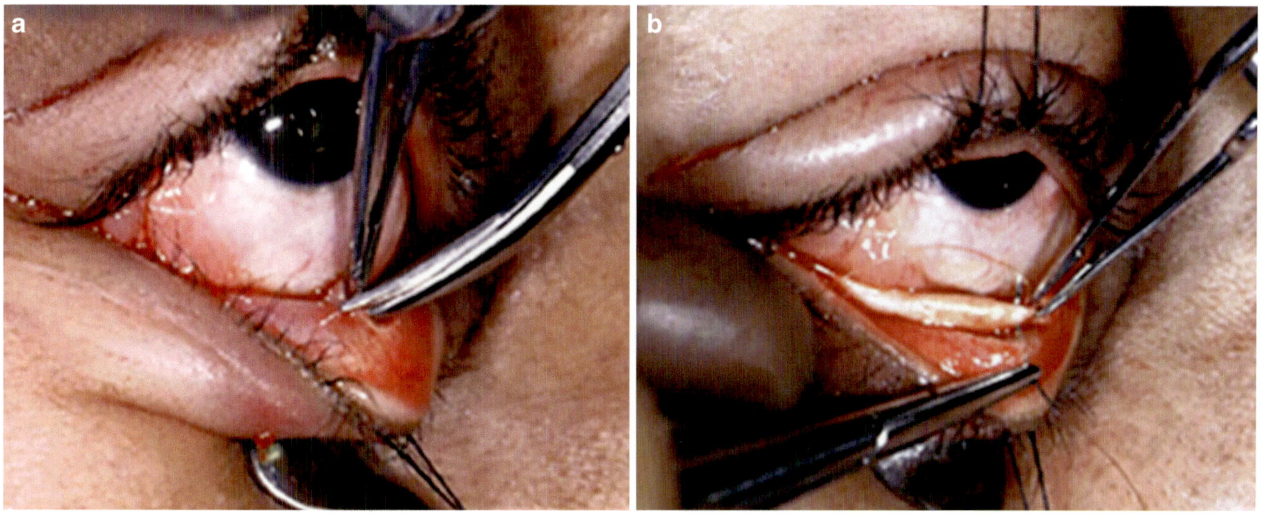

Fig. 11.24 Donor scleral graft. (**a**) The lower lid retractor is separated from the inferior tarsus. (**b**) A donor scleral graft is sutured between the tarsus and retractors

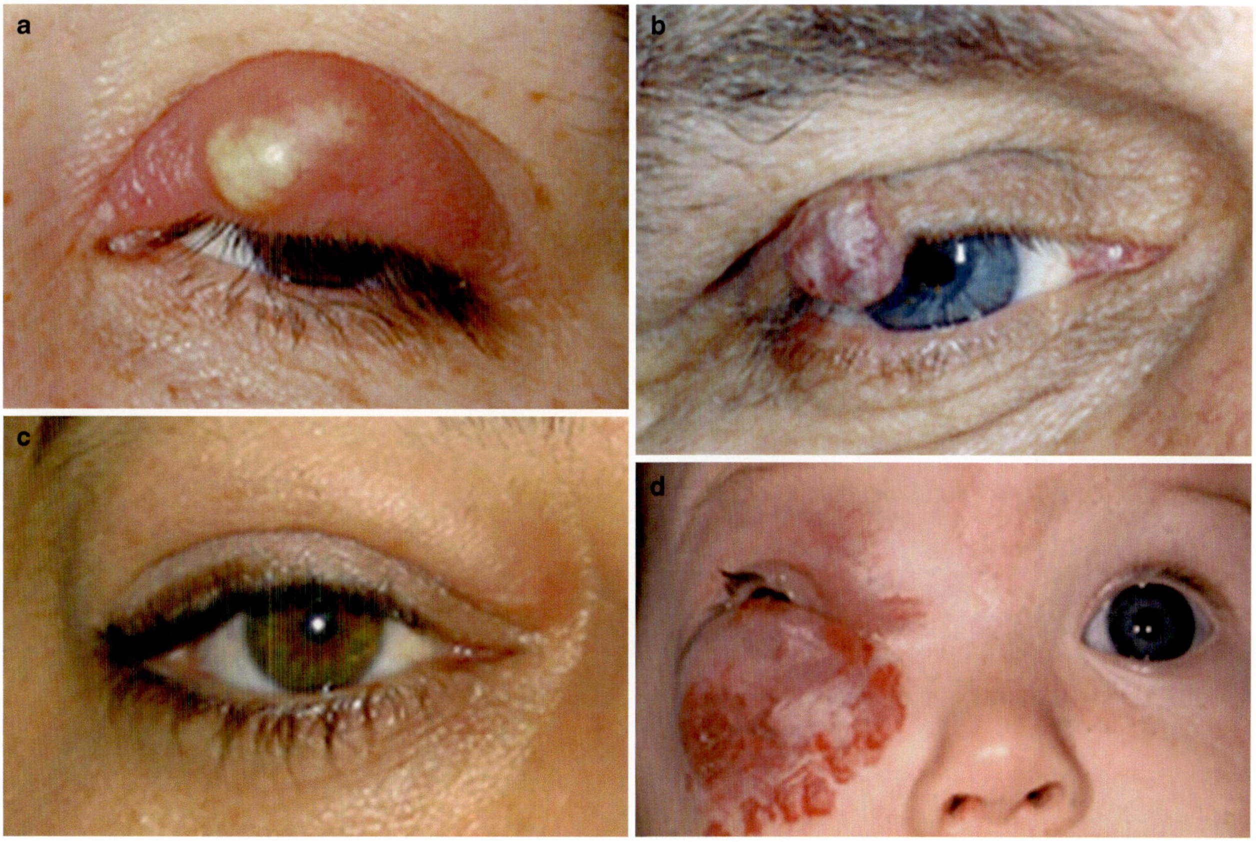

Fig. 11.25 Mechanical entropion. (**a**) Upper eyelid abscess. (**b**) Eccrine nodular adenoma. (Courtesy of Dr. Bettina Meekins). (**c**) Amyloidosis infiltrating the upper eyelid. (**d**) Capillary hemangioma

etry measurements in patient with and without involutional entropion. However, numerous other cases of mechanical entropion have been reported associated with enophthalmos from age-related fat atrophy [98], orbital trauma [99], lymphoma [100], and silent brain syndrome [101, 102].

Another form of marginal eyelid deformity that may be considered a special type of mechanical entropion is sometimes seen after eyelid surgery, particularly in the upper eyelid. This can follow excessive resection of the levator muscle or aponeurosis in congenital ptosis or following placement

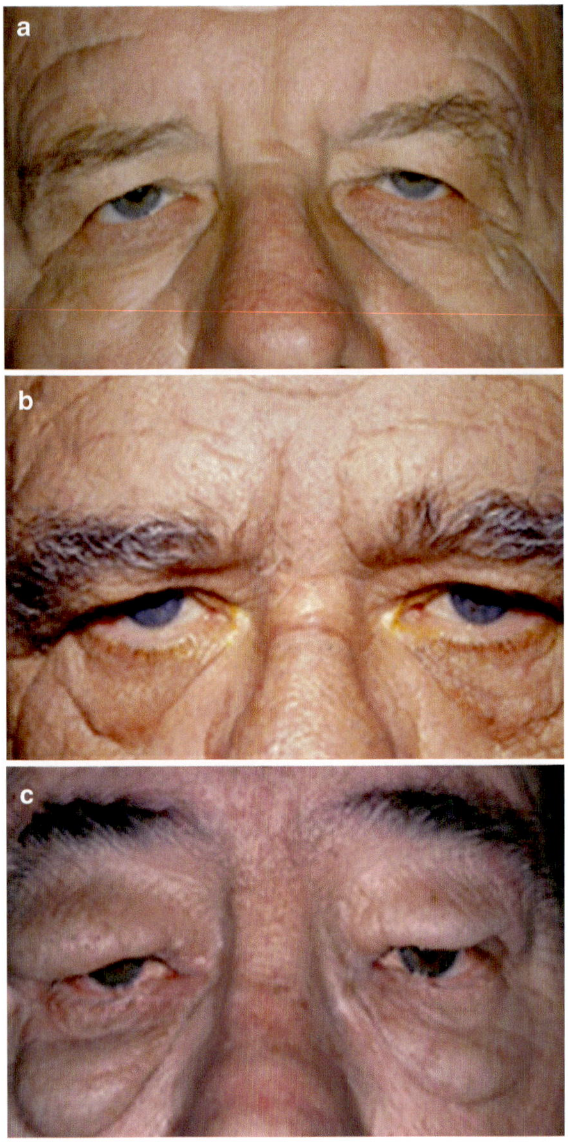

Fig. 11.26 Mechanical entropion. (**a**) Dermatochalasis. (**b**) Severe brow ptosis. (**c**) Chronic lymphedema

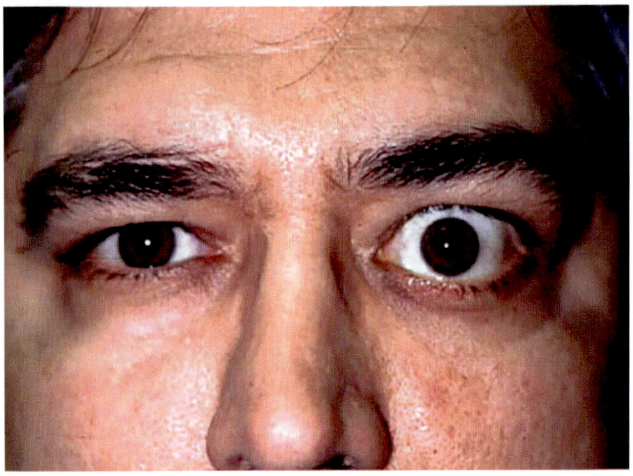

Fig. 11.27 Retraction of the left upper eyelid in Graves' disease with mechanical entropion of the lid margin

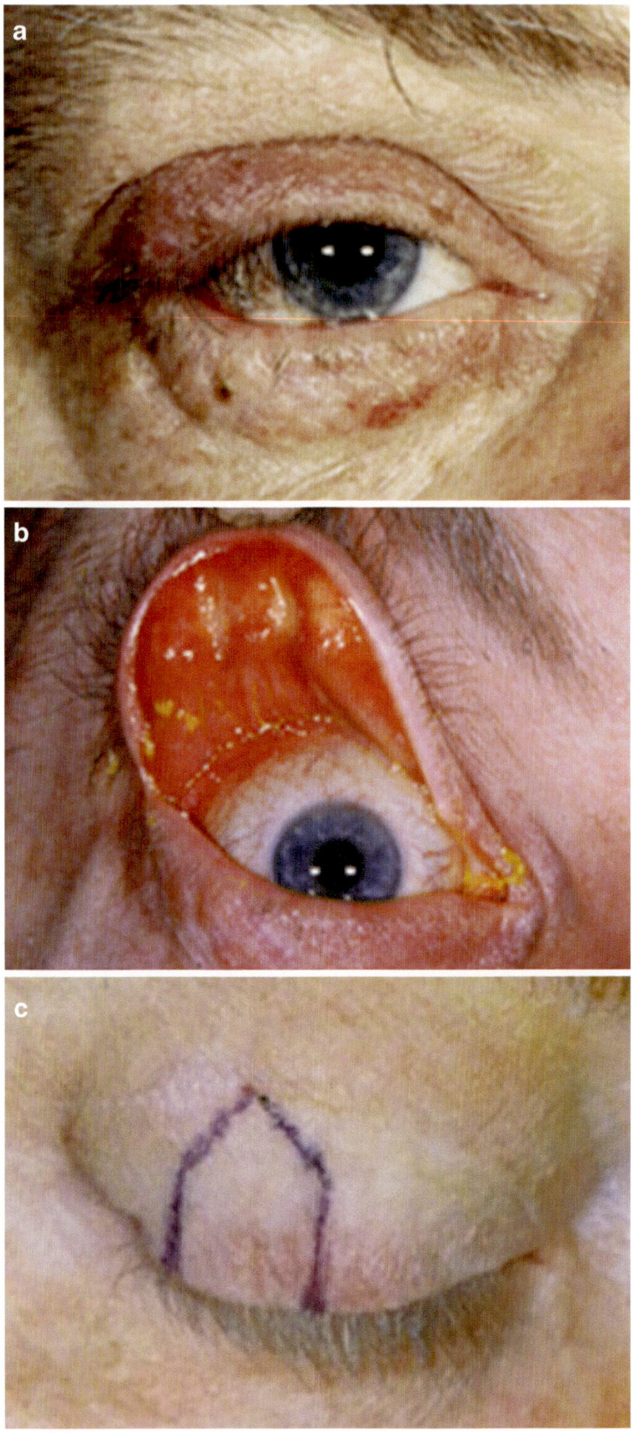

Fig. 11.28 (**a**) Floppy eyelid syndrome with entropion of the right upper eyelid from horizontal eyelid redundancy. (**b**) The eyelid is pulled upward to show the severe laxity. (**c**) The surgical plan marked to resect a wedge for shortening the lid

of the aponeurosis onto the lower mid-tarsus in acquired ptosis cases where the tarsal plate is thin and flexible [103]. The abnormal tension on the tarsus can deform the structure into an entropic configuration. Such cases are corrected by repositioning the aponeurosis to the upper border of the tarsus. In

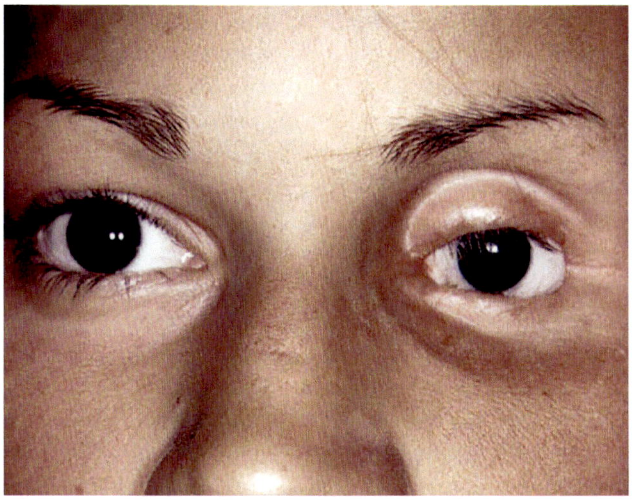

Fig. 11.29 Enophthalmos in an anophthalmic socket with mechanical entropion of the left upper eyelid

congenital ptosis corrected with a frontalis sling, placing the sling too close the upper tarsal border can mechanically rotate the upper tarsus outward and the marginal tarsus inward. In such cases, the elevating vector forces are direct upward and forward as the sling passes over the supraorbital brow ridge.

Goldberg et al. noted medial lower lid entropion in 20% of patients following orbital decompression, particularly those performed through a transantral approach [104]. They suggested that the cause was inferomedial displacement of the muscle cone resulting in transmission of a force vector along the capsulopalpebral fascia that intorts the lid.

Another form of lower eyelid mechanical entropion is associated with epiblepharon [105]. This condition occurs more commonly in young Asian patients, and the condition is more prevalent in patients with a high body mass index where cheek fat is greater [106]. About 90% of cases involve the lower eyelid [107], although a related anomaly can occur in the upper eyelid of Asian children [108]. The defect is caused by the absence or attenuation of the normal fascial adhesions between anterior and posterior lamellae. These normally allow the lamellae to move as a single unit. Without this fixation in patients with epiblepharon, the skin-muscle lamella rides up over the tarsus with a mechanical inward rotation of the eyelashes. This is more pronounced in downgaze when the condition involves the lower lid (Fig. 11.30). While hypertrophy of the orbicularis muscle had been postulated as a cause of this disorder, Kakizaki et al. failed to show any histological evidence of muscle hypertrophy in 41 cases of epiblepharon [109]. More than 50% of patients will show some degree of astigmatism, and 9% will develop amblyopia from this condition [110].

Conservative management is appropriate in younger patients with congenital epiblepharon. The condition usually resolves spontaneously during the second or third years of life associated with facial development. However, repair is necessary when there is significant corneal irritation. In such cases, treatment is done with refixation of the preseptal orbicularis muscle to the underlying capsulopalpebral fascia to form an eyelid crease. This may be achieved with full-thickness Quickert-Rathbun sutures (Fig. 11.30). As mentioned above, such sutures used for entropion in general trend offer only a temporary benefit, but in epiblepharon, the results typically last until the condition corrects itself with age. Woo et al. proposed an internal lamellar fixation procedure without an external crease that they felt was more cosmetically acceptable to Asian patients [111]. When the disorder persists into later childhood or even adulthood, a more permanent crease reformation procedure is preferred (3). Usually this is accomplished with excision of a small horizontal strip of the skin and orbicularis muscle with reformation of the eyelid crease by suturing muscle to the underlying orbital septum or tarsus (Fig. 11.31). Other

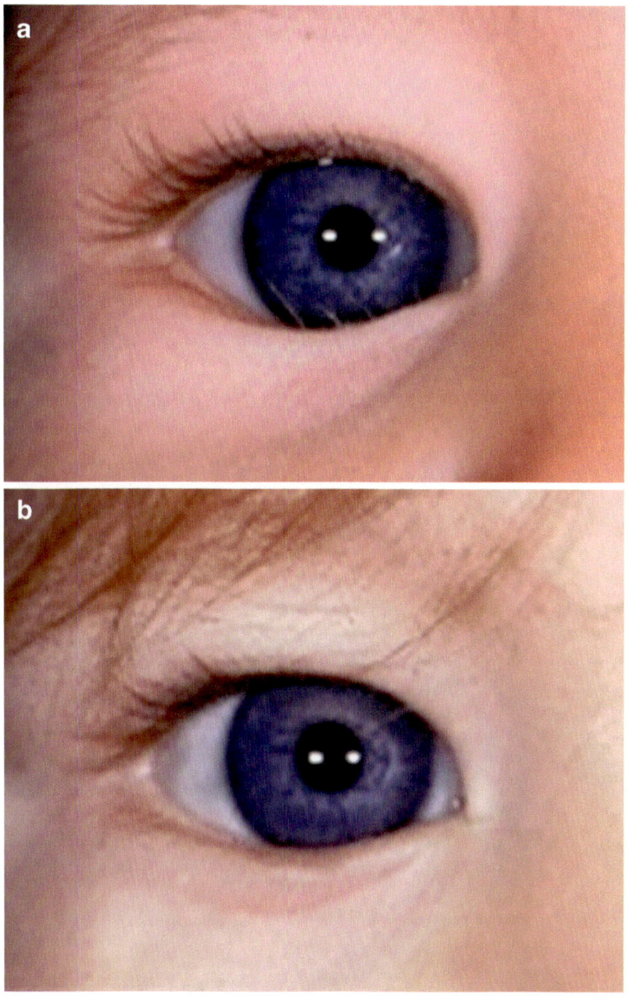

Fig. 11.30 (**a**) Congenital epiblepharon of the lower eyelids. (**b**) Surgical correction with full-thickness Quickert-Rathbun sutures to reform the eyelid crease

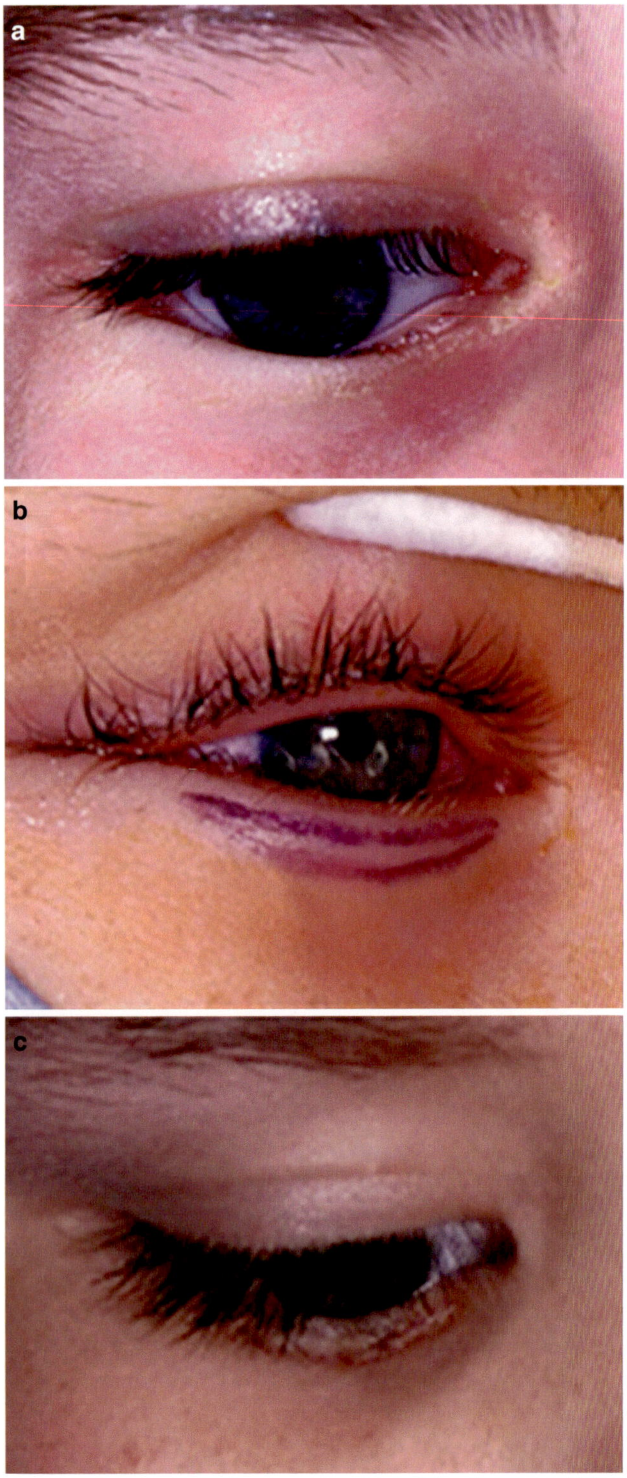

Fig. 11.31 (**a**) Epiblepharon in an older child. (**b**) Planned resection of a narrow horizontal strip of skin and orbicularis muscle. (**c**) The lower eyelid crease is reformed to unite the anterior and posterior lamellae

modifications of crease reformation have been described [112]. One approach is thermal cauterization of the orbital septum just below tarsus to create an adhesion between the septum and orbicularis muscle. In mild cases, eyelash rotation sutures can produce good results [113]. Another procedure is light cautery applied to the inferior tarsus, septum, and orbicularis muscle without rotation sutures [114].

Epicanthal folds are common in patients with epiblepharon. In such cases, an epicanthoplasty is often performed along with the epiblepharon repair. However, Asamura et al. reported good results in many patients, even without the need for simultaneous epicanthoplasty [115]. A less permanent approach was reported with the use of botulinum toxin into the medial lower eyelid orbicularis muscle with improvement of symptoms [116]. Because this condition usually resolves by age 2–3 years, this approach could avoid more invasive surgery, although injections into the lids of young children are not easy.

An acquired form of epiblepharon is seen in patients following eyelid surgery in which a subciliary skin-muscle flap has been elevated and normal fascial attachments related to the eyelid crease have been disrupted. It may also occur spontaneously, associated with involutional changes. Repair consists of reformation of the eyelid crease, generally through a direct skin incision approach.

Management of mechanical entropion must be directed at the source of pathology, with secondary repair of any residual eyelid malposition as necessary. Where there is excess skin or subcutaneous fat, blepharoplasty with or without debulking will help reorient the lid margin.

In some cases, as with benign or malignant mass lesions, resection may entail sacrifice of adjacent normal eyelid tissue. Repair may require some degree of eyelid reconstruction in order to reposition the eyelid into a normal orientation with the globe.

Spastic Entropion

Spastic entropion is an acute reflex spasm of the eyelids produced by hyperactivity of the orbicularis muscle. It is more commonly seen in response to ocular irritation or inflammation following ocular surgery such as cataract procedures [117]. With forced eyelid closure, the orbicularis muscle rides up and rotates the tarsal margin inward. The condition may be predisposed in patients with redundancy or disinsertion of the lower eyelid retractor complex and those with horizontal eyelid laxity. In most cases, this resolves with resolution of the inflammatory condition. Temporary symptomatic relief can be obtained with botulinum toxin into the lower eyelid orbicularis muscle [118].

Medical Therapy

No medical treatment will cure entropion. Some measures, however, can provide a temporizing effect. However, there are situations where surgery is declined by the patient or may not be appropriate because of the patient's general medical health. In addition, medical intervention can alleviate symptoms while the patient waits for definitive surgical repair.

Medical therapies are intended to relieve the discomfort of ocular surface irritation and foreign body sensation. They can also prevent corneal damage from abrasion by eyelashes and eyelid skin. The mainstay of such treatment consists of ocular lubrication with appropriate ointments or with a bandage or scleral contact lens. Treatment of blepharitis is appropriate with lid hygiene, topical antibiotics, and steroids. In some cases of involutional entropion, the lower eyelid can be held in a normal position with tape to the upper cheek. Temporary relief can be achieved with botulinum toxin into the pretarsal orbicularis muscle [55, 118], but this will have to be repeated about every 3 months.

Potential Complications of Surgery for Entropion

Overcorrection

Overcorrection of the eyelid margin or consecutive ectropion may be seen after any marginal rotation procedure (Fig. 11.32). When mild, observation is appropriate since this will often resolve with time. When significant and persistent, the cause is often related to excessive advancement of the capsulopalpebral fascia, reattachment of the retractors too high on the anterior tarsal surface, or uncorrected horizontal eyelid laxity. Including the orbital septum within the retractor sutures will also evert the lid margin. In some cases, revision surgery will be required to reposition the eyelid margin.

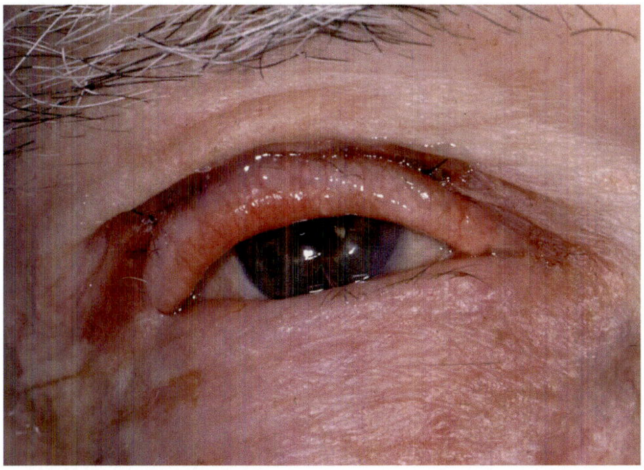

Fig. 11.32 Slight overcorrection of the upper eyelid after entropion repair

Hematoma

There is much controversy regarding the continuation of anticoagulation for minor surgical procedures. Most surgical societies these days recommend continuation of medically indicated anticoagulation for low-risk procedures, such as most eyelid surgeries. For those patients on prophylactic aspirin therapy without specific medical indications, discontinuation 7–10 days prior to surgery is not unreasonable. Intraoperative hemostasis must be assured with meticulous cautery. When an eyelid hematoma does occur, it is usually self-limiting and resolves with conservative management. If bleeding is significant, the wound is re-explored with evacuation of the hematoma and cautery of bleeding vessels. Rarely, a drain may be placed.

Eyelid Retraction

Eyelid retraction without entropion or ectropion can be seen when the eyelid is excessively tightened horizontally or when the capsulopalpebral fascia is tucked too much. It can also follow from incorporation of the orbital septum into the retractor sutures. When recognized early, retraction is corrected with revision of the surgery and replacement of the inappropriate sutures.

Lateral Canthal Angle Rounding or Dystopia

This sometimes occurs with lateral canthal tendon tightening procedures. When the tendon or tarsal strip is sutured to the orbital rim or anterior to it rather than inside the rim, the canthal angle can be pulled away from the globe. Rounding of the canthus occurs if the acute angle is not reformed by suturing the upper and lower lid edges together when repairing the incision.

References

1. Kirkwood BJ, Kirkwood RA. Trichiasis: characteristics and management options. Insight. 2011;36:5–9.
2. Wolfley D. Excision of individual follicles for the management of congenital distichiasis and localized trichiasis. J Pediatr Ophthalmol Strabismus. 1987;24:22–6.
3. Dutton JJ. Atlas of oculoplastic and orbital surgery. Philadelphia: Lippincott Williams & Wilkins; 2013. p. 7–24.
4. Dutton JJ. Atlas of clinical and surgical orbital anatomy. 2nd ed. London: Elsevier Saunders; 2011. p. 129–64.
5. Kakizaki H, Malhotra R, Selva D. Upper eyelid anatomy an update. Ann Plast Surg. 2009;63:336–43.
6. Kakizaki H, Malhotra R, Madge SN, Selva D. Lower eyelid anatomy: an update. Ann Plast Surg. 2009;63:344–51.
7. Kakizaki H, Takahashi Y, Ichinose A, et al. Lateral canthal anatomy: a review. Orbit. 2012;31:279–85.

8. Beigi B, Kashkouli MB, Shaw A, Murthy R. Fornix fat prolapse as a sign for involutional entropion. Ophthalmology. 2008;115: 1608–12.
9. Faria-E-Sousa SJ, de Paula Gomes Vieira M, Silva JV. Uncovering intermittent entropion. Clin Ophthalmol. 2013;7:385–8.
10. Benger R, Musch DC. A comparative study of eyelid parameters in involutional entropion. Ophthal Plast Reconstr Surg. 1989;5: 281–7.
11. Khan IJ, Ghauri AJ, Hodson J, et al. Defining the limits of normal conjunctival fornix anatomy in a healthy south Asian population. Ophthalmology. 2014;121:492–7.
12. Kemp EG, Collin JR. Surgical management of upper lid entropion. Br J Ophthalmol. 1986;70:575–9.
13. Dailey RA, Harrison AR, Hildebrand PL, Wobig JL. Levator aponeurosis disinsertion in congenital entropion of the upper eyelid. Ophthal Plast Recon Surg. 1999;15:360–2.
14. Alsuhaibani AH, Bosley TM, Goldberg RA, Al-Faky YH. Entropion in children with isolated peripheral facial nerve paresis. Eye. 2012;26:1095–8.
15. Tomita K, Tsurui H, Otsuka S, et al. Ocular findings in 304 children with down syndrome. Nihon Ganka Gakkai Zasshi. 2013;117:749–60.
16. Hiles DA, Wilder LW. Congenital entropion of the upper lids. J Pediatr Ophthalmol. 1969;6:157–61.
17. Zak TA. Congenital primary upper eyelid entropion. J Pediatr Ophthalmol Strabismus. 1984;21:69–73.
18. Kettesy A. Entropion in infancy caused by folding of the tarsus; report of a case. Arch Ophthal. 1948;39:640–2.
19. Naik MN, Honavar SG, Bhaduri A, Linberg JV. Congenital horizontal tarsal kink; a single-center experience with 6 cases. Ophthalmology. 2007;114:1564–8.
20. Sires BS. Congenital horizontal tarsal kink: clinical characteristics from a large series. Ophthal Plast Reconstr Surg. 1999;15:355–9.
21. El-Mulki S, Laeson J, Taylor D. A new and simple procedure for correction of congenital tarsal kink. J Pediatr Ophthalmol Strabismus. 1998;35:172–3.
22. Lucci LM, Fukumoto WK, Alvarenga LS. Trisomy 13: a rare case of congenital tarsal kink. Ophthal Plast Reconstr Surg. 2003;19:408–10.
23. Unal M, Tunc M, Konuk O. Severe congenital horizontal tarsal kink without levator aponeurosis disinsertion. Ophthal Plast Reconstr Surg. 2003;19:79–81.
24. McElvanney AM, Adhikary HP, Ridgway AE, et al. Congenital tarsal kink: a rare cause of neonatal corneal ulcers. Eye. 1994;8: 702–3.
25. Demirel S, Firat C, Firat PG. Modified temporary eyelid margin suture for correction of congenital horizontal tarsal kink: a novel surgical technique. Ophthal Plast Reconstr Surg. 2012;29:300–2.
26. Biglan AW, Buerger GF Jr. Congenital horizontal tarsal kink. Am J Ophthalmol. 1980;89:522–4.
27. Tenzel RR, Miller GR, Rubenzik R. Cicatricial upper lid entropion. Treated with banked scleral graft. Arch Ophthalmol. 1975;93:999–1000.
28. McCarthy RW. Lamellar tarsoplasty – a new technique for correction of horizontal tarsal kink. Ophthalmic Surg. 1984;15:859–60.
29. Bosniak S, Hornblass A, Smith B. Re-examining the tarsal kink syndrome: considerations of its etiology and treatment. Ophthalmic Surg. 1985;16:437–40.
30. Aziz S, Bhatt PR, Lavy T, Dutton G. A simple correction for congenital tarsal kink syndrome associated with distichiasis. J AAPOS. 2006;10:281–2.
31. Salour H, Owji N, Razavi ME, Zeaei H. Tarsal kink syndrome associated with congenital corneal ulcer. Ophthal Plast Reconstr Surg. 2003;19:81–3.
32. Price NC, Collin JR. Congenital horizontal tarsal kink: a simple surgical correction. Br J Ophthalmol. 1987;71:204–6.
33. Yuksel D, Kosker M. The surgical treatment of congenital tarsal kink syndrome associated with corneal ulcer. Ophthalmic Surg Lasers Imaging. 2011;42:e126–8.
34. Damasceno RW, Osaka MH, Dantes PE, Belfort R Jr. Involutional entropion and ectropion of the lower eyelid: prevalence and associated risk factors in the elderly population. Ophthal Plast Reconstr Surg. 2011;27:317–20.
35. Bashour M, Harvey J. Causes of involutional ectropion and entropion – age-related tarsal changes are the key. Ophthal Plast Reconstr Surg. 2000;16:131–41.
36. Awan MA, Chandha V, Gonzalez P, et al. Small tarsal plates causing recurrent lower lid entropion in a young adult. Eye. 2009;23:2129–30.
37. Babuccu O. An alternative approach for involutional entropion: a preliminary study. Lasers Med Sci. 2012;27:1009–12.
38. Leibovitch I. Lateral wedge resection: a simple technique for repairing involutional lower eyelid entropion. Dermatol Surg. 2010;36:1412–8.
39. Roberts MA, Baddeley P, Sinclair N, Lane CM. The lower lid diamond: a simple entropion repair to correct both horizontal and lower-lid retractor laxity. Ophthal Plast Reconstr Surg. 2012;28:44–6.
40. Anderson RL, Gordy DD. The tarsal strip procedure. Arch Ophthalmol. 1979;97:2192–6.
41. Della Rocca DA. The lateral tarsal strip: illustrated pearls. Facial Plast Surg. 2007;23:200–2.
42. Olver JM, Barnes JA. Effective small-incision surgery for involutional lower eyelid entropion. Ophthalmology. 2000;107:1982–8.
43. Quickert MH, Rathbun E. Suture repair of entropion. Arch Ophthalmol. 1971;85:304–5.
44. Zoccali G, Orsini G, Giuliani M. Entropion correction using a modified Quickert technique. Graefes Arch Clin Exp Ophthalmol. 2013;251:2821–2.
45. Jang SY, Choi SR, Jang JW, et al. Long-term surgical outcomes of Quickert sutures for involutional lower eyelid entropion. J Craniomaxillofac Surg. 2014;42:1629–31.
46. Park MS, Chi MJ, Baek SH. Clinical study of single-suture inferior retractor repair for involutional entropion. Ophthalmologica. 2006;220:327–31.
47. Caldato R, Launde-Pimentel R, Sabrosa NA, et al. Role of reinsertion of the lower eyelid retractor on involutional entropion. Br J Ophthalmol. 2000;84:606–8.
48. Erb MH, Uzcategui N, Dresner SC. Efficacy and complications of the transconjunctival entropion repair for lower eyelid involutional entropion. Ophthalmology. 2006;113:2351–6.
49. Ben Simon GJ, Molina M, Schwarcz RM, et al. External (subciliary) vs internal (transconjunctival) involutional entropion repair. Am J Ophthalmol. 2005;139:482–7.
50. Kakizaki H, Chan WO, Takahashi Y, Selva D. Overriding of the preseptal orbicularis oculi muscle in Caucasian cadavers. Clin Ophthalmol. 2009;3:243–6.
51. Rabinovitch A, Allard FD, Freitag SK. Lower eyelid involutional entropion repair with lateral tarsal strip and infraciliary rotation sutures: surgical technique and outcomes. Orbit. 2014;33:184–8.
52. Ranno S, Sacchi M, Gilardi D, et al. Retractor plication versus retractor plication and lateral tarsal strip for eyelid entropion correction. Eur J Ophthalmol. 2014;24:141–6.
53. Scheepers MA, Singh R, Ng J, et al. A randomized trial comparing everting sutures with everting sutures and a lateral tarsal strip for involutional entropion. Ophthalmology. 2010;117:352–5.
54. Ding J, Chen F, Zhai W, et al. Orbicularis oculi muscle transposition for repairing involutional lower eyelid entropion. Graefes Arch Clin Exp Ophthalmol. 2014;252:1315–8.

55. Dutton JJ, Fowler AM. Botulinum toxin in ophthalmology. Surv Ophthalmol. 2007;52:13–31.
56. Deka A, Saikia SP. Botulinum toxin for lower lid entropion correction. Orbit. 2011;30:40–2.
57. Carruth BP, Meyer DR. Linear IgA bullous dermatosis: an unusual cause of upper eyelid cicatricial entropion. Ophthal Plast Reconstr Surg. 2013;29:e151–4.
58. McNab AA. Lacrimal canalicular obstruction associated with topical ocular medications. Aust N Z J Ophthalmol. 1998;26:219–23.
59. D'Ostroph AO, Dailey RA. Cicatricial entropion associated with chronic dipivefrin application. Ophthal Plast Reconstr Surg. 2001;17:328–31.
60. Custer PL, Kent TL. Observations on prostaglandin orbitopathy. Ophthal Plast Reconstr Surg. 2016;32:102–5.
61. Malhotra R, Yau C, Norris JH. Outcomes of lower eyelid cicatricial entropion with grey-line split, retractor recession, lateral-horn lysis, and anterior lamella repositioning. Ophthal Plast Reconstr Surg. 2012;28:134–9.
62. Elder MJ, Bernauer W. Cryotherapy for trichiasis in ocular cicatricial pemphigoid. Br J Ophthalmol. 1994;78:769–71.
63. Dutton JJ, Tawfik HA, DeBacker CM, Lipham WJ. Direct internal eyelash bulb extirpation for trichiasis. Ophthal Plast Reconstr Surg. 2000;16:142–5.
64. Wojno TH. Lid splitting with lash resection for cicatricial entropion and trichiasis. Ophthal Plast Reconstr Surg. 1992;8:287–9.
65. Ross AH, Cannon PS, Selva D, Malhotra R. Management of upper eyelid cicatricial entropion. Clin Exp Ophthalmol. 2011;39:526–36.
66. Ahmed RA, Abdelbaky SH. Short term outcome of anterior lamellar repositioning in treating trachomatous trichiasis. J Ophthalmol. 2015;2015:568363.
67. Dunnington JH, Regan EF. Ziegler cautery puncture for noncicatricial entropion. Am J Ophthalmol. 1966;61:1090–2.
68. El-Kasaby HT. Cautery for lower lid entropion. Br J Ophthalmol. 1992;76:532–3.
69. Koreen IV, Taich A, Elner VM. Anterior lamellar recession with buccal mucous membrane grafting for cicatricial entropion. Ophthal Plast Reconstr Surg. 2009;25:180–4.
70. Mameletzi E, Hamedani M, Majo F, Guex-Crosier Y. Clinical manifestations of mucous membrane pemphigoid in a tertiary center. Klin Monatsbl Augenheilkd. 2012;229:416–9.
71. Bleyen I, Dolman PJ. The Wies procedure for management of trichiasis or cicatricial entropion of either upper or lower eyelids. Br J Ophthalmol. 2009;93:1612–5.
72. Rosbach J, Khaleghi-Zand F, Pitz S. Patient satisfaction after transverse blepharotomy (Wies procedure) in the management of senile entropion – a postoperative analysis. Klin Monatsbl Augenheilkd. 2014;231:3–5.
73. Nasr AM. Eyelid complications in trachoma. I. Cicatricial entropion. Ophthalmic Surg. 1989;20:800–7.
74. Cheung D, Sandramouli S. Consecutive ectropion after the Wies procedure. Ophthal Plast Reconstr Surg. 2004;20:64–8.
75. Baylis HI, Cies WA, Kamin DF. Overcorrection of the Wies procedure. Ann Ophthalmol. 1977;9:744–8.
76. Serin D, Buttanri IB, Karslioglu S, et al. The efficacy of the combined procedure in involutional entropion surgery: a comparative study. Korean J Ophthamol. 2013;27:405–8.
77. Dutton JJ, Tawfik HA, DeBacker CM, Lipham WJ. Anterior tarsal V-wedge resection for cicatricial entropion. Ophthal Plast Reconstr Surg. 2000;16:126–30.
78. Stephenson CM, Brown BZ. The use of tarsus as a free autogenous graft in eyelid surgery. Ophthal Plast Reconstr Surg. 1985;1:43–50.
79. Mannor GE, Mathers WD, Wolfley DE, Martinez JA. Hard-palate mucosa graft in Stevens-Johnson syndrome. Am J Ophthalmol. 1994;118:786–91.
80. Swamy BN, Benger R, Taylor S. Cicatricial entropion repair with hard palate mucous membrane graft: surgical technique and outcomes. Clin Exp Ophthalmol. 2008;36:348–52.
81. Wójcicki P, Kobus K. Treatment of entropion using mucous membrane and cartilage grafts from the nasal septum. Klin Ocz. 2006;108:431–3.
82. Chen J, Wang Z, Gu J. Management of cicatricial entropion of the upper lid using acellular human dermal allograft. J Plast Reconstr Aesthet Surg. 2008;61:610–4.
83. Gu J, Wnag Z, Sun M, et al. Posterior lamellar eyelid reconstruction with acellular dermis allograft in severe cicatricial entropion. Ann Plast Surg. 2009;62:268–74.
84. Bee YS, Alonzo B, Ng JD. Review of AlloDerm acellular human dermis regenerative tissue matrix in multiple types of oculofacial plastic and reconstructive surgery. Ophthal Plast Reconstr Surg. 2014; Epub ahead of print.
85. Cho WK, Park JW, Park MR. Surgical correction of Hallermann-Streiff syndrome: a case report of esotropia, entropion, and blepharoptosis. Korean J Ophthalmol. 2011;25:142–5.
86. Camera JG, Nguyen LT, Sangalang-Chuidian M, et al. Involutional lateral entropion of the upper eyelid: a new physical finding in Asian patients. Arch Ophthalmol. 2002;120:1682–4.
87. Al-Faky YH, Salih MA, Mubarak M, Al-Rikabi AC. Bilateral congenital entropion with cutis laxa. Pediatr Dermatol. 2014;31:e82–4.
88. Shah-Desai SD, Collins AL, Tyers AG. Surgical correction of entropion and excess upper eyelid skin in congenital cutis laxa: a case report. Orbit. 1999;18:53–8.
89. Ma'luf RN, Ghazi N, Ghanim MN, Tawal AN. Involutional type entropion in a child with cutis laxis. Br J Ophthalmol. 2000;84:1432–3.
90. Yazici B, Toka F, Cömez AT. Anatomical characteristics and surgical treatment of bilateral congenital upper eyelid entropion in an infant with neonatal progerioid syndrome. Ophthal Plast Reconstr Surg. 2014;30:e164–6.
91. Shah-Desai S, Sandy C, Collin R. Lax eyelid syndrome or 'progeria' of eyelid tissues. Orbit. 2004;23:3–12.
92. Collin JR. Blepharochalasis. A review of 30 cases. Ophthal Plast Reconstr Surg. 1991;7:153–7.
93. Heydenrych LG, Aldous CM, Giles R, et al. Cerebrospinal fluid in the upper eyelid: an "abscess" of a different kind. Ophthalmology. 2014;132:1485–6.
94. Raina J, Foster JA. Obesity as a cause of mechanical entropion. Am J Ophthalmol. 1996;122:123–5.
95. Lin SL, Liang SS. Evaluation of adverse reactions of aponidine hydrochloride ophthalmic solution. J Ocul Pharmacol Ther. 1995;11:267–78.
96. McNab AA. Floppy eyelid syndrome and obstructive sleep apnea. Ophthal Plast Reconstr Surg. 1997;13:98–114.
97. Kersten RC, Hammer BJ, Kulwin DR. The role of enophthalmos in involutional entropion. Ophthal Plast Reconstr Surg. 1997;13:195–8.
98. Fonseca Junior NL, Lucci LM, Rehder JR. The role of senile enophthalmos in involutional entropion. Arq Bras Oftalmol. 2007;70:6306.
99. Chen CT, Huang F, Chen YR. Management of posttraumatic enophthalmos. Chang Gung Med J. 2006;29:251–61.
100. Beden U, Sonmez B, Kandemir B, Erkan D. Bilateral simultaneous primary orbital lymphoma presenting with unilateral enophthalmos. Ophthal Plast Reconstr Surg. 2008;24:145–7.
101. Bernardini FP, Rose GE, Cruz AA, Priolo E. Gross enophthalmos after cerebrospinal fluid shunting for childhood hydrocephalous: the "silent brain syndrome". Ophthal Plast Reconstr Surg. 2009;25:434–6.

102. Chen JJ, Cohen AW, Wagoner MD, Allen RC. The "silent brain syndrome" creating a severe form of the "giant fornix syndrome". Cornea. 2012;31:1065–7.
103. Shafi FK, Mehta P, Ahluwalia HS. Upper lid entropion post ptosis correction: is tarsal buckling the cause? Orbit. 2012;31: 246–8.
104. Goldberg RA, Christenbury JD, Shorr N. Medial entropion following orbital decompression for dysthyroid ophthalmopathy. Ophthal Plast Reconstr Surg. 1988;4:81–5.
105. Levitt JM. Epiblepharon and congenital entropion. Am J Ophthalmol. 1957;44:112–3.
106. Hayasaka Y, Hayasaka S. Epiblepharon with inverted eyelashes and high body mass index in Japanese children. J Pediatr Ophthalmol Strabismus. 2005;42:300–3.
107. Kim JS, Jin SW, Hur MC, et al. The clinical characteristics and surgical outcomes of epiblepharon in korean children: a 9-year experience. J Ophthalmol. 2014;2014:156501.
108. Choo CT, Chan CM, Fong KS. Surgical management of upper lid epiblepharon. Eye. 1998;12:623–6.
109. Kakizaki H, Takahashi Y, Kang H, et al. No histological evidence of orbicularis oculi muscle hypertrophy in congenital epiblepharon. Clin Exp Ophthalmol. 2013;41:167–71.
110. Peechawal P, Amrith S, Wong I, Sundar G. Refractive changes in epiblepharon. Am J Ophthalmol. 2007;143:835–9.
111. Woo KI, Yi K, Kim YD. Surgical correction for lower li epiblepharon in Asians. Br J Ophthalmol. 2000;84:1407–10.
112. Wladis EJ. Transconjunctival epiblepharon repair. Ophthal Plast Reconstr Surg. 2014;30:271–2.
113. Lee H, Park M, Lee TE, Baek S. Surgical correction of epiblepharon using thermal cauterization of the orbital septum and lash-rotating sutures. J Craniofac Surg. 2010;21:1069–71.
114. Chang M, Lee TS, Yoo E, Baek S. Surgical correction for lower lid epiblepharon using thermal contraction of the tarsus and lower lid retractor without lash rotating sutures. Br J Ophthalmol. 2011;95:1675–8.
115. Assamura S, Kakizaki H, Shindou E, et al. What is the best strategy for Asians with involutional entropion? J Craniofac Surg. 2014;25:972–5.
116. Chen CY, Nava-Castaneda A. Successful treatment of lower eyelid epiblepharon by injection of botulinum toxin A in patients under two years old. Nepal J Ophthalmol. 2013;5:177–81.
117. Levine MR, Enlow MK, Terman S. Spastic entropion after cataract surgery. Ann Ophthalmol. 1992;24:195–8.
118. Winterhoff J, Köhler S, Laskawi R. Botulinum toxin for the treatment of spastic entropion. Case report. HNO. 2013;61:665–7.

Lower Eyelid Ectropion and Retraction

12

Adam J. Cohen

Lower eyelid ectropion is a common albeit complex issue in some cases and stems from a variety of etiologies.

The most common ectropion, involutional (age-related), results from horizontal eyelid laxity stemming from canthal tendon and pretarsal orbicularis weakness.

Congenital ectropion mostly involves the lower eyelid and occurs infrequently and is secondary to vertical shortening of anterior lamellar segment. Microphthalmos, buphthalmos, blepharophimosis, Down syndrome, and ichthyosis can be related to congenital ectropion.

Cicatricial ectropion is secondary to anterior and/or posterior lamellar scarring. This type of ectropion usually occurs with eyelid retraction and warrants repair of both the ectropion and retraction to have a satisfactory surgical outcome. Postsurgical changes, trauma, burns, and chronic integument inflammation are the most common etiologies.

Mechanical ectropion may occur with lid tumors, such as neurofibromas, that evert the lower lid pulling it away from the globe.

Neuropraxic ectropion is a secondary cranial nerve dysfunction with secondary orbicularis oculi weakening. Etiologies such as Bell's palsy, posterior fossa tumors, otic herpes zoster infection, parotid neoplasia, and iatrogenic following surgery.

Anatomy

The orbicularis oculi muscle (OOM) function is a key component of eyelid position homeostasis. The OOM is described as having orbital and palpebral sections with the palpebral section further delineated into preseptal and pretarsal.

Laterally the pretarsal OOM attaches to the lateral orbital tubercle via the lateral canthal tendon. This tendon plays a key role in eyelid position, hence the use of lateral strip in the overwhelming cases of lower eyelid repositioning.

Medially the frontal process of the maxilla serves as the anchoring site for anterior pretarsal OOM via the anterior crus of the medial canthal tendon, while the posterior pretarsal orbicularis inserts into the posterior lacrimal crest. The small strip of pretarsal muscle at the lid margin forms the gray line and is also known as the muscle of Riolan.

Evaluation

Patients can present with epiphora secondary to decreased tear pump function resultant from punctal malposition and eyelid laxity, ectropion, entropion, and retraction. Additionally patients may experience ocular irritation and keratopathy secondary to lagophthalmos and have aesthetic concerns.

Lower eyelid laxity can be ascertained with the snap test. A lower eyelid with normal laxity should snap back into normal immediately when down and away from the eye. The more delayed in returning to a normal position, the more lax the eyelid. Usually grading is 0–4, with 0 as normal and 4 as severe laxity.

Lateral canthal laxity can be assessed by stretching the eyelid medially – if the lateral canthal is displaced medially by more than 2 mm, this is considered abnormal. A grading system of 0–4 is used similar to the snap test.

Medial canthal laxity is tested by lateral displacement of the eyelid. If more than 1 mm of displacement of the punctum is found, this is considered abnormal. Again a grading system of 0–4 is used.

If patients present with epiphora and nasolacrimal duct patency is found pointing to the etiology of tear pump dysfunction, then a dye disappearance test is useful to confirm tear pump failure once dry eye or keratopathy has been excluded.

Examination should include measurement of marginal reflex distances (MRD) 1 and most importantly 2. Lower

A. J. Cohen (✉)
Eyelid & Facial Plastic and Reconstructive Surgery, Chicago and Glenview, IL, USA
e-mail: acohen@theartofeyes.com

A. J. Cohen, C. N. Burkat (eds.), *Oculofacial, Orbital, and Lacrimal Surgery*, https://doi.org/10.1007/978-3-030-14092-2_12

eyelid retraction option accompanies ectropion; hence, the MRD2 is essential as is determining if lagophthalmos exists.

Inspection of the anterior lamella is crucial to detect the amount of skin deficiency so that a myocutaneous cheek flap or skin graft may be considered for repair of the ectropion and retraction.

The posterior lamella should be inspected for cicatricial changes and conjunctival scarring. If present, placement of a posterior lamellar graft and or fornix reconstruction may be necessary for maximal repair.

Ectropion and retraction following eyelid surgery may be the result of internal eyelid scarring. This middle scarring usually occurs between the lower eyelid retractors and septum. Removal of this scar tissue is often necessary for maximal eyelid repositioning.

Treatment

Management of ectropion is usually surgical, but the use of preoperative topical and injectable steroids may be indicated if cicatricial changes exist.

The most commonly used surgical procedure is lateral canthoplasty for horizontal tightening of the eyelid (Fig. 12.1a–c). The surgeon should be cognizant of eyelid retraction that can worsen following lateral canthoplasty or proptosis that can lead to iatrogenic retraction.

Other procedures such as bipolar conjunctival coagulation is ideal for localized medial ectropion or ectropion with a diffusely floppy tarsus. This modality can be used with or without eyelid tightening procedures (Fig. 12.2a–c). A medial spindle procedure and permanent medial tarsorrhaphy are options with later less favored because of aesthetic issues. Whichever technique is employed, care must be taken to avoid damage to the lacrimal system; a lacrimal probe passed through the proximal lacrimal system into the nasolacrimal sac can aid in localization for avoidance of lacrimal structures.

Tarsorrhaphy can be used as a temporary or permanent procedure for repair of ectropion in selected patients. Temporary tarsorrhaphy is often used during used of a skin graft or placement of posterior lamellar graft for placing the eyelid on cephalad stretch.

If the ectropion is due to an anterior lamellar deficiency, retraction and cicatricial changes are usual. If mild deficiency exists, a myocutaneous cheek advancement flap with periosteal and/or drill-hole fixation (Fig. 12.3) can be used for addressing the deficiencies. If moderate to severe tissue deficiency exists, a full-thickness skin graft is necessary for correction of the malposition. Both the myocutaneous flap and skin graft are usually combined with a lateral canthoplasty and temporary tarsorrhaphy that is opened in 5–7 days to optimize eyelid repositioning (Fig. 12.4a–d).

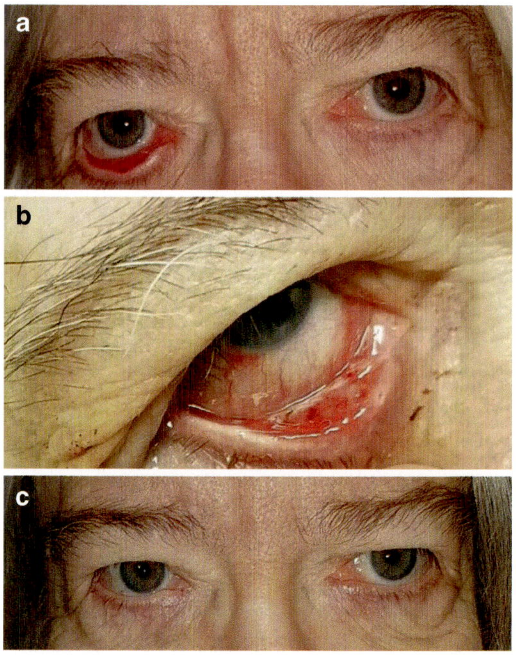

Fig. 12.2 (**a**) Right lower eyelid ectropion secondary to diffuse tarsal laxity. (**b**) Conjunctival wounds following bipolar coagulation and lateral canthoplasty. (**c**) Right eyelid following lateral canthoplasty and bipolar tarsal conjunctival bipolar coagulation

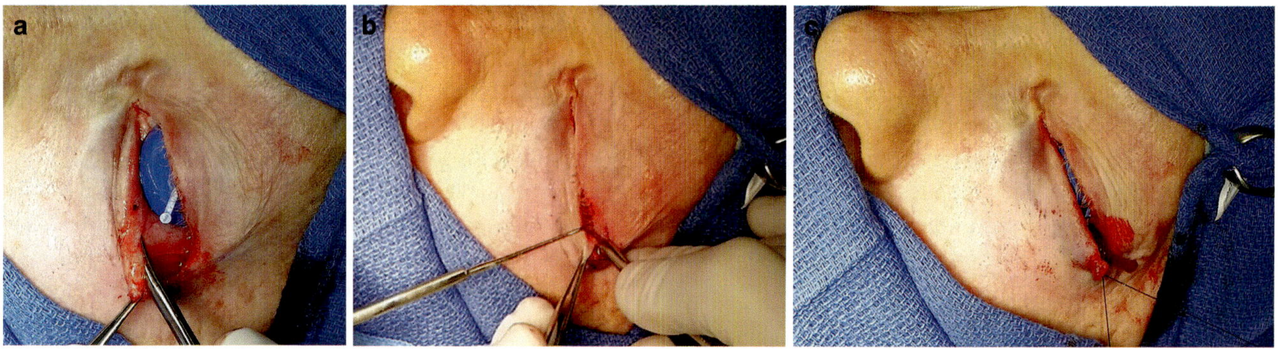

Fig. 12.1 (**a**) Cantholysis following canthotomy. (**b**) Creation of lateral tarsal strip. (**c**) Suture passed in horizontal mattress fashion through lateral tarsal strip

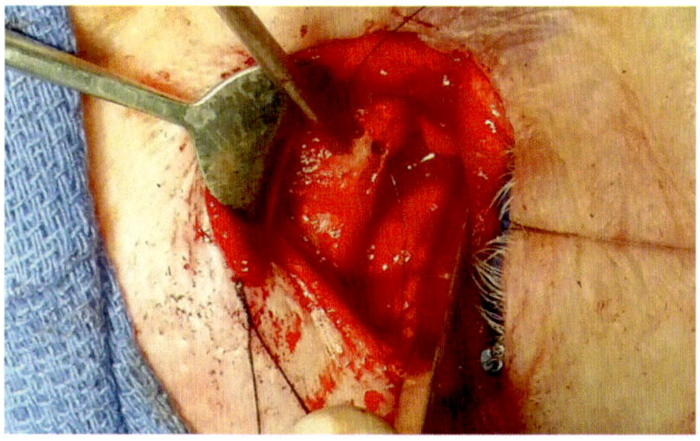

Fig. 12.3 Anterior maxillary face/inferior orbital rim drill with passage of suture for fixation of myocutaneous cheek flap

If cicatricial eyelid margin changes are present with posterior lamellar scarring and deficiency, a posterior lamellar graft is necessary with or without an amniotic tissue overlay. Grafting material options are numerous including hard palate, nasal turbinate, conchal cartilage, and various allogenic materials composed of decellularized extracellular matrix scaffolding (Fig. 12.5a–c).

Complications included persistent eyelid malposition, tearing, prolonged edema, and lagophthalmos. Other issues include symblepharon formation and keratopathy secondary to mechanical irritation from exposed forniceal sutures or graft malposition. Skin graft necrosis and rarely blindness can occur.

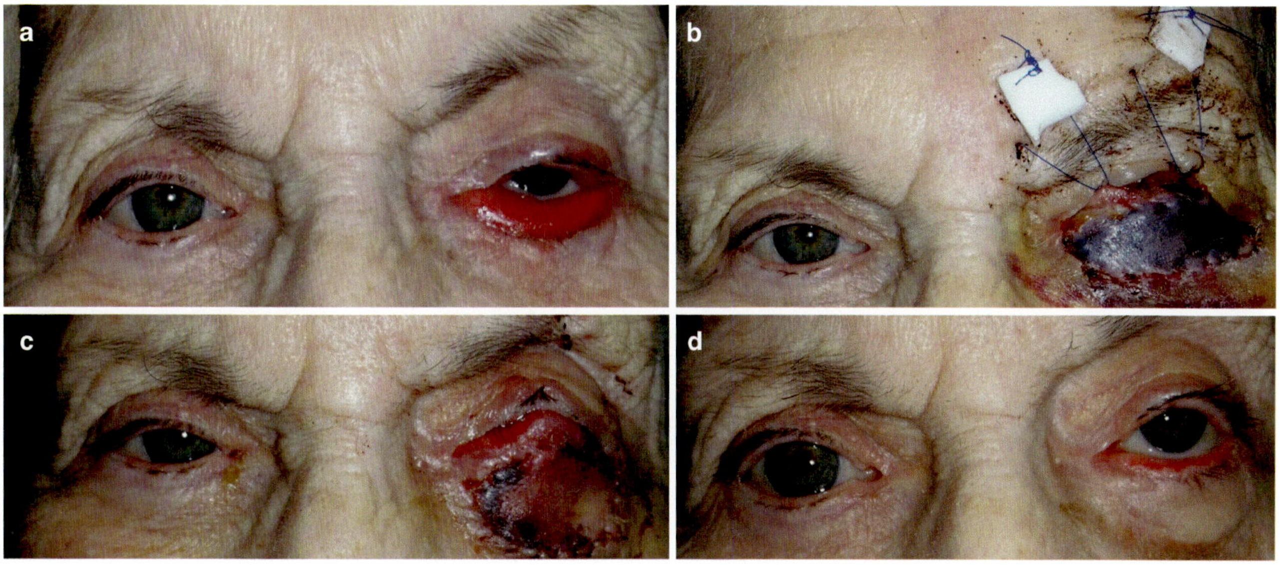

Fig. 12.4 (**a**) Severe left lower ectropion with anterior and posterior lamellae deficiency and cicatricial changes. (**b**) Status post repositioning with full-thickness skin graft, posterior lamellar graft, lateral canthoplasty, temporary tarsorrhaphy, and eyelid margin intraoperative steroid infiltration. (**c**) Release of temporary tarsorrhaphy well-healing skin graft. (**d**) Postoperative result with residual eyelid margin keratinization

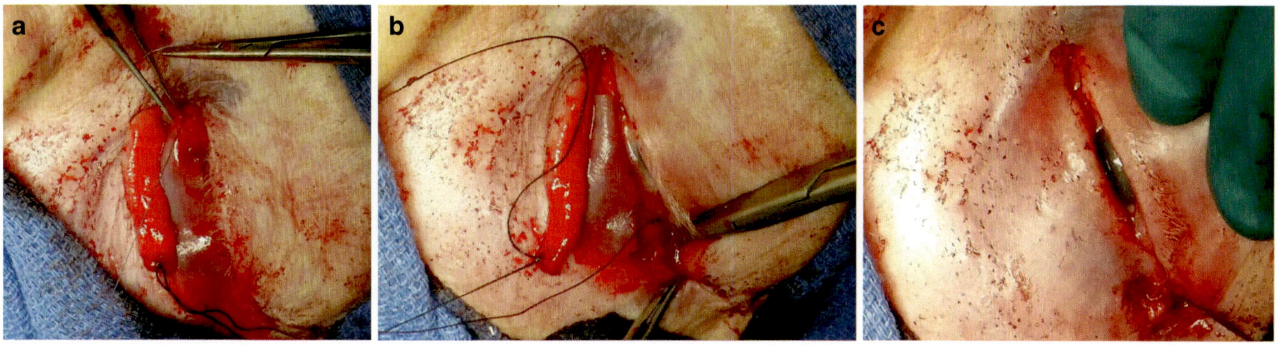

Fig. 12.5 (**a**) Securing decellularized extracellular matrix posterior lamellar spacer graft to inferior tarsal border superiorly and the conjunctiva inferiorly. (**b**) Posterior lamellar graft completely sewn into position and passing of suture needles through the periosteum of the lateral orbital rim for completion of lateral canthoplasty. (**c**) Intraoperative result after reforming the lateral canthus

13 Eyelid Retraction

Peter W. MacIntosh and Aaron Fay

Abbreviations

FTSG	Full-thickness skin graft
LF	Levator function
LTS	Lateral tarsal strip
MRD1	Margin reflex distance 1
MRD2	Margin reflex distance 2
PF	Palpebral fissure
SS	Scleral show
CCR	Central corneal light reflex

Introduction

The term "eyelid retraction" can be applied to either an upper or a lower eyelid. The upper eyelid is considered retracted if the upper eyelid margin is higher than normal, while the lower eyelid is considered retracted if the eyelid margin is lower than normal. Several etiologies can lead to eyelid retraction, the most common being thyroid eye disease or Graves' orbitopathy.

Patients with eyelid retraction may complain of a "big eye" or a "startled look." Furthermore, they may complain of dry eye or foreign body sensation due to ocular surface exposure or tearing due to a retracted lower eyelid position that does not adequately direct tears to the lacrimal drainage system.

While some forms of retraction may be addressed with conservative measures such as lubrication, others will require surgery for definitive management. The surgical approach to eyelid retraction depends on the eyelid affected and the specific etiology, and most have excellent outcomes.

P. W. MacIntosh (✉)
Department of Ophthalmology, University of Illinois, Chicago, IL, USA

A. Fay
Department of Ophthalmology, Harvard Medical School, Boston, MA, USA

Relevant Anatomy

The main function of the eyelids is to protect and help lubricate the cornea. The upper eyelid functions like a squeegee, moving up and down to distribute tears across the cornea and wipe away debris. The lower eyelid, on the other hand, remains mostly static and supports the tear film and cornea.

The upper eyelid is comprised of several layers. The inferior 10 mm of the upper eyelid from external to internal consists of the (1) skin, (2) orbicularis oculi muscle, (3) tarsus, and (4) conjunctiva (Fig. 13.1). The levator muscle is responsible for most of the elevator function of the upper eyelid and is innervated by cranial nerve III. The levator muscle is continuous with the levator aponeurosis which attaches to the superior 2/3 of the anterior surface of tarsus. The sympathetically innervated Müller's muscle contributes approximately 2 mm of additional lift to the upper eyelid and attaches to the superior margin of tarsus. The levator aponeurosis fans out nasally and temporally to attach to the entire width of tarsus.

The lower eyelid is comprised of layers analogous to those in the upper eyelid: the (1) skin, (2) orbicularis oculi muscle, (3) tarsus, and (4) conjunctiva (Fig. 13.1). There is no precise analogue to the levator muscle, however. The analogue to the Müller's muscle is the inferior tarsal muscle. There is a close relationship between the inferior rectus muscle and the lower eyelid retractors, and care should be taken when dissecting in this plane.

Clinical Features and Ancillary Tests

The approach to the management of eyelid retraction depends first on some basic measurements of the eyelids as well as measures of corneal exposure and health. These measurements are also important for the insurers to document the severity of retraction and its effect on overall eye health to justify insurance coverage for proposed corrective procedures.

A. J. Cohen, C. N. Burkat (eds.), *Oculofacial, Orbital, and Lacrimal Surgery*, https://doi.org/10.1007/978-3-030-14092-2_13

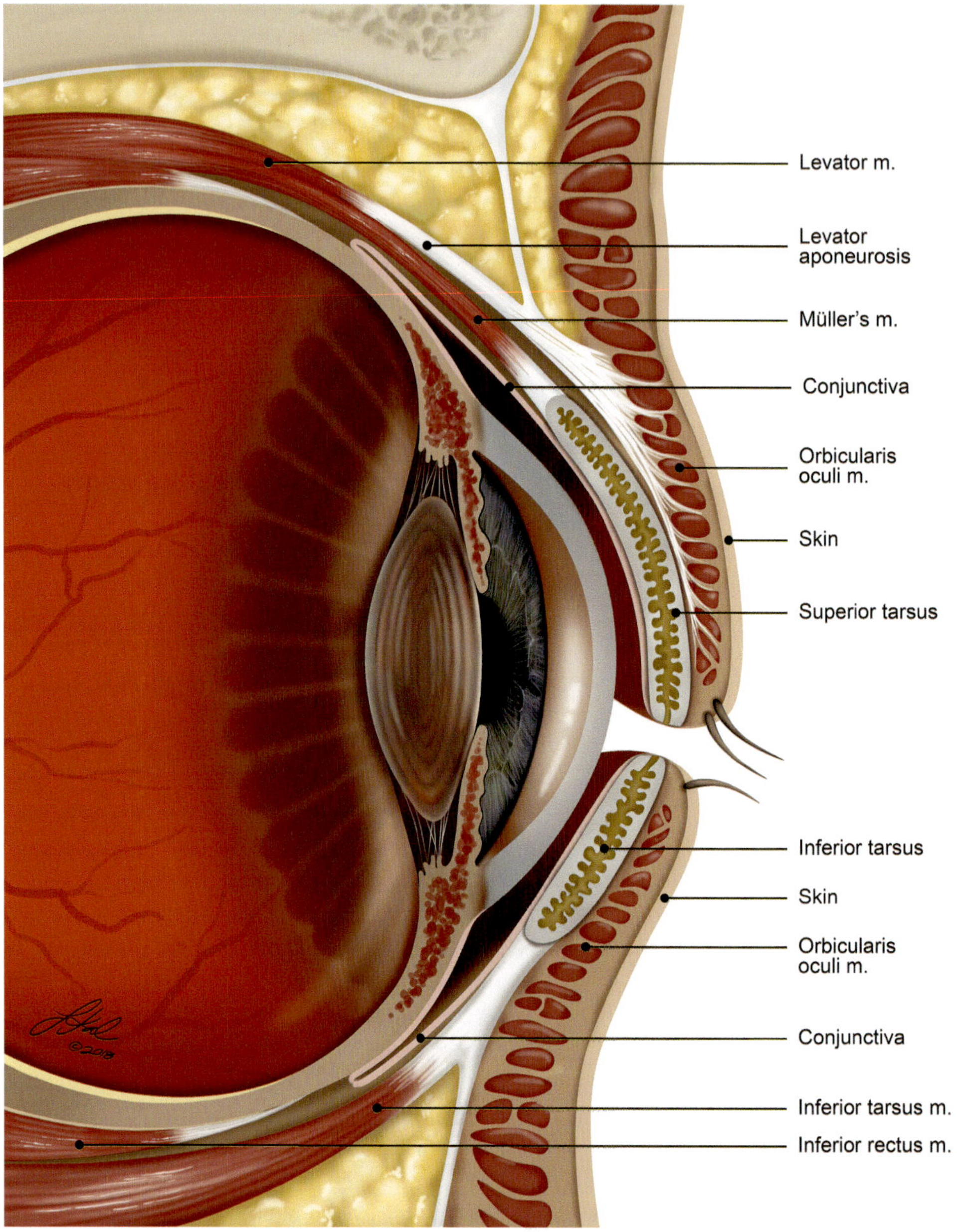

Fig. 13.1 Upper and lower eyelid anatomy

The upper eyelid position is measured with the margin reflex distance 1, or MRD1. MRD1 is a measure from the central corneal light reflex (CCR) to the upper eyelid margin. Normal MRD1 is 4 mm, which is usually about 1 mm below the superior limbus. Margin reflex distance 2, or MRD2, is a similar measurement for the lower eyelid and is measured from the CCR to the lower eyelid margin. MRD2 is normally 5 mm, which is about at the inferior limbus. Upper or lower eyelid retraction is defined by an increased MRD1 or MRD2, respectively (Fig. 13.2a). As MRD1 and MRD2 increase, the eyelid margin moves away from the limbus, exposing sclera, also called "scleral show" (Fig. 13.2b). Combining MRD1 and MRD2 results in the total palpebral fissure (PF) height, which is usually 9 mm. Levator function (LF) is a measure of the upper eyelid excursion from full down-gaze to full up-gaze and is normally 15 mm (Table 13.1 and Fig. 13.3).

Lagophthalmos is defined as an eyelid that cannot close fully and should be differentiated from lid lag, which is defined as a delay in the upper eyelid moving down as the eye looks down. Lid lag is a common finding in thyroid eye disease, where it is called Graefe's sign.

Patients with visually significant ptosis may recruit their frontalis muscle to elevate their brows in an attempt to also elevate their ptotic eyelid. In a patient with unilateral ptosis, recruiting the entire frontalis muscle will elevate the ptotic eyelid but may also elevate the other normal eyelid, giving it a retracted appearance. Immobilizing the frontalis muscle when evaluating the eyelids can help distinguish this form of

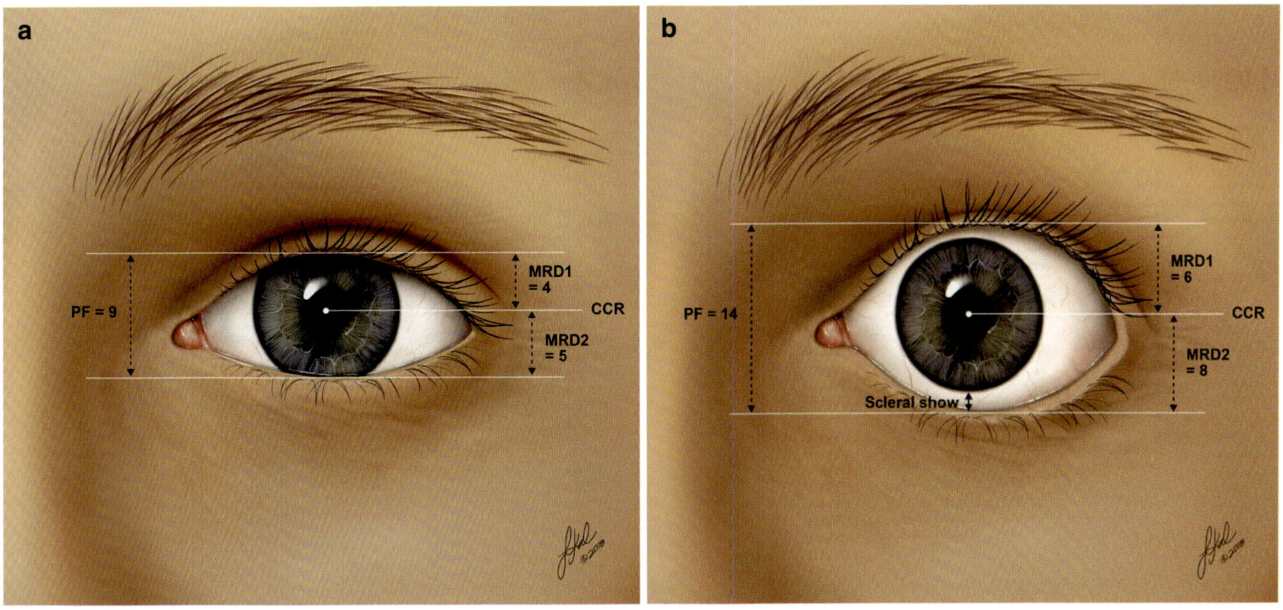

Fig. 13.2 (**a**) Normal eyelid measurements. (**b**) Example eyelid measurements in upper and lower eyelid retraction

Table 13.1 Eyelid measurements

Abbreviation	Definition	Normal value (mm)
MRD1	Margin reflex distance 1	4–4.5
MRD2	Margin reflex distance 2	5
PF	Palpebral fissure height	9
LF	Levator function	15
SS	Scleral show	0

pseudoretraction from true retraction. The treatment of this type of pseudoretraction would be contralateral ptosis surgery, rather than ipsilateral retraction surgery. Some patients may have frontalis overaction unrelated to ptosis, but this may also result in unilateral or bilateral pseudoretraction.

An important cause of eyelid retraction is proptosis, and the most common cause of proptosis in adults is thyroid eye (Graves') disease. Eyelid retraction is most commonly caused by Graves' disease due to fibrosis of the levator muscle and aponeurosis, but proptosis is an independent cause of retraction that is due to the mechanics of the globe moving anteriorly and forcing the eyelids to retract to accommodate the anteriorly displaced globe. Proptosis is most commonly measured with exophthalmometry, such as Hertel. Normal difference between the two eyes is usually less than 2 mm. The normal values for Hertel measurements are listed in Table 13.2.

The cornea is one of the most sensitive tissues in the human body due to its dense innervation with sensory nerve fibers from the long ciliary nerves, which in turn derive from the first division of the trigeminal nerve. This high level of sensation provides a protective function for the cornea, since even minor trauma results in pain that will elicit a protective response, such as eyelid closure. Patients with poor corneal sensation may be less able to protect the cornea from desiccation, minor trauma, infection, and ultimately perforation.

Corneal sensation can be grossly tested in the clinic with a cotton wisp from a cotton-tip applicator without applying topical anesthetic. Each quadrant of the cornea is tested and recorded as normal, reduced, or absent.

The Cochet-Bonnet esthesiometer is a device that can record the pressure applied to generate sensation in mm/gm. It should be tested in each of the four quadrants similar to the cotton-tip test.

Corneal exposure can cause excessive evaporation of tears and poor corneal tear coverage, which may result in exposure keratopathy and exposure conjunctivitis. Exposure keratopathy may cause a dry, gritty, or foreign body sensation as well as conjunctival injection. Left unchecked, keratopathy may advance to corneal ulceration and perforation, which is a medical emergency.

Skin type is an important consideration when assessing eyelid retraction, particularly of the lower eyelid. Patients with fair skin of low Fitzpatrick skin type are most susceptible to aging and sun-related skin changes that can cause contraction and shortening of the lower eyelid and cheek skin and anterior eyelid lamella, resulting in cicatricial lower eyelid retraction. On the other hand, as we age, the lower eyelid and its medial and lateral canthal tendons may become lax resulting in the eyelid sagging with lower eyelid retraction. This lower eyelid laxity may result in ectropion or entropion which can impair normal tear flow across the cornea to the tear drain system, leading to epiphora.

Certain eye drops may be the cause of retraction. Phenylephrine stimulates the sympathetically innervated Müller's muscle and can elevate the eyelid by about 2 mm. In

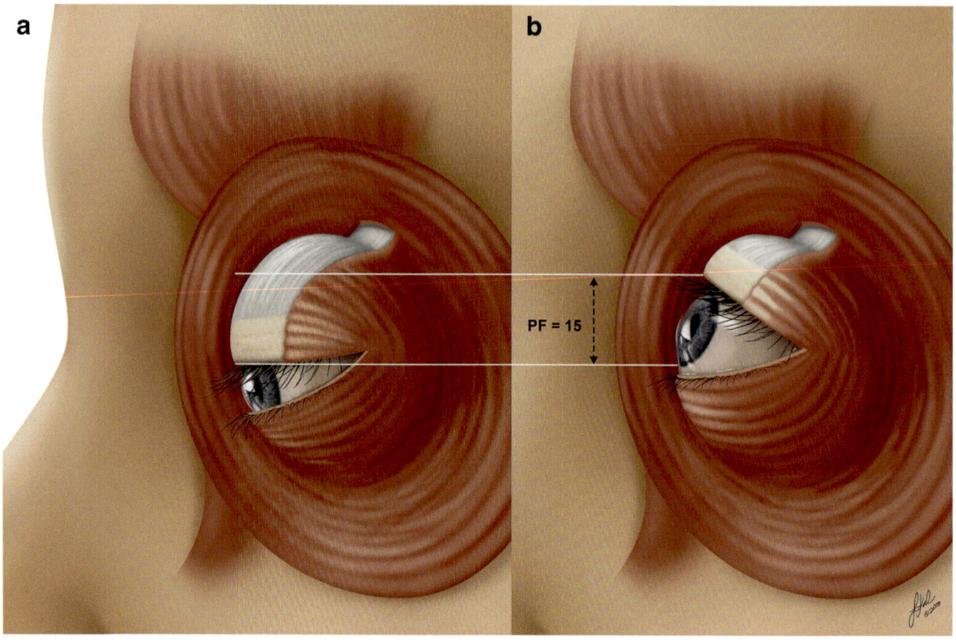

Fig. 13.3 Measuring levator function

Table 13.2 Mean exophthalmometry readings in adults [1]

	Caucasian	Black
Men (mm)	16.5	18.5
Women (mm)	15.4	17.8

fact, the phenylephrine test is used to determine if a patient is a good candidate for conjunctivomullerectomy surgery to correct for mild ptosis. As such, phenylephrine for dilation may also cause eyelid retraction, and this should be taken into consideration when evaluating the eyelids of a patient after dilation with phenylephrine. Similarly, unilateral phenylephrine may mask ipsilateral ptosis, cause ipsilateral retraction, or mask contralateral retraction.

Etiology

(a) Upper eyelid retraction

- Thyroid eye disease is the most common cause of eyelid retraction in adults. It is postulated to be caused by contraction of the levator muscle due to inflammation and fibrosis, although some studies suggest involvement of additional layers of the eyelid. This fibrosis is exacerbated between the lacrimal gland fascia and levator, contributing to the lateral flare that is commonly seen in these patients. Increased sympathetic tone to Müller's muscle may also contribute to retraction.
- Scarring either from previous eyelid surgery or trauma may contribute to a retracted state of the eyelid.
- Iatrogenic retraction may occur secondary to superior rectus muscle surgery. This finding is due to fascial connections between the superior rectus and the levator muscle in the upper eyelid. Superior rectus recession surgery may cause ipsilateral upper eyelid retraction, while superior rectus resection may cause ipsilateral upper eyelid ptosis. If this ptosis is visually significant, the patient may compensate with frontalis muscle and eyebrow recruitment to elevate the lid and, due to Hering's law (see below), may develop contralateral upper eyelid retraction.
- Hering's law of equal innervation states that there is equal and simultaneous innervation to yoked muscles, including the levator muscles. As a result, if one eyelid is ptotic relative to the other, and the patient attempts to elevate the ptotic lid with frontalis and brow elevation, both the ptotic and normal eyelid will be elevated by the same amount, resulting in the ptotic lid being brought to a higher, less ptotic position and the contralateral eyelid being artificially retracted.
- Parinaud's dorsal midbrain syndrome is a neurological syndrome due to a pretectal lesion in the posterior commissure that can cause eyelid retraction (Collier's sign) as part of the syndrome that also includes pupillary light-near dissociation and convergence retraction nystagmus. The etiology of the lesion depends on patient age, but obstructive hydrocephalus is most common in infants, a pineal mass in toddlers and young children, and strokes and hemorrhage are the most frequent cause in adults.

- Facial nerve paralysis is classically associated with lagophthalmos due to loss of orbicularis oculi muscle function. In addition, many of these patients also have upper eyelid retraction due to overaction of the levator muscle that is no longer countered by the orbicularis oculi muscle.
- Congenital eyelid retraction is relatively rare and should be considered a diagnosis of exclusion. These patients often undergo extensive evaluation to elicit a cause, most importantly for thyroid disease. Most patients present for evaluation of abnormal appearance. Unlike in adults, corneal pathology is rare in young children, even with exposure.

(b) Lower eyelid retraction

- Lower eyelid retraction, like upper eyelid retraction, may be most commonly secondary to thyroid eye disease.
- Involutional changes are another leading cause. As the tissues around the eyes age, they become lax. The lower eyelid is hung like a hammock between the medial and lateral canthal tendons, and as the tendons become lax with age, the eyelid tends to retract due to the effects of gravity, and may progress to ectropion or entropion.
- Iatrogenic lower eyelid retraction is most common from previous cosmetic lower eyelid blepharoplasty. Aggressive removal of skin can cause anterior lamellar shortage, putting the cheek and lower eyelid skin on stretch, which results in retraction. Retraction may be further exacerbated in patients with lower eyelid laxity, where the eyelid cannot resist the additional tension from tight lower eyelid skin.
- Similar to the upper eyelid, vertical (inferior rectus) muscle surgery may result in eyelid position changes due to its fascial associations with the capsulopalpebral fascia. Inferior rectus recession may result in ipsilateral lower eyelid retraction.
- The "actinic midface syndrome" refers to skin changes from aging and sun exposure that are most pronounced in patients with lower Fitzpatrick skin types. These patients develop taught, inelastic midface skin that contracts. Similar to patients with overaggressive lower eyelid skin blepharoplasties, the actinic midface syndrome can result in lower eyelid retraction that is exacerbated by lower eyelid laxity.
- Congenital lower eyelid retraction, as described above for the upper eyelid, is rare and a diagnosis of exclusion.
- Facial paralysis can cause retraction of the lower eyelid, but the etiology is different than for paralytic upper eyelid retraction. In the lower eyelid, the orbicularis oculi muscle is needed for normal tone and to balance the action of the capsulopalpebral fascia. Loss of the muscle results in an inability to keep tension on the lower eyelid against the globe, and the eyelid retracts with the force of gravity, and this may also progress to ectropion.

Management

General Treatments

Conservative

The main goal of treating patients with eyelid retraction is to manage corneal exposure. In patients with minimal exposure and no signs of corneal decompensation, this goal can be achieved easily with lubrication. Lubrication can be prescribed as an artificial tear eye drop, and/or a lubricating ointment. These medications can be used up to four times daily, and preservative-free drops can be used even more frequently. The ointments are thick and can cause blurry vision, so are best for overnight use, since they dissolve slowly and thus protect the eye overnight, but are dissolved by the morning, and so no longer cause blurry vision.

Moisture chamber glasses are another option, which function by preventing evaporation of tears from the ocular surface. The main drawback is the cumbersome nature of these devices.

Medical tape can be used to tape the eyelids closed overnight or even during the day if tolerated. The retracted lower eyelid that is due to laxity or paralysis may be supported with horizontal tape below the eyelid on a superior vector toward the lateral brow.

In patients with lower eyelid retraction due to overaggressive blepharoplasty with scar tissue formation, massage and silicone gel sheets may be beneficial to break up the scar tissue and lessen the effect of the scar on retraction [2].

Patching is generally not recommended for patients with eyelid retraction and corneal exposure. If the patch is placed incorrectly or if the eyelids open for any other reason under the patch, it could lead to corneal abrasion from the patch itself.

Semi-surgical

Filler injections have been described by some authors both to augment the lower eyelid and to treat upper eyelid retraction, although this is an off-label use of the product. A prospective study of hyaluronic acid injection into the levator plane in eight patients with upper eyelid retraction for Graves' orbitopathy showed an MRD1 decrease from 5.6 to 5 mm at 156 months [3]. In the lower eyelid, filler may be used to restore lost volume in patients with age-related volume loss or to support the eyelid in patients with facial paralysis. Filler would not be typically indicated to repair other causes of eyelid retraction such as scarring, anterior lamellar deficiency from previous blepharoplasty, or actinic midface syndrome.

Basic steps for upper eyelid filler injection:

1. Topical numbing medication.
2. Insert the needle transconjunctivally into the levator plane.
3. Inject approximately 0.3–0.4 ml of hyaluronic acid.

Tarsorrhaphy is a procedure that sutures the eyelids together. The tarsorrhaphy may be temporary with partial-thickness eyelid margin bites that incorporate tarsus for stability. Usually a silk or nylon suture is used for durability but easy removal when desired. Temporary tarsorrhaphy is ideal for patients with Bell palsy who are expected to regain eyelid function in a few weeks, and the sutures can be removed at that time. Tarsorrhaphy can also be performed permanently, by denuding the posterior eyelid margins in the upper and lower eyelids and suturing upper and lower eyelid tarsus together. These will heal together and form a permanent closure for any desired length of the eyelid. Permanent tarsorrhaphy is ideal for patients with poor prognosis who need eyelid closure to prevent ulceration, but who do not need advanced, cosmetically appealing interventions.

Temporary tarsorrhaphy technique (Fig. 13.4):

1. Use 4-0 or 6-0 permanent suture (e.g., nylon or silk).
2. Pass the suture through a bolster fashioned from suture packing foam or butterfly tubing.
3. Pass the suture through the lower eyelid skin superiorly to exit through the tarsus (Fig. 13.4a).
4. Pass the suture in cerclage fashion through the upper eyelid tarsus, exiting several millimeters away (Fig. 13.4b).
5. Pass the suture through the lower eyelid tarsus, and exit in the skin at parallel to the initial pass (Fig. 13.4c).
6. Tie the suture over the bolster (Fig. 13.4d).

Permanent tarsorrhaphy technique (Fig. 13.5):

1. Measure and mark the location and amount of eyelid to be closed.
2. Grasp the lower eyelid with forceps, and cut along the gray line with a number 11 Bard-Parker blade (Fig. 13.5a).
3. Using Wescott scissors, sharply dissect the orbicularis/skin lamella from the tarsus (Fig. 13.5b).
4. Cut a strip of epithelium from the superior border of tarsus in the area for the tarsorrhaphy to denude it (Fig. 13.5c).
5. Perform the same procedure for the opposing segment of upper eyelid.
6. Grasp the upper eyelid tarsus, and pass a 6-0 polyglactin suture partial thickness through its anterior surface to exit at the free margin (Fig. 13.5d).
7. Pass the suture through the free margin of the opposing eyelid to exit through the anterior tarsus partial thickness. Place as many sutures as needed approximately 2–3 mm apart (Fig. 13.5e).
8. Sutures can be passed through the anterior skin/orbicularis lamella for a two-layer closure, if desired (Fig. 13.5f).

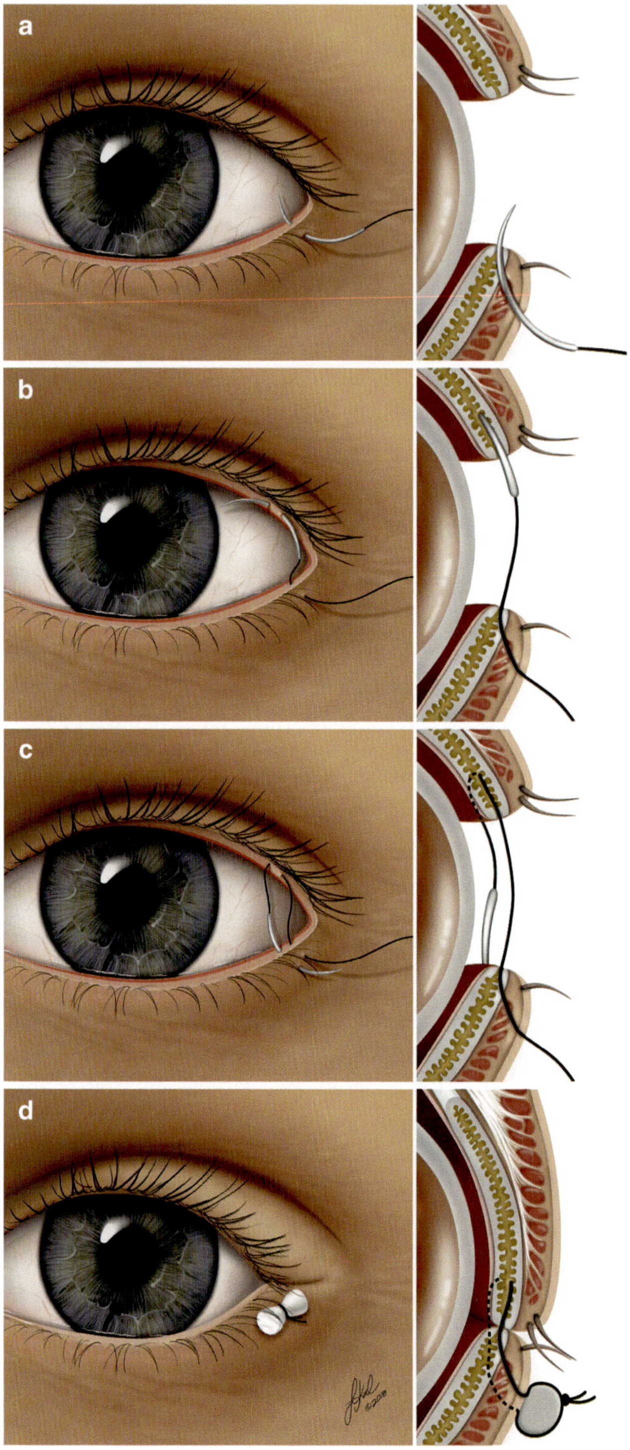

Fig. 13.4 Temporary tarsorrhaphy

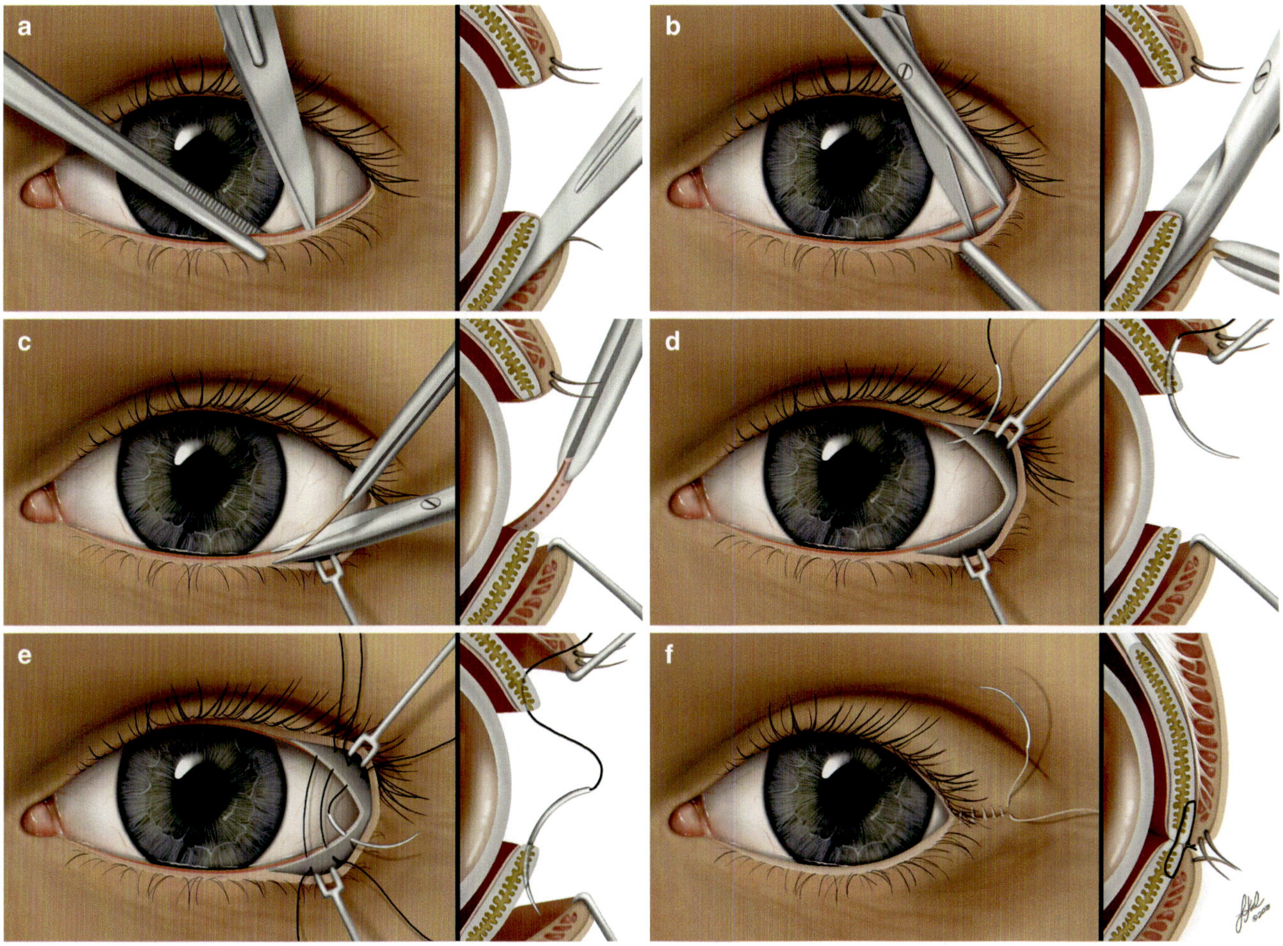

Fig. 13.5 Permanent tarsorrhaphy

Surgical

Full-thickness skin grafting (FTSG) is a useful surgical technique to restore anterior lamellar deficiency from scarring, actinic midface syndrome, or overaggressive upper or lower eyelid blepharoplasty. The eyelid skin is the thinnest in the body, and ipsilateral or contralateral upper eyelid skin is the best match and thus best suited for FTSG for eyelid repair. Other suitable skin can be harvested from the post- or preauricular, supraclavicular, and upper inner arm areas.

Full-thickness skin grafting technique (Fig. 13.6):

1. Make a horizontal incision in the skin. Use the eyelid crease in the upper eyelid or a subciliary incision or prior scar incision in the lower eyelid (Fig. 13.6a).
2. Allow the tissues to relax into the desired position, and measure the amount of skin deficiency (Fig. 13.6b).
3. Transfer this measurement to the donor skin site marking out the skin to remove in an ellipse (Fig. 13.6c).
4. Incise around the donor skin with a scalpel (Fig. 13.6c).
5. Dissect the full-thickness skin graft with sharp dissection.
6. Transfer the donor skin to the recipient site (Fig. 13.6d).
7. Suture the graft in place with interrupted 6-0 nylon or chromic gut sutures.
8. Close the donor site with interrupted 6-0 nylon, gut or fast-absorbing plain gut sutures.
9. Apply a pressure dressing to the newly grafted site.

Treatments for Upper Eyelid Retraction

Botulinum toxin may be used for upper eyelid retraction to weaken the levator muscle and Müller's muscle to cause a mild degree of ptosis. The advantages of botulinum toxin are that it is minimally invasive and reversible, since the effect will wear off in 3–4 months. However, it may be difficult to titrate the correct dose to achieve the desired amount of ptosis, and it may not be effective for retraction secondary to fibrosis as seen in thyroid eye disease.

The gold standard for upper eyelid retraction is the blepharotomy. This surgery can be performed through an eyelid crease incision or from a transconjunctival approach.

Transconjunctival blepharotomy technique (Fig. 13.7):

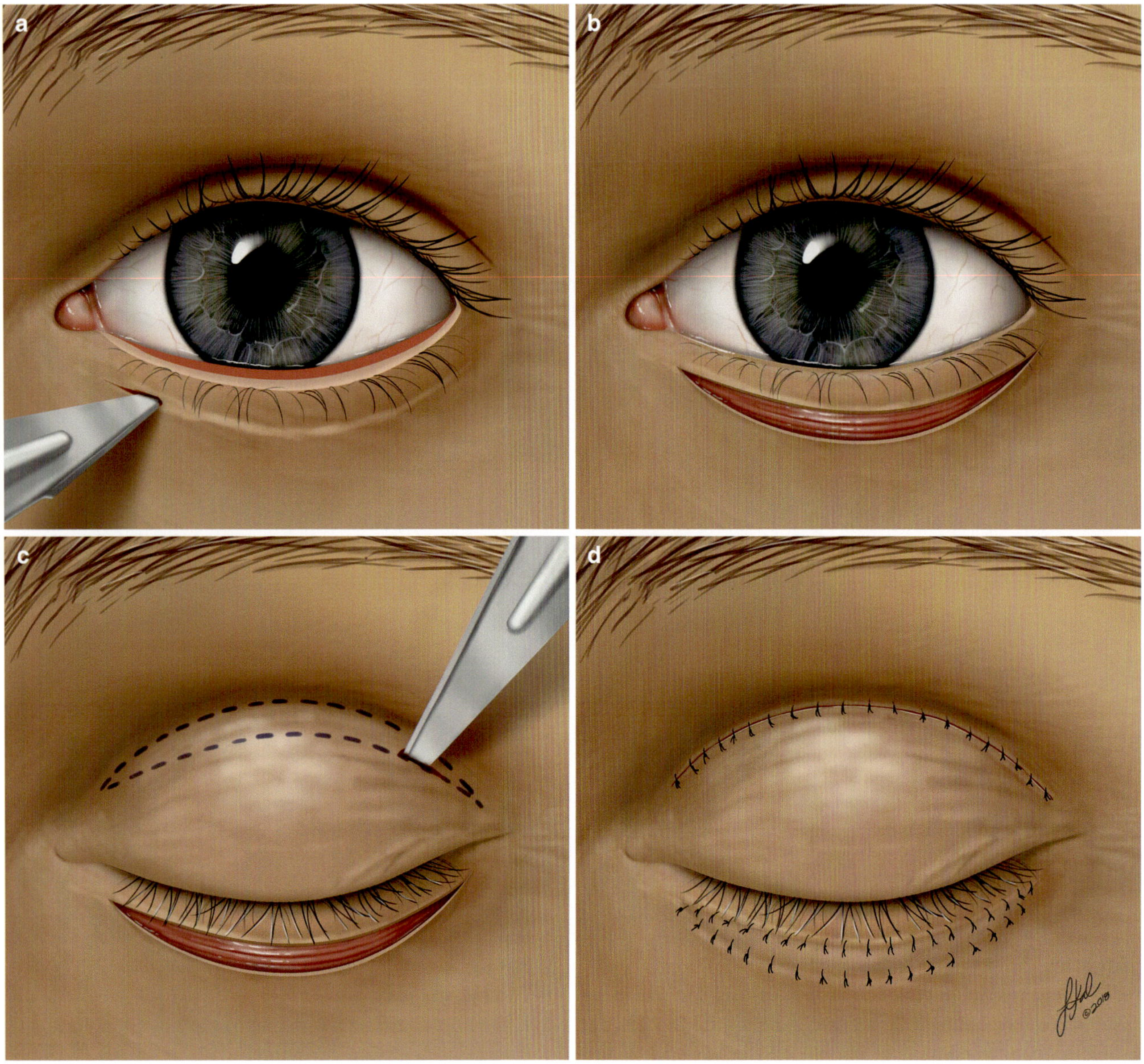

Fig. 13.6 Full-thickness skin graft harvesting technique

1. Place a 4-0 silk traction suture in the upper eyelid margin (Fig. 13.7a).
2. Evert the upper eyelid over a Desmarres retractor (Fig. 13.7b).
3. Inject local anesthesia in the subconjunctival space (Fig. 13.7b).
4. Identify the superior border of tarsus, and make an incision in the conjunctiva just superior to that, avoiding the peripheral vascular arcade (Fig. 13.7c).
5. Carry the incision nasally and laterally (Fig. 13.7d).
6. Continue the dissection through Müller's muscle and levator muscle.
7. Continually check the height of the eyelid to identify additional tissue to transect.
8. A central bridge of conjunctiva, Müller's muscle, and/or levator muscle may be left if needed for eyelid contouring, but often this is not necessary.

Eyelid skin crease blepharotomy technique (Fig. 13.8):

1. Mark the upper eyelid crease and inject with local anesthesia (Fig. 13.8a).
2. Make an incision in the upper eyelid crease skin, extending nasally and temporally (Fig. 13.8b).
3. Dissect through the orbicularis to tarsus inferiorly and the levator aponeurosis superiorly (Fig. 13.8c).
4. Sharply dissect the levator muscle from the tarsus (Fig. 13.8d).
5. Sharply dissect the Müller's muscle from the superior border of tarsus (Fig. 13.8e).
6. Leave the conjunctiva intact.
7. Close the skin crease incision with 6-0 fast-absorbing plain gut suture (Fig. 13.8f).
8. You can optionally also close the orbicularis muscle plane, if needed.

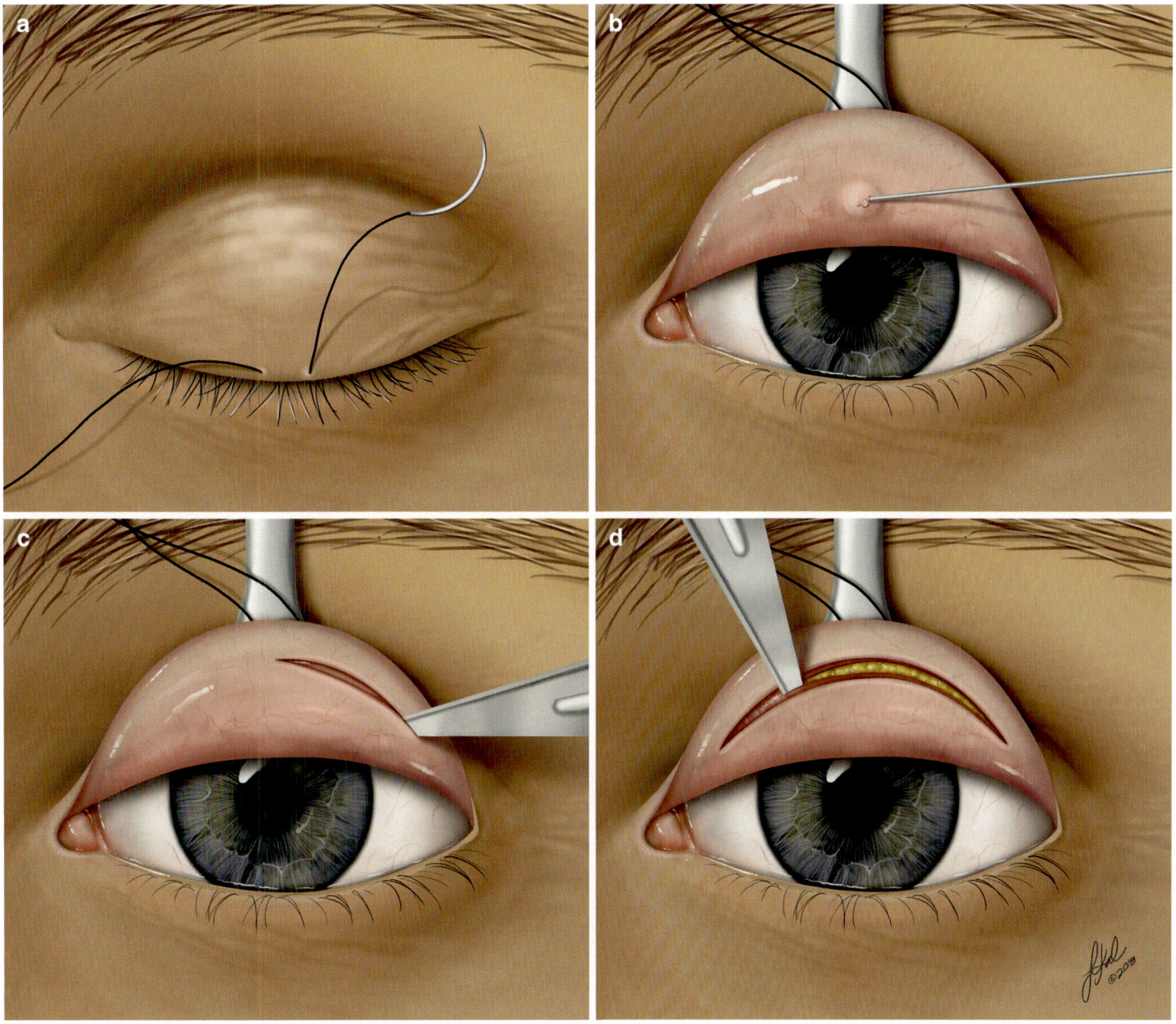

Fig. 13.7 Transconjunctival blepharotomy technique

Particular attention should be given to vertically incise/release the lateral levator-tarsus attachments in patients with thyroid eye disease in order to correct the lateral flare seen in that condition.

Some variations on this surgery include inserting spacer materials such as temporalis fascia, fascia lata, cartilage, pericardium, or sclera between the superior border of tarsus and the Müller's muscle to prevent the deeper layers of eyelid from fusing back together. Alternatively, the spacer can be placed laterally to help address lateral flare.

The levator muscle alone may be recessed to correct upper eyelid retraction. Hang-back sutures may be added that can be adjusted to prevent overcorrection and postoperative ptosis. Recently, the graded Müller's muscle resection has been described for patients with upper eyelid retraction from Graves' orbitopathy and showed a statistically significant decreased in the MRD1 from 5.7 to 4 mm [4]. Often the levator muscle dissection needs to extend up to the superior fornix in order to recess the eyelid adequately.

Upper eyelid weights (gold or platinum) have also been used to weigh down the retracted upper eyelid. The size of the weight should be measured preoperatively to determine the correct weight to achieve the desired goal.

Upper eyelid weight for eyelid retraction technique (Fig. 13.9):

1. Mark the upper eyelid crease and inject with local anesthesia (Fig. 13.9a).
2. Make an incision in the upper eyelid crease skin, extending nasally and temporally (Fig. 13.9b).
3. Dissect through the orbicularis to tarsus inferiorly (Fig. 13.9c).
4. Bare the tarsus down toward the cilia but leaving the inferior 2 mm undisturbed (Fig. 13.9c).

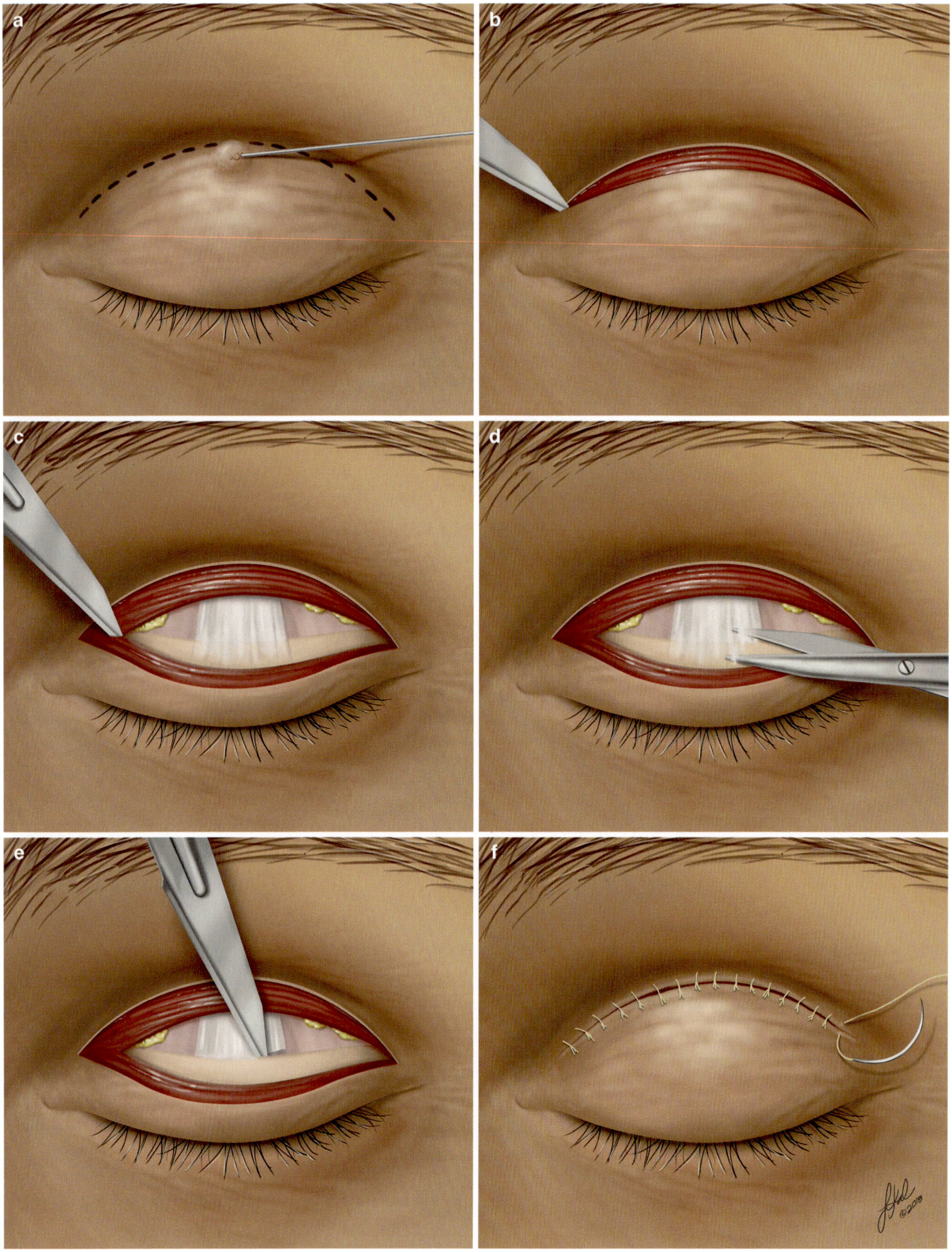

Fig. 13.8 Eyelid crease blepharotomy technique

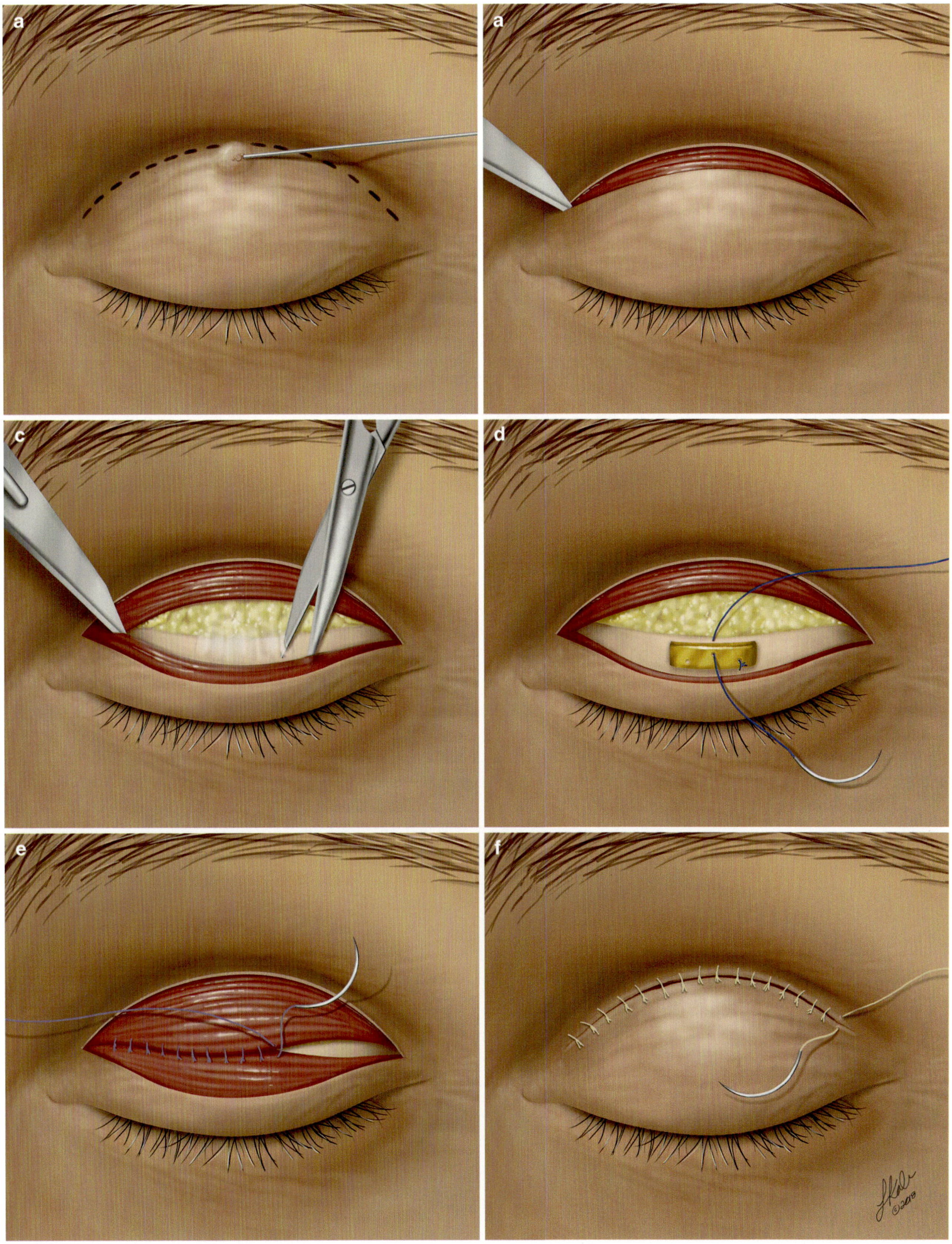

Fig. 13.9 Upper eyelid gold weight load

5. Place the predetermined weight against the tarsus, and suture into place with 6–0 prolene sutures, anchoring them partial thickness to the tarsus (Fig. 13.9d).
6. Close the orbicularis over the implant with 6-0 polyglactin sutures (Fig. 13.9e).
7. Close the skin with 6-0 fast-absorbing plain gut sutures (Fig. 13.9f).

Weights have the advantage of being easy to place and also easily removed if they are no longer needed or if a different weight is needed. On the other hand, they rely on gravity to close the eyelid, and in a supine position may not fully close the eyelid, and, in some cases, can pull the eyelid open depending on the vectors. Furthermore, they add bulk to the eyelid and may be cosmetically unappealing to some patients.

The palpebral spring, custom made of titanium alloy, is another implant that has been classically used to treat paralytic lagophthalmos, but it can also be used to treat upper eyelid retraction (Fig. 13.10).

Palpebral spring for upper eyelid retraction technique:

1. Mark the upper eyelid crease with a "lazy S" extension over the lateral orbital rim, and inject with local anesthesia.
2. Make an incision in the upper eyelid crease as marked.
3. Dissect through the orbicularis to tarsus inferiorly and to the superior orbital rim superiorly. Take care to leave the levator muscle intact.
4. Custom design the spring from a titanium alloy to generate the desired amount of tension.
5. Suture the superior arm to the periosteum just inside the superior orbital rim.
6. Suture the fulcrum to the lateral orbital rim periosteum.

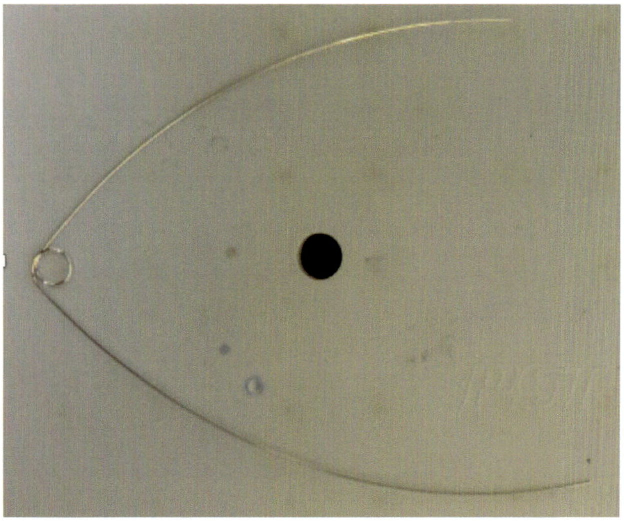

Fig. 13.10 Custom palpebral spring device

7. Turn the end of the palpebral arm into a closed circle with a diameter of 4 mm.
8. Fashion a 5×5 mm pouch out of a polyethylene sheet, and place the lower palpebral arm into this pouch.
9. Suture the polyethylene pouch to the tarsus.
10. Make final adjustments to the spring tension to ensure adequate closure and pressure against the cornea.
11. Close the orbicularis over the spring with 6-0 polyglactin suture.
12. Close the skin with 6-0 fast-absorbing plain gut suture.

A small levator advancement can be added to counteract the mild amount of ptosis that can result from the procedure. The spring has the advantage over an eyelid weight of not relying on gravity for its function; rather it uses a spring mechanism built into its fulcrum to store energy and close the eyelid. Both eyelid weights and springs can create a few millimeters of ptosis, but this ptosis is often beneficial in treating eyelid retraction or exposure. In the past years, eyelid springs have become less widely used due to complications of extrusion and exposure through the eyelid tissues.

Treatments for Lower Lid Retraction

Lower eyelid retraction treatment depends on the etiology of the retraction. As discussed above, anterior lamellar shortage from previous blepharoplasty or actinic midface syndrome requires treatment with full-thickness skin grafting. This treatment may be cosmetically unappealing to the patient who is experiencing this complication after a cosmetic lower eyelid blepharoplasty, but if upper eyelid skin is available for grafting, this should be used since it is the best skin match for this anatomic location.

Patients with retraction from lower eyelid laxity or paralysis will benefit from a horizontal eyelid tightening procedures such as lateral tarsal strip (LTS) to correct the laxity. A midface suborbicularis oculi lift is sometimes a helpful addition to further support the LTS. An alternative to traditional LTS is passive suspension of the lower eyelid with periosteal flap or fascia lata graft. Additional discussion on the importance of the lateral canthal tendon and options for management are covered in a separate chapter of this text.

Lateral tarsal strip technique (Fig. 13.11):

1. Inject the lateral canthus and lower eyelid with local anesthesia.
2. Perform a lateral canthotomy and inferior cantholysis (Fig. 13.11a, b).
3. Separate the anterior orbicularis and skin lamella from the posterior tarsus and conjunctiva lamella laterally to create the tarsal strip of appropriate size (Fig. 13.11c).

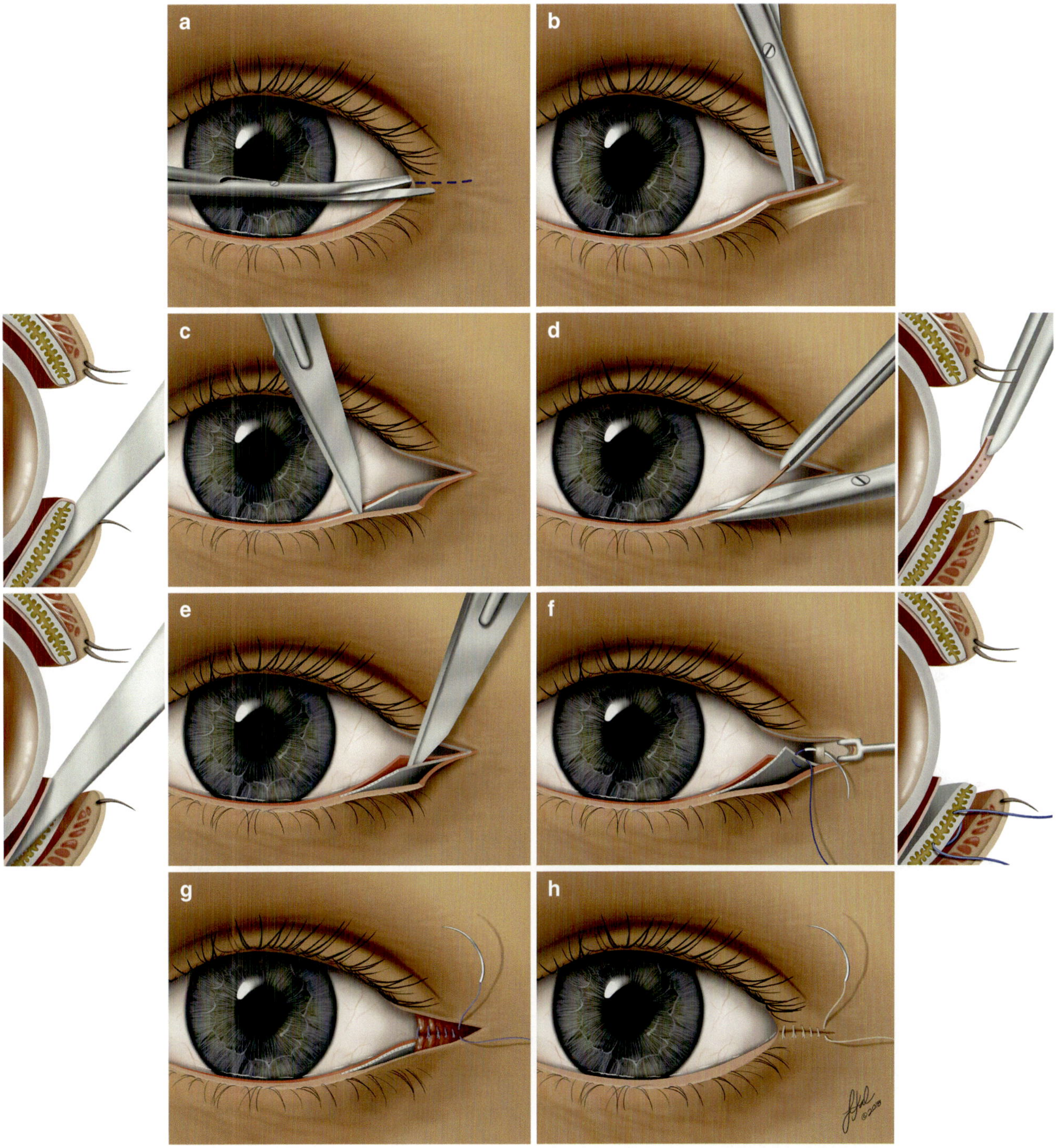

Fig. 13.11 Lateral tarsal strip procedure

4. Denude the eyelid margin from the posterior lamella segment with Wescott scissors (Fig. 13.11d).
5. Denude the palpebral conjunctiva from the tarsal strip by scraping with a blade, although many surgeons may not perform this step (Fig. 13.11e).
6. Pass a double armed 4–0 prolene or polyester fiber suture horizontal mattress style through the tarsal strip (Fig. 13.11f).
7. Pass the suture through the periosteum just inside the lateral orbital rim at Whitnall's tubercle (Fig. 13.11f). One to two sutures can be placed to secure the tarsal strip.
8. Alternatively, for paralytic or recurrent retraction, a small burr hole can be drilled in the lateral orbital rim at Whitnall's tubercle to anchor the tarsal strip with nonabsorbable sutures.

9. The sharp lateral canthal angle is reformed by closing the upper and lower eyelid margin with a buried 6-0 polyglactin suture.
10. Close the orbicularis over the lateral orbital rim with 6-0 polyglactin sutures (Fig. 13.11g).
11. Close the lateral canthal skin with 6-0 fast-absorbing gut suture (Fig. 13.11h).

Passive lower eyelid suspension with periosteal flap or fascia lata graft (Fig. 13.12):

1. A nasal skin incision is made down to the nasal bone (Fig. 13.12a).
2. The periosteal flap is harvested from the lateral orbital rim with its base left intact at Whitnall's tubercle. It is rotated 180° to be fed in a pretarsal plane along the lower eyelid margin with a Wright needle (Fig. 13.12b).
3. Alternatively, fascia lata is harvested from the leg with a stripper and is passed in a pretarsal plane along the length of the eyelid with a Wright needle.
4. For the fascia lata, the temporal end can be fed through a burr hole made in the lateral orbital rim near Whitnall's tubercle and then sutured to the periosteum lateral to the rim.
5. It is important to have a posterior vector on the eyelid to keep it apposed to the globe, and pulling the fascia lata through a burr hole helps to achieve this goal.
6. The nasal end of the periosteal flap or fascia lata graft is secured to bone with a mini anchor screw (Fig. 13.12c).

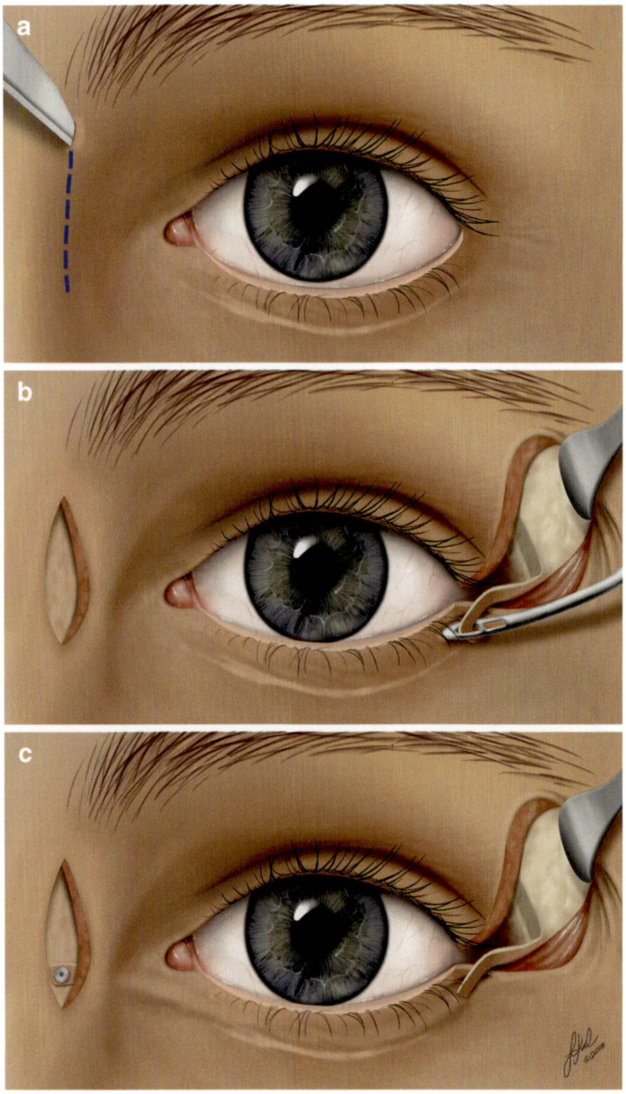

Fig. 13.12 Lower eyelid suspension periosteal flap technique

The passive suspension approach has the advantage over LTS of better addressing medial canthal dystopia but may result in ectropion or entropion since the eyelid "hangs" on the fascia lata, rather than supporting tarsus itself, although this can be mitigated by suturing the sling to tarsus. Addition of a midface lift may also help augment the tissues that sag due to paralysis or aging changes.

Patients with middle and posterior lamellar deficiency will benefit most from spacers placed in those planes. Similarly, patients with lower eyelid retraction from proptosis are best treated with lower eyelid spacers to elevate the eyelid since horizontal tightening can worsen the retraction in these cases. Appropriate spacer materials include autologous hard palate, tarsus (from the ipsilateral or contralateral upper eyelid), acellular human dermis (Alloderm), split-skin derived acellular collagen matrix (Xenoderm), bioengineered eyelid spacer (Tarsys), and ear or nasal cartilage.

Transconjunctival lower eyelid spacer grafting technique (Fig. 13.13):

1. Place a 4-0 silk traction suture in the lower eyelid margin (Fig. 13.13a).
2. Evert the lower eyelid over a Desmarres retractor (Fig. 13.13b).
3. Inject local anesthesia in the subconjunctival space (Fig. 13.13b).
4. Identify the inferior border of tarsus, and make an incision just inferior to that in the conjunctiva and lower eyelid retractors (Fig. 13.13c).
5. Dissect the conjunctiva off the inferior retractor layer (Fig. 13.13d).
6. Suture the spacer inferiorly to the retractors and superiorly to the inferior border of tarsus (Fig. 13.13e).
7. The conjunctiva is left retracted to prevent any undue traction on the eyelid that may compromise the result.

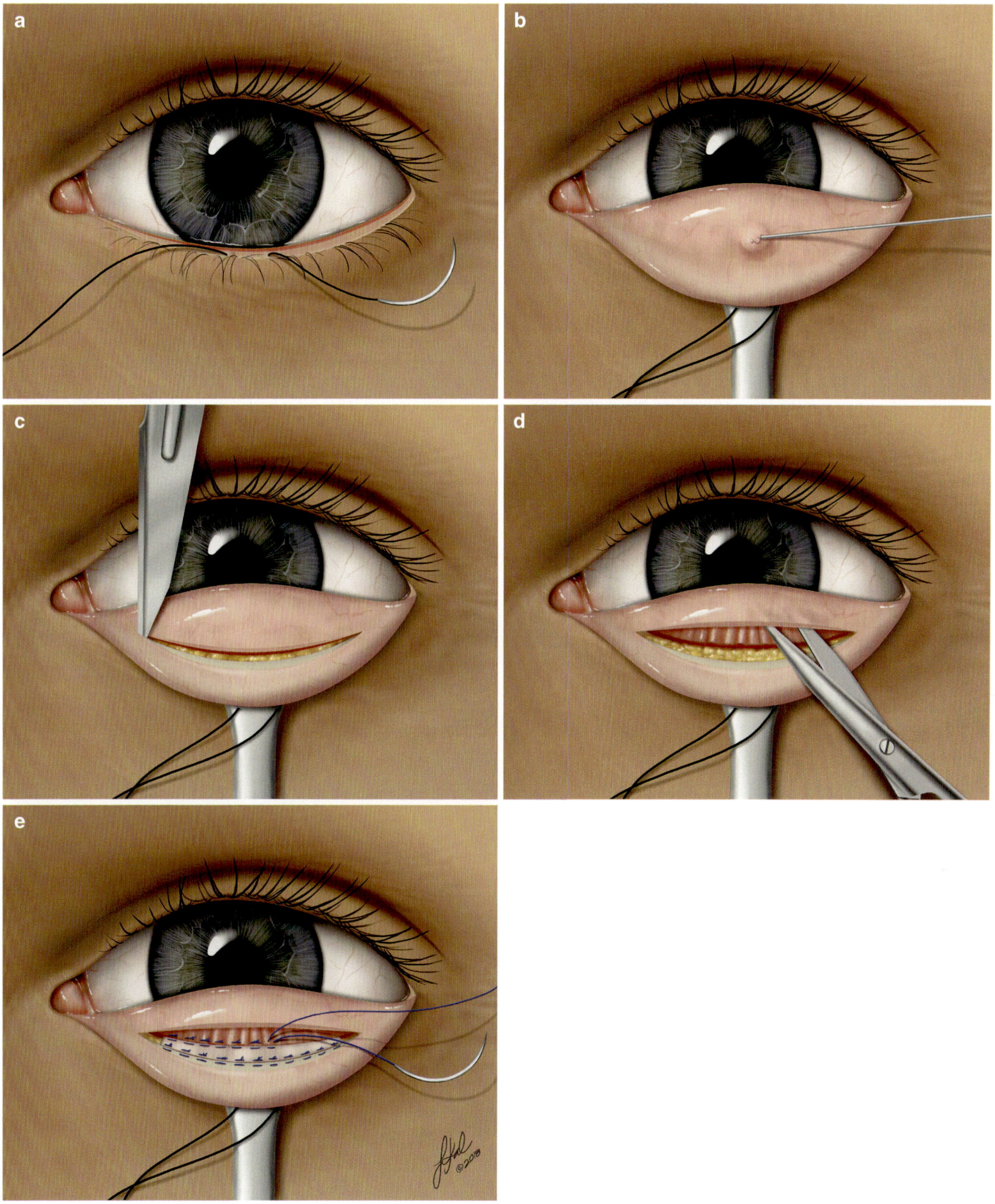

Fig. 13.13 Transconjunctival spacer graft technique

Complications of Treatment

Common complications after retraction surgery are over- and undercorrection. Overcorrection in the upper eyelid repair may result in ptosis that may be visually significant. Undercorrection may leave the patient with corneal exposure or cosmetically undesirable retraction. Eyelid contour issues may also arise, particularly in patients with thyroid eye disease and lateral eyelid flare. Some surgeons advocate preserving the central conjunctival bridge to minimize the risk of eyelid contour flattening.

Other postoperative concerns include ecchymosis, edema, chemosis, asymmetry, and need for additional surgeries. In some cases, failure to improve the retraction may be due to choosing the wrong surgical technique. Particularly in patients with lower eyelid retraction after blepharoplasty, a surgeon may attempt to correct the retraction without a full-thickness skin graft in order to avoid a cosmetically noticeable graft. However, posterior lamellar surgery will not correct an anterior lamellar deficiency.

Extrusion is a known complication of any spacer implant and must be monitored for. Cartilage grafts were very popular throughout the 1990s but have fallen out of favor due to complications from disintegration and extrusion [5].

References

1. Migliori ME, Gladstone GJ. Determination of the normal range of exophthalmometric values for black and white adults. Am J Ophthalmol. 1984;98(4):438–42.
2. Fulton JE Jr. Silicone gel sheeting for the prevention and management of evolving hypertrophic and keloid scars. Dermatol Surg. 1995;21:947–51.
3. Kohn JC, Rootman DB, Liu W, et al. Hyaluronic acid gel injection for upper eyelid retraction in thyroid eye disease. Ophthal Plast Reconstr Surg. 2014;30:400–4.
4. Ribeiro SFT, Garcia DM, Leal V, et al. Graded Mullerectomy for correction of Graves' upper eyelid retraction. Ophthalmic Plast Reconstr Surg. 2014;30:384–7.
5. MacIntosh PW, Jakobiec FA, Stagner A, et al. Failed cartilaginous grafts in the eyelid: a retrospective clinicopathological analysis of 5 cases. Ophthal Plast Reconstr Surg. 2016;32(5):347–53.

Eyelid Malignancies

14

Preamjit Saonanon

Eyelid malignancies can cause anatomical deformity and visual impairments. Eyelid malignancy can arise from the epidermis or adnexal organs and represents around 5–10% of all skin malignancies [1]. The most frequent lesion worldwide is basal cell carcinoma (85–90%) followed by squamous cell carcinoma (SCC) in Caucasians, whereas sebaceous carcinoma is the second most common eyelid malignancy in Asians [2, 3]. Other less common malignant lesions of the eyelid include malignant melanoma and Merkel cell carcinoma. Aging changes and epithelial damage from excessive exposure to UV light are known predisposing factors, particularly in light-skinned individuals. A history of periorbital radiation, previous skin lesions, smoking, and immunosuppression are also important and need to be elicited. Typical clinical features that are suggestive of malignancy include slow, painless growth with destruction of normal eyelid architecture and madarosis (loss of eyelashes) (Fig. 14.1). However, malignant neoplasms can also present with rapid growth, or be associated with pain in some instances. Regional lymph node palpation, including the preauricular and submandibular area, should be performed for evidence of metastasis. A thorough evaluation for systemic metastasis to the liver, lung, brain, and bone marrow should be performed in patients with sebaceous carcinoma and malignant melanoma, and can be coordinated with the appropriate oncologist.

Orbital invasion is rare except in neglected cases and may present with extensive eyelid involvement, facial disfigurement, proptosis, limitation of extraocular motility (EOM), decreased visual acuity, and optic nerve compromise.

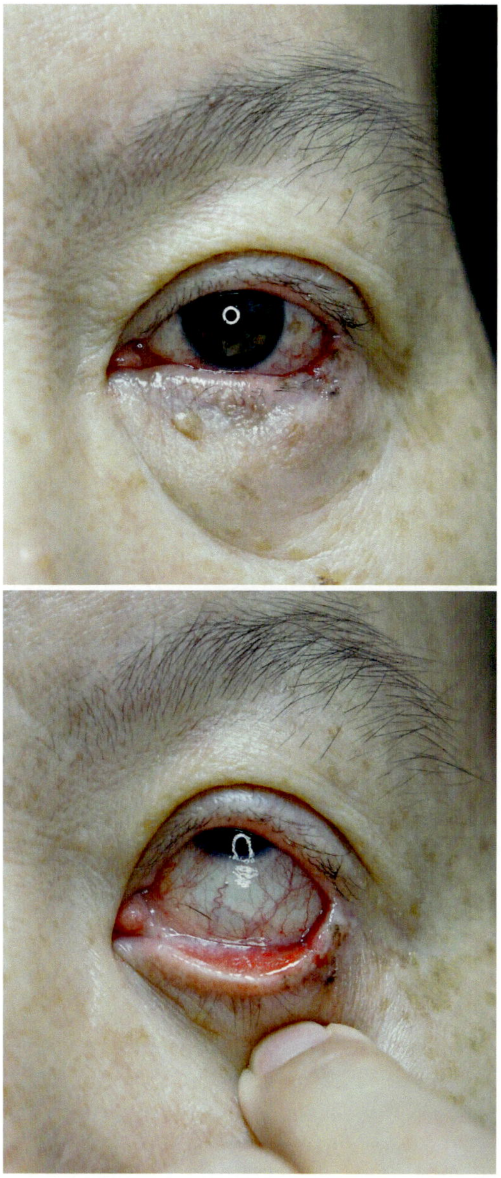

Fig. 14.1 Photos demonstrate typical clinical signs of basal cell carcinoma (left lower eyelid) with destruction of normal eyelid architecture and loss of eyelashes (madarosis)

P. Saonanon (✉)
Department of Ophthalmology, Faculty of Medicine, Chulalongkorn University, Bangkok, Thailand

Department of Ophthalmology, King Chulalongkorn Memorial Hospital, Thai Red Cross Society, Bangkok, Thailand

A. J. Cohen, C. N. Burkat (eds.), *Oculofacial, Orbital, and Lacrimal Surgery*, https://doi.org/10.1007/978-3-030-14092-2_14

An incisional biopsy is essential to confirm any clinically suspicious malignant lesion. Complete tumor removal or excisional biopsy with simple eyelid reconstruction is appropriate for diagnosis and treatment in small lesions that do not involve the eyelid margin. Surgical complete excision with histologic control of the margins is the gold standard treatment for all eyelid malignancies. Adjuvant therapies such as radiation, chemotherapy, and targeted therapies are outside the scope of this chapter, and are used primarily for unresectable lesions or metastasis.

The current AJCC (American Joint Committee on Cancer) guidelines for eyelid carcinoma and skin melanoma referenced in this chapter are from the seventh edition, published in 2009. The eighth edition was launched in 2016, but not yet in general use. The eyelid malignancies discussed in this chapter will be:

- Basal cell carcinoma
- Squamous cell carcinoma
- Sebaceous carcinoma (also termed sebaceous cell carcinoma, sebaceous adenocarcinoma)
- Malignant melanoma
- Merkel cell carcinoma

Basal Cell Carcinoma

Basal cell carcinoma (BCC) accounts for 85–90% of eyelid malignancy in Western case series with the incidence of 15.7 per 100,000 population in the United States [1]. BCC typically occurs in light-skinned adults, between 40 and 79 years old. Younger individuals with BCC tend to have more aggressive disease with higher recurrence and rarely may be associated with basal cell nevus syndrome (Gorlin-Goltz syndrome) or xeroderma pigmentosum. Sixty-five percent of eyelid BCC occur on lower eyelids, followed by the medial canthus (15%), upper eyelid (15%), and lateral canthus (5%).

Pathogenesis

A. Environmental Factors

Ultraviolet (UV) light exposure, especially during the first two decades of life, is the main predisposing factor to BCC. UV light stimulates the production of carcinogenic cellular changes which increase the chance of DNA mutations and deactivated tumor suppressor genes. The most mutagenic wavelengths are 290–320 nm in the UVB spectrum. Light-skinned individuals (Fitzpatrick types I and II), who typically burn rather than tan, are at highest risk of UV burns and DNA mutations. Smoking, prior ionizing radiation, arsenic, and coal tar exposure are also believed to cause carcinogenic effects [4].

B. Immunosuppression

Immunosuppression, such as reported in acquired immune deficiency syndrome (AIDS) and organ transplantation, yields 21 and 10 times higher incidence (respectively) of BCC, although the pathogenesis is not fully understood.

C. Genetics

Basal cell nevus syndrome is an autosomal dominant syndrome which, in some cases, is due to a mutation of PTCH1 (patched) gene on chromosome 9q22.3. An abnormal PTCH1 cannot suppress the sonic hedgehog pathway, thus resulting in uncontrolled cellular proliferation. This multisystem syndrome is associated with multiple BCC lesions in younger patients, typically during the second and third decades of life. Associated findings include skeletal anomalies, palmar and plantar keratinizing pits, odontogenic keratocysts, and central nervous system abnormalities, such as medulloblastoma and intellectual disability (Fig. 14.2). Note that this gene mutation can also be present in BCC without basal cell nevus syndrome, which allows for targeted therapy for BCC [5].

Clinical Features

There are four major subtypes of basal cell carcinoma (Fig. 14.3):

- *Nodular* or *noduloulcerative BCC* is the most common type occurring on the eyelid. It is characterized as a painless, typically slow-growing, pearly or waxy nodule, with rolled or heaped-up borders. Central ulceration, fine telangiectasias, loss of eyelid margin architecture, and madarosis are also typical findings. Secondary melanosis can occur in pigmented BCC and mimic a nevus or malignant melanoma.
- *Morpheaform (infiltrative or sclerosing) BCC* is less common but associated with a poorer prognosis. It appears as a pale yellow or skin-colored, thick indurated plaque with ill-defined margins. Loss of eyelid margin architecture is usually present due to infiltration in surrounding tissues.
- *Superficial BCC* usually arises on trunk and extremities. It appears as an erythematous patch or plaque with scale, which can often lead to misdiagnosis as psoriasis or fungal infections.
- *Mixed lesions* have features of more than one subtype.

Management

The rate of orbital invasion and metastasis in basal cell carcinoma is extremely low except in neglected or recurrent cases. The risk of local recurrence is less than 1% after complete

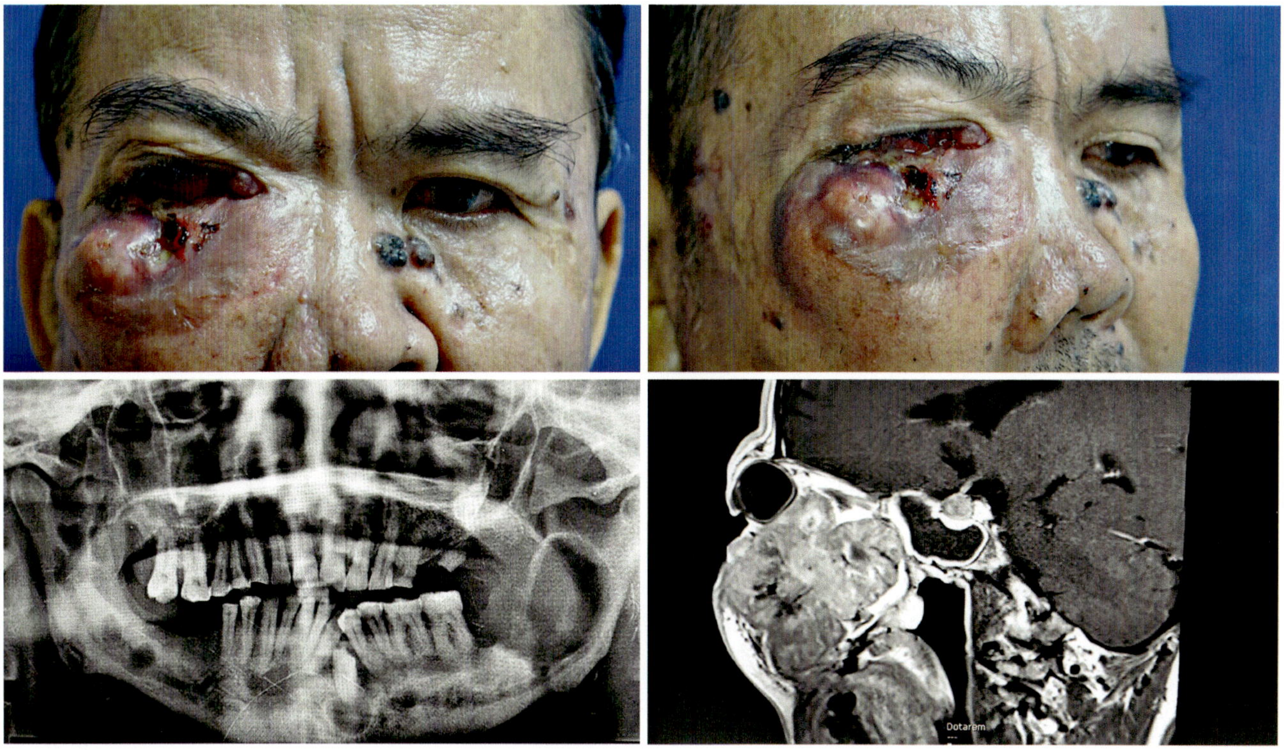

Fig. 14.2 Basal cell nevus syndrome (Gorlin-Goltz syndrome) with multiple recurrent periorbital basal cell and squamous cell carcinoma with right orbital and maxillary sinus invasion. Plain radiograph reveals multiple odontogenic keratocysts, seen as multiple various-sized intraosseous cystic-like lesions with expansile bony contouring of the mandible. MRI shows extensive involvement of the lesion occupying the entire right maxillary sinus and inferior aspect of the right orbit

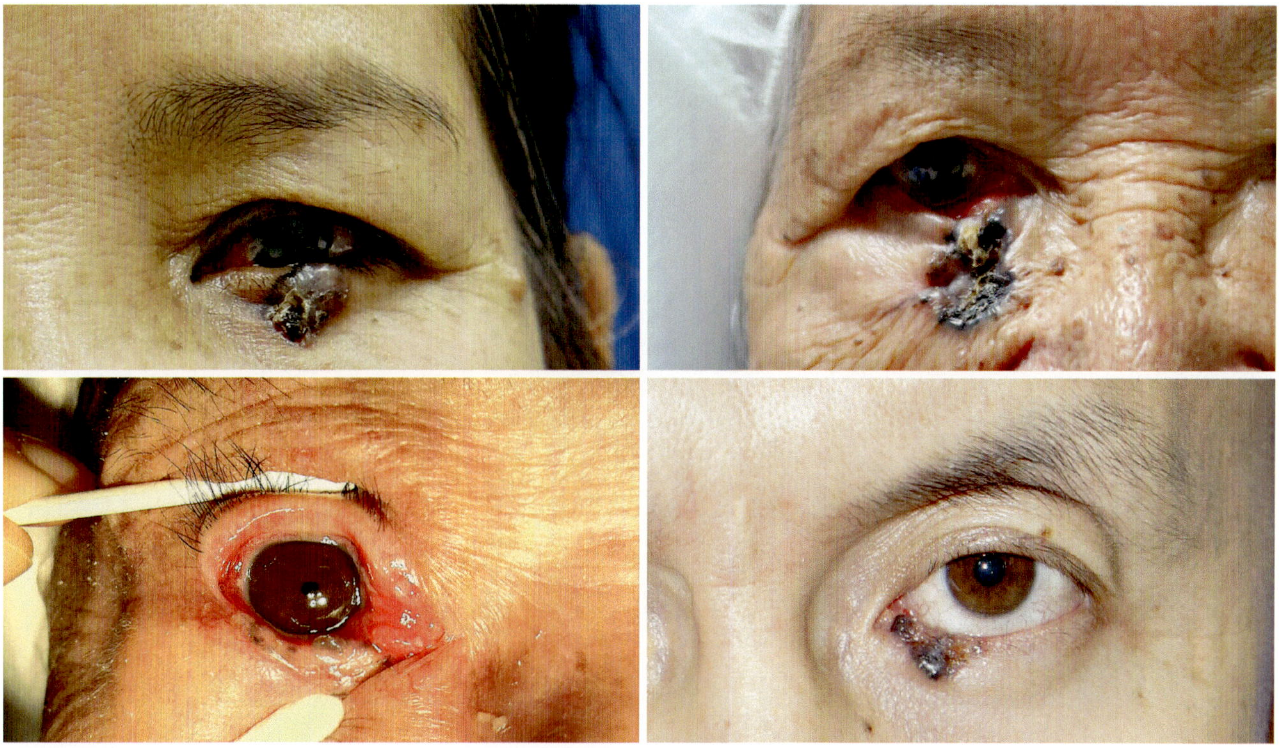

Fig. 14.3 Clinical features of basal cell carcinoma: left upper photo demonstrates left lower eyelid nodular type of BCCA with pigmentation. Right upper photo demonstrates noduloulcerative-type BCCA involving the right lower eyelid and tear trough area, with secondary cicatricial ectropion. Left lower photo shows a plaque-like lesion with ill-defined margins, consistent with morpheaform BCCA of the right lower eyelid. Total involvement of the entire eyelid is evidenced by loss of eyelid margin architecture and madarosis. Right lower photo demonstrates mixed type BCCA in the medial canthal area, involving the inferior punctum and canaliculus

tumor removal, with higher risk in medial canthal lesions and morpheaform subtypes.

The first line treatment is complete excision with histologic control of the margins using frozen section or Mohs micrographic surgery. Mohs micrographic surgery has become a common method of managing both BCC and SCC as it preserves the greatest amount of adjacent normal tissue. It is most beneficial in large, recurrent, medial canthal, and/or morpheaform lesions [6]. Although studies vary, the usual surgical margin in eyelid lesions is usually 2 mm beyond the clinically apparent tumor. Eyelid reconstruction is performed when all surgical margins are free of tumor. Other treatment modalities, including local radiotherapy, cryotherapy, CO_2 laser removal, and photodynamic therapy are associated with high rates of recurrence and poorer cosmetic results. These modalities may be considered as a palliative treatment in unresectable BCC or in poor surgical candidates.

Pharmacological therapy, including imiquimod and vismodegib, has demonstrated promising results in managing eyelid BCC in the past decade [7]. Imiquimod acts as an "immune response modifier" by augmenting the host immune response via stimulation of toll-like receptors 7 and 8. Imiquimod cream 5% was approved for the treatment of genital warts, actinic keratosis, and superficial BCC. Several case series have reported more than 80% complete resolution in both resectable and unresectable BCC, with topical imiquimod alone. Large BCC tumors without deep tissue infiltration, in which complete excision would cause significant local morbidity, can be good candidates for topical imiquimod. A recent study in large eyelid BCC demonstrated histological results of 89.5% tumor-free biopsy at 3 months after a regimen of once daily, 5 times a week application for 8–16 weeks [8]. Reversible local side effects include conjunctivitis, keratitis, foreign body sensation, lacrimation, decreased vision, and ectropion.

Vismodegib, a hedgehog pathway inhibitor, is approved for locally advanced or metastatic BCC [9]. Case series have shown that oral vismodegib is an effective and well-tolerated treatment in locally advanced and metastatic BCC, especially in basal cell nevus syndrome. Although with promising results, the high cost of the medication is a limitation for more widespread use. Vismodegib inhibits a hedgehog pathway without affecting underlying gene mutation; thus long-term therapy is required to suppress cell proliferation. Discontinuation of vismodegib in basal cell nevus syndrome has been reported to result in recurrent BCC; thus life-long medication may be necessary.

Pathology

Histopathological features of nodular BCC include nests (clusters) of basal cells with peripheral palisading cells in the epidermis with dermal invasion. Crack, or retraction artifact, is another pathognomonic feature due to loss of adherence of tumor cells to the surrounding stroma (Fig. 14.4). In the morpheaform subtype, thin cords of basaloid cells with peripheral radiation, also referred to as Indian-fire pattern, are seen.

Squamous Cell Carcinoma

Squamous cell carcinoma (SCC) accounts for 10% of eyelid malignancy and is more locally aggressive. The most common sites involved are the lower eyelids and medial canthus. SCC can invade directly to periocular nerves, referred to as perineural invasion (8–14%), or metastasize to regional lymph nodes (10–24%) [10].

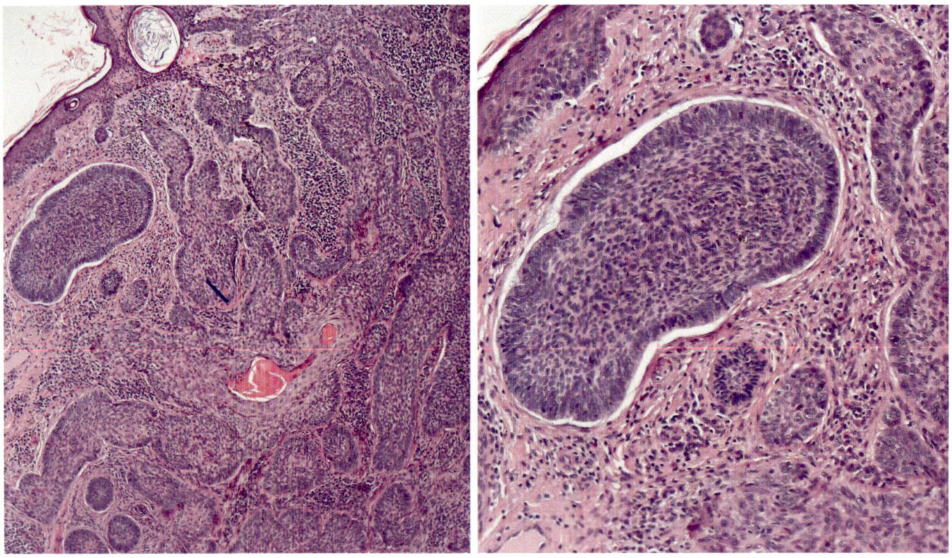

Fig. 14.4 Histopathologic features of nodular BCC include nests of blue basaloid cell in the epidermis, with disruption of basement membrane and dermal invasion. High-power field shows the pathognomonic features of peripheral palisading and crack artifact

Pathogenesis

Squamous cell carcinoma (SCC) can arise spontaneously, or more commonly at sites of actinic keratosis or other preexisting skin lesions such as radiation dermatitis, Bowen's disease (SCC in situ), chronic inflammatory lesions, and xeroderma pigmentosum. The most significant risk factor is exposure to UV light especially in lighter-skinned individuals. Smoking, exposure to chemicals, immunosuppression, human papillomavirus infection, and acquired immune deficiency syndrome are also more frequent risk factors for SCC [11].

Clinical Features

There are two major subtypes of SCC – differentiated and undifferentiated:

1. *Differentiated SCC* presents as a slow-growing, painless papule or nodule, with overlying keratinization, scaling, and central ulceration, resembling BCC.
2. *Undifferentiated SCC* can present as a soft, fleshy, or granulomatous mass (Fig. 14.5). A large erythematous base or surrounding scaly lesion or actinic keratosis may help in clinical diagnosis.

Perineural invasion can cause characteristic pain or numbness of the periocular area, which is not typically seen in BCC. Orbital invasion in neglected cases can present as proptosis, epiphora, diplopia, and visual loss.

Management

In general, management is similar to BCC; however, a wider surgical margin of 3–4 mm is recommended due to its more aggressive nature. According to the AJCC criteria, the category of eyelid cancer at presentation correlates with the risk of nodal metastasis and local recurrence in SCC [12]. A large retrospective cohort study recommended sentinel lymph node biopsy or stricter nodal surveillance for SCC tumors categorized as T2b or greater (tumor >10 mm in greatest dimension or involving full thickness of eyelid). For recurrent tumors or concern for orbital involvement, orbital CT scan or MRI is recommended, and orbital exenteration for local control may be indicated. A multidisciplinary tumor board is beneficial in determining the most appropriate management plan for the patient.

Targeted therapies, with epidermal growth factor receptor (EGFR) inhibitors, are approved and available for inoperable head and neck SCC. However, at present, efficacy and tolerability of these medications in periocular SCC are still insufficient, and further studies are necessary.

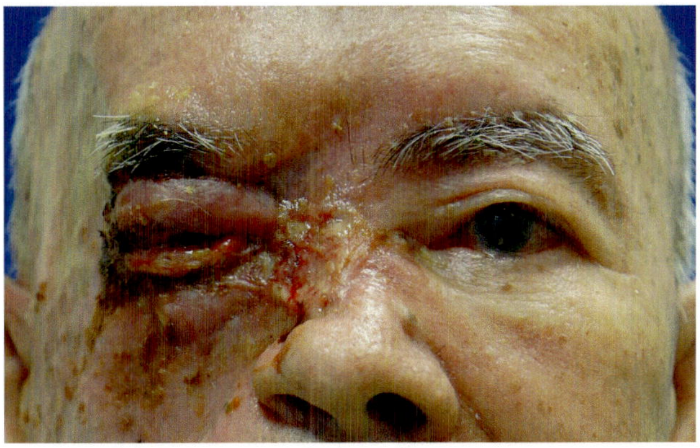

Fig. 14.5 Squamous cell carcinoma, undifferentiated subtype, presenting as a soft, fleshy, granulomatous-like mass involving the right periorbital area and nasal area. Photo shows local invasion with orbital involvement and recurrence after multiple surgical excisions and radiation

Pathology

SCC is characterized by anaplastic squamous cells that replace the normal epidermis, disruption of the epithelial basement membrane, and tumor extension to the dermal layer. It can present with well-differentiated cells with intercellular bridges, hyperkeratosis, and dyskeratosis or as poorly differentiated cells that cannot be distinguished from other malignancies (Fig. 14.6).

Sebaceous Carcinoma

The incidence of sebaceous carcinoma (previously termed sebaceous cell carcinoma, sebaceous adenocarcinoma) varies greatly among ethnicity, representing less than 5% of eyelid malignancy in Caucasians but as high as 37% in Asians [12]. This difference reflects the very low rate of BCC and SCC in Asian populations, rather than a true increased risk of sebaceous carcinoma in Asians. Sebaceous carcinoma can arise from meibomian glands, the glands of Zeis, or sebaceous glands of the caruncle. The most common site involved is the upper eyelid, which reflects the higher number of meibomian gland and glands of Zeis. The intraepithelial (pagetoid) tumor growth and multicentric behavior of sebaceous carcinomas limit the accuracy of clinical tumor evaluation, and therefore, may result in higher tumor recurrences. Rates of regional nodal metastasis (20–30%), systemic metastasis (8–67%), and disease-related mortality (3–41%) are also the highest among eyelid malignancies [12, 13].

Pathogenesis

Sebaceous carcinoma is more common in elderly females >50 years. In a patient with multiple sebaceous adenomas or

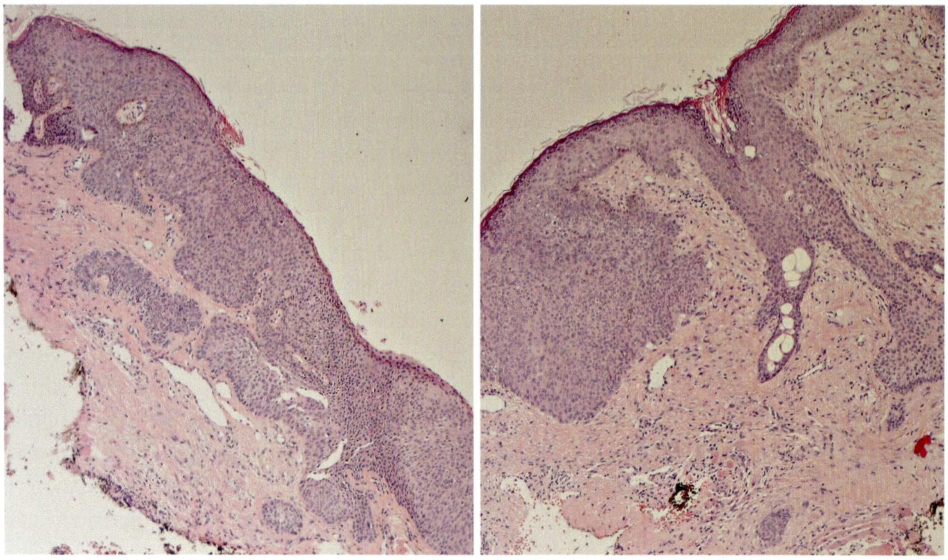

Fig. 14.6 Histopathologic features of SCC include anaplastic squamous cells that replace the normal epidermis, disruption of the epithelial basement membrane, and tumor extension to the dermal layer. The irregularly thick epidermis demonstrates normal to full-thickness dysplasia, with involvement of sebaceous and eccrine glands

carcinomas or in a young patient with sebaceous carcinoma, further evaluation for the possibility of Muir-Torre syndrome should be considered. Muir-Torre syndrome is an autosomal dominant cancer syndrome with an increased risk of colon and genitourinary tract cancer and thus requires long-term follow-up.

Clinical Features

There are two common presentations of sebaceous carcinoma – eyelid nodules and diffuse eyelid thickening with inflammation.

1. Eyelid nodular cancer, arising from the glands within the tarsal plates, can resemble an internal hordeolum or chalazion (Fig. 14.7). Yellowish content with telangiectasias can be more visible with eyelid eversion. Sebaceous carcinoma should be suspected in all cases of recurrent chalazia, especially in the elderly, and warrants biopsy.
2. Diffuse eyelid thickening with inflammation can also resemble chronic blepharitis or meibomian gland disease (Fig. 14.8). Highly suspicious features include unilateral involvement, uneven thickening of tarsal plate, and madarosis. Intraepithelial spread can extend to and involve both bulbar and palpebral conjunctiva and present as papillary conjunctivitis.

Management

Full-thickness eyelid incisional or punch biopsy should be performed in all suspicious cases of recurrent chalazia or chronic blepharitis. Histologic misdiagnosis of sebaceous carcinoma is common if the specimen is a superficial skin biopsy or from only the content of incision and curettage. Containing a portion of adjacent normal eyelid tissue within the specimen to examine the transitional area is also advised. Tissue can be placed in formalin as usual, but communication with pathologist is necessary as routine tissue processing with xylene can wash out fat content and lead to misdiagnosis.

Wide excision of at least 4 mm margin and margin control by frozen section or Mohs micrographic surgery is the treatment of choice for sebaceous carcinoma. However, due to intraepithelial spread and multicentric origins, conjunctival map biopsy is recommended in cases of conjunctival involvement. Intraepithelial spread can be managed with double freeze-thaw cryotherapy or topical mitomycin-C eye drops.

According to the AJCC criteria, T category eyelid cancer at presentation significantly correlates with risk of nodal metastasis, distance metastasis, and disease-specific survival rates in sebaceous carcinoma. Like SCC, T2b or greater lesions (tumor >10 mm in greatest dimension or involving full thickness of eyelid) correlate with a higher risk of nodal metastasis and local recurrence, requiring sentinel lymph node biopsy and long-term surveillance [13]. Orbital exenteration may be indicated in recurrent cases or cases with orbital invasion.

Pathology

Sebaceous carcinoma is characterized by abnormal proliferations of sebaceous cells with vacuolated cytoplasm (Fig. 14.9), best visualized by special staining such as Oil Red O or Sudan black. Careful evaluation for intraepithelial involvement to the conjunctival epithelium and dermal appendages should be studied. Some

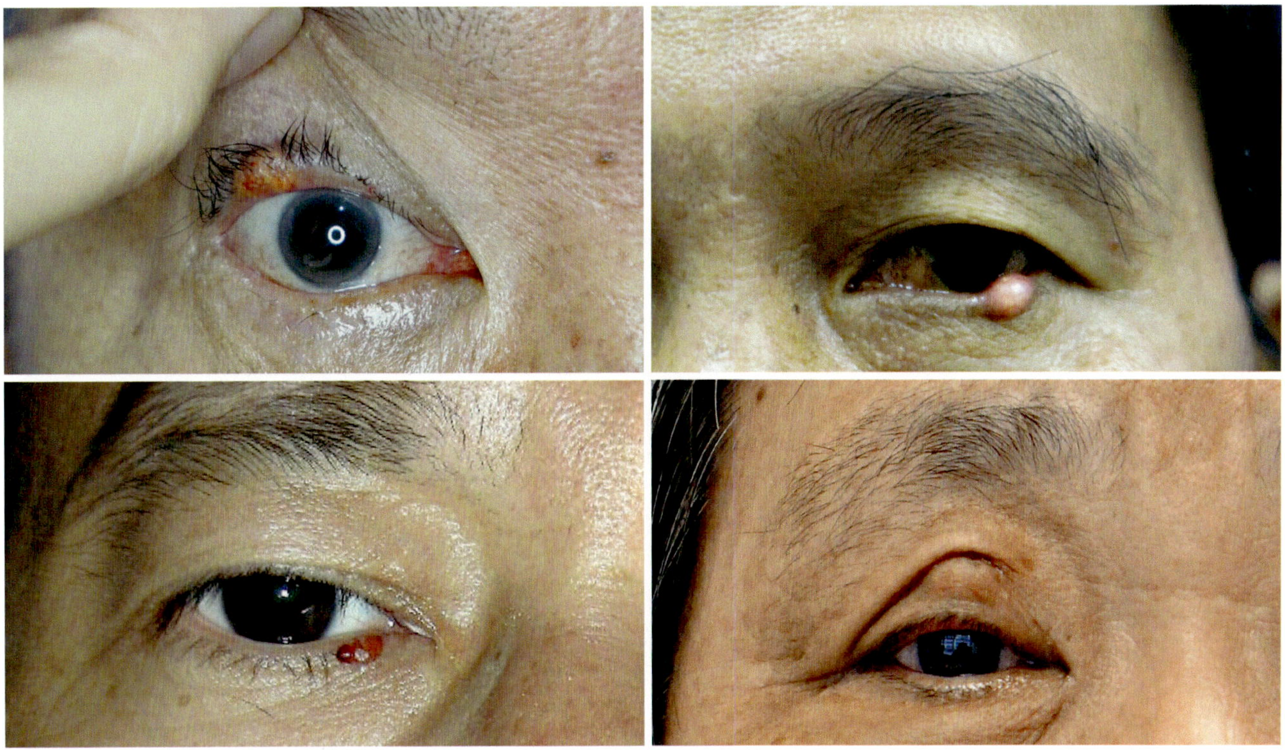

Fig. 14.7 Clinical features of sebaceous carcinoma can mimic benign lesions. Early presentations of eyelid sebaceous carcinoma can resemble a common internal hordeolum, chalazion, or epidermoid/sebaceous cyst. Incisional or excisional biopsy with pathological examination is indicated in all cases with recurrent lesions, particularly in the elderly population

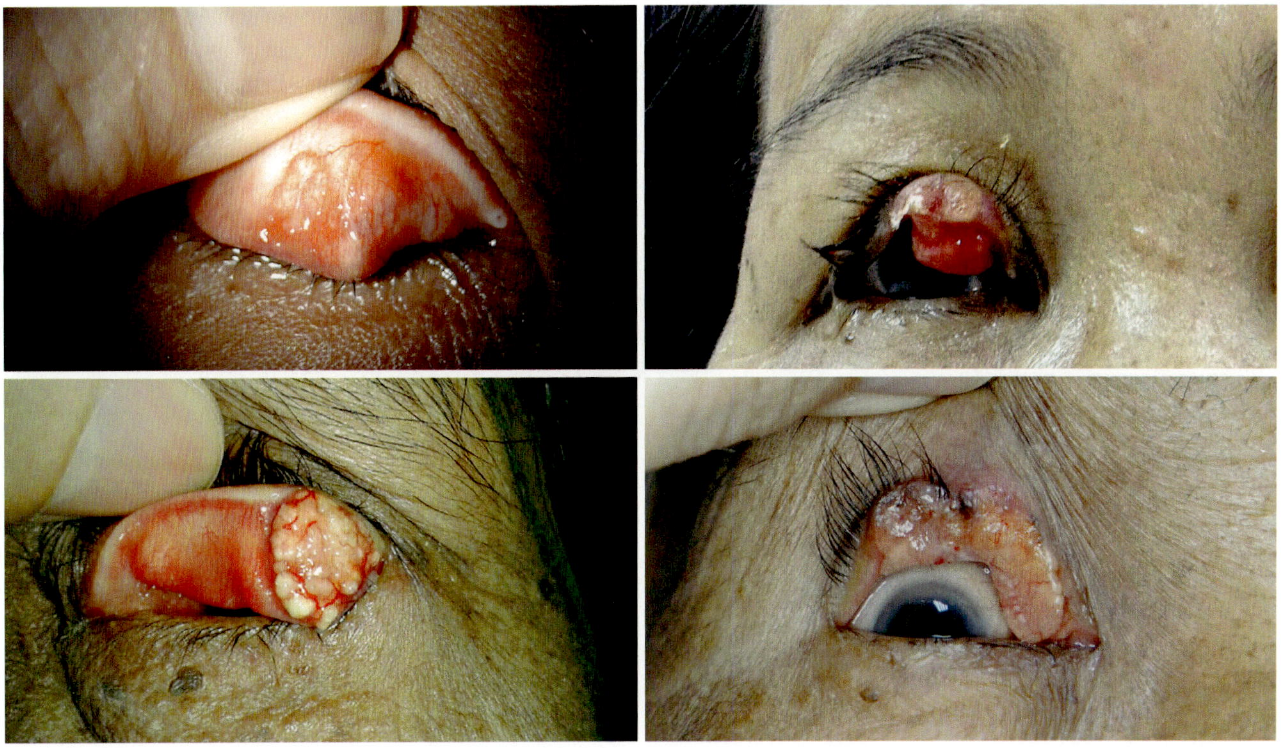

Fig. 14.8 Clinical features of advanced sebaceous carcinoma include obvious involvement of the tarsal plate and eyelid margin destruction. Conjunctivitis can be present and may warrant conjunctival map biopsies to search for pagetoid tumor spread and skip lesions

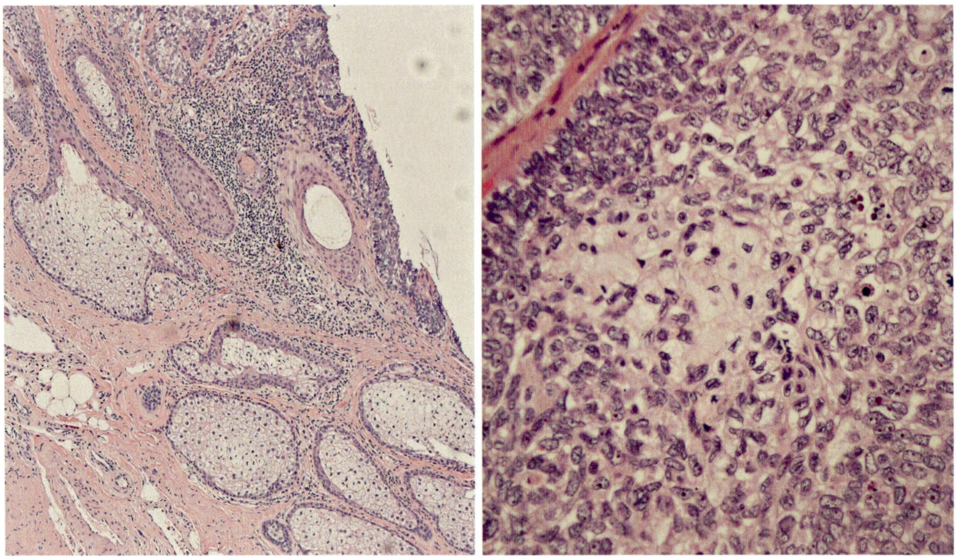

Fig. 14.9 The histopathology of sebaceous carcinoma is characterized by abnormal proliferation of sebaceous cells with vacuolated cytoplasm. High-power field demonstrates sebaceous and basophilic cells with both atypical nuclei and frequent mitoses

immunohistochemistry studies have suggested that adipophilin can be a sensitive and reliable marker for sebaceous carcinoma, and help differentiate it from mimicking lesions.

Malignant Melanoma

Malignant melanoma accounts for less than 1% of eyelid lesions, but 10% of nodal metastasis risk [1]. It can develop de novo or from pre-existing hyperpigmented lesions, such as benign nevus, dysplastic nevus, and lentigo maligna (melanoma in situ). It presents most frequently on the lower eyelid and can invade the orbit by neural invasion.

Pathogenesis

Melanoma can arise spontaneously or, more commonly, at sites of benign or dysplastic nevi and lentigo maligna. The most significant risk factor is exposure to UV light, especially in Caucasians. Ingestion of arsenic containing fluids and exposure to insecticides have been associated with an increased risk of melanoma.

Clinical Features

The American Cancer Society developed a popular mnemonic "ABCDEs" to serve as a guideline for the diagnosis of malignant melanoma (Fig. 14.10). "A" stands for *a*symmetrical shape, "B" stands for irregular *b*order, "C" stands for uneven *c*olor, "D" stands for *d*iameter larger than 6 mm, and "E" stands for *e*volving nature of the lesion. Any acquired pigmented lesion after the second decade of life, or any change in size except during puberty and pregnancy, should be considered suspicious for melanoma.

There are four forms of malignant melanoma: lentigo maligna melanoma, nodular melanoma, superficial spreading melanoma, and acral lentiginous melanoma. Only the first three occur in the periocular region.

1. Lentigo maligna melanoma is the most common form of eyelid melanoma, occurring in approximately 30–50% of patients with lentigo maligna. Lentigo maligna, also known as precancerous melanosis, is a premalignant melanocytic lesion, characterized by a macule that has slow enlargement, uneven coloration, and irregular borders. It usually occurs on the malar region and extends to the eyelid and conjunctival surface. Histopathology demonstrates abnormal cells isolated to the epidermis. With malignant transformation, it can present as a pigmented nodule within a larger macule due to invasive vertical growth into the dermis (Fig. 14.11).
2. Nodular melanoma can arise from nevi and present as a variably pigmented, often black, nodule with possible ulceration and bleeding. Thickness of the lesion often represents vertically invasive growth, and indicates poorer prognosis.
3. Superficial spreading melanoma is by far the most common subtype, accounting for 70–80% of all melanomas particularly in Caucasians. This relatively flat lesion is most often seen in areas of sun exposure in young individuals and can also arise in a previously benign mole or as a new lesion. It demonstrates varying colors of tan, brown, black, red, blue, or white. Superficial spreading melanoma has a prolonged radial growth phase during which the lesion remains thin, until it penetrates into the dermis and becomes elevated. Although it can occur anywhere on the body, it most often occurs on the trunk, legs, or upper back.

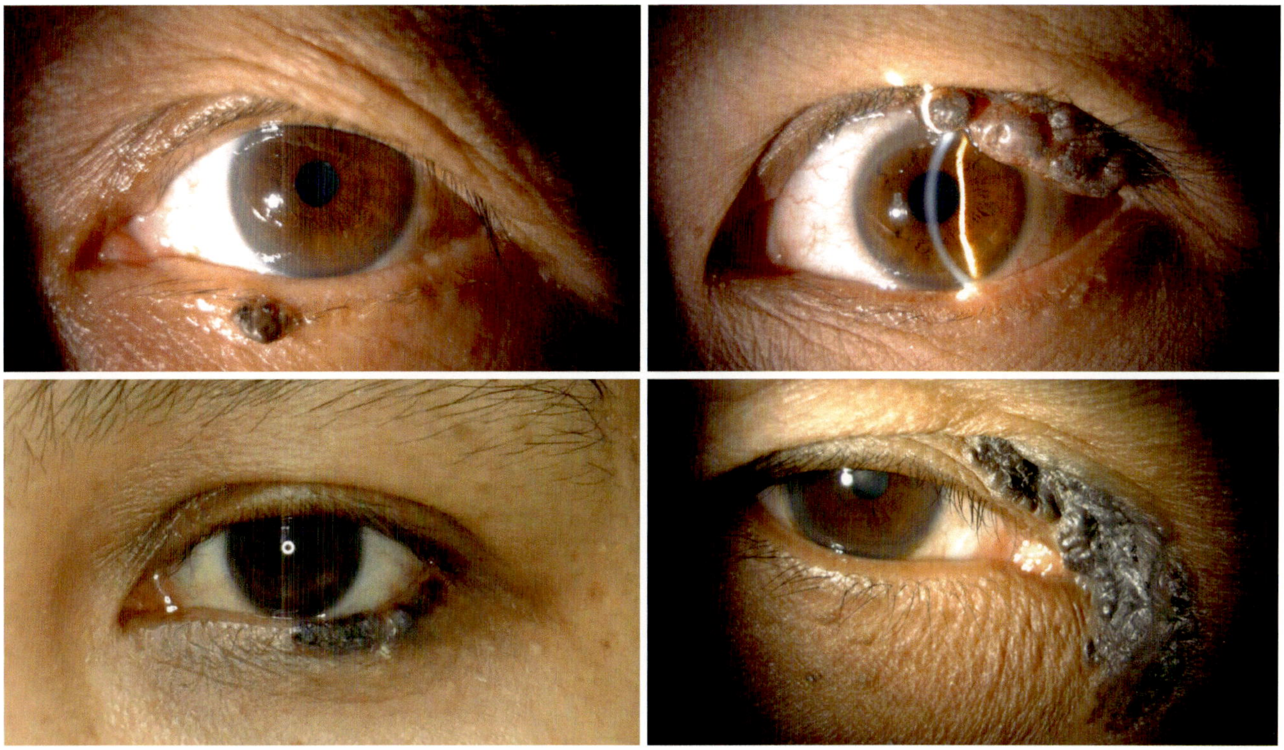

Fig. 14.10 Clinical differences of benign nevus and malignant melanoma. Upper images demonstrate a typical benign nevus of the eyelid margin. These lesions are often present since childhood and have an even brown color with no change in size or eyelid margin destruction. The presence of eyelashes growing through the mass is also suggestive signs of a benign lesion. The lower images show malignant melanoma with darker, irregular colors within the lesions, loss of eyelashes, and increase in size over months

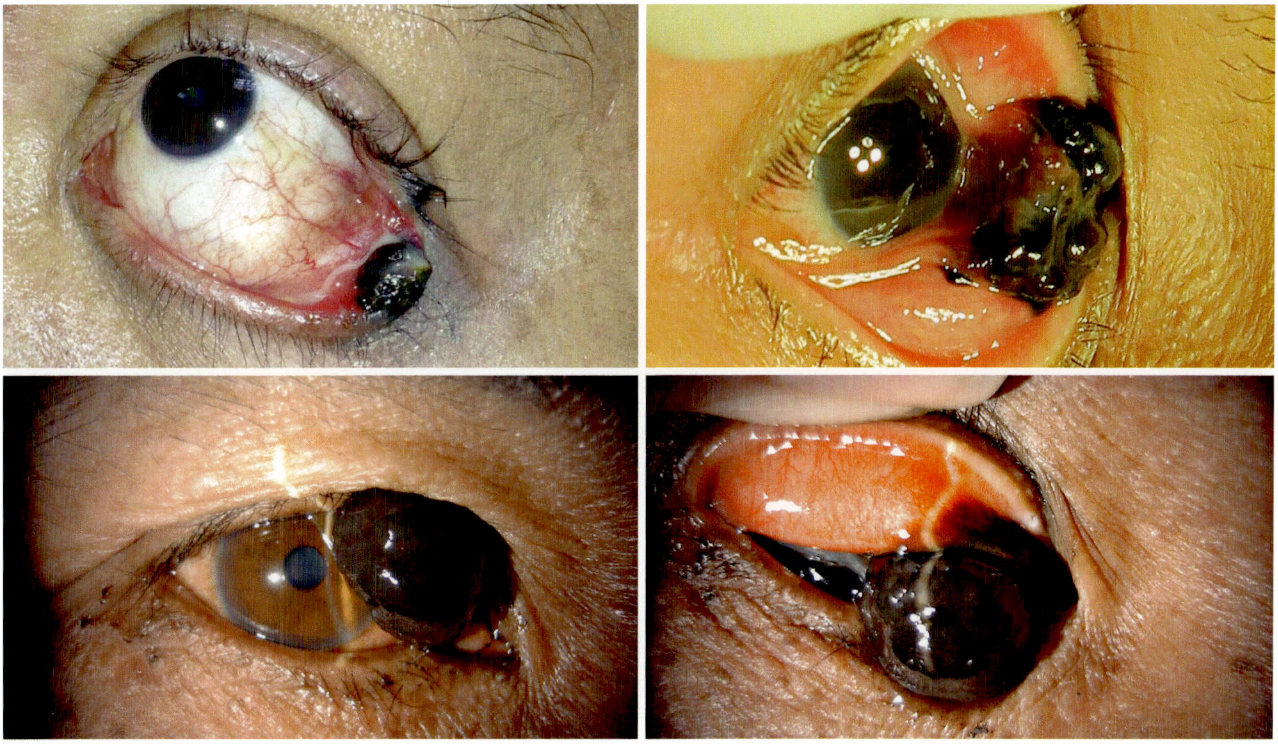

Fig. 14.11 Malignant melanoma (MM) arising from a premalignant lesion. Left upper image shows lentigo maligna melanoma with a hyperpigmented macule at the lateral canthus underlying the nodular lesion. Right upper image shows MM arising from primary acquired melanosis of the conjunctiva which later involved both upper and lower eyelids. Lower images show MM arising from the palpebral conjunctiva of the upper eyelid

Management

Incisional biopsy is indicated in all suspicious pigmented lesions. The AJCC criteria for eyelid melanoma are different from eyelid carcinoma. For cutaneous melanoma, T category is based on three independent histologic prognostic factors: Breslow thickness, the presence of ulceration, and the presence of mitotic figures. As increased tumor thickness is associated with lower 5- and 10-year survival rates, full-thickness lesion biopsy at its thickest portion should be determined using a skin punch or scissors. AJCC T category of T2b (tumor 1.01–2.00 mm with ulceration) or greater is correlated with a higher risk of nodal metastasis requiring sentinel lymph node biopsy or closer nodal surveillance [12, 14]. The long-term value of sentinel lymph node biopsy is still controversial; however, long-term follow-up is mandatory as malignant melanoma can metastasize years later.

Wide surgical excision and histopathological margin control using permanent sections are recommended for melanoma. Frozen section may cause erroneous results due to tissue processing without bleaching. Contrary to other cutaneous melanoma, margins of less than 1 cm are usually employed in eyelid melanoma in the interest of tissue preservation for lid functioning. Currently, there is no accepted standard recommendation for the optimal excisional margin for eyelid melanoma. The Collaborative Eyelid Skin Melanoma Group Report suggests a surgical margin of 5 mm when feasible [15].

For lentigo maligna, 5% imiquimod cream has been demonstrated to be effective and tolerable in the periocular area. Several case series describing adjuvant treatment of conjunctival involvement or primary acquired melanosis (PAM) with interferon-alpha2b ophthalmic solution have been promising. These topical medications are options for local control of melanoma in situ and may allow globe preservation in cases of extensive superficial involvement. With orbital invasion, orbital imaging is necessary and exenteration should be considered. A multidisciplinary tumor board is beneficial in determining the most appropriate management plan for the patient.

Pathology

Histopathologic examination of malignant melanoma is characterized by a proliferation of atypical melanocytes in the epidermis with disruption of epithelial basement membrane and tumor extension to dermis layers. A pre-existing nevus can sometimes be seen as a well-circumscribed nest of mature melanocytes surrounding the area of atypia. Special stains such as HMB-45 and Melan-A (MART-1) can be used to confirm melanocytic origin, and to assess the surgical margins and extent of lesion (Fig. 14.12).

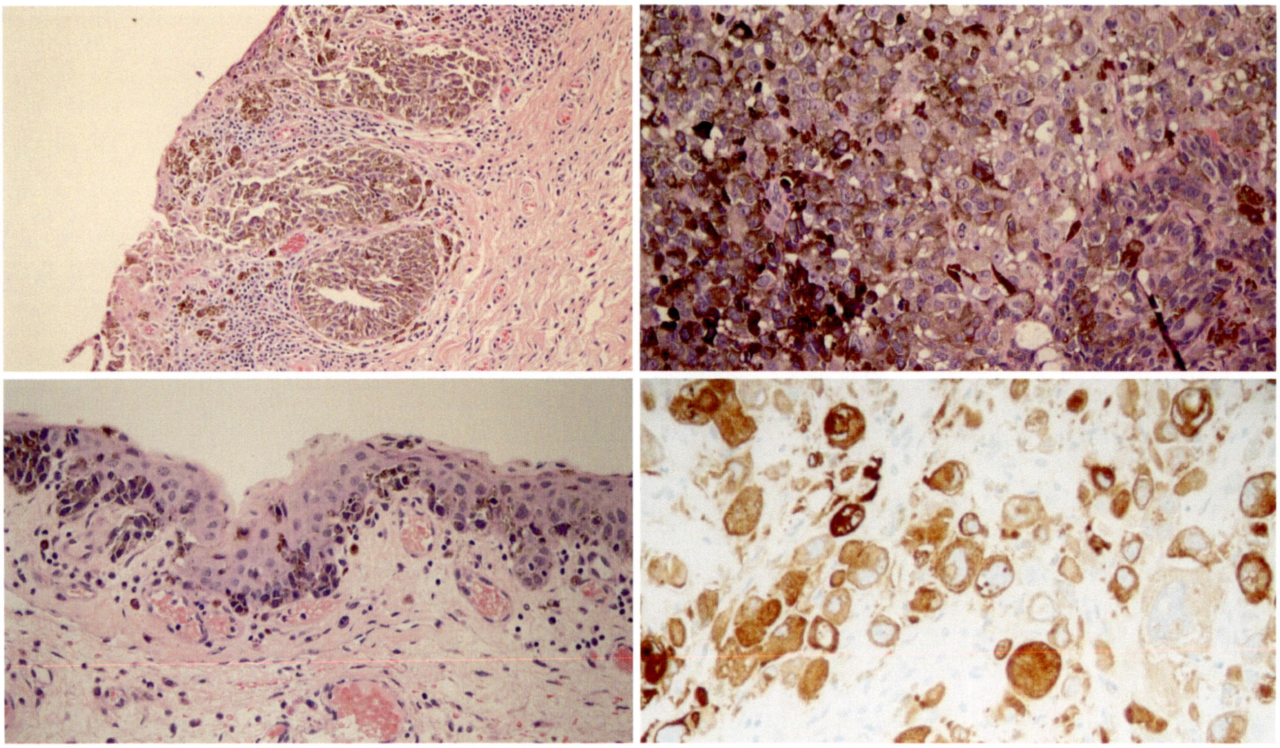

Fig. 14.12 Histopathological examination of malignant melanoma is characterized by a proliferation of atypical melanocytes in the epidermis with disruption of epithelial basement membrane and tumor extension to dermis (left upper). High-power field demonstrates numerous large pleomorphic cells with high nuclear to cytoplasm ratio and abundant mitotic figures (right upper). Left lower image shows primary acquired melanosis with severe atypia, with pleomorphic cells with high nuclear to cytoplasmic ratio and melanin pigment granules occupying the conjunctival epithelium. Right lower image demonstrates positive Melan-A staining for melanocytes

Merkel Cell Carcinoma (Cutaneous Neuroendocrine Carcinoma)

Merkel cell carcinoma involving the eyelid encompasses approximately 10% of all Merkel cell carcinoma cases, and typically involves the upper eyelid [16]. Although it is a rare type of skin malignancy, it is an aggressive tumor with a local recurrence rate of approximately 10% and a 19% rate of distant metastasis, often within the first few years after initial diagnosis [17].

Pathogenesis

Merkel cell carcinoma arises from Merkel cells, which are specialized neuroendocrine receptors that mediate touch sensation of the skin and mucosa. It can present anywhere on the body surface, including the eyelids. Common risk factors include a history of excessive sun exposure, including artificial light (tanning beds) and ultraviolet A therapy for psoriasis, prior infection with polyomavirus, chronic immunosuppression from leukemia or organ transplantation, and HIV infection [12].

Clinical Features

Eyelid Merkel cell carcinoma usually presents as a painless, rapidly growing, erythematous or violaceous nodule close to the eyelid margin. Similar to other skin malignancies, it has a predilection for older patients with fair skin. The classic clinical appearance is a reddish-purple, dome or sausage-shaped nodular lesion with telangiectasias. In the early stage, it can sometimes resemble an internal hordeolum or chalazion, and result in delayed diagnosis.

Management

Biopsy should be performed in all suspicious lesions. Wide excision and margin control by frozen section or Mohs micrographic surgery is the treatment of choice, when possible. There is a specific category of the AJCC criteria for cutaneous Merkel cell carcinoma; however, the T classification for cutaneous Merkel cell carcinoma may be impractical for eyelid lesions. For cutaneous Merkel cell carcinoma, the T1 category includes tumors $\leq$2.00 cm, and T2 tumors measure 2.01–5.00 cm. As the eyelid is approximately 3 cm wide, almost all cases will be categorized in the T1 category. Therefore, for eyelid Merkel cell carcinoma, staging based on the AJCC criteria for eyelid carcinoma may be more appropriate with better prognostic value. AJCC T category of T2b (tumor 1.01–2.00 mm with ulceration) or greater is correlated with a higher risk of nodal metastasis requiring sentinel lymph node biopsy or closer nodal surveillance [12, 17].

Pathology

The histopathology of Merkel cell carcinoma is characterized by poorly differentiated cells with round to oval nuclei and abundant mitotic activity. The densely basophilic tumor cells usually arrange in lobules, sheets, or nests in the dermal layer. Frequently, the tumor will demonstrate involvement of the overlying epidermis, as well as invade the subcutaneous fat. The cell outlines often mold together or resemble lymphocytes, and necrosis and lymphovascular invasion are common. Less commonly, in situ squamous cell carcinoma or sarcomatoid differentiation may be seen in Merkel cell carcinoma or in the overlying skin. Immunohistochemistry may demonstrate positivity for CK-20 proteins.

Summary

In summary, a complete description of all surgical and medical treatment options is outside the scope of this chapter, but the surgeon should be highly cognizant of these skin malignancies that can occur in the periorbital region.

References

1. Cook BE Jr, Bartley GB. Epidemiologic characteristics and clinical course of patients with malignant eyelid tumors in an incidence cohort in Olmsted County, Minnesota. Ophthalmology. 1999;106:746–50.
2. Deprez M, Uffer S. Clinicopathological features of eyelid skin tumors: a retrospective study of 5504 cases and review of literature. Am J Dermatopathol. 2009;3:256–62.
3. Watanabe A, Sun MT, Pirbhai A, et al. Sebaceous carcinoma in Japanese patients: clinical presentation, staging and outcomes. Br J Ophthalmol. 2013;97:1459–63.
4. Margo CE, Waltz K. Basal cell carcinoma of the eyelid and periocular skin. Surv Ophthalmol. 1993;38:169–92.
5. Honavar SG, Shields JA, Shields CL, et al. Basal cell carcinoma of the eyelids associated with Gorlin-Gorltz syndrome. Ophthalmology. 2001;108:1115–23.
6. Malhotra R, Huilgol SC, Huynh NT, et al. The Australian Mohs database, part II: periocular basal cell carcinoma outcome at 5-year follow-up. Ophthalmology. 2004;111:631–6.
7. Silverman N, Shinder R. What's new in eyelid tumors. Asia Pac J Ophthalmol. 2017;6:143–52.
8. de Macedo EM, Carneiro RC, de Lima PP, et al. Imiquimod cream efficacy in the treatment of periocular nodular basal cell carcinoma: a non-randomized trial. BMC Ophthalmol. 2015;15:35.
9. Sekulic A, Migden MR, Oro AE, et al. Efficacy and safety of vismodegib in advanced basal-cell carcinoma. N Engl J Med. 2012;366:2171–9.
10. Faustina M, Diba R, Ahmadi MA, et al. Patterns of regional and distant metastasis in patients with eyelid and periocular squamous cell carcinoma. Ophthalmology. 2004;111:1930–2.
11. Donaldson MJ, Sullivan TJ, Whitehead KJ, et al. Squamous cell carcinoma of the eyelids. Br J Ophthalmol. 2002;86:1161–5.
12. Ford J, Thakar S, Thuro B, et al. Prognostic value of the staging system for eyelid tumors in the 7th edition of the American Joint Committee on Cancer Staging manual. Ophthal Plast Reconstr Surg. 2017;33:317–24.

13. Esmaeli B, Nasser QJ, Cruz H, et al. American Joint Committee on Cancer T category for eyelid sebaceous carcinoma correlates with nodal metastasis and survival. Ophthalmology. 2012;119:1078–82.
14. Yin VT, Warneke CL, Merritt HA, et al. Number of excisions required to obtain clear surgical margins and prognostic value of AJCC T category for patients with eyelid melanoma. Br J Ophthalmol. 2014;98:1681–5.
15. Esmaeli B, Youssef A, Naderi A, et al. Collaborative Eyelid Skin Melanoma Group. Margins of excision for cutaneous melanoma of the eyelid skin: the Collaborative Eyelid Skin Melanoma Group Report. Ophthal Plast Reconstr Surg. 2003;19:96–101.
16. Missotten GS, de Wolff-Rouendaal D, de Keizer RJ. Merkel cell carcinoma of the eyelid review of the literature and report of patients with Merkel cell carcinoma showing spontaneous regression. Ophthalmology. 2008;115:195–201.
17. Herbert HM, Sun MT, Selva D, et al. Merkel cell carcinoma of the eyelid: management and prognosis. JAMA Ophthalmol. 2014;132:197–204.

Upper Eyelid Reconstruction

15

Morris E. Hartstein

The upper eyelid is a very specialized and critical structure, providing protection for the cornea and the globe. With defects in the upper eyelid, it is crucial to not only restore the missing or injured anatomy but also to make sure that physiologic function is preserved, specifically, the excursion or mobility of the eyelid and its protective function, especially against dry eye. Reconstructive considerations in a full-thickness eyelid defect include providing tarsus or a substitute to provide for stability of the eyelid margin as well as being in contact with the cornea. If skin is to be reconstructed, it will need to be thin and redundant enough to allow for eyelid closure but also flexible enough to allow for eyelid opening. Finally, palpebral fissure opening needs to be taken into account [1, 2].

Compared to the lower eyelid where generally the lid can be made extremely taut, in the upper lid, this may lead to ptosis. In the upper eyelid, it is crucial to have a non-keratinizing epithelial lining to avoid any irritation of the cornea. In the lower eyelid, this is less crucial, and even non-keratinizing surface may be used such as a hard palate graft. The tarsal plate in the lower eyelid is only about 4 mm in vertical height, whereas it is about 10 mm in the upper eyelid and therefore requires more attention during reconstruction. A defect in the upper eyelid from tumor excision or trauma usually requires prompt attention to prevent dry eye or corneal injury [1, 2].

Upper eyelid defects may result from trauma, tumor excision, or congenital malformation such as coloboma. Many of these defects can be closed primarily in young and older patients (Fig. 15.1a, b). In older patients where there is usually significant horizontal laxity, defects comprising even 50% of the upper eyelid can be closed primarily, especially when combined with lateral canthal release. While the eyelid at first may appear tight and ptotic, over the course of the first few weeks postoperatively, the tension will relax, and eyelid aperture will enlarge (Fig. 15.2a, b). Advantages of direct closure include avoiding the need of a graft or flap, staged procedures, and most importantly preserved continuity at the lash line [1].

Reapproximating the eyelid margin is the crucial step during full-thickness repair, especially at the tarsus. Closure is best facilitated when there is a vertical tarsal incision. In tumor excision, this can be created when excising the tumor. In trauma cases, it may be necessary to excise additional tissue to create vertical edges which are better for repair. The vertical height of the tarsus is about 10 mm in the upper eyelid and should be excised along its full height in order to achieve good reapproximation at the eyelid margin. This is not a place to be conservative with incisions.

The eyelid margin wound edges can initially be reapproximated using forceps or a temporary suture to see if there is enough "give" to allow closure. If there is slight tension preventing full reapproximation, then a lateral cantholysis can be performed. A lateral canthotomy is performed initially using a 15 blade or sharp scissors. The superior crus of the lateral canthal tendon is then divided using Westcott scissors until the eyelid is "released" and the lid margin can be closed without tension. There are several techniques for lid margin closure, but the most important aspect of the repair is to ensure that the tarsus, lash line, and meibomian glands are lined up properly. The author prefers to place two vertical mattress sutures of either 6-0 Vicryl or 6-0 silk sutures. The first mattress suture is placed through the tarsal plate, and a similar mattress suture is placed just anterior to the first suture. When these sutures are tied, it should provide good eversion at the lid margin. The tarsal plate then needs to be closed along its length superiorly. This is done by placing several interrupted 6-0 Vicryl sutures partial thickness through the tarsus, beneath the orbicularis. If the tarsus is not closed fully along its length, this can cause notching at the lid margin. The skin is closed using 6-0 Vicryl, plain, or silk sutures. The lid margin sutures are cut long

M. E. Hartstein (✉)
Department of Ophthalmology, Assaf Harofeh Medical Center, Tel Aviv University-Sackler School of Medicine, Tel Aviv, Israel

A. J. Cohen, C. N. Burkat (eds.), *Oculofacial, Orbital, and Lacrimal Surgery*, https://doi.org/10.1007/978-3-030-14092-2_15

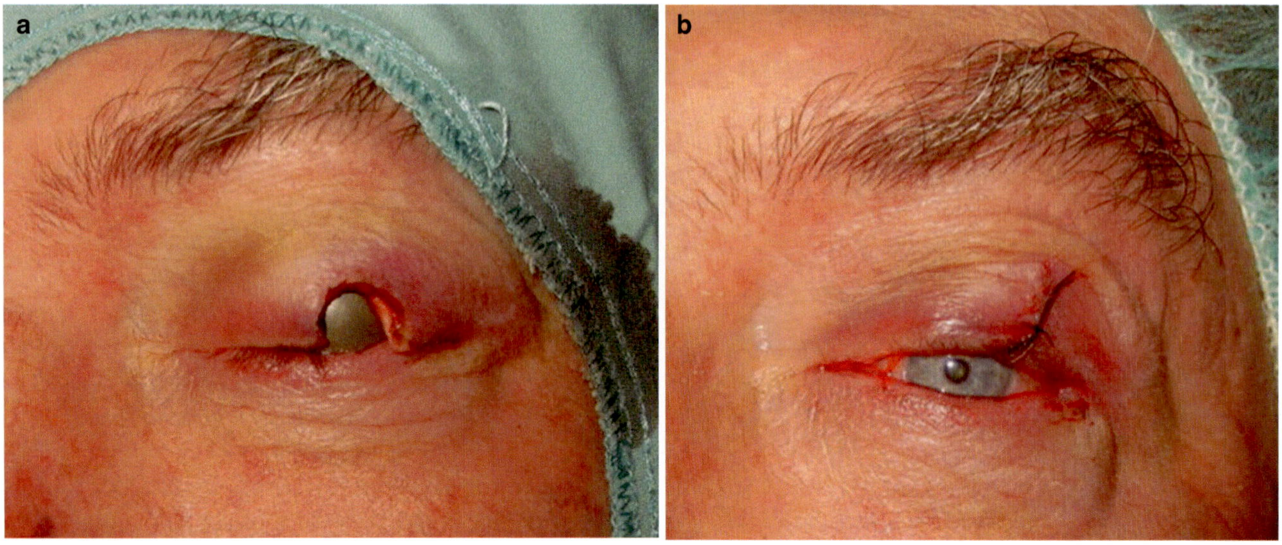

Fig. 15.1 Upper eyelid defect (**a**) that can be closed primarily (**b**) without the need for additional flaps

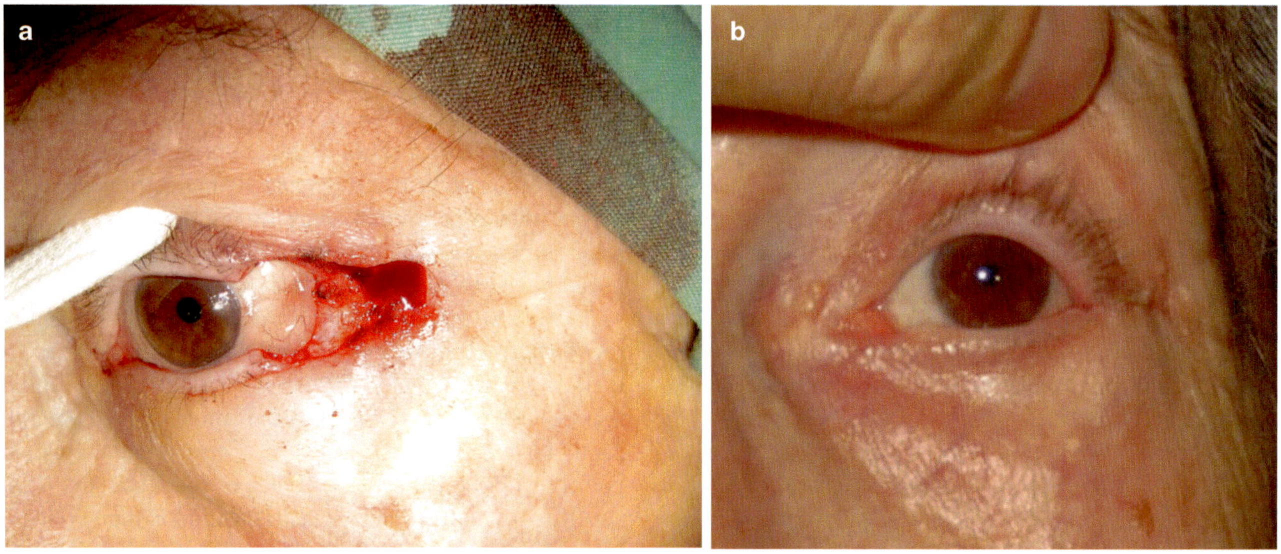

Fig. 15.2 Complex upper and lower eyelid and lateral canthal defect (**a**). After surgical repair, the eyelid may initially appear tight and ptotic (**b**)

and tied down under a more anterior skin suture to prevent irritation of the cornea [3].

In the case of a traumatic injury to the upper lid, it will often appear as if there is loss of tissue (Fig. 15.3a, b). This is because the upper lid is naturally under some tension in order to conform to the globe with blinking and closure. In most trauma cases, there is no true tissue loss—rather, the eyelid edges have just pulled apart due to release of the normal lid tension. Thus, in most cases, the wound edges, including the tarsus, can just be sutured together. If the tarsus is highly irregular from the laceration, a minimal amount of tissue may be excised vertically in order to produce a more regular edge to suture. The lid margin is then closed in similar fashion as described above.

In cases with a full-thickness lid margin defect which cannot be closed primarily even with lateral canthal release, a semicircular or Tenzel flap may be used [4, 5]. First, the upper lid defect is prepared as outlined above with vertically straight edges, perpendicular to the lid margin. A semicircular line is outlined, beginning at the lateral canthus and arching inferiorly (Fig. 15.4a, b). Using a 15 blade, an incision is made along the demarcated line and the flap undermined with scissors underneath the orbicularis layer. The superior crus of the lateral canthal tendon is lysed, thereby allowing complete mobilization of the lateral portion of the upper lid. Once the lateral lid is free, the lid margin defect can be closed as outlined above. Additional undermining of the flap can be carried out as needed for further mobilization medially. The underside of the flap is sutured to the lateral orbital rim periosteum, thereby creating a new lateral canthus. Care should be taken to place the lid on some tension with this suture as the lid will relax over time. Conjunctiva may be undermined

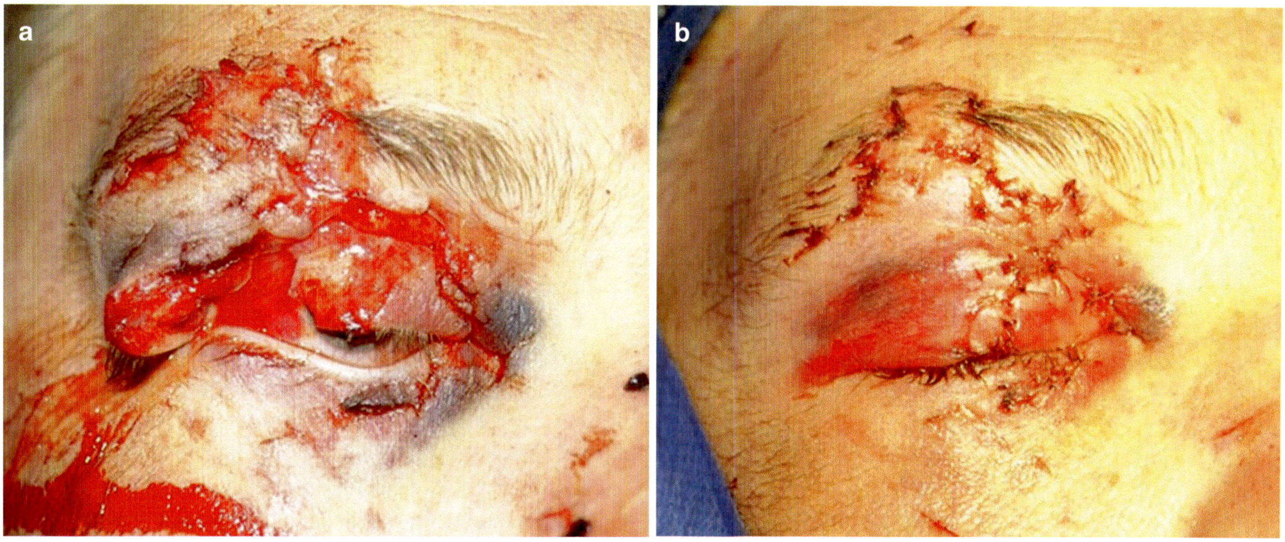

Fig. 15.3 Traumatic injury to the upper eyelid will often appear as if there is loss of tissue (**a**). Reconstruction with meticulous repair can typically demonstrate the presence of all eyelid tissue (**b**)

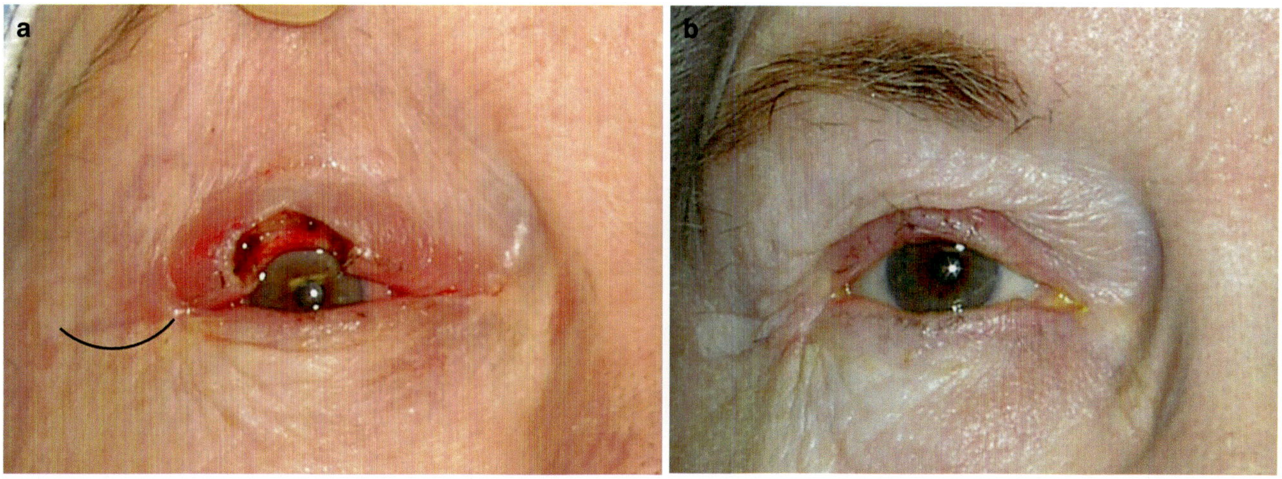

Fig. 15.4 The Tenzel flap is marked in a semicircular fashion from the lateral canthus (**a**). Eyelid shape and function are preserved after healing (**b**)

at the lateral aspect of the lid in order to advance it to cover the flap posteriorly; however, this step is often not necessary. The flap incision can be closed with interrupted 6-0 silk or prolene sutures.

In cases where primary closure is not possible, and when even a semicircular flap may not provide enough tissue for closure, the sliding Hughes-type flap may be employed [6–8]. This is a useful flap when a lid-sharing procedure such as a Cutler-Beard is not yet necessary or desired. The technique begins in similar fashion to the Hughes' tarsoconjunctival flap (Fig. 15.5). Once the Hughes flap is mobilized, instead of swinging it down into the lower lid, the flap is rotated either medially or laterally into the area of the defect. The donor tarsus can be slightly smaller than the defect to allow for slight tension on the lid when the flap is sutured into place. The tarsus is anchored into position to provide posterior lamella. The anterior lamella can be reconstructed either by mobilizing a small skin-muscle flap from an adjacent tissue or by using a full-thickness skin graft since the sliding flap is on a vascularized pedicle (Fig. 15.6a–d).

Large defects encompassing nearly the entire upper eyelid can be reconstructed with the Cutler-Beard bridge flap [9–11]. Although not often employed or necessary, this flap is very useful for reconstructing the entire upper lid by utilizing a full-thickness flap from the lower lid on the same side. It is important to check that the patient has good vision in the fellow eye since this flap will occlude the operated eye for a significant period of time. The flap is begun by outlining a rectangle 4–5 mm inferior to the lower lid margin in order to preserve the vascular supply and the viability of the lid margin. A 15 blade is used to make a full-thickness incision through the outlined flap. Vertical incisions are made perpendicular to the first cut. On the conjunctival side, dissection is carried out to the fornix and on the skin side, undermining is carried out over the cheek. Once the flap is totally dissected free, the conjunctiva can

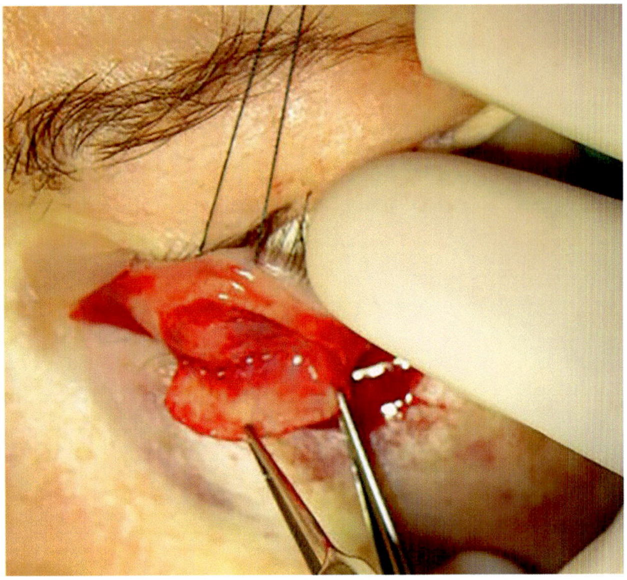

Fig. 15.5 The sliding Hughes tarsoconjunctival flap utilizes an upper eyelid flap that is rotated either medially or laterally into the defect of the same upper eyelid. The first step is creating a tarsoconjunctival flap

be dissected off the skin-muscle flap separately, pulled through beneath the lower lid margin bridge, and then sutured into place in the area of the upper lid defect. At this point, it should be noted that the upper lid does not contain any tarsus. It is possible at this stage to harvest a graft of cartilage or hard palate graft (HPG) and place it anterior to the conjunctiva as a tarsal replacement. However, despite the lack of tarsus, these lids can often do quite well, and a graft can always be placed secondarily after healing. The skin-muscle portion of the flap is then advanced under the lid margin bridge and secured into place in the area of the defect under slight tension. If necessary, additional undermining can be carried out to allow the skin-muscle flap to advance easily into the defect. The flap is allowed to heal for a period of 6–8 weeks. Early separation of the flap may lead to contracture from inadequate vascular supply. When separating the flap, an incision is made about 2 mm inferior to where the upper lid margin should be. A groove director or moistened cotton-tip applicator is placed beneath the flap to protect the eye during flap separation. A 15 blade may be used to begin the incision to divide the flap which is

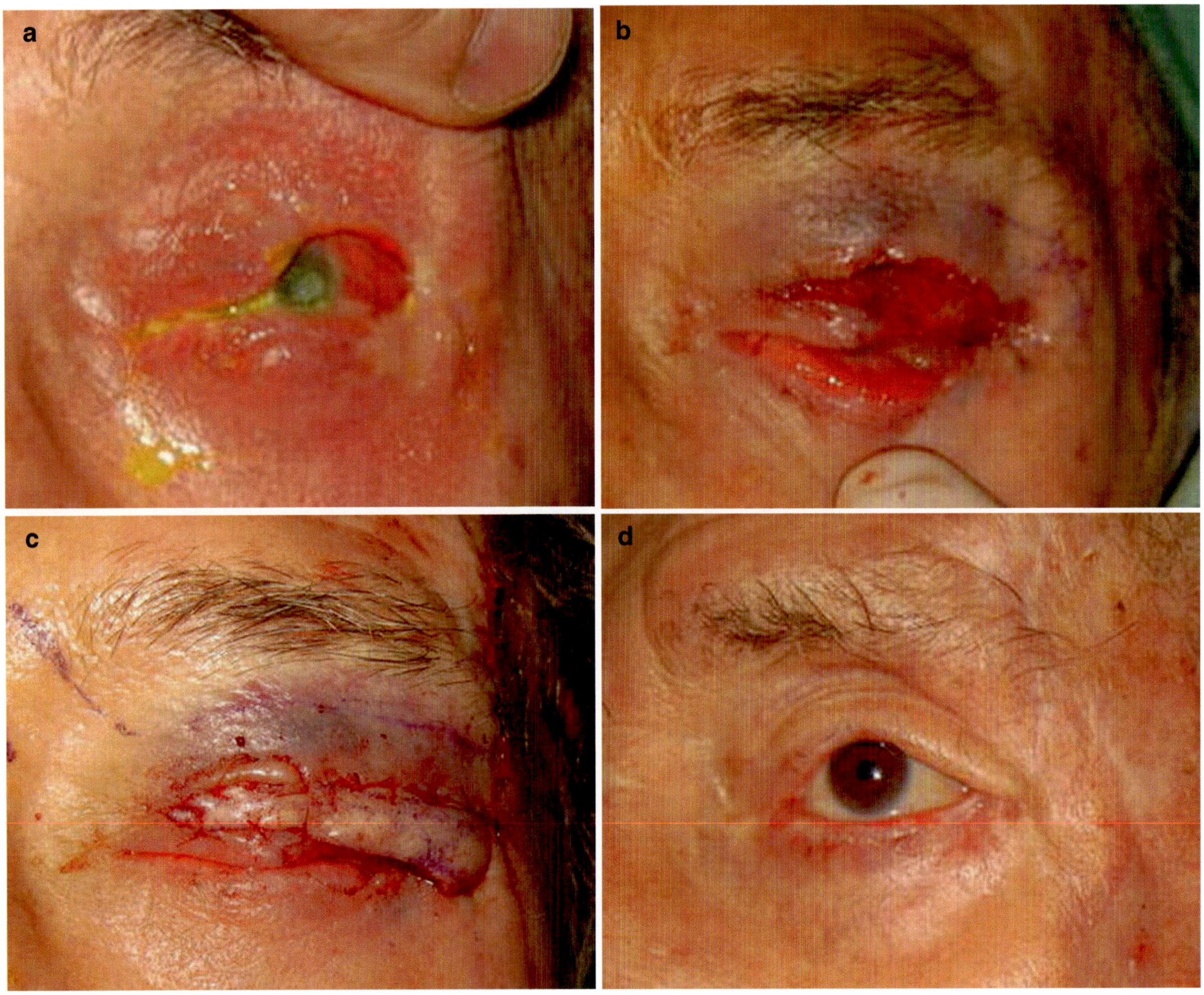

Fig. 15.6 The sliding Hughes tarsoconjunctival flap: (**a**) large centrolateral left upper eyelid defect; (**b**) the upper eyelid tarsoconjunctival flap is dissected from the medial upper eyelid and pulled laterally into the defect and sutured to the periosteum; (**c**) the temporal skin flap is rotated to create the anterior lamella over the tarsoconjunctival flap; (**d**) healed upper eyelid 9 months following surgery

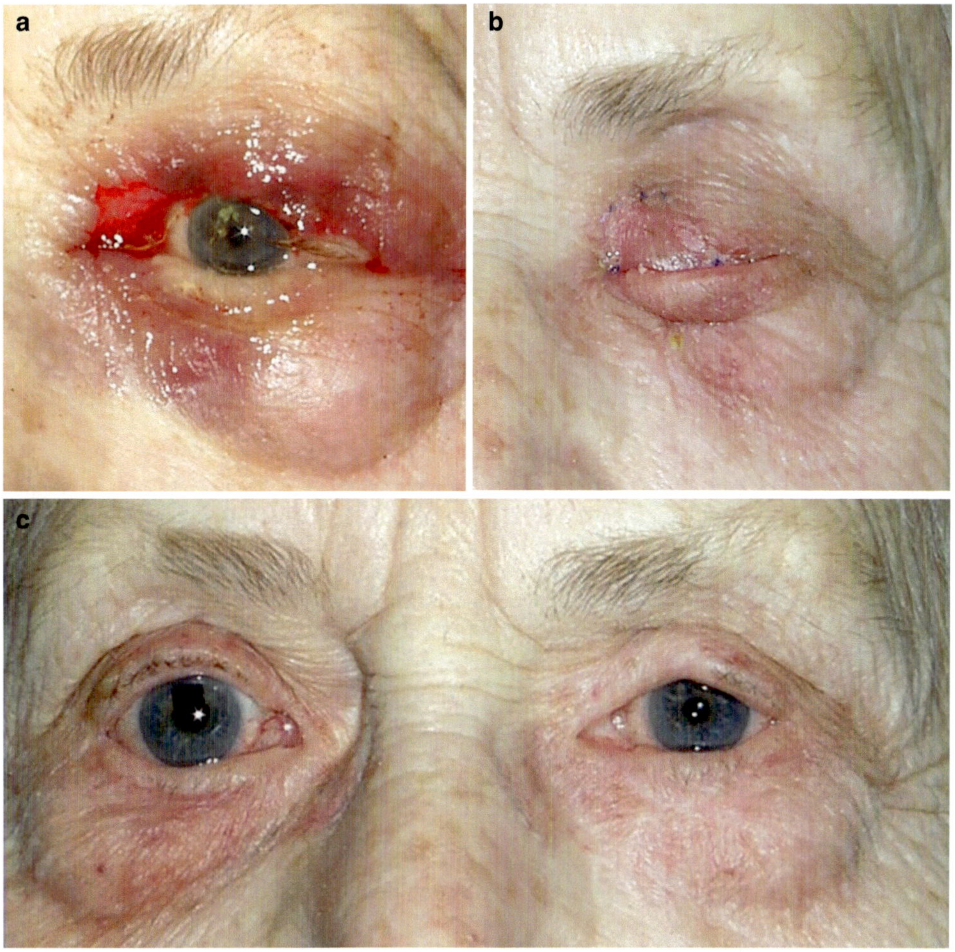

Fig. 15.7 Cutler-Beard procedure: (**a**) large defect encompassing nearly the entire upper eyelid; (**b**) the lower eyelid skin-muscle flap is advanced posterior to the eyelid margin bridge and secured into place in the area of the defect; (**c**) postoperative result several months after opening the bridge flap

completed with scissors. Once divided, 1–2 mm of skin and muscle from the edge of the flap is excised, leaving a free edge of conjunctiva. The conjunctival edge can be rotated to cover the new lid margin and prevent corneal erosions from the lid margin skin abutting the cornea. In the lower lid, the inferior portion of the lid margin bridge is de-epithelialized in preparation for return of the skin-muscle flap (Fig. 15.7a–c).

As a result of tumor excision and/or reconstruction or as a result of trauma (chemical injury), the upper eyelid may suffer from vertical shortening but with an intact lid margin. There may be associated trichiasis or distichiasis (Fig. 15.8a). In order to lengthen the posterior lamella, a graft such as cartilage, Alloderm, or hard palate is required [1, 12, 13]. The author prefers HPG as it undergoes minimal shrinkage and is well tolerated. Although HPG is a technically keratinizing epithelium, it usually will not adversely affect the cornea when placed in the upper lid. The lid is everted, which can sometimes be difficult due to the shortage of tarsus. A posterior incision is made through the remaining tarsus about 3–4 mm above the lid margin. The tarsus is dissected until it is free and allowed to recess superiorly toward the fornix (Fig. 15.8b). HPG is then harvested and placed in a moistened saline sponge. Hemostasis is achieved at the donor site on the hard palate using Monsel's solution and then Surgicel packing. Cautery is kept to a minimum so as not to cause excessive damage to the underlying perichondrium. The HPG graft is then sutured into place between the recessed tarsal edge and the eyelid margin, thereby lengthening the eyelid vertically (Fig. 15.8c). Mattress sutures are placed to quilt the graft to the overlying soft tissues (Fig. 15.8d). Often a ring conformer is placed during the healing period (Fig. 15.8a–d).

In summary, most upper eyelid defects can be closed primarily or with cantholysis. For larger size defects, the semicircular or sliding tarsoconjunctival flaps can be used. For extremely large defects, the Cutler-Beard flap may be employed although this requires occlusion of the eye. It is important to consider what will replace both tarsus and skin when managing full-thickness upper lid defects and to be attuned to the special function the upper lid has with respect to the globe. Whenever possible, adjacent tissue-containing normal tarsus, orbicularis, and eyelid skin should be utilized. Finally, in cases with large defects and when adjacent tissue is not available, tissue may be recruited from the temporal region or the median forehead.

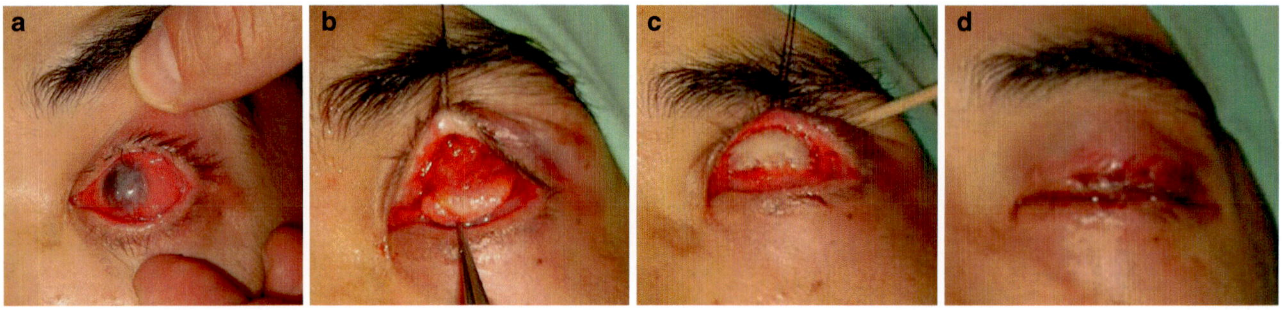

Fig. 15.8 Upper eyelid with vertical shortening but an intact eyelid margin due to a chemical injury (**a**). The tarsus is dissected until it is free and allowed to recess superiorly toward the fornix (**b**). The hard palate graft is then sutured into place between the recessed tarsal edge and eyelid margin, resulting in vertical lengthening of the lid (**c**). Mattress sutures are placed to quilt the graft to the overlying soft tissues (**d**)

References

1. Wesley RE, McCord CD Jr. Reconstruction of the upper eyelid and medial canthus. In: McCord Jr CD, Tannenbaum M, Nunnery WR, editors. Oculoplastic surgery. 3rd ed. New York: Raven Press; 1995. p. 99–117.
2. Dutton JJ. Upper eyelid reconstruction. In: Vol II, Dutton JJ, editors. Atlas of ophthalmic surgery. St. Louis: Mosby; 1992. p. 168–85.
3. Bowman P, Fosko S, Hartstein ME. Periocular reconstruction. Semin Cutan Med Surg. 2003;22:263–72.
4. Tenzel RR, Stewart WB. Eyelid reconstruction by the semicircle flap technique. Ophthalmology. 1978;85(11):1164–9.
5. Tenzel RR. Reconstruction of the central one half of an eyelid. Arch Ophthalmol. 1975;93(2):125–6.
6. Hughes WL. Reconstruction of the lid. Am J Ophthalmol. 1945;28:1203.
7. Leone CR Jr. Tarsal conjunctival advancement flaps for upper eyelid reconstruction. Arch Ophthalmol. 1983;101:945.
8. Malik A, Shah-Desai S. Sliding tarsal advancement flap for upper eyelid reconstruction. Orbit. 2014;33(2):124–6.
9. Cutler N, Beard C. A method for partial and total upper lid reconstruction. Am J Ophthalmol. 1955;39:1–7.
10. Rahmi D, Mehmet B, Ceyda B, Sibel O. Management of the large upper eyelid defects with cutler-beard flap. J Ophthalmol. 2014;2014:424567.
11. Yoon MK, McCulley TJ. Secondary tarsoconjunctival graft: a modification to the Cutler-Beard procedure. Ophthal Plast Reconstr Surg. 2013;29(3):227–30.
12. Sinkin JC, Yi S, Wood BC, Kwon S, Gavaris LZ, Gavaris PT, Rogers GF, Sauerhammer TM. Upper eyelid coloboma repair using accessory preauricular cartilage in a patient with goldenhar syndrome: technique revisited. Ophthal Plast Reconstr Surg. 2017;33:e4–e7.
13. Hayek B, Hatef E, Nguyen M, Ho V, Hsu A, Esmaeli B. Acellular dermal graft (AlloDerm) for upper eyelid reconstruction after cancer removal. Ophthal Plast Reconstr Surg. 2009;25(6):426–9.

Lower Eyelid Defect: Reconstructive Options

16

Qiang Kwong, Naresh Joshi, and Richard Scawn

Introduction

Eyelid reconstruction, following tumor excision or trauma, has the primary purpose of regaining the protective globe function afforded by the eyelids. Inadequate eyelid position or function may result in corneal exposure and potential vision compromise [1, 2]. Secondary reconstructive goals include restoration of lacrimal function, comfort, and aesthetics.

The eyelid protective function is nearly exclusively carried out by the upper eyelid [3]. This is because the lower eyelid usually sits relatively stationary at the inferior limbus and upon lid closure, the upper eyelid orbicularis contracts to cover the cornea. This is also sometimes supplemented by upturning of the globe in patients with an intact Bell's phenomenon.

Patients with a limited Bell's reflex, abnormal globe position, or dysmotility, however, may rely on the presence of the lower lid for partial corneal coverage. In the presence of a functioning upper lid and normal cornea status including sensation, the lower eyelid has more limited functionality. Thus, reconstruction of the lower eyelid is therefore primarily to restore aesthetic and lacrimal function. Conversely, in the presence of compromised upper eyelid, a lower eyelid reconstruction will be functional.

Q. Kwong · N. Joshi · R. Scawn (✉)
Oculoplastic and Craniofacial Service, Chelsea and Westminster Hospital, London, UK
e-mail: naresh.joshi@chelwest.nhs.uk; oculoplastics@richardscawn.com

Principles of Lower Eyelid Reconstruction

Techniques for lower eyelid defects can also be divided into four broad types.

A combination of techniques may be required in many reconstructions [3].

1. Direct closure with or without tissue undermining
2. Healing by secondary intention (laissez-faire)
3. Grafts
4. Local/regional flaps
   (a) Random
   (b) Pedicle

A useful approach to reconstruct the lower eyelid is to consider the anterior and posterior lamella separately. The "reconstructive ladder" concept popularized in general plastic surgery offers a good basis. Working up the ladder of reconstructive complexity considers the simplest procedure to achieve the optimal result without tissue tension or distortion [4].

Repair of the Anterior Lamella

Direct Closure with or Without Undermining

If possible, direct closure should be attempted for small- to medium-sized defects as this tends to provide the best aesthetic result. As long as there is minimal tension in the tissues, this would typically be the preferred technique. The lower eyelid, however, tends to have little tissue laxity, so undermining is usually required in order to mobilize the surrounding cheek tissues.

The tissue plane through which one is undermining is very important, in order to prevent damage to the neurovascular network in this area.

A. J. Cohen, C. N. Burkat (eds.), *Oculofacial, Orbital, and Lacrimal Surgery*, https://doi.org/10.1007/978-3-030-14092-2_16

Anatomical location	Plane of dissection
Within orbital rims	Suborbicularis/preseptal
Outside orbital rims	Subcutaneous

Although one is typically taught that tissues should be closed with the resultant scar parallel to natural skin creases, this does not apply when the defect is nearer to the lower eyelid margin. This is because any vertical tissue tension can easily result in lower eyelid malposition and cicatricial ectropion. Therefore, any defect close to the eyelid margin should be closed horizontally, resulting in a vertical scar.

To prevent tension at the skin level, anchoring sutures are used to attach the deep tissues of the undermined tissues to a firm anchoring point such as the periosteum over the inferior or lateral orbital rims. A suture such as a 4-0, 5-0, or 6-0 absorbable, polyglactin (Vicryl) suture could be used. Layered closure should be performed with 4-0, 5-0, or 6-0 absorbable sutures for the deep tissue, followed by skin closure with 6-0 absorbable or nonabsorbable, interrupted, or continuous sutures.

If there is any concern for possible tissue tension on the wound edges, lower eyelid horizontal tightening and/or a "Frost" suture to the eyebrow for 48 hours should be performed to prevent postoperative lower eyelid retraction.

Healing by Secondary Intention (Laissez-Faire)

The entire or partial defect can be left to granulate on its own in some instances. The disadvantages for this method are the longer healing period and possible increased risk of wound infection. The patient is advised to keep the wound clean and to apply topical antibiotic ointment regularly. In younger patients, the scarring is often more obvious with a less predictable aesthetic outcome. This is generally more suitable for smaller defects away from the eyelid margin. Granulation of the wound leads to contraction, and the closer the defect is to the eyelid margin, the more likely this may cause eyelid margin malposition. However, others have described using it particularly for medial canthal defects where webbing can be caused by flaps.

Myocutaneous Flaps

For larger anterior lamellar defects, myocutaneous advancement flaps are generally preferable to skin grafts. Flaps in the periocular area have better color and texture match than grafts and are therefore preferable aesthetically. Other advantages to a flap include having its own blood supply and innervation, which tend to result in better postoperative healing and functioning.

When designing a periocular flap, a key concept is to avoid vertical tension on the eyelid to avoid postoperative retraction and ectropion. Keep to the appropriate plane of dissection to ensure preserved vascularity and innervation of the flap. Consider overcorrecting the flap height to avoid postoperative wound contraction that may pull the tissues inferiorly. Flaps for the lower eyelids should ideally be designed with the point of rotation above an imaginary line drawn from medial to lateral canthus.

If postoperative eyelid malposition is a risk based on the size of the defect and proximity to the eyelid margin, additional procedures are indicated, such as anchoring sutures, horizontal eyelid tightening, or a Frost suture.

Note that in some cases, portions of the posterior lamella may need to be excised even if the defect primarily involved the anterior lamella. This is to prevent bunching of the posterior lamella with repositioning of the myocutaneous flap or if the anterior lamella is under a lot of tension. This is particularly true if the anterior lamellar defect involves the thin pretarsal tissue. Often these defects involve the eyelid margin, skin, and pretarsal orbicularis muscle layers, but portions of the tarsal plate may remain. In order to optimally recreate a smooth eyelid contour and avoid tarsal bunching, the tarsus in the region of the defect may need to be wedge resected, to allow the tissues to line up well for closure.

Heteropalpebral Flap Technique

A particularly useful flap is the heteropalpebral flap, where the skin flap is taken from the upper eyelid anterior lamella and transposed to the lower eyelid. The vascular supply remains in the lateral canthal tissue where the flap rotates from the upper to lower eyelid. This is best used for middle to lateral lower eyelid defects as the blood supply to the tip of the flap tends to be too weak to reach over to the medial eyelid.

- The upper eyelid skin (or skin-muscle) flap is marked in the eyelid crease with the base above the level of the lateral canthus (Fig. 16.1)
- The outer base of the flap should widen as much as possible to increase vascular supply
- The skin marking continues from the flap base at the angle to the lower eyelid subciliary line blending into the lateral eyelid defect
- The flap base should be above the level of the lateral canthus to reduce risk of postoperative ectropion
- Local anesthetic is injected (10 ml mixture of 4 ml 0.5% bupivacaine +adrenaline 1:200000; 4 ml lignocaine + adrenaline 1:80,000; 4 ml dexamethasone 3.3 mg/ml)
- Skin preparation
- Sterile drape
- Corneal shield lubricated with ophthalmic ointment

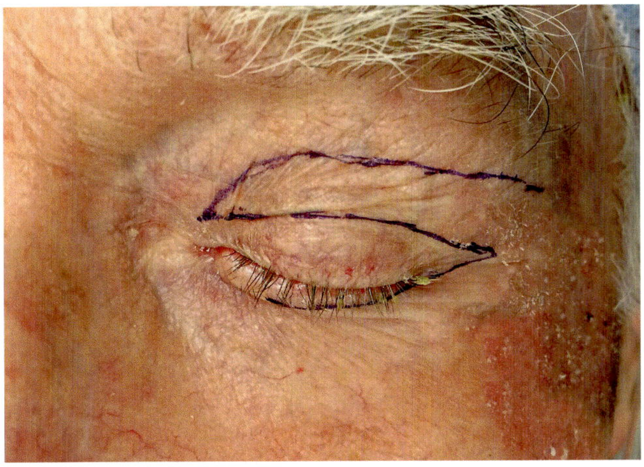

Fig. 16.1 In the heteropalpebral flap technique, the upper eyelid skin (or skin-muscle) flap is marked in the eyelid crease and subciliary line, with the widened flap base above the level of the lateral canthus. (Image courtesy of Cat Nguyen Burkat, MD FACS)

- 5-0 silk vertical traction suture to lower eyelid
- A #15 Bard Parker blade or monopolar cutting needle is used to incise the skin markings
- Westcott scissors are used to elevate the skin flap from the upper eyelid
- Minimize cautery to the flap to avoid compromising vascular supply
- Be sure to release the lateral tissues widely to freely rotate the base of the flap
- Undermine the subciliary skin with scissors if needed to open the anterior lamella from the lateral canthus to the skin defect
- Consider a lateral lower eyelid canthopexy or tarsal strip, if laxity exists
- Rotate the upper eyelid flap down to fill in the defect in the lower eyelid anterior lamella (Fig. 16.2)
- Donor upper eyelid site is closed with 6-0 polypropylene (PROLENE) or fast gut sutures
- The flap is sutured into the lower eyelid defect with running sutures
- Deep quilting sutures can be applied with 5-0 polyglactin or nylon to ensure attachment of the flap to the deep tissue or lateral rim periosteum
- 5-0 polypropylene (PROLENE) traction Frost suture is passed through the lower margin and tied superiorly above the eyebrow to apply vertical traction in the initial postoperative period
- Antibiotic ointment is placed on the sutures
- Pressure bandage can be applied if indicated

Postoperative management:

- Pressure bandage and traction suture are removed after 48 hours

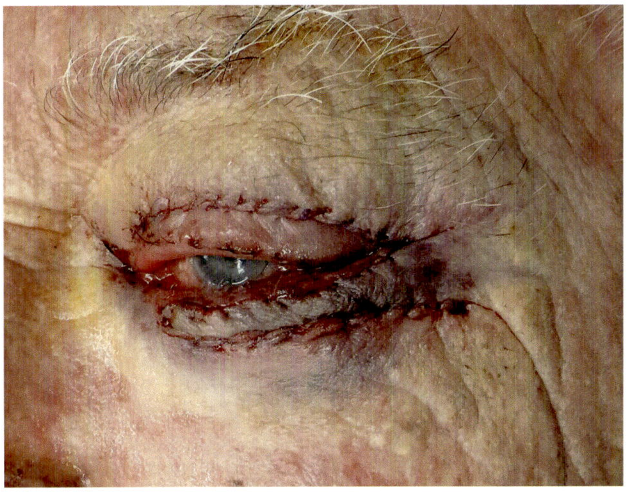

Fig. 16.2 The upper eyelid flap is rotated into position into the subciliary defect of the lower eyelid. (Image courtesy of Cat Nguyen Burkat, MD FACS)

- Commencement of topical lubricant 3 times daily and nighttime topical antibiotic ointment for 4 weeks
- Follow-up in 7–10 days for suture removal

Forehead Flap Technique

Another useful, albeit more complex, flap used in oculoplastic anterior lamellar reconstruction is the paramedian forehead flap. This flap tends to be most useful for extensive medial canthal or medial lower eyelid defects.

This is a two-staged procedure with the first stage creating and transferring the paramedian forehead flap into the defect and the subsequent second stage involving division of the pedicle. The second stage typically is performed 4–8 weeks later once the distal flap has developed its own blood supply at the recipient site.

Stage 1 (Figs. 16.3, 16.4, 16.5, and 16.6)

- Using Doppler ultrasonography, the path of the contralateral supratrochlear artery is marked from its origin at the superior orbital rim and extending superiorly
- Estimate the length of pedicle flap required by using a flexible material (such as gauze) to measure the distance between the base of the pedicle to the defect
- Ensure sufficient length of the pedicle to arch over the nasal bridge (Fig. 16.3)
- Mark the edges of the pedicle on either side of the artery ensuring a pedicle width of at least 1.5 cm
- Create a card or plastic template of the defect, and mark on the template the superior, inferior, lateral, and medial (nasal) sides of the defect (Fig. 16.3)

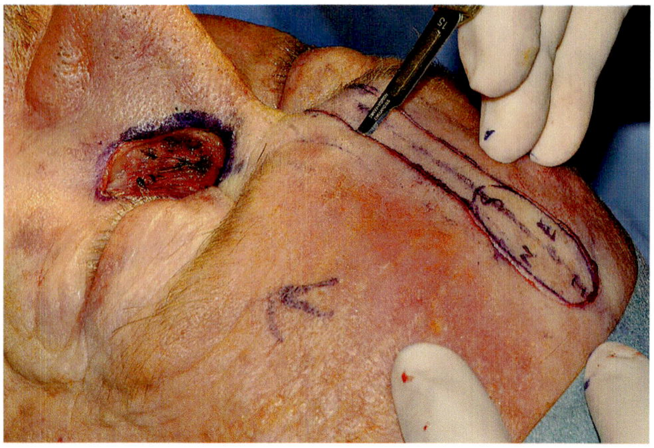

Fig. 16.3 Forehead flap: Design of the flap to ensure good vascular supply and different thicknesses along the flap

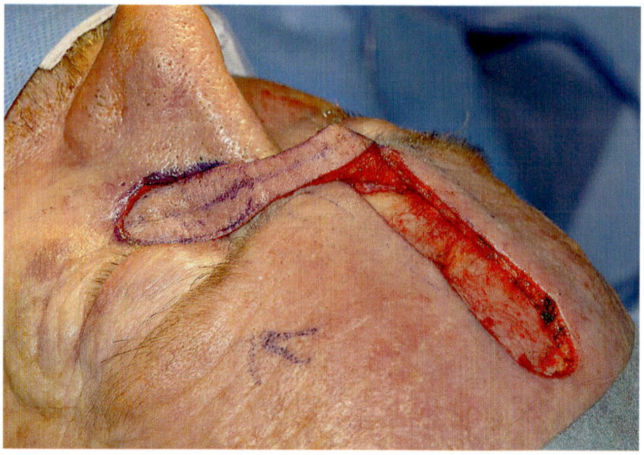

Fig. 16.4 Forehead flap: Allow sufficient length of the pedicle to allow easy placement of flap into defect

- Using this template, transfer the size, shape, and orientation onto the flap skin
- Make sure the orientation is correctly marked, incorporating a 180° rotation
- Local anesthetic is injected
- Skin preparation
- Sterile drape
- Corneal shield lubricated with ophthalmic ointment
- Incise skin and subcutaneous tissue with a #15 Bard Parker blade
- Dissect the flap and its pedicle with Westcott scissors
- The flap thickness varies depending on the distance from the pedicle base:
  - For the distal 1/3, dissect as deep as the anterior frontalis muscle surface
  - For the middle 1/3, dissect in the supraperiosteal layer
  - For the proximal 1/3, dissect in the subperiosteal layer
- Rotate the flap into the recipient defect site (Fig. 16.4)
- Close the forehead defect with deep 4-0 PDS, Monocryl, or polyglactin sutures (Fig. 16.5)
- Close skin with 5-0 polypropylene (PROLENE) interrupted sutures (Fig. 16.6)
- Consider thinning the distal end of the flap to match thickness of defect
- Suture flap into defect with interrupted 6-0 polyglactin to suture to the posterior lamella of the eyelid, and/or place deep sutures from the posterior flap to the nasal wall periosteum (Fig. 16.6)
- In some cases, the forehead can be left to heal by secondary intention if unable to be closed directly

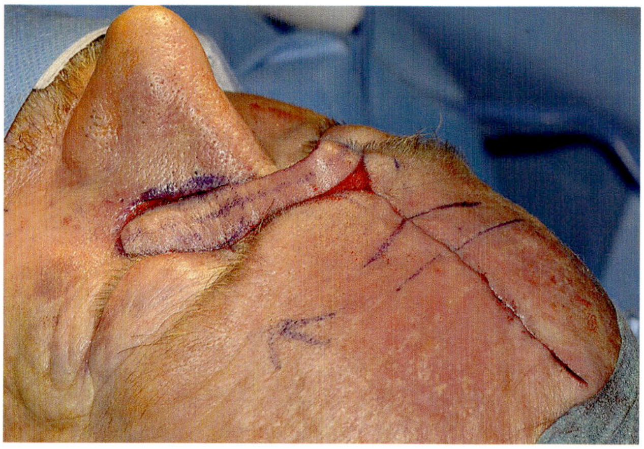

Fig. 16.5 Forehead flap: The forehead defect is closed with deep and superficial sutures

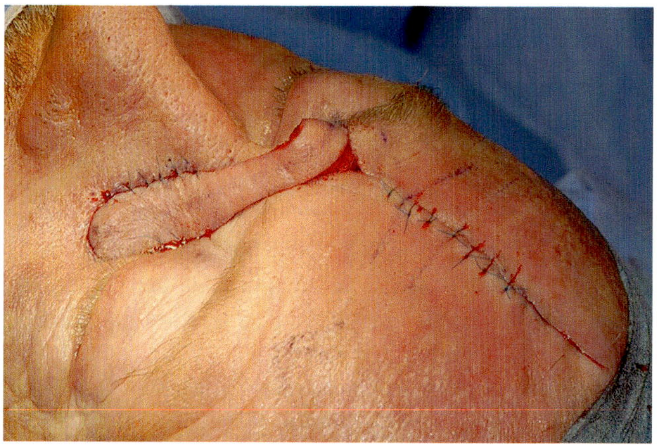

Fig. 16.6 Forehead flap: The distal flap is sutured into the defect

Postoperative management:

- Apply calcium alginate wound matrix dressing onto forehead wound to aid healing by secondary intention, if required
- Wrap paraffin gauze dressing (Jelonet) around the pedicle of the flap
- Assess distal end in several hours as may need leaching or pricking to prevent venous congestion
- Follow-up in 1 week for suture removal

Stage 2

- Confirm that an independent blood supply has developed for the flap by tying a gauze/suture/glove finger around the pedicle tightly and observing the flap for pallor
- Inject local anesthetic into the flap base while observing the flap tip to ensure no blanching occurs
- Once sure that cutting the pedicle will not result in distal flap necrosis, incise the pedicle
- Trim any residual pedicle to allow both the base and tip of the flap to fill the defects
- The distal flap can be thinned to match the contour of the adjacent tissue, if required

Skin Graft

If the use of a myocutaneous or cutaneous advancement flap is not possible due to size or location, then a skin graft can be an appropriate option.

Skin grafts are either full-thickness or split-thickness. As the names suggest, full-thickness grafts contain both the epidermis and dermis with associated skin appendages, whereas split-thickness grafts leave the deep dermis with appendages at the donor site. Therefore, full-thickness grafts transfer any hair follicles to the recipient site. Also, full-thickness donor sites require closure, thus limiting the size of any graft taken; whereas split-thickness graft donor sites are not closed.

Most periorbital skin grafts are full-thickness as they tend to contrast less postoperatively and have better skin color and texture matching. Split-thickness grafts, on the other hand, tend to be reserved for very large defects, as the donor site does not require direct closure.

Typical donor graft sites for full-thickness skin grafts include:

- Upper eyelid (ipsilateral/contralateral)
- Preauricular
- Retroauricular
- Inner upper arm
- Clavicular
- Groin

Full-Thickness Skin Graft Harvesting

- Use a plastic or card template over the defect to mark out the size of the desired donor graft (oversize slightly to compensate for shrinkage) (Fig. 16.7)
- Mark out the graft on the donor site skin using the template
- Local anesthetic injection
- Incise donor site skin with a #15 Bard Parker blade or monopolar cutting needle
- Harvest the graft by dissection between the skin and subcutaneous fat (Fig. 16.8)
- Once graft is harvested, use Westcott spring scissors to thin the posterior fatty surface to reveal white dermis without creating buttonholes

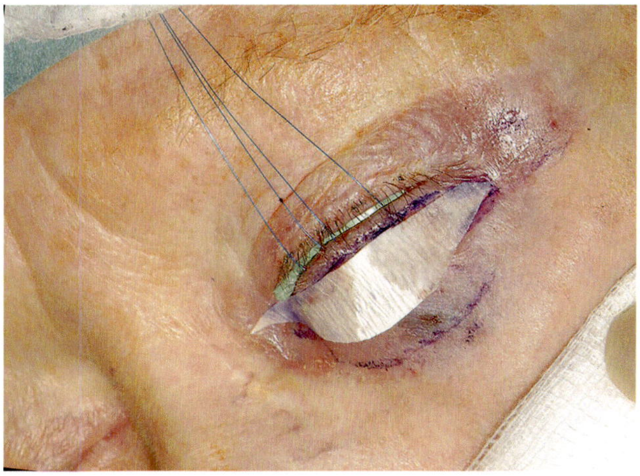

Fig. 16.7 A 5-0 polypropylene (PROLENE) traction suture is placed into the lower eyelid, and a template made of the size and shape of the defect

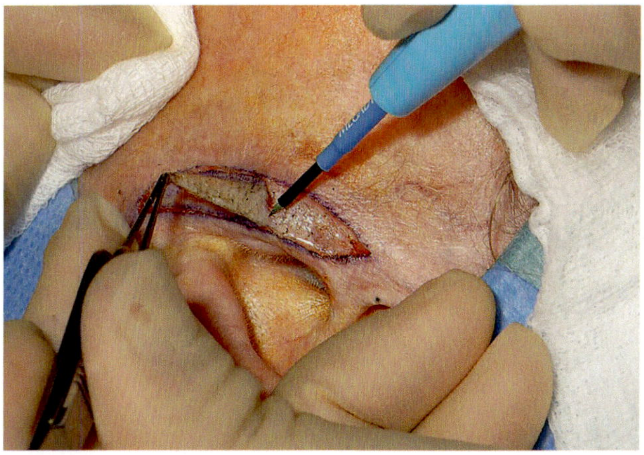

Fig. 16.8 Skin-only dissection of underlying subcutaneous fat is performed

- Close donor site with 5-0 or 6-0 polyglactin (Vicryl) subcutaneous sutures and cutaneous 6-0 polypropylene (PROLENE) (Fig. 16.9)
- Suture graft into defect with running 6-0 absorbable or nonabsorbable sutures
- Use 5-0 polyglactin (Vicryl) quilting sutures to anchor the graft down to deeper tissue (Fig. 16.10)
- Several small incisions can be made within the central graft to allow for egress of serosanguinous fluid below the graft
- Use a traction suture to place superior traction on the lower eyelid (Frost tarsorrhaphy), and use Steri-Strips to keep in place (Fig. 16.10)
- Antibiotic ointment placed on donor/graft site and ocular surface
- Paraffin gauze dressing and pressure bandage to graft site, if desired

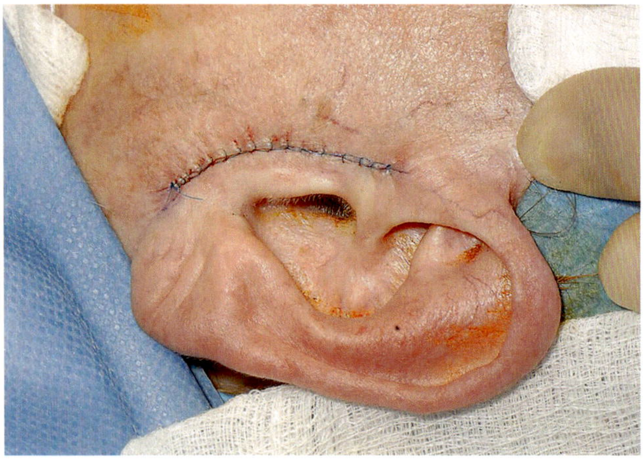

Fig. 16.9 Donor site is closed with 5-0 polyglactin (Vicryl) subcutaneous and continuous interlocking 6-0 polypropylene (PROLENE)

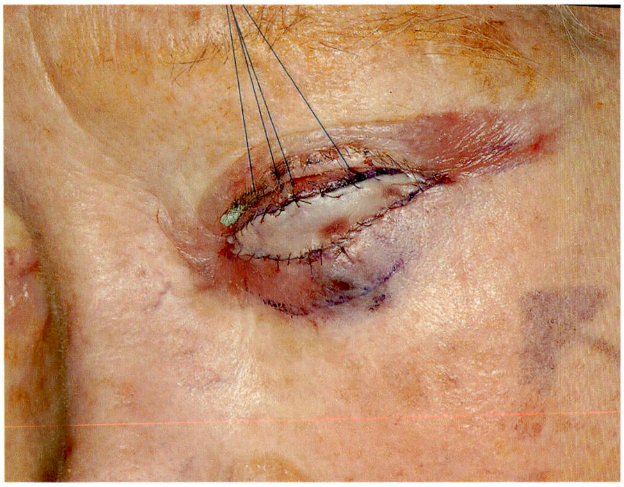

Fig. 16.10 The graft is sutured into the defect with running 6-0/7-0 polyglactin (Vicryl) or gut sutures, and quilting sutures are placed in the central graft to anchor the graft down to deeper tissues. The lower eyelid is placed on superior vertical traction during healing

Postoperative management:

- Eye pad and traction suture removed after 48 hours
- Commencement of topical antibiotic ointment 3 times daily and at night
- Follow-up in 7–10 days for donor site suture removal

Posterior Lamella Reconstruction

Full-thickness eyelid margin involvement will require reconstruction of the posterior lamella (tarsus and conjunctiva).

The technique used will depend on a number of factors:

1. Extent of the lower eyelid margin defect
2. Laxity of the adjacent tissues
3. Location of the defect along the eyelid

Determining which surgical technique is indicated can be considered in a graded fashion. Smaller defects or defects in tissues with great elasticity may just require direct closure. In contrast, longer defects or defects in tissues with little laxity (such as in a young patient) may require the use of lateral canthal release, advancement flap, or even a graft. The following algorithm should be only considered a guide, as differences in tissue laxity can greatly affect the procedure selected. From simple to more complex techniques:

1. Direct closure (defect is <25% of total eyelid length but can greater in lax tissue)
   (a) Irregular wound is converted to a pentagonal shape for optimal tissue reapproximation
2. Direct closure with lateral canthal release (defect is 25–50% of total eyelid length)
3. Semicircular rotation flap/Tenzel flap (defect is 50–75% of total eyelid length)
4. Tarsoconjunctival (Hughes) flap (defect is 75–90% of total eyelid length)
5. Free tarsal and/or mucous membrane graft

Defects <25% of Total Eyelid Margin Length

If possible, the first method of repair to consider is *direct closure*. Traditionally, this has been suggested to be appropriate for defects <25% of the total eyelid length. However, this depends on how easily the wound edges can be opposed. In older patients with more horizontal tissue laxity, full-thickness margin defects much greater than 25% can sometimes be repaired with direct layered closure. To allow easier tissue closure, the wound edges should be trimmed to sharp regular edges or the wound converted to a pentagonal shape.

Direct Closure Full-Thickness Defect Technique

- Local anesthetic injection
- Skin preparation
- Sterile drape
- Corneal shield lubricated with ophthalmic ointment
- Using toothed Adson forceps to gently grasp the two sides of the defect, the edges of the eyelid defect are reapproximated to ensure satisfactory apposition without tension
- Eyelid margin sutures are placed in the gray line and eyelash line using buried vertical mattress, or buried interrupted, 6-0 polyglactin sutures
- Slight eversion of the eyelid margin is desired
- Rotate suture knots and tails away from the ocular surface
- Tarsus is next sutured with 2–3 interrupted, 6-0 polyglactin (Vicryl) sutures, with the first placed just under the eyelash line for margin strength
- Tarsal sutures are horizontal and partial thickness to avoid corneal abrasion
- Inferior retractor layer is closed with 6-0 polyglactin sutures if defect extends further
- Orbicularis muscle closure with 6-0 polyglactin buried sutures
- Skin closure

Postoperative management:

- Eye pad, if placed, is removed after 24 hours
- Commencement of topical antibiotic ointment 3 times daily and at night
- Follow-up in 7–10 days for skin suture removal

Defects 25–50% of Total Eyelid Margin Length

For defects between 25% and 50%, it is unlikely that direct closure without tissue release is sufficient, unless significant pre-existing laxity exists. If the tissues are still under tension when the edges are reapposed, the next step is to release the lower eyelid via a lateral canthotomy and cantholysis, in conjunction with pentagonal eyelid margin closure.

Canthotomy and Cantholysis with Direct Closure Full-Thickness Technique

- Local anesthetic injection
- Skin preparation
- Sterile drape
- Corneal shield lubricated with ophthalmic ointment
- Horizontal skin incision made at lateral canthus using #15 scalpel blade or monopolar needle
- Lateral canthotomy made using straight scissors aiming toward the lateral orbital rim and cutting tissue overlying the lateral orbital rim to allow separation of upper and lower eyelid
- Inferior cantholysis:
  - Pull the cut lateral lower eyelid away from the globe to place the inferior tendon on traction
  - Aim along the inferolateral orbital rim between the skin and conjunctiva
  - Use the closed end of Westcott or straight iris scissors to strum the band of tissue connecting the inferior tarsus to the orbital rim
  - Selectively cut these bands (inferior limb of canthal tendon) to completely release the eyelid
  - Lower eyelid should be able to move freely toward the defect
- Eyelid margin full-thickness closure is performed as above

Defects 50–75% of Total Eyelid Margin Length

If the above steps are not sufficient, the next surgical option is a semicircular, myocutaneous, rotation flap, also known as the Tenzel flap (Figs. 16.11 and 16.12) [5].

The advantage of this technique is that it is a single-stage reconstruction, which makes it preferable in patients with poor vision in the fellow eye (who would otherwise have difficulty with eyelid-sharing techniques that occlude the visual axis).

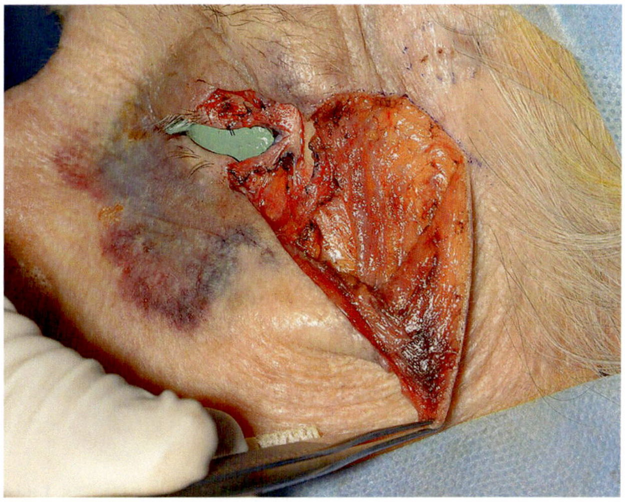

Fig. 16.11 A Tenzel myocutaneous flap is fashioned, taking care to avoid the facial nerve branch approximately 20 mm from the lateral canthus

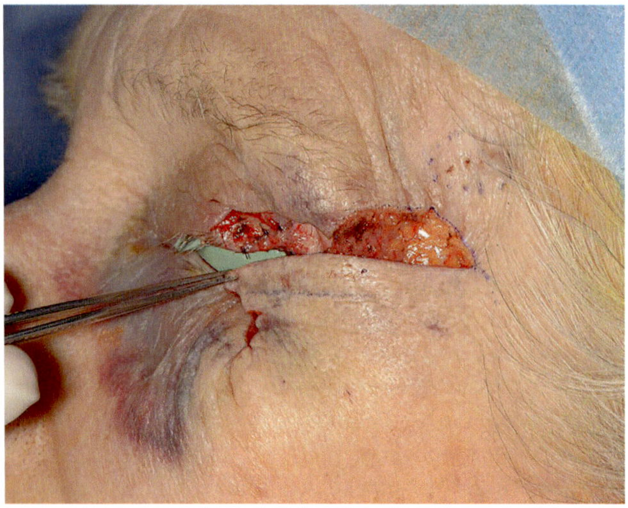

Fig. 16.12 The Tenzel myocutaneous flap is attached to the lateral portion of the residual lower eyelid

Semicircular Tenzel Flap Technique (Figs. 16.11 and 16.12)

- Local anesthetic injection
- Skin preparation
- Sterile drape
- Corneal shield lubricated with ophthalmic ointment
- Skin incision is marked, extending from lateral canthus superolaterally – keep within the periorbital skin staying medial to the lateral border of eyebrow (Fig. 16.11)
- Avoid the frontal nerve branch of the facial nerve as it crosses zygomatic arch
- Incise skin and lateral canthal angle
- Create a skin-muscle flap by undermining with tenotomy scissors between the orbicularis and superficial temporal fascia
- Perform a lateral canthotomy (see above)
- Perform cantholysis of the inferior limb of the canthal tendon
- Perform direct closure of eyelid margin defect edges (see above) (Fig. 16.12)
- Reform the lateral canthus by suturing the advanced flap to the lateral orbital rim periosteum with 5-0 polyglactin (Vicryl) suture
- Mobilize the inferolateral conjunctiva to line the posterior surface of the flap and suture with 7-0 polyglactin (Vicryl) to the flap eyelid margin
- Skin closure with 6-0 polypropylene (PROLENE) or fast-absorbing plain gut suture

Postoperative management – see above

Defects >75% of Total Eyelid Margin Length

For larger lesions which the Tenzel flap cannot close, the tarsoconjunctival flap shared from the upper eyelid (Hughes procedure [6]) is typically preferred for creation of the posterior lamella. The anterior lamella is reconstructed either with a myocutaneous advancement flap or skin graft. This is a two-stage procedure that requires coverage of the visual axis of the surgical side for at least a few weeks.

The tarsoconjunctival flap may not be optimal in patients with limited vision in the contralateral eye, in which case a free tarsal graft may be more appropriate. This would necessitate a myocutaneous advancement flap, rather than a skin graft, for anterior lamella reconstruction as the underlying tarsal graft would not have its own blood supply.

Tarsoconjunctival Hughes Flap Technique

Stage 1 (Figs. 16.13 and 16.14)

- Local anesthetic injection
- Skin preparation
- Sterile drape
- Corneal shield lubricated with ophthalmic ointment
- Upper eyelid traction with 5-0 polypropylene (PROLENE) or silk suture through gray line
- Eversion of upper eyelid over a Desmarres retractor to expose entire posterior tarsus
- An adequately sized tarsoconjunctival flap is marked, ensuring a 4–5 mm scaffold of tarsus is left adjacent to the margin for structural integrity of upper eyelid (Fig. 16.13)
- Horizontal dimension of the flap should be slightly smaller than the lower eyelid defect to allow for horizontal tightening of the lower eyelid

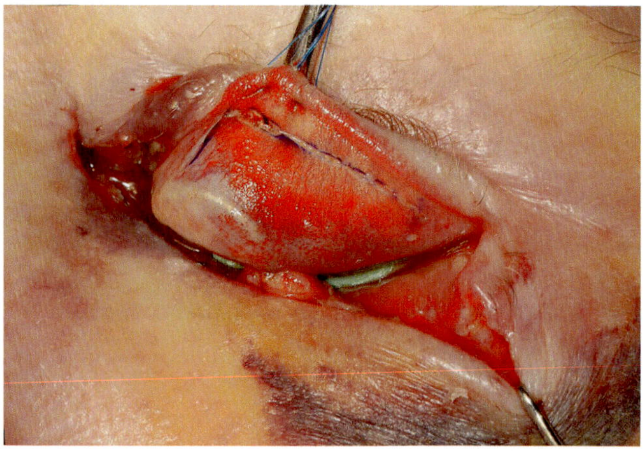

Fig. 16.13 Hughes flap, stage 1: Fashioning of the tarsoconjunctival flap, leaving a 4–5 mm tarsal scaffold adjacent to the eyelid margin

- Tarsus is incised horizontally with a #15 blade scalpel
- Dissection of pretarsal plane and relaxing vertical incisions on both sides are performed with Westcott scissors
- The tarsoconjunctival flap is dissected off the bed of Müller's muscle up to the superior fornix
- Avoid buttonholes in conjunctiva
- Suture flap to residual lower eyelid tarsus with multiple 6-0 or 7-0 polyglactin sutures (Fig. 16.14)
  - By undersizing the horizontal flap length, this tightens the lower eyelid to avoid postoperative ectropion
- Repair the anterior lamella either with an advancement flap or skin graft
- Avoid corneal abrasion by sutures along superior skin graft
- Antibiotic ointment is placed on sutures
- Pressure eye patch, if desired
- Allow sufficient time to elapse before division of the flap in order to allow local vascularization of new lower eyelid tissue (at least 3 weeks)

Stage 2

- Local anesthetic injection to flap
- Use Westcott or iris scissors to divide the conjunctiva a few millimeters above the superior tarsal edge (Fig. 16.15a, b)
- Care is taken to avoid damaging the underlying cornea – a thin malleable retractor can be slid behind the flap to protect the cornea
- The residual frond of conjunctiva is then sutured forward with 7-0 polyglactin (Vicryl) to the anterior lamella, which ensures that the new eyelid margin is lined with conjunctiva (Fig. 16.16)
- This also prevents hairs from the anterior lamella from irritating the cornea
- The base of the flap is trimmed off the posterior eyelid superiorly to minimize the risk of postoperative eyelid retraction

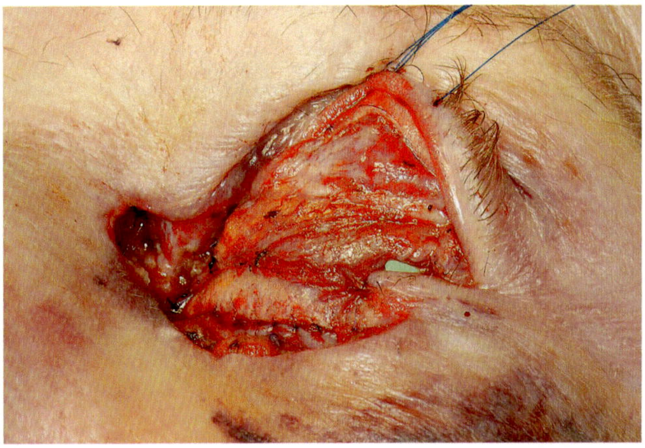

Fig. 16.14 Hughes flap, stage 1: Flap is sutured into the residual lower eyelid defect

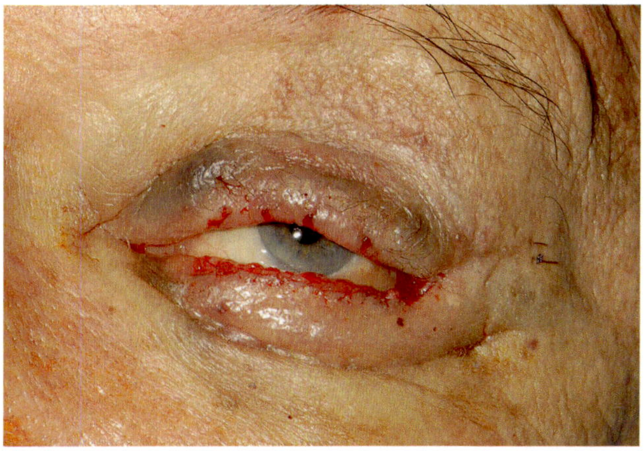

Fig. 16.16 Hughes flap, stage 2: Frond of conjunctiva is then sutured to the skin with 7-0 polyglactin (Vicryl), ensuring that the new eyelid margin is covered in conjunctiva

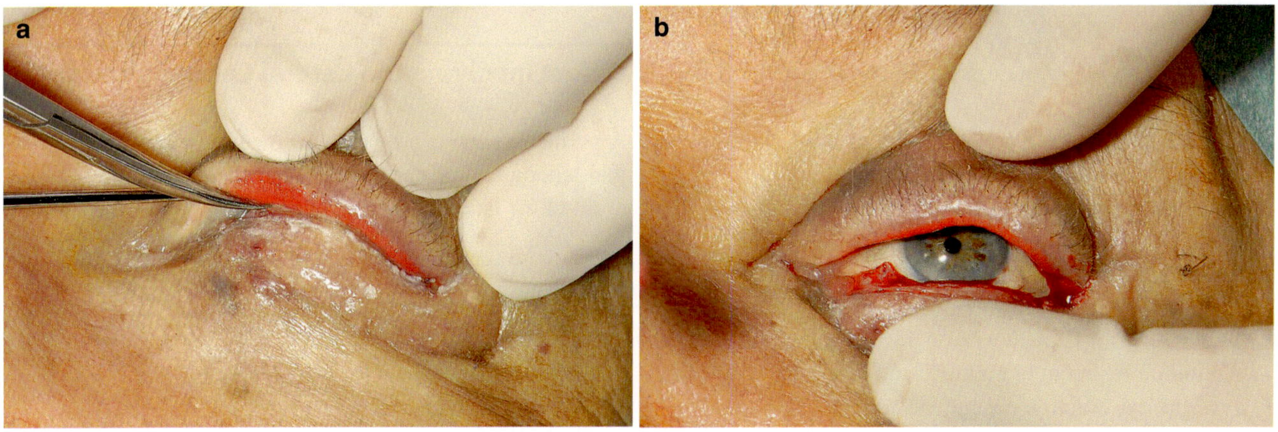

Fig. 16.15 Hughes flap, stage 2: Flap is divided (**a**), leaving a short frond of conjunctiva (**b**)

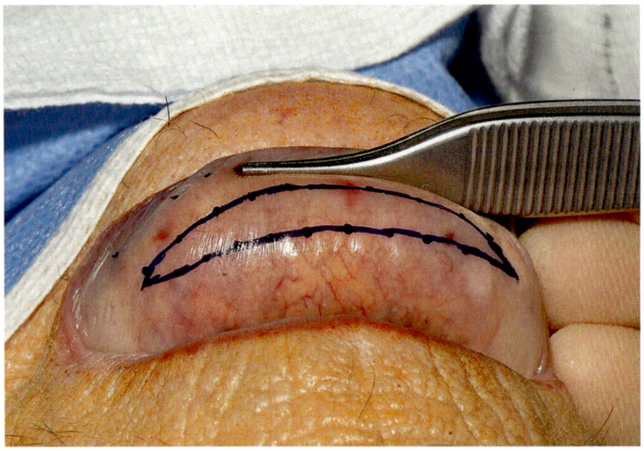

Fig. 16.17 Mucous membrane graft harvesting: The donor graft size is marked on the mucosa, taking care to avoid the salivary papillae

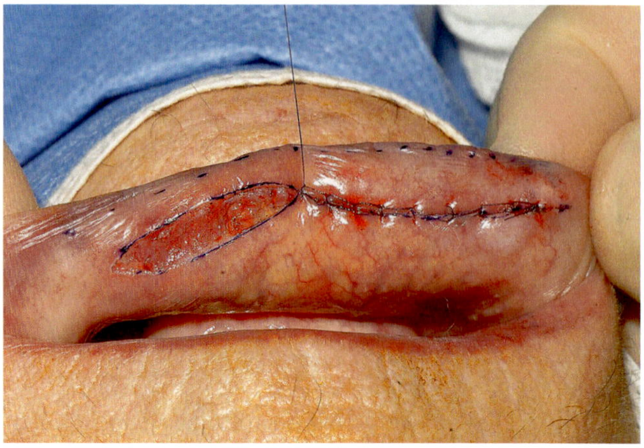

Fig. 16.18 Mucous membrane graft harvesting: Donor site is closed with deep 5-0 polyglactin (Vicryl) sutures, followed by continuous running locking 6-0 polyglactin (Vicryl) sutures

Mucous Membrane Graft

If the posterior lamellar defect is extensive or an appropriate tarsal flap or graft is not available, one can use a mucous membrane graft. This is also useful for reconstruction of the posterior lamella from conjunctival scarring or shortened fornices. Typically, the inner cheek or lower lip buccal mucosa are harvested for use in eyelid reconstruction.

Mucous Membrane Graft Technique

- Cleanse the donor buccal mucosal site
- Mark out the donor graft size using a template measured out over the defect (slightly oversize to compensate for shrinkage)
- Mark out the graft on the buccal mucosa (inner cheek or lower lip) using the template (Fig. 16.17)
- Avoid injury to the lip frenulum and the salivary papillae
- Local anesthetic injection
- Incise mucosa with a #15 Bard Parker blade or monopolar cutting needle
- Harvest the graft in submucosal plane and place on wet saline gauze
- Close donor site with deep 5-0 polyglactin (Vicryl) subcutaneous sutures
- Close mucosa with 5-0 polyglactin or mild chromic gut running locking sutures (Fig. 16.18)
- Use Westcott scissors to thin the posterior aspect of the graft, being careful not to create buttonholes (Fig. 16.19)
- Suture graft into defect with running 6-0 or 7-0 polyglactin (Vicryl) suture
- Repair anterior lamella with an advancement flap
- Antibiotic ointment to graft site and ocular surface
- Pressure eye patch, if desired

Postoperative management:

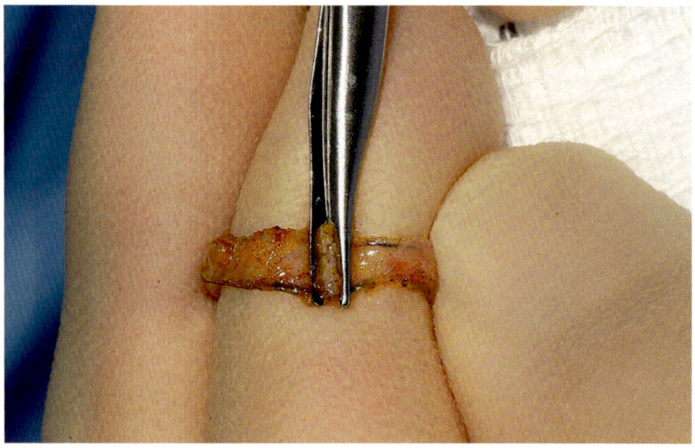

Fig. 16.19 Mucous membrane graft harvesting: The fatty posterior aspect of the graft is thinned with Westcott scissors

- Eye pad removed after 48 hours
- Commencement of topical antibiotic ointment 3 times daily and at night

Defect Involving the Lateral Canthal Tendon

A periosteal flap can be used to reconstruct the lateral canthal tendon and posterior lamella if the defect involves part or all of the lateral canthal tendon.

Periosteal Flap Technique

- Local anesthetic injection
- Skin preparation
- Sterile drape
- Corneal shield lubricated with ophthalmic ointment

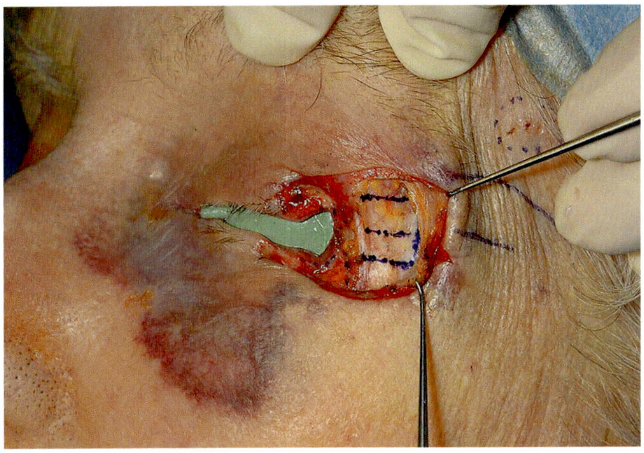

Fig. 16.20 Periosteal flap technique: The periosteum of the lateral orbital rim is exposed and a rectangular, wide flap is marked to create length for the deficient lateral canthal tendon

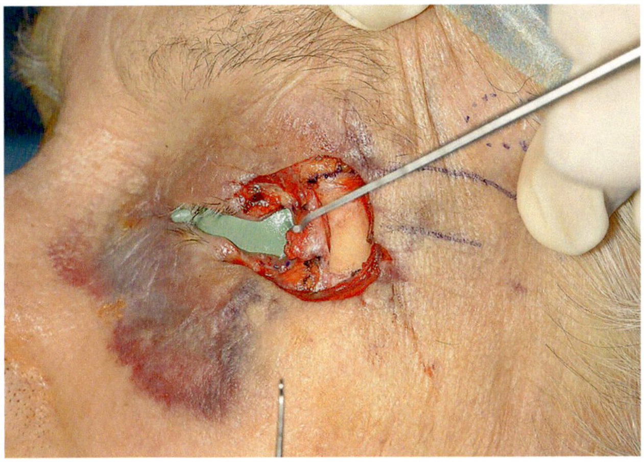

Fig. 16.21 Periosteal flap technique: The periosteal flap is carefully elevated off the underlying bone and flipped into the eyelid defect. Here the flap is divided to repair both the upper and lower eyelid defects

- Lateral orbital rim is exposed, being careful not to damage the periosteum
- The rectangular flaps are drawn onto the lateral rim periosteum, ensuring that the base of the flap is above the medial canthus (Fig. 16.20)
- Flap is based along the lateral orbital rim
- Ensure a sufficient length of flap is drawn to cover the defect (oversize slightly)
- Vertical height of the flap should be at least 8–10 mm
- Using a sharp #15 blade, the incision is made through periosteum
- The flap is elevated with a periosteal (freer) elevator to the lateral rim (Fig. 16.21)

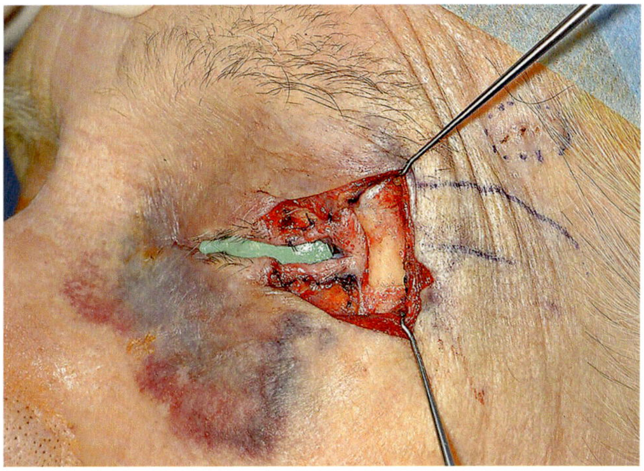

Fig. 16.22 Periosteal flap technique: Periosteal flap is sutured to the lateral edge of the residual tarsus

- Suture flap to the residual lower eyelid tarsus with multiple 6-0 polyglactin sutures (Fig. 16.22)
- Suture the inferior border of the flap to the residual conjunctiva/mucosal flap
- Repair anterior lamella either with an advancement flap or full-thickness skin graft
- Antibiotic ointment to sutures

Summary

In conclusion, detailed knowledge of the various reconstructive options, as well as following the general principle of repairing anatomic structures without tension, will yield the most optimal functional and aesthetic results.

References

1. Huggins AB, Latting MW, Marx DP, Giacometti JN. Ocular adnexal reconstruction for cutaneous periocular malignancies. Semin Plast Surg. 2017;31(1):22–30.
2. Nerad JA. Techniques in ophthalmic plastic surgery: a personal tutorial. USA: Saunders; 2009.
3. Saha K, Joshi N. Eyelid reconstruction. In: Farhadieh RD, Bulstrode NW, Cugno S, editors. Plastic and reconstructive surgery: approaches and techniques. New Jersey: Wiley-Blackwell; 2015.
4. Simman R. Wound closure and the reconstructive ladder in plastic surgery. J Am Col Certif Wound Spec. 2009;1(1):6–11.
5. Tenzel RR, Stewart WB. Eyelid reconstruction by the semicircle flap technique. Ophthalmology. 1978;85(11):1164–9.
6. Hughes WL. Reconstructive surgery of the eyelids. Adv Ophthalmic Plast Reconstr Surg. 1986;5:25–87.

Medial Canthal Defect: Reconstructive Options

17

Chau Pham, Peter W. MacIntosh, and Aaron Fay

Abbreviations

5-FU	5-Fluorouracil
BTXA	Botulinum toxin A
CT	Computed tomography
MRI	Magnetic resonance imaging

Introduction

Medial canthal defects range from congenital problems such as telecanthus and epicanthal folds to large defects resulting from trauma and tumor resection. The medial canthus is a small, yet complex, area that represents the confluence of several anatomic units that affect the structure and function of the ocular and lacrimal apparatus. As a result, the reconstruction of this area requires special attention and skill. The following chapter will provide a focused review of the relevant anatomy and a broad overview of the clinical entities specific to the medial canthus and offer approaches to management of more commonly encountered defects.

Relevant Anatomy

Medial canthal anatomy is complicated due to its intimate association with the lacrimal apparatus. The medial canthal tendon is split into anterior and posterior crura that wrap around the lacrimal sac. The posterior crus is the most important for maintaining eyelid apposition to the globe, and it forms from an amalgamation from the nasal end of the upper and lower eyelids and travels posterior to the lacrimal sac to insert on the posterior lacrimal crest. The anterior crus forms similarly to the posterior but travels anterior to the lacrimal sac to insert onto the anterior lacrimal crest (Fig. 17.1) [1, 2].

The canalicular system, likewise, runs just adjacent to the medial canthal tendon and can easily be damaged by trauma to or during repair of this area. The upper and lower eyelids have puncta at their nasal end that form the opening to the upper and lower canaliculi. The puncta are typically adjacent to the plica semilunaris with the upper punctum located slightly more medial than the lower punctum. The lower canaliculus travels inferiorly for 2 mm before turning 90° to travel 10 mm nasally into the lacrimal sac. The upper canaliculus travels superiorly for 2 mm, turns 90°, and then travels 10 mm nasally into the lacrimal sac (Fig. 17.2). Greater than 90% of the population has a common canaliculus that connects the upper and lower canaliculi before entering the lacrimal sac [3–5]. Understanding of this anatomy is critical to successful repair of defects involving the canaliculus and/or the medial canthus. Identification of the canalicular system using nasolacrimal duct probes and subsequent intubation if indicated can aid in identification of landmarks, prevent damage to canalicular structures, and preserve structure and function during medial canthal repair.

The medial canthus is about 2 mm below the lateral canthus, and this allows for tears to be directed toward the puncta. Repair of this area should aim to preserve this anatomic relationship in order to optimize cosmesis and function.

The angular artery is most commonly a terminal branch of the facial artery (although it has been found to occasion-

C. Pham · P. W. MacIntosh (✉)
Department of Ophthalmology, University of Illinois, Chicago, IL, USA

A. Fay
Department of Ophthalmology, Harvard Medical School, Boston, MA, USA

A. J. Cohen, C. N. Burkat (eds.), *Oculofacial, Orbital, and Lacrimal Surgery*, https://doi.org/10.1007/978-3-030-14092-2_17

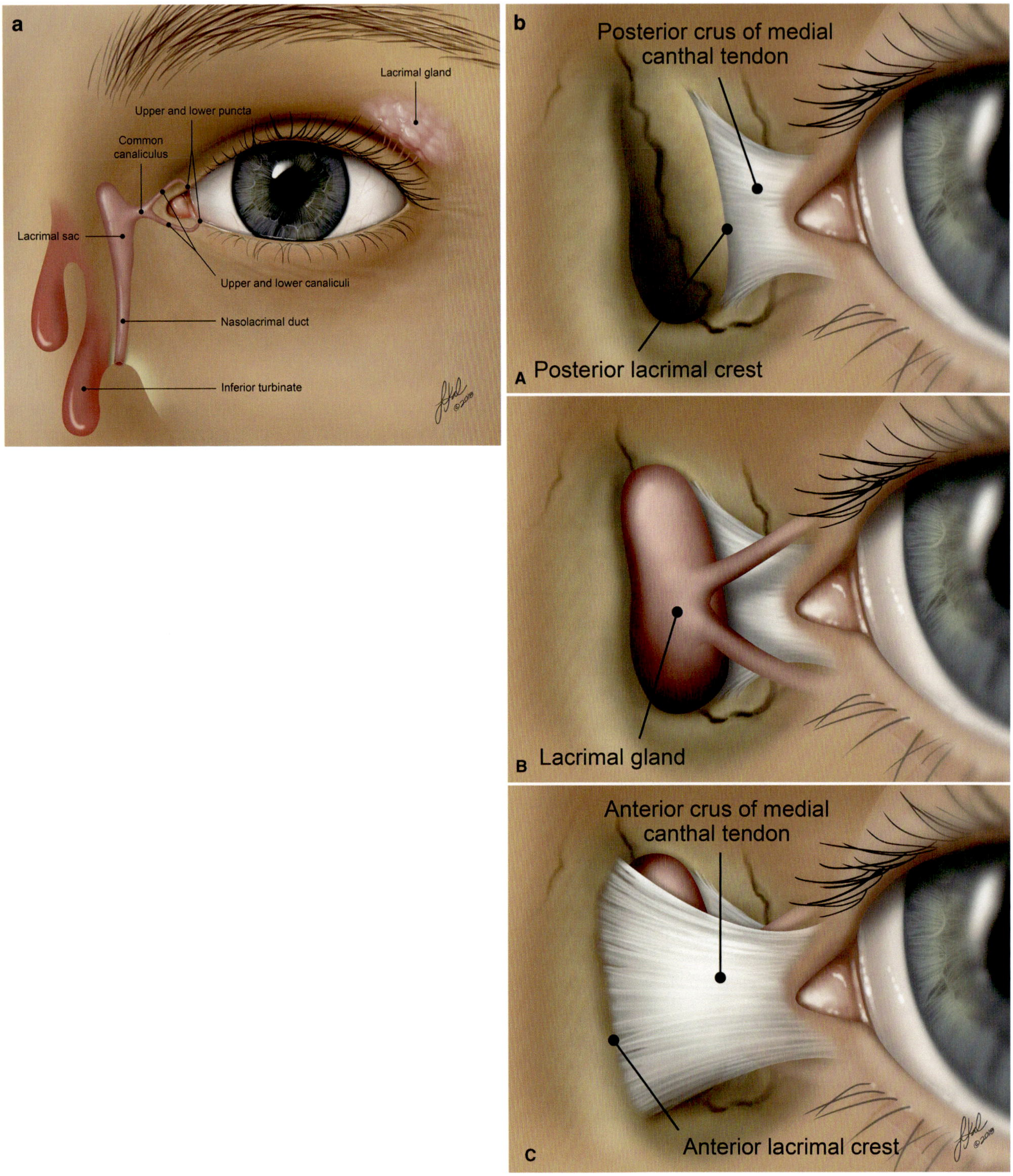

Fig. 17.1 Medial canthal tendon/lacrimal sac complex

ally arise as a branch of the ophthalmic artery). It arises from a branch point of the lateral nasal artery and ascends from alongside the nasolabial fold or the ala of the nose to the medial canthal area. Incisions and dissections carried out in this area should be mindful of this artery and its possible anatomic variants [6, 7].

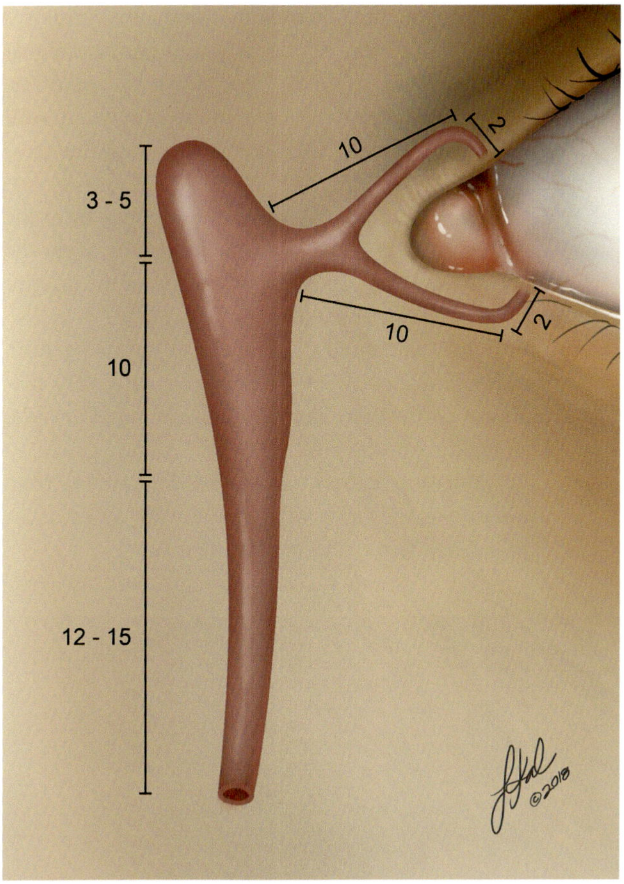

Fig. 17.2 Canalicular system and measurements

Clinical Features and Ancillary Tests

The assessment of medial canthal defects is primarily focused on evaluation of visual function, eyelid function, and patency of the lacrimal system. Ocular function should be evaluated first and foremost – particularly in the setting of trauma. Open globe injuries should be fully evaluated and repaired prior to any repair of the medial canthal area. The assessment of congenital medial canthal abnormalities in the pediatric population should be carried out in concert with a pediatric ophthalmologist to assess for strabismus and screen for amblyopia.

The eyelids protect and lubricate the globe and cornea and play an important role in the operation of the lacrimal pump. Medial lagophthalmos, rounding of the canthal angle, and poor apposition of the lid to globe can be signs of medial canthal tendon avulsion and should raise suspicion for canalicular injury. The presence or absence of entropion, ectropion, and cicatricial changes and assessment for presence and amount of tissue loss can aid in surgical planning. The assessment of orbicularis tone and Bell's reflex can help mitigate complications related to corneal exposure.

The approach to the management of medial canthal defects largely depends on the patency of the lacrimal drainage system. Evaluation of the puncta and nasolacrimal probing and irrigation are the first steps in the evaluation of the lacrimal system. If patent, the repair can proceed with direct closure, a graft, or a flap. If it is not patent, then reconstruction must include repair of the canaliculus to prevent postoperative tearing.

Canalicular probing and irrigation:

1. Find the puncta and dilate with a punctal dilator if necessary.
2. Pass a 0-00 Bowman probe into the canaliculus, directing it first superiorly or inferiorly and then carefully medially toward the lacrimal sac, and a "hard stop" to evaluate if the passage way is patent.
3. To test the patency of the nasolacrimal duct, the probe is then directed inferiorly, posteriorly, and laterally.
4. If the probe becomes visible in the wound, the canaliculus is lacerated and will need to be repaired. If resistance is met, either the probe is in the incorrect tract or there is an obstruction – withdraw the probe and gently redirect to avoid canalicular injury.
5. Irrigation may be used as an adjunct to, or instead of, probing to evaluate the canaliculus. Irrigation fluid will be visible in the wound if the canaliculus is lacerated. Staining the irrigation fluid with fluorescein can aid in visualization.

Should probing and irrigation reveal a lacerated canaliculus, repair should proceed with intubation. Should there be an obstruction, repair may require a separate bypass procedure such as a dacryocystorhinostomy or a conjunctivodacryocystorhinostomy, which are discussed in separate chapters.

Because of the complex anatomy of the medial canthal region, imaging can be an important adjunct to assessment of this region. The bony attachments of the medial canthal tendon are the anterior and posterior lacrimal crest and as such can be disrupted by medial orbital wall, LeFort type II, and LeFort type III fractures. The management of medial canthal injuries can vary depending on presence or absence of fractures; thus thorough evaluation with computed tomography (CT) scanning with fine maxillofacial and/or orbital cuts is recommended, especially in the setting of trauma. When assessing defects associated with tumors, magnetic resonance imaging (MRI) is the preferred modality and can better delineate soft tissue abnormalities than CT. MRI can be particularly important in assessment and surgical planning for excision of lacrimal sac neoplasms and in distinguishing between clinical entities such as dacryocele and encephalocele or meningocele. MRI is also the preferred imaging modality in children where limitation of radiation exposure is desired.

Etiology

As alluded to the introduction, the etiology of medial canthal defects encompasses a wide range of conditions. The following discussion is not meant to be an exhaustive description of the topic but instead aims to be a broad overview of defects that may commonly be encountered by the oculoplastic and facial plastic surgeon. Medial canthal defects can be broadly grouped into the following categories: (1) congenital malformations/variations, (2) traumatic defects, and (3) defects related to tumor excision. The discussion of the etiology of medial canthal defects will follow this categorization, and likewise the discussion of management to follow will parallel this taxonomy.

A. Abnormalities of the medial canthal area can arise as anatomic variation or as congenital malformations. These can occur as an isolated phenomenon or as part of a syndromic developmental abnormality. Epicanthal folds are one of the most commonly encountered medial canthal abnormalities. They are folds of the skin that extend vertically or obliquely from the upper or lower eyelid toward the medial canthal area. They are divided into four subtypes (Fig. 17.3) [8, 9]:

1. Epicanthus tarsalis: epicanthal fold arising from the tarsal fold of the upper lid that partially covers the inner canthus and terminates in the skin of the inferior portion of the inner canthus.
2. Epicanthus palpebralis: epicanthal fold arising from the upper lid above the tarsus that runs inferiorly, partially covers the inner canthus, and terminates near the lower margin of the orbit.
3. Epicanthus supraciliaris: epicanthal fold arising from the brow that runs inferiorly, partially covers the inner canthus, and terminates near the tear sac.

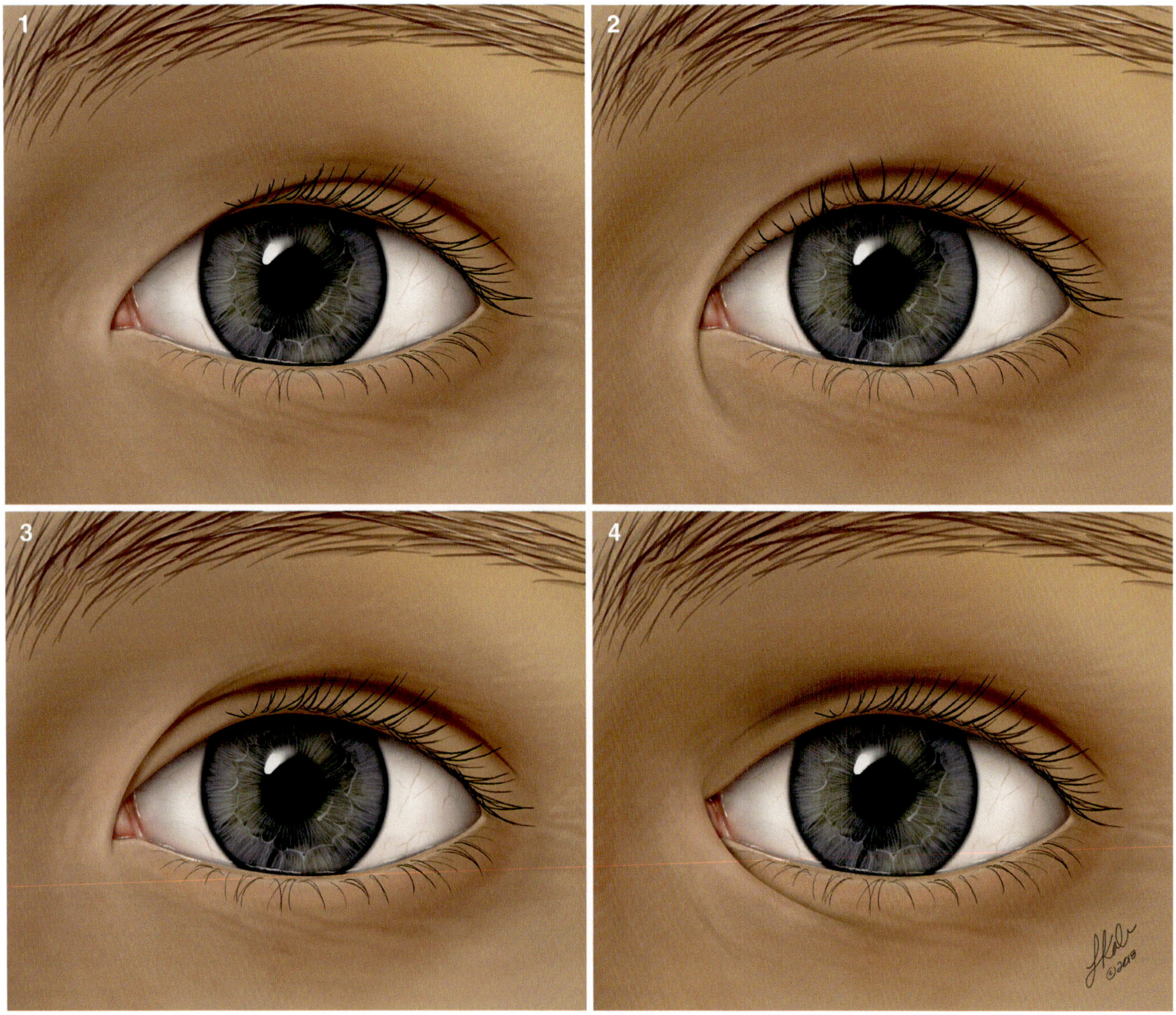

Fig. 17.3 Epicanthus types

4. Epicanthus inversus: epicanthal fold arising from the lower lid that runs superiorly, partially covers the inner canthus, and terminates in the skin of the superior portion of the inner canthus.

The average distance between medial canthi in an adult can vary from 32 mm in Caucasians to 37 mm in those of Chinese descent [10]. Distances that exceed these measurements are considered abnormal. When accompanied by a normal interpupillary distance, this condition is referred to as telecanthus and can arise independently as an anatomical variant or occur in conjunction with other eyelid abnormalities such as blepharophimosis syndrome, Down syndrome, fetal alcohol syndrome, or Waardenburg syndrome. Telecanthus can also be acquired following traumatic facial injuries resulting in the avulsion or laceration of the medial canthal tendon, with widening of the medial soft tissues rather than the bony orbits. When an increased intercanthal distance is accompanied by a widened interpupillary distance, this condition is referred to as hypertelorism. Hypertelorism represents a lateralization of the medial orbital wall and orbit and can be seen in craniosynostosis syndromes and craniofacial dysplasias [8, 9].

B. Direct or indirect injury to the eyelids or face is more commonly observed in young adults and children but is also observed in older adults in the setting of mechanical falls. Traumatic medial canthal defects can be broadly grouped into injuries involving the soft tissues only and those involving bony fractures. Soft tissue injuries can be further subdivided into those involving the canalicular system and those that do not. The most common cause of canalicular laceration is blunt force from fists, while in children dog bites were the most common cause [11]. The lower canaliculus is more commonly injured, and injury of the upper canaliculus should increase suspicion for an open globe injury [12].
C. The close approximation of vital structures within the medial canthal area necessitates great care in tumor resection, and a Mohs microsurgical approach is recommended if possible to preserve as much normal tissue as possible. Even with microsurgical techniques, removal of the skin or lacrimal sac tumors from the medial canthal area may result in rather large defects involving multiple facial structures (e.g., eyelid, nose, and cheek) and may require sacrificing of all or part of the lacrimal apparatus. Superficial tumors may not affect the deeper lacrimal drainage system but deeper ones may. Care should be taken to preserve the lacrimal drainage system whenever possible.

Management

The approach to management of medial canthal defects should proceed with the following goals in mind: (1) prevention of amblyopia in children, (2) maintenance of eyelid position and function, (3) preservation of the lacrimal system, and (4) cosmesis. Optimal outcomes may require a staged approach or multidisciplinary intervention, particularly in cases of congenital defects.

A. Congenital abnormalities:
Epicanthoplasty with or without repair of telecanthus: Care must be taken to avoid damage to the lacrimal system. Consider inserting Bowman probes into canaliculi in order to ensure preservation. There are many approaches to epicanthoplasty and many authors recommend selection of technique be based on degree of epicanthal fold: Z-plasty, modified Z-plasty, and Y-V plasty are suited for mild epicanthus or epicanthus tarsalis, while Mustarde or modifications are better for severe cases or epicanthus inversus [13]. Correction can be limited to superficial repair of epicanthal folds or can be combined with repair of congenital or acquired telecanthus. A further discussion of repair of telecanthus using miniscrews or miniplates can be found in the section on traumatic repair.

Park Z-plasty (Fig. 17.4) [14, 15]:

1. A dot (point A) is marked on the epicanthal fold that approximates the medial-most extent of the lacrimal lake.
2. Point B is placed where the epicanthal fold joins the skin of the medial canthus or the lower eyelid.
3. Point D is the actual medial-most extent of the lacrimal lake (point A is the surface representation of point D and should align as one point when viewed from the front).
4. A double eyelid crease is marked and carried medially toward point A running parallel to the eyelid margin.
5. An oblique line starting from point A running 45° from horizontal in a superomedial direction toward the glabella. The intersection of this line with the double crease line is point C.
6. The triangle EAC is excised.
7. The flap EABD is lifted, rotated, and sutured in place.
8. This can be incorporated with a double eyelid crease procedure.

Y-V plasty [16]:

1. A small Y-shape is drawn along the edge of the epicanthal fold horizontally from the medial canthus to the desired point of the medial canthus.
2. Incisions are made with a scalpel, and the skin is dissected from subcutaneous tissue and orbicularis.
3. The medial canthus is advanced medially, the redundant skin is excised, and the skin is closed using 6-0 plain gut or 6-0 Prolene suture.

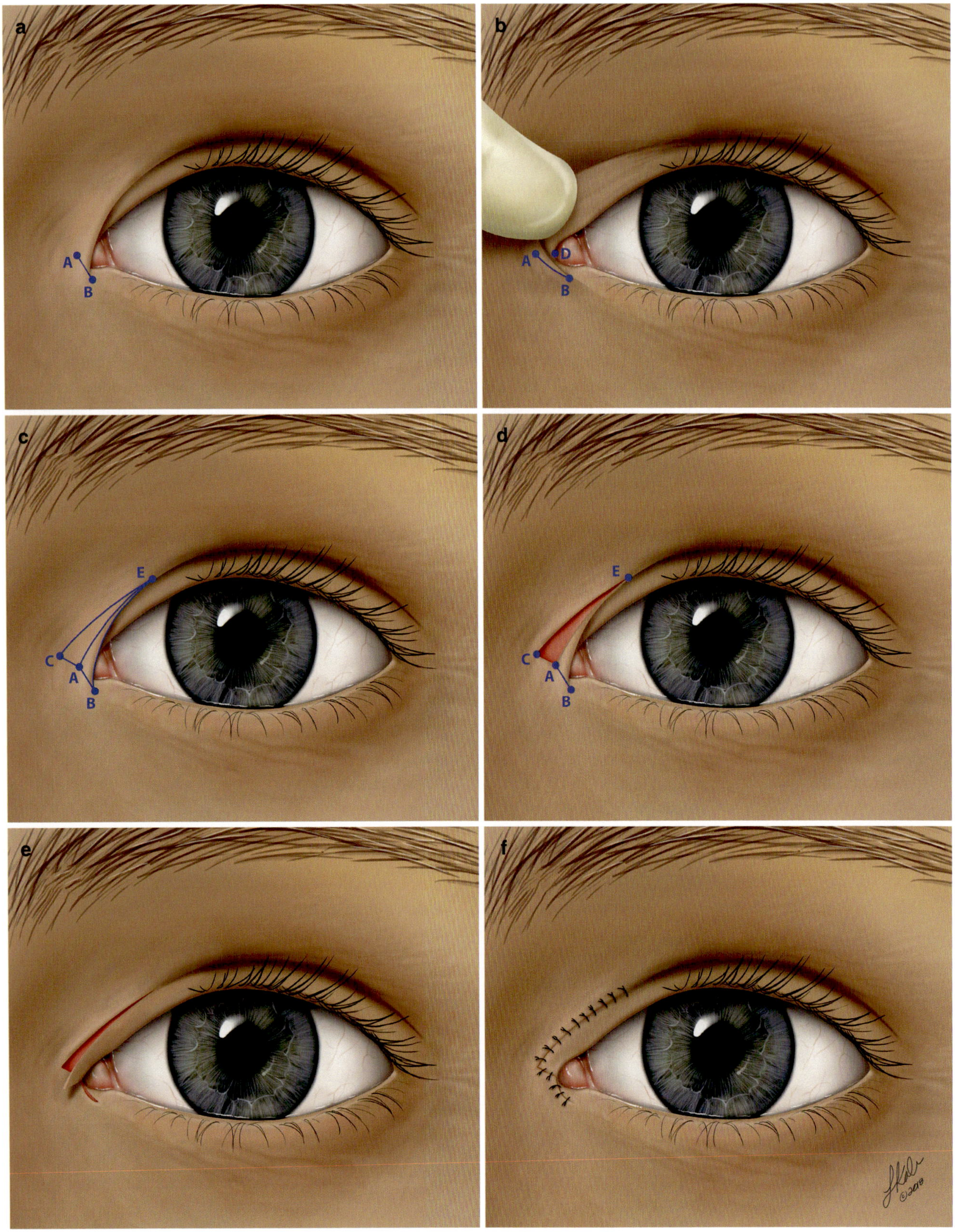

Fig. 17.4 Park Z-epicanthoplasty

Kim et al. describe a canthopexy technique using obliquely oriented transnasal wiring accomplished through the Y-V plasty incision [17]:

1. The medial orbital wall is accessed via the Y-V incision.
2. The contralateral nasal recession is incised, and dissection is carried out to the medial orbital wall. Drill holes are made from this point to the contralateral anterior and posterior lacrimal crests of the affected orbit.
3. A 2-0 wire is passed through the medial canthal tendon of the affected side and then through the holes to the contralateral side.
4. The wire is pulled and tightened.
5. Once satisfactory positioning of the medial canthus is confirmed, the skin is closed.

Mustarde four flap with medial canthopexy (Fig. 17.5) [18, 19]:

1. Mark the site of the desired new medial canthus.
2. Pull the skin medially to obliterate any fold, and mark the position of the actual canthus.
3. These two marks are joined by a horizontal line.
4. The center of this horizontal line is identified, and two vertical lines oriented at 60° from this point are drawn extending superotemporal and inferotemporal.
5. From the distal extent of these vertical lines, backcuts at a 45° angle are made.
6. Paramarginal incisions are made from the point of the actual canthus.
7. Incisions are made with a scalpel dissection and undermining carried out to level of the orbicularis medially, while dissection down to periosteum is performed at the site of the new canthus.
8. The medial tendon complex is identified and is affixed to the periosteum at the new canthus site using a 4-0 nonabsorbable suture (the original description uses silk) in a mattress fashion.
9. Once proper canthal position is confirmed, the cutaneous flaps are transposed and sutured into place using 6-0 plain gut suture.

B. Traumatic injury to the medial canthus usually results in an avulsion injury. In these types of injuries, there is usually no tissue loss, and a graft or flap will not typically be necessary. Instead, the main issue is laceration of the canaliculus, typically at the distal canaliculus or common canaliculus. If nasolacrimal duct probing reveals a patent canalicular system, repair may proceed primarily. If the canaliculus is determined to be lacerated, it must be repaired first, and then attention can be turned to repair of the medial canthal tendon [20–22]. When there is no concurrent medial wall fracture, repair is as simple as reattachment of the cut ends. In the setting of concomitant medial wall fracture, repair may need to proceed in conjunction with plating and transnasal wiring.

Canalicular repair:

1. Feed a silicone stent through the punctum, and retrieve from the proximal cut end of the canaliculus. Options include mono- and bicanalicular stents – the former only intubates upper or lower canaliculi, and the latter intubates the entire lacrimal system.
2. Find the distal cut end of the canaliculus. This task may be aided with a strong head light to evaluate the distal end of the laceration for a small, white annulus that represents the distal canaliculus.
3. Pass the silicone stent into the distal canaliculus. Mini monocanalicular stents do not need to be retrieved in the nose, but the standard ones do. The advantage of the standard stents retrieved in the nose is that traction on the stent via the nose can help to reapproximate the medial canthal tendon to aid repair. Smaller lacerations may be sufficiently treated with mini monocanalicular stents.
4. Suture the canaliculus with a double armed 7-0 polyglactin suture. Grasp the edge of the lacerated canaliculus, and pass an arm of the suture, skirting along the silicone tube and into the canaliculus and coming out through the wall. Repeat from the opposite cut end with the opposite arm.
5. Repeat #4 in a second location 180° around the canaliculus.
6. Once both sutures are placed, they may be tied.
7. The soft tissue and skin may then be closed around the repaired canaliculus.

Medial canthal avulsion repair:

1. Identify the proximal end of the medial canthal tendon.
2. Identify the distal posterior crus of the medial canthal tendon.
3. Suture tendon to posterior crus with 5-0 polyglactin suture.
4. Additional deep sutures may be placed if needed.
5. Close the skin.

If there is loss of tissue (as can happen in tumor resection), and all or part of the medial canthal ligament is missing, a nasal periosteal flap can be elevated and used for medial canthal tendon reconstruction. A modification of this technique using periosteum for medial canthopexy and tarsal reinforcement was described by Cardim et al. [21, 22]. Disadvantages to this technique include increased risk of damage to lacrimal structures (should they be intact) during elevation of the periosteal flap.

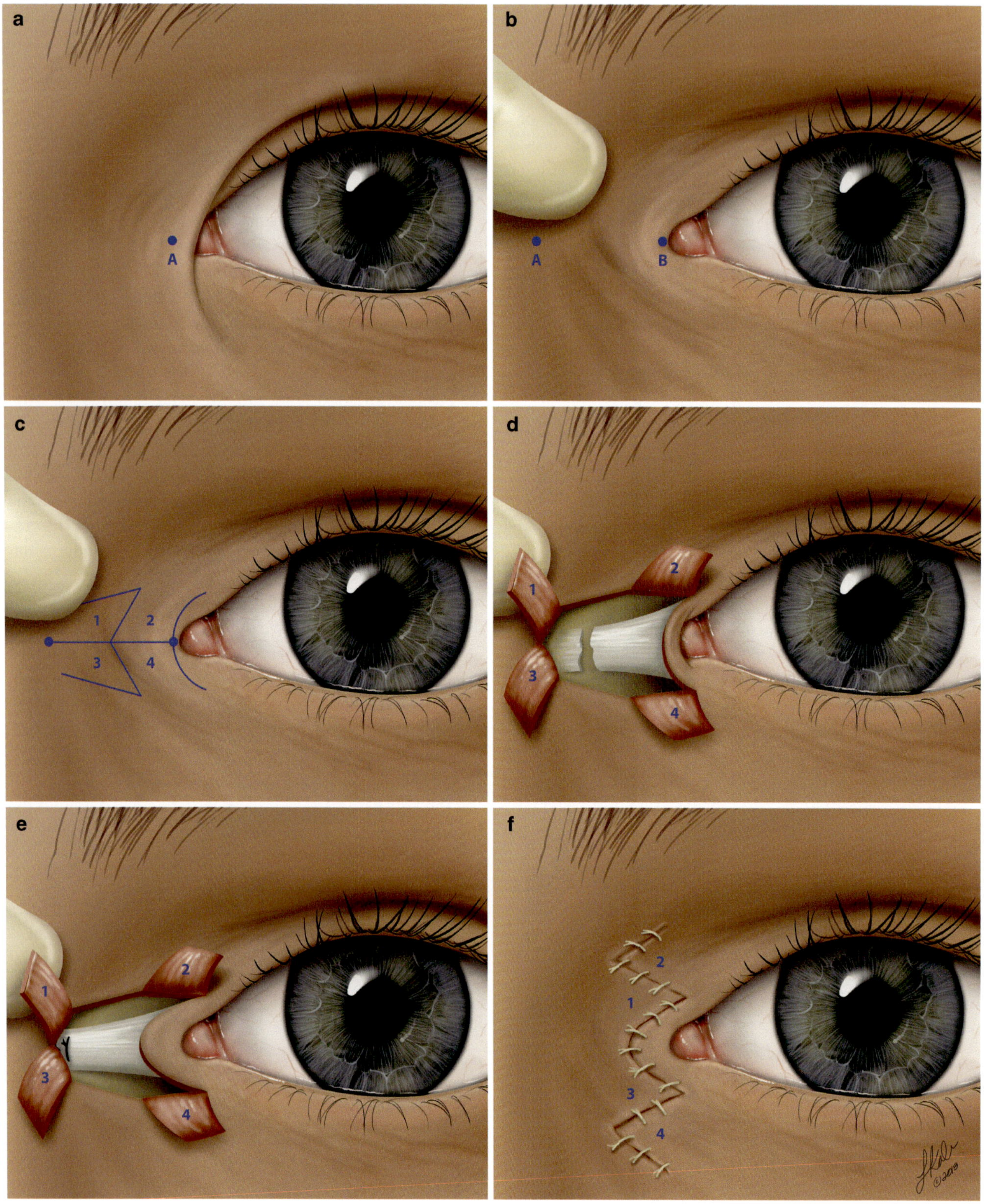

Fig. 17.5 Mustarde four flap epicanthoplasty

Alternatives to the periosteal flap include transnasal wiring, use of miniplates or cantilevered miniplates, and fixation using microscrews [23–31]. Wiring and microplate techniques are advantageous when the naso-orbital-ethmoid (NOE) complex is displaced or disfigured; however these techniques are beyond the scope of this chapter and discussed elsewhere in this text.

Medial canthal repair using nasal periosteum [21, 22]:

1. Dissection is carried out down to the nasal orbital rim.
2. A pedicle with the base located at the natural insertion of the medial canthal tendon is marked along the anterior orbital rim.
3. The pedicle of periosteum is incised using Bovie cautery using a Colorado tip or a scalpel blade.
4. The periosteum is carefully elevated using a periosteal elevator, taking care not to amputate or narrow the base of the pedicle.
5. The periosteum can then be rotated and sutured to the tarsus or the proximal cut end of the canthal tendon using 5-0 polyglactin suture.

Microscrew/miniplate fixation [31]:

1. The site of the desired medial canthus is marked.
2. A reverse Y-incision is made, which later will be closed into a "V" shape as with a "Y-V" flap.
3. Dissection is carried out to the medial orbital wall, and the periosteum is dissected to expose the anterior and posterior lacrimal crest.
4. If there is good bony support along the medial orbital wall, self-driving titanium microscrews can be driven into the bone. Should there be a weak or absent medial wall, a malleable microplate can be affixed across the weak area secured in place deep to the orbital rim.
5. 3-0 wire suture is first attached to the stump of the medial canthal ligament and then attached to the microscrew or plate. The wire is then twisted and tightened until the canthus is secured and in a satisfactory position.
6. The wire is then trimmed, and repair can proceed with closure of soft tissue using 5-0 Vicryl for deeper structures and 6-0 plain gut or Prolene sutures for skin.

C. Medial canthal defects from tumor excision may have various presentations that require different techniques for repair. Small defects may be repaired with simple undermining of the skin and small adjacent tissue flaps. This type of repair is preferred if possible since neighboring skin will best match the missing skin [32]. Larger defects involving only the anterior lamella may require grafts or flaps for adequate closure. Defects involving full-thickness medial upper and/or lower eyelids require reconstruction of both anterior and posterior lamella.

Adjacent tissue transfer flap: When the defect is next to an area of skin laxity where the tension of closure would not compromise eyelid function, closure of the defect can be accomplished by horizontal advancement of adjacent tissue. This technique has the advantages of skin matching as well as a native blood supply but relies on the presence of enough skin laxity to achieve tension-free closure with a favorable scar. Contraindications include the presence of active infection or tumor [33].

1. Grasp the skin edge with forceps.
2. Using Westcott scissors, bluntly and sharply dissect the skin from the underlying orbicularis.
3. Horizontal relaxing incisions may be made in the skin to create an H-plasty and permit the opposing flaps to slide together.
4. Avoid vertical tension on the eyelid to prevent ectropion or retraction.
5. Suture the orbicularis muscle and subcutaneous layers with interrupted 6-0 polyglactin suture.
6. Suture skin edges with 6-0 fast gut or Prolene sutures.

Rotational flap: These flaps have the advantage of mobilizing a large area of tissue with a wide native vascular base to repair defects without adequate adjacent skin laxity for primary closure or use of an advancement flap. This technique can require extensive cutting and dissection beyond the area of the defect. Knowledge of neurovascular anatomy can help prevent compromise of blood vessels or nerves.

The primary defect can be thought of as a part of a larger circle where adjacent tissue is rotated into the area of defect around a fulcrum. Many approaches to repair of the medial canthal area using rotational flaps have been described including transnasal rotational flaps, transnasal advancement flaps, bilobed variants, rhomboid flaps, modified transposition, and upper lid myocutaneous flap [34–39]. Regardless of technique chosen, the goal is to achieve adequate coverage of the defect with scar lines falling along natural skin tension lines while optimizing skin and hair matching.

Infraglabellar bilobed transnasal flap (as described by Mehta et al.*)*: This flap is constructed from the infraglabellar dorsum and contralateral nose (Fig. 17.6).

1. The bilobed flap is marked starting with a line that emanates perpendicularly from the superior-most aspect of the defect. This line is carried across the dorsum of the nose following natural skin tension lines to form the primary lobe. The diameter of the primary lobe should be comparable in size to the vertical height of the defect.
2. The smaller secondary lobe utilizes tissue from the contralateral nose and is slid/rotated into the primary lobe defect.

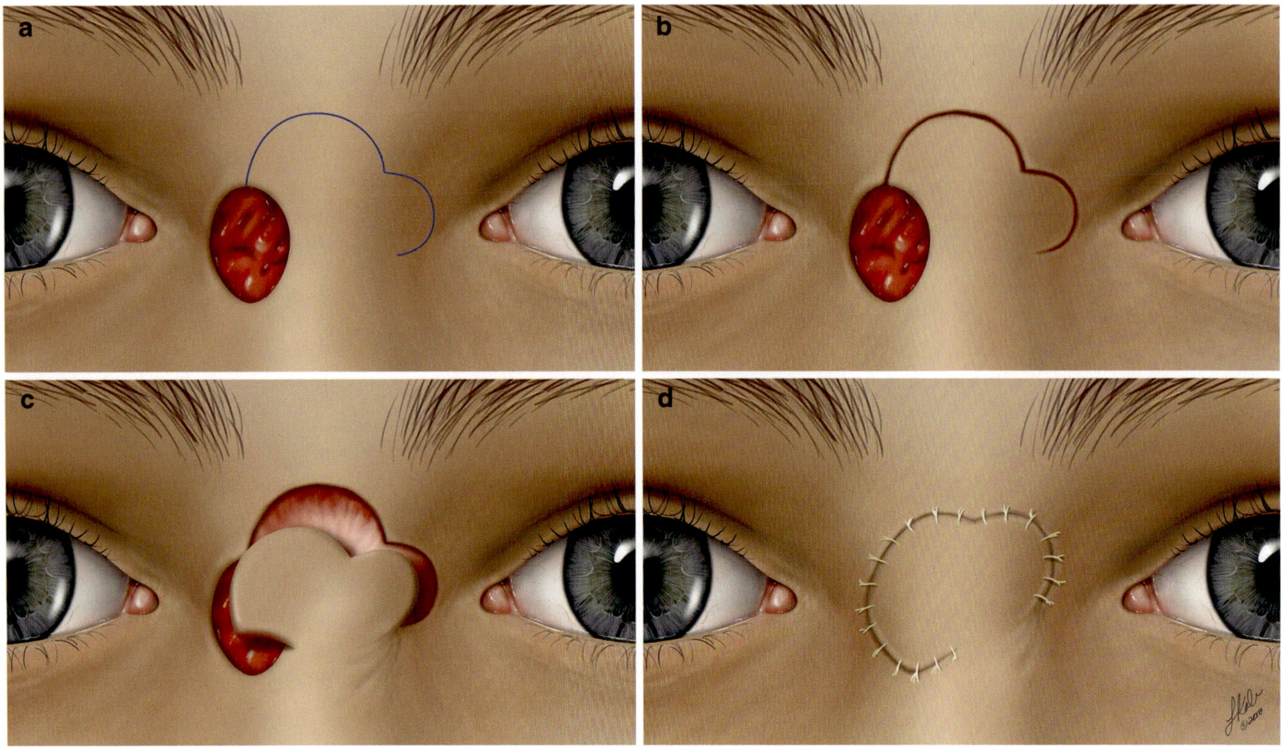

Fig. 17.6 Bilobed transnasal flap (Mehta)

3. Local infiltrative anesthesia with an epinephrine-containing anesthetic mixture is given.
4. Skin incisions are made using a scalpel, and the flap is undermined and mobilized to the level of the subcutaneous fat.
5. The flap is rotated into place, and interrupted deep sutures using 5-0 Vicryl may be placed to secure the flap.
6. Skin closure is done in an interrupted fashion using 6-0 plain gut or 6-0 Prolene.
7. The area is padded with nonstick dressings, and it is recommended to affix bolsters to provide adequate compression during initial healing.

Rhomboid flap (as described by Ng et al.) (Fig. 17.7):

1. Although most Mohs defects are oval in shape, this technique visualizes the defect as a rhomboid shape with the long axis oriented vertically.
2. The flap is marked starting with a line directed from the middle of the defect horizontally across the dorsum of the nose. The length of this line should approximate half the vertical height of the defect.
3. A line oriented at 60° and extending from the end of the horizontal line is drawn.
4. Local infiltrative anesthesia with an epinephrine-containing anesthetic mixture is given.
5. Skin incisions are made using a scalpel, and the flap is undermined and mobilized to the level of the subcutaneous fat. The edges of the recipient site are also undermined.
6. The flap is rotated into place, and interrupted deep sutures using 5-0 Vicryl may be placed to secure the flap. The underside of the flap should be anchored to the periosteum to reform the concave contour of the medial canthal area.
7. Skin closure is done in an interrupted fashion using 6-0 plain gut or 6-0 Prolene.
8. The area is padded with nonstick dressings, and it is recommended to affix bolsters to provide adequate compression during initial healing.

Pedicle/interpolation flap: The pedicle flap can be used when there is insufficient tissue or mobility preventing primary closure as can happen with wide excisions of tumor in the nasal area. This technique often requires a staged approach with division and inset occurring weeks after initial repair. The paramedian forehead flap can be used for reconstruction of the medial canthal area in conjunction with nasal defects [40, 41]. Larger defects may require longer pedicles that extend toward the hairline – care should be taken to avoid transfer of hair to the recipient site (Fig. 17.8).

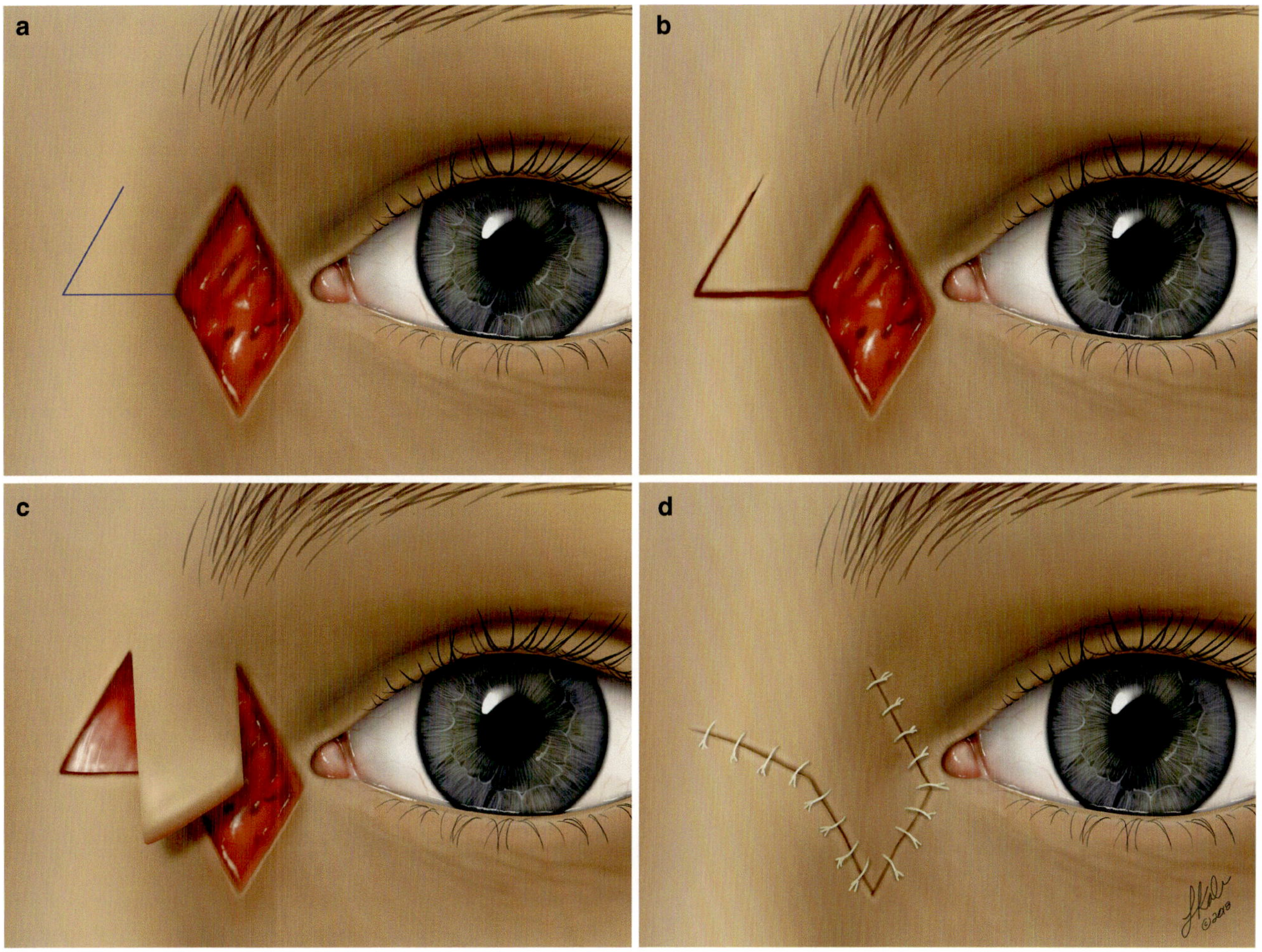

Fig. 17.7 Rhomboid flap (Ng)

1. Identify the supratrochlear artery on the same side as the majority of the defect to be repaired. A Doppler probe may be used to help localize the artery, but it is most often located 2 cm lateral to the midline.
2. The base of the pedicle is marked out over the supratrochlear artery measuring 1.5 cm in width.
3. Outline the cutaneous defect by squaring off the corners. Form a template of the defect from thin foam or paper. The template should match exactly the size of the defect and not be oversized.
4. Position the template with the superior edge of the defect facing inferiorly on the forehead skin, centered 2 cm lateral to the midline, in line with the supratrochlear artery identified above. Place the inferior edge of the template at the frontal hairline.
5. Confirm the pedicle is long enough to permit rotation into the defect.
6. Local infiltrative anesthesia is administered using and anesthetic mixture containing epinephrine.
7. The marked pedicle is initially incised with a scalpel and then dissected and elevated beginning at the distal end. The distal end of the pedicle should be thinned to best match tissue thickness at the recipient site.
8. The pedicle is then rotated, inset into the recipient site, and secured using 5-0 Vicryl. The underside of the flap may be anchored to the periosteum to reform the concave contour of the medial canthal area.
9. Skin closure is done in an interrupted fashion using 5-0 or 6-0 plain gut or Prolene.
10. Significant undermining of the surrounding donor site should be undertaken in order to generate adequate laxity for closure. Donor site closure proceeds with judicious deep closures, and then skin closure can be accomplished with permanent nonabsorbable suture in an interrupted fashion.
11. For patient convenience and comfort, nonabsorbable dressing can be placed between the pedicle tissue bridge and normal skin, or the posterior, raw edge of the pedicle can be covered with a full-thickness skin graft.
12. Division and inset of the graft can occur as early as 10–14 days after the 1st stage, although some authors recommend waiting 3–4 weeks for full vascularization.

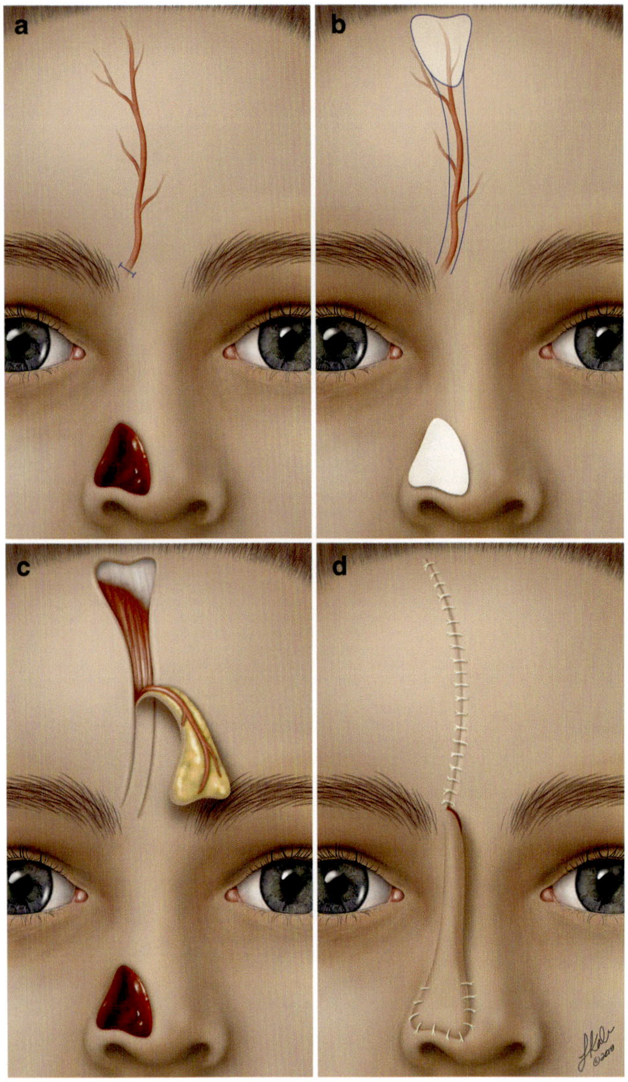

Fig. 17.8 Paramedian pedicle flap

If the primary defect cannot be fully covered using flaps, remaining small defects can be covered with grafts.

Full-thickness skin graft: Both the epidermis and dermis are transplanted from one location to another on the same individual. The benefit of the full-thickness graft is that blood vessels and accessory glands are transplanted with the graft. These grafts tend to have less contracture than split-thickness grafts and are more likely to grow with the individual when performed in a child. This graft does require a small, well-vascularized, and clean defect and is relatively contraindicated in smokers [42].

1. The wound bed should be clean and free of infection, tumor, or necrotic tissue and have adequate blood supply.
2. Donor site selection should attempt to best match the morphologic characteristics of the recipient site. Skin thickness, color, and presence of hair should all be considered. For periocular recipient sites, grafts are most commonly obtained from the ipsilateral or contralateral upper eyelid and posterior auricular, supraclavicular, or inner upper arm.
3. Measure the size of the defect and transfer this to the donor site. The area to be excised is usually oversized slightly to account for contracture.
4. An ellipse-shaped incision is made with a blade, and the full-thickness graft is freed from the donor site making certain to remove residual adipose tissue.
5. The graft may be "pie-crusted" to allow for egress of underlying fluid and to prevent seroma formation.
6. The graft is secured to the recipient site using 6-0 plain or mild chromic gut suture.
7. A bolster should be fashioned out of a nonadherent material and secured over the grafted area to ensure good approximation between graft and wound bed.

Split-thickness skin graft: The epidermis and partial-thickness dermis are transplanted from one location to another on the same individual. This graft requires a less than ideal recipient bed and can cover a larger area than a full-thickness graft. But because it is subject to more contracture, less resistant to subsequent radiotherapy, and often less than ideal skin color matching, this type of graft is often more functional than cosmetic and does not often play a role in medial canthal reconstruction.

Conjunctival autograft: Because of the intimate association between the medial canthal area and the ocular surface, a conjunctival autograft may be required to maintain apposition of a nonkeratinized surface to the globe. Most commonly described in the setting of pterygium surgery, the natural redundancy and presence of stem cells make ipsilateral autograft an excellent source of mucosa to cover a medial canthal defect [43]. Donor site selection requires a normal healthy conjunctiva.

1. After measurement of the defect, an appropriate number of clock hours are marked along the limbus opposite the side of the defect (usually superotemporal).
2. A peritomy is made, and a conjunctival flap is lifted by making relaxing incisions posteriorly. The conjunctiva is carefully dissected from underlying Tenon's layer using Westcott scissors. Non-toothed forceps are typically used to avoid damage to the delicate tissue.
3. The graft is then freed, and the donor site can either be left bare to heal primarily or amniotic membrane can be applied.
4. The graft is brought to the wound bed and is affixed either using 7-0 chromic or 7-0 Vicryl suture in a buried interrupted fashion. A braided absorbable is preferred if the site is to be in close proximity to the cornea as the suture is softer and causes less keratopathy and discomfort.

Scar Prevention and Management

Scar formation, particularly on the face, is of particular concern to both surgeon and patient. Wound healing is a complex process that involves inflammation, proliferation, and remodeling – a process that is dynamic and can occur over 6 months or longer. Some determinants of scar formation such as skin tension and vascular supply can be mitigated by surgical technique, while others such as patient age and skin type can be taken into account during preoperative counseling.

Incisions should be made along natural skin tension lines when possible, and the five "A's" of surgical technique should be followed: asepsis, absence of tension, accurate approximation, avoidance of raw surface, and atraumatic tissue handling. Judicious use of cautery and undermining should be used to ensure good vascularization, nonabsorbable sutures should be removed in the first week, and traction tape and/or sutures can be utilized to minimize traction on a healing incision [44, 45].

Some degree of scar formation is inevitable. Conservative measures such as massage have anecdotal success though a review of the literature found the quality of studies and the evidence to be weak [46]. Intralesional steroid has been used alone or in conjunction with 5-fluorouracil (5-FU) in hypertrophic scars as well as keloids. In the face, 2.5–20 mg/mL of triamcinolone with or without 0.9 mg (50 mg/mL) of 5-FU is injected directly into the body of the scar taking care to avoid injection into the skin or fat as this can result in depigmentation and atrophy [44, 45, 47]. Laser technology has been used alone and in conjunction with other treatments to mitigate scar formation as well as decrease the appearance of scars once they form. Laser-assisted skin healing uses elevated temperature to modify the wound healing process by stimulating heat shock proteins, while pulsed dye laser interferes with microcirculation and vascularization of the scar [45].

The use of botulinum toxin A (BTXA) in both prevention of scar formation and the lessening of scar appearance has been of particular interest. BTXA can prevent formation of scar by decreasing traction and tension by paralysis of opposing muscles. Additionally, laboratory and animal studies have shown it to inhibit fibroblasts and decrease intralesional collagen thickness and disorder in hypertrophic scars [48]. Some authors have found BTXA to be equally effective and better tolerated than intralesional steroid in the treatment of keloids [49]. Dosing protocols vary, and published studies use 1-5 U of BTXA per 1 cm^3 of tissue. A meta-analysis and literature review found promise of its use in scar prevention and management, but both concluded that more high-quality studies with better stratification and larger number of patients were needed [50, 51].

Finally, topical silicone gel or gel sheets have been shown in some studies to reduce the degree of scarring in a number of studies. The advantages of silicone are that it is applied topically and thus is noninvasive and well tolerated. It can also be applied to irregular surfaces and moving parts and can cover any size scar [52–54].

References

1. Turvey TA, Golden BA. Orbital anatomy for the surgeon. Oral Maxillofac Surg Clin. 2012;24(4):525–36.
2. Robinson TJ, Stranc MF. The anatomy of the medial canthal ligament. Br J Plast Surg. 1970;23(1):1–7.
3. Zoumalan CI, Joseph JM, Lelli GJ, Segal K, Adeley A, Kazim M, Lisman R. Evaluation of the canalicular entrance into the lacrimal sac: an anatomical study. Ophthal Plast Reconstr Surg. 2011;27(4):298–303.
4. Anand S, Hollingworth K, Kumar V, Sandramouli S. Canaliculitis: the incidence of long-term epiphora following canaliculotomy. Orbit. 2004;23:19–26. 32.
5. Zaldívar RA, Bradley EA. Primary canaliculitis. Ophthal Plast Reconstr Surg. 2009;25:481–4.
6. Kim YS, Choi DY, Gil YC, Hu KS, Tansatit T, Kim HJ. The anatomical origin and course of the angular artery regarding its clinical implications. Dermatol Surg. 2014;40(10):1070–6.
7. Lee HJ, Won SY, O J, Hu KS, Mun SY, Yang HM, Kim HJ. The facial artery: a comprehensive anatomical review. Clin Anat. 2018;31(1):99–108.
8. Foster JA, et al. Basic and clinical science course: section 7. San Francisco: American Academy of Ophthalmology; 2016–2017.
9. Lueder GT, et al. Basic and clinical science course: section 6. San Francisco: American Academy of Ophthalmology; 2016–2017.
10. Le TT, Farkas LG, Ngim RC, Levin LS, Forrest CR. Proportionality in Asian and North American Caucasian faces using neoclassical facial canons as criteria. Aesthetic Plast Surg. 2002;26(1):64–9.
11. Kennedy RH, May J, Dailey J, Flanagan JC. Canalicular laceration. An 11-year epidemiologic and clinical study. Ophthal Plast Reconstr Surg. 1990;6(1):46–53.
12. Naik MN, Kelapure A, Rath S, et al. Management of canalicular lacerations: epidemiological aspects and experience with mini-monoka monocanalicular stent. Am J Ophthalmol. 2008;145(2):375–80.
13. Kim CY, Lee SY. Structural and cosmetic outcomes of medial epicanthoplasty: an outcome study of three different techniques. J Plast Reconstr Aesthet Surg. 2015;68(10):1346–51.
14. Park JI, Park MS. Park Z-epicanthoplasty. Facial Plast Surg Clin North Am. 2007;15(3):343–52.
15. Yoo WM, Park SH, Kwag DR. Root z-epicanthoplasty in asian eyelids. Plast Reconstr Surg. 2002;109(6):2067–71.
16. Kao YS, Lin CH, Fang RH. Epicanthoplasty with modified Y-V advancement procedure. Plast Reconstr Surg. 1998;102:1835e41.
17. Kim TG, Chung KJ, Kim YH, Lim JH, Lee JH. Medial canthopexy using YV epicanthoplasty incision in the correction of telecanthus. Ann Plast Surg. 2014;72(2):164–8.
18. Mustarde JC. Epicanthus and telecanthus. Br J Plast Surg. 1963;16:346e56.
19. Yoon K. Modification of Mustardé technique for correction of epicanthus in Asian patients. Plast Reconstr Surg. 1993;92:1182e6.
20. Ricca AM, Kim AK, Chahal HS, Shriver EM. Nasolacrimal stents: an introductory guide. EyeRounds.org. posted January 29, 2018; Available from: http://EyeRounds.org/tutorials/Stents/
21. Leibsohn JM, Hahn F. Medial canthal tendon reconstruction with nasal periosteum. Ophthalmic Plast Reconstr Surg. 1992;8(1):35–40.
22. Cardim VL, Bazzi K, dos Santos Silva A, e Silva MG, dos Santos FM, Salomons RL, e Silva AD, Dornelles RD. Canthopexy and

tarsal reinforcement using a periosteal flap. Revista Brasileira de Cirurgia Plástica. 2013;28(1):36–40.
23. Converse JM, Smith B. Naso-orbital fractures and traumatic deformities of the medialcanthus. Plast Reconstr Surg. 1966;38:147–62.
24. Mustarde JC. Repair and reconstruction in the orbital region: a practical guide. London: Churchill Livingstone; 1966.
25. Tessier P. Plastic surgery of the orbit and eyelids. Baltimore: Masson; 1981.
26. McCarthy J, Jelks G, Valauri A, Wood-Smith D, Smith B. The orbit and zygoma. Philadelphia: W.B. Saunders; 1990.
27. Howard GR, Nerad JA, Kersten RC. Medial canthoplasty with microplate fixation. Arch Ophthalmol. 1992;110(12):1793–7.
28. Shore JW, et al. Repair of telecanthus by anterior fixation of cantilevered miniplates. Ophthalmology. 1992;99(7):1133–8.
29. Callahan A, Callahan MA. Fixation of the medial canthal structures: evolution of the best method. Ann Plast Surg. 1983;11:242–5.
30. Sharma V, Nemet A, Ghabrial R, et al. A technique for medial canthal fixation using resorbable poly-L-lactic acid–polyglycolic acid fixation kit. Arch Ophthalmol. 2006;124(8):1171–4.
31. Qin Y, Li D, Chen T. Management of the delayed traumatic medial telecanthal deformity. Aesthet Surg J. 2010;30(4):516–21.
32. Hayano SM, Whipple KM, Korn BS, Kikkawa DO. Principles of periocular reconstruction following excision of cutaneous malignancy. J Skin Cancer. 2012;2012:438502.
33. Baker SR, Baker SR. Local flaps in facial reconstruction. 3rd ed. Philadelphia: Elsevier; 2007.
34. Custer PL. Transnasal flap for medial canthal reconstruction. Ophthalmic Surg. 1994;25(9):601–3. PMID 7831002.
35. Sciscio A, Joshi N. The transnasal advancement flap: a technique for medial canthal area defects. Orbit. 2001;20(2):141–7.
36. Mehta JS, Olver JM. Infraglabellar transnasal bilobed flap in the reconstruction of medial canthal defects. Arch Ophthalmol. 2006;124(1):111–5.
37. Ng SGJ, Inkster CF, Leatherbarrow B. The rhomboid flap in medial canthal reconstruction. Br J Ophthalmol. 2001;85:556–9.
38. Rajabi MT, Hosseini SS, Rajabi MB, Tabatabaie SZ. A novel technique for full thickness medial canthal reconstruction; playing with broken lines. J Curr Ophthalmol. 2016;28(4):212–6.
39. Jelks GW, Glat PM, Jelks EB, Longaker MT. Medial canthal reconstruction using a medially based upper eyelid myocutaneous flap. Plast Reconstr Surg. 2002;110:1636–43.
40. Kim JH, Kim JM, Park JW, Hwang JH, Kim KS, Lee SY. Reconstruction of the medial canthus using an ipsilateral paramedian forehead flap. Arch Plast Surg. 2013;40(6):742–7. PMID 24286048.
41. Correa BJ, Weathers WM, Wolfswinkel EM, Thornton JF. The forehead flap: the gold standard of nasal soft tissue reconstruction. Semin Plast Surg. 2013;27(2):96–103.
42. Thornton JF. Skin grafts and skin substitutes. In: Selected readings in plastic surgery. 2004;10(1):1–24.
43. Kenyon KR, Wagoner MD, Hettinger ME. Conjunctival autograft transplantation for advanced and recurrent pterygium. Ophthalmology. 1985;92(11):1461–70.
44. Son D, Harijan A. Overview of surgical scar prevention and management. J Korean Med Sci. 2014;29(6):751–7.
45. Liu A, Moy RL, Ozog DM. Current methods employed in the prevention and minimization of surgical scars. Dermatol Surg. 2011;37(12):1740–6.
46. Shin TM, Bordeaux JS. The role of massage in scar management: a literature review. Dermatol Surg. 2012;38(3):414–23.
47. Darougheh A, Asilian A, Shariati F. Intralesional triamcinolone alone or in combination with 5-fluorouracil for the treatment of keloid and hypertrophic scars. Clin Exp Dermatol. 2009;34(2):219–23.
48. Xiao Z, Qu G. Effects of botulinum toxin type a on collagen deposition in hypertrophic scars. Molecules. 2012;17(2):2169–77.
49. Shaarawy E, Hegazy RA, Abdel Hay RM. Intralesional botulinum toxin type a equally effective and better tolerated than intralesional steroid in the treatment of keloids: a randomized controlled trial. J Cosmet Dermatol. 2015;14(2):161–6.
50. Prodromidou A, Frountzas M, Vlachos DE, Vlachos GD, Bakoyiannis I, Perrea D, Pergialiotis V. Botulinum toxin for the prevention and healing of wound scars: a systematic review of the literature. Plast Surg. 2015;23(4):260–4.
51. Zhang DZ, Liu XY, Xiao WL, Xu YX. Botulinum toxin type a and the prevention of hypertrophic scars on the maxillofacial area and neck: a meta-analysis of randomized controlled trials. PLoS One. 2016;11(3):e0151627.
52. Puri N, Talwar A. The efficacy of silicone gel for the treatment of hypertrophic scars and keloids. J Cutan Aesthet Surg. 2009;2(2):104–6.
53. Poston J. The use of the silicone gel sheeting in the management of hypertrophic and keloid scars. J Wound Care. 2000;9:10–2.
54. Suetake T, Sasai S, Zhen YX, Tagami H. Effects of silicone gel sheet on the stratus corneum hydration. Br J Plast Surg. 2000;13:157–9.

Part II

Oculofacial

Introduction to Brow Lifting

18

Bradford W. Lee, Brian C. Tse, Benjamin P. Erickson,
and Don O. Kikkawa

Brow Aesthetics and the Aging Brow

The height, shape, and configuration of the eyebrows are a defining feature of a person's appearance, and the dynamic movement of the eyebrows plays an important role in expressing human emotion. There is great diversity in the appearance of the brows among youthful individuals, and the brows should complement and be harmonious with the surrounding structures.

In spite of such variation, youthful brows tend to share certain characteristics that vary by gender and ethnicity. Youthful brows rest at or above the superior orbital rim and are higher in women and lower in men. In terms of configuration, youthful female brows are naturally thinner and more arched with the tail of the brow oftentimes located higher than the head of the brow, whereas male brows are thicker with denser brow cilia and have a more horizontal configuration. Compared to Caucasian brows, Asian brows of both genders are typically higher set and more arched than their Caucasian counterparts (Fig. 18.1).

Youthful brows and faces also have fuller, more volumized facial fat pads. Youthful brows typically have fullness beneath the tail of the brow in the region of the retro-orbicularis oculi fat (ROOF) and robust soft tissue support along the region of the corrugator muscles. The superior sulcus is also fuller in youth where the brows meet the eyelids. Nearby, a healthy volume of muscle and fat in the temporalis fossa help to camouflage the lateral orbital rim where the brow transitions into the temple.

With age, everything that characterizes the youthful brow and face deflates and descends. As the brow complex descends and falls below the orbital rim, it can cause the appearance of heavy eyelids with excess eyelid skin that functionally occludes the superior visual fields. The lateral brow becomes ptotic and accentuates temporal eyelid hooding due to unopposed brow depressor action from orbicularis oculi, since the frontalis muscle often does not extend laterally enough to elevate the lateral brow. The ROOF devolumizes, the superior sulcus hollows, and the temporalis muscle and temporal fat atrophy to unmask the superior and lateral orbital rim. This "skeletonization" of the brow and periorbital region is a common and prominent finding among patients in their eighth and ninth decades of life (Fig. 18.2).

Trends in brow aesthetics over the past two decades have shown an appreciation for the importance of volume in brow rejuvenation. While brow lifts in the past may have dramatically lifted the brows and created secondary hollowing of the superior sulci, modern brow rejuvenation techniques aim to modestly raise the brows and volumize the tissues of the brows and their surrounding structures. Cosmetic facial surgeons now recognize that unnatural splaying of the heads of the brows via overaggressive transection of the corrugator muscles is likewise not a youthful or natural look. In the modern era of aesthetics, dermal fillers and volume augmentation combined with brow-shaping and lifting via surgery and neurotoxins can achieve supe-

None of the authors have any financial interest to disclose.

B. W. Lee (✉)
Division of Oculofacial Plastic and Reconstructive Surgery, Bascom Palmer Eye Institute, Department of Ophthalmology, University of Miami Miller School of Medicine, Miami, FL, USA

Division of Oculofacial Plastic and Reconstructive Surgery, UC San Diego Department of Ophthalmology, Shiley Eye Institute, La Jolla, CA, USA
e-mail: blee@miami.edu

B. C. Tse · B. P. Erickson
Division of Oculofacial Plastic and Reconstructive Surgery, Bascom Palmer Eye Institute, Department of Ophthalmology, University of Miami Miller School of Medicine, Miami, FL, USA

D. O. Kikkawa
Division of Oculofacial Plastic and Reconstructive Surgery, UC San Diego Department of Ophthalmology, Shiley Eye Institute, La Jolla, CA, USA

Division of Plastic Surgery, UC San Diego Department of Plastic Surgery, La Jolla, CA, USA

A. J. Cohen, C. N. Burkat (eds.), *Oculofacial, Orbital, and Lacrimal Surgery*, https://doi.org/10.1007/978-3-030-14092-2_18

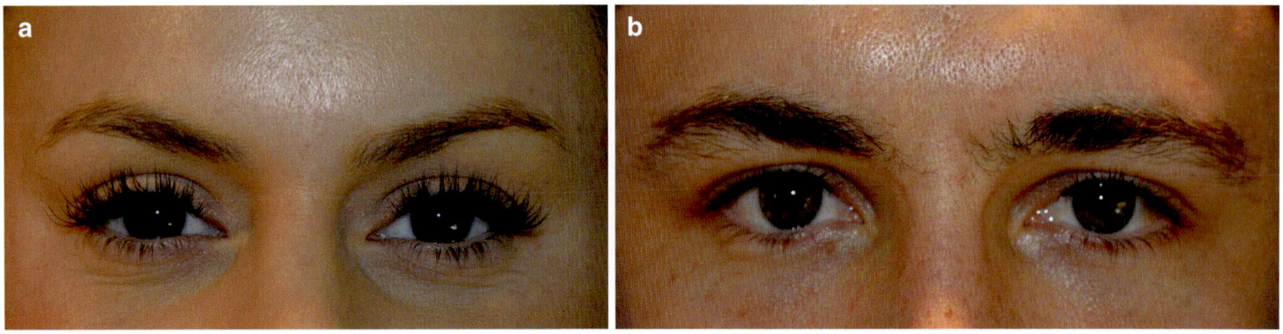

Fig. 18.1 Youthful Caucasian female brows (**a**) and youthful Caucasian male brows (**b**)

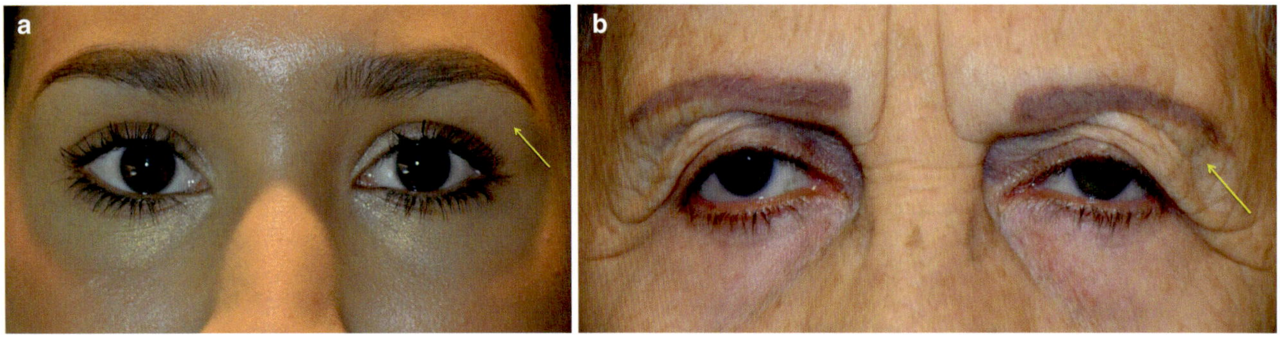

Fig. 18.2 (**a**) Youthful brows resting at or above the orbital rim with a graceful arch and fullness of the brow fat pad beneath the tail of the brow (arrow). (**b**) Aged brows with lateral brow ptosis and deflation of the brow fat pad beneath the tail of the brow (arrow)

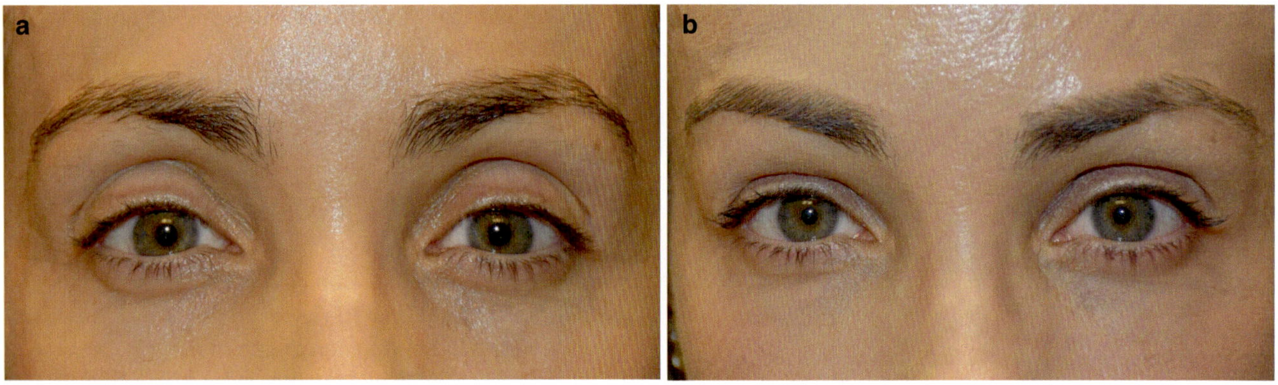

Fig. 18.3 (**a**) Age-related hollowing of the brow fat pad and superior sulcus. (**b**) The same patient after brow rejuvenation using neurotoxins and fillers to volumize and contour the brow shape for a natural and youthful appearance

rior results that were previously not possible. In such a way, patients undergoing brow rejuvenation procedures today look more natural and youthful without a postsurgical or surprised look (Fig. 18.3).

Anatomical Planes of the Upper Face

The upper third of the face is demarcated by the hairline superiorly and the eyebrows and glabella inferiorly. There are five layers to the scalp, starting most superficially with the skin, subcutaneous connective tissue, galea aponeurotica, loose areolar tissue, and periosteum (pericranium). The skin of the forehead is the thickest skin on the face and contains many sebaceous and sweat glands. The subcutaneous tissue is highly vascularized and composed mainly of adipose tissue and fibrous septae. The vertically oriented frontalis muscle of the forehead is the sole brow elevator, arising from the inferior border of the galea aponeurotica of the scalp. The galea aponeurosis envelops the frontalis muscle, with the deeper layer firmly attaching to the supraorbital rim and contributing to the arcus marginalis (Fig. 18.4).

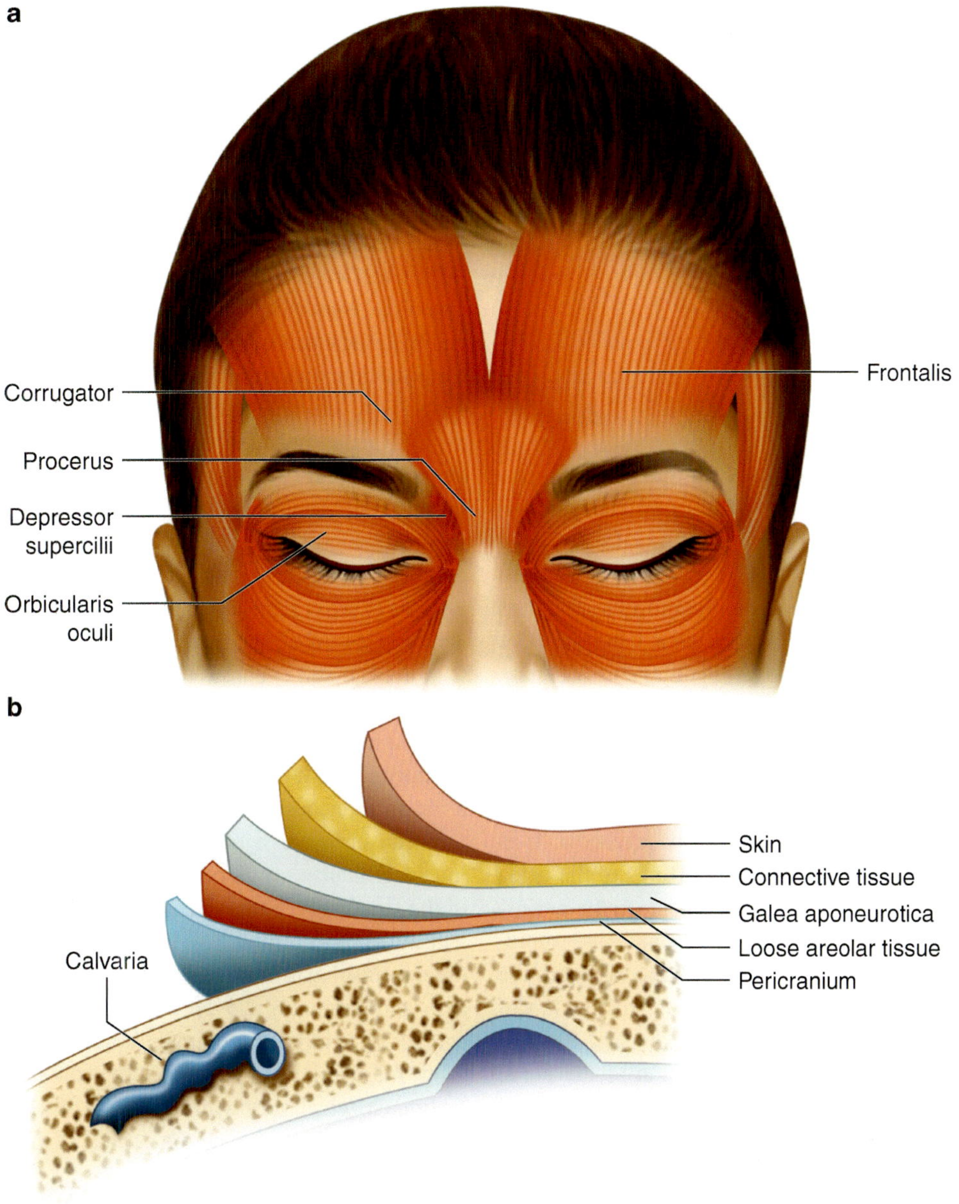

Fig. 18.4 (**a**) shows the frontalis muscle, the sole brow elevator. Also shown are the brow depressors, which include the corrugator supercilii, depressor supercilii, procerus, and orbicularis oculi. (**b**) shows the layers of the forehead centrally

The frontalis muscle interdigitates with the brow depressors inferiorly, namely, the corrugator supercilii, depressor supercilii, procerus, and orbicularis oculi. The paired corrugator muscles arise from the superomedial orbital rim and run superolaterally, becoming more superficial as they insert into the brow skin. Contraction of these muscles leads to vertical glabellar folds. The procerus muscle sits between the corrugator muscles, originating from the nasal bone and inserting into the glabella and mid-forehead. Procerus contraction leads to horizontal glabellar folds. While the orbicularis oculi's primary function is to close the eyelids, the orbital portion of the muscle arises from the medial canthal tendon, runs in a circumferential manner around the orbital rim, interdigitates with the frontalis and corrugator supercilii muscles, and inserts laterally onto the zygoma. The orbital portion of the orbicularis oculi contributes to forced closure of the eyelids and brow depression, and contraction creates the "crow's feet."

Between the galea and periosteum is loose connective tissue that is a natural glide plane that can be utilized during brow and forehead surgery. At the periosteal level, three retaining ligaments have been identified [1]. The inferomedial retaining ligament is 12 mm lateral to midline at the

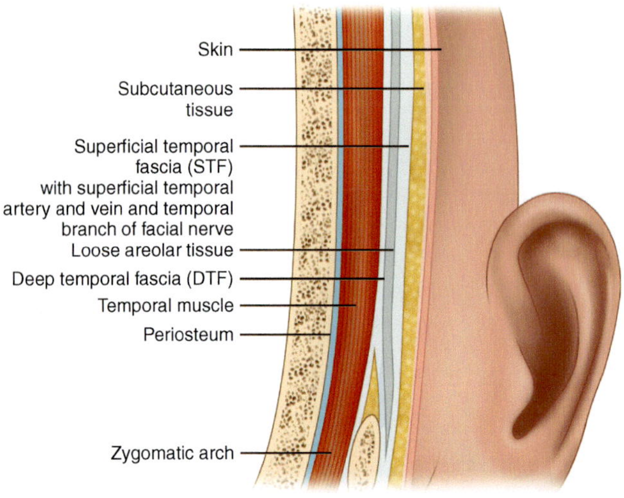

Fig. 18.5 Facial diagram showing layers of the temporal scalp

superior orbital rim. The superomedial retaining ligament is 13 mm lateral to midline and 10 mm above the superior orbital rim. The superotemporal retaining ligament is 23 mm lateral to midline and 10 mm above the orbital rim. Surgically releasing these attachments promotes effective brow and forehead elevation.

The retro-orbicularis oculi fat (ROOF) is located inferior to the brow cilia and gives volume to the eyebrow. It is enveloped by the anterior and posterior portions of the galea aponeurotica. The ROOF has deep attachments to the periosteum of the supraorbital rim. The supraorbital and supratrochlear nerves track superiorly in the plane between the ROOF pad and the periosteum. The superficial division of the supraorbital nerve enters the frontalis muscle 2–3 cm above the supraorbital rim. The deep division of the nerve runs superiorly and obliquely between the periosteum and galea aponeurotica. At the level of the mid-forehead, the deep division runs 0.5–1.5 cm medial to the superior temporal line in a parallel fashion [2]. Inferiorly, the ROOF can extend onto the preseptal surface of the eyelid, as it is continuous with the posterior orbicularis fascia.

The brow cilia orientation varies depending on location. Medial and inferior brow cilia grow superotemporally, whereas superior brow cilia grow inferotemporally.

Neurovascular Anatomy of the Brow and Forehead

Sensory innervation to the medial forehead is derived from the supraorbital nerve (approximately 29 mm lateral to midline) and supratrochlear nerve (approximately 16 mm lateral to midline), which are both branches of the ophthalmic division of the trigeminal nerve [3]. Similarly, blood supply to the medial forehead is from the supraorbital and supratrochlear arteries, both branches of the ophthalmic artery. The supraorbital nerve, artery, and vein exit the skull via either a supraorbital notch or foramen. The lateral forehead receives sensory input from the lacrimal, zygomaticofacial, and auriculotemporal nerves, which run beneath the frontalis muscle. Blood supply to the lateral forehead is from the superficial temporal and zygomaticotemporal arteries (Fig. 18.5).

The layers of the temporal scalp include skin, subcutaneous tissue, superficial temporal fascia (STF), deep temporal fascia (DTF), and temporalis muscle. The STF is a continuation of the superficial musculoaponeurotic system (SMAS) in the midface and the galea aponeurotica of the scalp. Both the superficial temporal artery and frontal branch of the facial nerve run within the STF. A loose areolar tissue plane separates the STF from the DTF and is the safest dissection plane when operating in the temporal region to avoid injury to the facial nerve. The DTF is located superficial to the temporalis muscle and inserts on the superior temporal line and zygomatic arch. The conjoined tendon is located anteriorly along the superior temporal line and consists of the confluence of the STF, galea aponeurotica, DTF, and central forehead periosteum.

Forehead and eyebrow function are supplied by the facial nerve (cranial nerve VII). The facial nerve exits the tympanomastoid foramen approximately 1.5 cm inferior to the external auditory canal. Within the parotid gland, the nerve divides into its main branches, with the temporal branch innervating the forehead and upper eyelid and the zygomatic branch innervating the orbicularis oculi of the lower eyelid. The buccal branch of the facial nerve innervates the orbicularis oris, buccinators, and zygomaticus muscles. The temporal branch runs in an oblique fashion across the zygoma, crossing the zygomatic arch approximately 2.5 cm lateral to the lateral canthus. It courses superiorly, approximately 1 cm lateral to the tail of the brow, following Pitanguy's line. To avoid injury to the temporal branch, which runs within the STF, dissection in this region is carried out deeply along the surface of the DTF.

History and Clinical Evaluation of the Brow and Upper Face

A careful preoperative assessment will help to ensure selection of an appropriate brow procedure to meet the needs of each patient. When obtaining a clinical history, one should elicit information regarding prior facial surgery, as well as dry eye symptoms and treatments. While it is rare to induce significant lagophthalmos with conservative brow lifting endpoints – which focus more on contour and fullness rather than absolute height [4–6] – the risk is certainly greater in the setting of prior aggressive blepharoplasty, particularly if orbicularis was excised. The risk of postoperative exposure-related symptoms is also significantly increased if concomitant blepharoplasty is planned.

In order to better understand a patient's true brow morphology, one should also inquire regarding eyebrow shaping

Table 18.1 Relative indications and contraindications of brow lifting techniques

	Relative indications	Relative contraindications	Benefits	Risks
Direct	Bushy brows (typically male)	Thin or plucked brows (female)	Simple	Potential to create an arched brow contour in men
	Desire for robust visual improvement	Low tolerance for visible scars	Robust and durable lift due to brow tissue excision	Visible scar
	Marked lateral brow ptosis			
Mid-forehead	Prominent forehead rhytides	Low tolerance for visible scars	Creates pseudo-rhytides in cases of paralytic brow ptosis	Visible scar
	Unilateral paralytic brow ptosis			Poor cosmesis
Pretricheal/ Trichophytic	Prominent forehead rhytides	Baldness or receding hairline	Reduces forehead rhytides	Potentially limited hairstyles
	High hairline/long forehead with hairline concealed by hairstyle	Low hairline/short forehead	Lowers the hairline	Potentially visible scar
	Desire for cosmetic forehead rejuvenation		Surgical access for brow depressor weakening	Potential cutaneous numbness or paresthesias
Coronal	Prominent forehead rhytides	Baldness, thinning hair, or receding hairline	Reduces forehead rhytides	Raises the hairline
	Low hairline/short forehead	High hairline/long forehead	No facial scar	Cutaneous numbness or paresthesias
	Desire for cosmetic forehead rejuvenation		Surgical access for brow depressor weakening	Potential alopecia
Endoscopic	Mild to moderate brow ptosis	Heavier brow and forehead tissues	No facial scars	Potential alopecia
	Thinner brow and forehead tissues	Extensive brow ptosis, cutaneous laxity, and prominent forehead rhytides	Facilitates brow contouring	Potential facial nerve injury
	Desire for cosmetic forehead rejuvenation	Baldness, thinning hair, or receding hairline	Surgical access for brow depressor weakening	Complications associated with suspension mechanism (e.g., implant, plate, screw, bone tunnels)
Internal browpexy	Mild to moderate lateral brow ptosis	Prominent medial brow ptosis	Easily performed via blepharoplasty incision	Questionable durability due to tenuous periosteal fixation
	Concomitant upper lid blepharoplasty procedure	Marked brow ptosis and forehead cutaneous laxity	Volumizes brow fat pad	Unable to correct medial brow ptosis
			Enables brow contouring	
Neurotoxin and dermal fillers	Mild brow ptosis	Need for durable correction	Excellent brow contouring ability	Not covered by insurance
	Desire for brow contouring	Marked brow ptosis obstructing vision	Can address deflation of the brow fat pad	Need for maintenance treatments
	Brow fat pad deflation/ superior sulcus hollowing		Nonsurgical with minimal downtime	Risk of intravascular complication with fillers (e.g., blindness, skin necrosis)

techniques (e.g., electrolysis, threading, or waxing), tattooing, and prior use of injectables, such as hyaluronic acid dermal fillers, autologous fat, and neurotoxins. With brow shaping, one should attempt to determine whether hair removal techniques have been temporary or permanent. History of neurotoxin administration within the past 4 months should also be elicited, as injections to the frontalis, orbicularis, and glabella impact the apparent height and contour of the brows [7, 8]. Hairstyle preferences should be elicited as the wearing of bangs helps to conceal certain incisions, such as the pretrichial incision.

Particularly with male patients, one should elicit any family history of pattern baldness, as well as any personal history of hairline recession, hair transplantation, or hair loss treatments, such as finasteride or topical minoxidil. It is important to emphasize in the informed consent process that future changes in the hairline or hair density may unmask the incisions created by coronal, pretrichial, or even endoscopic brow surgery.

Assessment of the height and contour of the resting brows with respect to the supraorbital ridge is a key aspect of the presurgical evaluation. Having patients close their eyes and relax the forehead allows one to evaluate the natural resting position of the brows by overcoming the sometimes insuppressible drive to activate the frontalis muscle and clear the visual axis in cases of prominent brow ptosis, ptosis, or der-

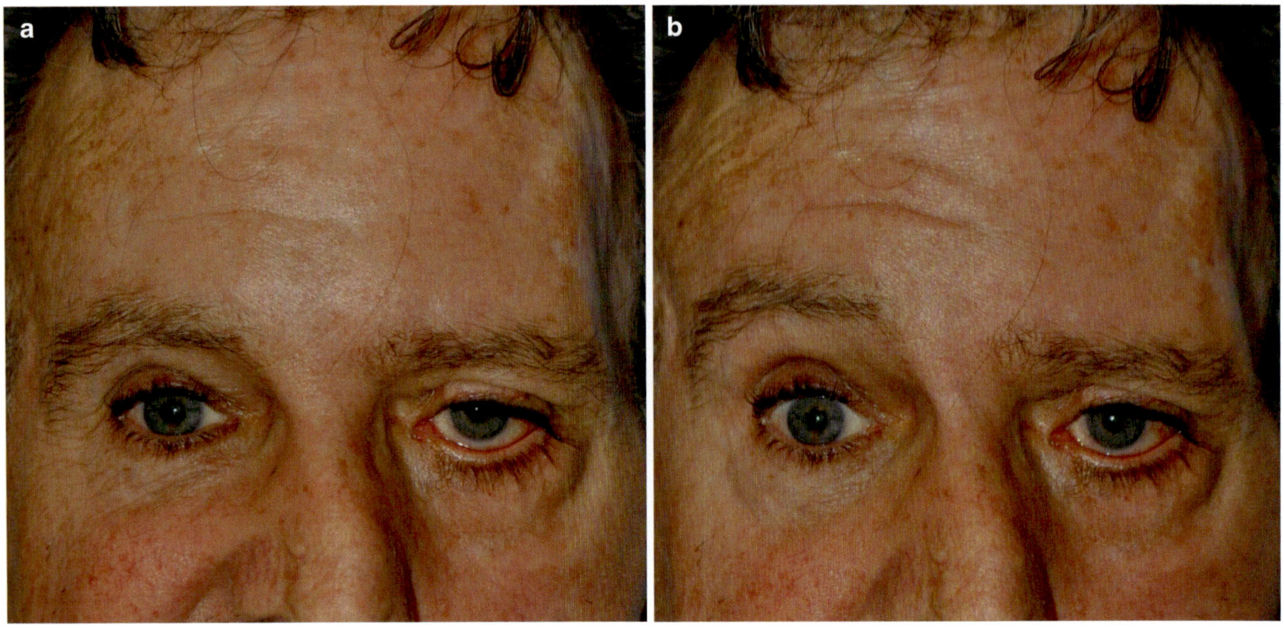

Fig. 18.6 (**a**) Left-sided facial nerve palsy resulting in left brow ptosis and absence of left-sided forehead rhytides (**a**). The asymmetry of brow height and forehead rhytides is even more apparent with attempted elevation of the brows (**b**)

matochalasis. In addition to considering the generally accepted gender ideals of brow shape and position, one should consider patients' individual preferences as well as their own youthful brow configurations and how these have changed with age. Obtaining facial photos from prior decades of life can help determine how the process of "descent and deflation" has affected the individual patient (Table 18.1).

Brow shaping and tattooing can significantly impact the natural height and contour of the brow, and evidence of these procedures should be sought on exam regardless of the clinical history provided. The transition between thicker brow and glabellar skin to thinner eyelid skin should be clinically apparent regardless of prior removal of eyebrow cilia. Determining the location of this transition zone is particularly important when attempting to distinguish the relative contributions of brow ptosis and dermatochalasis to eyelid fold prominence and temporal hooding. Assessment of natural brow hair color, density, and distribution is also important in determining whether supraciliary incisions can be effectively disguised following direct browplasty.

A preoperative assessment of brow symmetry at rest and with dynamic elevation with appropriate photographic documentation is essential, and any asymmetries should be discussed. Many individuals have some degree of asymmetry, and this can often be addressed to some degree with differential lifting. Asymmetries due to underlying differences in morphology of the supraorbital ridge and bony calvarium are more difficult to correct [9, 10]. Patients should be counseled that persistence of some degree of asymmetry does not constitute an adverse surgical result. Similarly, brow asymmetry due to a facial nerve palsy is challenging to correct due to the absence of dynamic elevation and muscle tone (Fig. 18.6).

Manual lifting of the brow complex is an important part of the clinical evaluation and simulates the effect a brow lift will have on eyelid crease height, eyelid fold configuration, and superior sulcus fullness. It thus helps the surgeon to formulate a global strategy for periocular rejuvenation that may also include upper eyelid blepharoplasty, soft tissue reduction and sculpting, or volume augmentation.

Prominent horizontal forehead rhytides and redundant forehead tissue are signs of chronic frontalis overaction that can result from brow ptosis. If forehead rhytides are a concern to the patient, a pretrichial brow lift can effectively ameliorate these if an amenable hairline is present. In patients with prominent forehead rhytides, mid-forehead lifting can also be considered, since prominent forehead rhytides can help to camouflage the appearance of the resulting depressed scar [11].

Forehead length and hairline configuration are other important metrics to assess. Both coronal and endoscopic forehead lifting will raise the hairline and lengthen the vertical height of the upper face. This may be advantageous in patients with short foreheads and low hairlines but should be approached with caution in patients with long foreheads and high hairlines [10]. Pretrichial or trichophytic incisions can be used for patients who would benefit from maintaining or reducing the vertical dimension of the forehead. The surgeon should also review the implications of a proposed brow lift technique for range of hairstyles. For instance, a patient with bangs may be a good candidate for a pretrichial lift but should be counseled that pulling the hair back may reveal the pretrichial incision line.

Conclusion

There are many surgical and nonsurgical approaches to brow lifting and forehead rejuvenation that will be covered in the ensuing chapters. There is a wide variety of brow configurations that can look natural and aesthetically pleasing on the appropriate patient. The various options and their advantages and disadvantages should be discussed with patients and tailored to their individual anatomy and personal preferences. Brow lifting can dramatically improve a patient's appearance, and proper discussion and planning will help achieve a satisfactory result for both patient and surgeon.

References

1. Sullivan PK, Salomon JA, Woo AS, Freeman MB. The importance of the retaining ligamentous attachments of the forehead for selective eyebrow reshaping and forehead rejuvenation. Plast Reconstr Surg. 2006;117:95–104.
2. Knize DM. A study of the supraorbital nerve. Plast Reconstr Surg. 1995;96:564–9.
3. Jeong SM, Park KJ, Kang SH, et al. Anatomical consideration of the anterior and lateral cutaneous nerves in the scalp. J Korean Med Sci. 2010;25(4):517–22.
4. Briceño CA, Zhang-Nunes SX, Massry GG. Minimally invasive surgical adjuncts to upper blepharoplasty. Facial Plast Surg Clin North Am. 2015;23(2):137–51.
5. Drolet BC, Phillips BZ, Hoy EA, Chang J, Sullivan PK. Finesse in forehead and brow rejuvenation: modern concepts, including endoscopic methods. Plast Reconstr Surg. 2014;134(6):1141–50.
6. Kiang L, Deptula P, Mazhar M, Murariu D, Parsa FD. Muscle-sparing blepharoplasty: a prospective left-right comparative study. Arch Plast Surg. 2014;41(5):576–83.
7. Ahn MS, Catten M, Maas CS. Temporal brow lift using botulinum toxin A. Plast Reconstr Surg. 2000;105(3):1129–35; discussion 1136–9.
8. Carruthers A, Carruthers J. Eyebrow height after botulinum toxin type A to the glabella. Dermatol Surg. 2007;33(Suppl 1):26–31.
9. Macdonald KI, Mendez AI, Hart RD, Taylor SM. Eyelid and brow asymmetry in patients evaluated for upper lid blepharoplasty. J Otolaryngol Head Neck Surg. 2014;43(1):36.
10. Angelos PC, Stallworth CL, Wang TD. Forehead lifting: state of the art. Facial Plast Surg. 2011;27(1):50–7.
11. Huijing MA, van der Lei B. Gull wing midforehead lift: when a poor man's forehead lift becomes the treatment of choice for brow ptosis. Ann Plast Surg. 2010;64(6):713–7.

Cutaneous Approaches to Brow Lifting

19

Bradford W. Lee, Ashley M. Crane, Kimberly D. Tran, and Don O. Kikkawa

Introduction

The brows play an important role in facial aesthetics by manifesting facial expressions and by framing the eyes and the eyelids. Brow ptosis is defined as brows that rest below the supraorbital ridge and can compromise vision via obstruction of the superior visual fields. Brow ptosis also confers an aged facial appearance by causing eyelid pseudo-ptosis and accentuating the appearance of dermatochalasis. Most brow ptosis is involutional in origin, arising from gravitational descent, chronic repetitive brow depression, and age-related changes in collagen and elastin. Less commonly, brow ptosis can be caused by facial nerve palsy or cicatricial changes beneath the brow(Fig. 19.1) [1].

Cutaneous approaches to brow lifting utilize the excision of redundant cutaneous tissues to powerfully and durably lift the brows. The oculofacial surgeon strives to conceal incisions along the junctions of the cosmetic units of the face at the superior border of the brow, the hairline, within a deep forehead rhytid, or within hair-bearing scalp [2]. This chapter will discuss the various cutaneous methods of brow lifting, including the direct supraciliary, mid-forehead, pretrichial/trichophytic, coronal, and temporal approaches. Choosing the ideal procedure requires evaluating the height and contour of the brows, brow cilia thickness and density, the forehead, hairline, overall facial proportions, and patient aesthetic preferences (see chapter entitled "Introduction to Brow Lifting") (Fig. 19.2).

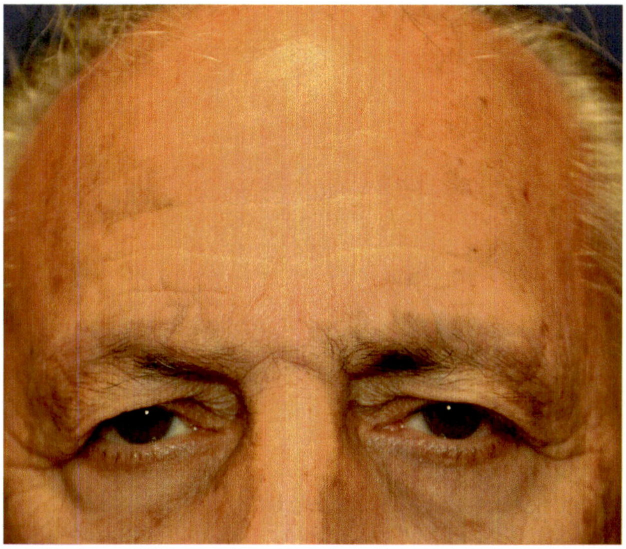

Fig. 19.1 This patient with involutional brow ptosis has brows that rest below the supraorbital ridge, particularly laterally. The brow ptosis exacerbates the appearance of upper lid dermatochalasis and eyelid ptosis, and compensatory frontalis overaction has resulted in deeply etched forehead rhytides

None of the authors have any financial interest to disclose.

B. W. Lee (✉)
Division of Oculofacial Plastic and Reconstructive Surgery, Bascom Palmer Eye Institute, Department of Ophthalmology, University of Miami Miller School of Medicine, Miami, FL, USA

Division of Oculofacial Plastic and Reconstructive Surgery, UC San Diego Department of Ophthalmology, Shiley Eye Institute, La Jolla, CA, USA
e-mail: blee@miami.edu

A. M. Crane · K. D. Tran
Division of Oculofacial Plastic and Reconstructive Surgery, Bascom Palmer Eye Institute, Department of Ophthalmology, University of Miami Miller School of Medicine, Miami, FL, USA

D. O. Kikkawa
Division of Oculofacial Plastic and Reconstructive Surgery, UC San Diego Department of Ophthalmology, Shiley Eye Institute, La Jolla, CA, USA

Division of Plastic Surgery, UC San Diego Department of Plastic Surgery, La Jolla, CA, USA

A. J. Cohen, C. N. Burkat (eds.), *Oculofacial, Orbital, and Lacrimal Surgery*, https://doi.org/10.1007/978-3-030-14092-2_19

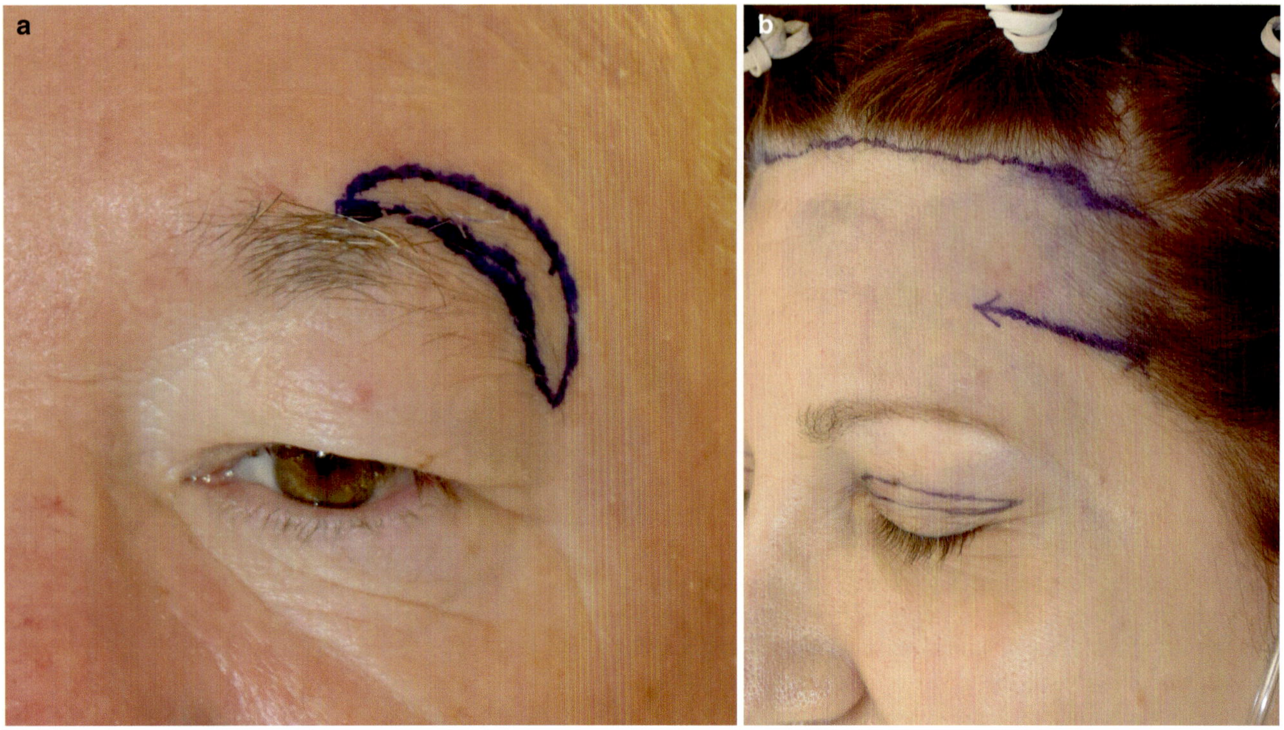

Fig. 19.2 (**a**) Markings for a temporal direct supraciliary brow lift (**a**) and a pretrichial/trichophytic brow lift (**b**) place the incision at the junction of the cosmetic units of the face. In Fig. 19.2a, the cutaneous excision is limited to the lateral 2/3 of the brow. In Fig. 19.2b, the incision is marked just behind the hairline in an irregularly irregular fashion that follows the natural hairline. A transverse arrow is marked approximately 2 cm above the brow, indicating the territory of the temporal branch of the facial nerve

Direct Supraciliary Brow Lift

The direct brow lift involves excising an ellipse of the skin and subcutaneous tissue just above the highest brow cilia. While the tissue removed can be extended across the entire length of the brow, many surgeons (including the authors of this chapter) prefer to keep the incision hidden in the lateral aspect of the brow to avoid more prominent scarring in the medial region. The skin of the medial brow and glabellar region is thicker and has more sebaceous glands than that of the lateral brow, resulting in a more prominent scar. Moreover, incisions located in the glabellar region are within the aesthetic center of the face, which attracts more attention due to focus on the periocular region.

The direct brow lift is probably the most straightforward and effective technique for alleviating temporal hooding and peripheral visual field obstruction due to lateral brow ptosis. It is well suited to male patients with thick, bushy eyebrows that help to camouflage the incisions. Advantages of this procedure include its simplicity and ability to excise tissue directly above the brow for a controlled and durable lift. The main disadvantages are risk for visible scarring at the surgical site and a potentially unnatural brow contour [3].

Technique: An ellipse of the skin just above the superior brow cilia is marked to approximate the desired height and contour of the brow after surgery. The ellipse is drawn such that the greatest vertical height of the ellipse corresponds to the area of greatest brow ptosis (usually laterally). When marking the ellipse, patients should be sitting in an upright position with their eyes closed to facilitate complete frontalis relaxation. At multiple points along the brow, the brow is manually lifted to the desired height at or above the superior orbital rim. A surgical marking pen is then positioned overlying the superior brow cilia, and the brow is allowed to descend to its resting position inferiorly. The marking pen is touched to the skin after allowing the brow to descend. Connecting these marks in a curvilinear fashion demarcates the superior border of the ellipse to be excised, whereas the inferior border of the ellipse conforms to the superior brow cilia.

Local anesthetic (e.g., 2% lidocaine with 1:100,000 epinephrine) is infiltrated into the surgical site. The marked ellipse is incised with a #15 Bard Parker blade taking care to bevel the incision superiorly and parallel to the brow cilia follicles. After the incision is completed, a subcutaneous dissection plane is created, and the excised tissue is removed with Westcott scissors or monopolar cautery, taking care to avoid excessive cautery near the superior brow cilia. Care should be taken in the region of the supraorbital nerve to avoid inadvertent injury. Once hemostasis has been achieved, the subcutaneous tissues are closed with buried, interrupted 5-0 Vicryl (polyglactin) or Monocryl sutures, and the skin is closed in a running or running horizontal mattress fashion using a 5-0 Prolene (polypropylene) suture. The running

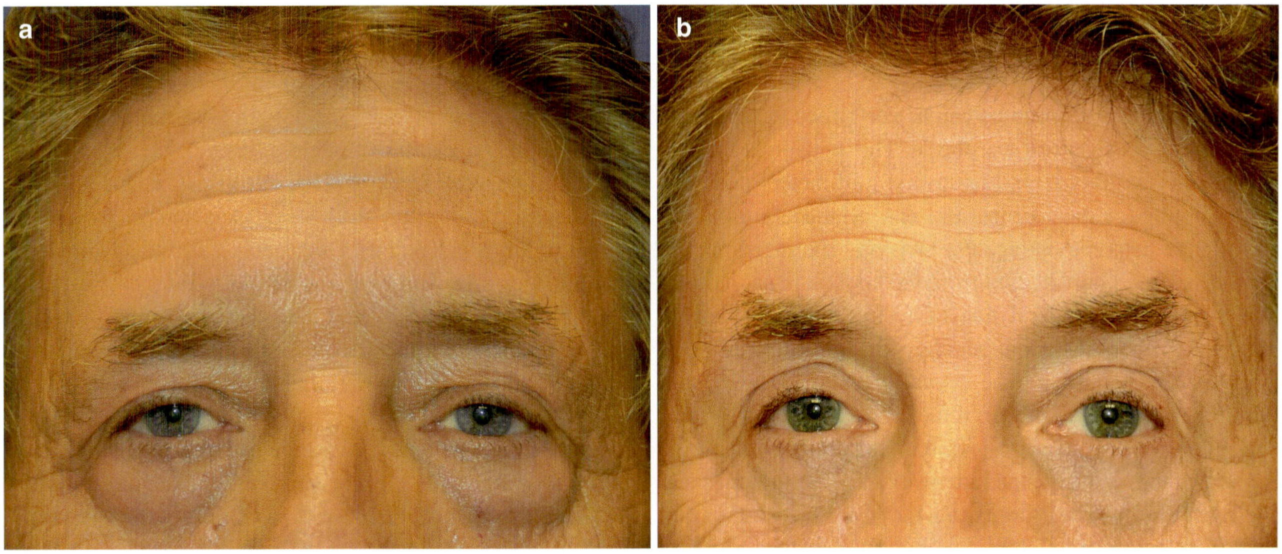

Fig. 19.3 Before (**a**) and after (**b**) a direct supraciliary temporal brow lift, along with upper and lower lid blepharoplasty. Notice the improvement in lateral brow ptosis and maintenance of a horizontal masculine brow contour postoperatively. The incisions are visible but are camouflaged reasonably well by the horizontal forehead rhytides

horizontal mattress stitch everts the edges of the incision to help mitigate formation of a depressed scar. Sutures are removed at the end of the first postoperative week (Fig. 19.3).

Mid-forehead Brow Lift

Mid-forehead brow lifting involves excising the skin and subcutaneous tissues through an incision made within mid-forehead rhytides to conceal the incision. This technique is useful for patients with deeply etched forehead rhytides and patients with male-pattern baldness who are not ideal candidates for brow lifting methods that utilize hair-bearing scalp or the hairline. Typically, the ideal candidates are men with deep forehead rhytides or patients with paralytic brow ptosis with asymmetrically smooth foreheads on the paralytic side [2]. In the latter situation, an incision or incisions can be created to resemble the contralateral forehead rhytides.

As with direct brow lifting, the closer proximity of the tissue excised with respect to the brows provides a more effective vertical lift, and the mid-forehead brow lift can further address medial brow ptosis and tissue laxity across the entire horizontal extent of the forehead. However, in the authors' experience, the mid-forehead incision is commonly noticeable and can be difficult to conceal, as the incision is not at the junction of the cosmetic facial units. There can also be associated forehead hypesthesia if the cutaneous dissection is carried too deeply. For these reasons, the mid-forehead lift may not be an ideal choice for the majority of patients.

Technique: The incision line or lines are chosen based on the location of deep forehead rhytides. One continuous incision can be made following a long transverse rhytid. If two separate incisions are made, one on each side, they can be centered on rhytides at different heights on the forehead, which can help camouflage the incisions. An ellipse of the skin to be excised is marked centered on the chosen rhytid or rhytides. Local anesthetic with epinephrine is infiltrated subcutaneously, and a #15 Bard Parker blade is used to create the incisions through the skin and subcutaneous tissue. The ellipse of skin is excised using Westcott scissors or cutting monopolar cautery. Some surgeons will dissect more inferiorly to visualize and myotomize the brow depressors (i.e., the corrugators and procerus). With deeper dissection, care should be taken to avoid injury to the supraorbital nerve. Hemostasis is achieved with electrocautery. The deep tissues of the forehead are closed with buried 5-0 Vicryl or Monocryl (poliglecaprone) sutures, and the skin is closed in a running horizontal mattress fashion with 5-0 Prolene suture. Sutures are removed at the end of the first postoperative week.

Pretrichial or Trichophytic Brow Lift

The pretrichial or trichophytic brow lift has the ability to elevate the entire brow complex, reduce forehead cutaneous laxity, and effectively efface forehead rhytides. It is also the only brow lifting procedure that lowers the hairline, compared to the coronal and endoscopic approaches that elevate the hairline. Most men and women do not desire an elevated hairline that gives the appearance of a long forehead. The procedure requires a long incision at the hairline and is ideal for patients with high hairlines and long foreheads and those who wear their hair in a way that would conceal the incision. Disadvantages of this procedure are the potential for a visible scar, potential limitation of hairstyles that reveal the hairline incision, forehead hypesthesia, and the development of a more visible scar in the setting of progressive hairline recession [4, 5].

Technique: This procedure can be performed under monitored sedation or general anesthesia. The incision is marked just anterior to (pretrichial) or several millimeters posterior to (trichophytic) the hairline and can be made irregularly irregular to help camouflage the incision. The incision runs approximately 3 cm laterally from the midline in each direction toward the temporal line of fusion and can then be extended further laterally either along the hairline or running into hair-bearing scalp. The lateral extent of the incision should correspond to the tail of the brow. The hair and forehead is prepped, and local anesthetic containing epinephrine is injected along the planned incision line. Dilute tumescent anesthesia is infiltrated throughout the planned region of dissection in the forehead. Some surgeons will further administer supraorbital and supratrochlear nerve blocks to augment regional anesthesia.

A #15 Bard Parker blade is used to incise the skin along the previous markings, and in the case of a trichophytic incision, the incision should be acutely beveled such that the deep follicles of the anterior most hair shafts can later grow up through or even anterior to the incision. A subcutaneous dissection plane is created taking care not to injure the frontalis muscle and the sensory nerves of the forehead. This also allows effective undermining of the skin and effacement of forehead rhytides. Gentle bipolar cautery is used for hemostasis, particularly near the incision where excessive cautery may damage the hair follicles. Dissection is carried down inferiorly, and the skin should be intermittently redraped to assess the amount of brow elevation and effacement of rhytides possible based on the extent of dissection.

Some surgeons may dissect in a deeper subgaleal plane between the periosteum and galeal fascia and then transition to a subperiosteal plane in the central forehead region to transect the corrugator and procerus. However, this increases the risk of forehead hypesthesia, can result in unnatural splaying of the distance between the medial brows, and is not something that the authors of this chapter routinely perform.

Once the desired brow elevation can be achieved based on elevation of the skin flap, the appropriate amount of the skin can be excised from the skin flap in a beveled fashion and typically measures about 1.5–2.0 cm in vertical height. The incision is closed with deep 5-0 Monocryl sutures to reduce tension on the skin incision. A running horizontal mattress 6-0 Prolene suture is used to close the skin at the hairline, and if the incision is carried posteriorly on the sides into hair-bearing scalp, the scalp can be closed with staples. Topical antibiotic ointment can then be applied. No drain is needed, and staples and sutures can be removed between 7 and 10 days postoperatively or left several days longer in patients with diabetes, a recent smoking history, use of immunosuppressive medications, advanced age, or other risk factors for delayed wound healing (Fig. 19.4).

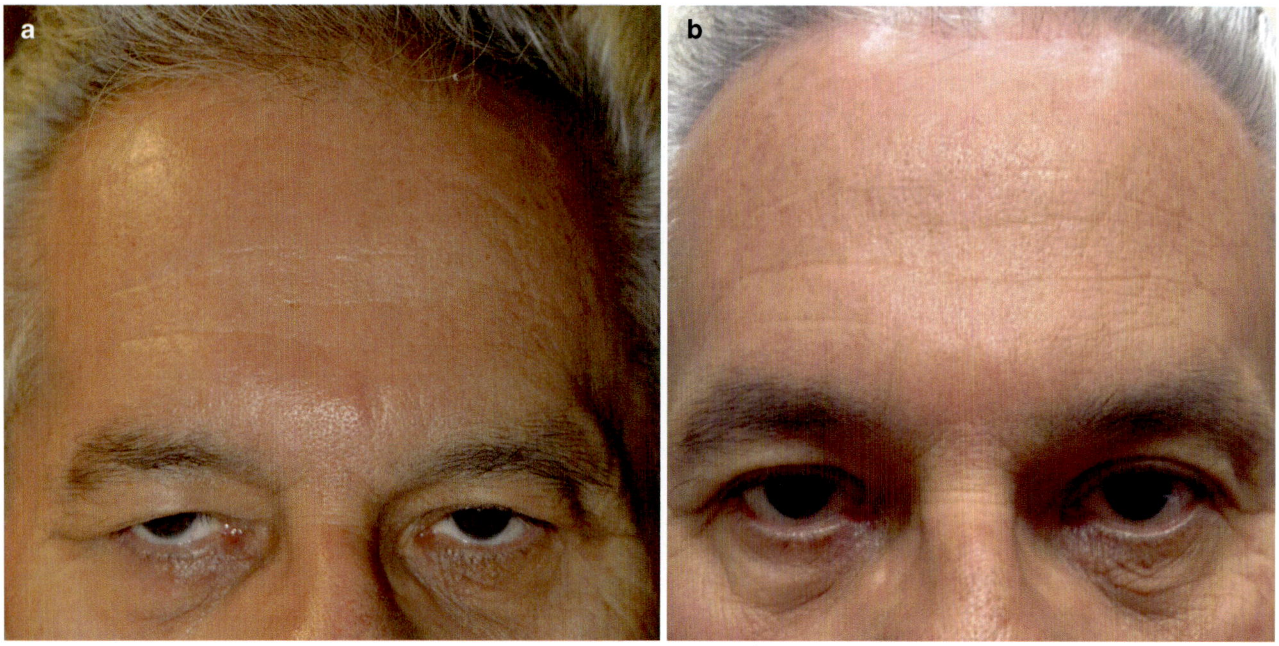

Fig. 19.4 Below are photos before (**a**) and after (**b**) a pretrichial brow lift with bilateral upper lid blepharoplasty. Notice the improvement of brow ptosis across the entire extent of the brow with improvement in forehead rhytides. This surgery was performed in a subcutaneous dissection plane with no division of the corrugators or procerus muscle. Postoperatively, there was no forehead numbness

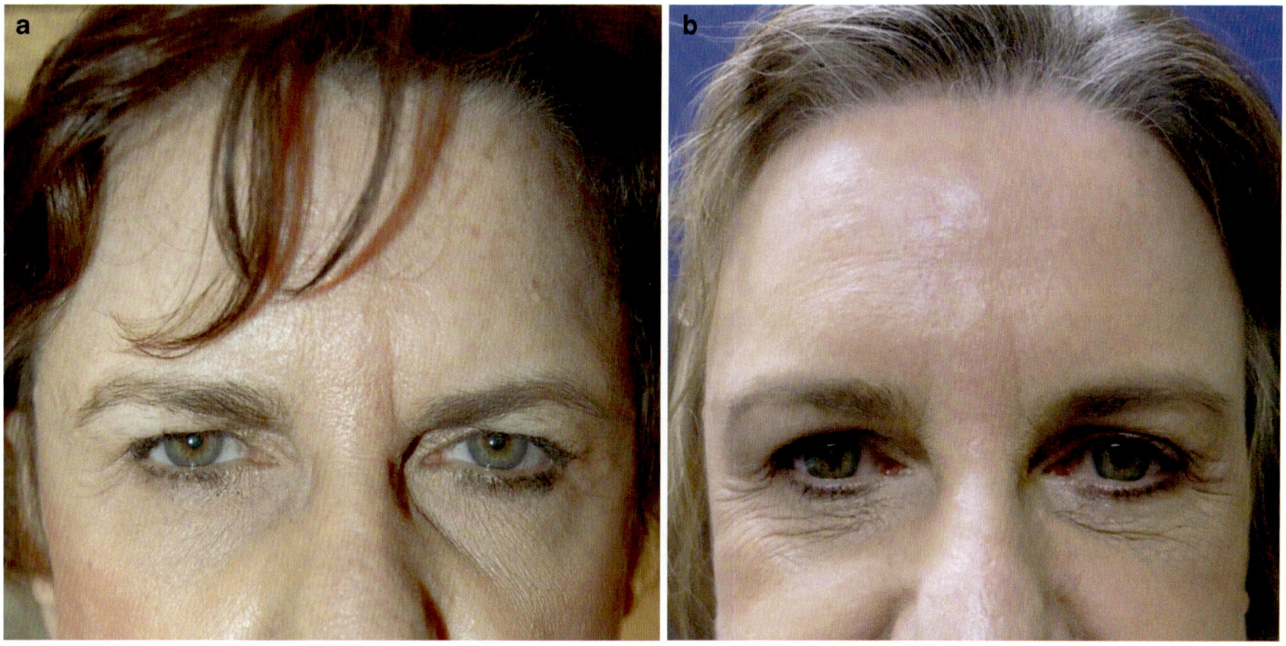

Fig. 19.5 Before (**a**) and after (**b**) a coronal brow lift. Notice the improvement of brow ptosis across the entire extent of the brow with mild elevation of the hairline

Coronal Brow Lift

The coronal brow lift elevates tissues from the eyebrows to the hairline via an incision within the hair-bearing scalp that leaves no facial scar. It is ideally suited for patients with significant brow ptosis, forehead rhytides, thick hair density, and a normal to low hairline. This procedure requires an ear-to-ear incision placed posterior to the hairline with excision of scalp tissue anterior to the incision. Potential disadvantages include raising the hairline, significant loss of hair-bearing scalp, alopecia, a visible scar in patients with thinning hair, and hypesthesia or paresthesia in the supraorbital nerve distribution [1].

Technique: This procedure is typically performed under monitored anesthesia care or general anesthesia. The incision is marked along a meridian running from ear to ear and located approximately 4–6 cm behind the hairline. The incision is marked in a straight or curvilinear pattern. The hair is prepped, and local anesthetic containing epinephrine is injected along the planned incision line. Dilute tumescent anesthesia can be infiltrated throughout the planned region of dissection running down to the superior orbital rim.

The incisions are made with a #15 Bard Parker blade down to the subgaleal plane centrally and the deep temporalis fascia laterally. Raney clips can be placed on the incision edges to assist with hemostasis. Dissection is carried down inferiorly and can transition to a subperiosteal plane in the central forehead approximately 2 cm above the superior orbital rim to help avoid injury to the supraorbital and supratrochlear nerves. The arcus marginalis is released at the superior orbital rim, and once again, there is the option of dividing the corrugators and procerus muscles to weaken the brow depressors. Once the forehead is completely mobilized, the anterior scalp flap is redraped superiorly and redundant tissue is excised, taking care to avoid excessive tension on the incision that can cause alopecia. The galea is closed with 4-0 Vicryl sutures, and the scalp incision can be closed with staples. A drain can optionally be placed and left within the incision for the first 24 hours. Antibiotic ointment is placed on the incision, and a Kerlix wrap is applied. The wrap is removed on POD 1, and staples are removed at POD 7–10. Scalp hypesthesia may be present initially but typically improves gradually over the first several months (Fig. 19.5).

Temporal Brow Lift

There are numerous ways to perform a temporal brow lift, and the direct supraciliary brow lift, trichophytic brow lift, and coronal brow lift all have temporal variants. The benefits of performing temporal brow lifts, in comparison to their full counterparts, are that the incisions are shorter, lateralized, and away from the sensory innervation of the forehead. The incisions are more concealed from the aesthetic center of the face, but the temporal variant cannot address medial brow ptosis or central forehead rhytides.

The authors' preferred temporal brow lift is performed posterior to the hairline in the temporal region with the scalp incision oriented parallel to the tail of the brow with the midpoint of the incision located along the pretragal line [6]. Dissection is performed in the plane running above the deep temporalis fascia, which avoids the temporal branch of the facial nerve contained within the superficial temporalis fascia. The deep temporalis fascial plane is transitioned to a subperiosteal plane at the superotemporal orbital rim to allow complete release of the arcus marginalis. The temporal flap is then elevated, and an ellipse of redundant tissue can be excised. The flap is then supraplaced and anchored to the deep temporalis fascia using 3-0 Maxon (polyglyconate) suture. The scalp incision is closed with staples that can be removed in 7–10 days postoperatively.

Conclusion

Among the various cutaneous techniques for brow lifting, each procedure has different relative indications and contraindications and must be individualized to effectively improve aesthetics and visually limit brow ptosis. Each of these brow lifting techniques relies on excision of redundant tissue, but each has a different risk profile, level of invasiveness, and capacity for upper facial rejuvenation. A comprehensive evaluation and discussion of the pros and cons of each method will help the patient and physician choose the appropriate procedure for the patient.

References

1. Arneja JS, Larson DL, Gosain AK. Aesthetic and reconstructive brow lift: current techniques, indications, and applications. Ophthal Plast Reconstr Surg. 2005;21:405–11.
2. Kersten RC, Kulwin DR. Direct, midforehead, and pretrichial browplasty. In: Tse DT, editor. Color atlas of oculoplastic surgery. 2nd ed. Philadelphia: Lippincott Williams & Wilkins; 2011. p. 136–48.
3. Tyers AG. Brow lift via the direct and trans-blepharoplasty approaches. Orbit. 2006;25(4):261–5.
4. Bidros RS, Salazar-Reyes H, Friedman JD. Subcutaneous temporal browlift under local anesthesia: a useful technique for periorbital rejuvenation. Aesthet Surg J. 2010;30(6):783–8.
5. Niamtu J 3rd. The subcutaneous brow- and forehead-lift: a face-lift for the forehead and brow. Dermatol Surg. 2008;34(10):1350–61; discussion 1362.
6. Kikkawa DO, Miller SR, Batra MK, Lee AC. Small incision nonendoscopic browlift. Ophthal Plast Reconstr Surg. 2000;16:28–33.

Endoscopic Forehead Lifting with Fat Grafting

20

Francesco P. Bernardini, Alessandro Gennai, and Brent Skippen

Introduction: The Role of the Eye

Scientific studies have proven the central role of the eyes in aesthetic facial rejuvenation. Nguyen HT et al. used an eye-tracking system to demonstrate that age and fatigue judgments are related to preferential attention toward the eye region. Consequently, aesthetic surgery to the eye region may be one of the most effective interventions in enhancing the overall appearance of an individual [1]. A recent prospective study on 72 female patients with an average age of 48, which represents the bulk of the aesthetic population worldwide, showed that 74.6% of these patients felt that their first sign of aging occurred in the eyes, 26.7% in the neck, and only 12.6% in the cheeks [2]. Among this female group, 78.8% of patients expressed interest in improving the appearance of their eyes, 28.8% the cheeks, and lips only 15% [2]. Facial beauty is linked to the eyelid fissure, and studies have demonstrated that attractive Caucasian faces have a relatively narrower eye fissure width compared to the average Caucasian face [3]. It is not just the medical literature but also fashion magazines across the world which strongly reinforce this issue, showing on their covers beautiful models who have especially attractive eyes. This is not just a new trend of the western world as beauty has been represented similarly by classic painters throughout history. It is also of extreme relevance in all parts of the world independent of race.

It is worthwhile to acknowledge art before science especially as painters have been among the first to recognize and represent graphically the signs of periocular age beautifully. In "Old Man with a Gold Chain," it is remarkable that a man wearing a hat and sporting a beard which hides much of his face, Rembrandt (art museum, Chicago), was able to represent old age by specifically focusing on features of the periocular region. Here the aging changes of the lower and upper eyelids are beautifully represented. In the upper subunit of the periocular region, forehead and eyebrow descent is prominent, especially laterally, causing deepening of the upper sulcus and dermatochalasis with lateral hooding. In the lower complex, volume defects such as infraorbital and orbitomalar grooves, V-shaped deformity and orbital fat prolapse are prominent, as well as signs of lower eyelid laxity, such as inferior scleral show, horizontal shortening of the eyelid fissure, rounding of the lateral corner. Additionally, signs of eyelid skin laxity, including both skin excess or just laxity, and static and/or dynamic skin rhytides are prominent. Finally, the cheek appears flattened due to loss of malar support.

On the other hand, the master's school was able to represent magisterially the periocular signs of youth and beauty that we as surgeons should strive to emulate as the final result of our surgery: a smooth eyelid/cheek transition, a short lower eyelid, long horizontal fissure ending with an acute lateral angle, with an almond-shaped eyelid fissure and tight skin. The cheek appears full and the zygomatic arch is well represented with a strong malar projection. In the upper complex, the forehead shows no wrinkles, the eyebrows are high, arched with a higher tail, and thick, with a well-represented retro-orbicularis oculi fat (ROOF) giving the eyebrow anterior projection; the upper sulcus is full and the tarsal platform show (TPS) well represented but relatively low. We need science to give us a better understanding of the transformation that occurs to our face; as we age volume plays a major role in this respect.

In a previous publication, we retrospectively reviewed our patient population who underwent endoscopic face lifting and fat grafting at the same time and discovered that it was composed similarly to that of Sobanko et al. [4]. Among the 400 patients of the study, 85% were female and 77% were aged between 40 and 55 [4]. The aging process that occurs in this age group affects the center of the face, represented by the periocular region and the mouth. In the same paper, we defined the concept of the periocular aesthetic unit, the

F. P. Bernardini · A. Gennai · B. Skippen (✉)
Oculoplastica Bernardini, Genova, Italy
e-mail: info@brentskippen.com.au

A. J. Cohen, C. N. Burkat (eds.), *Oculofacial, Orbital, and Lacrimal Surgery*, https://doi.org/10.1007/978-3-030-14092-2_20

impact of volume loss, and the tissue descent in the aging process and proposed a treatment algorithm [4]. It is clear that as surgeons dedicated to the periocular region we should consider more than just the eyelids. If it is true that the eyelids are the closest to the eye, we have come to learn that what happens to the eyelids during the aging process is affected by what happens to the tissues around them. Schematically, one can define the periocular aesthetic unit as being formed by the superior complex (SC), which includes the forehead, eyebrow, and upper eyelid; by the inferior complex (IC), formed by the lower eyelid and cheek; and finally, by the lateral complex (LC), formed by the temple, malar mound, and lateral canthus. If we expand our view to the perioral unit we are now looking at the whole center of the face, which deserves our focus as surgeons.

We have tried to diagrammatically represent the impact of changes that occur in the center of the face as depicted graphically in Fig. 20.1. Descent has a greater impact on the superior complex as the tissues that form it are affected by gravity and the continuous effects of strong protractor muscles, notably the corrugator, depressor supercilii, procerus, and orbicularis oculi which act synergistically. Volume loss plays a relevant role especially at the level of the eyebrow fat, where there is thinning of the eyebrow, deepening of the upper sulcus and loss of eyelid support with dermatochalasis. At the level of the lateral complex lies the temporalis fossa, stuck between the temporal crest superiorly and the zygomatic arch inferiorly, which has no room to descend and

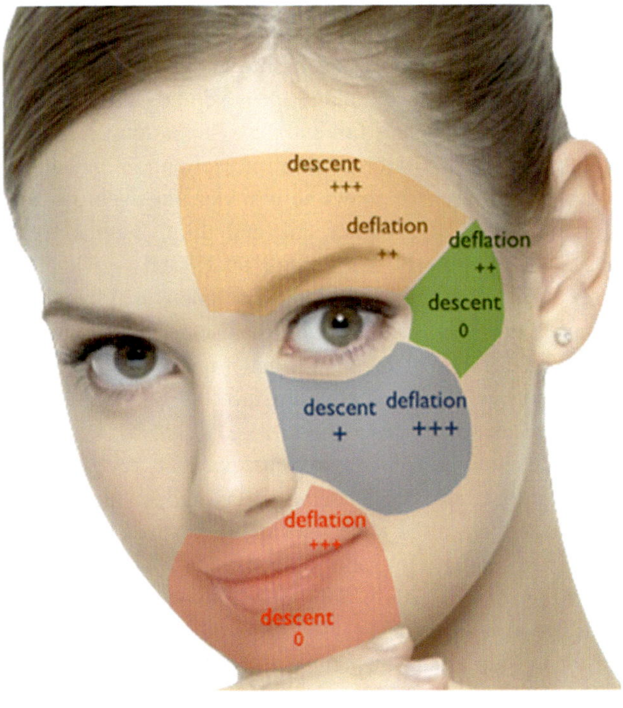

Fig. 20.1 Impact of age-related changes occurring in the center of the face

its aging is determined exclusively by volume loss. Volume loss also plays a major role at the level of the inferior complex along with some effects of gravity on the cheek. Finally, no descent occurs at the level of the perioral unit; instead, volume loss alone causes the age-related changes. Based on this review of the aging changes to our areas of concern, it is intuitive that in order to achieve the most natural rejuvenation one should aim to restore the position of the descended tissues, mainly the superior complex and partly the inferior complex, and restore the volume loss in those areas at the same time.

In the past, aesthetic surgeons have dedicated their best efforts to rejuvenation of the contours of the face, the periphery as opposed to the center, offering variably satisfying results at the price of long scars, extensive dissection, and strong horizontal traction with unnatural effects. When evaluating patients for aesthetic rejuvenation, attention is immediately drawn to the periocular aesthetic unit, based on the patient's requests and desires; however, evaluation of all areas starting from the forehead to neck is important in order to make the best attempt to blend all key aesthetic facial units in the final outcome. Compared to the past, skin and fat are removed much less from the eyelids, as surgeons have realized that removing tissue can accentuate aging. Vertically repositioning the descended tissues seems to be the most anatomically correct way of facial rejuvenation as it corrects the natural, vertical vector of aging. This is especially true for the superior complex and partially for the inferior complex. However, for as much as tissues can be lifted up, there is still a lack of the natural, three-dimensional volume restoration that can be offered by autologous fat grafting. Fat grafting, such as with the superficial enhanced fluid fat injection (SEFFI) technique, also aids in skin regeneration.

Skin atrophy and volume loss have been recognized as two of the major factors involved in facial aging, contributing to formation of facial rhytids, skeletonization, and pseudo-descent of the midface. Early signs of facial aging involving the periocular and perioral areas include thinning of the eyebrows, deepening of the superior sulcus, infraorbital hollows, atrophy of the midface, nasolabial folds, marionette lines, and lip atrophy. In the past, surgeons have focused on the anatomical structures of the periocular region individually, correcting eyebrow ptosis, upper dermatochalasis, lower lid bags or tear trough deformities, and malar descent/atrophy individually or in variable combinations. Knowledge of the factors that occur during the aging process of the face have significantly evolved over the years and there is now an opportunity to systematically address this area of interest, the periocular region, as a single aesthetic unit. With respect to aesthetic units, two previous studies attempted to systematically address the aesthetic units of the face. Ramirez proposed an endoscopic approach for the aesthetic rejuvenation of the central oval of the face. He reported excellent results in over 500 cases with a low complication rate [5]. Citarella et al. also described a systematic approach to the entire face with a 91% satisfaction rate, combining endoscopic lifting with middle third and cervical transposition of the superficial muscular aponeurotic system (SMAS) to address the aging face [6]. These reports suggest that a systematic approach to the aesthetic unit offers a higher satisfaction rate.

Surgical Steps of Endoscopic Dissection: Anatomical Basis

Key Steps

1. Blind dissection
2. Temporal dissection with clear visualization of all anatomical landmarks
3. Malar and zygomatic dissection
4. Frontal dissection for full periosteal release
5. Tension free dissection
6. Fixation
    1. Paramedian
    2. Deep temporal
    3. Malar
    4. Bicoronal

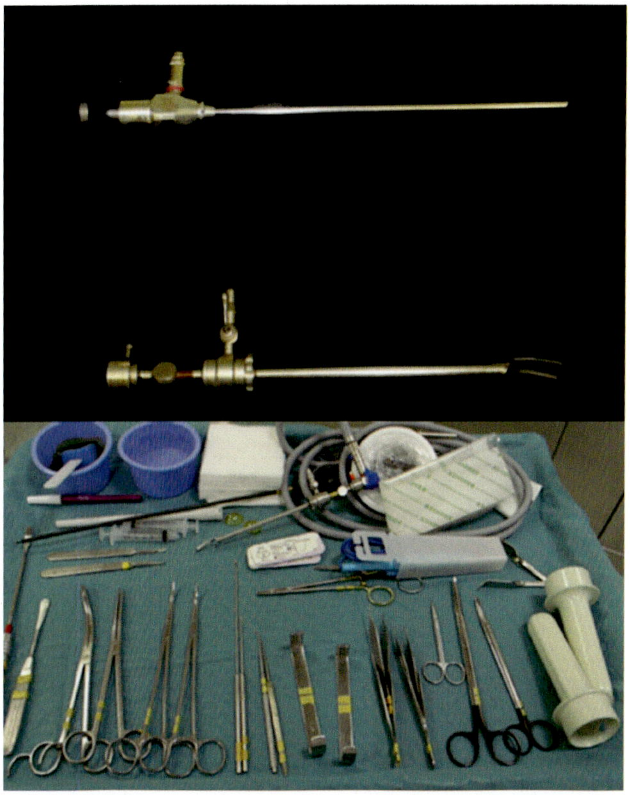

Fig. 20.2 Surgical instruments required for endoscopic dissection

Surgical Instrumentation

There are multiple dedicated surgical instruments (Fig. 20.2), but the single most important is the endoscopic elevator that slides on the fiber optic, which allows the surgeon to elevate the tissues while viewing with one hand.

Areas of Blind Dissection

With the patient under intravenous sedation and given a Klein type of local anesthesia, the initial dissection is performed to prepare for the endoscopic view (Fig. 20.3); it is necessary to form the physical space in order to have an optimal view with the endoscope, and this preparatory part can be performed blindly and quickly. In the frontal part, blind dissection is performed under the periosteum, trying to maintain an intact periosteum. This maneuver will create an optical pocket up to the "safety area," located 2 cm above the superior orbital rim. Special care needs to be taken not to elevate the conjoint tendon (frontotemporal fusion line) from frontal to temporal as this maneuver may break the temporalis muscle. The lateral extension will be up to the temporal crest laterally and 2–3 cm posterior to the hairline. In the temporalis area an optical pocket is created blindly and the dissection plane lies above the superficial plane of the deep temporal fascia. From the temporal dissection the conjoint tendon (temporal fusion line) can be safely elevated and the frontal and lateral pockets can be joined. In the temporomalar area, the dissection can be performed only with an endoscope to allow for optimal visualization.

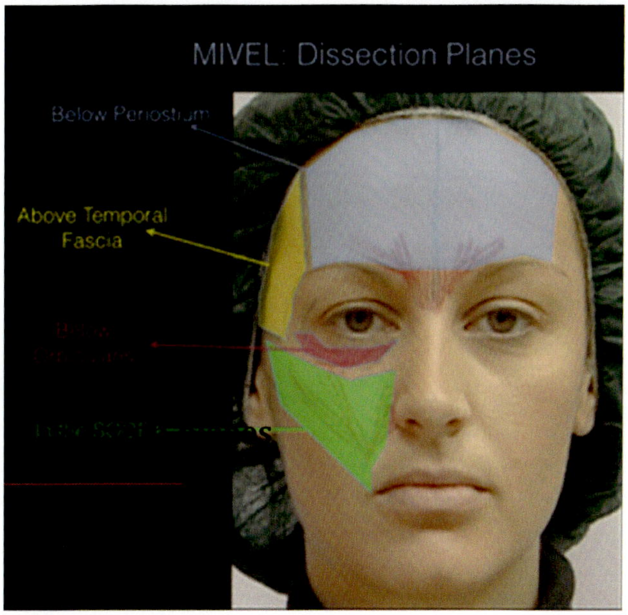

Fig. 20.3 MIVEL dissection planes for endoscopic visualization

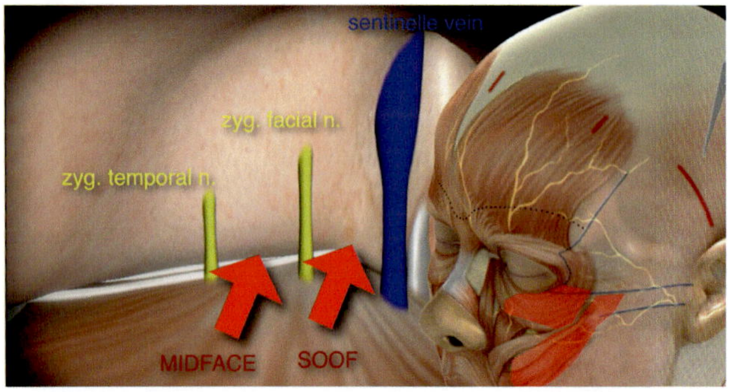

Fig. 20.4 Diagram showing the anatomical landmarks utilized under endoscopic visualization to safely dissect the SOOF and midface

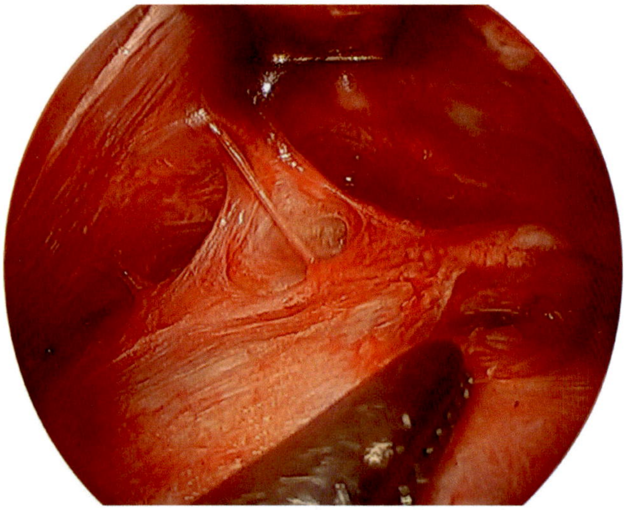

Fig. 20.5 Optical pocket to localize key anatomical landmarks corresponding to the ones depicted in Fig. 20.4

Endoscopic Dissection: General Points

After blind dissection is completed and a single optical pocket formed in the frontal and temporal area (Fig. 20.5), it is then time to enter with the endoscope. The first area to enter with the fiber optic of the endoscope is the temporal area; it is imperative that every single strand of the superficial temporal fascia is elevated so that further dissection can be extended above the deep temporal fascia; the facial nerve will remain above the instruments the entire time if the right plane is maintained; additionally, the more "tissue" which can be elevated, the more protected the frontal branch of the facial nerve will be.

Aiming toward these anatomical landmarks:

1. Sentinel vein
2. Zygomaticofacial nerve
3. Zygomaticotemporal nerve

Temporal Endoscopic Dissection

While bluntly dissecting the temporal area in the plane of the temporalis fascia and aiming toward the lateral eyelid corner, the sentinel vein can be easily seen and isolated. This is the first landmark and ideally it is initially preserved. Lateral to the sentinel vein, further blunt dissection reveals a neurovascular bundle, the zygomaticofacial nerve and vein. Lateral to this bundle lies the zygomaticotemporal vein and nerve. The three of them act like electrical posts above which runs the frontal branch of the facial nerve. Once the landmarks are clearly visible, one can elect where to dissect; laterally to the sentinel vein, between it and the zygomaticofacial bundle, the sub-orbicularis oculi fat (SOOF) will be entered next, while between the zygomaticofacial and zygomaticotemporal bundle, the path to the midface will be found. Medial to the sentinel vein lies the lateral retinaculum and the lateral canthal tendon. In order to consider the dissection complete it is necessary to free the tissue across the entire length of the zygomatic arch, elevate the SOOF, and release the lateral retinaculum.

Frontal Endoscopic Dissection

In the frontal part, the plane will be subperiosteal all the time. Always try to preserve the integrity of the periosteum until the orbital rim. Once the orbital rim is reached, coming from laterally to medially and bluntly elevating the periosteum, the supraorbital neurovacular bundle will be encountered. All the strands of periosteum need to be elevated at each side of the nerve and also behind it. This is because the periosteum is very strong and even small residual bands will prevent easy forehead flap upward mobilization. Beyond the supraorbital nerve, dissection will be aimed toward the glabella, elevating and dissecting the corrugator and procerus muscles; in between the muscle fibers of the corrugator muscles lies the supratrochlear nerve (Fig. 20.6).

Background

In the past, too much emphasis was given to the strength of the fixation, with the idea that strong fixation was necessary to pull the tissues up against gravity. Thus, the use of bone tunnels, Endotines, and stronger screws were popularized. On the other hand, use of these fixation devices was associated with limited dissection especially of the temporal area, the lateral retinaculum, and the medial frontal periosteum. The most important factor is to achieve a complete tension-free flap that includes the forehead, temporal area, lateral retinaculum, SOOF, and zygomatic arch. Once everything from the scalp to the mouth is free, fixation can be achieved with simple, safe, and affordable sutures. The role of fixation is to help maintain the dissected tissues in the right position until they adhere into their new position by fibrosis. The time necessary to allow scar fixation is most likely less than the time of suture reabsorption. Fixation with permanent devices is unnecessary, nor is excision of scalp tissue which can cause alopecia and visible scars, and does not add any particular value to the deep fixation.

The authors used fixation with Endotine forehead implants in more than 300 patients before switching to suture fixation, which has been now used in more than 200 patients [4]. The amount of elevation and the stability of fixation have been comparable in the short and long term. Suture fixation also reduces the risk of complications. In the Endotine group, displacement of the device from the site of implantation was observed in 11 cases, causing a visible asymmetrical result in three patients, while 8 patients experienced exposure or infection of the device. In three cases the Endotine was removed – one upon getting exposed and infected and two for prolonged (>12 months) visibility/palpability of the implant. The Endotine implant was visible in front of the hairline in 15 patients, while it was palpable by the majority of the patients even after 9 months. The implant broke at the time of placement in six patients, while five cases of bleeding related to the bone trephination were encountered. In the suture fixation group by contrast, none of the patients experienced complications or referred any complaint other than a noticeable bulging of the skin folds of the forehead in the first 2 weeks, of which they were informed in advance.

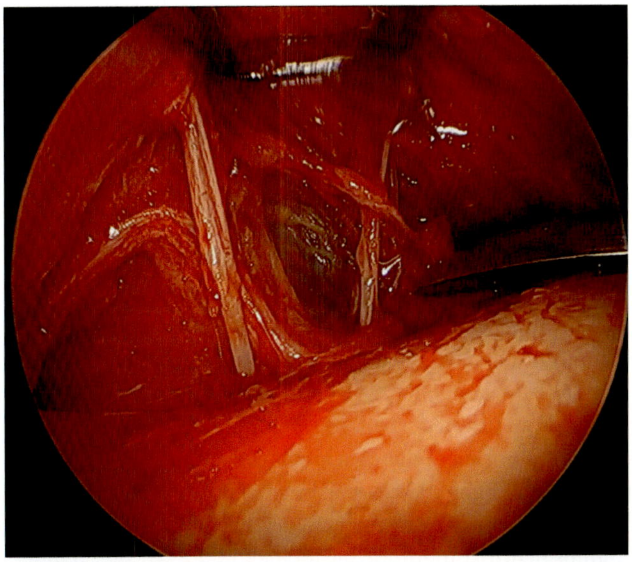

Fig. 20.6 Complete periosteal dissection until the supraorbital and supratrochlear nerves

Paramedian Fixation

The *Gennai stitch* is utilized for paramedian fixation, which determines the highest point of the eyebrow (see Fig. 20.7).

1. Two small horizontal stab wound incisions are made in the forehead at the same level, one on each side, below the paramedian incisions and the Reverdin needle is passed from the forehead incision under the scalp to exit at the paramedian incision.
2. The needle is loaded with the suture and brought back at the forehead incision.
3. The tip of the Reverdin needle is then used to grasp the tissue below the skin at the forehead incision and to pass the suture needle below the scalp and out at the paramedian incision again, where the suture needle is freed from the Reverdin needle.
4. The suture needle grasps the tissues deep to the skin at the posterior edge of the paramedian incision.
5. All the deep tissues between the two incisions are brought together by tightening the suture, thus creating a temporary fold of redundant skin between the forehead and scalp incisions.

Role of Paramedian Fixation

Once a tension-free flap has been achieved, the tissue must be held in the new position. The shape of the eyebrow can also be altered based on the fixation position. In order to achieve a natural appearance of the superior complex (forehead/eyebrow/upper lid), the different shapes of the natural feminine eyebrow should be considered and carefully inspect the patient's old pictures. The aim is to raise the tail of the

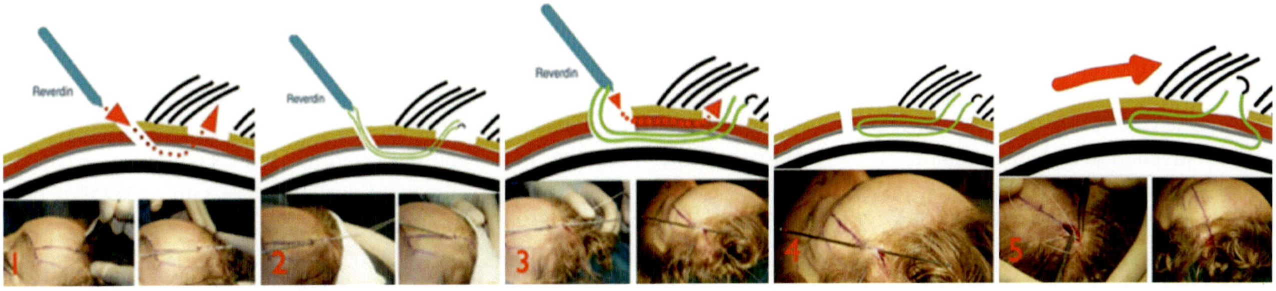

Fig. 20.7 Paramedian fixation with the Gennai stitch

eyebrow while at the same time raising the body of the eyebrow until the final shape is a naturally arched eyebrow ending with an elevated tail. The more lateral in respect to the midline of the forehead that the paramedian fixation is placed, the greater the effect on the tail. The closer the fixation is placed to the midline, the stronger the effect on the body or the head of the eyebrow. On average the paramedian fixation is placed 5 cm from the midline in a female patient and 4 cm in a male. Also, the lower the entry point on the forehead the stronger the pull of the fixation and the larger the skin fold resulting on the forehead. Therefore, a heavier forehead, such as a male forehead, would require a stronger pull, resulting in a more visible skin fold.

Deep Temporal Fixation

Temporal fixation of the deep subcutaneous tissues of the elevated flap to the deep temporal fascia is performed with a 3-0 polyglactin (Vicryl) suture. This fixation elevates at once the tail of the eyebrow, the temporozygomatic area, and along to the corner of the eyelids, thereby elongating the eyelid fissure.

Bicoronal Fixation

This fixation is used to enhance the effect of elevation of the tail of the eyebrow and is used in about 50% of patients. It is performed with a 2-0 polyglactin (Vicryl) suture.

Superficial Enhanced Fluid Fat Injection (SEFFI)

Skin atrophy and volume loss have been recognized as two of the major factors involved in facial aging, contributing to the formation of facial rhytids, skeletonization, and pseudodescent of the midface. Early signs of facial aging involving the periocular and perioral areas include thinning of the eyebrows, deepening of the superior sulcus, infraorbital hollows, atrophy of the midface, nasolabial folds, marionette lines, and lip atrophy. Some volume defects, such as tear trough deformities and a deep upper eyelid sulcus, can be iatrogenic following an overly aggressive excisional blepharoplasty or may have a constitutional basis and be evident since adolescence or early adulthood.

Volume restoration of the face is regarded as a key step in facial rejuvenation and may be addressed with autologous fat transfer. Traditionally, autologous fat grafting is based on Coleman's harvesting technique with a 2 mm side-port cannula, followed by fat injection in the deep pre-periosteal plane with a blunt cannula [7, 8]. Because of the limitations of this technique, which include unpredictable fat survival and the potential for visible lumpiness, various authors have recently focused their attention on micro-fat grafting.

Reported advantages of micro-fat grafting include the possibility of treating the periocular area with a superficial implant using syringe needles and the presence of a higher content of stem cells compared to the traditional Coleman technique [9–11]. The micro-fat preparations proposed so far are based on various fat processing methods that take place upon completion of the traditional harvesting technique, and use either collagenase digestion or manual emulsification. Strict legal limitations regulate the use of collagenase in humans, while manual centrifugation affects adipocyte viability.

The author's technique, called superficial enhanced fluid fat injection (SEFFI), consists of directly harvesting "micro"-fat using "micro" side-port cannulas, without the need for further fat processing [4, 9, 10]. The resulting fat, rich in stem cells and viable adipocytes, is subsequently enhanced and rendered fluid by adding autologous platelet-rich plasma (PRP) and injected superficially with syringe needles. Based on clinical observations in a large series of patients, SEFFI has proven to be a safe and effective method for replacing volume loss and correcting skin atrophy of the entire face, including the periocular and perioral regions. Recently more importance has been given to contour improvements and tissue regeneration in addition to volume restoration. In facial rejuvenation, correcting volume loss is not limited to volume restoration, but also includes contour reshaping and skin regeneration, specifically in the periocular area. This is the reason for considering various "types" of fat which can offer more options based on the rejuvenation goals. SEFFI simultaneously provides volume restoration, contour enhancement, and skin regeneration [9, 10]. If a larger volume of fat needs to be restored, then the larger 0.8 mm SEFFI will be harvested. For more delicate areas, either the finer 0.5 mm or 0.3 mm SEFFI are more appropriate [9, 10].

A major advance in the micro-fat evolution has been the finding that disruption of fat lobules improved the viability of the adipocytes [12], in contrast to Coleman's hypothesis that preserving the lobular structure of the fat was essential for its survival [13]. Moscatello and co-workers proved that the greater surface area of the disrupted fat lobules on the recipient bed significantly improved fat survival after injection [14], confirming Nguyen's similar findings in mice [15]. A higher stromal vascular fraction (SVF) has been demonstrated in other micro-fat grafting techniques that involve fat disruption as part of the procedure [16, 17]. The SVF contains adipocyte-derived stem cells (ADSC), pre-adipocytes, hematopoietic, endothelial, and smooth muscle cells [18, 19]. These factors may be involved in prolonging fat graft survival and providing skin regeneration. PRP enhancement is useful as it may have a positive role in skin regeneration, increasing fat grafting survival and improving wound cosmesis [20–23]. It also provides the necessary fluidity to the SEFFI, allowing an easy exit from small needles under minimal digital pressure.

The growing literature is focused on the role of "micro-fat" and "nano-fat." The micro-fat options proposed so far are based on traditional fat harvesting using large side-port cannulas, followed by various modalities of fat processing to disrupt the large fat lobules harvested. For example, Tonnard proposed manual fat emulsification to achieve a nano-fat solution rich in SVF and consequently ADSCs, but void of viable adipocytes [16]. Consequently, the indications of nano-fat are reportedly limited to skin regeneration and do not include volume restoration. Youn et al. reported on intradermal eyelid injection of collagenase digested fat to correct periocular dark circles [24]. The use of collagenase is time consuming and has strict legal restrictions in humans, since the enzymatic digestion potentially affects the normal collagen in the injection sites. On the other hand, Trivisonno et al. have shown that harvesting fat with a microcannula carried a twofold increase in ADSC content compared to traditional harvesting cannulae [11]. The authors believe that it is the diameter of the side ports rather than that of the cannula which determines the size of the harvested fat lobules. The authors have previously reported their preliminary experience with fat harvested with a 1 mm side-port cannula and implanted superficially with a needle, with excellent results [4].

With respect to the recent micro-fat evolution, SEFFI is unique as it does not require further fat processing; the size of the fat lobules harvested are determined at the origin by the size of the side ports. This is important as the smaller the fat lobules are, the more superficially the micro-fat can be implanted with a reduced risk of visible irregularities in the more delicate facial areas. Since the adipocytes are much smaller compared to the size of the side ports, their integrity is preserved as histological examination has confirmed, thus they can effectively provide volume correction.

SEFFI: Histological Evidence

The fat harvested from a healthy patient with cannulae of three different size ports (0.5 mm, 0.8 mm, and 2 mm) was examined histologically after centrifugation and mock injection. Hematoxylin and eosin stains (H&E) demonstrated mature viable adipocytes, with intact cell walls and visible nuclei equally represented in the three different specimens. A well-represented stromal component was noted between adipocytes, without signs of cell necrosis (Fig. 20.8). The adipocyte size ranged from 0.03 mm to 0.13 mm and was independent of the size of the harvesting cannula used.

Fat Preparation

Instruments

The following instruments are required: the harvesting cannulae are the most important part of the set, with aspirating holes with diameters of 0.8 mm, 0.5 mm, and 0.3 mm. Manual aspiration of fat is performed with a 10 cc syringe mounted alternatively with different multi-perforated side-port cannulae. The cannulae were 20 cm long, with a 2 mm diameter and side ports of either 0.3 mm, 0.5 mm, or 0.8 mm (see Fig. 20.9). Preferred harvesting sites for structural fat are the fat-rich areas such as the suprapubic region, the hips, trochanteric, and the medial part of the knee. Fat centrifugation for 1 minute at 2000 rpm, with an estimated gravitational force of 448 g, is an optional step in the process. The PRP is obtained by withdrawing blood from the patient's vein into four 4.5 mL citrate-containing Vacutainer tubes and centrifuging at 1000 rpm for 2 minutes. The concentrated PRP is taken with a sterile syringe and mixed with the fat to obtain a final concentration of 20% of the total fat harvested. The end result of this process is an enhanced, fluid fat that can be injected with a small syringe needle under minimal digital pressure (Fig. 20.9). The choice of needle size is based on the smallest size that allows easy exit flow under minimal pressure in order to facilitate uniform distribution of the fat, even though 0.3 SEFFI is small enough to exit through 25 gauge needles.

Fat Injection

The finer 0.3 mm and 0.5 mm SEFFI are injected using multiple 1 cc syringes mounted with 25 gauge or 23 gauge needles at the level of the orbicularis oculi muscle of the upper eyelid sulcus, eyebrow, lower eyelid, tear trough, infraorbital hollows, and subdermally in the perioral area. The 0.8 mm SEFFI is injected using 3 cc syringes mounted with 21 gauge needles in the subdermal layer of the temporal fossa, eyebrow, malar mound, zygomatic arch, and mandible line. In the lips, the 0.8 mm SEFFI is injected in the orbicularis oculi muscle.

Surgical Results (Figs. 20.10, 20.11, 20.12, 20.13, and 20.14)

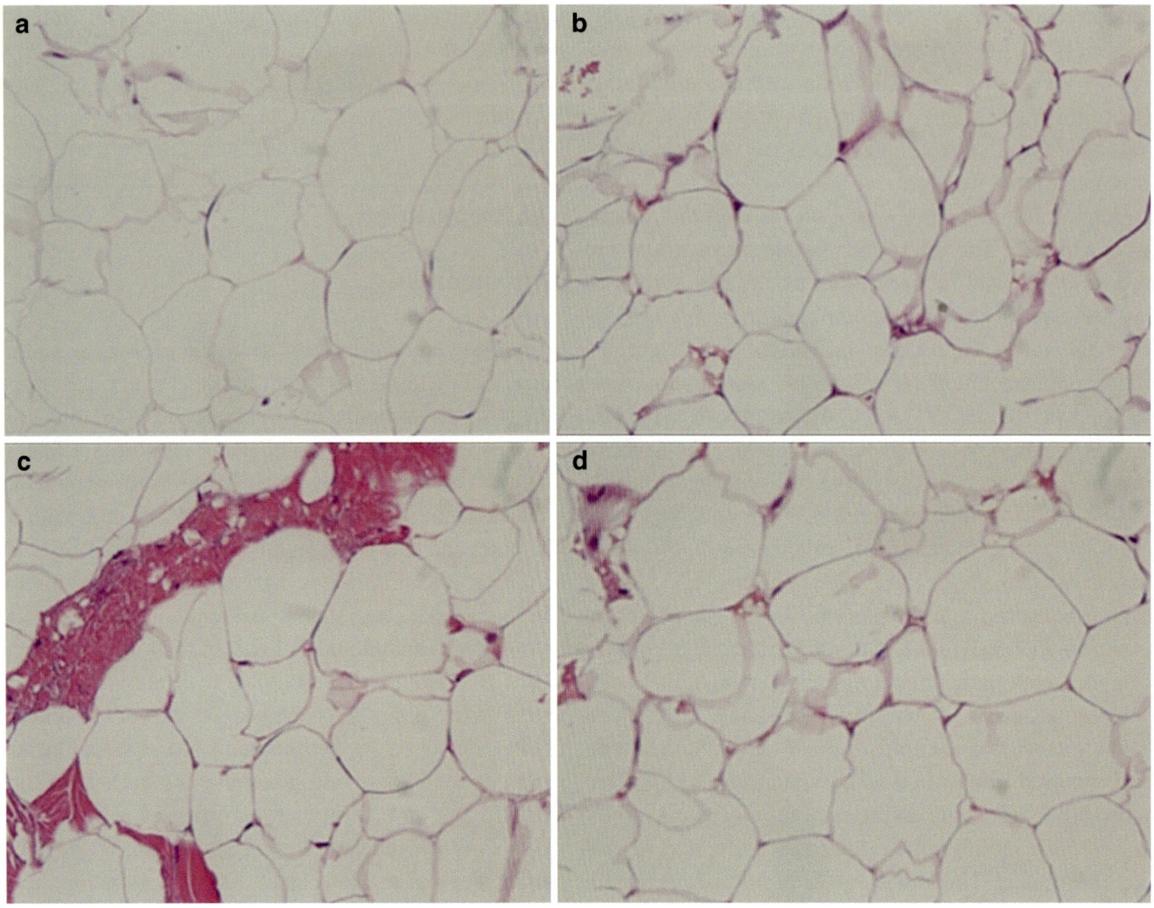

Fig. 20.8 Histological view of fat harvested using SEFFI cannulae

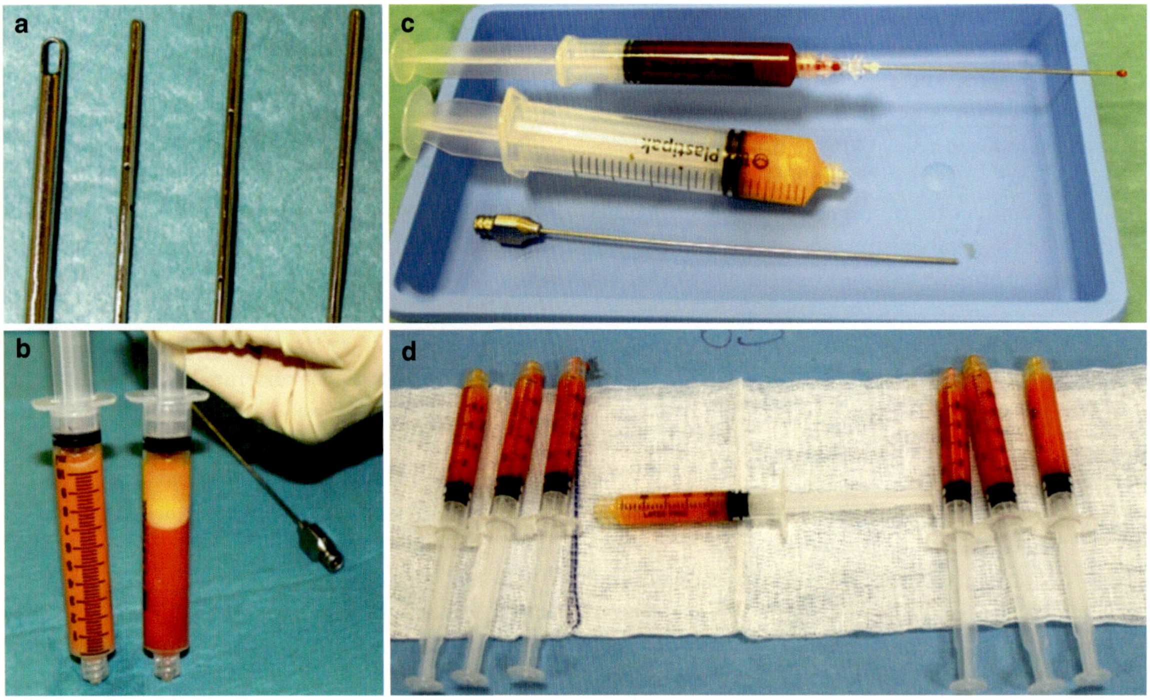

Fig. 20.9 Preparation of SEFFI

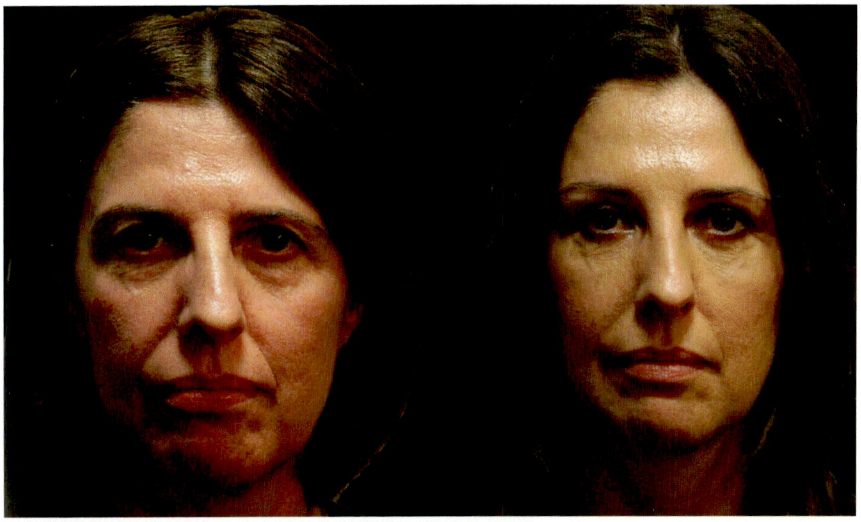

Fig. 20.10 46-year-old female: results of MIVEL + SEFFI

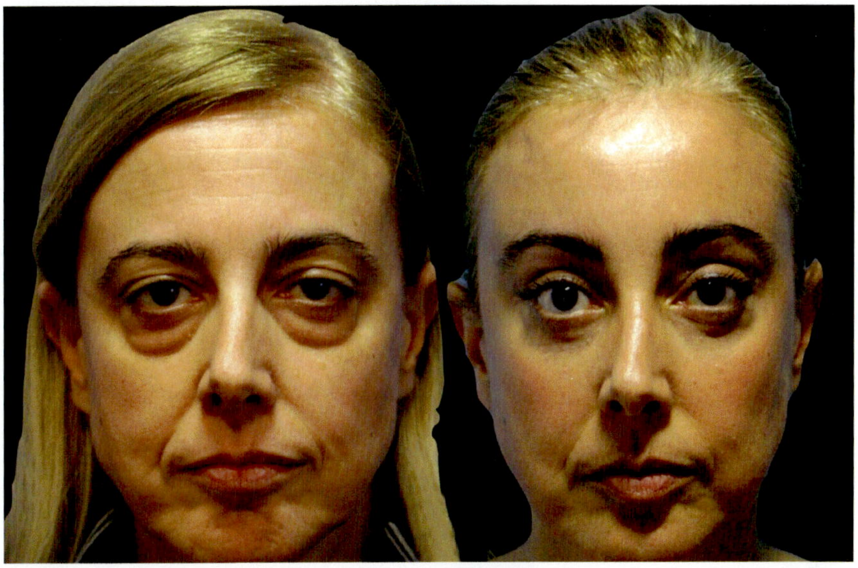

Fig. 20.11 48-year-old female: results of MIVEL + SEFFI

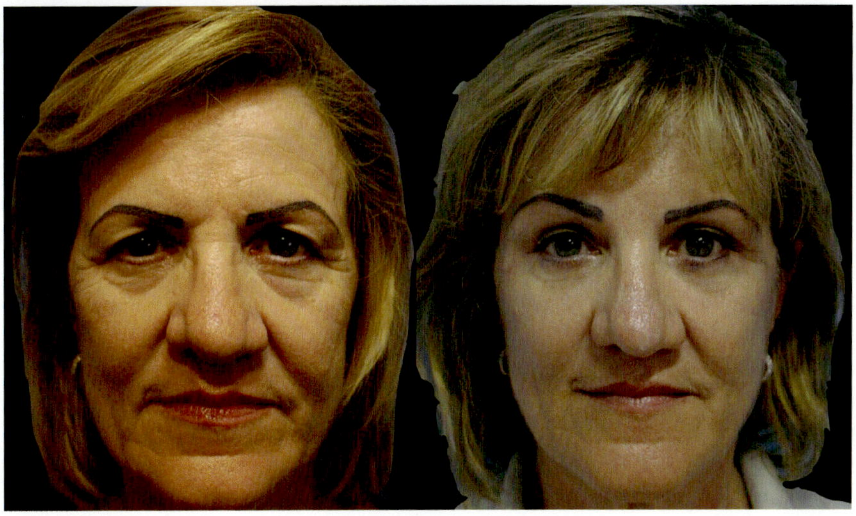

Fig. 20.12 56-year-old female: results of MIVEL + SEFFI

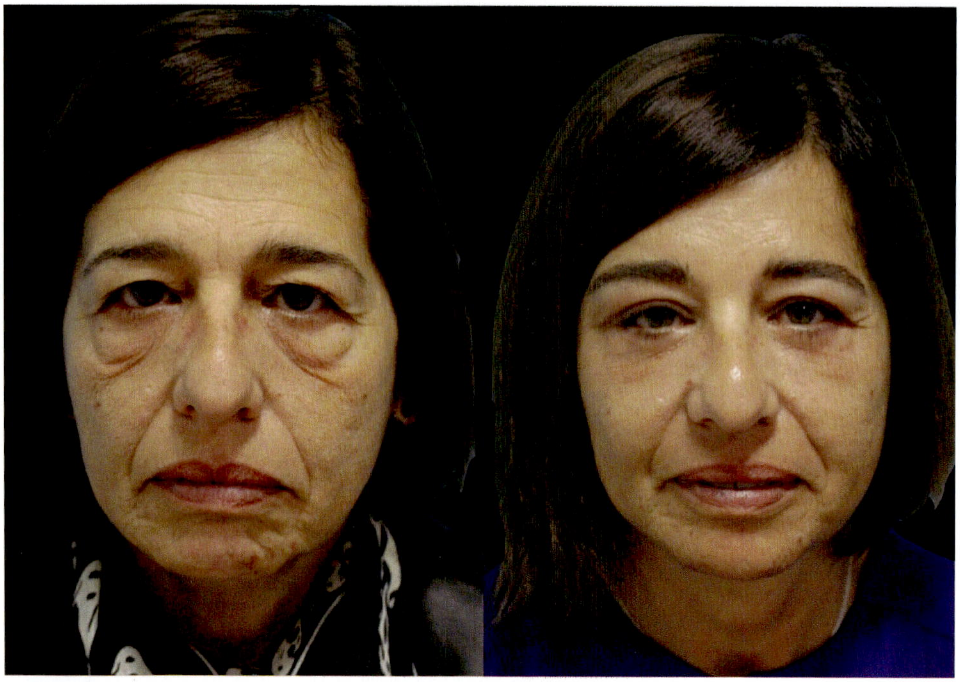

Fig. 20.13 59-year-old female: results of MIVEL + SEFFI

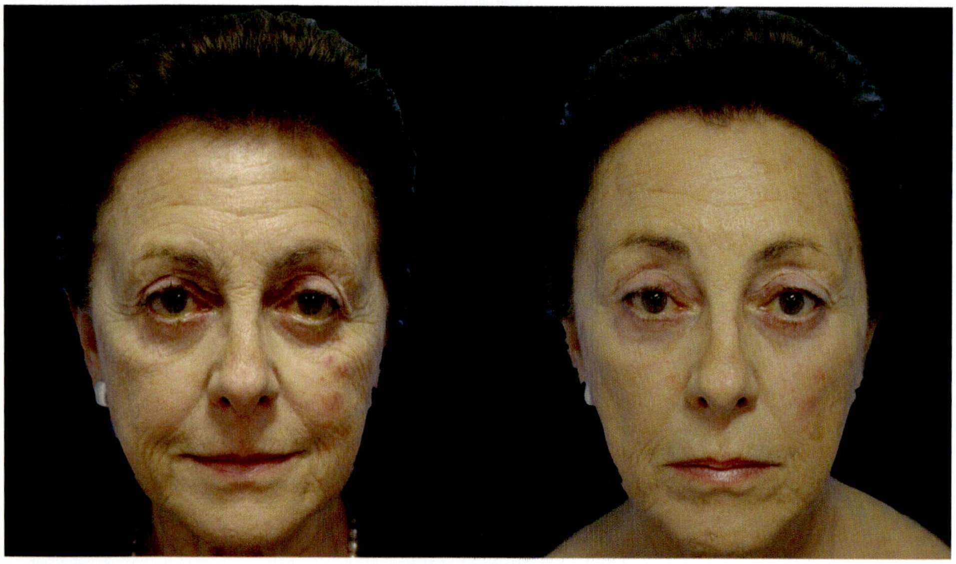

Fig. 20.14 67-year-old female: results of MIVEL + SEFFI

Conclusions

A systematic approach to aesthetic units carries a high satisfaction rate. With the goal of rejuvenating the periocular region, the authors advocate approaching this area as a unit rather than with individual isolated techniques that can achieve only limited improvements. MIVEL (minimal incisions vertical endoscopic lifting) is a scarless technique that respects the vertical vector of tissue descent. As much as tissues can be lifted, a three-dimensional rejuvenation of the periocular aesthetic unit can only be achieved if associated with volume restoration. Conservative removal of skin and/or fat in the eyelids is part of this general wider approach and can be effectively utilized when indicated.

References

1. Nguyen HT, Isaacowitz DM, Rubin PA. Age- and fatigue-related markers of human faces: an eye-tracking study. Ophthalmology. 2009;116(2):355–60.
2. Sobanko JF, Taglienti AJ, Wilson AJ, Sarwer DB, Margolis DJ, Dai J, Percec I. Motivations for seeking minimally invasive cos-

metic procedures in an academic outpatient setting. Aesthet Surg J. 2015;35(8):1014–20.
3. Rhee SC, et al. Biometric study of eyelid shape and dimensions of different races with references to beauty. Aesthetic Plast Surg. 2012;36:1236–45.
4. Bernardini FP, Gennai A, Izzo L, Devoto MH. Minimal incisions vertical endoscopic lifting and fat grafting as a systematic approach to the rejuvenation of the periocular esthetic unit. Ophthal Plast Reconstr Surg. 2013;29:308–15.
5. Ramirez OM. The central oval of the face: tridimensional endoscopic rejuvenation. Facial Plast Surg. 2000;16(3):283–98.
6. Citarella ER, Sterodimas A, Condé-Green A. Endoscopically assisted limited-incision rhytidectomy: a 10-year prospective study. J Plast Reconstr Aesthet Surg. 2010;63(11):1842–8.
7. Coleman SR. Facial recontouring with lipostructure. Clin Plast Surg. 1997;24:347–67.
8. Coleman SR, Grover R. The anatomy of the aging face: volume loss and changes in 3-dimensional topography. Aesthet Surg J. 2006;26(1S):S4–9.
9. Bernardini FP, Gennai A. Fluid fat injection for volume restoration and skin regeneration of the periocular aesthetic unit. JAMA Facial Plast Surg. 2016;18(1):68–70.
10. Bernardini FP, Gennai A, Izzo L, Zambelli A, Repaci E, Baldelli I, Fraternali-Orcioni G, Hartstein ME, Santi PL, Quarto R. Superficial enhanced fluid fat injection (SEFFI) to correct volume defects and skin aging of the face and periocular region. Aesthet Surg J. 2015;35(5):504–15.
11. Trivisonno A, Di Rocco G, Cannistra C, Finocchi V, Torres Farr S, Monti M, Toietta G. Harvest of superficial layers of fat with a microcannula and isolation of adipose tissue-derived stromal and vascular cells. Aesthet Surg J. 2014;34(4):601–13.
12. Derby BM, Dai H, Reichensperger J, Cox L, Harrison C, Cosenza N, Yang M, Bueno RA, Neumeister MW. Adipose-derived stem cell to epithelial stem cell transdifferentiation: a mechanism to potentially improve understanding of fat grafting's impact on skin rejuvenation. Aesthet Surg J. 2014;34(1):142–53.
13. Coleman SR. Structural fat grafting. 1st ed. St Louis: Quality Medical Publishing Inc; 2004. p. 30.
14. Moscatello DK, Schiavi J, Marquart JD, Lawrence N. Collagenase-assisted fat dissociation for autologous fat transfer. Dermatol Surg. 2008;34:1314–21.
15. Nguyen PS, Desouches C, Gay AM, et al. Development of micro-injection as an innovative autologous fat graft technique: the use of adipose tissue as dermal filler. J Plast Reconstr Aesthet Surg. 2012;65:1692–9.
16. Tonnard P, Verpaele A, Peeters G, Hamdi M, Cornelissen M, Declercq H. Nanofat grafting: basic research and clinical applications. Plast Reconstr Surg. 2013;132(4):1017–26.
17. Stuzin JM. Discussion: Nanofat grafting: basic research and clinical applications. Plast Reconstr Surg J. 2013;132:1027–8.
18. Dong Z, Peng Z, Chang Q. The survival condition and immunoregulatory function of adipose stromal vascular fraction (SVF) in the early stage of nonvascularized adipose transplantation. PLoS One. 2013;8(11):e80364.
19. Ong WK, Sugii S. Adipose-derived stem cells: fatty potentials for therapy. Int J Biochem Cell Biol. 2013;45:1083–6.
20. Fabi S, Sundaram H. The potential of topical and injectable growth factors and cytokines for skin rejuvenation. Facial Plast Surg. 2014;30:157–71.
21. Sommeling CE, Heyneman A, Hoeksema H, et al. The use of platelet-rich plasma in plastic surgery: a systematic review. J Plast Reconstr Aesthet Surg. 2013;66:301–11.
22. Azzena B, Mazzoleni F, Abatangelo G, et al. Autologous platelet-rich plasma as an adipocyte in vivo delivery system: case report. Aesthetic Plast Surg. 2008;32:155–8.
23. Blanton MW, Hadad I, Johnstone BH, et al. Adipose stromal cells and platelet-rich plasma therapies synergistically increase revascularization during wound healing. Plast Reconstr Surg J. 2014;123:56S–64S.
24. Youn S, Shin JI, Kim JD, et al. Correction of infraorbital dark circles using collagenase-digested fat cell grafts. Dermatol Surg. 2013;39:766–72.

Upper Blepharoplasty: Advanced Techniques with Fat Repositioning and Muscle Modification

21

John P. Fezza

Introduction

Upper eyelid blepharoplasty is one of the oldest and most effective cosmetic surgeries. Simply removing a fold of redundant skin can improve appearance and in some cases expand peripheral vision. Astute surgeons have evolved from purely skin excision to an appreciation of three-dimensional curves of the face and lids. Certain highlights and shadows of the face are markers of youth, while others connote aging. Facial contours known as an ogee describe a convexity of the cheek sloping gently to a concavity of the submalar area. The face in fact is a double ogee with the most superior convexity the brows and the inferior concavity the lateral canthus. Likewise, the upper aesthetically pleasing upper eyelid is also an ogee or sigmoid curve in three dimensions. The lateral lid brow complex displays a convexity which gently slopes to a concavity of the medial upper lid. Understanding the subtleness the aesthetic upper lid curves is essential in tailoring the optimum blepharoplasty result. This concept of three-dimensional thinking has lead surgeons to progress from simply skin excisers to true facial sculptures.

Concepts of Upper Eyelid Beauty

The eyes are the first place people look, and the eyelids can convey many perceptions of a person from a tired, worn look to a bright, youthful appearance. As far back as the ancient Egyptians reports of surgically removing skin have been recorded along with the application of eyeliner to enhance the periorbital area. As we age predictable changes occur that typify the aging upper lid. There is a consistent contour shift which includes medial fullness from excess fatty herniation through a weakened septum. This is accompanied by a deflated, sunken lateral upper lid, with lateral lid-sub brow fat atrophy. In addition the thin lid skin is thin and lax, contributing to a redundant, hooded lateral lid typical of aging (Fig. 21.1). In order to counteract the aging changes in the upper lid, medial fat must be reduced while adding volume back laterally. Traditional upper lid blepharoplasty may not achieve true rejuvenation as purely removing skin can create a skeletonized appearance (Fig. 21.2). In fact earlier techniques described debulking lateral lid or brow fat to create more tarsal show [1–3]. This can accentuate a hollowed and

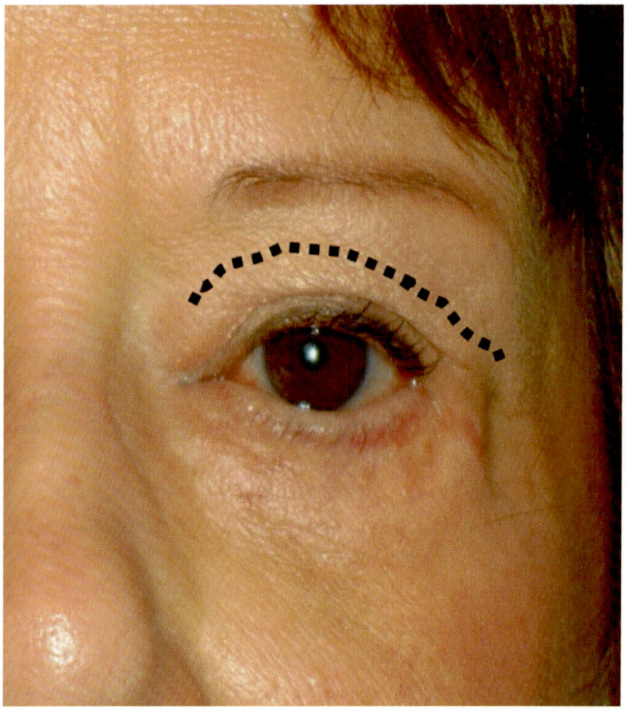

Fig. 21.1 The upper lid is characterized by predictable aging stigmata. This patient demonstrates the characteristic medial fat herniation, giving fullness to this area and a deflated lateral sub brow fat area with skin hooding. The soft tissues changes give a comma shape (black dotted line) seen in the aging upper lid in contrast to youthful sigmoid contours

J. P. Fezza (✉)
Center for Sight, Sarasota, FL, USA
e-mail: jfezza@centerforsight.net

A. J. Cohen, C. N. Burkat (eds.), *Oculofacial, Orbital, and Lacrimal Surgery*, https://doi.org/10.1007/978-3-030-14092-2_21

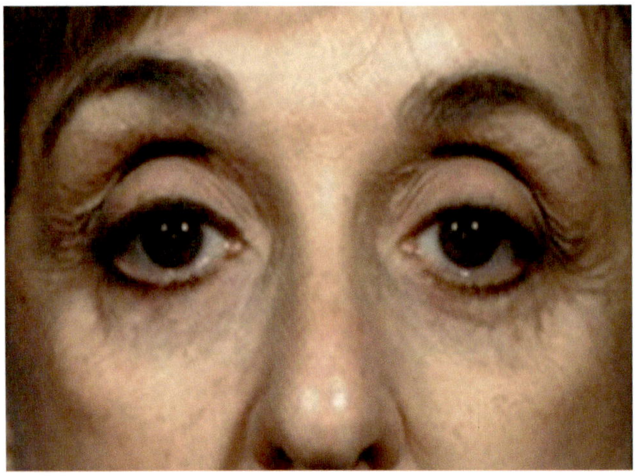

Fig. 21.2 This patient demonstrates the sequela of traditional blepharoplasty with a hollowed, sunken upper lid due to aggressive fat and tissue removal. The result is an aged and cadaveric appearance as opposed to a rejuvenated one

cadaveric, aged upper lid. The lids suffer from gravitational droop along with deflation and volume shifts. Modern facial and eyelid cosmetic surgery focuses on a three-dimensional appreciation of shape and has shifted away from tissue excision toward reinflation of tissues [4]. This more conservative approach allows for less soft tissue removal and is in accordance with fat preservation as is done in other areas of the face [5]. Volume should be maintained in the upper lateral lid to restore youthfulness [6].

The goal of an upper eyelid blepharoplasty is to restore aesthetically pleasing curves present in youth. An attractive upper lid is heralded by features of smooth skin, no redundant skin hooding, and no appreciable ptosis. The female lid should also have a fuller lateral sub brow area and a sculpted medial lid free of bulging fat herniation. Just as the face should exhibit an ogee curve of youth, so should the upper lid. This has not been assessed as critically in the upper lid. The ogee curve describes a convexity that gently transitions to a concavity. In the face an ogee refers to a rounder apple cheek that slopes to a concavity before reaching the jaw line. In the lid the ogee curve is also described as a sigmoid or "S"-shaped curve marked by a fuller, convex sub brow lateral upper lid that gently curves to a concave medial lid [7] (Fig. 21.3). Appreciation of the lid in three dimensions allows a perceptive surgeon to recreate a pleasing lid versus pure skin excision. An awareness of shadows and the integral play of light on eyelid contours give surgeons the ability to resculpt an old lid and transform it to a youthful one. Modern makeup artist recreates an attractive upper lid utilizing this concept of the sigmoid shape (Fig. 21.4). They use light colors over the lateral sub brow area to enhance this area to pop out while shadowing the medial lid to give the illusion of a curve and depth. In order to achieve this result, surgically all tissue layers must be addressed from the skin, muscle, and fat.

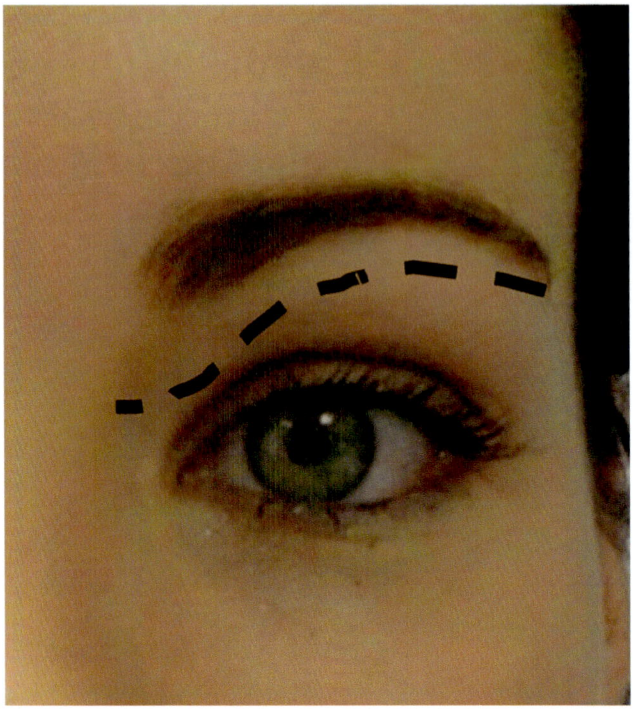

Fig. 21.3 A youthful upper lid topography has a sigmoid shape, which is a lateral convexity in the sub brow region that gently transitions to a medial concavity toward the nose. The sigmoid "S" shape is analogous to the ogee shape of a youthful face and is delineated by a black dotted line

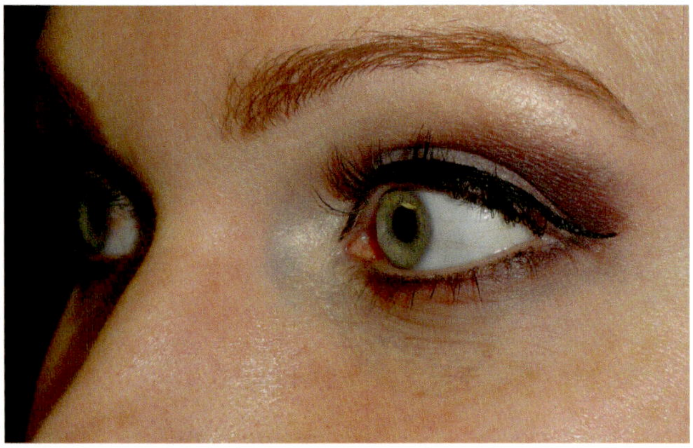

Fig. 21.4 Makeup artist recreates the upper lid sigmoid shape by using a palate of colors to give the illusion of medial shadowing and lateral prominence to the upper lid-sub brow region

Preoperative Patient Assessment

A thorough health history is essential. Adverse reactions to past surgeries or anesthesia are particularly important to note. A list of medicines and allergies with particular focus on blood thinners is critical to prevent postoperative hemorrhage. An ever-growing list of new blood thinners has provided debate on the necessities of stopping blood thinners and for how long in preparation to surgery. Clearance and advice from the internist or cardiologist may provide guidance on the safest approach to stopping these medications. If the septum is planned to be opened and fat manipulated, then stopping antiplatelet and anticoagulation medicine is recommended. If only the skin is to be excised in a functional case and the septum is left intact, then operating on a patient with blood thinners can be reasonable in most scenarios.

A tactile approach with palpation is important in assessing patient needs. The amount and quality of the excess skin should be recorded such as the difference between thin, crepe skin and doughy skin as they present different challenges. The pattern of hooding should be noted, as lateral hooding is easier to treat than medial webbing. The location and amount of fatty herniation should be documented, and retropulsion on the globe can help to further elucidate adipose characteristics. Downward lid excursion and mobility help to determine the degree of lid tightness and any potential restrictive components. The presence of abundant lateral fullness may be indicative of lacrimal gland ptosis or prominence, which may need to be addressed to prevent an unsightly lump postoperatively (Fig. 21.5). Large lacrimal glands may also be an indicator of disease, such as thyroid, sarcoid, or lymphoma. Importantly asymmetry should be recorded and the patient made aware of any differences between sides prior to surgery to avoid unhappy patients postoperatively.

The upper lid and brow are a continuum and should be addressed in this manner. Brow position and ptosis are essential in treating the upper lid. If brow ptosis or a sagging forehead is present, then a surgical brow lift or a chemical lift with botulinum neurotoxin can be discussed to enhance upper lid results. Eyelid ptosis should be recorded with MRD1 measurements, lid crease position, as well as levator function. Preexisting ptosis should be corrected at the time of blepharoplasty to avoid a sleepy postoperative appearance. There are many options to perform ptosis surgery, but with a blepharoplasty and external approach, levator advancement gives good results without making an additional internal incision. Detection of dry eyes will prepare the patients and surgeon alike for the need for postoperative therapy with drops, ointment, or punctual plugs. A history of dry eyes, blepharitis, rheumatoid disease, or Sjögren's can give forewarning to the development of corneal dryness. A history of LASIK also should be an alert that corneal sensation can be diminished and the blink reflex compromised leading to dry eyes. Lid closure, any lagophthalmos, and Bell's phenomenon should be assessed preoperatively. The inability of the eyes to roll upward and backward on forced lid closure is a warning sign of a poor Bell's phenomenon and potential compromised eye protection and dryness after upper lid surgery.

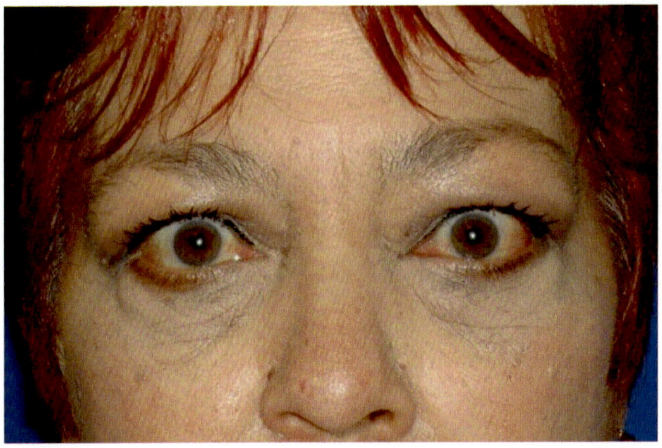

Fig. 21.5 While a modest lateral upper lid fullness of indicative of youth, an overly full lateral lid can be a sign of an enlarged lacrimal gland or systemic disease. This patient has thyroid eye disease with enlarged glands giving her unattractive lateral rubbery fullness to her upper lids. The assessment and treatment to address an unsightly lump in the lacrimal area are important in achieving a good surgical result. Tacking up a prolapsed gland should be considered if a lacrimal gland becomes ptotic with age. Gland resection should be avoided as it can lead to significant postoperative swelling and a dry eye

Surgical Markings

The importance of accurate preoperative markings cannot be overemphasized. Numbing drops should be placed initially to prevent blinking and unwanted lid movement and avoid smudging of the marker. A fine felt tip marker is used for drawing a spindle-shape area of tissue to be excised. The first line should be horizontal and low along the natural lid crease. In non-Asian women, the line should be about 9–10 mm above the lid margin and in men 7–8 mm (Fig. 21.6). These lid crease markings are lower than usually described as the lid crease migrates cephalad over time. An old upper lid incision that is placed too far superiorly looks unsightly as aging progresses (Fig. 21.7). Patients can be marked in any position but they are most comfortable lying supine. In this scenario the incision should wing up laterally approximately 1 cm past the lateral canthus to address the lateral skin hood. When the patient sits up, this lateral wing should fall into a natural lateral lid crease.

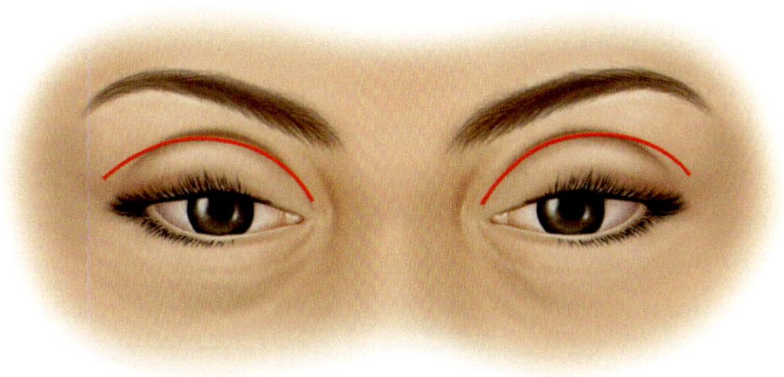

Fig. 21.6 Typical lid crease incision pattern. The crease should follow the patient's natural crease and be low, as the crease can migrate superiorly over time

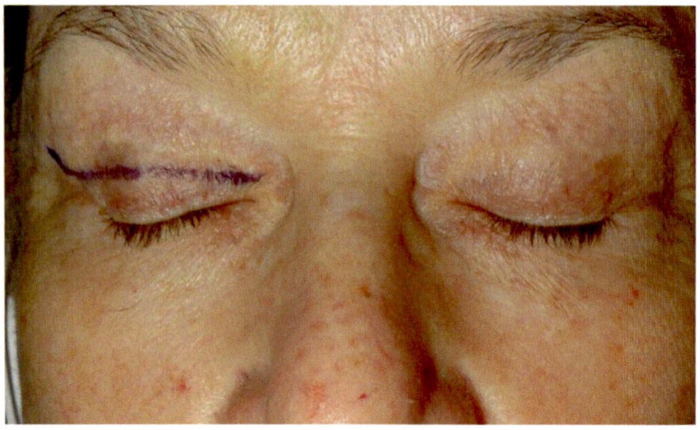

Fig. 21.7 A revision upper lid blepharoplasty on a patient who had surgery 20 years prior. Note the old scar has elevated to an unnaturally high position. The new marking is well below this to restore a proper lid crease

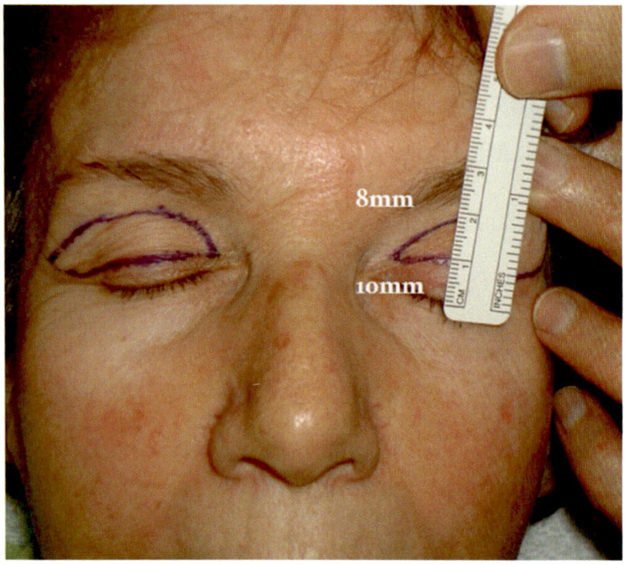

Fig. 21.8 It is important to leave enough skin to allow good eyelid closure. Leaving approximately 18–20 mm between the lower brow hairs and the upper lid margin is typically sufficient. This can easily be measured out with a ruler prior to skin excision

The upper marks of the incision are obtained by pinching the redundant skin together with fingers or gently a fine non-toothed forceps. The upper lid margin and lashes should evert slightly, but care should be taken to avoid aggressive skin excision. When the upper mark is made, lines can be made medially and laterally connecting to the inferior mark. Enough skin must be left behind to for easy eyelid closure. A simple rule is to leave 18 mm to 2 cm of skin behind from below the brows to the lid margin, and this can be measured with a flexible ruler (Fig. 21.8). This should be sufficient tissue for upper lid closure. A final step in the marking is to have the patient close their eyes and pull up on the brows, allowing an inspection from above to judge crease heights and symmetry of tissue to be removed (Fig. 21.9).

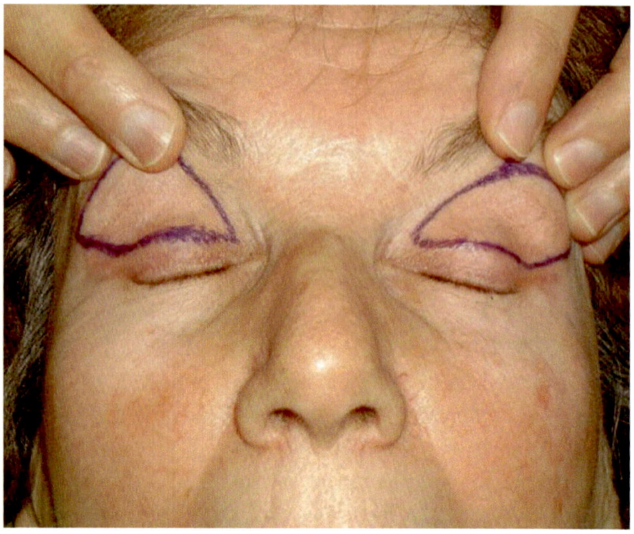

Fig. 21.9 A final step in marking is to have a patient close their eyes gently and pull up on the brows to assess lid crease symmetry and plan skin ellipse excisional areas

After sedation, xylocaine 2% with epinephrine is injected by making a superficial tissue wheel and avoiding an intramuscular injection, which can cause bleeding. Injections should be performed slowly from the side, avoiding injections downward over the brow which can direct a needle toward to globe (Fig. 21.10). Usually a total of 3 ccs of local provides adequate anesthesia. After the patient is prepped and draped and prior to cutting, additional numbing drops and shields can be placed over the eyes and the amount of extra tissue to be excised rechecked with forceps. Shields provide protection from light, improves safety, and decreases anxiety should a patient be awake.

The Sigmoid Blepharoplasty Procedure

The sigmoid blepharoplasty is an advanced surgical technique to achieve maximal aesthetic upper lid youthful topography. Cutting the excess skin can be performed with a variety of instruments. The monopolar cautery set on pure cut with a fine needle tip provides fine scarring results similar to a blade but with more efficiency and hemostasis. Maintaining a dry field is helpful in this vascular-rich area. Only the skin is removed while leaving the underlying orbicularis muscle bed intact (Fig. 21.11). This muscle allows fullness to be retained to counteract the natural forces of deflation that occurs with age. Next an orbiculectomy is performed medially by excising a strip of medial orbicularis muscle (Fig. 21.12). The effect is twofold. It allows a debulking of the medial lid to accentuate a concavity in this area as the muscle can contribute to unwanted fullness in this region. Similar concepts of selectively debulking orbicularis muscle

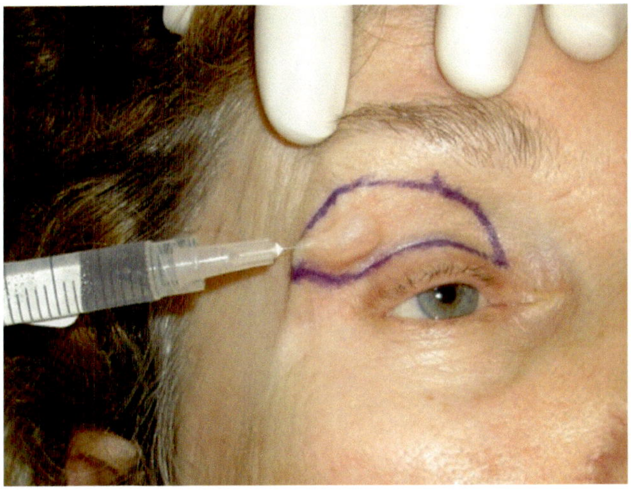

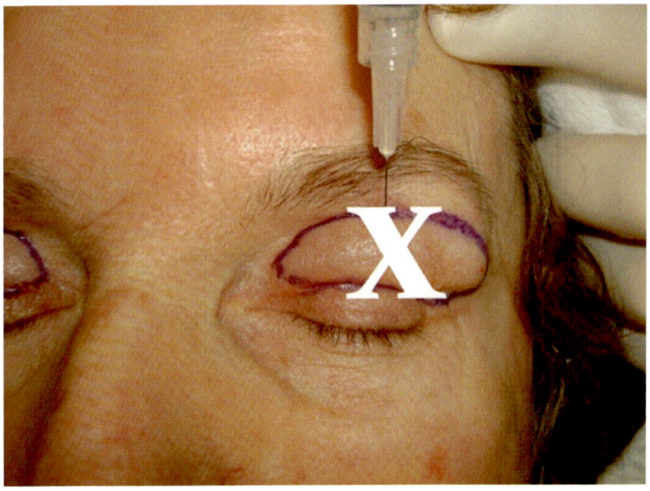

Fig. 21.10 Injecting local anesthesia should be performed with a small, 30 gauge needle creating a wheel of fluid under the skin and above the muscle. The injections should be done from the side and not above to avoid downward injections toward the globe, which can increase unwanted globe penetration with the needle

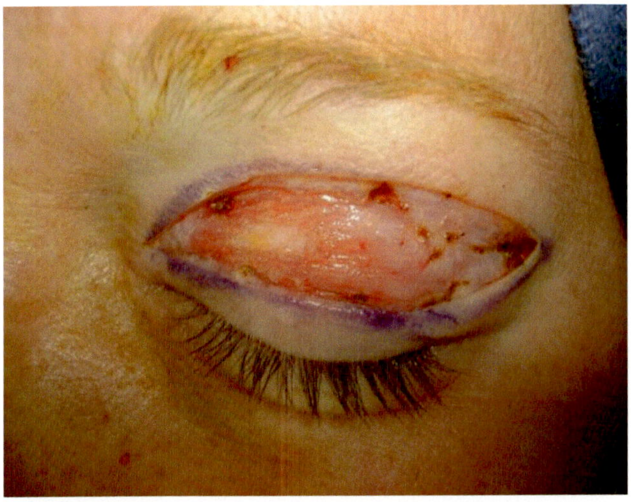

Fig. 21.11 In the sigmoid blepharoplasty, first only the skin is removed leaving orbicularis muscle intact. This maintains lateral fullness

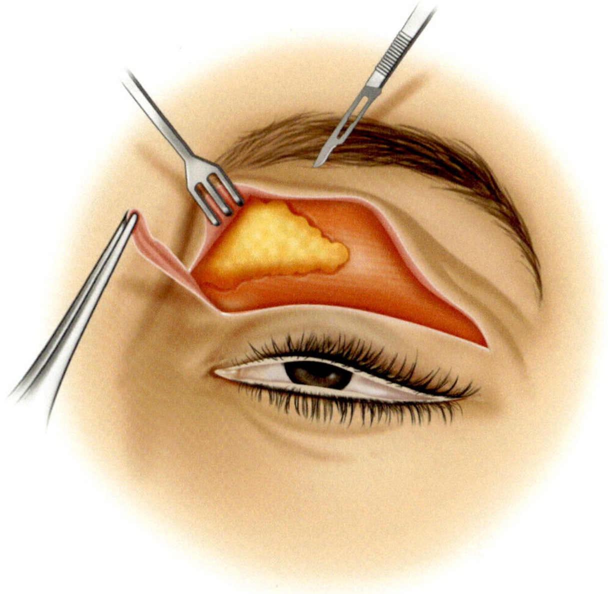

Fig. 21.12 Next a selective medial orbiculectomy is performed to debulk unwanted fullness in the medial lid. This also provides good access to medial fat

have been described in lower lid blepharoplasty to address unsightly orbicularis muscle hypertrophy [8]. Removing muscle also allows for easy access to the orbital septum, which can be opened to expose the fat. Only the medial fat is removed, and if necessary, the central pad can be debulked if excessive fat is present. The medial fat pad can become more prominent with aging, giving an unwanted fullness to the medial upper lid [9].The medial fat is distinct in its features as it is whiter in color and firmer in texture than the yellow softer pre-aponeurotic central pad. Removal of medial muscle and fat allows a more sculpted medial upper lid, without unwanted bulges or lumps. Fat is removed with a cutting cautery with meticulous hemostasis, without clamping as this may tear vessels and aggravate bleeding (Fig. 21.13). It is important to advise the anesthetist to turn down the oxygen to room air when using the cautery as the eyelid region poses a fire risk in the setting of high flow oxygen.

In order to establish upper lateral lid convexity, a 1 cm horizontal lateral orbiculotomy is created with a cutting monopolar device through the muscle to serve as a recipient bed for a fat graft (Fig. 21.14). The incision is placed in the vertical plane below the arch of the brow and serves to create both improved anterior lid projection and also brow support and lift. Medial upper lid fat is firm and has demonstrated a preponderance of progenitor stem cells

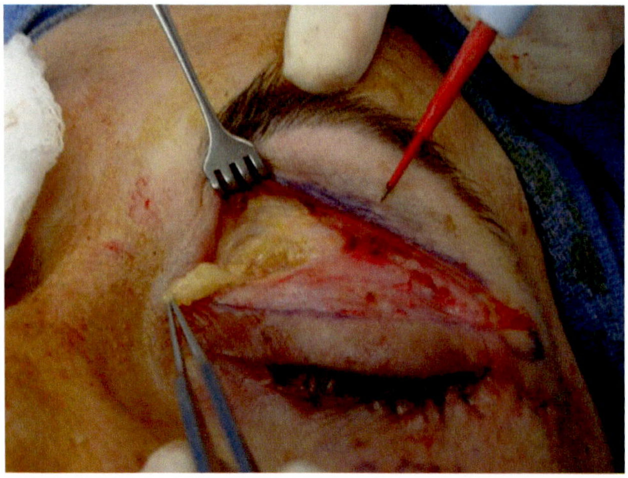

Fig. 21.13 Medial fat removal helps to achieve the desired gentle medial concavity. This is accomplished with a cutting cautery without clamping. Visualization and hemostasis of all bleeding vessels are important

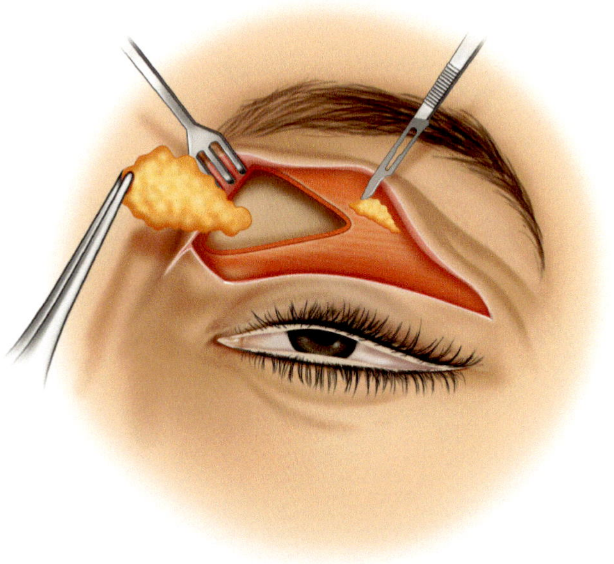

Fig. 21.14 A horizontal lateral orbiculotomy is performed below the brow arch as a recipient site for a fat graft

that serve as an excellent fat graft [10]. This free fat is placed into the orbiculotomy site of the lateral lid and is sutured below the muscle with a 6-0 plain suture (Fig. 21.15). The combination of this fat and the rich, encircling muscular blood supply creates a favorable environment for excellent fat graft take. The end result is a plump, augmented area of fullness in the lateral lid that creates tight skin and a convex contour.

The blepharoplasty wound is closed with a 7-0 monofilament running suture placed only in the skin edges, which is removed in 1 week (Fig. 21.16). The end result of the sigmoid blepharoplasty is the re-establishment of youthful lid contours with a full, convex lateral lid without hooding that gently slopes into a medial sculpted concavity. A bright-eyed appearance is achieved, as well as a platform to apply makeup in a youthful appearance. The brow support provided by the lateral lid fat graft prevents tissue descent and establishes a natural open lateral canthus look (Fig. 21.17a, b). Postoperative care involves ophthalmic

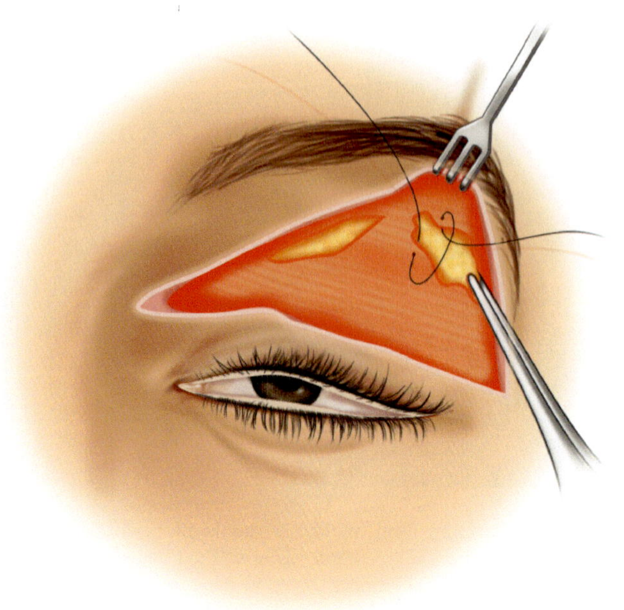

Fig. 21.15 The firm, white fat graft is taken from the medial lid where it has a robust supply of stem cells. It is placed into the orbiculotomy site laterally to achieve the desired lateral brow fullness and to support and raise the brow arch from below. The fat is sutured with 6-0 plain suture below the muscle pocket, and the fat take is excellent due to the robust blood supply in the muscle

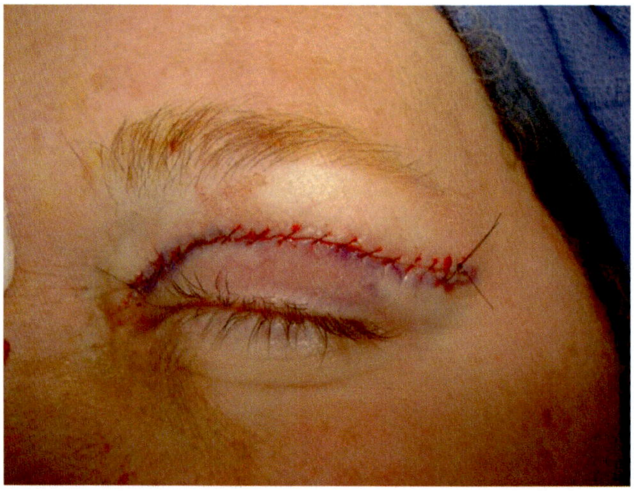

Fig. 21.16 The upper lid wound is closed with a running non-dissolving, monofilament 7-0 suture that is removed in 1 week. The suture is not tight, allowing the wound edges to "kiss" without tension. This promotes fine scar healing and avoids unwanted suture bumps

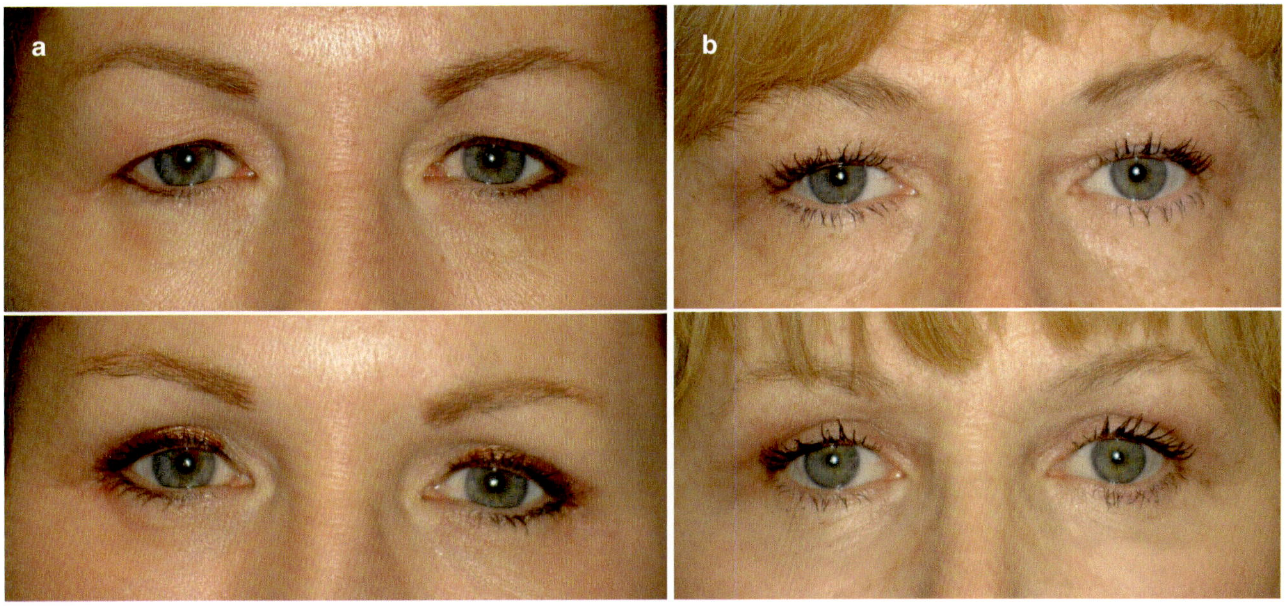

Fig. 21.17 (a) Result of a sigmoid blepharoplasty pre- and postoperatively. This patient had signs of aging lids, with characteristic medial fullness and lateral lid deflation and droop. The youthful sigmoid curve is restored postoperatively. Upper and lower lid blepharoplasty was performed. (b) Another result of a sigmoid blepharoplasty pre- and postoperatively. This patient had signs of aging lids, with characteristic medial fullness and lateral lid deflation and droop. The youthful sigmoid curve is restored postoperatively. Upper and lower lid blepharoplasty was performed

ointment twice a day for 2 weeks and cold packs to the eyes for the first 48 hours to reduce bruising.

Alternative Options for Upper Lid Blepharoplasty

There are many schools of thought on what an attractive upper lid should look like. Some of the discrepancy is based on cultural, geographical, or environmental influences. Certainly while the sigmoid approach provides a brighter-eyed, more youthful appearance, other options exist. Skin excision alone with keeping all muscle and fat intact has been described as a method to maintain lid fullness [11]. While this may provide good results in selected cases, fullness in and of itself is not the true goal. Youthful curves should be the priority of the blepharoplasty surgeon, with fullness selected for appropriate areas. Others describe using fat pedicle flaps to transpose from medial to lateral to reduce medial fullness and create lateral convexity [12]. The fat pedicle has an excellent take with an intact blood supply and is placed under the lateral orbicularis muscle's rich blood supply (Fig. 21.18a, b). The pre-aponeurotic fat is soft and may not be in sufficient quantity to give an abundant lateral fill however. Lastly transposing medial fat into the glabella area has been described to reduce medial fullness but also to lift deflated tissues between the medial brows in selected cases [13] (Fig. 21.19a, b).

Lateral Orbiculotomy

The orbicularis oculi is the most potent lateral brow depressor. Reducing some of its downward pull allows the frontalis muscle to lift more effectively. The orbicularis muscle acts like a rubber band encircling the eye. Incising the muscle full thickness (orbiculotomy) is analogous to cutting the constricting forces of a rubber band (Fig. 21.20a, b). The result is not only a smoothing of upper crow's feet wrinkles but a subtle lateral brow lift as would be seen with botulinum neuromodulator injection. The procedure is performed when the lateral brow is ptotic and deflated. As always the initial step of the blepharoplasty involves retaining lateral orbicularis muscle. The muscle is then incised with a monopolar cautery on a 45° angle, splitting the muscle and exposing the retro-orbicularis fat (Fig. 21.21). The muscle will splay, exposing the deep fat. Fat grafts from the medial lid can be placed into this area to maintain an elegant fullness and counteract the deflation forces of aging. It is important to understand that the fat pads around the orbital rims not only descend but also atrophy with time contributing to a sinking of the lateral brows over the lids. Importantly the fat grafts also act as a spacer graft separating and weakening this cut muscle and preventing reattachment (Fig. 21.22). The muscle is not sutured over the grafts in this scenario as the goal is to keep the muscle separated with diminished function. The fat provides increased lift from below and acts as a pillar of support (Fig. 21.23). The fat graft also adds youthful anterior projection to the sub brow region. This lateral sub brow

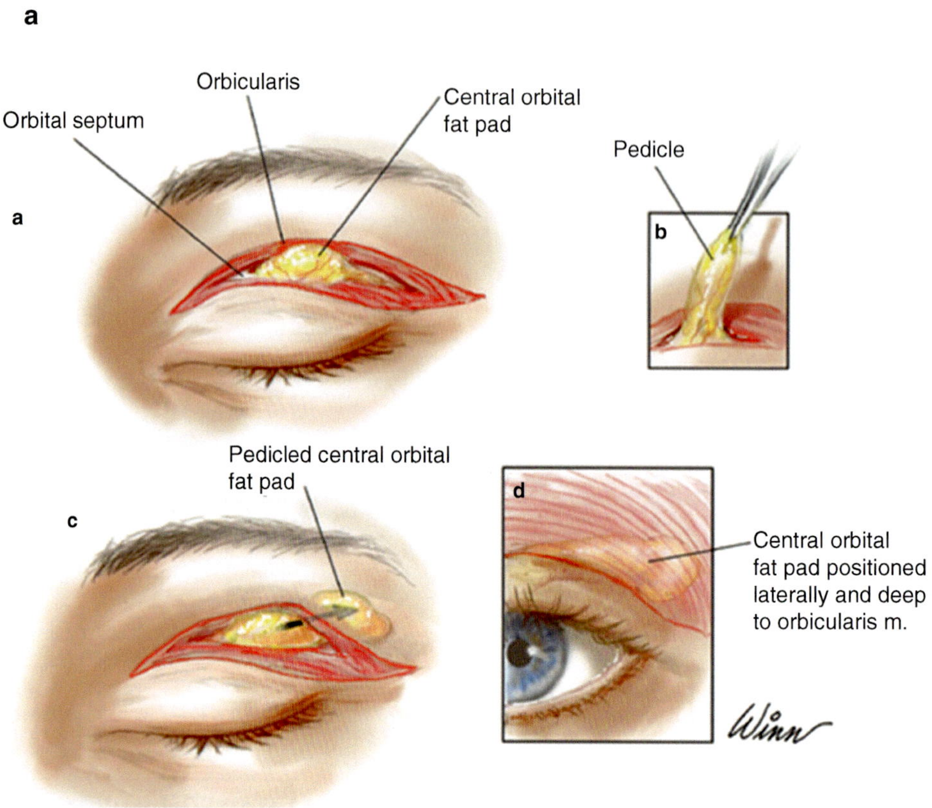

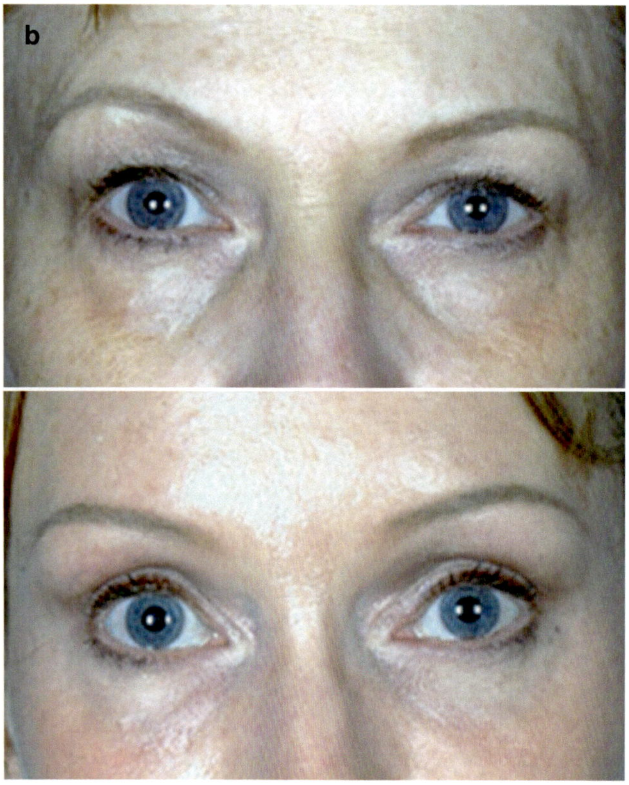

Fig. 21.18 (**a**) Sozer's upper blepharoplasty technique demonstrating a sliding lateral fat pedicle placed under the muscle from medial to lateral to achieve fullness. (**b**) Pre- and postoperative result of this surgery

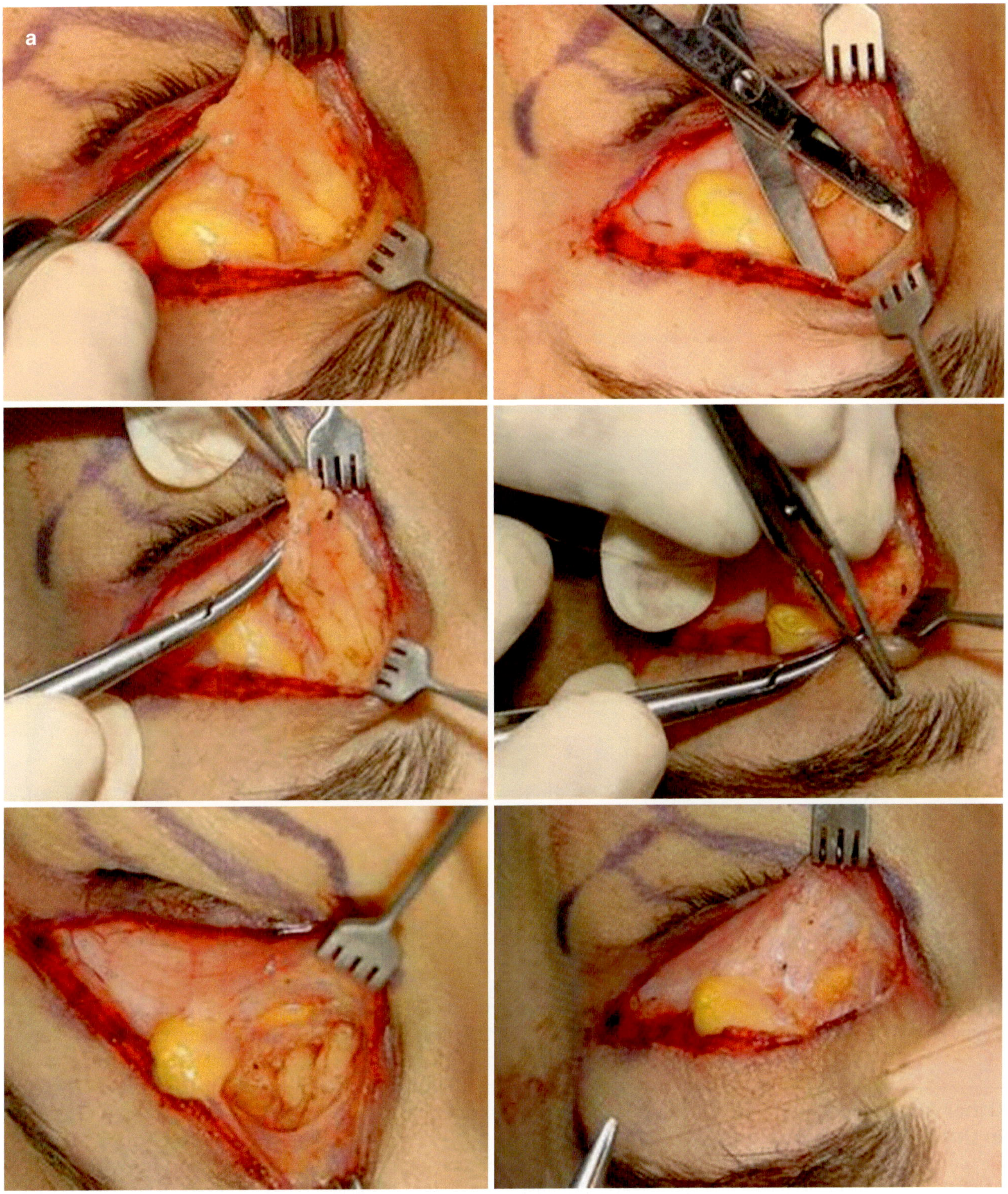

Fig. 21.19 (**a**) Massry's sliding medial fat pedicle to fill a deficient glabella region. (**b**) Pre- and postoperative results

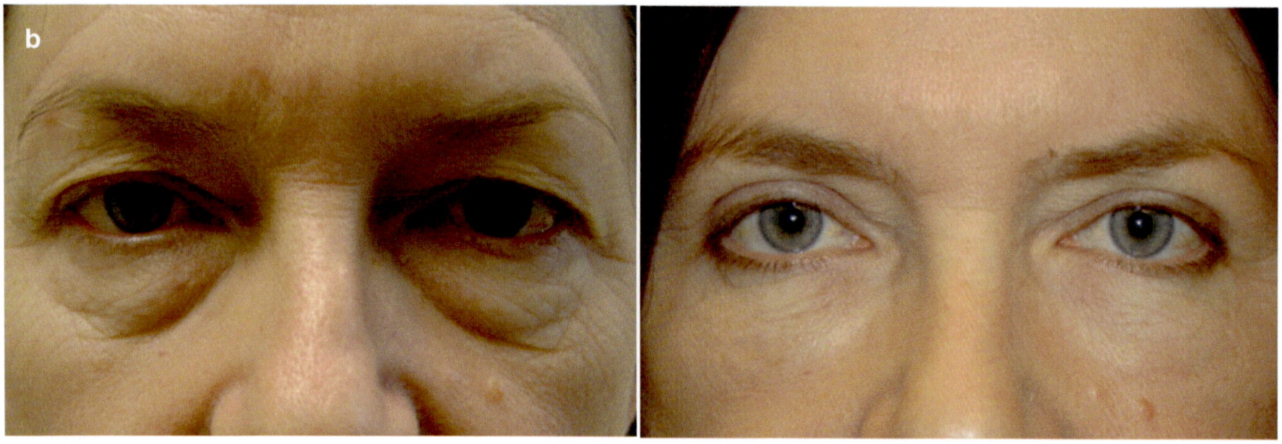

Fig. 21.19 (continued)

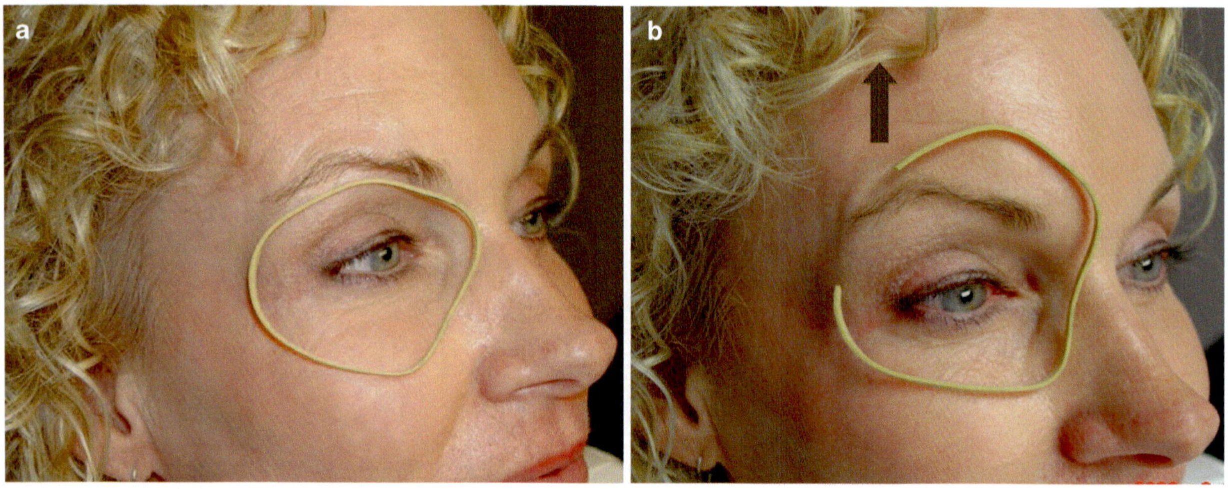

Fig. 21.20 (**a**) The orbicularis oculi muscle is like a rubber band encircling the eye. It is a powerful lateral brow depressor and creator of crow's feet wrinkles. (**b**) Releasing the muscle is analogous to severing the rubber band. The effect is to weaken the lateral brow depressor and allow the lateral brow to lift more unabated (upward arrow). It also helps in softening the upper laugh lines

fullness restores an upper face ogee curve, which is the convexity of the brow transitioning to a concavity of the lateral canthus best seen on a three quarter view (Fig. 21.24).

Other Advanced Muscle Modifications in Upper Lid Blepharoplasty

In cases of extreme lid asymmetry, where one eye is smaller and heavier with a lower brow, knowledge of facial muscle function can be helpful. Understanding the agonist/antagonist relationship of facial muscles can be helpful in achieving balance to the lids. While the orbicularis, corrugators, and procerus pull the brows down to close the eyes, the frontalis elevates the brows to open the eyes. Using this knowledge, orbicularis muscle can be removed on the smaller, heavier eye to decrease lid volume and lid depression while allowing the frontalis less effort in raising the brow on that side [14]. This maneuver improves eyelid contour and provides some added lift to a fuller side. This is analogous to treatment with neurotoxins, where depressor muscles are targeted to weaken to allow the elevators to lift unabated.

Debate has also surrounded the best method for eyelid closure. Certainly the finest suture ranging from a 6-0 to 7-0 size will yield the best results. Typically monofilament, nondissolving sutures are the least reactive and result in the finest scars. Some advocate dissolving plain suture for convenience as these do not have to be removed, but retained suture can result in irregularities such as suture bumps. Closure in the subcutaneous plain with a Prolene suture is attractive and easy to remove by clipping and pulling the sutures ends but can have a tendency to cause a whiter medial

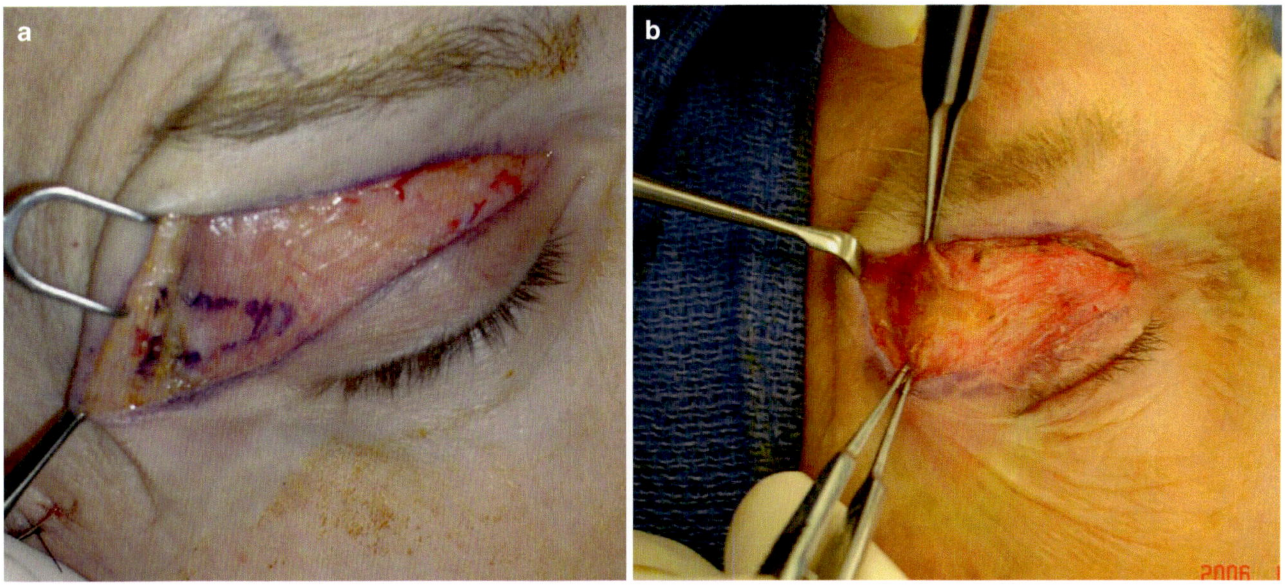

Fig. 21.21 (**a**) The right upper lid orbicularis muscle is marked at a 45° angle in the preparation for muscle incision. The blue marks outline the expected amount of muscle separation after severing the muscle full thickness. (**b**) A lateral orbiculotomy is initiated by incising the muscle full thickness exposing the underlying deep brow fat pad. This ensures effective lateral muscle release. The orbicularis is a tight sphincter muscle and will splay after incising, so no muscle has to be removed

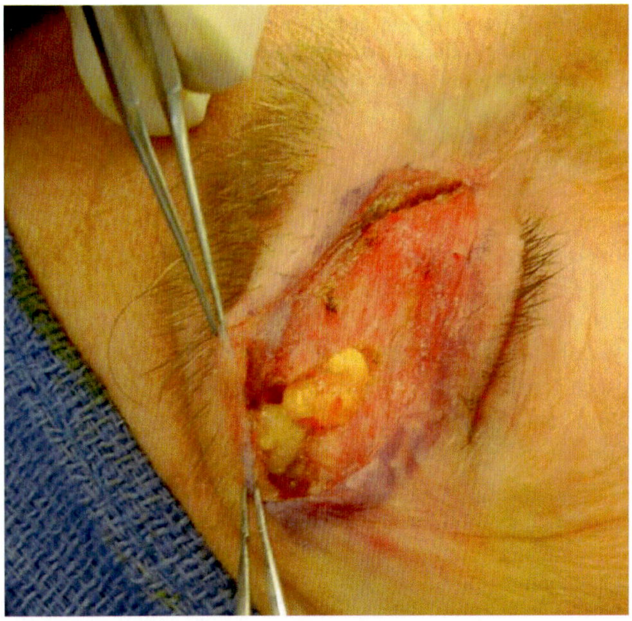

Fig. 21.22 Fat from the medial lid is placed into to the area between the split muscle to add back volume and act as a spacer graft so the muscle will not reattach. The muscle is not sutured over the fat as is done in a sigmoid procedure, because the intention is to weaken the muscle and suturing it back together would restrengthen the muscle

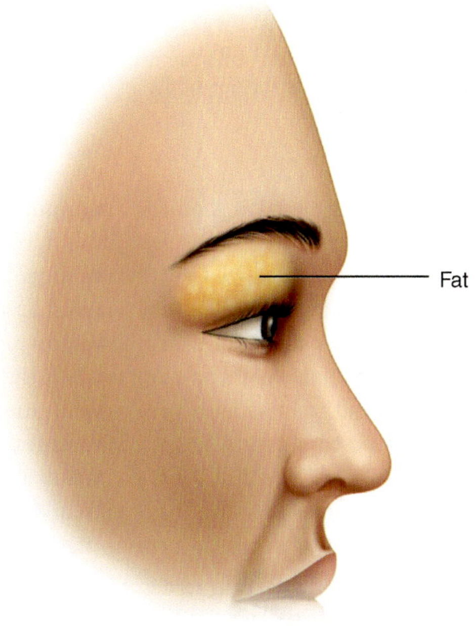

Fig. 21.23 The fat graft also adds volume to the lateral sub brow area and provides lateral brow lift and support. The lateral orbiculotomy procedure with fat grafting creates a youthful and arched lateral brow. The fat graft also improves anterior brow projection and counteracts the effects of deflation and sinking that can be problematic on the lateral brow

scar. Interrupted sutures are accurate but can be time-consuming and result in more suture cysts. The running suture is fast, effective, and predictable in most hands.

The creation of a lid crease during closure has not received as much attention as in the past [15]. Formation of a crisp upper lid crease can be appealing for those individuals that desire a more defined crease or to address asymmetry. In reality most individuals do not have sharp or deep upper lid creases, but a softer line instead. In order to recreate a defined

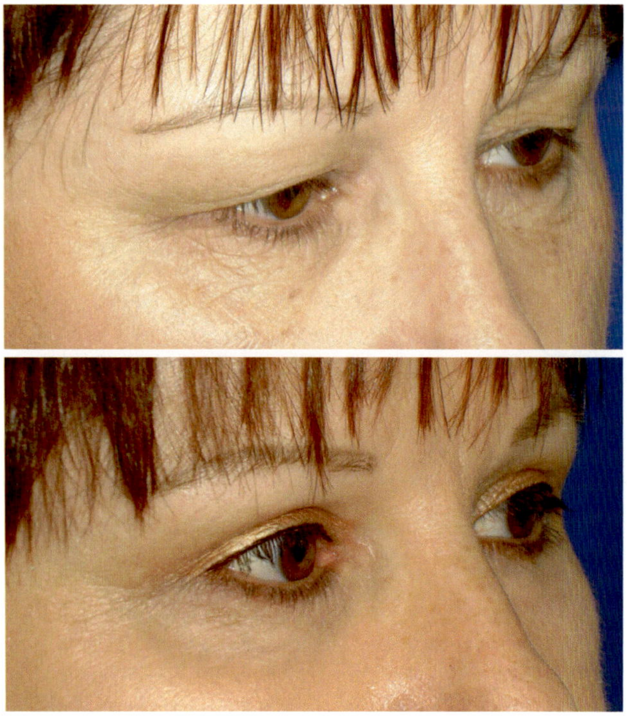

Fig. 21.24 A youthful face is actually a double ogee with the superior convexity at the lateral brow descending into the more concave lateral orbit. The classic ogee of the face is lower and describes the relationship between a convex midface and a concave submalar area. A three quarter view demonstrates restoration of the upper ogee using the lateral orbiculotomy technique

crease closure of the wound, it should involve a suture bite of the upper skin and orbicularis muscle, followed by a bite of levator aponeurosis and finalized by a bite of the lower orbicularis and skin. Care should be taken to avoid purchase of the orbital septum as this may cause unwanted tether and lagophthalmos. In this author's opinion, rarely is this type of closure needed, and most patients benefit by closing skin to skin. Creating a crease contradicts general surgical principles of wound closure which involve good wound eversion under minimal tension to achieve maximal scar camouflage. Usually forming symmetrical lid creases starts with well-designed matching crease incision lines. In cases of asymmetry, eyelid ptosis is often the culprit of a higher crease, and ptosis should be corrected at the time of blepharoplasty. Despite the preferred method of closure, the wounds should "kiss" and approximate without tension as swelling will cause delayed wound tension.

Corrugator Removal Through the Upper Lid Approach

The glabella and brow region are contiguous with the upper lids and should be assessed when looking at the upper lids. The "11" lines of the glabella are a result of the persistent

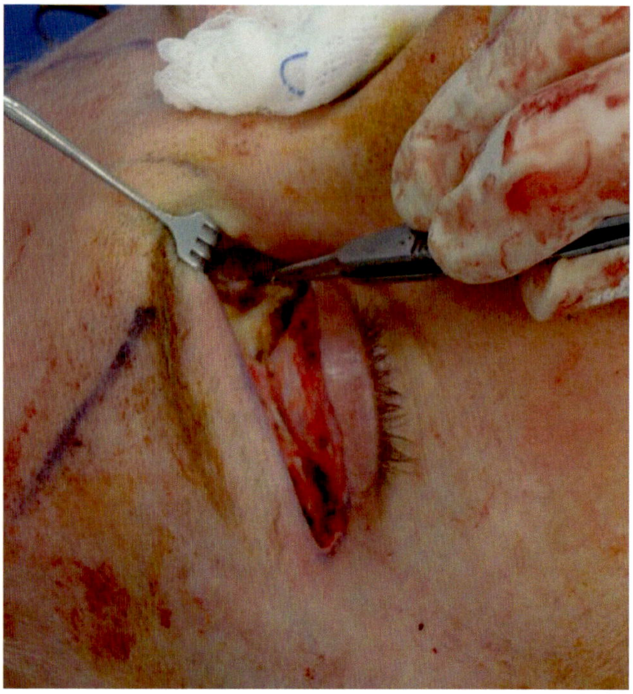

Fig. 21.25 The upper eyelid incision provides close and easy access to the glabella muscles. A dissection plane upward toward to superior orbital rim between the orbicularis muscle and the septum leads to the corrugator muscle. Once identified, the corrugators can be grasped with a forceps and a section of the muscle belly removed with cautery

horizontal movements of the corrugators muscles. These muscles can be weakened with injectable neuromodulators or surgery. The transblepharoplasty approach to the corrugators is a convenient access to modify these depressor muscles [16, 17]. Access through the upper lids is a much shorter distance than from the scalp approach in a brow lift. During an upper lid blepharoplasty, the monopolar cautery can be used to create a dissection plane below the medial orbicularis oculi muscle and above the septum. Small rakes can help to provide excellent exposure by pulling the skin/orbicularis muscle flap upward over the superior orbital rim. The deep, finger-like corrugator muscles can be identified and divided. Grasping the corrugator muscle with a heavy forceps and delivering it downward into view help to isolate the muscle (Fig. 21.25). Due to the glabella's rich bold supply, it is helpful to first cauterize on either side of the muscle belly with a bipolar cautery before severing the muscle full thickness with a monopolar cutting cautery. The medial head is strongly attached to the frontal bone, and elevation with a periosteal elevator is helpful. An elevator can be passed from one upper lid incision exiting the other side to ensure full release of the muscles (Fig. 21.26).

Removing a section of muscle is more effective than simply cutting it. Aggressive extirpation should be avoided as this can cause unwanted tissue indentation and medial spaying of the brows. One disadvantage of the transblepharoplasty approach is the lateral corrugators are difficult to

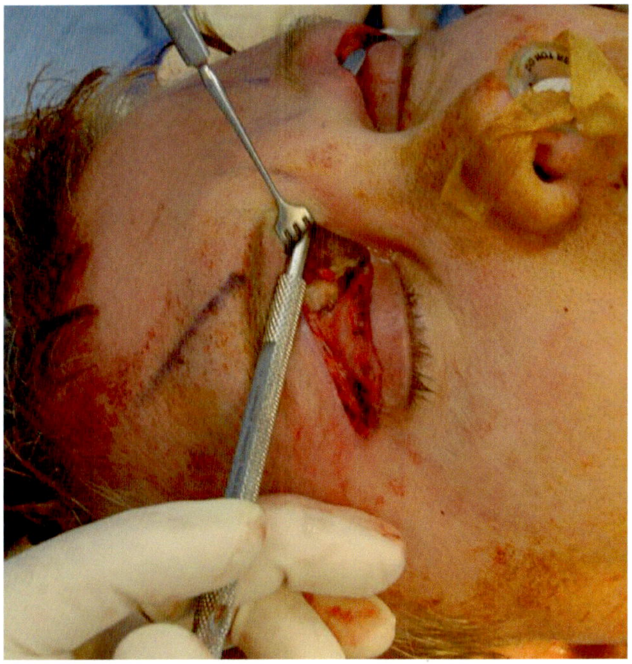

Fig. 21.26 The medial head of the corrugators are extremely adherent to the frontal bone. A periosteal elevator helps to achieve full medial release. The elevator can be passed from one eyelid incision and exit the other, ensuring full flap elevation

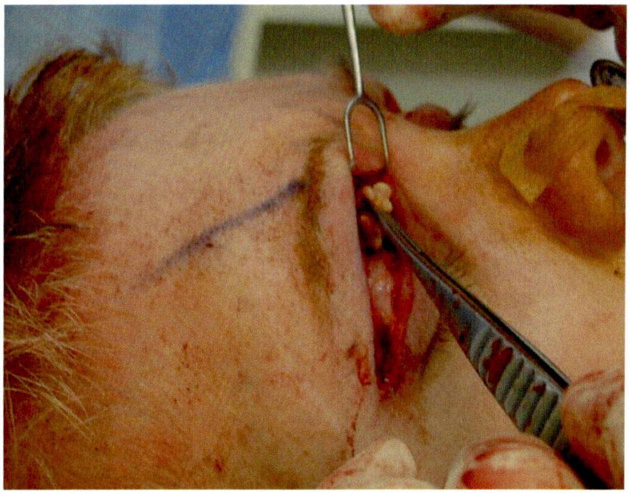

Fig. 21.27 Fat grafts can be placed from the blepharoplasty incisions below to fill any void created from glabella muscle removal and to act as a spacer graft to prevent corrugator reattachment

remove as the supraorbital neurovascular bundle blocks full exposure, so some lateral muscle function will remain. It is important preoperatively to mark and know the two neurovascular bundles that exit the superior orbit and innervate the forehead. The supra-trochlear neurovascular bundle is 1.6 mm lateral to the midline, and the supraorbital bundle is 2.6 mm lateral to the midline and can be palpated as a notch in the superomedial orbit. This will help to avoid damage to these delicate structures. Muscle removal can also cause a tissue void that may benefit from fat grafts placed from the upper lid incision (Fig. 21.27). Again the grafts act to add back lost volume but also function as a spacer graft to prevent corrugator reattachment.

Conclusions

Concepts of eyelid beauty are evolving. Regardless, the goal of upper lid blepharoplasty is to recreate a youthful appearance. This involves an appreciation of aesthetically appealing curves and a restoration of the sigmoid or ogee curve. The sigmoid shape refers to a medial concavity achieved by muscle and fat sculpting and a convex lateral lid formed by retaining muscle and adding fat grafts. The result is recreating a youthful upper lid ogee that transitions from a medial concavity to a lateral convexity. This approach addresses the two most common complaints of traditional upper blepharoplasty: residual nasal fullness and excess lateral hooding. The crux of upper blepharoplasty is retaining volume and appreciating the value of utilizing fat as a tool to augment results. An understanding of the eyelid muscles and their function can allow for finesse in fine-tuning asymmetry. Whatever approach is utilized, moderation and an appreciation of aesthetic contours should guide surgical judgment. Most importantly as in most surgeries, preoperative planning and precise markings are the key to achieving an excellent result.

References

1. May JW Jr, Fearon J, Zingarelli P. Retro-orbicularis oculus fat (ROOF) resection in aesthetic blepharoplasty: a 6-year study in 63 patients. Plast Reconstr Surg. 1990;86:682–9.
2. Owsley JQ Jr. Resection of the prominent lateral fat pad during upper lid blepharoplasty. Plast Reconstr Surg. 1980;65:4–9.
3. Persichetti P, Di Lella F, Delfino S, Scuderi N. Adipose compartments of the upper eyelid: anatomy applied to blepharoplasty. Plast Reconstr Surg. 2004;113:373–8.
4. Hudson DA. A paradigm shift for plastic surgeons: no longer focusing on excising excess skin. Plast Reconstr Surg. 2000;106:497–9.
5. Rohrich RJ, Coberly DM, Fagien S. Current concepts in aesthetic upper blepharoplasty. Plast Reconstr Surg. 2004;113:32e–42e.
6. Gulyas G. Improving lateral fullness in the upper eyelid. Aesthet Plast Surg. 2006;30:641–8.
7. Fezza J. The sigmoid upper eyelid blepharoplasty: redefining beauty. Ophthal Plast Reconstr Surg. 2012;28(6):446–51.
8. Loeb R. Necessity for partial resection of the orbicularis oculi muscle in blepharoplasties in some young patients. Plast Reconstr Surg. 1977;60:176–8.
9. Oh SR, Chokthaweesak W, Annunziata CC. Analysis of eyelid fat changes with aging. Ophthal Plast Reconstr Surg. 2011;27:348–51.
10. Korn BS, Kikkawa DO, Hicok KC. Identification and characterization of adult stem cells from human orbital adipose tissue. Ophthal Plast Reconstr Surg. 2009;25:27–32.
11. Fagien S. Advanced rejuvenative upper blepharoplasty: enhancing aesthetics of the upper periorbita. Plast Reconstr Surg. 2002;110(1):278–91.

12. Sozer SO, Agullo FJ, Palladino H, et al. Pedicled fat flap to increase lateral fullness in upper blepharoplasty. Aesthet Surg J. 2010;30:161–5.
13. Massry GG. Nasal fat preservation in upper blepharoplasty. Ophthal Plast Reconstr Surg. 2011;27:352–5.
14. Fagien S. The role of the orbicularis oculi muscle and the eyelid crease in optimizing results in aesthetic upper blepharoplasty: a new look at the surgical treatment of mild upper eyelid fissure and fold asymmetries. Plast Reconstr Surg. 2010;125:653–66.
15. Putterman AM, Urist MJ. Reconstruction of the upper eyelid crease and fold. Arch Ophthalmol. 1976;94:1941–54.
16. Guyuron B, Michelow B, Thoms T. Corrugator supercilii muscle resection trough blepharoplasty incision. Plast Reconstr Surg. 1995;95:691–6.
17. Paul MD. Subperiosteal transblepharoplasty forehead lift. Aesthet Plast Surg. 1996;20:129–34.

Complications of Blepharoplasty

22

Alison B. Callahan and Richard D. Lisman

Blepharoplasty is one of the most common aesthetic surgeries performed by a variety of surgical specialists. While minor variations in technique exist, in general, the procedures are relatively straightforward. However, as with any surgical procedure, complications can arise and range from minor aesthetic nuances to vision-threatening emergencies. Proper screening and perioperative management can help to prevent many of these complications. This article offers a comprehensive and up-to-date summary of complications arising from upper and lower eyelid blepharoplasties based on recent peer-reviewed literature and the professional experience of the authors.

Vision Loss

Vision loss is the most serious and thus feared complication of upper or lower eyelid blepharoplasty. It occurs most commonly from retrobulbar hemorrhage, which occurs at a frequency of 0.04–0.05% [1, 2]. Associated permanent vision loss has been found in large case series review to occur at a frequency of 0.0045% [2]. This corresponds to a 1 in 2000 risk of hemorrhage and 1 in 10,000 risk of permanent vision loss from hemorrhage. The vast majority of hemorrhages (96%) occur within the first 24 hours of surgery [2], though hemorrhage as late as 9 days postoperatively has been reported [3]. Pain and pressure are the most common presenting complaints, and examination reveals decreased visual acuity, afferent pupillary defect, proptosis, impaired extraocular motility, and elevated intraocular (and intraorbital) pressure (Fig. 22.1a, b). Increased intraorbital and intraocular pressures result in ischemic damage to the optic nerve and/or retina.

Treatment begins first and foremost with prevention. Preoperative evaluation should always elicit risk factors such as hypertension, vascular disease, and anticoagulation. In particular, one must take care when asking about anticoagulants as patients often omit medications such as a baby aspirin, fish oil, vitamin E, or other supplements if not specifically asked about these entities. Discontinuing these medications with ample time to clear their anticoagulant effect is most prudent for these elective, often cosmetic procedures. Given the propensity for hemorrhages to occur within the first 24 hours of surgery, the authors advise avoiding restarting anticoagulants during this period if possible. Newer anticoagulants such as the direct factor Xa inhibitors that lack robust clinical data for perioperative management pose a particular challenge, though recent case reports have aided in the field's collective experience [4]. Intraoperatively, control of hemostasis is critical, and meticulous hemostasis is the only condition in which a case should be concluded. The use of antiemetics and antitussives can limit Valsalva maneuvers postoperatively. Many advocate elevating the head of the bed and use of ice compresses, though scientific data neither supports nor refutes this common practice. The use of occlusive patching was not found to reduce the incidence of retrobulbar hemorrhage [2]. Some surgeons still prefer occlusive patching to prevent postoperative edema [5], though the current authors believe its benefits do not outweigh the risk of delayed diagnosis of hemorrhage.

When retrobulbar hemorrhages do occur, prompt diagnosis and treatment can still result in favorable outcomes. Glaucoma medications may be used to treat nonprogressive hemorrhages when intraocular pressure is slightly elevated. However, when bleeding threatens the visual system or is uncontrolled and worsening, surgical therapy is required. This incision should be opened widely through the orbital

A. B. Callahan
Tufts Medical Center, Ophthalmology, Boston, MA, USA
e-mail: acallahan1@tuftsmedicalcenter.org

R. D. Lisman (✉)
Ophthalmology/Plastic Surgery, NYU School of Medicine, New York, NY, USA

Ophthalmology/Plastic Surgery, Manhattan Eye, Ear and Throat Hospital, New York, NY, USA
e-mail: drlisman@lismanmd.com

A. J. Cohen, C. N. Burkat (eds.), *Oculofacial, Orbital, and Lacrimal Surgery*, https://doi.org/10.1007/978-3-030-14092-2_22

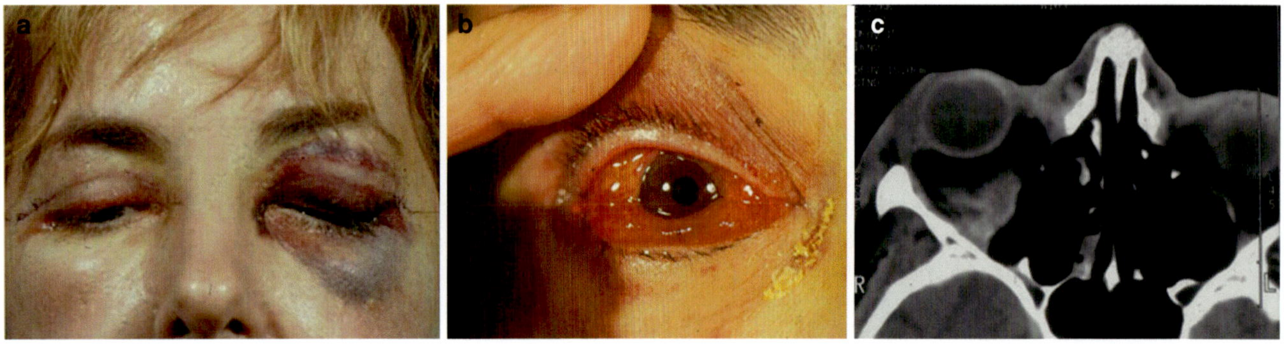

Fig. 22.1 Retrobulbar hemorrhage producing ecchymosis after a frontal nerve block during transcutaneous blepharoplasty (**a**) and retrobulbar hemorrhage in a hypertensive patient demonstrating sudden proptosis and chemosis (**b**). Imaging demonstrates a posterior orbital hemorrhage (**c**)

septum to allow for evacuation of clot and identification and treatment of bleeding areas. In particularly severe or unresponsive cases, a lateral canthotomy and cantholysis may be performed. If these measures still fail, non-contrast CT should be obtained and a floor decompression considered for a posterior, organized hemorrhage (Fig. 22.1c). Profound vision loss has been reported to recover after even 24 hours, and therefore treatment interventions should remain aggressive for at least that time period [6].

Although retrobulbar hemorrhage is the most common cause of vision loss following blepharoplasty, other vision-threatening complications have been reported including globe perforation, acute angle closure, and ischemic optic neuropathy. Inadvertent globe penetration can result from any periocular procedure, and therefore care must be used during both injection of local anesthetic and throughout the procedure [7, 8]. The use of protective corneal shields aid in the prevention of perforating globe injuries; however, such complications are reported even in the context of their use [9]. If such an injury occurs, it should be considered an ophthalmic emergency necessitating emergent evaluation and treatment (Fig. 22.2). Rare reports of acute angle closure causing vision loss in the setting of blepharoplasty have also been documented in the literature [9, 10]. It is thought to be related to the use of mydriasis secondary to the use of anesthetics, dark adaptation during patching, or increased anxiety in the setting of a predisposed eye (e.g., axial hypertropia). Finally, cases of perioperative optic neuropathies in the absence of orbital hemorrhage have been attributed to posterior ischemia [11, 12].

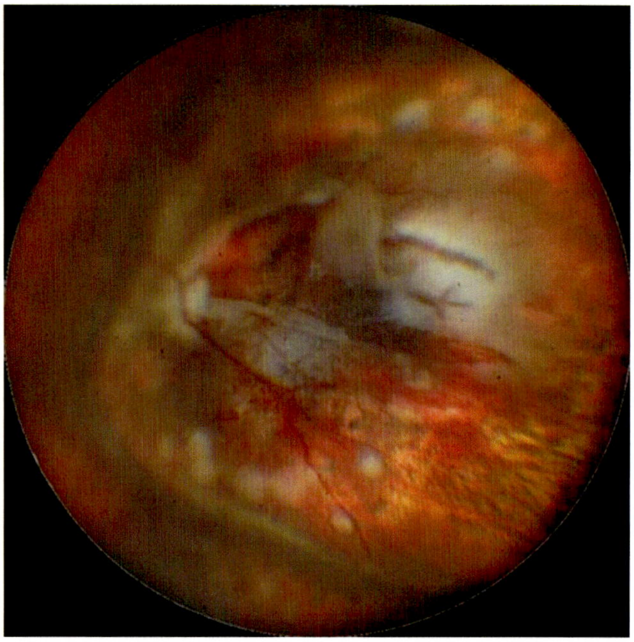

Fig. 22.2 A retinal flap tear with tractional retinal detachment is present after inadvertent corneal perforation during injection for an upper eyelid blepharoplasty. The patient also suffered from a traumatic cataract secondary to lenticular penetration

Infection

The eyelid is privileged to have a rich vascular supply, and, consequently, postoperative infections are exceedingly uncommon. Nevertheless, infectious complications can and do arise including preseptal cellulitis, orbital cellulitis, and necrotizing fasciitis (Fig. 22.3) [13, 14, 15]. Such infections can result in permanent vision loss, meningitis, or even death. Early recognition is enabled by contrast-enhanced computed tomography and clinical examination focused on such things as the presence of orbital signs or, in the case of necrotizing fasciitis, uncharacteristically rapid progression with eventual tissue cyanosis. Some surgeons used perioperative and/or postoperative prophylactic antibiotics in an effort to reduce the risk of postoperative infections, but others feel the risk of an antibiotic reaction outweighs the risk of a postoperative infection in an otherwise sterile operation. While there is scientific evidence to support the use of perioperative intravenous antibiotics when implanting a foreign body, scientific evidence and consensus are otherwise lacking [16, 17]. The authors do not routinely use prophylactic

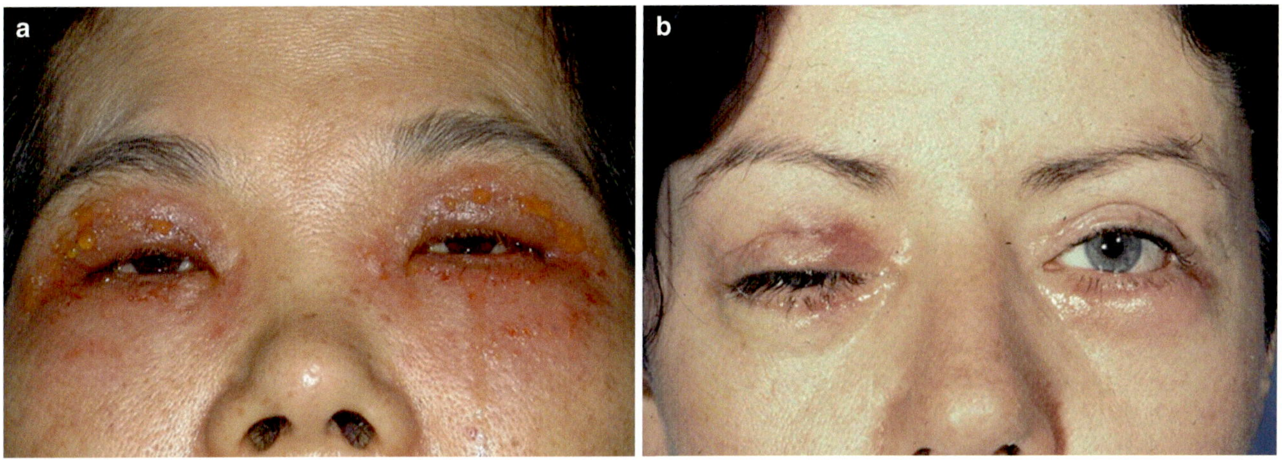

Fig. 22.3 Early bilateral preseptal cellulitis demonstrating bilateral eyelid edema and erythema (**a**), pseudomonas cellulitis with associated abscess formations 3 days after blepharoplasty (**b**)

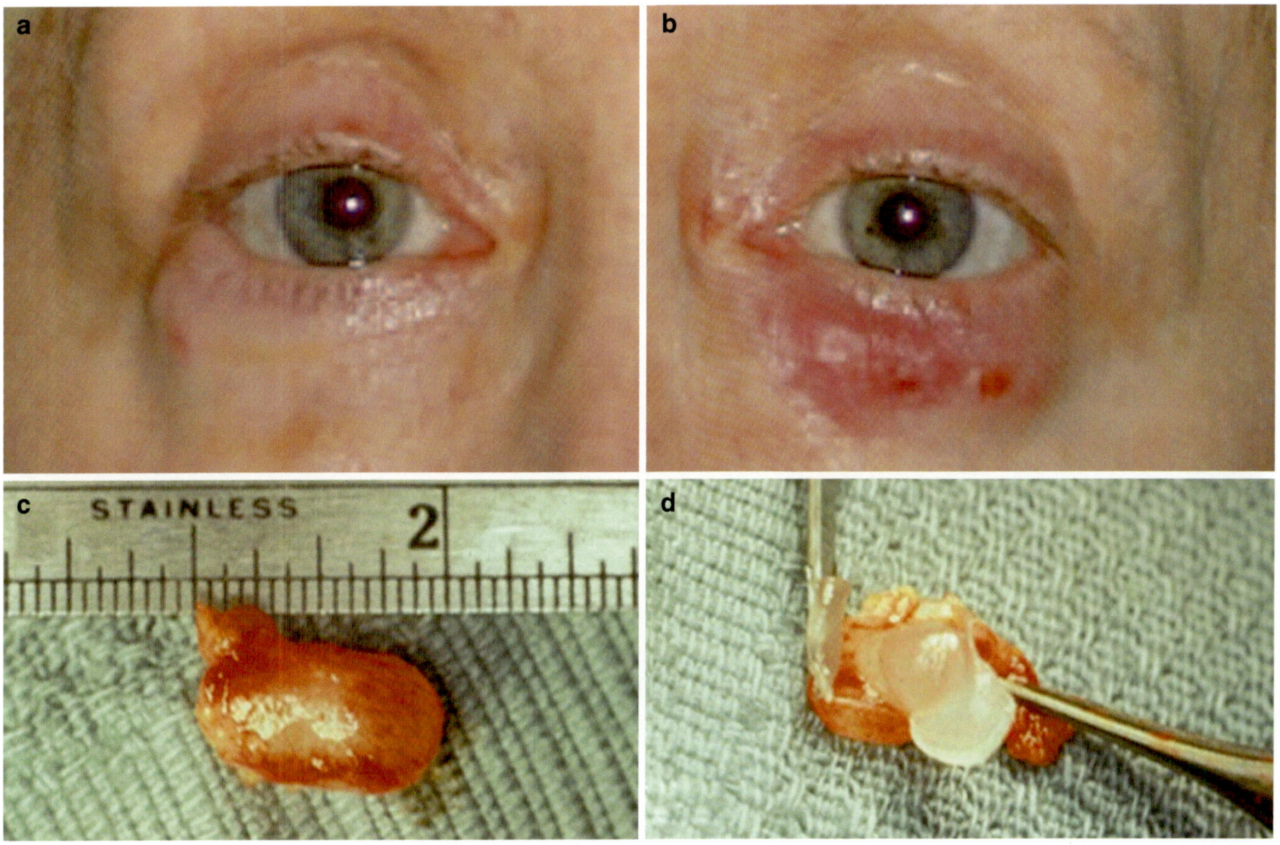

Fig. 22.4 Left lower eyelid erythema and "lumpy" edema occurring 10 days postoperatively (**a**), excised, encapsulated ointment granuloma (**b**), opening of the capsule reveals its oily contents with chemical analysis consistent with ophthalmic ointment (**c**)

antibiotics, but rather prefer to implement them only when there is a specific risk factor for infection, such as an immunocompromised patient.

On occasion, ophthalmic lubricant can be introduced into the deeper eyelid tissues via an open transconjunctival wound. A granulomatous reaction in the early or mid-postoperative period can ensue and mimic an atypical infection (Fig. 22.4) [18]. Such ointment granulomas are best avoided by judicious use of ophthalmic lubricants when leaving conjunctival wounds open without closure. When they do occur, intralesional steroids and/or definitive surgical excision are recommended.

Ocular Surface Decompensation

One of the eyelid's primary functions is to guard the ocular surface and to produce and maintain a moist environment. Consequently, it is of no great surprise that disruptions of the ocular surface are a well-known complication of both upper and lower eyelid blepharoplasties. Injury to the ocular surface as a result of blepharoplasty has many etiologies including corneal abrasion, lagophthalmos, lower eyelid malposition, unmasking thyroid disease, or simply exacerbating a preexisting propensity toward dry eye disease. Approximately 10% of patients will experience dry eye following blepharoplasty, but only 2% will have symptoms that persist beyond 2 months [19]. The risk of postoperative ocular surface disorders can be reduced by appropriate screening during initial examination. Inquiring about a history of dryness, the use and frequency of artificial tears and history of prior laser refractive surgery can help assess for a predisposition toward dryness that likely would be worsened to some degree by blepharoplasty. Examination should also note any punctate staining, the presence or absence of a good Bell's reflex, as well as any preexisting upper or lower eyelid retraction or lower eyelid laxity.

Corneal Abrasions

Corneal abrasions may be avoided with careful attention to lubricating and/or protecting the corneal surfaces throughout surgery. If they do occur, however, they are treated with an antibiotic ointment to prevent bacterial superinfection and should resolve within 24 hours. Persistent signs or symptoms should prompt repeat ophthalmic examination.

Lagophthalmos

Lagophthalmos occurs frequently during the postoperative period, usually transiently as a result of postoperative pain, guarding, incomplete closure following local anesthetic to the orbicularis, or tethering from dressings such as Steri-Strips (3M, St. Paul, MN). Temporary lagophthalmos in the immediate postoperative period due to the causes listed above is usually amenable to lubrication with artificial tears and ointment at bedtime. However, lagophthalmos that persists in the late postoperative period is most often the result of over-resection of skin or incorporation of the orbital septum in skin closure resulting in retraction. Exposure due to inadequate eyelid closure is further worsened in the presence of a poor Bell's phenomenon (Fig. 22.5). If conservative lubrication and massage therapy fail, or if severe keratopathy or thinning necessitates intervention, surgical options include elevation of the lower eyelid to narrow the aperture from below, skin grafting to replace the deficient anterior lamella, release of orbital septal adhesions, or full-thickness blepharotomy.

Lower Eyelid Retraction/Malposition

Lower eyelid malposition is a common complication following lower eyelid blepharoplasty, more frequently encountered with transcutaneous approaches. In addition to a suboptimal aesthetic, lower eyelid malposition and eyelid retraction can cause decompensation of the ocular surface through excess exposure. Lid malposition is the result of an imbalance in lower eyelid forces. Abnormal negative vectors can result from excessive skin resection, cicatrization of the anterior and middle lamellae, and lateral canthal dystopia. Patients with a negative vector preoperatively may also be predisposed to lower eyelid retraction.

The incidence of lower eyelid malposition following transcutaneous blepharoplasty ranges in the literature from 3% to 32% and is well-known to occur in even the most skilled surgical hands [20, 21, 22]. By contrast, the transconjunctival approach circumvents many of these complications by avoiding an anterior and/or middle lamellar wound prone

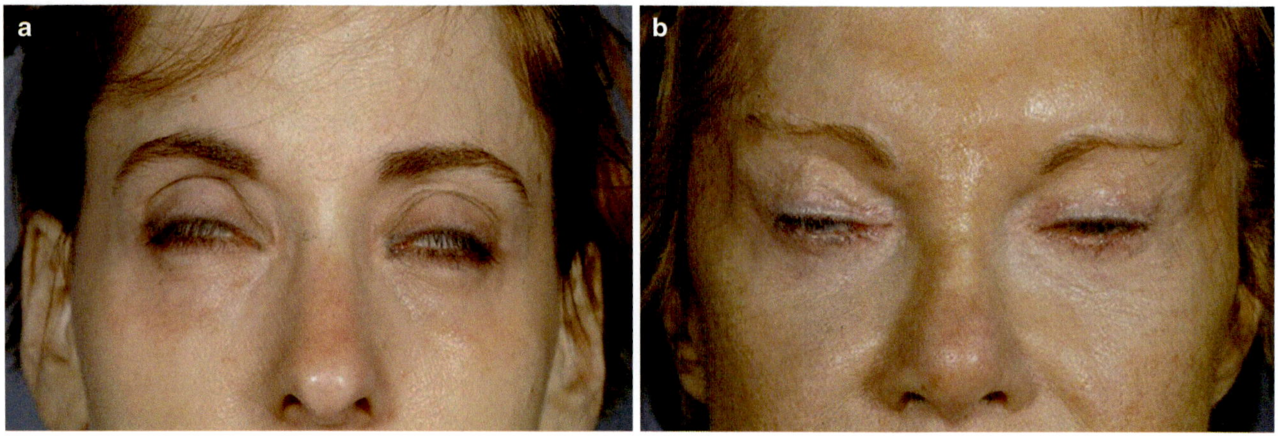

Fig. 22.5 The difference between a good (**a**) and poor (**b**) Bell's reflex is shown. Patients with a poor Bell's phenomenon are at increased risk for corneal epitheliopathy

to contracture and thereby retraction. Indeed, most series examining complications of transconjunctival blepharoplasty report the absence of lower lid retraction complications [19, 20, 21]. Interestingly, a recent article examining margin reflex distance 2 following transconjunctival blepharoplasty found the lower lid actually slightly *elevates* following surgery [23]. However, other complications such as granuloma formation are more common in transconjunctival blepharoplasty (Fig. 22.4) [20, 21], and the conjunctival approach in isolation does not address the excess skin and overriding orbicularis that are more common findings in the aged patient. As an alternative, many advocate the use of laser resurfacing [24] or chemical peels [25] for skin tightening in conjunction with transconjunctival blepharoplasty.

Preoperative identification of patients at risk for developing lower eyelid retraction is important, including globe prominence or myopia, hypoplasia of the malar eminence, and lower eyelid laxity. Laxity should be addressed at the time of surgery with tightening. Skin resections, when utilized, should be judicious.

Excessive skin resection inducing lower eyelid retraction is a well-recognized complication of transcutaneous lower eyelid blepharoplasty, which can induce ocular discomfort, chronic irritation, and exposure keratopathy in addition to an undesirable appearance. If recognized early in the postoperative period, sutures can be removed on day 2 or 3 and the wound gaped to allow for subsequent granulation. While not ideal cosmetically, it is sometimes still preferable over a severe ectropion requiring later skin grafting. Massage is needed throughout granulation to counter the inherent forces of contracture. A similar gaping technique may also be applied to upper eyelid retraction due to over-resection (Fig. 22.6). Unfortunately, not all anterior lamellar deficiency is recognized in the early postoperative period, but rather becomes evident in the late postoperative period. In these cases, one may observe lower eyelid movement/retraction upon opening of the mouth (Fig. 22.7). Surgical repair at this juncture often requires replacement of skin via a skin graft, frequently in conjunction with tarsal resuspension (Fig. 22.8a, b). Tarsal suspension may sometimes be performed in isolation in patients who do not wish to receive a skin graft, though patients should be counseled that this intervention may fail then ultimately requiring a skin graft (Fig. 22.8c, d).

Cicatrization of the middle lamellae can also cause additional downward force creating lower eyelid retraction. It may be diagnosed by attempting to stretch the central eyelid superiorly over the limbus. If resistance is encountered

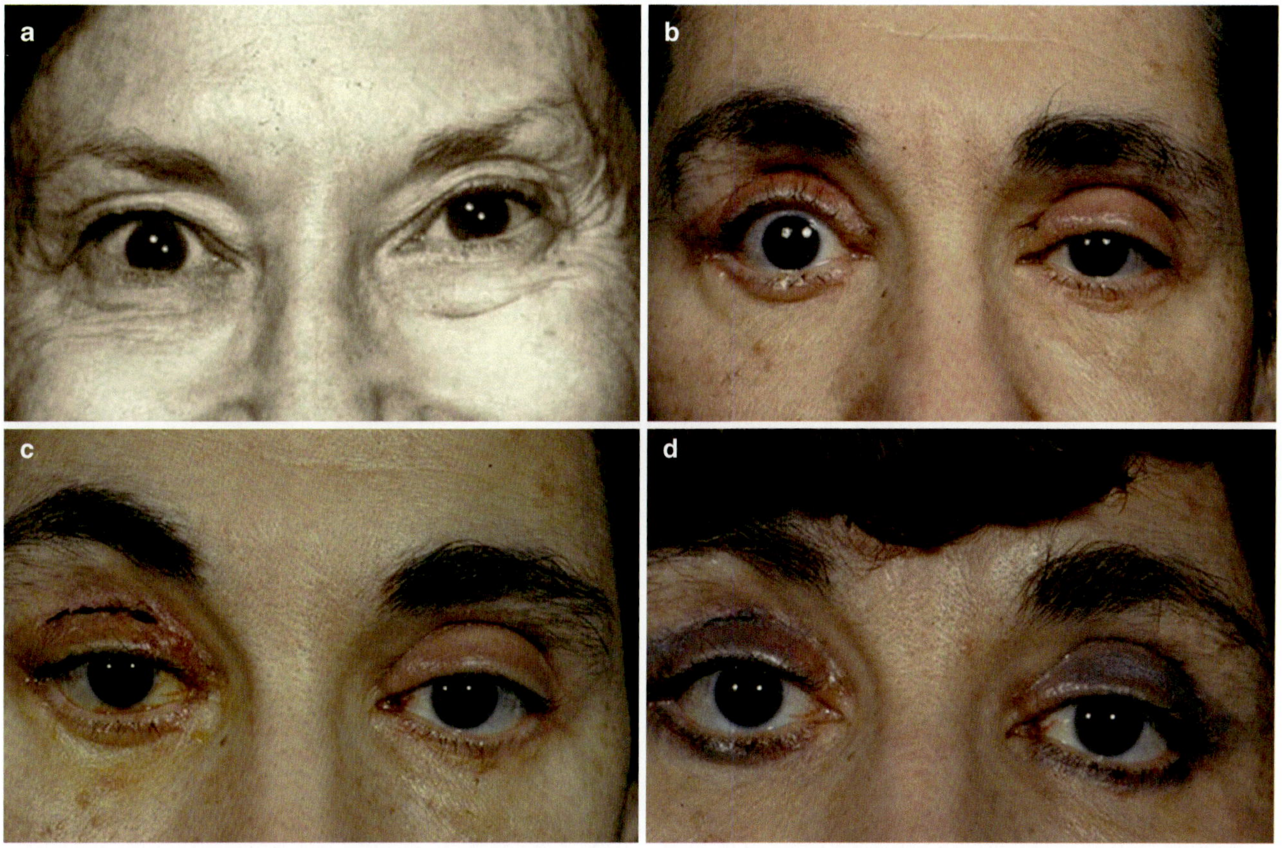

Fig. 22.6 A patient with undiagnosed thyroid ophthalmopathy with right upper eyelid retraction proceeds with upper lid blepharoplasty. Preoperative photograph (**a**) demonstrates mild asymmetry of the palpebral fissures with apparently minimal right upper eyelid retraction. One week postoperatively (**b**) the retraction is obvious and the wound is opened (**c**). After granulation, the appearance is reasonably symmetric at 3–4 weeks postoperatively (**d**)

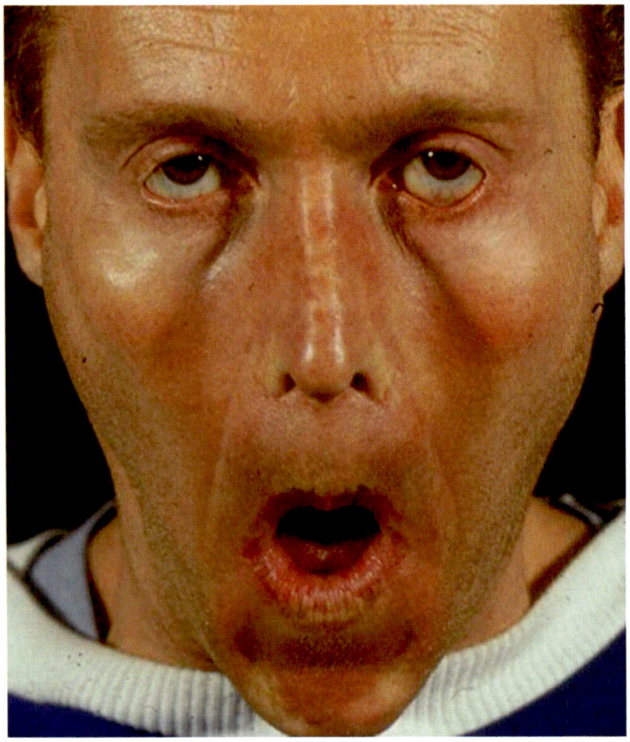

Fig. 22.7 Cicatricial lower eyelid retraction from excessive skin excision and anterior lamellar deficiency is best diagnosed by having the patient open their mouth and observing inferior excursion of the lower lids

prohibiting elevation, it is likely that adhesions at the level of the capsulopalpebral fascia and orbital septum are at least in part contributing to the overall lid malposition. Mild lid retraction may be managed conservatively with upward stretch, massage, and topical steroid ointment. When conservative measures fail, surgical repair requires lysis of the adhesions often in conjunction with a lateral fixation procedure. Occasionally, posterior lamellar lengthening may be necessary to fully correct the retraction. Hard palate, ear cartilage, and acellular dermis have all been used with success as posterior lamellar spacer grafts to help correct lower eyelid retraction following blepharoplasty (Fig. 22.8e, f) [26, 27].

Lateral canthal dystopia is most often the consequence of failure to address a preoperatively loose lower eyelid. The term "fishmouthing" has been used by some to describe the appearance of the postblepharoplasty eyelid with dehisced lateral canthal tendon [28]. In addition to the appearance of an aberrant blink, it also causes ocular discomfort and dry eye, underscoring the importance of preoperative evaluation of lateral canthal support. It should also be noted, however, that it is also possible to "misplace" a canthus while tightening it. This is less common with lateral retinacular suspension in which the canthus or canthal angle is never incised, but an unnatural vector is still achievable even with this minimal procedure.

Unmasking Prior Conditions

Finally, the unmasking of preexisting conditions can also lead to ocular surface breakdown following blepharoplasty. It is increasingly common, particularly in the cosmetically oriented population, to encounter patients who have had laser in situ keratomileusis (LASIK). Patients who have undergone LASIK have been found at increased risk of developing postoperative keratopathy following blepharoplasty [29]. Also worth mentioning is the patient with undiagnosed thyroid ophthalmopathy who undergoes blepharoplasty that unmasks eyelid retraction and keratopathy (Fig. 22.6). Proper screening for preexisting dry eye symptoms, history of LASIK, or other systemic illnesses predisposing to dryness (e.g., Sjogren's) as well as a careful examination for stigmata of thyroid ophthalmopathy will help to select appropriate surgical candidates and tailor one's surgical plan to avoid later complications.

Ptosis

While upper eyelid retraction is far more common, ptosis can occur following blepharoplasty. Often subtle levator dehiscence is present preoperatively but undiagnosed [30] as patients with extensive dermatochalasis can mask a reduced marginal reflex distance (Fig. 22.9). Postoperative ecchymosis or edema can also induce a mechanical ptosis. Most often, this resolves with time as the fluid and hemorrhage resorb and can be aided by cool compresses and a small burst of oral steroids if more significant. However, if the ptosis persists after resolution of the edema, it is possible that the edematous state precipitated levator attenuation. Persistent edema and its treatment are addressed elsewhere in the chapter.

Epiphora

Epiphora can arise from a number of etiologies and is, in fact, often multifactorial. As described in great length above, abnormalities leading to ocular surface decompensation (corneal abrasions, lagophthalmos, lower eyelid malposition, and preexisting propensities toward dry eye) will all cause epiphora. Additionally, an impaired lacrimal pump, punctal malposition, and canalicular damage can also cause epiphora. The superficial and deep heads of the medial canthal tendon (extensions of the pretarsal and preseptal orbicularis muscle) straddle the lacrimal sac and are responsible for pumping tears into a normally functioning lacrimal system. Postsurgical alteration in the action of these muscles can lead to a (usually) temporary pump dysfunction. If the problem persists, one should assess the patient for punctal malposition and lacrimal system obstruction, both of which would require additional surgery to correct.

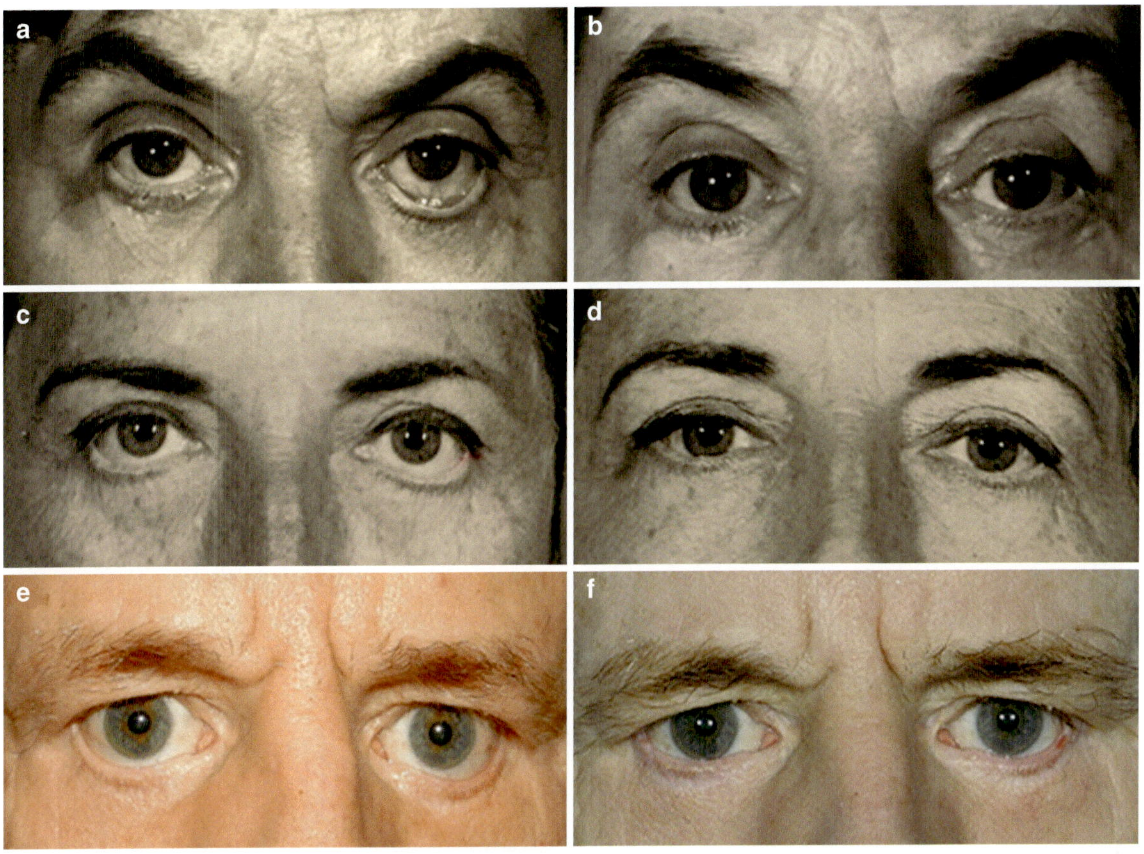

Fig. 22.8 Severe left lower eyelid retraction and ectropion following blepharoplasty before and after surgical repair with full-thickness posterior auricular skin graft and tarsal suspension (**a**, **b**); postblepharoplasty left lower eyelid retraction before and after surgical correction with tarsal suspension alone (**c**, **d**); bilateral postblepharoplasty lower eyelid retraction before and after surgical correction with bilateral hard palate grafts and tarsal suspension (**e**, **f**)

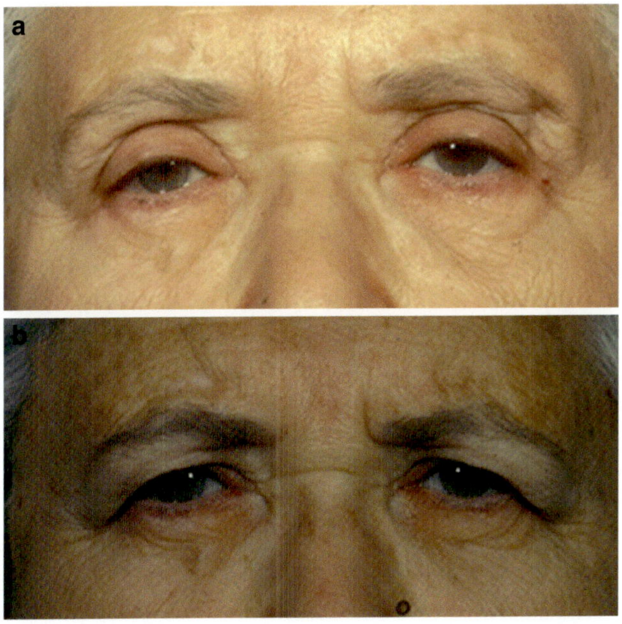

Fig. 22.9 Preoperative photo of a patient with concomitant dermatochalasis and aponeurotic ptosis (**a**) who underwent upper eyelid blepharoplasty without addressing the underlying ptotic eyelids (**b**). Not the residual blepharoptosis in the postoperative photo (**b**)

Chemosis

Conjunctival edema can result from a combination of inflammation and poor lymphatic drainage. Inflammation can occur intraoperatively or postoperatively and may be triggered by surgical trauma, allergy, infection, or underlying medical disorders such as renal failure and thyroid eye disease. Its increased occurrence has also been associated with blepharoplasties in which concomitant canthoplasty or canthopexy is performed [31]. Ultimately, the concern over chemosis is primarily related to its potential corneal sequelae. As edematous conjunctiva balloons around the cornea (due to its insertion at the limbus), tears are prevented from adequate dispersion on the corneal surface and can lead to dellen formation or keratopathy. If significant chemosis is observed intraoperatively, one may consider conjunctival plication or cutdown. Conservative treatment with artificial tears and ointment is usually sufficient (Fig. 22.10). However, more severe or refractory cases may be treated with topical phenylephrine (vasoconstriction), topical steroid, or even oral steroid. Rarely, 24 hour patching, a temporary lateral tarsorrhaphy, conjunctival cutdowns, or cauterization may be needed [30,

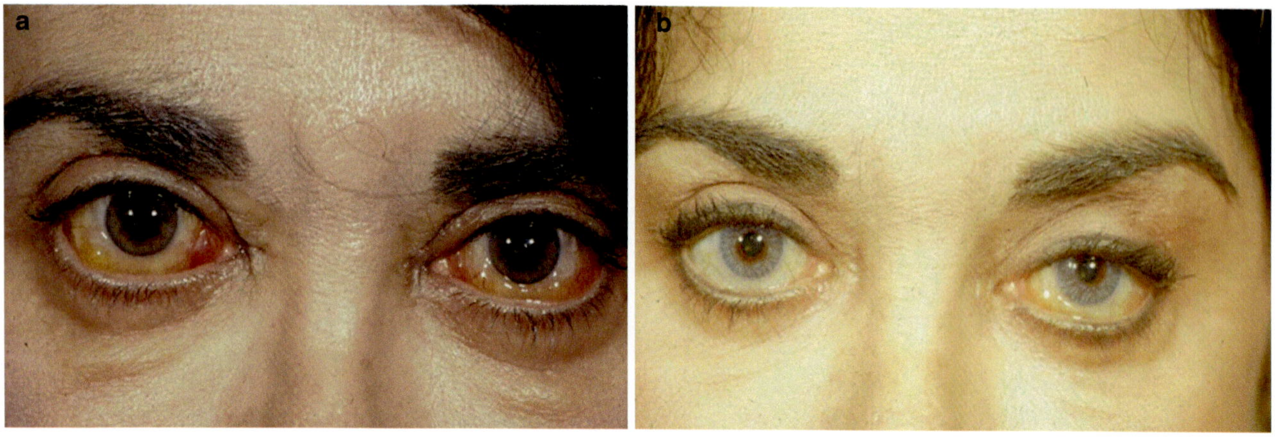

Fig. 22.10 A patient with chronic renal failure who developed postoperative chemosis following lower eyelid blepharoplasty (**a**). Lubrication and time allowed significant resolution of the chemosis over 6 months. Note that mild persistent chemotic conjunctiva is present and can be a management problem in patients with underlying thyroid or renal disease (**b**)

32]. More recently, radiowave needling has been used with success as a form of drainage and coagulation [33]. While significant variation in the use of these modalities exists from surgeon to surgeon, algorithms for the treatment of post-blepharoplasty chemosis have been proposed [28].

Strabismus

Diplopia is an uncommon yet potentially debilitating complication of blepharoplasty [34, 35]. Its causes are manifold and often transient. Disruption of the normal tear film commonly occurs following blepharoplasty and can cause intermittent monocular diplopia that clears with blinking. Alternatively, temporary muscle dysfunction can be caused by muscle contusion, hematoma, or edema. More persistent diplopia may, indeed, be the result of iatrogenic muscle injury (Fig. 22.11). Fat adherence syndrome has also been reported to mimic an inferior oblique injury following blepharoplasty [36]. Although the inferior oblique is most commonly associated with postblepharoplasty diplopia due to its susceptible location, injury to the inferior rectus and superior oblique is also possible [37, 38]. Damage may be the result of direct injury to the muscle or secondary to aggressive cautery which may cause thermal injury and microvascular compromise. In a large series of transconjunctival lower eyelid blepharoplasties, the overall risk of persistent strabismus following blepharoplasty was found to be approximately 0.2% [39].

Prevention of this complication involves, most importantly, experience with the anatomy of the extraocular muscles, particularly the inferior oblique's location between the nasal and central fat pads. Judicious use of cautery is also advocated [40]. The muscle may be visualized and avoided during surgery. Alternatively, if excising fat in a suspicious

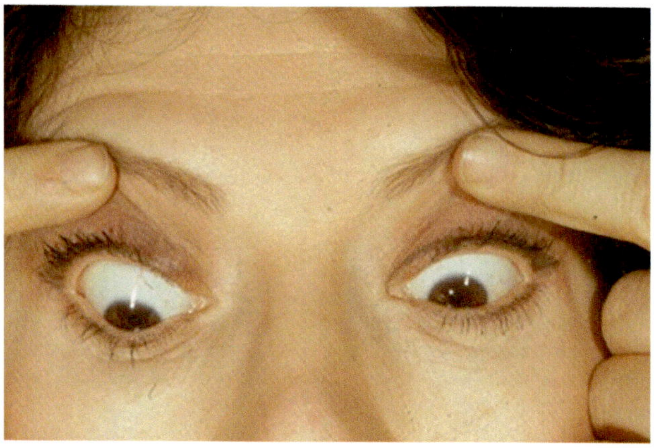

Fig. 22.11 Example of a patient with inferior oblique paresis following transconjunctival blepharoplasty

anatomic location, pulling on the fat prior to excision may reveal globe movement signifying proximity of the muscle that should be either bluntly dissected free of its attachments or avoided altogether.

Even in the setting of suspected iatrogenic muscle injury, initial treatment of postoperative diplopia is conservative. Often, the diplopia will resolve or improve. Fresnel prisms can help temporize the misalignment until it is clear that the misalignment is static. At this point, if diplopia persists, surgical correction should be considered, although successful treatment may be challenging [41].

Scarring/Pigmentation

While blepharoplasty skin incisions are typically well-concealed within the natural creases of the eyelid, any wound has the potential to cause pigmentation or texture changes.

Although rare, when these complications do arise, one may consider the supplemental use of dermabrasion, laser, intralesional kenalog, or 5-fluorouracil injections, depending on the type of scarring and baseline pigment of the skin [42]. While dermabrasion is decreasing in its use with the advent of laser resurfacing, it continues to be a reliable option in the nonpigmented patient for smoothing contours and matching skin tones. Intralesional kenalog continues to be used in the revision of hypertrophic scars, though is limited by its known side effects of hypopigmentation and soft tissue atrophy. A more recent trend toward the use of 5-fluorouracil injections for scar modification has shown promising results without associated hypopigmentation or atrophy but instead carries its own side effect profile that includes hyperpigmentation [43, 44, 45]. Surgical scar revision is rarely necessary but also always a viable option.

Persistent Pretarsal Edema and Malar Bags/ Festoons

Persistent edemas in the form of both pretarsal edema and malar bags or festoons are some of the more challenging postblepharoplasty complications to treat. In the case of persistent pretarsal edema, there are unfortunately no good predictors of its occurrence to be avoided in one's preoperative evaluation. Treatment modalities are also limited. The authors often first try an oral steroid. Intralesional steroid injection may also be considered; however, if some combinations of excess inflammatory response or poor lymphatic drainage are at play, an injection of any type may trigger the former and add to the fluid load of the latter. The authors have observed some successful intralesional treatments, and so, with appropriate patient counseling, it is certainly an option. Although not a definitive treatment of the underlying problem, persistent edema can also be treated with oral diuretics with potassium replacement (e.g., furosemide 40 mg) with the permission of the patient's primary care physician. This can provide significant, and relatively immediate, aesthetic benefit for those wishing to improve the edema for an important event.

Malar bags are similarly troublesome in their management. However, unlike pretarsal edema, there is often some evidence of malar bags or festoons that can be appreciate preoperatively. The best prevention of malar bags is thus to diagnose them preoperatively and recognize patients at increased risk. While the exact mechanism of malar mounds continues to be debated, it is most likely multifactorial including attenuated orbicular muscle (either due to senile change or chemodenervation [46]), orbitomalar stretching and descent of the lid/cheek junction, malar edema accumulation [47], and impaired lymphatic drainage. Patients with findings should be questioned about a history of thyroid disease, renal dysfunction, sinusitis, and allergies. Particularly in light of recent trends in injectable therapy, patients should be specifically asked whether they have ever had filler injected into their lower eyelids, as this has been associated with festoons, presumably due to a combination of the material's hydrophilicity as well as impaired lymphatic outflow [48]. Patients at increased risk for fluid accumulation should be counseled preoperatively of this risk and treated with intraoperative intravenous and postoperative oral steroids. Furosemide in the early postoperative period can also be helpful in reducing lymphatic load and ultimate accumulation (Fig. 22.12).

Treatment interventions for persistent festoons are varied, which the authors would argue reflects the absence of a modality that predictably treats this problem. Nonsurgical options include the use of laser resurfacing to create a controlled burn, which, if deep enough, may theoretically scar down the potential space in which fluid is collecting [49]. Recently, intralesional tetracyclines have also been used as a nonsurgical means of treating festoons [50]. Tetracyclines are well-known for their sclerosing properties and are used in the treatment of lymphatic malformations. Their use in festoons is based upon the notion that altered lymphatic drainage is contributing to their formation. The authors have similarly used intralesional doxycycline, which is more readily available through most hospital pharmacies and in our small (not-yet-reported) series of cases has similar effects to tetracycline (Fig. 22.13).

Surgical approaches are manifold and include liposuction, orbicularis suspension, skin muscle flaps, midface lifts, and direct excision [51, 52]. Treatment algorithms have been proposed [49], though consensus is still very much lacking.

Complications Associated with Concomitant Use of Injectables

With the increasing use of injectable agents in aesthetic facial rejuvenation, it is important to understand how these adjunctive procedures can affect and, in some occasions, complicate blepharoplasties. As mentioned above, malar edema can occur following periorbital injection and should be noted preoperatively and considered if performing concomitant procedures. Certain fillers are more hydrophilic than others and can be selected against in patients at particular risk. Also as briefly referenced in the preceding sections, neurotoxin to the lower eyelids has been associated with the formation of festoons [45]. The proposed mechanism for this finding is decreased orbicularis tone causing impaired muscular pumping action and, ultimately, accumulated lymphedema. Finally, one should always inquire about prior use of neurotoxin in the forehead and brow during preoperative evaluation for upper eyelid blepharoplasty as this can directly

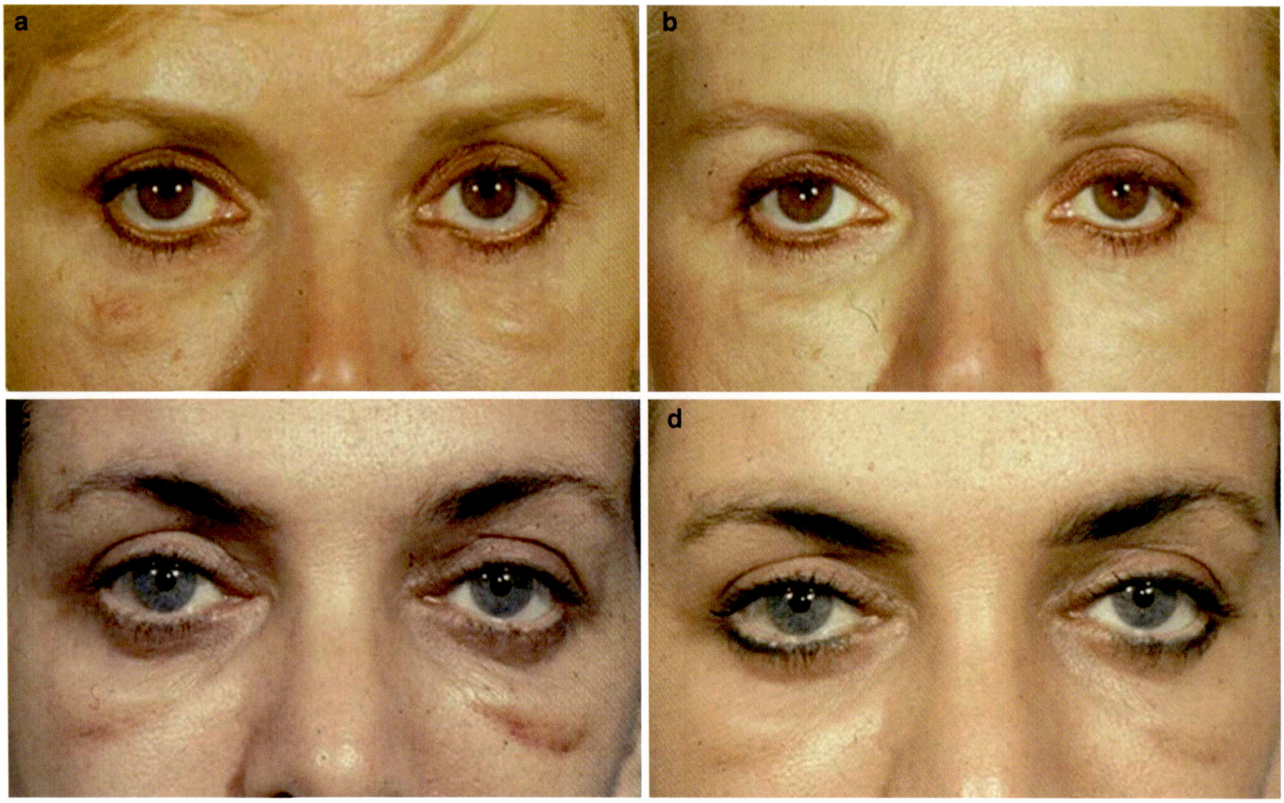

Fig. 22.12 Pre-treatment (**a**, **c**) and posttreatment (**b**, **d**) examples of malar bags responding to diuretic therapy. Each patient was treated with furosemide and potassium replacement

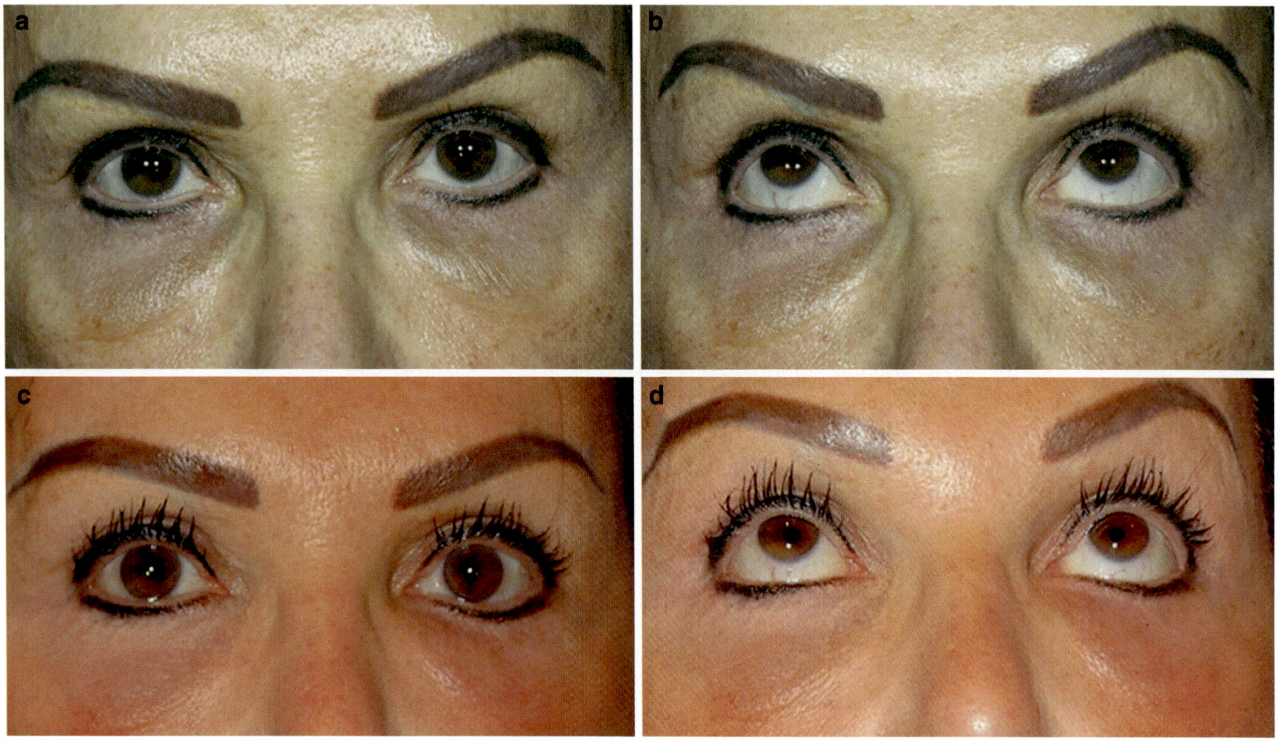

Fig. 22.13 Pre-treatment primary (**a**) and upgaze (**b**) demonstrate significant bilateral festoons. Two months after one injection of intralesional doxycycline (10 mg/ml × 1 ml to each festoon) demonstrates interval improvement (**c**, **d**)

affect brow position and thereby the amount of dermatochalasis. Some patients may be on a consistent and stable schedule of injections, maintaining their brow at a certain position. Those patients should merely be counseled that the evaluation is based on this brow position and any future surgery should be performed on whatever regimen they use (provided they are happy with the result and intend to continue). Other patients, however, may have had a new injection pattern or may not plan to continue with injections, in which case both the evaluation and surgery should be performed once the neurotoxin has completely worn off.

Summary

Although blepharoplasty is a commonly performed and relatively straightforward procedure, even the most gifted of surgeons will encounter complications. Careful preoperative evaluation, meticulous surgical decision-making, and prompt recognition and treatment of adverse events will minimize their occurrence and magnitude.

References

1. DeMere M, Wood T, Austin W. Eye complications with blepharoplasty or other eyelid surgery. Natl Surv Plast Reconstr Surg. 1974;53(6):634–7.
2. Hass AN, Penne RB, Stefanyszyn MA, Flanagan JC. Incidence of postblepharoplasty orbital hemorrhage and associated visual loss. Ophthal Plast Reconstr Surg. 2004;20(6):426–32.
3. Teng CC, Reddy S, Wong JJ, Lisman RD. Retrobulbar hemorrhage nine days after cosmetic blepharoplasty resulting in permanent visual loss. Ophthal Plast Reconstr Surg. 2006;22(5):388–9.
4. Liu CY, Samimi DB, Tao JP. Hemorrhagic complications of rivaroxaban after eyelid surgery. Ophthal Plast Reconstr Surg. 2016;32(1):74.
5. Anderson RL, Georgescu D, Vagefi MR, McMullan TF, Burroughs JR, McCann JD. To patch or not to patch? That is the question. Arch Facial Plast Surg. 2007;9(4):290–2.
6. Lee KY, Tow S, Fong KS. Visual recovery following emergent orbital decompression in traumatic retrobulbar haemorrhage. Ann Acad Med Singap. 2006;35(11):831–2.
7. Parikh M, Kwon YH. Vision loss after inadvertent corneal perforation during lid anesthesia. Ophthal Plast Reconstr Surg. 2011;27(5):e141–2.
8. Darlington JK, Lee WB, Schwab IR. Corneal perforation during laser blepharoplasty. Ophthalmic Surg Lasers Imaging. 2006;37(4):327–9.
9. Bleyen I, Rademaker R, Wolfs RC, van Rij G. Acute angle closure glaucoma after oculoplastic surgery. Orbit. 2008;27(1):49–50.
10. Haverals K, Augustinus A, Hondeghem K. Bilateral acute angle-closure glaucoma after blepharoplasty. Bull Soc Belge Ophtalmol. 2010;316:59–61.
11. Kordic H, Flammer J, Mironow A, Killer HE. Perioperative posterior ischemic optic neuropathy as a rare complication of blepharoplasty. Ophthalmologica. 2005;219(3):185–8.
12. Good CD, Cassidy LM, Moseley IF, Sanders MD. Posterior optic nerve infarction after lower lid blepharoplasty. J Neuroophthalmol. 1999;19(3):176–9.
13. Chiu ES, Capell BC, Press R, Aston SJ, Jelks EB, Jelks GW. Successful management of orbital cellulitis and temporary visual loss after blepharoplasty. Plast Reconstr Surg. 2006;118(3):67e–72e.
14. Goldberg RA, Li TG. Postoperative infection with group A beta-hemolytic Streptococcus after blepharoplasty. Am J Ophthalmol. 2002;134(6):908–10.
15. Lazzeri D, Agostini T. Eyelid and periorbital necrotizing fasciitis as an early devastating complication of blepharoplasty. Plast Reconstr Surg. 2010;126(3):1112–3.
16. Kuipers T. Prophylactic antibiotics in plastic and reconstructive surgery. Plast Reconstr Surg. 2000;105:815–6.
17. Fay A, Nallasamy N, Pemberton JD, Callahan A, Wladis EJ, Nguyen J, Durand ML, New England Oculoplastics Society Study Group. Prophylactic postoperative antibiotics for enucleation and evisceration. Ophthal Plast Reconstr Surg. 2013;29(4):281–5.
18. Belinsky I, Patel P, Charles NC, Lisman RD. Ointment granulomas following sutureless transconjunctival blepharoplasty: diagnosis and management. Ophthal Plast Reconstr Surg. 2015;31(4):282–6.
19. Hamawy AH, Farkas JP, Fagien S, Rohrich RJ. Preventing and managing dry eyes after periorbital surgery: a retrospective review. Plast Reconstr Surg. 2009;123(1):353–9.
20. Baylis HI, Long JA, Groth MJ. Transconjunctival lower eyelid blepharoplasty. Technique and complications. Ophthalmology. 1989;96(7):1027–32.
21. Perkins SW, Dyer WK 2nd, Simo F. Transconjunctival approach to lower eyelid blepharoplasty. Experience, indications, and technique in 300 patients. Arch Otolaryngol Head Neck Surg. 1994;120(2):172–7.
22. Pacella SJ, Nahai FR, Nahai F. Transconjunctival blepharoplasty for upper and lower eyelids. Plast Reconstr Surg. 2010;125(1):384–92.
23. Segal KL, Patel P, Levine B, Lisman RD, Lelli GJ. The effect of transconjunctival blepharoplasty on margin reflex distance 2. Aesthet Plast Surg. 2016;40(1):13–8.
24. Carter SR, Seiff SR, Choo PH, Vallabhanath P. Lower eyelid CO(2) laser rejuvenation: a randomized, prospective clinical study. Ophthalmology. 2001;108(3):437–41.
25. McKinney P, Zukowski ML, Mossie R. The fourth option: a novel approach to lower-lid blepharoplasty. Aesthet Plast Surg. 1991;15(4):293–6.
26. Li TG, Shorr N, Goldberg RA. Comparison of the efficacy of hard palate grafts with acellular human dermis grafts in lower eyelid surgery. Plast Reconstr Surg. 2005;116(3):873–8; discussion 879–80.
27. Baylis H, Perman K, Fett DR, Sutcliffe RT. Autogenous auricular cartilage grafting for lower eyelid retraction. Ophthal Plast Reconstr Surg. 1985;1(1):23–7.
28. McCord CD, Miotto GC. Dynamic diagnosis of "fishmouthing" syndrome, an overlooked complication of blepharoplasty. Aesthet Surg J. 2013;33(4):497–504.
29. Korn BS, Kikkawa DO, Schanzlin DJ. Blepharoplasty in the post-laser in situ keratomileusis patient: preoperative considerations to avoid dry eye syndrome. Plast Reconstr Surg. 2007;119(7):2232–9.
30. Lowry JC, Bartley GB. Complications of blepharoplasty. Surv Ophthalmol. 1994;38(4):327–50.
31. McCord CD, Kreymerman P, Nahai F, Walrath JD. Management of postblepharoplasty chemosis. Aesthet Surg J. 2013;33(5):654–61.
32. Weinfeld AB, Burke R, Codner MA. The comprehensive management of chemosis following cosmetic lower blepharoplasty. Plast Reconstr Surg. 2008;122(2):579–86.
33. Woo KI, Choi CY. High-frequency radiowave electrosurgery for persistent conjunctival chemosis following cosmetic blepharoplasty. Plast Reconstr Surg. 2014;133(6):1336–42.
34. Hayworth RS, Lisman RD, Muchnick RS, Smith B. Diplopia following blepharoplasty. Ann Ophthalmol. 1984;16(5):448–51.
35. Syniuta LA, Goldberg RA, Thacker NM, Rosenbaum AL. Acquired strabismus following cosmetic blepharoplasty. Plast Reconstr Surg. 2003;111(6):2053–9.

36. Jameson NA, Good WV, Hoyt CS. Fat adherence simulating inferior oblique palsy following blepharoplasty. Arch Ophthalmol. 1992;110:1369.
37. Wesley RE, Pollard ZF, McCord CD Jr. Superior oblique paresis after blepharoplasty. Plast Reconstr Surg. 1980;66(2):283–6.
38. Harley RD, Nelson LB, Flanagan JC, Calhoun JH. Ocular motility disturbances following cosmetic blepharoplasty. Arch Ophthalmol. 1986;104(4):542–4.
39. Ghabrial R, Lisman RD, Kane MA, Milite J, Richards R. Diplopia following transconjunctival blepharoplasty. Plast Reconstr Surg. 1998;102(4):1219–25.
40. Ortiz-Basso T, Vigo R, Prémoli EJ. Horizontal diplopia following upper blepharoplasty. Case Rep Ophthalmol. 2014;5(3):289–91.
41. Mazow ML, Avilla CW, Morales HJ. Restrictive horizontal strabismus following blepharoplasty. Am J Ophthalmol. 2006;141(4):773–4.
42. Kerwin LY, El Tal AK, Stiff MA, Fakhouri TM. Scar prevention and remodeling: a review of the medical, surgical, topical and light treatment approaches. Int J Dermatol. 2014;53(8):922–36.
43. Gupta S, Kalra A. Efficacy and safety of intralesional 5-fluorouracil in the treatment of keloids. Dermatology. 2002;204:130–2.
44. Ledon JA, Savas J, Franca K, Chacon A, Nouri K. Intralesional treatment for keloids and hypertrophic scars: a review. Dermatol Surg. 2013;39(12):1745–57.
45. Yoo DB, Azizzadeh B, Massry GG. Injectable 5-FU with or without added steroid in periorbital skin grafting: initial observations. Ophthal Plast Reconstr Surg. 2015;31(2):122–6.
46. Goldman MP. Festoon formation after infraorbital botulinum A toxin: a case report. Dermatol Surg. 2003;29:560–1.
47. Pessa JE, Garza JR. The malar septum: the anatomic basis of malar mounds and malar edema. Aesthetic Surg J. 1997;17:11–7.
48. Petris C, Eviatar J, Lisman R. Filler problems: complications of periocular injection. In: Foad Nahai, editor. Problems in oculoplastic surgery: a repair manual. Thieme, New York: CRC Press; 2018.
49. Scheiner AJ, Baker SS. Laser treatment of festoons. In: Massry G, et al., editors. Master techniques in blepharoplasty and periorbital rejuvenation. New York: Springer; 2011.
50. Perry JD, Mehta VJ, Costin BR. Intralesional tetracycline injection for treatment of lower eyelid festoons: a preliminary report. Ophthal Plast Reconstr Surg. 2015;31(1):50–2.
51. Liapakis IE, Paschalis EI. Liposuction and suspension of the orbicularis oculi for the correction of persistent malar bags: description of technique and report of a case. Aesthet Plast Surg. 2012;36:546–9.
52. Kpodzo DS, Nahai F, McCord CD. Malar mounds and festoons: review of current management. Aesthet Surg J. 2014;34(2):235–48.

23 Blepharoplasty in Asian Patients

Michael T. Yen

Introduction

Asian blepharoplasty is a term that has greater meaning than simply upper eyelid blepharoplasty in an Asian patient [1]. Historically in Western countries, the term has often referred to changing the appearance of the Asian eyelid to an Occidental eyelid [2]. This could often be achieved with the creation of a high eyelid crease and deep superior sulcus and elimination of the epicanthal fold. However, as aesthetic surgery has become more popular in Asian countries, the term now often refers to creating a "double-eyelid" appearance [1–4]. Furthermore, with the globalization of cultures and interracial relationships, traditional "Asian" eyelid features are becoming more prevalent in many regions of the world where the patients may not consider themselves to be of Asian heritage. Therefore, it is perhaps more appropriate to think of Asian blepharoplasty as surgery in an upper eyelid that has these traditionally "Asian" features characterized by an epicanthal fold, lower eyelid crease, and supratarsal fullness.

As with most surgical procedures, the key steps in successful Asian blepharoplasty occur before the first skin incision is made. The most important part of the preoperative assessment is to determine the aesthetic goals of the patient. An Occidental eyelid appearance can often result in patient dissatisfaction despite perfectly successful surgery. While this may be the desired appearance for some patients, many Asian patients do not desire the deep superior sulcus and high eyelid crease that is often associated with the Occidental eyelid. Yet when some Asian patients present for surgical evaluation, they express their desire for the "double-eyelid" appearance to be synonymous with the Occidental eyelid. Discordant expectations between surgeon and patient can often be avoided with a thorough and thoughtful preoperative discussion with the patient that identifies their unique anatomical features and their desired postoperative appearance. This can be challenging if cultural or language barriers limit the preoperative discussion but must be accomplished if a successful outcome is to be achieved. The patient's aesthetic goals will also dictate the surgical parameters such as the position of the eyelid crease, size of the supratarsal fold, degree of fullness in the superior sulcus, and the extent of the epicanthal fold. Additionally, differences in eyelid shape, height, contour, and anatomy require an individualistic, rather than "cookbook," approach to surgery.

Anatomy of the Asian Eyelid

Comparisons of the characteristic Asian and Occidental upper eyelids underscore significant variations in anatomy [5]. In the Occidental eyelid, the levator aponeurosis and orbital septum intersect and insert on the superior aspect of the tarsus, some 8–10 mm above the lid margin. At a similar height, anterior projections of the levator attach to the overlying dermis creating a well-defined lid crease. In the Asian eyelid, the levator likewise inserts on the superior aspect of the tarsus. The septum, however, inserts more inferiorly along the anterior surface of the tarsus, and the anterior projections of the levator to the dermis occur closer to the eyelid margin or may be absent. Preaponeurotic orbital fat is allowed to descend further inferiorly creating a fuller eyelid appearance. In addition, there is more subcutaneous fat in the Asian eyelid, while in Caucasians and African-Americans, there is essentially no subcutaneous fat (Fig. 23.1). An additional feature of the Asian upper eyelid is a prominent epicanthal fold (Fig. 23.2). The epicanthus tarsalis gives the eyelid a unique and distinct appearance, and retention of the epicanthal fold is often necessary to

M. T. Yen (✉)
Cullen Eye Institute, Baylor College of Medicine, Houston, TX, USA

Alkek Eye Center, Baylor College of Medicine, Houston, TX, USA
e-mail: myen@bcm.edu

A. J. Cohen, C. N. Burkat (eds.), *Oculofacial, Orbital, and Lacrimal Surgery*, https://doi.org/10.1007/978-3-030-14092-2_23

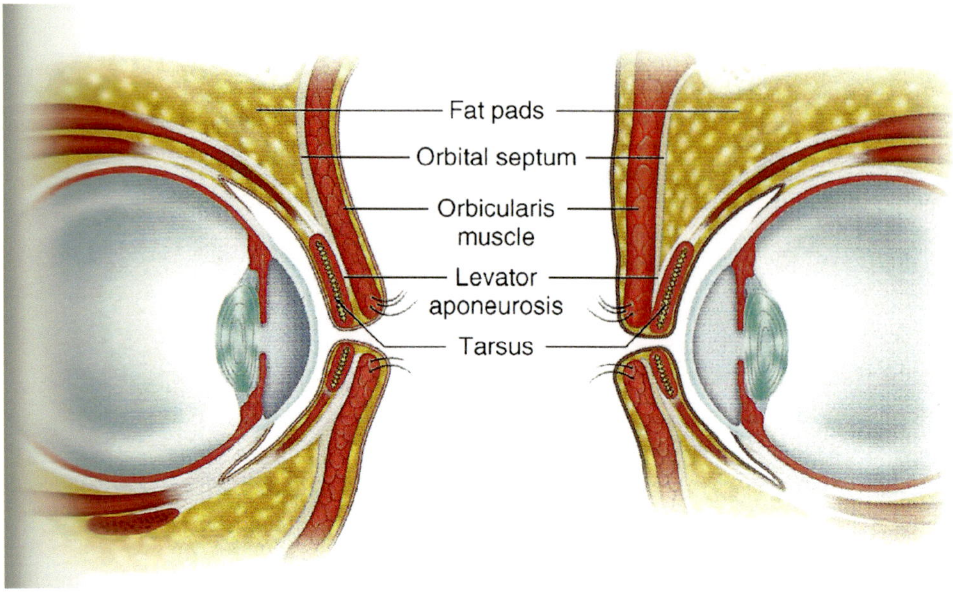

Fig. 23.1 Anatomical differences between the Asian (right side) and Occidental eyelid (left side). In the Asian eyelid, the orbital septum attaches to the anterior tarsal surface allowing preaponeurotic fat to extend more inferiorly and creating a fuller appearance. Additionally, there is more subcutaneous fat in the Asian eyelid. (Figure from Hartstein ME, Massry GG, Holds JB, eds. Pearls and Pitfalls in Cosmetic Oculoplastic Surgery, Fig. 40.5, page 137, Springer)

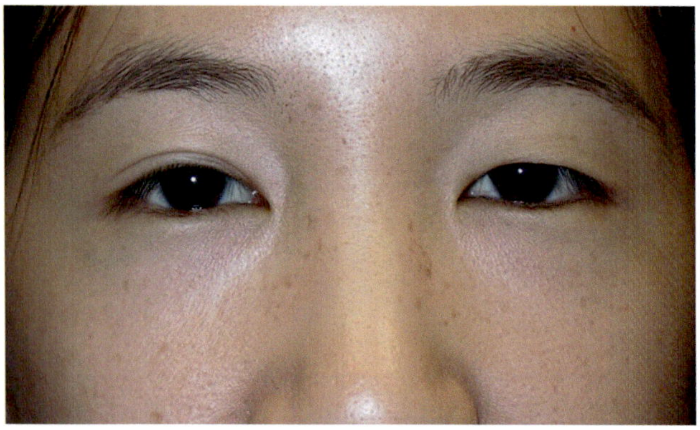

Fig. 23.2 The epicanthal fold gives the Asian eyelid its unique and distinctive appearance. In this patient with congenital asymmetry of the eyelid crease, both the double eyelid (right upper eyelid) and single eyelid (left upper eyelid) still retain an Asian appearance due to the epicanthal fold

retain an Asian eyelid appearance. The epicanthal fold can override the medial canthus and caruncle and give the impression of a widened nasal bridge, although true telecanthus is not present.

Even among Asian patients, there are different configurations to the eyelid anatomy. Type I Asian eyelids are characterized by an eyelid crease with a pretarsal platform that gives a double-eyelid appearance. Type II eyelids are characterized by an eyelid crease, but the pretarsal platform is covered by the supratarsal fold that extends to the eyelid margin. This results in a single-eyelid appearance in primary gaze. Type III eyelids are characterized by a very low or no eyelid crease and a single-eyelid appearance. Recognizing the correct anatomical configuration is necessary before determining the appropriate surgical technique for eyelid surgery (Fig. 23.3).

Surgical Technique

The technical steps of surgery in the Asian eyelid are no different than in the Occidental eyelid. However, in Asian blepharoplasty, particular attention should be given to the placement of the eyelid crease incision, the amount of skin excision and fat contouring, and determining the need for epicanthoplasty. These factors are determined mostly by the patient's aesthetic goals and expectations, though underlying anatomical factors may also dictate the specific surgical approach or technique utilized (Table 23.1).

Creating the Eyelid Crease

The first decision in Asian blepharoplasty is to determine if an eyelid crease can be created by the suture technique versus an open incisional technique. Often, when the only goal is to create or modestly elevate the eyelid crease and no skin excision is required, using the suture technique is adequate. This non-incisional technique was originally described in 1896 by Mikamo where three full-thickness silk sutures were placed through the upper eyelid and removed after 4–6 days [6]. The success of this procedure is dependent on adhesions developing to firmly fixate the skin at the lid crease line down to the underlying tarsus or levator. The development of these adhesions can be enhanced with the use of absorbable sutures, such as 6-0 chromic gut suture, as they stimulate a more significant inflammatory response compared to permanent sutures. Additionally, passing the suture for the full width of the eyelid crease, either as separate interrupted sutures or with a running horizontal mattress, allows greater control of the resulting eyelid crease contour.

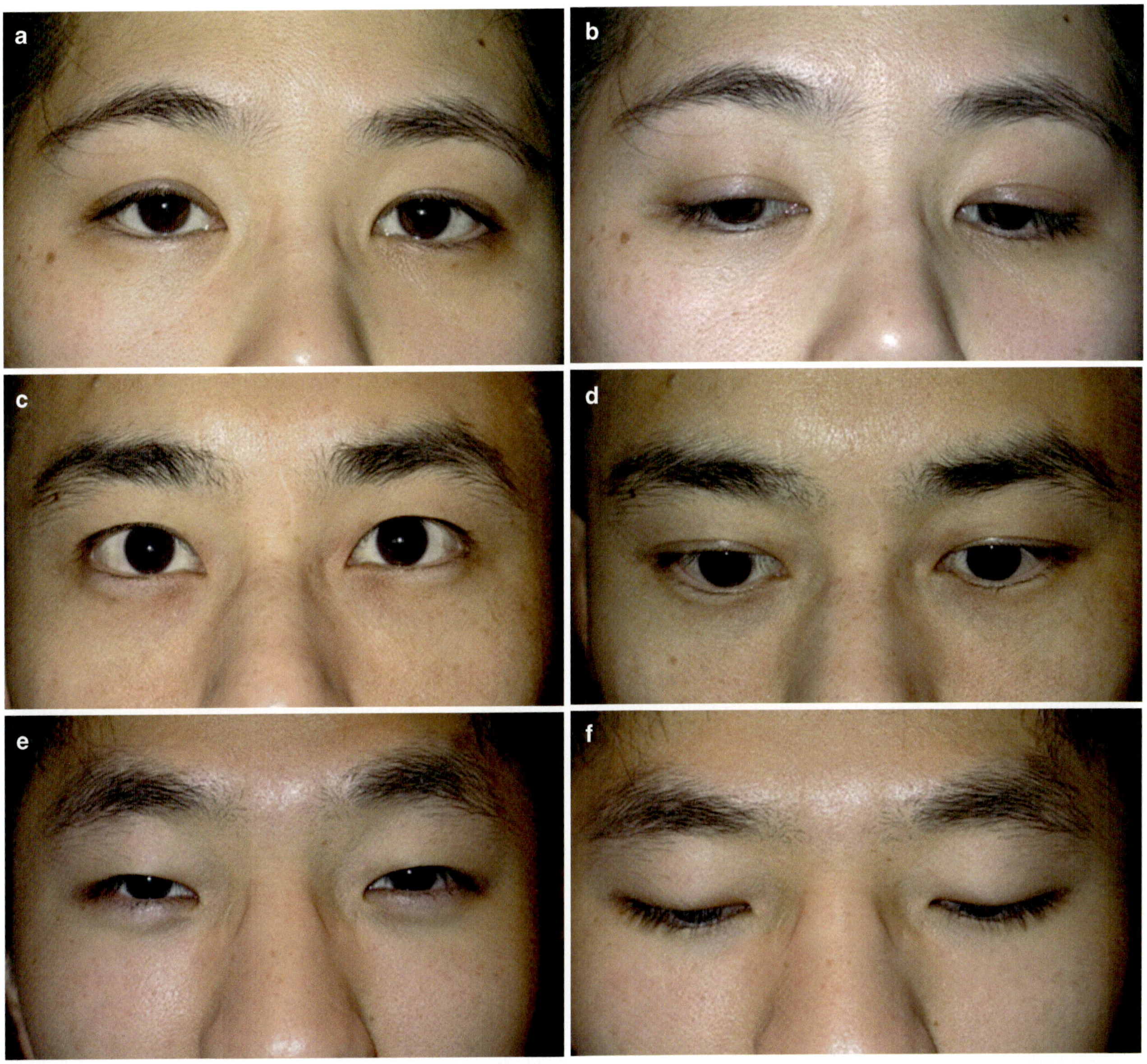

Fig. 23.3 Three anatomical configurations of the Asian eyelid. (**a**) Type I: The Asian double eyelid with the pretarsal eyelid distinctly visible. (**b**) In downgaze, the eyelid crease is visible in the Asian double eyelid. (**c**) Type II: The Asian single eyelid with crease. Note that the supratarsal fold extends down to the eyelid margin. (**d**) In downgaze, the eyelid crease is visible in the Asian single eyelid with crease. (**e**) Type III: The Asian single eyelid without crease. Note that there is no supratarsal fold as the eyelid crease is nonexistent or very low toward the eyelid margin. (**f**) In downgaze, no eyelid crease is identifiable in the Asian single eyelid without crease

Table 23.1 Suggestions for Asian blepharoplasty based on eyelid anatomy

Eyelid anatomy	Typical surgical goals	Surgical technique	Lid crease position	Skin excision	Fat excision	Epicanthal fold
Type I	Make double eyelid more visible, raise lid crease, or reduce size of supratarsal fold	Suture or incisional technique	Use existing crease or position slightly higher	Small skin excision	Minimal fat excision	Epicanthoplasty may be required depending on how high the lid crease is positioned and how much skin is excised
Type II	Make double eyelid visible and reduce size of supratarsal fold	Incisional technique usually required	Use existing crease or position slightly higher	Moderate skin excision	Minimal fat excision	Epicanthoplasty usually required to soften or eliminate epicanthal fold
Type III	Create an eyelid crease and double eyelid	Suture or incisional technique with longer-lasting sutures	Low, approximately 3–5 mm above lid margin	Usually no skin excision or minimal skin excision	No fat excision	Epicanthoplasty usually not required unless lid crease incision placed higher

The advantage of the non-incisional technique is a short operative time, minimal bruising, faster postoperative recovery, and minimal scarring. This procedure is most appropriate for younger patients where age-related dermatochalasis is minimal and skin excision is not required. The suture technique is not appropriate, however, when fatty contouring or skin excision is required or when significant elevation of the eyelid crease or a high placement of the eyelid crease is desired as this could potentially result in excessive accentuation of the epicanthal fold [4].

When an open incisional approach is to be performed, a critical step in blepharoplasty surgery occurs before anesthetic injection or skin incisions are made, this being the marking of the eyelid. Typically, in type I or type II Asian eyelids, the natural eyelid crease is marked representing the inferior incision location. Even if a truly Occidental eyelid appearance with a high lid crease and deep superior sulcus is desired, an incision located within the natural crease minimizes the likelihood of developing multiple eyelid creases or skin folds after blepharoplasty. However, there are exceptions to this when the surgeon and patient may wish to create an alternate lid crease position such as when the creases are asymmetric between the two eyelids. In type III Asian eyelids, where the lid crease is very low or nonexistent, a new location for the eyelid crease must be determined. Usually a low position for the incision, approximately 3–4 mm above the eyelid margin, will achieve a desirable "double-eyelid" appearance without excessive accentuation of the epicanthal fold (Fig. 23.4). As a general rule, it is easier to raise rather than lower a lid crease; therefore caution must be taken in placement of the incision as an excessively high eyelid crease will often look unnatural in an Asian patient.

Upper Eyelid Skin Excision

Once the eyelid crease incision marking is made, the surgeon must determine the amount of eyelid skin to remove and make the superior marking. Due to the typically lower eyelid crease position in the Asian eyelid, more skin needs to be retained on the eyelid to allow for adequate eyelid closure, and therefore less supratarsal skin should be excised compared to blepharoplasty in an Occidental eyelid (Fig. 23.5). With an eyelid crease close to the lid margin, even a small amount of redundant skin can creep over the lid margin or obscure the eyelash base and give the appearance of untreated dermatochalasis. Aggressively removing excess skin in this situation has the potential to produce significant lagophthalmos. The amount of skin excised is ultimately determined by the underlying eyelid configuration and the desired postoperative appearance. For example, no skin excision or minimal skin excision is typically necessary when a "double-eyelid" appearance is desired in a type III eyelid.

Fat Excision and Contouring

Due to the lower descent of preaponeurotic fat, the Asian eyelid is typically characterized by fullness in the superior sulcus. Excessive fat excision during blepharoplasty can result in notable deepening of the superior sulcus, a smaller supratarsal fold, and loss of the "double-eyelid" appearance. In most cases of Asian blepharoplasty, only minimal fat contouring is advisable to allow visualization and access to the underlying levator aponeurosis. In older patients, age-related fat prolapse may necessitate additional fat excision and contouring. However, caution is advised to avoid removing too much fat which may

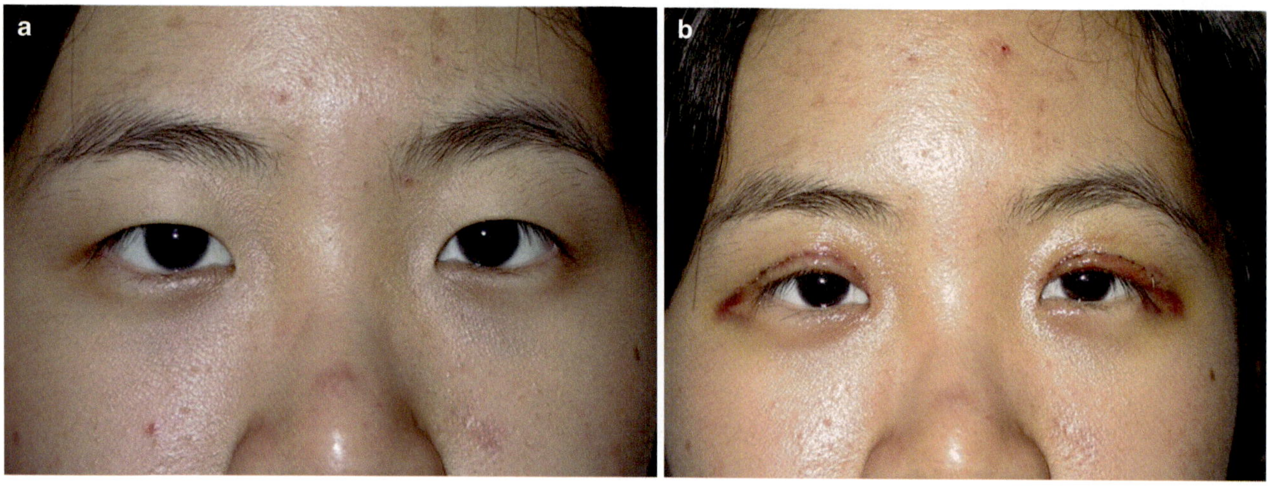

Fig. 23.4 (**a**) Type III Asian eyelid with no lid crease before blepharoplasty. (**b**) After incisional blepharoplasty now with double-eyelid appearance. The low eyelid crease incision was created at 3 mm, and no epicanthoplasty was needed

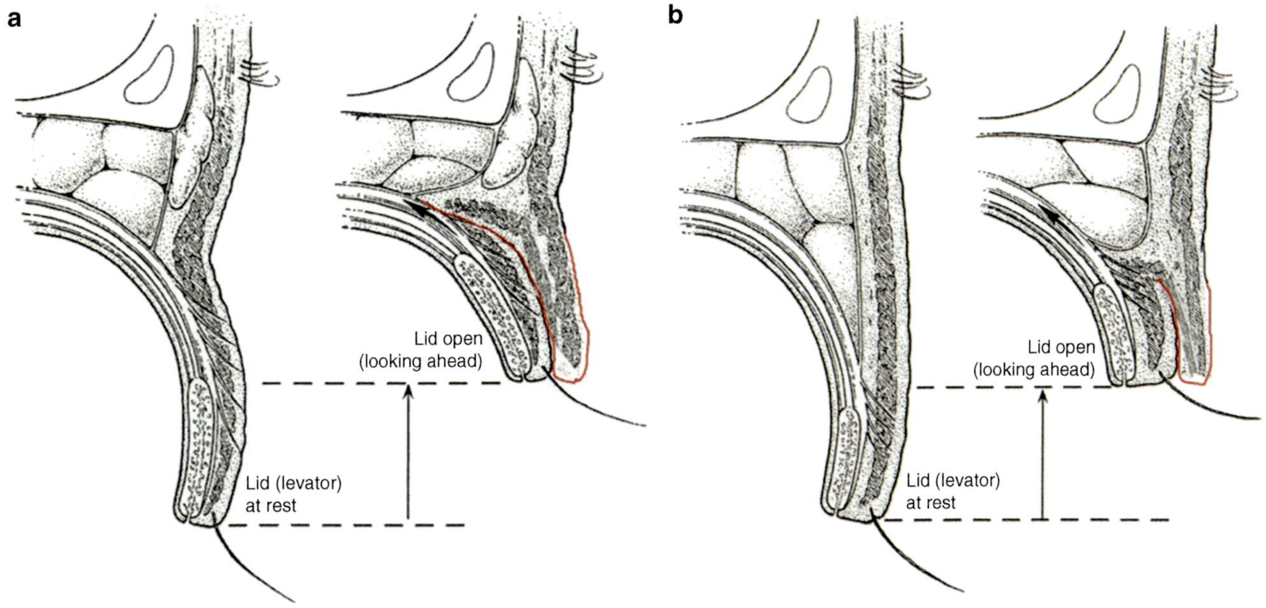

Fig. 23.5 Schematics demonstrating the amount of excisable skin (outlined in red) above the eyelid crease incision when the supratarsal fold extends to the eyelid margin in (**a**) an Occidental eyelid and (**b**) an Asian eyelid. Note that despite a similar size of the supratarsal fold, due to the lower eyelid crease position in the Asian eyelid, there is less excisable skin

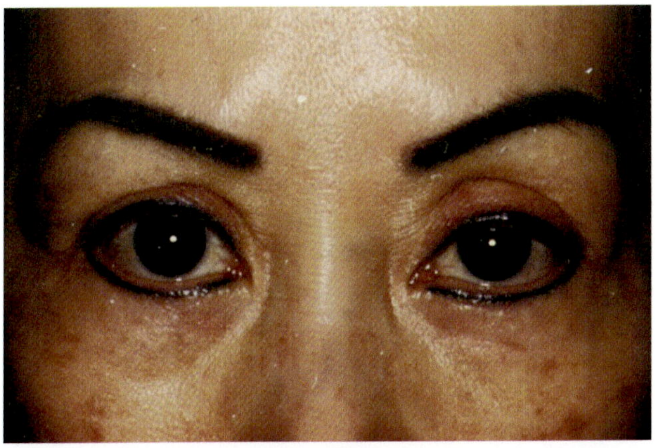

Fig. 23.6 High eyelid crease and deep superior sulcus after Asian blepharoplasty with excessive fat excision

result in excessive deepening of the superior sulcus and loss of the Asian eyelid characteristics (Fig. 23.6). If an aesthetically unacceptable amount of residual fat remains after blepharoplasty, this can be easily contoured and excised in a separate procedure; however, if excessive fat is removed during the primary blepharoplasty procedure, postoperative volume augmentation can be challenging and unpredictable.

The Epicanthal Fold

The final feature of the Asian eyelid that requires attention during blepharoplasty surgery is the epicanthal fold. Depending on the underlying eyelid anatomy, the placement of the eyelid crease, and the amount of skin excision, epicanthoplasty may or may not be necessary. Since most Asian patients still desire some Asian eyelid features after blepharoplasty, complete elimination of the epicanthal fold is usually not necessary. However, blepharoplasty can often accentuate the epicanthal fold, and softening the fold may be necessary to achieve a more natural postoperative appearance.

Epicanthoplasty can be performed by a number of ways. Common procedures include various modifications of Z-plasty and Y-V advancement procedures [7–9]. In these approaches, flaps are elevated and transposed to bring additional length to the medial canthal region and allow the epicanthal fold to be flattened. These transposition-style procedures are very effective and powerful and should be considered when complete elimination or significant softening of the epicanthal fold is desired (Fig. 23.7). A disadvantage of all of these transposition procedures, however, is that they require multiple incisions in the medial canthus skin that sometimes may result in noticeable scarring. An alternative approach is the subcutaneous epicanthoplasty which allows softening of the epicanthal fold with minimal risk of medial canthal scarring [10, 11]. The tissue beneath the epicanthal folds is undermined, and the excess fibro-fatty tissue is debulked (Fig. 23.8). A dissolvable suture is then used to fixate the fold deep into the medial canthal tissues, flattening and softening the epicanthal fold. This is an effective technique that does not require the complexity of transposition flaps required with other techniques of epicanthoplasty, but the subcutaneous approach is not as powerful of a procedure and may not be adequate for very prominent epicanthal folds or when complete elimination of the fold is desired.

Closing the Eyelid Crease Incision

To create a well-defined eyelid crease, the most important step occurs in the closure of the incision. The normal eyelid crease is formed from anterior projections from the levator as it approaches the superior tarsal edge. Similarly, when surgically altering the lid crease position, the levator must be involved in the closure. To create a deep and defined eyelid crease, the suture closure of the incision should be passed through the inferior skin edge and imbricate the levator before exiting through the superior skin edge. Thus the wound will be tacked down to and move with the levator, allowing for secure adhesions to form and creating a long-lasting well-defined eyelid crease.

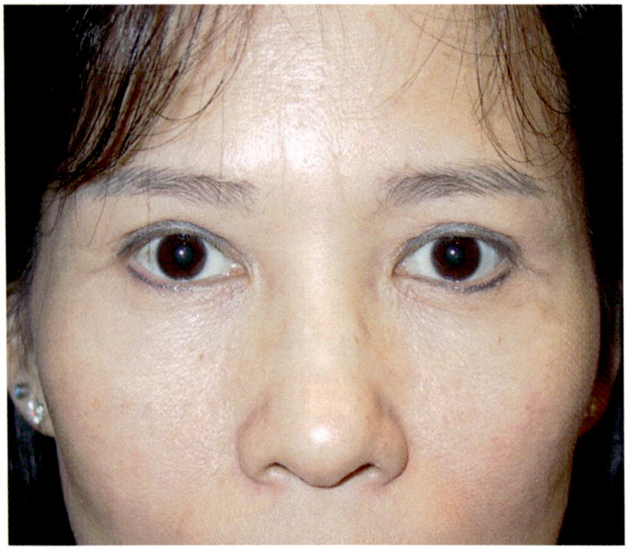

Fig. 23.7 Complete elimination of the epicanthal fold after Asian blepharoplasty with a modified Z-epicanthoplasty

Proper placement of this levator fixation is crucial, as securing the skin to the levator too superiorly or inferiorly can interfere with levator function producing eyelid ptosis or retraction. Furthermore, the location where the skin is secured to the levator will also determine the contour of the eyelid crease, and uneven fixation may result in an unnatural lid crease appearance. Intraoperative assessment by having the patient look up and down intermittently during closure will ensure proper placement of the sutures and illustrate the new lid crease.

Summary

In summary, Asian blepharoplasty has become a popular aesthetic procedure worldwide. Particular attention should be given to the placement of the eyelid crease incision, the amount of skin excision and fat contouring, and determining the need for epicanthoplasty. These factors are determined mostly by the patient's aesthetic goals and expectations, though underlying anatomical factors may also dictate the specific surgical approach or technique utilized. The most critical component of the procedure, however, is the preoperative communication between patient and surgeon to determine the desired goals and expectations of eyelid surgery.

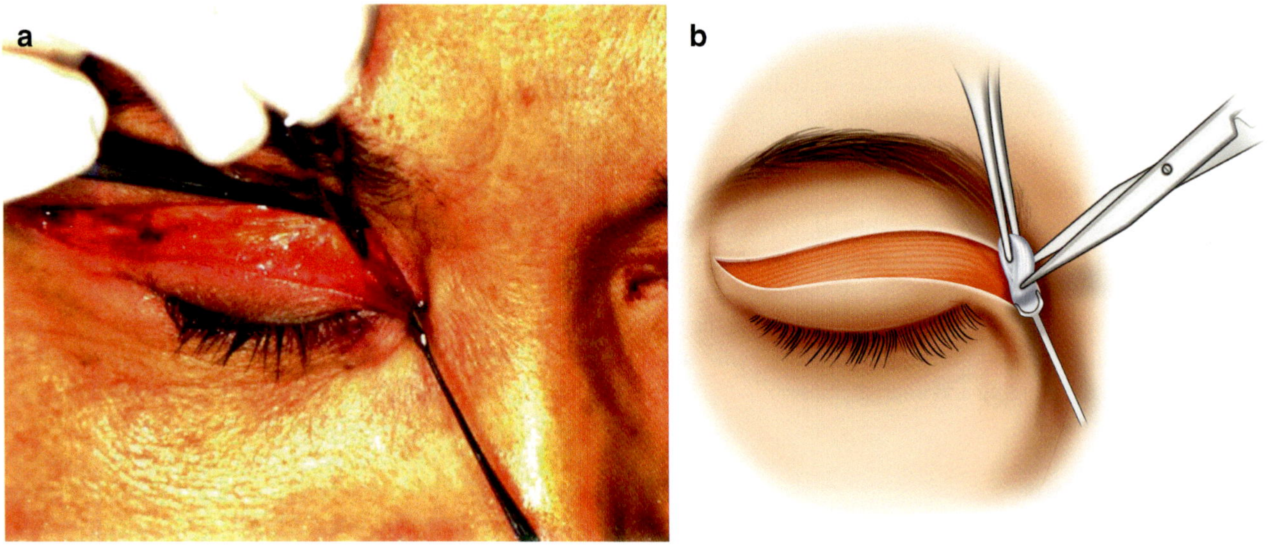

Fig. 23.8 Subcutaneous epicanthoplasty. (**a**) Through the medial portion of the eyelid crease incision, the subcutaneous tissues are dissected away from the overlying skin and excised. (**b**) Line art of the subcutaneous epicanthoplasty

References

1. Chen WP, Park JD. Asian upper lid blepharoplasty: an update on indications and technique. Facial Plast Surg. 2013;29:26–31.
2. Fakhro A, Yim HW, Kim YK, Nguyen AH. The evolution of looks and expectations of Asian eyelid and eye appearance. Semin Plast Surg. 2015;29(3):135–44.
3. Jinghe Z, Huifant X, Lihong W, et al. Three mini-incision double-eyelid blepharoplasty. Ann Plast Surg. 2014;72:141–4.
4. Yoon HS, Park BY, Oh KS. Tarsodermal suture fixation preceding redundant skin excision: a modified non-incisional upper blepharoplasty method for elderly patients. Arch Plast Surg. 2014;41:398–402.
5. Doxanas MT, Anderson RL. Oriental eyelids – an anatomic study. Arch Ophthalmol. 1984;102:1232–5.
6. Mikamo M. Mikamo's double-eyelid operation: the advent of Japanese aesthetic surgery. 1896. Plast Reconstr Surg. 1997;99:664–9.
7. Yi SK, Paik HW, Lee PK, et al. Simple epicanthoplasty with minimal scar. Aesth Plast Surg. 2007;31:350–3.
8. Park JI. Modified Z-epicanthoplasty in the Asian eyelid. Arch Facial Plast Surg. 2000;2:43–7.
9. Zhao YQ, Luo DA. Modified Y-V epicanthoplasty with raised medial canthus in the Asian eyelid. Arch Facial Plast Surg. 2010;12:274–6.
10. Yen MT, Jordan DR, Anderson RL. No-scar Asian Epicanthoplasty: a subcutaneous approach. Ophthal Plast Reconstr Surg. 2002;18:40–4.
11. Yen MT. Medial epicanthoplasty using the skin redraping method. Plast Reconstr Surg. 2007;120:1740.

Complications of Asian Upper Blepharoplasty and Their Solutions

24

Preamjit Saonanon and Cat Nguyen Burkat

Asian blepharoplasty, also known as "double eyelid" surgery or eyelid crease fixation, is among one of the most popular cosmetic procedures in Asia. Approximately 40–90% of Asians, especially East and Southeast Asians, possess "single eyelids" with an absent or poorly defined eyelid crease. Due to significant differences in eyelid anatomy between Caucasian and Asian eyes, one cannot perform optimal Asian eyelid surgery from Western textbooks alone. Major differences between Caucasian and Asian eyelids include the presence of subcutaneous or submuscularis fat (SMFAT) which manifests as puffier eyelids, the lower position of a transverse ligament which limits levator excursion, and the absent/low eyelid crease due to orbital septum fusion lower on the levator aponeurosis [1–3].

To avoid upper blepharoplasty complications in the Asian patient, several distinct portions of the eyelid should be appreciated during the examination. First, the medial eyelid should be evaluated for the presence and severity of the epicanthal fold. Second, the central eyelid should be assessed for eyelid crease type and presence of asymmetric margin reflex distances (MRD_1) or blepharoptosis. Eyelid crease type in Asians can be subcategorized into three types: single eyelid, partial eyelid crease, and double eyelid. Third, the lateral eyelid can be examined for whether the lateral canthus runs parallel, upward, or downward as compared to the medial canthus. Failure to recognize these subtleties and/or inadequate discussion with the patient preoperatively can result in postsurgical dissatisfaction [4].

P. Saonanon (✉)
Department of Ophthalmology, Faculty of Medicine, Chulalongkorn University, Bangkok, Thailand

Department of Ophthalmology, King Chulalongkorn Memorial Hospital, Thai Red Cross Society, Bangkok, Thailand

C. N. Burkat
Department of Ophthalmology and Visual Sciences, University of Wisconsin-Madison, Madison, WI, USA
e-mail: cburkat@wisc.edu

Blepharoptosis and Eyebrow Ptosis

Undesirable results after cosmetic upper blepharoplasty or double eyelid surgery commonly occur due to undetected pre-existing blepharoptosis. Diagnosis of frank blepharoptosis is usually unproblematic but occasionally can be difficult to recognize in certain situations:

- Mild unilateral blepharoptosis: The eyelid crease will become more evident in a ptotic eyelid, and a patient may present with asymmetric eyelid creases and request double eyelid surgery on the normal eye in order to create similarity between the sides. However, performing unilateral eyelid crease fixation will result in a persistent asymmetrical MRD_1 (Fig. 24.1).
- Bilateral blepharoptosis: In individuals with a single eyelid configuration, a smaller palpebral fissure is commonly seen due to either the hooding pretarsal skin fold or true blepharoptosis. Lifting the overhanging skin fold to appreciate true MRD_1 is mandatory to detect underlying blepharoptosis. The normal MRD_1 in Asians is approximately 3–4 mm, and blepharoptosis should be addressed if MRD_1 is less than 2.5 mm. Performing blepharoplasty alone without repairing aponeurotic ptosis will result in high eyelid creases and a drowsy appearance.
- Compensatory eyebrow elevation and deep superior sulcus: In patients with marked ptosis, an exaggerated high eyebrow position usually presents as a compensatory mechanism due to superior visual field obstruction. This can also be seen in mild ptosis, presenting as a high eyebrow position or hollow superior sulcus with normal MRD_1. Patients are usually unaware of their eyebrow height and rather focus only on the hollow upper eyelid appearance. Managing this group of patients with volume augmentation will temporary improve the eye socket appearance but may later result in more ptosis. Phenylephrine testing can be useful to document improvement of the hollow superior sulcus and demonstrate the postoperative outcome of ptosis surgery to the patient (Fig. 24.2). Eyebrow suppression by the examiner hand tends to be less useful to illustrate this.

A. J. Cohen, C. N. Burkat (eds.), *Oculofacial, Orbital, and Lacrimal Surgery*, https://doi.org/10.1007/978-3-030-14092-2_24

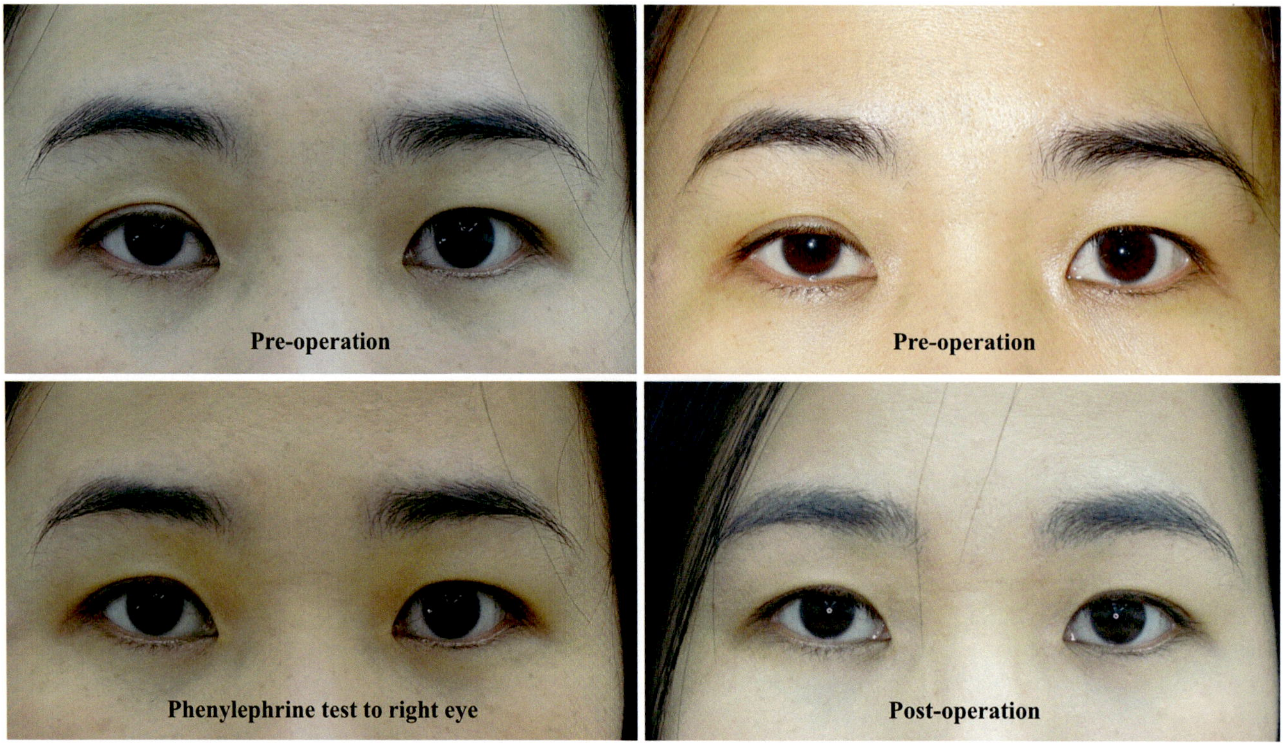

Fig. 24.1 A patient presents with asymmetric eyelid creases, requesting upper blepharoplasty surgery on the left side. However, the upper images demonstrate asymmetric MRD_1 from mild right upper eyelid ptosis. The left lower image shows improved MRD_1 symmetry after instillation of topical phenylephrine to the right eye; therefore, the appropriate surgery was a right conjunctivo mullerectomy (1 month postoperatively in right lower image)

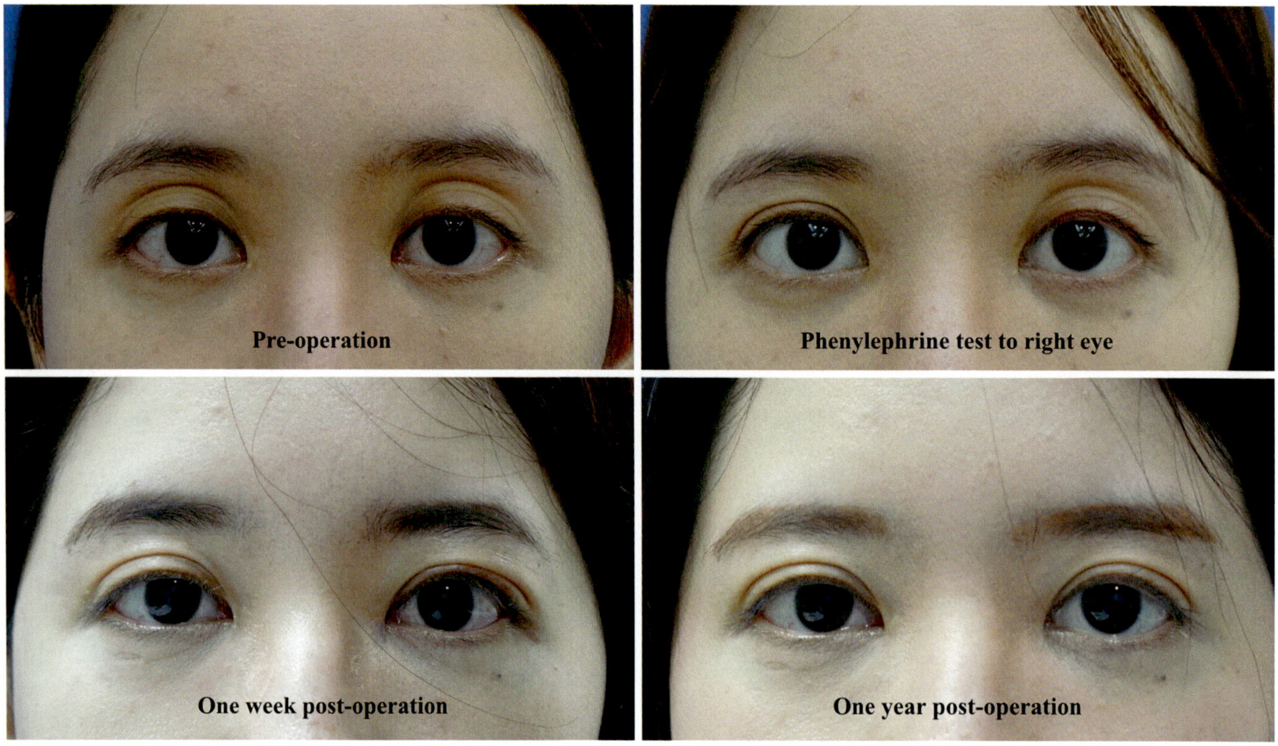

Fig. 24.2 Young patient has hollow superior sulci due to compensatory eyebrow elevation from mild bilateral blepharoptosis. Exam demonstrated absence of eyelid creases but normal MRD_1, and the patient was suggested elsewhere to undergo volume augmentation with fat grafting. After instillation of topical phenylephrine to the right eye, the exam showed a formed eyelid crease and skin fold, resolved socket hollowness, and a lower eyebrow position. Bottom images were 1 week and 1 year after bilateral conjunctivo mullerectomy surgery

Complications

Common complications after cosmetic upper blepharoplasty or double eyelid surgery include:

1. Asymmetric eyelid creases
2. High eyelid crease deformity (westernized appearance to Asian eyelid)
3. Bifid crease (multiple crease)
4. Lagophthalmos
5. Eyelash eversion/ectropion
6. Visible or hypertrophic scarring

As the eyes are the most expressive and recognizable area of the face, patients with surgical complications or suboptimal results will seek medical attention and be highly motivated to undergo corrective surgery. There is no practical guideline for the most suitable time for revision surgery; however, many surgeons will typically observe for 3 months or more for complete wound maturation and scar formation prior to considering revision. Candidates for revisional procedures need to also understand the process of corrective and reconstructive surgery and be realistic with regard to the expected outcome, as additional surgery may sometimes improve but not completely correct their concerns.

Asymmetric Eyelid Creases

Asymmetric eyelid creases can result from:

1. Asymmetric skin markings

Even minimal differences after surgery can be noted easily by patients and cause undue stress. Creating truly identical eyelid creases is impossible, and patients should be counseled that similar, but not identical, eye appearances can be expected postoperatively. To optimize symmetry, meticulously measure the location of the eyelid crease, which can sometimes be asymmetric prior to surgery, and note the prominence of the epicanthal fold. The skin can be gently stretched during the preoperative marking for accurate measurements, and the markings should be made prior to local anesthetic infiltration. The eyelid crease incision, or medial blepharoplasty crescent, should blend precisely into the epicanthal fold to avoid abnormal creases or webbing.

2. Undetected preoperative blepharoptosis

This is a relatively common etiology of patients who seek corrective surgery for presumed asymmetric creases. Preexisting unilateral or bilateral asymmetrical ptosis will become more noticeable after blepharoplasty. Upper blepharoplasty may also unmask underlying ptosis that was not previously noted due to the full skin fold; therefore, careful preoperative MRD_1 measurements with gentle elevation of the hooding skin are essential. Blepharoptosis can then be managed by appropriate ptosis surgery options depending on levator function and ptosis severity (Fig. 24.3). Iatrogenic blepharoptosis from previous aggressive blepharoplasty with high eyelid crease fixation, and/or injury to the levator complex, is more challenging and requires careful communication with the patient. In addition, previous manipulation of the levator aponeurosis, such as by levator tucking procedures with multiple sutures, will result in thick fibrosis of the distal levator aponeurosis. Correction of ptosis will then typically require scar debulking and external levator advancement.

High Eyelid Crease Deformity (Westernized Appearance to Asian Eyelid)

The traditional approach to "double eyelid surgery" in the past was to change the Asian eye to look Caucasian, and therefore a high eyelid crease was deemed necessary. Now, it is universally accepted that each ethnicity has its own unique beauty and, therefore, aggressive transformation would result in an unnatural facial appearance (Fig. 24.4) [5]. Furthermore, the levator aponeurosis and its excursion in the gliding zone can be compromised by high eyelid crease fixation sutures, thus resulting in iatrogenic blepharoptosis. In addition, excessively high crease fixation will result in scar formation between the levator aponeurosis and skin, which can potentially change the vector force of the levator complex from vertically to the tarsus to horizontally to the skin (Fig. 24.5). The scar may also limit levator excursion and sometimes result in a dull, aching discomfort around the orbit when looking upgaze. In general, it is strongly discouraged to create high eyelid creases in a patient with Asian eyelids, with the desired eyelid crease typically at 4–7 mm above the eyelid margin.

It is important to note that it is typical for the eyelid creases to appear slightly higher in the initial postoperative period due to edema. This prominent pretarsal edema occurs due to the dissection and excision of a strip of subcutaneous tissue from the inferior incision that is performed to create definition of the eyelid crease. Once the edema resolves in several months, the eyelid creases will soften to the lower height that was marked.

Other causes of eyelid creases that are too high include:

- Patient request: A patient may specifically request a higher than natural-appearing eyelid crease, as the eyes will look more defined with heavy makeup and on photos. However, an unnatural appearance without makeup, and

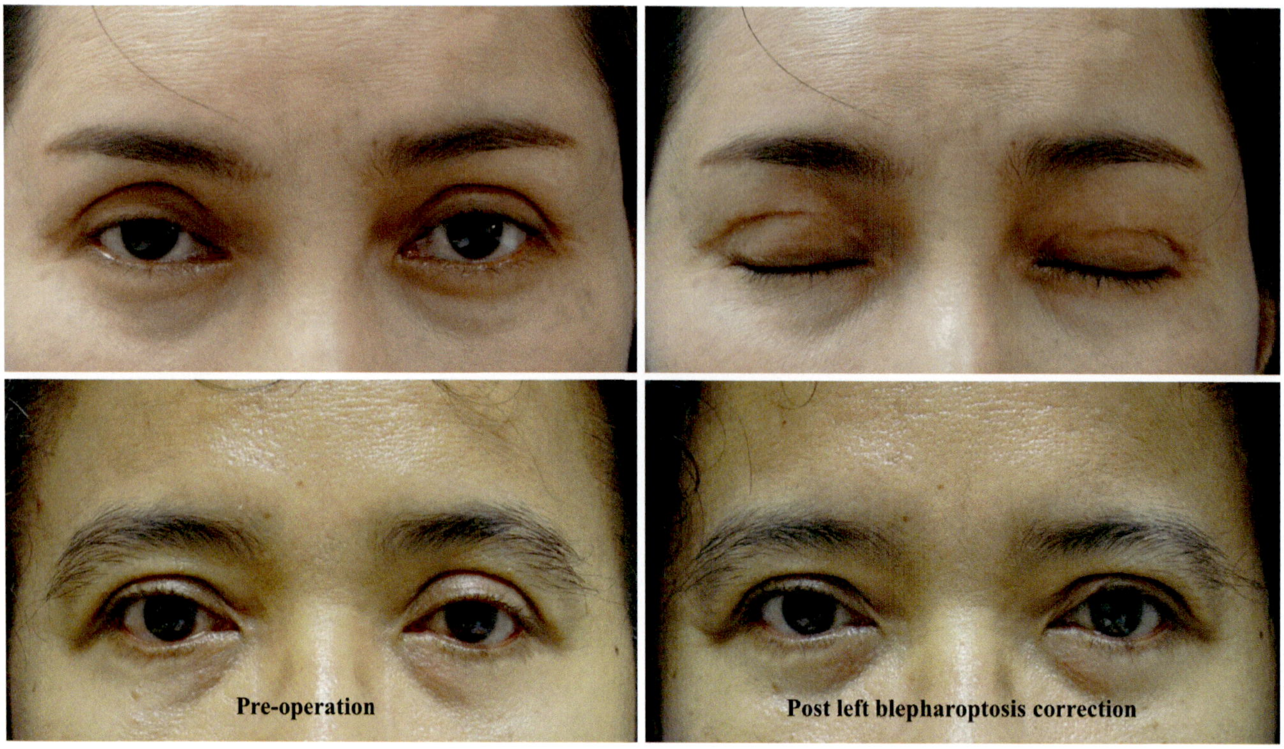

Fig. 24.3 Two patients with asymmetric eyelid creases. The upper images illustrate marked asymmetric placement of the eyelid crease skin incisions and blepharoptosis of the right eye. The patient in the lower images has a higher left eyelid crease due to blepharoptosis, with resolution of the asymmetric creases after left upper eyelid ptosis correction

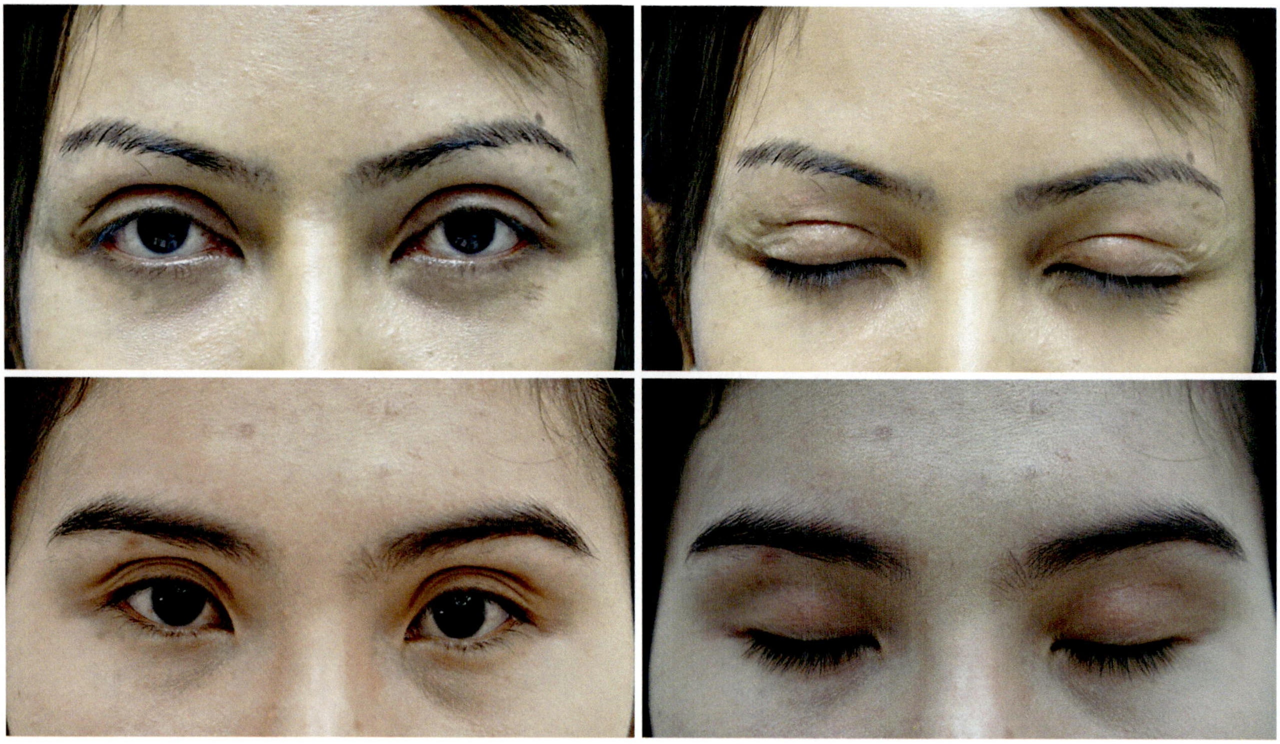

Fig. 24.4 High eyelid crease deformity or westernized look of Asian eyelids, seen in two patients

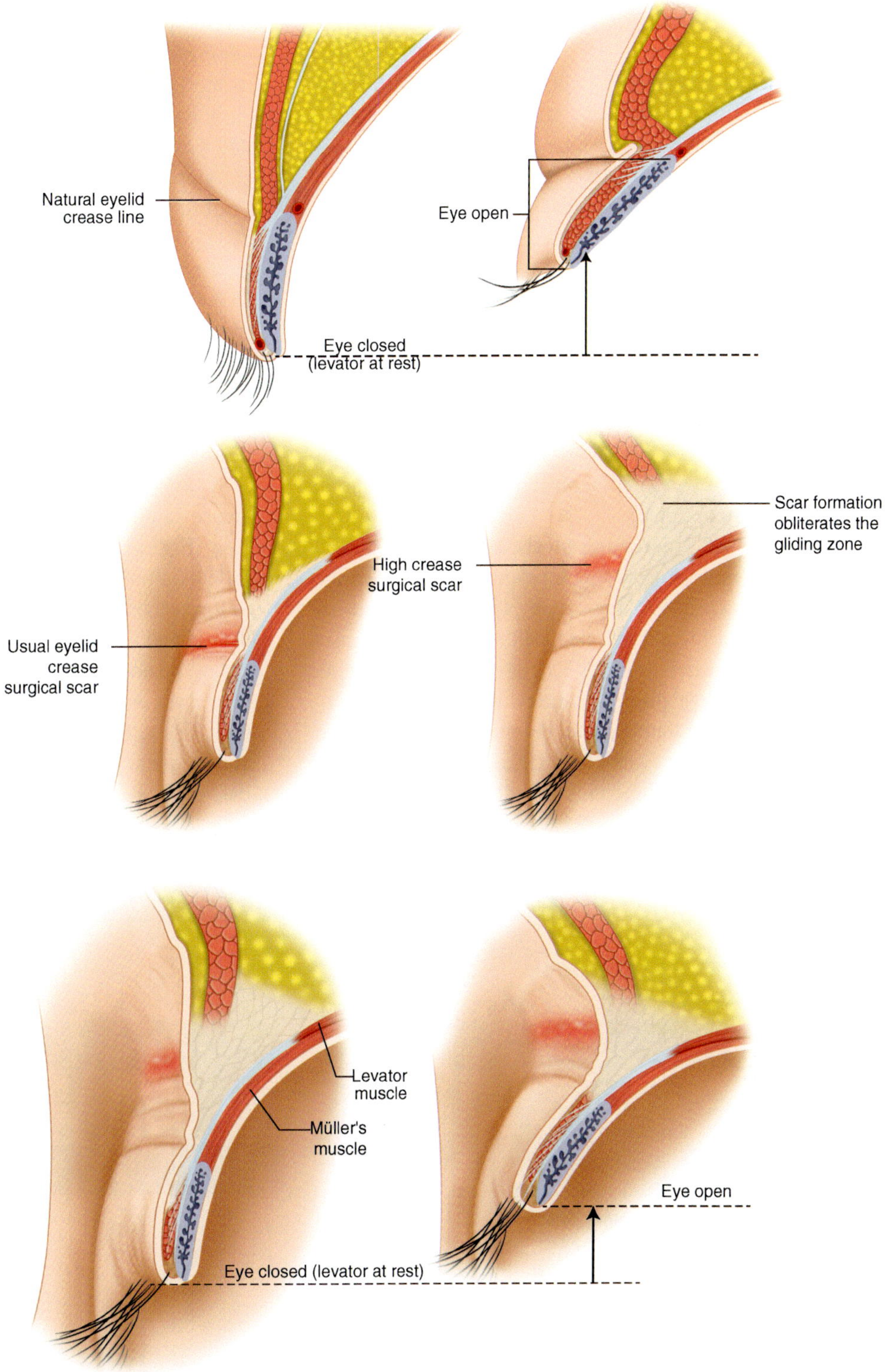

Fig. 24.5 High eyelid crease fixation-induced blepharoptosis. In eyes without previous surgery, levator muscle runs horizontally from the orbital apex and reaches the Whitnall's ligament where it turns 90° down to reach tarsal plate (upper left). Preaponeurotic fat creates a gliding zone for the levator muscle and its aponeurosis to move freely. When levator muscle contracts, levator aponeurosis pulls pretarsal skin to form eyelid crease and pulls tarsal plate up to open the eye (upper right). With optimal height placement of eyelid crease fixation sutures, scar formation occurs only along the inferior levator aponeurosis, and the gliding zone is preserved (middle left). Levator aponeurosis and its excursion in the gliding zone can be compromised in high eyelid crease fixation and result in surgical-induced blepharoptosis. When crease fixation is placed too high and significant scar forms, the levator muscle and aponeurosis fuse to the eyelid skin (middle right). Extensive scar formation between the levator aponeurosis and skin can alter the levator force direction from vertically to the tarsus to horizontally to the skin, thus compromising eyelid opening (lower)

lessening of their ethnic contours, should be thoroughly discussed and documented. The patient should bring in photos of others that have the eyelid configuration and appearance that they desire. Cosmetic upper blepharoplasty should deliver natural looking outcomes which should be emphasized by the surgeon.

- Poor patient selection: Small incision or suture fixation double eyelid surgery should be preserved for younger individuals without skin redundancy or puffy eyelids. These minimally invasive techniques fold up skin without removal, and are therefore not suitable for patients with excess skin. If performed in these patients, the fixation sutures tend to be placed higher in order to compensate for the redundant skin, thus resulting in abnormally high creases.

- Imprecise skin marking: In elderly individuals with severe wrinkles and skin redundancy, failure to gently stretch the upper eyelid skin during the marking process may result in an eyelid crease that is too high once the pretarsal skin stretches after eyelid crease fixation.

Management of a high eyelid crease (Fig. 24.6):

A postoperative elevated crease in an Asian eyelid can be very challenging to correct, and therefore avoidance of this complication is optimal.

- However, if noted, one first needs to determine whether the high eyelid crease is secondary to concurrent blepharoptosis, which can then be managed by the appropriate ptosis surgery options.
- If there was no pre-existing ptosis, one should evaluate for clinical signs of levator compromise. With placement of these high crease tacking sutures, the levator aponeurosis, or even the levator muscle itself, can be compromised as discussed earlier. Signs of levator compromise include MRD_1 lower than prior to surgery, eyelid retraction on downgaze, lagophthalmos, and inability to pinch the eyelid skin up from the eyelid. If MRD_1 is normal, there is no lagophthalmos, and the skin is not adherent to the levator; a lower-position eyelid crease can be achieved by marking the desired lower eyelid crease and removing intervening scar tissue (Fig. 24.7). However, if any signs of levator compromise are present, revision surgery typically involves lysis of scar, external levator advancement, and possible tissue grafting to prevent readhesion. It is recommended to allow for at least 3–6 months of healing prior to surgical revision.
- To lower the eyelid crease, the desired natural eyelid crease is first marked, at 4–7 mm above the eyelid margin. The skin between the higher previous surgical scar and the new crease needs to be excised. It is critical that the residual amount of sub-brow skin measures a minimal of 12–15 mm in order to prevent lagophthalmos. Therefore, the potential of this surgery depends on the level of the desired eyelid crease and the residual amount of sub-brow skin. In patients with more skin laxity, a lower eyelid crease can be thus achieved as they have more sub-brow skin (Fig. 24.8). In contrast, a young patient with very little skin redundancy may be limited in revision surgery to lower the eyelid crease if the intervening skin between the old and new creases cannot be safely excised. In those cases, the new eyelid crease may require compromise and placed not as low as desired, in order to avoid lagophthalmos. In some patients with skin shortage, eyelid massage and frequent pinching of eyelid skin may help lengthen the sub-brow skin.

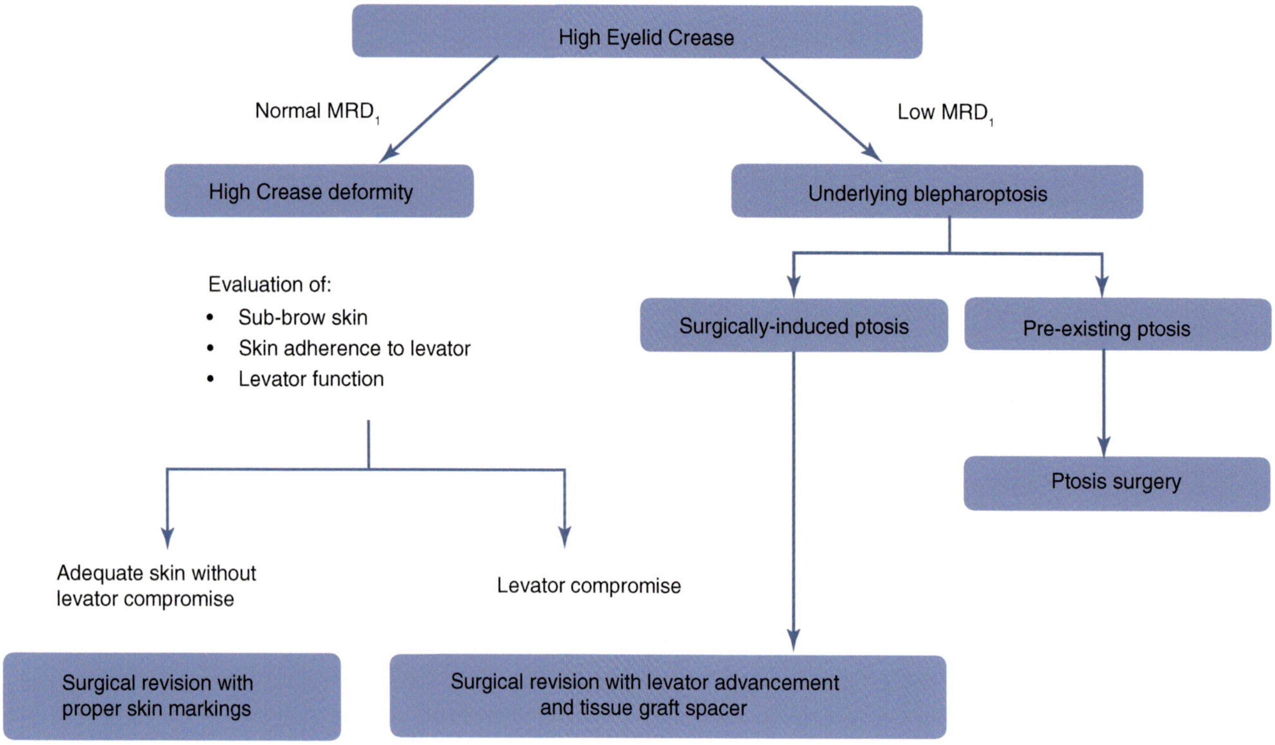

Fig. 24.6 Flow chart for managing a high eyelid crease deformity

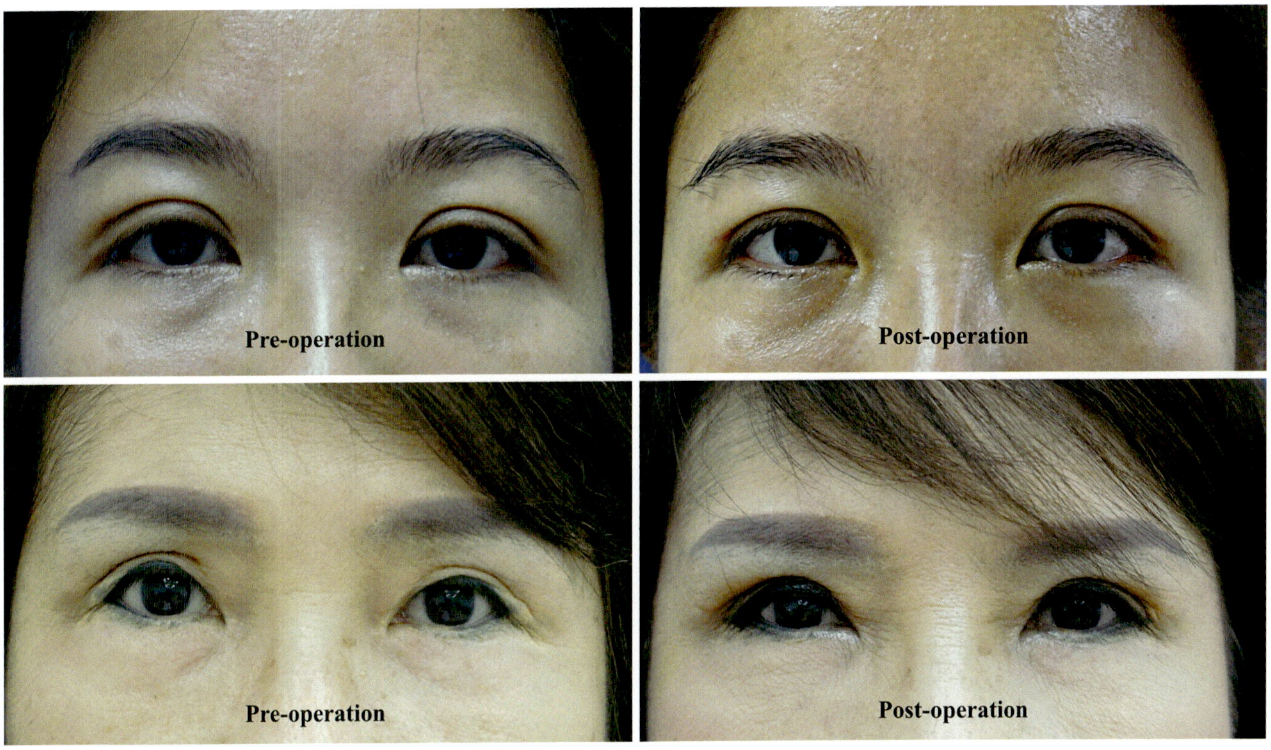

Fig. 24.7 High eyelid creases in an Asian patient typically result in an unnatural and drowsy eye appearance. Redundant pretarsal skin in a young patient (top images are pre- and post-revision blepharoplasty) will result in bulging/fullness of the pretarsal area or a sausage-like appearance. In older patients, pretarsal skin redundancy manifests as large skin folds and wrinkles

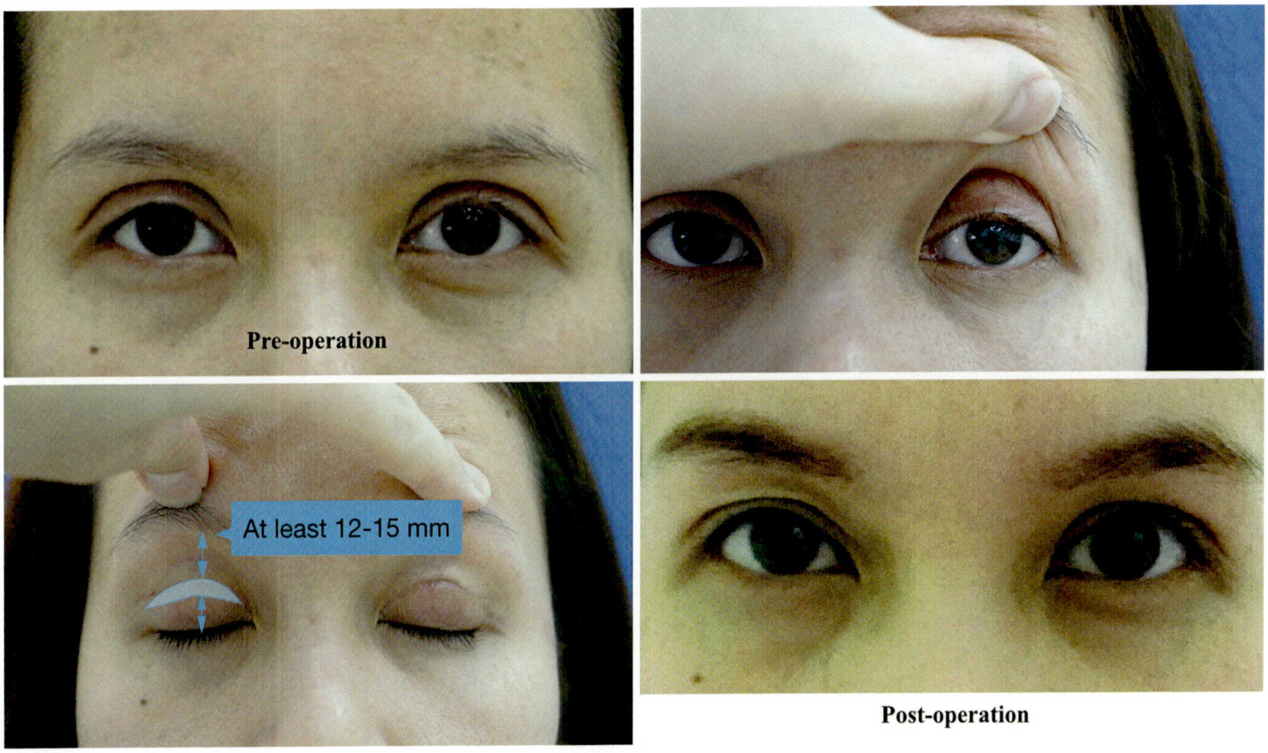

Fig. 24.8 In cases with high eyelid crease fixation, the skin is often tightly fused to the levator aponeurosis, and the skin cannot be pinched up from the posterior lamella (top right image). To lower the eyelid crease, skin inferior to the previous surgical scar needs to be excised (area in blue). It is important to preserve a minimum of 12–15 mm residual sub-brow skin to avoid lagophthalmos. Therefore, surgical revision is dependent on the height of the desired eyelid crease and the available amount of sub-brow skin. Bottom right image demonstrates the postoperative result after bilateral scar revision with external levator advancement and fascia lata grafting

Surgical technique for a high eyelid crease:

- First, the desired eyelid crease is carefully marked, making sure it is a natural height for the Asian eyelid and also symmetric to the contralateral side.
- An ellipse of skin is marked with the superior marking incorporating the previous surgical scar and the inferior line being the new eyelid crease.
- The markings should be drawn prior to local anesthetic infiltration as this will distort the eyelid tissues.
- Upon flap excision, care should be taken to remove only the skin and most superficial scar tissue, to avoid injury to the levator aponeurosis with deeper excision.
- Next, careful dissection with Westcott scissors or a microdissection needle is performed to separate the levator aponeurosis from adhesions to the overlying septum, orbicularis, or skin.
- It is critical to continue the dissection superiorly up to Whitnall's ligament, as failure to separate the entire length of the levator complex will result in an unresolved high lid crease, thus resulting in triple eyelid creases. Complete scar release can be checked by holding the eyelid skin inferiorly and having the patient look up. Limitation of eyelid excursion or visible transmission of an upward pull to the eyelid skin indicates inadequate scar release, with more tissue dissection necessary.
- Once the levator complex is released adequately from adhesions, the new eyelid crease is created by posterior fixation sutures attaching the inferior incision to the pretarsal tissue or levator aponeurosis just above the tarsal plate. Gently lifting the pretarsal tissue superiorly guides the placement height of these posterior tacking sutures.
- Finally, the gliding zone is re-established with the residual preaponeurotic fat. This step is most successful if the preaponeurotic fat is abundant enough to allow for inferior transposition over the dissected levator complex and sutured to the subcutaneous tissue at the skin edge. If there is insufficient preaponeurotic fat, tissue grafting with fascia lata, temporalis fascia, or dermis fat is needed to prevent readhesion of the levator aponeurosis to the skin (Fig. 24.9).

Bifid Crease

Either end of the surgical incision can sometimes heal with a bifid, or Y-shaped, skin fold crease (Fig. 24.10). The medial canthal skin is typically the hardest part to mark due to prominent epicanthal folds in younger individuals and skin redundancy in elderly patients. Proper tapering of the skin marking is critical and difficult to master. Conservative excision and

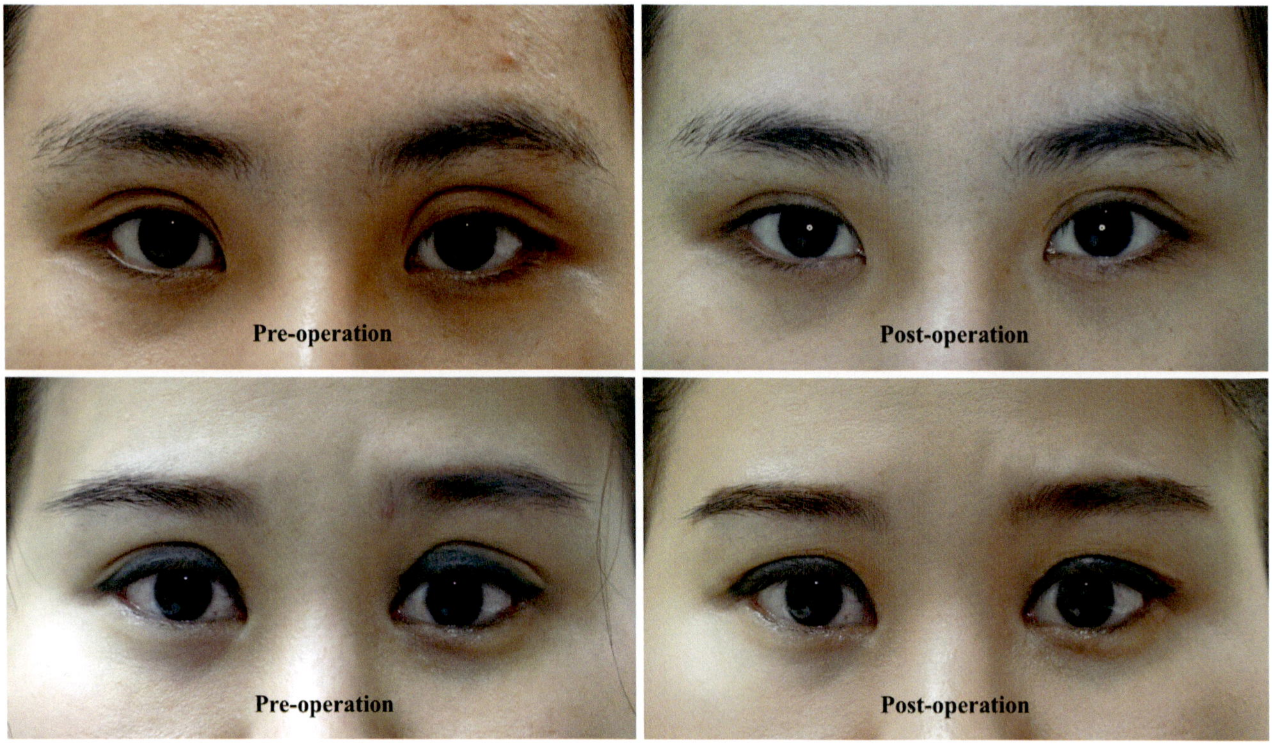

Fig. 24.9 Preoperative and postoperative results in two patients. The patient in the top images underwent bilateral scar revision with external levator advancement and fascia lata grafting on the left side due to levator compromise. Bottom images demonstrate improvement after bilateral scar revision with repositioning of preaponeurotic fat

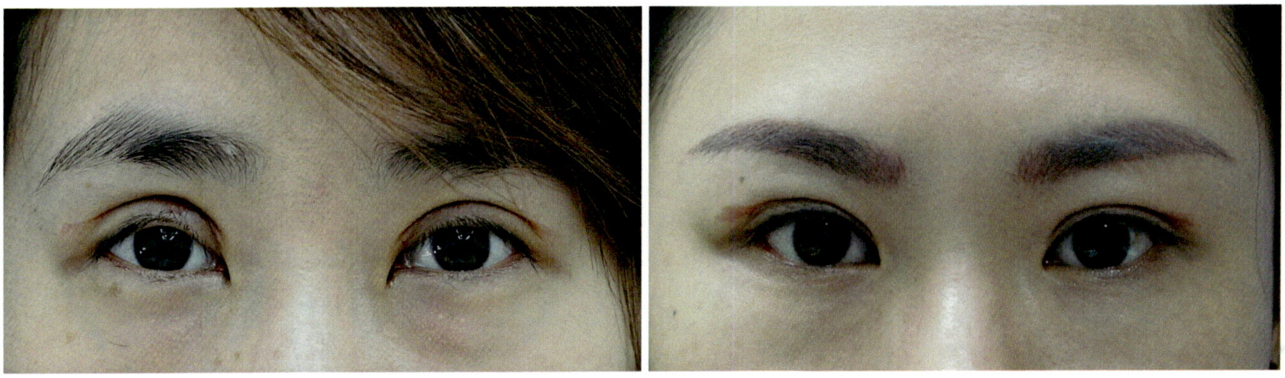

Fig. 24.10 Bifid crease of the medial canthal (left image) and lateral canthal (right image) areas as a result of redundant skin and suboptimal eyelid crease fixation points

additional skin removal at the end of surgery after all fixation sutures are placed is one technique to adjust the proper amount of skin removal. In younger patients, the epicanthal fold often limits the height and curvature of the eyelid crease and can be troublesome in the open blepharoplasty technique. Some surgeons avoid the bifid crease complication by performing small-incision or suture fixation blepharoplasty solely. Ideally, surgeons should master both open and closed surgical techniques and utilize small-incision surgery only in cases with thin and minimal eyelid skin redundancy. In older individuals with severe dermatochalasis, bifid creases or multiple wrinkles at the medial incision line are common and therefore should be discussed with the patient preoperatively.

A bifid crease at the lateral canthus occurs due to improper placement of the lateral eyelid crease fixation suture. Most Asian eyelids have a sickle or triangular-shaped tarsal plate, with a tapered medial and lateral end. If the eyelid crease suture is fixated along the superior tarsus, this will result in a crease that tapers both medially and laterally. Although a nasally tapered eyelid crease is desirable, most people prefer a subtle flare to the lateral aspect to give the illusion of wider eyes. Eyelid eversion can be performed to check the tarsal plate shape, as well as to ascertain that the fixation sutures are not in full thickness through the tarsus. Therefore, in Asian eyelids with a sickle or triangular-shaped tarsus, ideal placement of the lateral crease fixation suture should be more medial than usual and can be placed just adjacent to the central fixation suture.

Management of bifid crease complications requires surgery to excise the appropriate redundant tissue, followed by proper positioning of the eyelid crease fixation sutures. Asking the patient to look up and down can also demonstrate whether the bifid crease has been obliterated properly.

Lagophthalmos

Mild lagophthalmos is common in the early postoperative period as the eyelids swell and usually resolve with time.

Persistent lagophthalmos can be due to:

- Aggressive skin removal: In less experienced surgeons, overly aggressive skin removal can cause not only cosmetic problems but threaten vision from exposure keratitis. The remaining sub-brow skin after skin markings should measure at least 15 mm in younger patients and 10–12 mm in older patients. Topical lubrication with frequent drops and ointment is essential, with consideration of a bandage contact lens for severe keratopathy. If corneal integrity is at risk, release of scar with placement of a full-thickness skin graft or skin flap may be indicated.
- Excessive orbicularis oculi muscle removal: In older patients with severe dermatochalasis, removal of skin including the orbicularis oculi might result in removal of all the preseptal orbicularis portion, thus resulting in incomplete eyelid closure. Although it is common to excise a strip of pretarsal orbicularis muscle and underlying subcutaneous/submuscular fat from the inferior incision edge to help create a more defined and longer-lasting crease, it is generally preferable to be conservative with orbicularis muscle excision. In Asian individuals with pre-existing hollowness to the superior sulcus, retaining the pretarsal and preseptal orbicularis muscle contributes more volume to restore a youthful appearance. If lagophthalmos is secondary to orbicularis oculi removal rather than skin shortage, supportive measures with topical lubrication and ointment or taping the eyelid closed at night is usually adequate.

Eyelash Eversion and Ectropion

The eyelid margin can evert and result in visibility of the white meibomian gland line if the crease fixation sutures are placed too high. As mentioned previously, the point of the eyelid crease fixation should lie exactly at the level of the inferior skin edge. In other words, the inferior skin edge should be gently elevated until the pretarsal skin is smooth;

the fixation suture is then placed in the tarsus just at the site where the upper edge of the skin reaches.

- A fixation point that is too low on the tarsus will result in bulging of the pretarsal area or a sausage-like appearance due to collapse of the pretarsal skin. In older patients, the pretarsal skin redundancy will be evidenced as multiple skin wrinkles and potentially droop over the eyelash line. Women with these findings will typically complain that they are unable to place eyeliner accurately on the lash line due to the sagging skin.
- Fixation sutures that are placed too high may result in eyelash eversion and margin ectropion, particularly if preexisting horizontal lid laxity is present (Fig. 24.11). As a natural-appearing eyelid crease height in Asian individuals is 4–7 mm, on average, any attempt to tack an eyelid crease to the levator aponeurosis is generally too high. However, if the eyelid crease is intentionally placed at 8–10 mm, then crease fixation to the levator aponeurosis is an option.
- Eyelash eversion is also seen after combining blepharoplasty with levator advancement in Asian eyelids. After the levator aponeurosis is advanced and sutured to the tarsus, the terminal aspect of the aponeurosis should be preserved for eyelid crease fixation. The inferior redundant portion of the aponeurosis should only be removed in congenital ptosis repair where a large amount of levator aponeurosis/muscle is advanced. If eyelash eversion is seen after placing the eyelid crease fixation sutures, the tacking sutures should be removed and fixated more inferiorly. If concurrent levator advancement surgery is performed, and the crease fixation to the lowest margin of aponeurosis still causes eyelash eversion, the crease fixation sutures should be removed. The eyelid crease is then fixated to the underlying tarsal plate instead.

The best management of this complication is avoidance and early recognition. Once scarring has occurred, correction of eyelash eversion is more difficult and unpredictable. The eyelid crease is incised and all pretarsal scarring released with scissors to allow the anterior lamella to drape normally without upward pull on the eyelashes. However, even with complete scar lysis and separation of the anterior from the posterior lamella to the eyelid margin, the eyelashes often remain everted. Therefore, attempts to correct this finding can be considered in the appropriate patient if other revisional surgery is being performed as well; however, surgery to correct eyelash eversion alone often yields suboptimal outcomes.

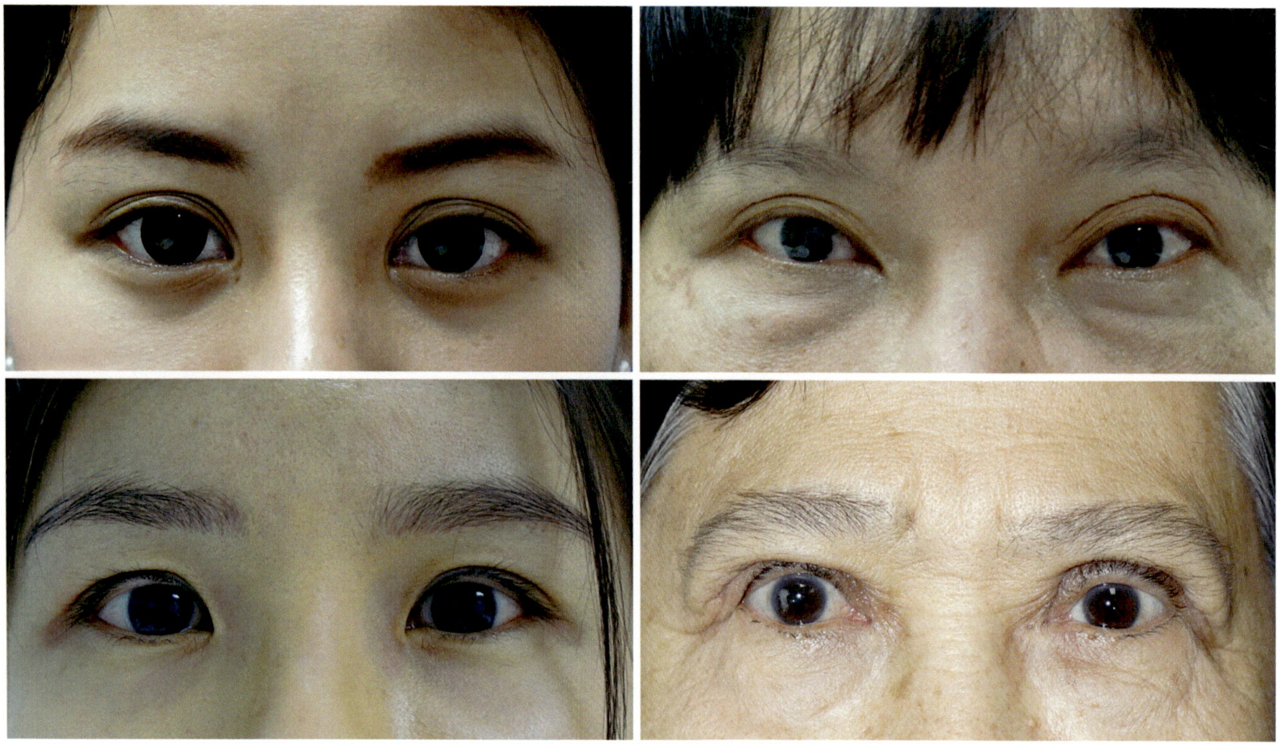

Fig. 24.11 Inaccurate positioning of eyelid crease fixation. The upper images illustrate redundant pretarsal skin that occurs when the eyelid crease skin incision is placed too high but then the eyelid crease is fixated too low. Redundant pretarsal skin causes wrinkle-like skin folds and sagging in young patients and persistence of pretarsal wrinkles in older individuals. The bottom photos demonstrate eyelash and eyelid margin eversion from fixation points that were placed too high after double eyelid surgery (bottom left) and levator advancement (bottom right)

Visible or Hypertrophic Scarring

Scar formation is a normal healing process, and the thin upper eyelid skin usually heals well without residual scar. However, in Asians or darker skin individuals, the scar can be pronounced. Redness and induration of a scar are typically most prominent 4–6 weeks postoperatively with normal healing. After maximum scar formation, it often becomes hyperpigmented, followed by gradual fading of color and softening of the induration. The complete wound healing process is 6 months, on average, which should be discussed with the patient preoperatively. Mild erythema of the scar can sometimes take up to 1 year to completely resolve. There are three main types of scars: hypertrophic, keloid, and atrophic scars. A true keloid is extremely rare on the eyelid area, but hypertrophic and atrophic scarring can form, even with good surgical technique. These occur most often in the medial and lateral canthal areas where skin is thicker (Fig. 24.12).

To minimize the risk of unsightly scar formation, meticulous attention to several key concepts in the closure is critical. There should be minimal tension on the skin layer, proper alignment of each tissue layer, and eversion of the wound edges. There is usually no tension on the eyelid incisions, unless aggressive skin excision was performed. Extension of the incision to the lateral canthal area for temporal hooding correction can leave a visible scar. The eyelid crease should also avoid crossing the level of the lateral canthal angle and may include a slight wing upward if needed to minimize the temporal holding. Closure of the orbicularis oculi and subcutaneous layer with buried sutures can decrease skin tension, thus minimizing scar. Good postoperative care can also help to decrease swelling and thus lessen skin tension during the early healing period.

The type of suture used in closure also has an effect on scar formation. In light-skin individuals, both absorbable and nonabsorbable sutures are acceptable for skin closure. In Asians or darker skin patients, a 6-0 to 8-0 monofilament nonabsorbable suture, such as nylon or polypropylene, is preferable as it causes the least skin reaction. The sutures are then removed in 5–10 days to avoid prolonged inflammation. However, in patients who are unable to tolerate suture removal, a 7-0 or 8-0 fast-absorbing suture is also acceptable. Similarly, minimizing thermal injury to the skin edges during surgery will also decrease the inflammatory response and deposition of fibrosis; therefore, incision of the skin flap may be performed with a 15-blade scalpel and scissors.

Scars typically fade by 6 months, although these can take up to 1 year in some patients. Scar hyperpigmentation can be treated with topical kojic acid or hydroquinone. In persistent bothersome scar discoloration, intense pulsed light or broad-spectrum light therapy can be effective, with extreme care to protect the globe during treatments.

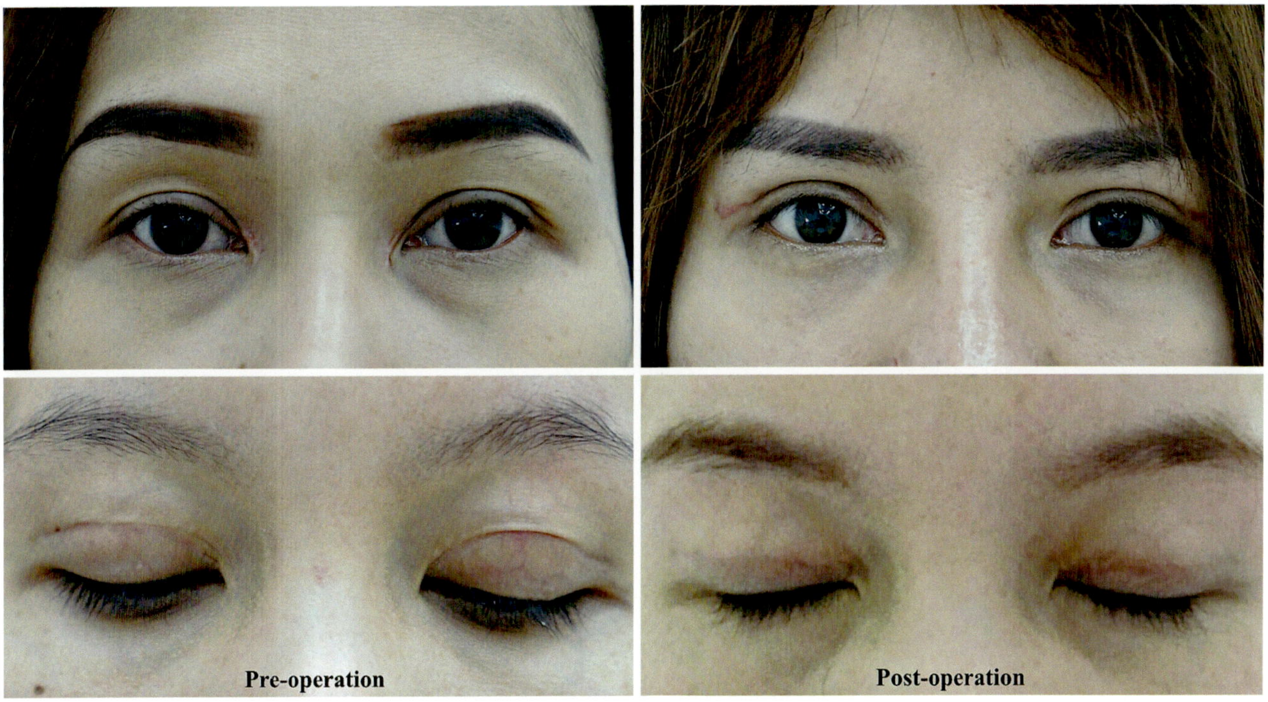

Fig. 24.12 Poor scar formation after upper blepharoplasty. To avoid poor scarring, proper alignment and minimal tension to the tissue layers, as well as wound edge eversion, are critical. The upper images show hypertrophic scarring at the medial and lateral canthal areas in two patients. The bottom images demonstrate improvement of a high crease deformity, with significantly less scarring, and pre- and post-revision with proper tissue alignment and skin closure

For hypertrophic scars, significant improvement can be seen with observation alone for 6 months. However, if necessary, intralesional steroid or 5-fluorouracil injection has been demonstrated to be effective in fibroblast suppression and to hasten scar remodeling [6]. Monthly injection of 0.1–0.4 ml of 40 mg/ml triamcinolone starting 1 month postoperatively can be given when obvious hypertrophic scarring is noted. Nevertheless, there is no literature to support that injections result in a superior result in the long term compared to observation alone. Residual elevated hypertrophic scars can also be flattened with ablative laser resurfacing but should be considered with caution as additional inflammation and pigmentary changes can subsequently occur.

Depressed scars are best avoided by wound edge eversion on surgical closure but, if present, may require scar excision or a combination of soft tissue filler augmentation with ablative laser resurfacing.

References

1. Ichinose A, Tahara S. Extended preseptal fat resection in Asian blepharoplasty. Ann Plast Surg. 2008;60:121–6.
2. Yuzuriha S, Matsuo K, Kushima H. An anatomical structure which results in puffiness of the upper eyelid and a narrow palpebral fissure in the Mongoloid eye. Br J Plast Surg. 2000;53:466–72.
3. Saonanon P. Update on Asian eyelid anatomy and clinical relevance. Curr Opin Ophthalmol. 2014;25:436–42.
4. Chen WP, editor. Asian blepharoplasty and the eyelid crease. 3rd ed. New York: Elsevier; 2015.
5. Kim KK, Kim W-S, Oh SK, Kim HS. High double eyelid fold correction using wide dual-plane dissection. Ann Plast Surg. 2017;78:365–70.
6. Ledon JA, Savas J, Franca K, et al. Intralesional treatment for keloids and hypertrophic scars: a review. Dermatol Surg. 2013;39:1745–57.

Lower Blepharoplasty: Skin-Muscle Flap Approach

25

Rakesh M. Patel and Allen M. Putterman

Lower blepharoplasty has evolved significantly over the last several decades from a volume-depleting procedure to a volume-preserving procedure. In the days past, the surgeon would remove significant amounts of fat with aggressive skin-muscle resection utilizing the skin-muscle flap approach. This led to a hollowed, surgical look that soon began to fall out of favor not to mention an unacceptably high incidence of lower eyelid retraction [1]. In the last two decades, lower eyelid blepharoplasty has progressed to a volume conservation procedure with more conservative resection of fat or repositioning of fat using a transconjunctival approach with skin maintenance using a separate method such as laser resurfacing, skin pinch, lateral orbicularis muscle or lateral canthal tightening, or excising skin laterally [2–4]. This maximally preserves orbital septum and infraciliary orbicularis muscle minimizing the risk of lower eyelid retraction and ectropion.

Nevertheless, in the appropriately selected patient, the skin-muscle flap lower eyelid blepharoplasty is an excellent procedure. The patient with significant lower eyelid dermatochalasis, cheek bags, and excess orbicularis oculi muscle will benefit from this approach.

Preoperative Evaluation

A key component in the examination of the patient who will undergo a skin-muscle flap lower eyelid blepharoplasty is evaluating for lower eyelid laxity. The surgeon should perform a snap test by gently pulling the lower eyelid away from the globe and assessing how quickly the eyelid snaps back to the eye upon release. In addition, the lid distraction test should be performed by pulling the lower eyelid away from the eye and measuring the distance from the globe to the eyelid. If there is a delay in the snap test or the lid distracts more than 6–8 mm away from the globe, lid laxity is present, and this must be addressed concurrently; otherwise, the patient is at high risk of developing lower eyelid retraction or ectropion postoperatively. Various lateral canthoplasty techniques are available to the surgeon to address lower eyelid laxity [5–7]. The senior author's preferred method has been performing a tarsal strip procedure or to plicate the lateral canthal tendon and orbicularis muscle to the lateral orbital wall [8, 9]. Whatever method chosen, the goal is to have a lower eyelid that sits tight against the globe to prevent postoperative eyelid malpositions as the wound heals.

Surgical Technique

The procedure is typically performed under local anesthesia with intravenous sedation although general anesthesia may be utilized if the patient desires. The patient's face is prepped with povidone-iodine 5% mixture and draped in the usual manner for major oculoplastic surgery. Topical tetracaine is applied to the eyes. Corneal shields are placed over the eyes bilaterally for protection, and so the patient does not have to see the procedure. A subciliary incision is marked by drawing a line approximately 1.5 mm below the eyelid margin from the punctum to 2–3 mm just past the lateral canthus. This line is then extended further temporally horizontally for approximately 1 cm. Local anesthetic consisting of 2% lidocaine with 1:100,000 epinephrine is injected subcutaneously throughout the lower eyelid. In addition, approximately 0.5–1.0 ml of local anesthetic is injected into the temporal, central, and nasal fat pads by passing a 25-gauge, 1.5 cm needle through the skin just above the inferior orbital rim taking care to point the needle in a downward direction to avoid the globe. The anesthetic is allowed to sit for several minutes to achieve maximal hemostatic effect.

R. M. Patel
Department of Ophthalmology, University of South Carolina and Prisma Health, Columbia, SC, USA

A. M. Putterman (✉)
University of Illinois College of Medicine, Chicago, IL, USA
e-mail: drputterman@drputterman.com

A. J. Cohen, C. N. Burkat (eds.), *Oculofacial, Orbital, and Lacrimal Surgery*, https://doi.org/10.1007/978-3-030-14092-2_25

A #15 Bard-Parker blade is used to make an incision through the skin in the previously demarcated area (Fig. 25.1). A 4-0 silk traction suture is placed through the lower eyelid skin, orbicularis, and superficial tarsus and clamped to the drapes superiorly placing the lower eyelid on tension. The surgeon grasps the lower wound edge reflecting the skin inferiorly and outwardly, while the Westcott scissor buttonholes the orbicularis muscle (Fig. 25.2). Blunt dissection is performed in the suborbicularis plane with the scissors, and the orbicularis is transected for the entire length of the wound with the scissor or cautery (Fig. 25.3). Blunt dissection is performed with a cotton-tip applicator beneath the orbicularis muscle to expose the fat pads (Fig. 25.4). An assistant uses a

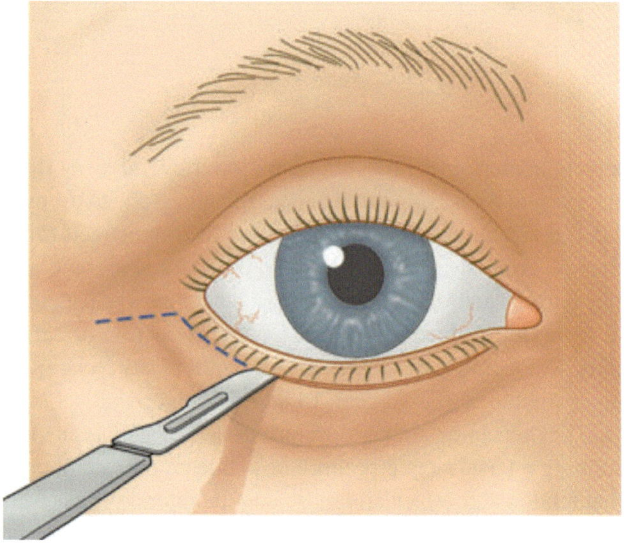

Fig. 25.1 Subciliary incision made with a #15 Bard-Parker blade and extended temporally past the lateral canthus. (The figures were published in *Putterman's Cosmetic Oculoplastic Surgery*, 4th edition edited by Steve Fagien. Page: 181–185 copyright Elsevier 2008)

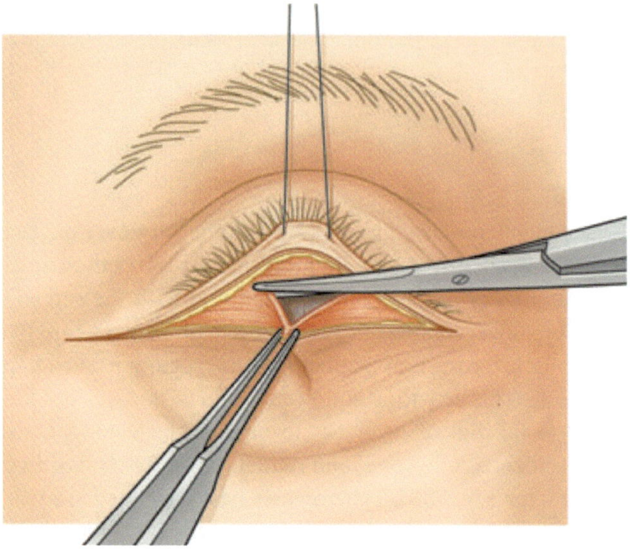

Fig. 25.3 The orbicularis is cut for the entire length of the wound with Westcott scissors. (The figures were published in *Putterman's Cosmetic Oculoplastic Surgery*, 4th edition edited by Steve Fagien. Page: 181–185 copyright Elsevier 2008)

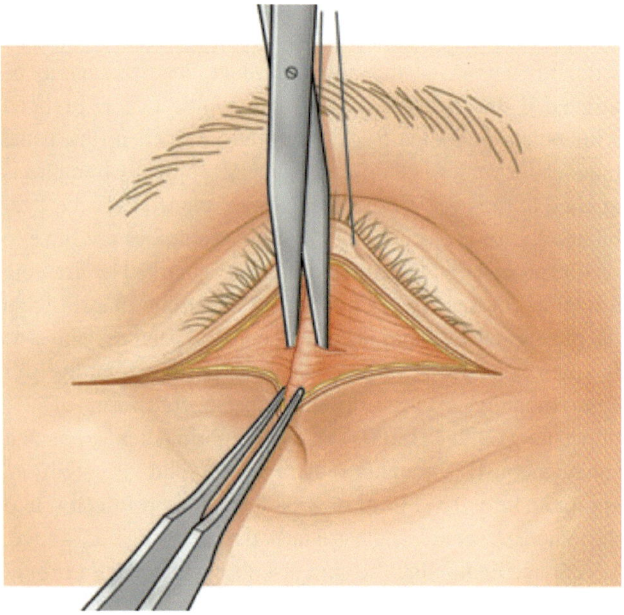

Fig. 25.2 Westcott scissors incise the orbicularis pointing the scissors inferiorly. (The figures were published in *Putterman's Cosmetic Oculoplastic Surgery*, 4th edition edited by Steve Fagien. Page: 181–185 copyright Elsevier 2008)

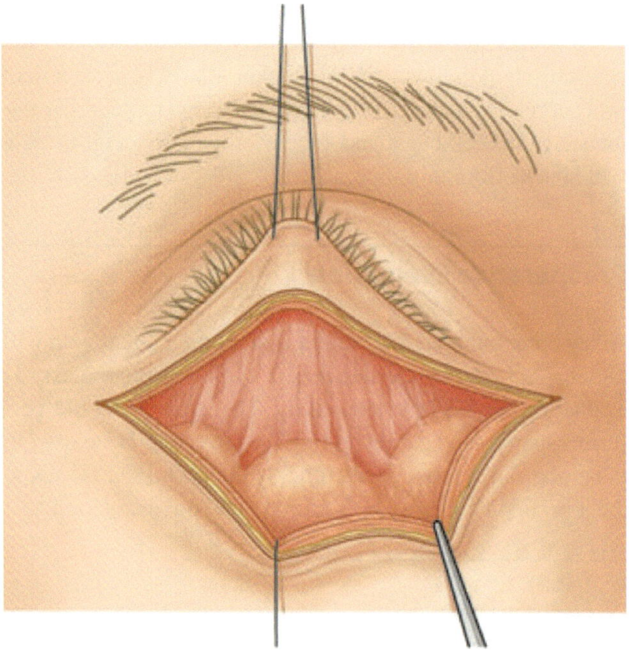

Fig. 25.4 The nasal, central, and temporal fat pads are visualized with blunt dissection. (The figures were published in *Putterman's Cosmetic Oculoplastic Surgery*, 4th edition edited by Steve Fagien. Page: 181–185 copyright Elsevier 2008)

Desmarres retractor to reflect the lower skin wound edge inferiorly to provide access to the fat pads.

Westcott scissors or disposable high-temperature cautery is used to buttonhole the suborbicularis fascia, orbital septum, and the fat capsule overlying the temporal fat pad. With gentle pressure on the globe, the fat pad prolapses forward. Toothed forceps may grasp the fat pad and cotton-tipped applicator used to bluntly dissect the fat pad free from any attachments. The fat may then be clamped with a straight hemostat flush with the inferior orbital rim, and a #15 Bard-Parker blade is used to shave the fat pad off the hemostat (Fig. 25.5). Cautery is applied to the fat stump with the hemostat still locked in place taking care to place two cotton tipped applicators underneath the clamp to protect the skin from the heat that is being conducted through the clamp. The hemostat is released while holding the fat stump with a toothed forceps, and the fat is inspected to ensure there is no bleeding before releasing the fat pad.

Often, there may be a second temporal fat pad that needs to be debulked as well [10]. Otherwise, one runs the risk of postoperative fullness of the temporal lower eyelid. The surgeon gently applies pressure to the globe to prolapse the second fat pad forward for conservative removal. Once the temporal fat has been adequately addressed, the central and nasal fat pads may be debulked in a similar manner if indicated. Care is taken to identify the inferior oblique muscle separating the nasal and central fat pads to prevent inadvertent injury to the muscle. For the patient with a nasojugal groove deformity, the nasal and central fat pads may be partially or completely repositioned into the subperiosteal or supraperiosteal plane to efface the groove [8, 11].

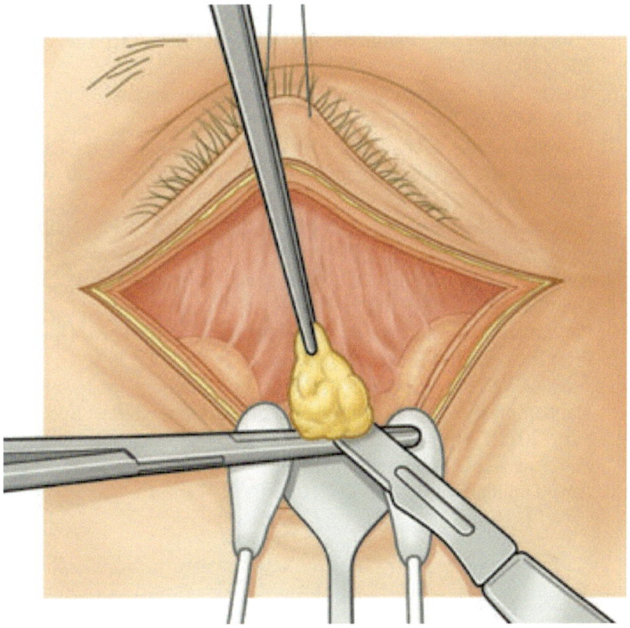

Fig. 25.5 The orbital fat pad is clamped with a straight hemostat and shaved with a #15 Bard-Parker blade. (The figures were published in *Putterman's Cosmetic Oculoplastic Surgery*, 4th edition edited by Steve Fagien. Page: 181–185 copyright Elsevier 2008)

Attention is then drawn to conservative skin-muscle resection portion of the procedure. The assistant uses a cotton-tipped applicator to apply moderate pressure to the globe by pushing on the scleral lens. This maneuver allows the lower eyelid to elevate comparable to the position of the lower eyelid in upgaze. A toothed forceps grasps the skin-muscle flap draping it over the incision in a superotemporal vector. The excess skin-muscle is then cautiously excised by removing a triangle of skin over the lateral canthal incision and another triangle of skin excised over the lower eyelid subciliary incision (Fig. 25.6). Again, care is taken to ensure skin and orbicularis removal is conservative to minimize anterior lamella shortage postoperatively that may lead to ectropion or lid retraction.

A 4–5 mm strip of orbicularis is excised over the distal edge of the skin-muscle flap and hemostasis maintained with cautery (Fig. 25.7). The excision of orbicularis helps prevent postoperative fullness at the incision site. In addition, in the patient with pretarsal fullness that is identified preoperatively, orbiculectomy will help minimize this. The skin edge is then closed by placing 2–3 interrupted 6-0 polyglactin 910 sutures at the lateral canthal wound. In addition, another 6-0 suture is placed at the temporal subciliary incision from the inferior skin edge to the inferior tarsal border to superior skin wound edge to prevent the skin from overriding the incision. The lateral canthus is then closed with a running 6-0 silk suture, and the subciliary incision is also closed with a separate running 6-0 silk suture (Fig. 25.8). The corneal protectors are removed and antibiotic ointment is placed on the incisions and the eyes.

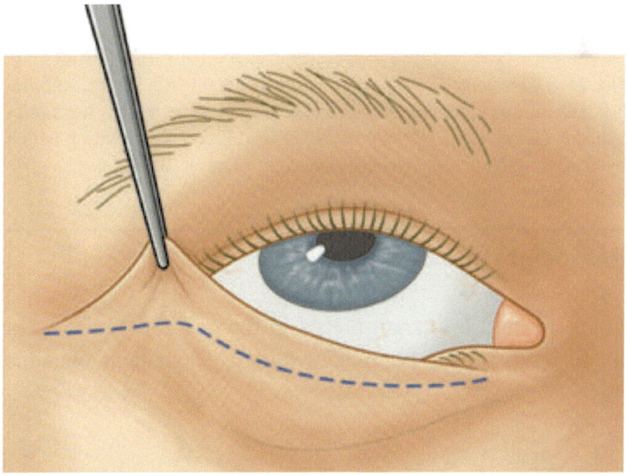

Fig. 25.6 Excess skin and muscle is draped over the incision and excised conservatively. (The figures were published in *Putterman's Cosmetic Oculoplastic Surgery*, 4th edition edited by Steve Fagien. Page: 181–185 copyright Elsevier 2008)

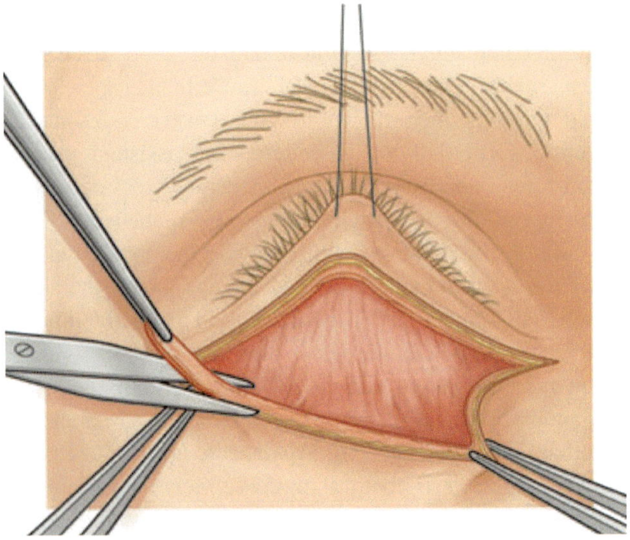

Fig. 25.7 A strip of orbicularis is excised for 4–5 mm from the skin flap. (The figures were published in *Putterman's Cosmetic Oculoplastic Surgery*, 4th edition edited by Steve Fagien. Page: 181–185 copyright Elsevier 2008)

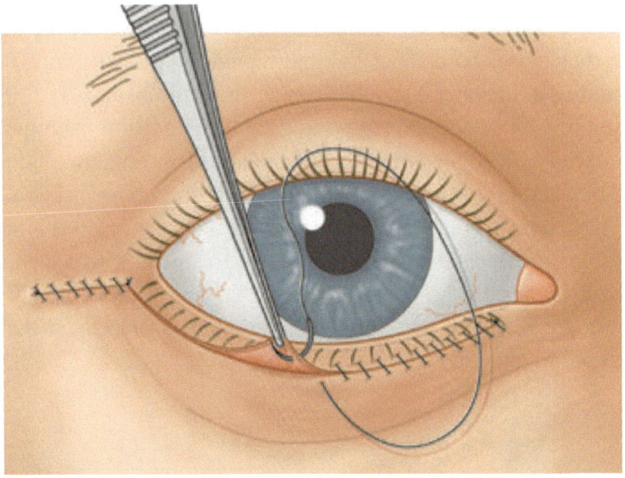

Fig. 25.8 The subciliary wound is closed with 6-0 silk suture. Another 6-0 silk suture closes the lateral canthal wound. (The figures were published in *Putterman's Cosmetic Oculoplastic Surgery*, 4th edition edited by Steve Fagien. Page: 181–185 copyright Elsevier 2008)

Postoperative Care

Frequent cold packs are placed to the eyes immediately in the recovery area to minimize swelling. The patient's head is also elevated on the stretcher decreasing venous return to the eyelids to further aid in reducing the swelling. The nurse checks the patients vision every 15–30 minutes to ensure the vision remains intact, pain is minimal, and there is no proptosis as these signs may indicate a retrobulbar hemorrhage. The incidence is low; however if identified, treatment must be instituted immediately consisting of suture removal and opening of the wounds. Any bleeding vessel is identified and cauterized and the wound then closed [12].

If the patient remains stable after a couple of hours, the patient may be discharged home with instructions to continue applying cold packs to the eyes and keeping the head elevated. The patient should also check his or her vision while at home to ensure they can at least count fingers a few feet from their face. The application of cold packs continues for the first 24 hours after surgery. Ointment is applied to the incisions and to the eye three times a day. The silk sutures are then removed on postoperative day 6 and the polyglactin 910 sutures removed approximately 2–3 weeks after surgery.

References

1. Schwarcz R, Fezza JP, Jacono A, Massry GG. Stop blaming the septum. Ophthal Plast Reconstr Surg. 2016;32(1):49–52.
2. Kim EM, Bucky LP. Power of the pinch: pinch lower lid blepharoplasty. Ann Plast Surg. 2008;60(5):532–7.
3. Hidalgo DA. An integrated approach to lower blepharoplasty. Plast Reconstr Surg. 2011;127(1):386–95.
4. Griffin RY, Sarici A, Ozkan S. Treatment of the lower eyelid with the CO2 laser: transconjunctival or transcutaneous approach? Orbit. 2007;26(1):23–8.
5. Georgescu D, Anderson RL, McCann JD. Lateral canthal resuspension sine canthotomy. Ophthal Plast Reconstr Surg. 2011;27(5):371–5.
6. Massry GG. Comprehensive lower eyelid rejuvenation. Facial Plast Surg. 2010;26:209–21.
7. Glat PM, Jelks GW, Jelks EB, et al. Evolution of the lateral canthoplasty: techniques and indications. Plast Reconstr Surg. 1997;100(6):1396–405.
8. Putterman AM. Cosmetic oculoplastic surgery. 3rd ed. Philadelphia: Saunders; 1999.
9. Anderson RL, Gordy DD. The tarsal strip procedure. Arch Ophthalmol. 1979;97(11):2192–6.
10. Putterman AM. The mysterious second temporal fat pad. Ophthal Plast Reconstr Surg. 1985;1(2):83–6.
11. Aakalu VK, Putterman AM. Fat repositioning in lower lid blepharoplasty: the role of titrated excision. Ophthal Plast Reconstr Surg. 2011;27(6):462.
12. Putterman AM. Temporary blindness after cosmetic blepharoplasty. Am J Ophthalmol. 1975;80(6):1081–3.

Lower Blepharoplasty: Transconjunctival Approach

26

Ana Filipa Duarte, Alice Varanda Pereira, and Martin H. Devoto

Introduction

Cosmetic lower blepharoplasty is one of the most common procedures in an oculoplastic surgeon practice. Several studies have shown that lower lid rejuvenation has a significant impact on age, attractiveness, and fatigue appearance [1, 2] and the vast majority of patients seeking cosmetic treatments address this area as the most desired for rejuvenation [3].

The progressive increase in blepharoplasty numbers in the last few decades has shown how this surgery can be rewarding but also challenging. Complications can be devastating and difficult to reverse [4], so the search for a technique that might fulfill all the requirements for safety and long-lasting results is far from over. Many techniques have been described, and trends have changed along the years. Lower blepharoplasty may be in fact a one to three-step procedure, encompassing orbital fat excision or transposition, skin treatment, and canthal support. In a recent survey on current trends in upper and lower eyelid blepharoplasty among the American Society of Ophthalmic Plastic and Reconstructive Surgery Members, 96% of surgeons reported using the transconjunctival approach for lower eyelid blepharoplasty; 80% included fat repositioning in their practice, mainly using the supraperiosteal plane; and 97% of the surgeons excised eyelid skin as needed, either using a pinch technique (79%), a skin-muscle (75%), or skin-only (61%) flap excision. Ninety-six percent of the surgeons added canthal suspension to the procedure, mainly by open canthoplasty, although closed canthopexies were also commonly performed [5].

This chapter highlights how the traditional blepharoplasty, using a myocutaneous flap and aggressive tissue resection (fat, skin, and muscle), has evolved to a more conservative technique. As surgeons realized that rejuvenation required volume enhancement more that tissue resection, modern facial surgery started to pursue a new and more cautious direction [6–8]. Nevertheless, it is difficult to establish a standard practice pattern for lower blepharoplasty, as each step of the procedure is planned according to individual findings and needs of each patient and framed as part of a global facial assessment. In this chapter we describe the fundamental aspects of the transconjunctival lower blepharoplasty with and without fat transposition. Surgical technique, its historical background, the complex anatomy of lower eyelid and evolving concepts of facial aging, as well as important preoperative, intraoperative, and postoperative aspects are described.

Historical Perspective: The Surgical Technique as an Adaptation of Contemporary Concepts of Face Aging

The traditional skin-muscle flap lower blepharoplasty, based on a transcutaneous approach with skin, muscle, and fat resection, was popularized by Rees in the 1970s [9]. For many years it was the standard procedure for rejuvenation of the lower eyelid; however, concerns then developed regarding long-term orbicularis muscle denervation, atrophy and eyelid malposition [10, 11], as well as aesthetic issues concerning rounding of the lateral canthus and periorbital hollowing [8]. As the interest about the genesis of age-related changes started to grow, and surgeons better understood the aging mechanisms, it was clear that aesthetic surgery, and specifically eyelid surgery, needed to be improved.

A. F. Duarte
Department of Ophthalmology, Centro Hospitalar de Lisboa Central, Lisbon, Portugal

Department of Ophthalmology, Hospital Cuf Descobertas, Lisbon, Portugal

A. V. Pereira
Plastic Reconstructive Surgery, Central Lisbon Hospital Center, Lisbon, Portugal

M. H. Devoto (✉)
Consultores Oftalmologicos, Ciudad de Buenos Aires, Argentina

A. J. Cohen, C. N. Burkat (eds.), *Oculofacial, Orbital, and Lacrimal Surgery*, https://doi.org/10.1007/978-3-030-14092-2_26

Aging changes become more evident during the fourth decade and involve all anatomic layers, from the skin to the bone [12–16]. Many authors have improved our knowledge, with two main currents existing nowadays for aging morphogenesis. Ligament attenuation and vertical soft tissue descent (the gravitational perspective) was the most widely accepted theory for many decades [17–20]. In 2000, Donofrio questioned its veracity and advocated the redistribution of facial fat (with alternate areas of atrophy/hypertrophy) as the primary factor for the "hill and valley" topography of the old face. The first arguments for a new volumetric theory were then proposed [21]. Later, Lambros superimposed and compared patient photos at two distant points in time and noticed that no descent of anatomical landmarks (such as moles and wrinkles) was seen and that the eyelid-cheek junction remained stable. Using objective data he demonstrated that aging changes of the midface were, as Donofrio had previously defended, caused mainly by anteroposterior shifts of volume in the facial fat compartments [22]. More recently, important anatomic studies from Rohrich et al. on facial fat compartments [23–27] also reiterated this phenomenon. Their findings, combined with imaging studies by other authors, added important information to this debate, demonstrating a distinct behavior between superficial and deep fat compartments, with a gradual enhancement of the first and deflation of the latter [12, 13].

The fact is that these two theories may not be mutually exclusive [26, 28]. Sagging of superficial fat occurs potentiated by a selective deflation of deep fat pads [13], causing what Rohrich had previously called "pseudoptosis" [27]. This is exacerbated by the age-related attenuation of the surrounding connective tissue and ligaments and bony volume loss. In light of this growing knowledge, surgeons have unquestionably changed our surgical and nonsurgical rejuvenation approaches. From a resective approach, we are now trying to recover the youthful enhanced facial contour. Within this background the transconjunctival lower blepharoplasty, with a lower rate of complications and a hidden incision, began to gain increasing popularity [29].

The transconjunctival approach for lower eyelid blepharoplasty was first described in 1924 by Bourget [30]. At the beginning it was used to excise fat [31, 32], becoming very popular in the 1990s [33]. A few years before, authors like Loeb [34], de la Plaza [35], and later Hamra [8, 36] and Mendelson [37] had already reported the efficacy of transcutaneous fat repositioning to the nasojugal fold to improve the eyelid-cheek transition. Instead of resecting the herniated orbital fat responsible for the double-convexity deformity and therefore risking a sunken lower eyelid appearance, the fat pads were slid over the inferior orbital rim creating a younger fuller and shorter eyelid. In 2000, two decades after the first description of transconjunctival fat removal, Goldberg described orbital fat transposition using a transconjunctival approach [38]. Since then, in parallel with a better understanding of the physical changes of facial aging, orbital fat repositioning, either in a supraperiosteal or subperiosteal plane, has become a widely accepted method, with a lower rate of complications and more natural results.

Lower Eyelid Anatomy: Important Aspects for Better Outcomes

The face should always be globally evaluated in any surgical procedure. More importantly, anatomic aspects of facial aging as a whole should always be kept in mind even when a single subunit procedure, such as an upper or lower blepharoplasty, is planned. Involutional changes have anatomic and functional repercussions, which are inseparable, demanding a thorough knowledge that goes beyond the simple anatomic topography of the periocular area.

From deep to superficial, the lower eyelid is divided into three lamellae: posterior, middle, and anterior lamella. Also, there are several anthropometric landmarks that become important when eyelid surgery is planned.

Anatomic Planes of the Lower Eyelid

The lower eyelid is divided into a posterior and an anterior lamella separated by the orbital septum (sometimes called the middle lamella). The anterior lamella is composed by skin in its most superficial plane (it is the thinnest skin of the body) and the orbicularis oculi muscle. The orbicularis muscle has two portions: the palpebral, formed by muscle fibers extending from the medial to the lateral canthus, and further subdivided in a pretarsal (anterior to the inferior tarsal plate) and preseptal (anterior to the orbital septum) subunits, and the orbital portion, formed by concentric fibers that extend anterior to the zygomatic and maxillary bones. The orbital septum is a thin fibrous lamina extending from the inferior arcus marginalis at the orbital rim up to about 5 mm below the tarsus, where it fuses with the capsulopalpebral fascia (the lower eyelid retractors). It separates orbital contents into a preseptal and a postseptal space. The posterior lamella is constituted by the inferior tarsus, lower eyelid retractors, and conjunctiva.

The lower eyelid retractors consist of the inferior tarsal muscle posteriorly, and the capsulopalpebral fascia anteriorly, a double sheet of connective tissue that extends from the fascia of the inferior rectus muscle, envelopes the inferior oblique muscle and continues superiorly reaching the tarsal plate [39]. This structure is the equivalent to the levator aponeurosis in the upper eyelid, and it also sends a few extensions that pass through the preseptal orbicularis muscle and reach the skin, contributing to the lower eyelid crease, a subtle line that extends 2 mm below the lash line medially and 5 mm laterally [40].

The inferior tarsus plate is a fibrous structure composed of dense connective tissue, measuring 4–5 mm in height, and lined on its posterior surface by the nonkeratinizing stratified columnar epithelium of the conjunctiva. The tarsus is secured to the orbital rim by the medial and lateral canthal tendons.

Tendons and Ligaments

The periorbital soft tissues (fat, muscle, skin) are interconnected by fibrous bands and attachments. The lateral canthal tendon (LCT) is a fundamental structure for eyelid anchorage and globe support [41]. Medially it is attached to the upper and lower tarsal plates by a superior and inferior crus, which insert as a single tendon in the Whitnall tubercle, located on the lateral orbital wall, approximately 3–5 mm posterior to the lateral orbital rim [42]. The LTC is located 2–4 mm above the level of the medial canthal tendon [43], allowing a 2–3° intercanthal tilt.

Anterior to the lateral canthal tendon, the lateral thickening attaches the orbicularis at the lateral orbital rim, extending inferiorly as a thinner structure called the orbicularis retaining ligament (ORL) or orbitomalar ligament [44]. Medially, the canthal tendon has an anterior and a posterior attachment inserted into the anterior and the posterior lacrimal crest, respectively. Each portion of the orbicularis (palpebral and orbital) inserts medially by a superficial and a deep head, which span the respective portion of the medial canthal tendon.

Finally, the Lockwood ligament is one of the suspensory structures of the inferior orbit. Laterally, it inserts onto Whitnall's tubercle, together with the lateral canthal tendon, and its lateral arcuate expansion divides the lateral from the central fat pads [44].

Fat Pads

Most of the orbital fat (60–70%) is located deep in the orbit, having little effect on the vertical position of the globe [41]. However, the more anterior postseptal orbital fat does have an important function on globe support. Manson et al. demonstrated that for every 2.5 ml of fat removed, the globe moves posteriorly by 2 mm and inferiorly by 1 mm [45]. The lower fat is organized into three compartments: lateral, central, and medial fat pads. The central and medial pads are separated by the inferior oblique muscle, while the lateral and central fat pads are almost continuous, being only separated by the arcuate expansion of Lockwood's ligament [46]. These are important landmarks during blepharoplasty surgery, and the inferior oblique muscle should always be identified during fat removal or transposition, in order to avoid injury and postoperative motility disturbances.

Inferior to the orbital rim, just posterior to the orbicularis, is the suborbicularis oculi fat pad (SOOF), which forms the roof of a triangular prezygomatic space. This space is limited inferiorly by the zygomatic ligament and superiorly by the ORL [47]. Rohrich et al. have shown that the SOOF is divided into a distinct lateral and medial area and also described another fat pad, the deep cheek fat, medial to the SOOF [25]. Aging changes of these components include gradual loss of fat and attenuation of ligaments and connective tissue, which explain the progressive ptosis of SOOF and the formation of "malar bags" or festoons [20].

The Nasojugal and Palpebromalar Grooves

The nasojugal groove or "tear trough" is a depression extending inferolaterally from the medial canthus to the vertical midpupillary line [47]. From there, parallel and slightly below the infraorbital rim extends the palpebromalar groove or eyelid-cheek junction [47]. These grooves become more visible with age, exacerbated by progressive malar volume loss. Together with the prolapse of orbital fat superiorly, and the malar mound inferiorly, this forms the "double-convexity" deformity. In 2009, Haddock demonstrated that these landmarks are explained in three distinct anatomic planes: in a superficial level (the difference in texture and thickness between the eyelid and cheek skin), in the subcutaneous plane (the transition between the palpebral and orbital portions of the orbicularis muscle), and in the deep, suborbicularis plane [48]. In the deeper plane, there are important differences to highlight for their surgical implications. Along the tear trough, the orbicularis muscle is directly attached to the maxillary bone, while laterally the ORL bridges the connection between the muscle and the bone. Both these landmarks form a continuous sulcus several millimeters below the orbital rim which should, as Haddock pointed out, be dissected and released prior to any fat transposition [48].

Innervation

Facial sensation is provided by the trigeminal nerve (V). The malar region, lower eyelid, cheek, nasal vestibule, and upper lip are innervated by the maxillary branch (V2). Motor innervation of the eyelid, on the other hand, has been a subject of debate. Motor nerve injury is usually a major concern in any midface surgery, as it may lead to lower eyelid retraction, ectropion and scleral show [10, 49]. For many years it was believed that vertical motor nerves entered the pretarsal muscle, originating from the zygomatic or buccal branches of the facial nerve [50, 51]. Such topography could explain those denervation-related complications, particularly during transcutaneous traditional blepharoplasty. The theory was called into question by McCord, who demonstrated no signs or symptoms of denervation after subciliary myocutaneous incisions [52]. That study, together with previous results after surgical denervation of the eyelids in patients with blepharospasm, created the intracanthal-extracanthal theory. This theory suggested that the medial intracanthal system, innervated by the buccal branch, was responsible for lower eyelid tone, while the extracanthal orbicularis muscle (zygomatic branch), transected during traditional blepharoplasty, would be less relevant for lower eyelid position [53].

A recent Korean study described a new model for lower eyelid innervation, proposing that the vertical suborbicularis nerves are actually sensory nerves. The motor route, originating from the facial zygomatic branch, would travel superiorly to the medial canthus through the anterior cheek, extending parallel or oblique to the orbicularis oculi muscle fibers while also projecting small branches to the medial upper eyelid [54]. The glabellar area, on the other hand, was not innervated by the zygomatic branch of the facial nerve but by the angular nerve that originated from the buccal branch. This work has unquestionably brought new insights to the motor and sensory innervation of the lower eyelid, allowing the definition of risk zones, such as the medial preseptal-pretarsal area of the lower eyelid and the premaxillary space lateral to the angular vein that may lead to damage to the eyelid sphincter function.

However, variations of these facial nerve branches do exist as noted in many other studies. That said, care should be taken in both cosmetic and reconstructive procedures, when operating in the medial area of both the inferior and superior eyelids.

Eyelid Vascularization

The eyelids are supplied by branches from the internal and external carotid artery network. These include the lateral and medial palpebral arteries (originating from the superficial temporal artery, lacrimal artery and other terminal branches from the ophthalmic artery), which anastomose with the zygomaticotemporal artery and transverse facial artery laterally, the infraorbital artery and medially the angular artery (a terminal branch of the facial artery lying 6–8 mm medial to the medial canthus). These anastomoses create the inferior marginal and superior peripheral palpebral arcades in the upper eyelid and, in the lower eyelid, a single vascular arcade adjacent to the margin.

The medial fat pad is usually associated with larger-caliber vessels, and care should be taken when fat is exposed and removed.

A recent study by Mendelson et al. has made important advances in the characterization of the lymphatic drainage of the conjunctiva and lower eyelid and thus its relationship with postoperative chemosis and edema [55]. They found interconnecting superficial and deep lymphatic pathways, draining laterally to the parotid nodes and medially to the submandibular nodes. Surgical damage, especially in the lateral lower eyelid, to both the superficial (traveling in the subcutaneous fat) and deep (located beneath the orbicularis muscle, around the ORL and into the SOOF) vessels may be the cause of postoperative edema and chemosis.

Anatomy of Aging

Throughout a lifetime, the human face undergoes changes that are fundamentally similar among races and genders. Even though there is interindividual variability, there are a few typical features that characterize the youthful face and that we, as blepharoplasty surgeons, must seek to reestablish.

In youth, the lower eyelid is tense and vertically short [56], its margin is at or slightly below the inferior corneal limbus, and the eyelid fissure is elongated with a positive tilt (slightly higher lateral canthus) [57, 58]. The eyelid-cheek transition is a smooth convexity, with a prominent malar area, and the skin is firm and unwrinkled. With age, due to dermal elastosis and collagen loss, wrinkles and a relative excess of skin appear [59], and this single convexity gradually transforms into a "double-convexity deformity" [8], or "hills and valleys" [60]. Anatomically, the prolapsed orbital fat superiorly is interrupted by a skeletonized inferior orbital rim, followed by an inferior convexity defined by the malar mound. This progressive demarcation of the tear trough and palpebromalar groove is related to a progressive laxity of the orbital septum and orbicularis oculi muscle, inferior orbital rim remodeling, attenuation of the suspensory eyelid ligaments, and selective deflation of the midface fat compartments [48, 61–63].

Progressive laxity of the lateral canthal tendon also results in gradual shortening of the horizontal eyelid fissure, rounding of the lateral canthal angle, and variable scleral show [58]. Therefore, these three key findings, when present, should be addressed for complete rejuvenation of the lower eyelid: the double-convexity deformity, skin excess, and lower eyelid laxity.

Preoperative Evaluation

As in any other cosmetic procedure, preoperative evaluation is of paramount importance both for the surgeon and for the patient. Patients, in general, desire the maximum improvement with minimal surgery. Although transconjunctival lower blepharoplasty may be very appealing as it leaves no visible scars, patients should be carefully selected and fully informed about the goals and limitations of this technique, otherwise the potential for postoperative dissatisfaction may be significantly high.

It is always helpful to have the patients demonstrate their specific concerns and desires for improvement while looking in a mirror. Also, the clinical findings and treatment options should be explained in detail, including the basic surgical strategy, necessary ancillary procedures, the expected aesthetic outcome, as well as treatment limitations and possible complications.

It is essential to ensure that the patients' expectations are realistic and that they are psychologically stable for the procedure. Every detail of the discussion should be fully documented.

Medical History

Obtaining a comprehensive history and physical examination is critical to tailoring the surgery to each individual patient. This will reduce the risk of complications, identify contraindications to the transconjunctival approach, and maximize the cosmetic and therapeutic aspects of the procedure.

The first step in a thorough evaluation includes a complete past ocular history, as well as a past medical history directed toward the identification of specific conditions that may increase the risk of complications.

General health conditions such as diabetes, hypertension, coagulopathy, thyroid, renal, cerebrovascular or cardiopulmonary diseases, active inflammation, or infection can affect the outcome by poor wound healing or increased bleeding.

Patients with a history of systemic inflammatory, autoimmune, or collagen vascular diseases, such as scleroderma, systemic lupus erythematous, periarteritis nodosa, Wegener's granulomatosis (granulomatous with polyangiitis), rosacea, rheumatoid arthritis, or Sjögren syndrome, are at greater risk for postoperative dry eye symptoms.

In addition, poorly controlled rosacea, pemphigoid, or sarcoidosis may predispose to scar contracture of the conjunctival fornix causing foreshortening and eyelid malposition.

Weak orbicularis oculi tone, or incomplete recovery of previous facial nerve palsy, may interfere with eyelid closure and also predispose the patient to dry eye complications and exposure keratopathy.

Hyperthyroidism or hypothyroidism should demonstrate 6–12 months of medical and clinical stability before elective cosmetic surgery. Patients with puffy eyelids will sometimes present to the oculoplastic surgeon with hyperthyroidism or euthyroid Graves' disease. If needed, blepharoplasty techniques should be modified to correct eyelid position or retraction and reduce the risk of inadequate corneal protection. However, thyroid hypofunction may cause a tendency for persistent eyelid edema in the perioperative period.

Patients with hypertension should medically optimize blood pressure at least 2 weeks prior to surgery to ensure a stable normotensive state. Other factors that influence bleeding tendencies should be identified and controlled before surgery. Any history of abnormal or easy bruising, prolonged clotting time, or family members with bleeding dyscrasia should be explored with appropriate coagulation profiles.

A full medication history must be documented, especially the use of antiarthritics, corticosteroids, aspirin, nonsteroidal anti-inflammatory medications, anticoagulants, and vitamin E, as patients will need to discontinue these medicines preoperatively for 1–2 weeks. Warfarin is generally held for 4–5 days preoperatively. Over-the-counter herbal medications, such as garlic, ginkgo biloba, or St. John's wort, should be discontinued, due to their effect on blood pressure and coagulation.

A history of cigarette, alcohol, and illicit drug use should also be elicited, as these may influence platelet function, skin quality, healing, and the patient's ability to follow appropriate postoperative instructions. Similarly, a past history of psychiatric or psychological disorders, as well as past litigation, is of paramount importance prior to proceeding with surgery.

Ophthalmic History

Past ophthalmologic history should always document any *previous eyelid surgery or trauma, dry eye, eyelid infection, chronic allergy or swelling*, the use of glasses or contact lenses, and changes in visual fields and/or visual acuity.

Patients should be questioned about symptoms of tearing, burning, gritty sensation or ocular discomfort, mucus production, eyelid crusting, and frequency of artificial tear use. These symptoms are suggestive of borderline or *inadequate tear production*, which may be aggravated after surgery.

The use of contact lenses and history of refractive surgery also predisposes patients to dry eyes and less tolerance to evaporative tear loss.In *laser* in situ *keratomileusis (LASIK)*, the flap disrupts corneal innervation, forming an anesthetic effect that suppresses tear production. These patients should avoid blepharoplasty for at least 6 months in order to allow the corneal incision adequate time to heal and to minimize the risk of superinfection in the event of *lagophthalmos* and dryness. Furthermore, ancillary procedures such as canthopexy can affect the refractive characteristics, cause mechanical irritation of the conjunctiva and cornea, or affect the corneal flap.

Other eye procedures, including glaucoma, retinal, strabismus, and cataract surgery, should be documented. History of *previous lower blepharoplasty* and the surgical approach should be noted, as well as any history of periocular trauma. Previous ocular or periocular intervention, including *soft tissue fillers*, may also potentially affect the result of lower eyelid surgery.

Every patient with a documented or suspected history of *glaucoma* must normalize intraocular pressure, as eyelid surgery may rarely precipitate and then mask the onset of acute closed-angle attack in susceptible eyes.

Chronic blepharitis may be exacerbated by blepharoplasty, and prophylactic therapy including systemic antibiotics may be warranted before surgery. Prophylactic antiviral agents may also be indicated before surgical procedures in patients who are predisposed to recurrent *herpes zoster* outbreaks.

Finally, although rare, *blepharochalasis* should be ruled out, particularly in women with repeated episodes of significant periorbital swelling. This eyelid disorder is caused by recurrent episodes of extreme edema, with longstanding stretching of the eyelid skin and septum, that eventually result in chronic puffy eyelids.

Physical Examination

The preoperative physical examination of a patient requesting lower blepharoplasty focuses on eyelid appearance and function as well as surrounding anatomy, which may need adjunctive procedures for best outcome. With the patient in the upright sitting position, the surgeon evaluates the aging changes in each layer, including the skin, muscle, fat pads, orbital fat, and bone. The entire face should be assessed, including facial appearance, symmetry, wrinkles, skin folds, scarring, and generalized skin texture changes.

Orbit and Malar Eminence

Assessment of the lower orbit and midface should include examining globe position relative to the bony orbital rim and malar eminence. When viewed from a lateral sagittal plane, there is normally 15–17 mm of globe projection as measured from the lateral orbital rim. Proptosis and enophthalmos correspond to the relative anterior and posterior displacement of the globe, respectively. Hertel exophthalmometry can be used to quantify the degree of ocular projection for documentation purposes.

Patients with a positive vector relationship have the most anterior projection of the globe lying behind the anterior projection of the malar eminence. A negative vector corresponds to globe projection extending more anteriorly than the malar eminence. Both prominent and deep-set eyes are at increased risk for complications. An excessively prominent globe may be secondary to malar hypoplasia and/or soft tissue proptosis. It is associated with poor lower eyelid support and higher risk for postoperative dryness and eyelid malposition if not addressed adequately. Even a transconjunctival approach in which only fat is transposed or removed may result in scleral show. Moreover, fat removal can sometimes accentuate an exophthalmic look. For severe cases with exposure problems, orbital rim or malar implants and lateral or inferior orbital decompression can improve aesthetic results.

In youth, the eyelid-cheek contour is a smooth single convexity from the tarsus to the cheek. Midface architecture changes with age, manifesting as deep tear troughs, festoons, malar mounds, and midfacial/facial ptosis. Concurrent or separate procedures may be necessary to address these problems specifically.

The ability to place the side of the finger into the bony furrow over the nasojugal grooves – tear trough test – suggests a potential benefit from tissue augmentation. Correction of this tear trough deformity can be addressed at the time of lower eyelid blepharoplasty through fat and orbicularis repositioning or fat grafts.

When laxity or stretching of the inferior orbital portion of the orbicularis oculi develops, the muscle may sag or form redundant folds known as festoons that are seen inferior to the bulges of herniated fat. True festooning must be differentiated from malar pads. These projections of the skin and fat in the area of the malar eminence represent altered orbicularis fibers that allow abnormal communication between subdermal and suborbicularis fat. Conventional transconjunctival blepharoplasty may reduce areas of fat bulging superior to the orbital rim, but it does not address the malar area, and separate procedures are needed to address these deformities. Patients must also be made aware that malar mounds and festoons can also worsen after lower blepharoplasty. Ptosis of the suborbicularis oculi fat (SOOF), orbicularis, and global midface may sometimes be addressed through transconjunctival midface elevation techniques.

Lower Eyelid

Focusing on the lower eyelid, it is critical to address each layer of the eyelid complex to ensure optimal outcomes in lower eyelid rejuvenation.

- *Dermatochalasis* is the excess of eyelid skin. Assessing for extra lower eyelid skin is best performed in upgaze with the mouth open (to allow for maximal excursion of the lower eyelid skin). The lower eyelid skin is then pinched with forceps until the eyelashes begin to evert. Patients must be informed that blepharoplasty alone will not improve fine rhytids and other skin quality issues around the eyes (e.g., texture, pores, sun-induced damage, pigmentary changes). The remaining eyelid skin that is not excised will still have its preoperative skin texture characteristics, which is often not intuitive to patients. Adjuvant resurfacing treatments, such as ablative (CO_2) lasers and chemical peels, are a good option for these skin issues and can have moderate skin tightening effect as well. In addition, bleaching creams and intense pulsed light therapy (broadband light) can improve abnormal hyperpigmentation. Dynamic creases in the lateral canthus and lower eyelid ("crow's feet") will also continue to require neuromodulation with botulinum toxin.

- *Herniated medial, central, and lateral lower eyelid fat pads*: Gentle retropulsion of the globe results in a distinct anterior movement of the fat pads, helping to differentiate them from other causes of eyelid fullness like edema or hypertrophic pretarsal orbicularis. Herniation of the medial and central fat pads is best tested with the patient eyes in an upward gaze, whereas looking upward and to the contralateral side accentuates the lateral fat.
- *Palpation of infraorbital rim and globe vector*: An excessive fat resection may contribute to a sunken eye appearance in the patient with a very prominent rim.
- *Eyelid margin inflammation*: Inflammatory changes and crusting along the eyelid margins or within the eyelashes may indicate blepharitis.
- *Malposition of eyelid and eyelashes* includes ectropion (turning out of the eyelid margin), entropion (turning in of the eyelid), retraction, and trichiasis. The presence of scleral show is objectively measured using the distance from the inferior corneal limbus to the lower eyelid margin. It is often associated with a prominent eye, lower eyelid laxity, and poor infraorbital support, defining patients at higher risk for postoperative complications.
- The *distraction and snapback tests* are useful in the preoperative identification of lower eyelid laxity and the need for a concurrent horizontal tightening procedure (tarsal strip, canthopexy). The eyelid distraction test is performed by grasping the lower eyelid and pulling it away from the globe. If the lower eyelid can be pulled more than 6–8 mm, horizontal laxity exists. In the snapback test, the eyelid is pulled down and then allowed to snap back to the globe. If significant laxity exists, the eyelid does not return to the globe until the next blink.
- *Position of the medial and lateral canthi*: A positive canthal tilt refers to a lateral canthus that is positioned superior to the medial canthus. A negative canthal tilt may indicate descent of the lateral canthus from disinsertion, laxity, or the presence of a prominent eye. Laxity of the lateral canthal tendon is the most common cause of lower eyelid laxity. Laxity of the medial canthal tendon is less frequent and is observed when the medial punctum can be displaced more than 4–5 mm laterally.

Ocular Examination

Finally, a baseline ocular examination should be performed to document visual acuity, slit lamp examination, motility, and the presence of Bell's phenomenon. The presence of an intact Bell's phenomenon is tested by gently forcing the upper eyelids open during tight closure. A normal Bell reflex, which is noted by upward globe rotation such that the cornea is covered under the upper eyelid, affords protection for the corneal surface in the event of incomplete eyelid closure after surgery. Baseline evaluation of ocular motility is important as diplopia can occur as a result of iatrogenic injury of the inferior oblique muscle.

Dry eye symptoms are frequent following blepharoplasty, and preoperative evaluation of the lacrimal system may direct surgical intervention and patient education. If any doubt exists regarding tear status, both basic and reflexive tear production should be assessed using Schirmer test strips or other appropriate tests. Visual fields and any further specific tests are also undertaken as necessary.

Photographic Documentation

Finally, standard photographs are taken of each patient. These are helpful in preoperative planning, as an intraoperative reference, and serve as a benchmark from which postoperative change can be determined. Recommended views include full-face lateral, oblique, and frontal views in primary, upgaze, and downgaze [64].

Surgical Technique

Transconjunctival blepharoplasty may be performed under conscious sedation or general anesthesia. With the patient in an upright, sitting position, a marking pen is used to mark the nasojugal groove. Tetracaine ophthalmic solution is instilled in each eye, and a corneal shield is placed. Two percent lidocaine with 1:100,000 units epinephrine and 0.5% bupivacaine in a 50:50 mixture is used for local anesthesia. A Desmarres retractor is used to expose the conjunctival area, and an incision is made 4–5 mm inferior to the tarsus using a Colorado needle (Fig. 26.1). Dissection is carried through the lower eyelid retractors and continued inferiorly behind the orbicularis muscle in a preseptal plane (Fig. 26.2). The infraorbital fat may be also accessed through a postseptal approach. In this case the incision is lower, 6–7.5 mm below the tarsus [65], keeping septal integrity and theoretically reducing the chance of mid-lamellar scarring [66]. This direct technique is a resective rather than repositioning approach and

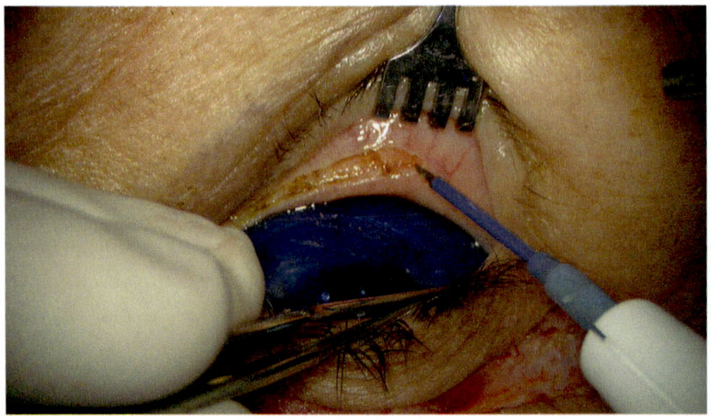

Fig. 26.1 A conjunctival incision is made, using a Colorado Needle, 4 mm below the lower tarsal edge

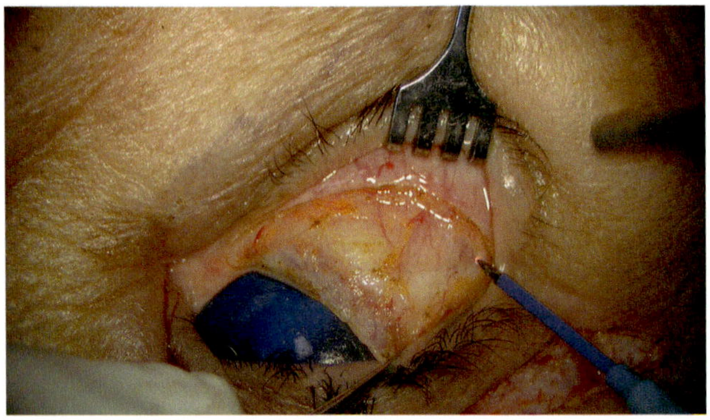

Fig. 26.2 The dissection is carried out in the postorbicularis/preseptal plane

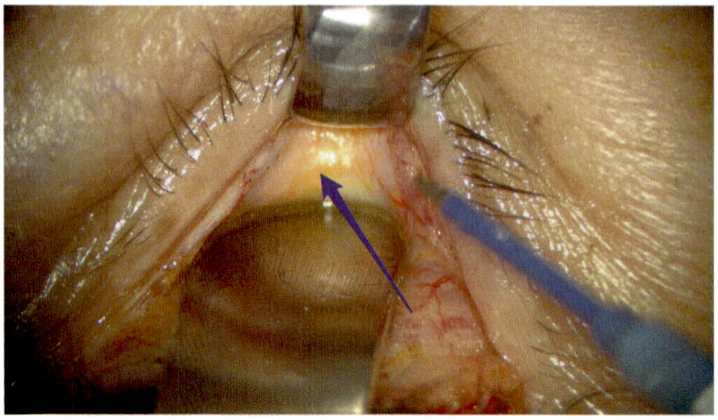

Fig. 26.3 Using an Araf elk retractor and a malleable retractor, the arcus marginalis is exposed (arrow)

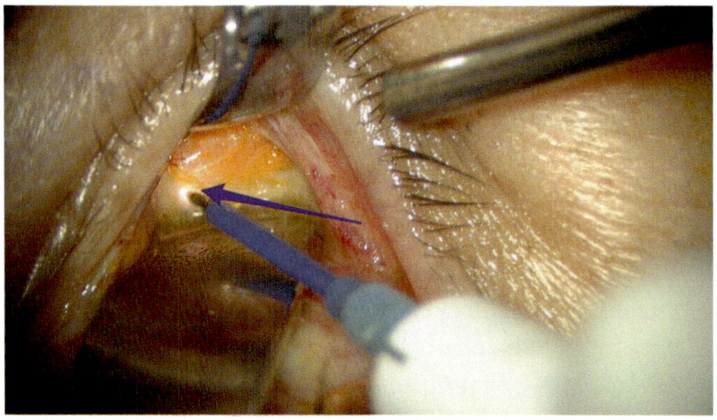

Fig. 26.4 The orbicularis is dissected off the rim in a preperiosteal plane

may be used in patients with prominent lower eyelid bags without a significant tear trough deformity [67].

A 4-0 silk traction suture is passed through the conjunctiva/retractors flap and secured to the head drape to aid in exposure of the fat pads. In the postseptal approach, gentle pressure on the globe helps the fat to herniate through the incision, which is then excised with the monopolar cautery. If the preseptal plane is preferred and the goal is fat repositioning, a Ragnell retractor is then used to retract the lower eyelid and a malleable retractor is placed over the fat pads to expose the arcus marginalis (Fig. 26.3). The dissection is carried out inferiorly in a preperiosteal plane (Fig. 26.4), releasing the attachments of the orbicularis muscle medially and the ORL (or orbitomalar ligament) laterally. It should extend about 10 mm beyond the inferior orbital rim (Fig. 26.5), with care to identify and protect the infraorbital neurovascular bundle. The lateral extension of the dissection depends on the planned extent of fat transposition. Some authors prefer to perform this dissection using tenotomy scissors in a spreading fashion [68].

With a Westcott scissors or the Colorado needle, the septum is opened inferiorly, close to the arcus marginalis (Fig. 26.6). The medial and central fat pads are carefully

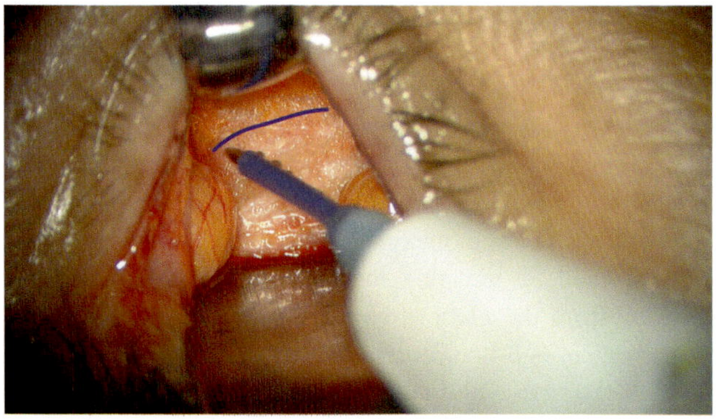

Fig. 26.5 Dissection to release the orbicularis muscle attachments and the orbitomalar ligament is carried out 10 mm inferiorly (Line)

dissected apart, showing the position of the inferior oblique muscle (Fig. 26.7). The medial fat pad is exposed and, with a help of a forceps, made into a pedicle through meticulous dissection of its fibrous attachments to the orbital septum, preserving its base (Fig. 26.8).

If the surgeon chooses to excise fat, it should be judicious in order to avoid a hollowed lower eyelid appearance (Fig. 26.9). The amount withdrawn from each area depends

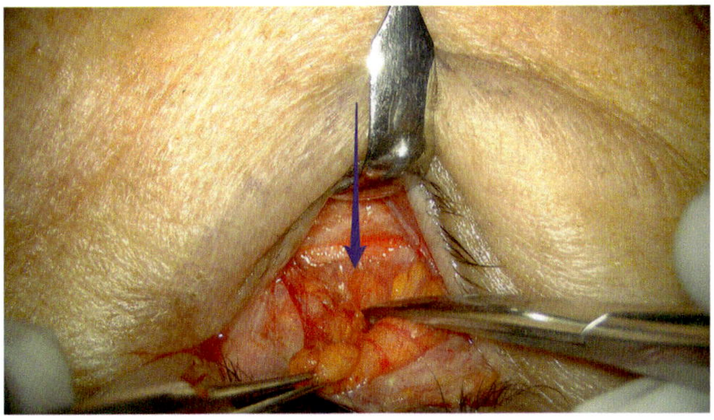

Fig. 26.6 The orbital septum is incised close to the arcus marginalis

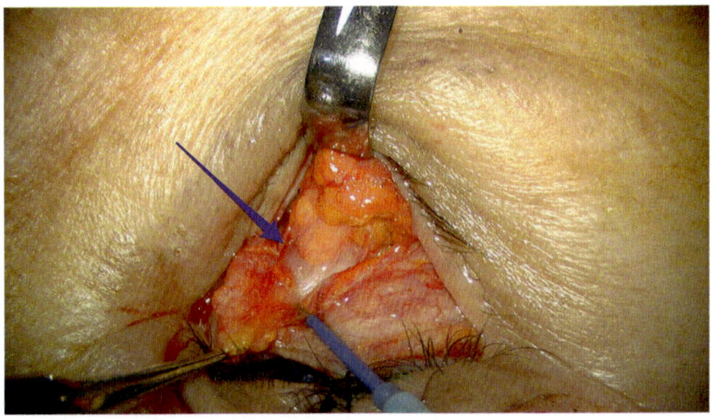

Fig. 26.7 The inferior oblique muscle is identified (arrow) between the medial and central fat pockets

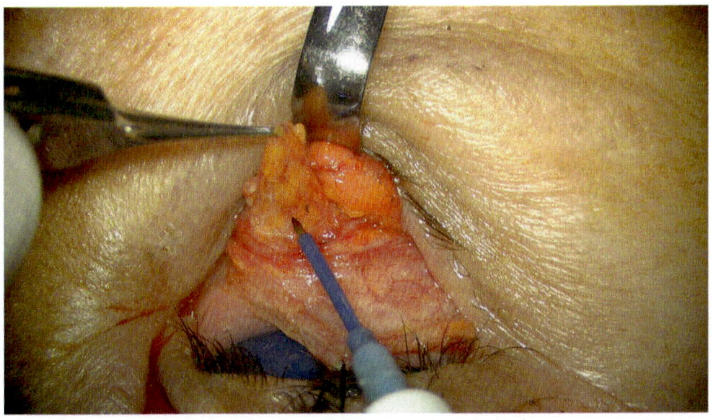

Fig. 26.8 Each fat pedicle is carefully dissected until it is freely mobile and does not retract the orbital septum or lower eyelid

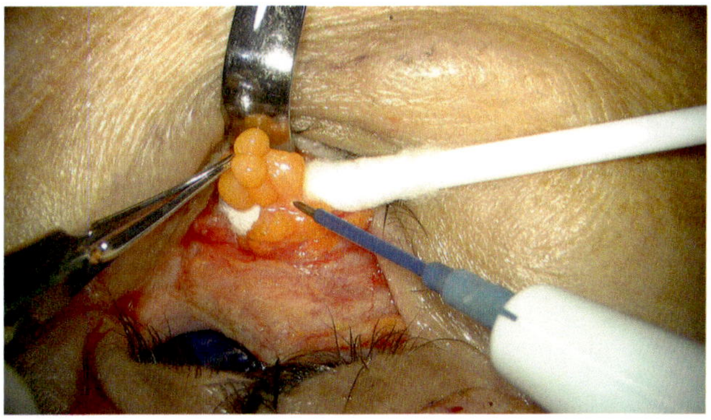

Fig. 26.9 Conservative fat resection is performed if needed

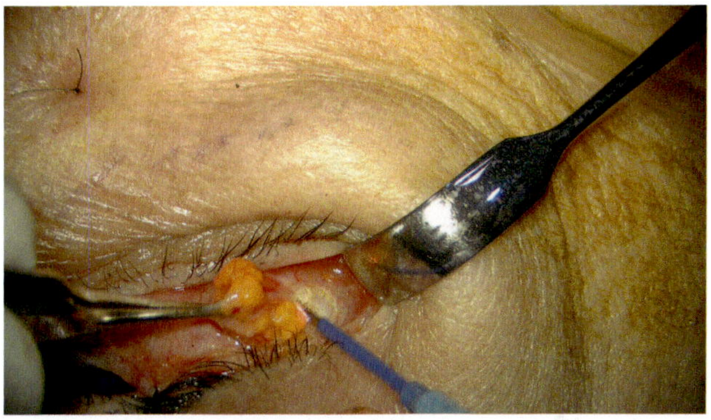

Fig. 26.10 The lateral fat pad is dissected

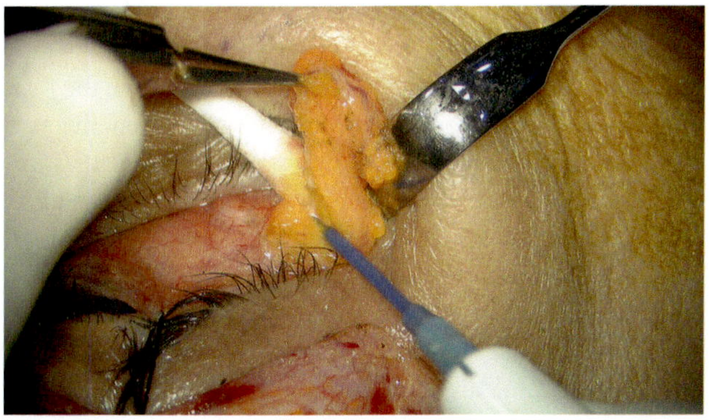

Fig. 26.11 Resection of the lateral fat pad is performed as planned preoperatively

on the preoperative evaluation. Fat can be grouped on a sponge, in order to compare the amount resected from each side. Careful hemostasis should be ensured. It is important to identify the inferior oblique muscle during fat manipulation to avoid iatrogenic injury. After a medial pedicle is created, the same steps described are performed in the central fat pad. Both the medial and central fat pads are grasped with forceps, and a "seesaw" movement is used in order to ensure free movement of the fat pads from the inferior oblique muscle. The lateral fat pad may be repositioned if indicated but is typically excised (Figs. 26.10 and 26.11).

An alternative to the supraperiosteal plane is to create a subperiosteal pocket into which the fat pads are slid [6, 69]. Using the Colorado needle, an incision is made along the arcus marginalis just below the inferior orbital rim. With a Freer elevator, the periosteum is carefully raised approximately 15 mm below the rim, around and with direct visualization of the infraorbital neurovascular bundle [48].

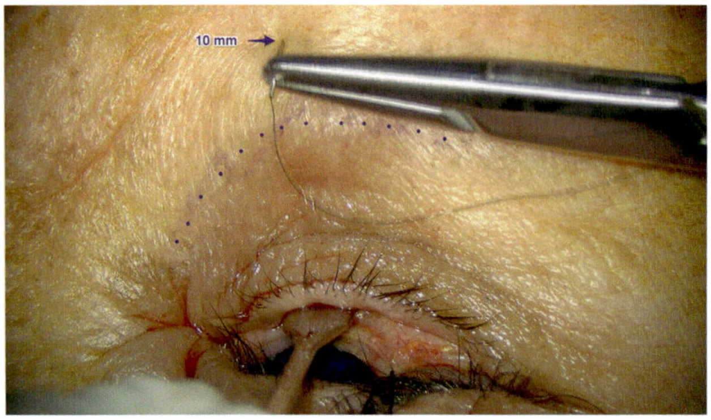

Fig. 26.12 A 5-0 nylon suture is passed from the skin deep under the dissected area, entering 10 mm below the previously marked location of the arcus marginalis or tear trough

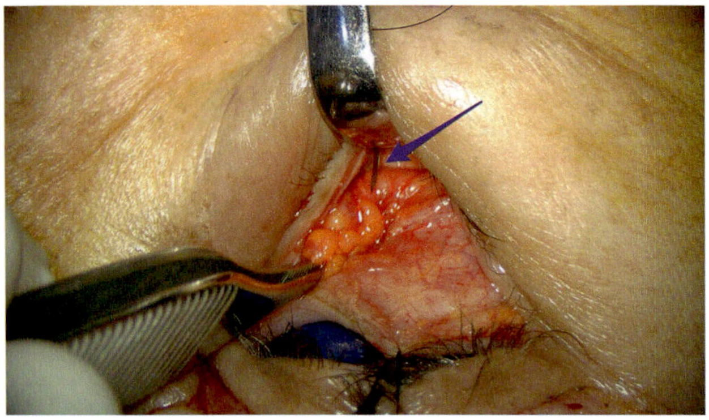

Fig. 26.13 The needle is retrieved under the orbicularis muscle in the desired plane (arrow)

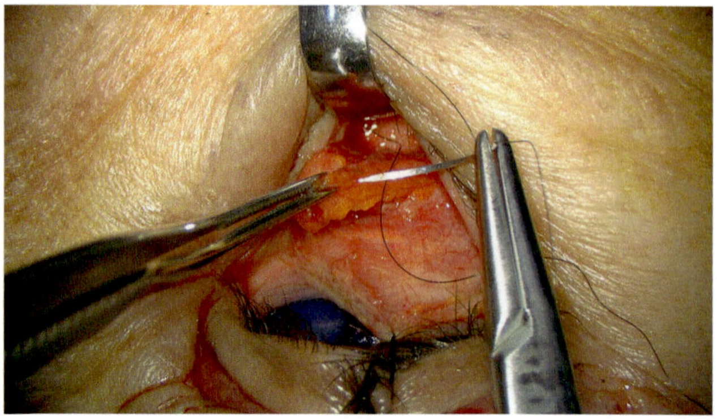

Fig. 26.14 The suture is passed through the tip of the fat pedicles

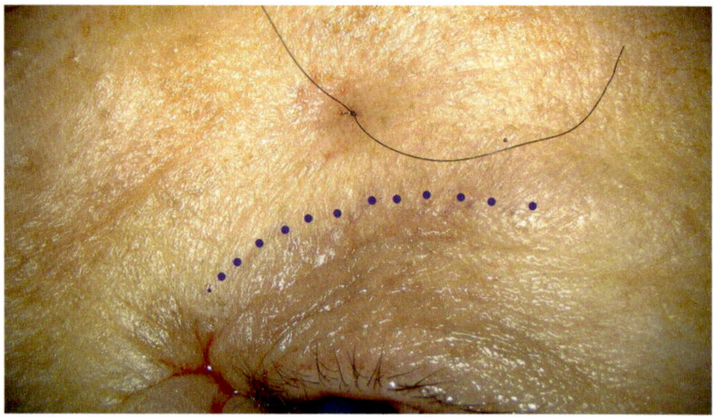

Fig. 26.15 The needle exits the skin and is tied loosely

Studies have not shown a significant difference in the final effacement of the tear trough deformity between the two techniques, with both demonstrating excellent results [68]. The supraperiosteal dissection is sometimes described as more traumatic when blunt dissection with scissors is used. The bruising and swelling may be minimized if meticulous dissection is carried out with a monopolar cautery. Also, the hypothesis of better fat survival in the subperiosteal plan has not yet been clinically confirmed. The supraperiosteal plan has the important advantage of directly releasing the orbicularis muscle attachments medially and the orbicularis retaining ligament (ORL) laterally, allowing better blending of the eyelid-cheek transition [7].

In both surgical approaches, a 5-0 nylon suture (Ethicon Mononylon Code 14501) is passed transcutaneously, approximately 10 mm under the previously placed skin mark at the tear trough (Fig. 26.12), exiting at the subperiosteal or supraperiosteal dissection plane (Fig. 26.13). The suture is then used to engage the tip of the fat pad (Fig. 26.14) and is passed back toward the skin, exiting just 4–5 mm lateral to the entry point. The suture is tied without tension (Fig. 26.15). The central fat pad is slid just inferolateral to the medial fat pad, and the lateral fat pad is, when indicated, transposed using the same technique. The result is the repositioning of the orbital fat pads over the inferior orbital rim, thus filling in the depression of the tear trough.

Another procedure, also called the septal reset, has also been advocated to improve the eyelid-cheek junction. After a preseptal dissection, the arcus marginalis is released, and a composite flap of septum and fat is sutured to the periosteum overlying the orbital rim [70, 71]. A canthopexy is performed prior to suturing, and the septum is fixated without tension.

The conjunctival incision may be closed with continuous or interrupted 6-0 polyglactin (Vicryl) sutures. Complications related to the incision, whether sutured closed or not, are very low [72].

Secondary Procedures

Skin Removal

Excess skin may be removed using a skin-only flap [69] or a pinch technique [73]. If a flap is chosen, a subciliary incision is made, and dissection exposes the pretarsal and preseptal orbicularis. The skin is then excised conservatively. Defenders of this technique, such as Hidalgo [69], believe

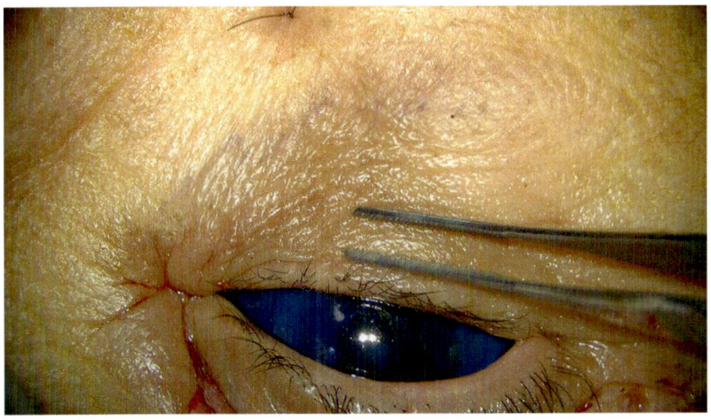

Fig. 26.16 A skin pinch of approximately 5 mm is prepared using a smooth Adson forceps

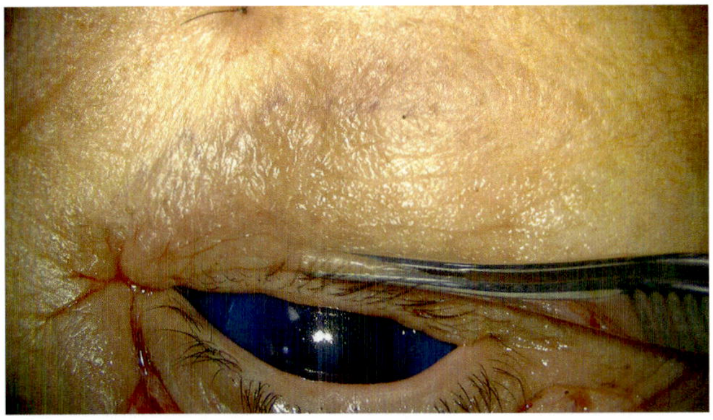

Fig. 26.17 The skin is pinched until a roll of skin stays elevated

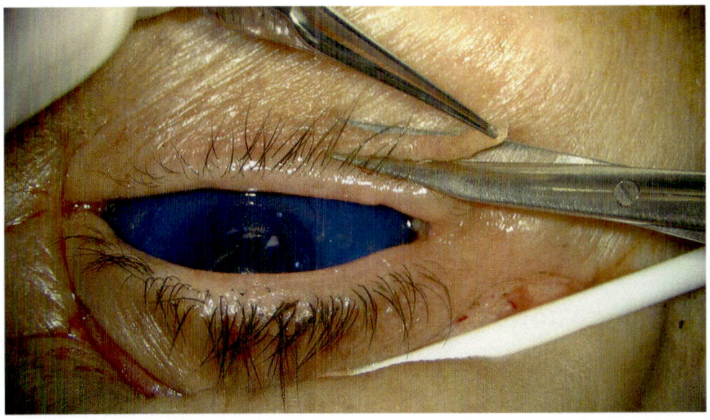

Fig. 26.18 The skin is excised close to the eyelash line using Westcott scissors without excising any orbicularis muscle

that this undermining allows a skin redraping over orbicularis with a more accentuated smoothening effect than other approaches. The skin pinch, on the other hand, is performed below the ciliary margin with the use of an Adson forceps (Figs. 26.16 and 26.17). A fold is created extending out to the crow's feet crease and then excised with a Westcott scissors without removing orbicularis muscle (Figs. 26.18 and 26.19). In both techniques, skin closure may be performed using a running 6-0 prolene or fast-absorbing plain gut suture. It is

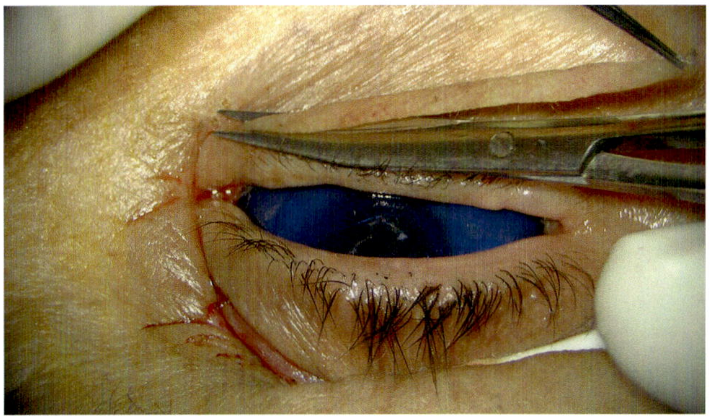

Fig. 26.19 The medial extent of the excision is the inferior punctum

important not to infiltrate an excessive amount of local anesthesia in order to remove a precise amount of skin, and care should be taken to avoid traction from the drapes as postoperative lower eyelid malposition may be caused by an overly aggressive skin resection. Resurfacing techniques with laser or chemical peel can also be used for skin texture improvement.

Canthal/Orbicularis Suspension

If lower eyelid laxity is identified, a lateral canthopexy/canthoplasty [74, 75] procedure should be added in order to prevent postoperative malposition or scleral show. For mild degrees of laxity (less than 6 mm of eyelid distraction), a closed canthopexy as described by Georgescu [76], Fagien [77], or Hamra [70] or orbicularis suspension techniques as reported by Lessa [78], Little [79], or Honrado [80] may be performed. The final vector of canthal suspension should be posterior, superior, and lateral in order to tighten the eyelid and avoid tenting of the canthus [81]. For greater degrees of laxity (greater than 6 mm of eyelid distraction), lateral canthoplasty with lateral cantholysis [75, 82] or a lateral tarsal strip procedure should be favored.

In patients with minimal/moderate laxity who undergo a skin pinch, we find the preseptal orbicularis suspension a very effective method for eyelid tightening. In this technique of orbicularis suspension, after skin pinch excision, a 5-0 polyglactin 910 suture (Ethicon Vicryl J 121) is passed through the periosteum inside the superolateral orbital rim (Fig. 26.20) (previously exposed through the upper blepharoplasty incision or, if this is not performed, through a 2 mm skin incision). The needle is passed under the orbicularis plane, exiting at the vertical halfway point of the skin pinch height (Fig. 26.21), and then reversed following the same path toward the upper rim periosteum (Fig. 26.22). This mattress suture essentially grasps the orbicularis plane, which is finally tied until a mild elevation of the lower eyelid is observed (Fig. 26.23).

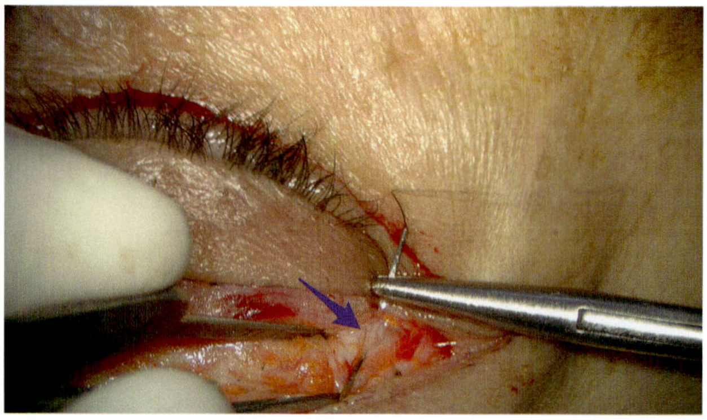

Fig. 26.20 A 6-0 polyglactin suture is passed through the periosteum above the canthal angle

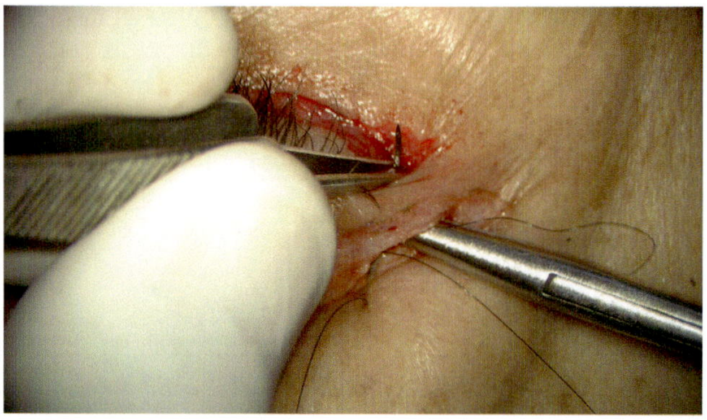

Fig. 26.21 The suture is passed to the lower lid under the orbicularis, exiting through the skin pinch excision

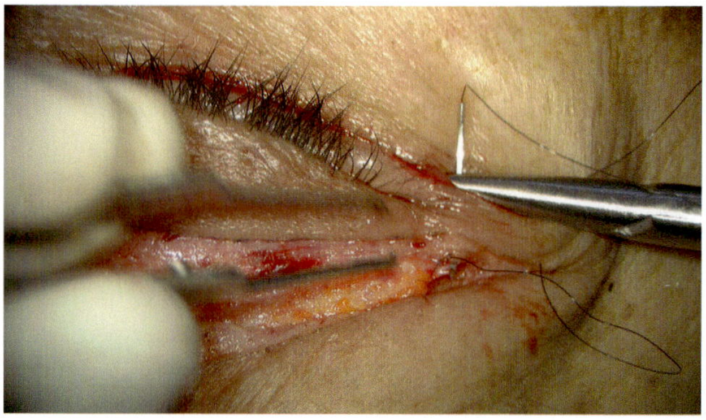

Fig. 26.22 The needle is reversed and passed back to the upper eyelid

Autologous Fat Augmentation

Some authors such as Rohrich [7, 83] propose the use of autologous fat transfer combined with transconjunctival fat resection in order to achieve a better and more predictable improvement of the midface contour. It should be highlighted, however, that the rate of fat graft absorption is not negligible [84], so this option may be less predictable and require additional procedures to add more fat. Alternatively, transposition of vascularized fat pedicles over the infraorbital rim may allow a higher rate of fat survival and may be supplemented with additional fat transfer if needed [85].

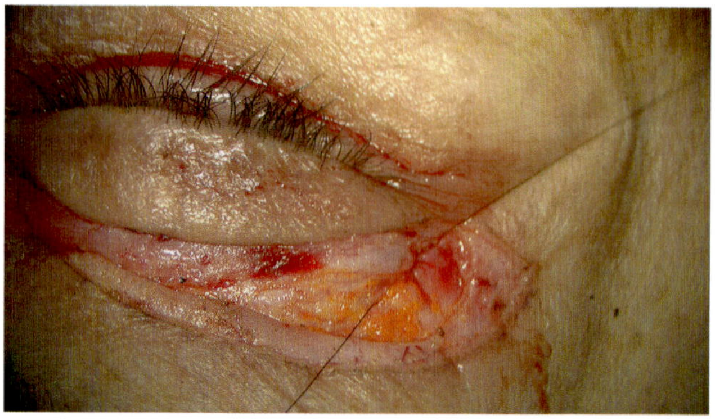

Fig. 26.23 The suture is tied with enough strength as to lift the lower eyelid a few millimeters

Postoperative Care

At the end of the procedure, the eyelids are taped 4 mm under the skin incision with a lateral and superior vector of pull. Patients are instructed to maintain a semi-upright position when resting for a few days and to apply local cold compresses for 48 hours. Antibiotic-steroid ophthalmic eye drops are used four times/day, together with frequent use of artificial tears. An antibiotic ointment is prescribed for any skin sutures. The patient is seen within the first few postoperative days to monitor visual acuity, motility, and the presence of edema and/or chemosis. Skin sutures are typically removed after 5–7 days.

Complications

Even the most experienced surgeon will eventually deal with postoperative complications following transconjunctival blepharoplasty and must be prepared to handle them. Many complications are avoidable through comprehensive preoperative evaluation, careful assessment, planning, meticulous surgical technique, and adequate patient education. Complications following blepharoplasty are either cosmetic, functional, or vision-threatening.

- Bleeding and Visual Impairment

The most devastating complication after blepharoplasty is visual loss. Although rare, the estimated incidence is 0.04%, and it may be caused by an orbital hemorrhage. The progressive expansion of a hematoma can result in compression of the optic nerve and its vascular supply, which can lead to permanent blindness. The risk of severe hematoma is thought to be theoretically lower following a transconjunctival approach if the incision is left open to allow drainage of any blood.

Retrobulbar hemorrhage occurs when the retroseptal compartment is violated and is thought to be related to (1) traction on orbital fat (medial fat pocket most commonly involved) disrupting the posterior orbital vessels, (2) retraction of an open vessel beneath the septum after fat release, (3) failure to recognize an open vessel because of vasospasm or epinephrine effect, (4) direct vessel trauma after local anesthetic injections beneath the orbital septum, and (5) rebleeding after closure resulting from any event that leads to an increased arteriovenous pressure, like a hypertensive peak or severe coughing or sneezing.

Significant bleeding can usually be minimized before surgery by optimizing coagulation profiles and normotensive status, during surgery through delicate tissue handling and meticulous hemostasis, and after surgery through head elevation, cold compresses, avoidance of strenuous activities, and appropriate analgesic support.

Should a hematoma develop, early recognition and treatment is essential for preservation of vision (retina can tolerate approximately 90 minutes of vascular occlusion before irreversible visual impairment). Avoiding occlusive-pressure dressings, instructing the patients to contact their surgeon in the event of alert signs, and maintaining accessibility during the postoperative interval facilitate early detection. Most hematomas occur within the early postoperative period and clinical signs include eye pain, mydriasis, progressive chemosis, proptosis, ophthalmoplegia, and decreased visual acuity.

Treatment, in the event of a retrobulbar hemorrhage, should be immediate decompression and hemostatic control with concomitant medical interventions. Staged decompressive strategy is instituted based on the severity of the hemorrhage and the degree of visual compromise. First, the wound is explored, and blood is evacuated. If signs of orbital compression persist, a lateral canthotomy with cantholysis is performed. As a last resort, bony orbital decompression may allow increased arterial perfusion pressure to the eye and optic nerve. Medical treatment includes intravenous diuretics, such as mannitol and acetazolamide, systemic corticosteroids, along with topical adrenergic blockers, head elevation, and possibly high-flow oxygen.

Small, superficial hematomas are relatively common, are typically self-limiting, and do not threaten vision. They usually result from bleeding from an orbicularis muscle vessel. Small hematomas may resolve spontaneously, although larger hematomas can be evacuated in the office, if indicated.

Although extremely rare, other possible causes of blindness after blepharoplasty are direct globe perforation, infection, and ocular circulation compromise by vasospasm or fat embolism after fat injection.

- Persistent edema and chemosis

Patients may occasionally experience persistent eyelid edema after transconjunctival blepharoplasty. This may cause the perception that the operation was inadequate or may lead to asymmetry. Early use of ice packs, external pressure with tape, and head elevation are indicated after the procedure and will reduce the amount of swelling significantly. Careful reassurance and close follow-up often comfort the patient during this period. For pronounced and/or persistent swelling, 5-fluorouracil (5-FU) injections with or without low-dose steroid have shown excellent results as a postsurgical inflammation/healing modulator without significant complications [86].

Chemosis is caused by the disruption of local lymphatic drainage. This may occur from physical trauma (conjunctival incision, irritation from swabs, or gauze pads) or chemical trauma (antibacterial agents used to sterilize the skin). Extensive edema may lead to conjunctival prolapse, which can be worrisome to the patient. This is managed by warm compresses, frequent lubrication, diuretics, topical steroid, eyelid exercises, and eyelid patching during sleep. Other options include incision for drainage or conjunctival cautery, although recurrence is not uncommon. Often it may take several months to resolve.

- Dry Eye Syndrome

Any patient may experience postsurgical dry eye, especially those with preoperative marginal tear production. Even without any skin resection, postoperative edema can lead to transient lagophthalmos, increasing globe exposure. Dryness may also be a sequel of cicatricial changes in the conjunctiva causing eyelid malposition. Patients may complain of foreign body sensation, burning, itching, discharge, and frequent blinking.

Most dry eye syndromes following blepharoplasty are temporary and resolve with topical lubricants applied on a regular basis. Should the symptoms persist, possible treatment options include eyelid taping at night or temporary/permanent punctal plugs.

- Epiphora

Blepharoplasty can cause a temporary reflex tear hypersecretion due to lagophthalmos, transient malposition of the lower eyelid, or direct corneal abrasion. Excessive tearing is also frequently caused by outflow obstruction secondary to edema that distorts or blocks the lacrimal drainage system or by an impairment of the lacrimal pump resulting from hypotonic orbicularis muscle, punctal eversion, temporary ectropion, or surgical trauma.

Outflow obstructions, secondary to a damaged inferior canaliculus, are preventable by keeping the conjunctival incision lateral to the punctum. Persistent postoperative punctal eversion can be managed by cauterization or diamond excision of the conjunctiva below the canaliculus followed by inverting sutures.

- Damage to the Cornea

Corneal abrasions or ulcerations may result from abrasive movements of instruments and sutures, inadvertent rubbing of the corneal surface with a gauze or cotton applicator, injudicious cauterization, chemical exposure to skin antiseptics, or postoperative desiccation as a result of lagophthalmos, ectropion, or preexistent dry eye syndrome. The best way to avoid direct intraoperative trauma to the cornea is to place corneal shields during surgery. They should be filled with lubricants/antibiotic ointment before insertion. Posterior conjunctival sutures may occasionally cause irritation, and rarely the transconjunctival approach may induce scarring that causes eyelid margin inversion with trichiasis.

Symptoms suggestive of corneal injury, such as pain, eye irritation, epiphora, and blurred vision, always warrant slit lamp observation with fluorescein staining. Appropriate measures for mechanical injury include topical antibiotic and artificial tears or ointments. Eye patching or bandage contact lenses may be necessary if the keratitis is painful.

- Infection

Periorbital infection as a result of blepharoplasty is rare, due to the extensive vascularity of the region. Nevertheless, once the orbital septum has been opened, pathogens can easily gain access to the deep orbital structures. A possible source of infection can be the nasolacrimal outflow system in patients with nasolacrimal duct stenosis in whom bacteria can multiply and reflux toward the conjunctiva.

Orbital cellulitis after blepharoplasty is very rare but may have devastating consequences. The causative organism is typically *Staphylococcus aureus*, and systemic antibiotics with possible hospital admission are warranted. If a true orbital abscess is identified by CT scanning, surgical drainage may be required.

- Asymmetry

One of the greatest challenges of lower blepharoplasty is achieving symmetry. A minor degree of self-limited asymmetry is common postoperatively and can be caused by edema, bruising, and asymmetric recovery times. The most common causes of persistent asymmetry post-transconjunctival blepharoplasty are uneven resection of the fat pads or an undiagnosed preoperative asymmetry.

If fat is removed rather than repositioned, the excised pieces should be placed on the operating table and labeled according to their location. The surgeon can compare the amounts of excised material to ensure equal removal. The preoperative photos may also be placed in the operating room so that it is clear which fat pads require treatment, as the local anesthetic will obscure the contour to some degree. Less often, asymmetry may result from scar contracture of the conjunctiva or eyelid malposition.

It is appropriate to wait at least 3–6 months, before any revision is undertaken, depending on the degree of severity and the patient dissatisfaction. Earlier surgical intervention on an immature scar bed with changing soft tissue profiles may lead to an inferior outcome.

- Inappropriate Fat Treatment

An overcorrection or undercorrection after fat resection can lead to hollowness or persistent fat prominence. Inappropriate fat management is less common with fat repositioning. Excessive fat resection in the lower eyelid must be avoided, as it results in a cosmetically displeasing look, with an accentuated tear trough deformity that contributes to a sunken eye appearance. A possible treatment solution for this situation is autologous fat transfer in very small amounts with cannulas or fine needles in one or more sessions, if necessary.

Inadequate fat removal may lead to irregular contour and persistent bulges. Often the lateral fat pocket is undercorrected and requires surgical revision for more complete resection or repositioning.

Fat grafting when performed in conjunction with lower blepharoplasty can also lead to contour irregularities. Fat granulomas are rare, occurring in less than 5% of cases, and may be treated with intralesional injections of low-dose steroid and, in some cases, surgical excision. If atrophy of the grafts is seen, mostly in older patients, further lipofilling sessions may be required.

- Eyelid Malposition

Lower eyelid laxity can lead to several postoperative complications including ectropion, entropion, retraction, inferior scleral show, and a round eye deformity (with excessive scleral exposure in the lateral and inferior portion of the palpebral fissure). Other causes of eyelid malposition include scarring of the orbital septum, persistent inflammation of the fat pockets, and, rarely, destabilization of the lower eyelid retractors (a potential yet uncommon complication of the transconjunctival approach). In order to prevent these complications, eyelid laxity and anatomical risk factors such as a preexisting negative vector should be identified, and a concomitant tightening procedure should be combined with the transconjunctival blepharoplasty.

Mild to moderate postoperative ectropion, scleral show, and lagophthalmos are often normal with healing and tend to be self-limited. They have been associated with eyelid loading from edema and local anesthetic impairment of orbicularis oculi function. Conservative treatment is usually adequate, as most cases resolve in several weeks to months. This includes management of dry eye symptoms with lubricants and local upward massages. The eyelids may be taped at night and skin tape used to pull the lower eyelid in a superolateral direction during the day. Fluorouracil (5-FU) injections, in combination with steroids, may also help facilitate the healing process [86]. If these measures are unsuccessful, surgical scar release and canthal suspension or even an autologous spacer may be needed in order to restore proper eyelid support. SOOF lifting or even anterior lamellar lengthening with a skin graft are also possible resources in cases of overaggressive skin resection.

- Diplopia

Temporary diplopia may occur from local anesthetic diffusion to the extraocular muscles. This typically resolves without treatment after several hours. Persistent diplopia may be secondary to direct or indirect (from edema or hemorrhage) injury to the inferior oblique (most common) or inferior rectus muscles during fat repositioning or removal. The risk of injury may be higher in secondary blepharoplasty.

Avoidance of diplopia requires careful hemostasis and the prevention of muscle trauma during fat manipulation. A conservative management with high-dose oral steroids generally allows most cases to resolve over time. Permanent muscle injury may, however, result from blind clamping or deep penetration of the fat pockets, electrocauterization, suture incorporation during closure, or Volkmann's ischemic contracture. Patients with refractory and incomplete recovery of muscle function should be referred to a strabismus specialist for evaluation and definitive treatment.

- Hyperpigmentation

Pigmentation of the lower eyelids may be present before surgery and should be documented. After blepharoplasty, this pigmentation may become more prominent and bothersome to the patient.

Postsurgical hyperpigmentation usually results from accentuation of preexisting pigmentation or from hemosiderin deposition after excessive bruising. This pigmentary change will usually resolve over several months. During the healing process, the use of sunscreens and direct sunlight avoidance is recommended, as these may lead to permanent pigmentary changes. Treatment options for refractory cases may include bleaching agents, chemical peels, or laser or light therapy.

Conclusion

Over the years the transconjunctival approach for lower blepharoplasty has become a preferred method for lower eyelid herniated fat and eyelid-cheek junction improvement. It avoids a visible incision and has been associated with a lower rate of postoperative malposition and scleral show. Also, additional procedures may be added in a graded way, including skin excision or resurfacing and lateral canthal support. Originally described as an alternative approach to the traditional muscle-skin flap for fat resection, transconjunctival blepharoplasty with fat transposition into the tear trough now occupies a prominent place in contemporary facial cosmetic rejuvenation.

References

1. Forte AJ, Andrew TW, Colasante C, Persing JA. Perception of age, attractiveness, and tiredness after isolated and combined facial subunit aging. Aesthet Plast Surg. 2015;39:856–69.
2. Nguyen HT, Isaacowitz DM, Rubin PA. Age- and fatigue-related markers of human faces: an eye-tracking study. Ophthalmology. 2009;116:355–60.
3. Sobanko JF, Taglienti AJ, Wilson AJ, et al. Motivations for seeking minimally invasive cosmetic procedures in an academic outpatient setting. Aesthet Surg J. 2015;35:1014–20.
4. Schwarcz RM, Kotlus B. Complications of lower blepharoplasty and midface lifting. Clin Plast Surg. 2015;42:63–71.
5. Kossler AL, Peng GL, Yoo DB, et al. Current trends in upper and lower eyelid blepharoplasty among American Society of Ophthalmic Plastic and Reconstructive Surgery Members. Ophthal Plast Reconstr Surg. 2018;34:37–42.
6. Massry GG, Hartstein ME. The lift and fill lower blepharoplasty. Ophthal Plast Reconstr Surg. 2012;28:213–8.
7. Rohrich RJ, Ghavami A, Mojallal A. The five-step lower blepharoplasty: blending the eyelid-cheek junction. Plast Reconstr Surg. 2011;128:775–83.
8. Hamra ST. Arcus marginalis release and orbital fat preservation in midface rejuvenation. Plast Reconstr Surg. 1995;96:354–62.
9. Rees TD, Dupuis CC. Baggy eyelids in young adults. Plast Reconstr Surg. 1969;43:381–7.
10. Griffin G, Azizzadeh B, Massry GG. New insights into physical findings associated with postblepharoplasty lower eyelid retraction. Aesthet Surg J. 2014;34:995–1004.
11. Maffi TR, Chang S, Friedland JA. Traditional lower blepharoplasty: is additional support necessary? A 30-year review. Plast Reconstr Surg. 2011;128:265–73.
12. Gosain AK, Klein MH, Sudhakar PV, Prost RW. A volumetric analysis of soft-tissue changes in the aging midface using high-resolution MRI: implications for facial rejuvenation. Plast Reconstr Surg. 2005;115:1143–52; discussion 1153–45.

13. Gierloff M, Stohring C, Buder T, et al. Aging changes of the midfacial fat compartments: a computed tomographic study. Plast Reconstr Surg. 2012;129:263–73.
14. Kahn DM, Shaw RB Jr. Aging of the bony orbit: a three-dimensional computed tomographic study. Aesthet Surg J. 2008;28:258–64.
15. Farkas JP, Pessa JE, Hubbard B, Rohrich RJ. The science and theory behind facial aging. Plast Reconstr Surg Glob Open. 2013;1:e8.
16. Shaw RB Jr, Katzel EB, Koltz PF, et al. Aging of the facial skeleton: aesthetic implications and rejuvenation strategies. Plast Reconstr Surg. 2011;127:374–83.
17. Stuzin JM, Baker TJ, Gordon HL. The relationship of the superficial and deep facial fascias: relevance to rhytidectomy and aging. Plast Reconstr Surg. 1992;89:441–9; discussion 450–41.
18. Gosain AK, Amarante MT, Hyde JS, Yousif NJ. A dynamic analysis of changes in the nasolabial fold using magnetic resonance imaging: implications for facial rejuvenation and facial animation surgery. Plast Reconstr Surg. 1996;98:622–36.
19. Mendelson BC, Jacobson SR. Surgical anatomy of the midcheek: facial layers, spaces, and the midcheek segments. Clin Plast Surg. 2008;35:395–404; discussion 393.
20. Lucarelli MJ, Khwarg SI, Lemke BN, et al. The anatomy of midfacial ptosis. Ophthal Plast Reconstr Surg. 2000;16:7–22.
21. Donofrio LM. Fat distribution: a morphologic study of the aging face. Dermatol Surg. 2000;26:1107–12.
22. Lambros V. Observations on periorbital and midface aging. Plast Reconstr Surg. 2007;120:1367–76; discussion 1377.
23. Rohrich RJ, Pessa JE. The fat compartments of the face: anatomy and clinical implications for cosmetic surgery. Plast Reconstr Surg. 2007;119:2219–27; discussion 2228–31.
24. Rohrich RJ, Pessa JE. The retaining system of the face: histologic evaluation of the septal boundaries of the subcutaneous fat compartments. Plast Reconstr Surg. 2008;121:1804–9.
25. Rohrich RJ, Arbique GM, Wong C, et al. The anatomy of suborbicularis fat: implications for periorbital rejuvenation. Plast Reconstr Surg. 2009;124:946–51.
26. Wan D, Amirlak B, Rohrich R, Davis K. The clinical importance of the fat compartments in midfacial aging. Plast Reconstr Surg Glob Open. 2013;1:e92.
27. Rohrich RJ, Pessa JE, Ristow B. The youthful cheek and the deep medial fat compartment. Plast Reconstr Surg. 2008;121:2107–12.
28. Buchanan DR, Wulc AE. Contemporary thoughts on lower eyelid/midface aging. Clin Plast Surg. 2015;42:1–15.
29. Marshak H, Dresner S. Transconjunctival lower blepahroplasty. In: Azizzadeh B, Murphy MR, Johnson CM, Massry GG, Fitzgerald R, editors. Master techniques in facial rejuvenation. Philadelphia: Saunders Elsevier; 2007. p. 89–98.
30. Bourguet J. Les hernies graisseuses de l'orbite: Notre traitement chirurgical. Bull Acad Nat Med. 1924;92:1227–32.
31. Tomlinson FB, Hovey LM. Transconjunctival lower lid blepharoplasty for removal of fat. Plast Reconstr Surg. 1975;56:314–8.
32. Tessier P. The conjunctival approach to the orbital floor and maxilla in congenital malformation and trauma. J Maxillofac Surg. 1973;1:3–8.
33. Dinner MI, Glassman H, Artz JS. The "no flap" technique for lower-lid blepharoplasty. Aesthet Plast Surg. 1992;16:155–8.
34. Loeb R. Fat pad sliding and fat grafting for leveling lid depressions. Clin Plast Surg. 1981;8:757–76.
35. de la Plaza R, Arroyo JM. A new technique for the treatment of palpebral bags. Plast Reconstr Surg. 1988;81:677–87.
36. Hamra ST. The role of orbital fat preservation in facial aesthetic surgery. A new concept. Clin Plast Surg. 1996;23:17–28.
37. Mendelson BC. Herniated fat and the orbital septum of the lower lid. Clin Plast Surg. 1993;20:323–30.
38. Goldberg RA. Transconjunctival orbital fat repositioning: transposition of orbital fat pedicles into a subperiosteal pocket. Plast Reconstr Surg. 2000;105:743–8; discussion 749–51.
39. Kakizaki H, Zhao J, Nakano T, et al. The lower eyelid retractor consists of definite double layers. Ophthalmology. 2006;113:2346–50.
40. Kikkawa DO, Kim JW. Lower-eyelid blepharoplasty. Int Ophthalmol Clin. 1997;37:163–78.
41. Pack S, Quereshy FA, Altay MA, Baur DA. Transconjunctival lower blepharoplasty. Atlas Oral Maxillofac Surg Clin North Am. 2016;24:147–51.
42. Gioia VM, Linberg JV, McCormick SA. The anatomy of the lateral canthal tendon. Arch Ophthalmol. 1987;105:529–32.
43. Ridgeway JM, Larrabee W. Anatomy for blepharoplasty and browlift. Facial Plast Surg. 2010;26:177–85.
44. Tan KS, Oh S-RO, Priel A, Korn BS, Kikkawa DO. Surgical anatomy of the forehead, eyelids, and midface for the aesthetic surgeon. In: Massry GG, Murphy MR, Azizzadeh B, editors. Master techniques in blepharoplasty and periorbital rejuvenation. New York: Springer; 2011.
45. Manson PN, Clifford CM, Su CT, et al. Mechanisms of global support and posttraumatic enophthalmos: I. The anatomy of the ligament sling and its relation to intramuscular cone orbital fat. Plast Reconstr Surg. 1986;77:193–202.
46. Tan KS, Oh S, Priel A, et al. Surgical anatomy of the forehead, eyelids, and midface for the aesthetic surgeon. In: Massry GG, Murphy MR, Azizzadeh B, editors. Master techniques in blepharoplasty and periorbital rejuvenation. New York: Springer; 2011. p. 11–23.
47. Mendelson BC, Muzaffar AR, Adams WP Jr. Surgical anatomy of the midcheek and malar mounds. Plast Reconstr Surg. 2002;110:885–96; discussion 897–911.
48. Haddock NT, Saadeh PB, Boutros S, Thorne CH. The tear trough and lid/cheek junction: anatomy and implications for surgical correction. Plast Reconstr Surg. 2009;123:1332–40; discussion 1341–32.
49. Codner MA, Wolfli JN, Anzarut A. Primary transcutaneous lower blepharoplasty with routine lateral canthal support: a comprehensive 10-year review. Plast Reconstr Surg. 2008;121:241–50.
50. Kim YK, Kim JW. Evaluation of subciliary incision used in blowout fracture treatment: pretarsal flattening after lower eyelid surgery. Plast Reconstr Surg. 2010;125:1479–84.
51. Ramirez OM, Santamarina R. Spatial orientation of motor innervation to the lower orbicularis oculi muscle. Aesthet Surg J. 2000;20:107–13.
52. DiFrancesco LM, Anjema CM, Codner MA, et al. Evaluation of conventional subciliary incision used in blepharoplasty: preoperative and postoperative videography and electromyography findings. Plast Reconstr Surg. 2005;116:632–9.
53. McCord CD, Walrath JD, Nahai F. Concepts in eyelid biomechanics with clinical implications. Aesthet Surg J. 2013;33:209–21.
54. Choi Y, Kang HG, Nam YS, et al. Facial nerve supply to the orbicularis oculi around the lower eyelid: anatomy and its clinical implications. Plast Reconstr Surg. 2017;140:261–71.
55. Shoukath S, Taylor GI, Mendelson BC, et al. The lymphatic anatomy of the lower eyelid and conjunctiva and correlation with postoperative chemosis and edema. Plast Reconstr Surg. 2017;139:628e–37e.
56. Fezza JP, Massry G. Lower eyelid length. Plast Reconstr Surg. 2015;136:152e–9e.
57. Shore JW. Changes in lower eyelid resting position, movement, and tone with age. Am J Ophthalmol. 1985;99:415–23.
58. van den Bosch WA, Leenders I, Mulder P. Topographic anatomy of the eyelids, and the effects of sex and age. Br J Ophthalmol. 1999;83:347–52.
59. Kligman AM, Zheng P, Lavker RM. The anatomy and pathogenesis of wrinkles. Br J Dermatol. 1985;113:37–42.
60. Naik MN. Hills and valleys: understanding the under-eye. J Cutan Aesthet Surg. 2016;9:61–4.
61. Owsley JQ, Roberts CL. Some anatomical observations on midface aging and long-term results of surgical treatment. Plast Reconstr Surg. 2008;121:258–68.

62. Chen YS, Tsai TH, Wu ML, et al. Evaluation of age-related intraorbital fat herniation through computed tomography. Plast Reconstr Surg. 2008;122:1191–8.
63. Richard MJ, Morris C, Deen BF, et al. Analysis of the anatomic changes of the aging facial skeleton using computer-assisted tomography. Ophthal Plast Reconstr Surg. 2009;25:382–6.
64. Flowers RS, Flowers SS. Precision planning in blepharoplasty. The importance of preoperative mapping. Clin Plast Surg. 1993;20:303–10.
65. Undavia S, Briceno CA, Massry GG. Quantified incision placement for postseptal approach transconjunctival blepharoplasty. Ophthal Plast Reconstr Surg. 2016;32:191–4.
66. Schwarcz R, Fezza JP, Jacono A, Massry GG. Stop blaming the septum. Ophthal Plast Reconstr Surg. 2016;32:49–52.
67. Hashem AM, Couto RA, Waltzman JT, et al. Evidence-based medicine: a graded approach to lower lid blepharoplasty. Plast Reconstr Surg. 2017;139:139e–50e.
68. Yoo DB, Peng GL, Massry GG. Transconjunctival lower blepharoplasty with fat repositioning: a retrospective comparison of transposing fat to the subperiosteal vs supraperiosteal planes. JAMA Facial Plast Surg. 2013;15:176–81.
69. Hidalgo DA. An integrated approach to lower blepharoplasty. Plast Reconstr Surg. 2011;127:386–95.
70. Hamra ST. The zygorbicular dissection in composite rhytidectomy: an ideal midface plane. Plast Reconstr Surg. 1998;102:1646–57.
71. Youn S, Shin JI, Kim JT, Kim YH. Transconjunctival subperiosteal fat reposition for tear trough deformity: pedicled fat redraping versus septal reset. Ann Plast Surg. 2014;73:479–84.
72. Mullins JB, Holds JB, Branham GH, Thomas JR. Complications of the transconjunctival approach. A review of 400 cases. Arch Otolaryngol Head Neck Surg. 1997;123:385–8.
73. Kim EM, Bucky LP. Power of the pinch: pinch lower lid blepharoplasty. Ann Plast Surg. 2008;60:532–7.
74. Linkov G, Wulc AE. Management of lower eyelid laxity. Atlas Oral Maxillofac Surg Clin North Am. 2016;24:153–9.
75. McCord CD, Boswell CB, Hester TR. Lateral canthal anchoring. Plast Reconstr Surg. 2002;112:222–36.
76. Georgescu D, Anderson RL, McCann JD. Lateral canthal resuspension sine canthotomy. Ophthal Plast Reconstr Surg. 2011;27:371–5.
77. Fagien S. Algorithm for canthoplasty: the lateral retinacular suspension: a simplified suture canthopexy. Plast Reconstr Surg. 1999;103:2042–53; discussion 2054–48.
78. Lessa S, Nanci M. Simple canthopexy used in transconjunctival blepharoplasty. Ophthal Plast Reconstr Surg. 2009;25:284–8.
79. Little JW, Hartstein ME. Simplified muscle-suspension lower blepharoplasty by orbicularis hitch. Aesthet Surg J. 2016;36:641–7.
80. Honrado CP, Pastorek NJ. Long-term results of lower-lid suspension blepharoplasty: a 30-year experience. Arch Facial Plast Surg. 2004;6:150–4.
81. Davison SP, Irio M, Oh C. Transconjunctival lower lid blepharoplasty with and without fat repositioning. Clin Plast Surg. 2015;42:51–6.
82. Jelks GW, Glat PM, Jelks EB, Longaker MT. The inferior retinacular lateral canthoplasty: a new technique. Plast Reconstr Surg. 1997;100:1262–70; discussion 1271–65.
83. Pezeshk RA, Sieber DA, Rohrich RJ. The six-step lower blepharoplasty: using fractionated fat to enhance blending of the lid-cheek junction. Plast Reconstr Surg. 2017;139:1381–3.
84. Boureaux E, Chaput B, Bannani S, et al. Eyelid fat grafting: indications, operative technique and complications; a systematic review. J Craniomaxillofac Surg. 2016;44:374–80.
85. Einan-Lifshitz A, Holds JB, Wulc AE, Hartstein ME. Volumetric rejuvenation of the tear trough with repo and Ristow. Ophthal Plast Reconstr Surg. 2013;29:481–5.
86. Yoo DB, Azizzadeh B, Massry GG. Injectable 5-FU with or without added steroid in periorbital skin grafting: initial observations. Ophthal Plast Reconstr Surg. 2015;31:122–6.

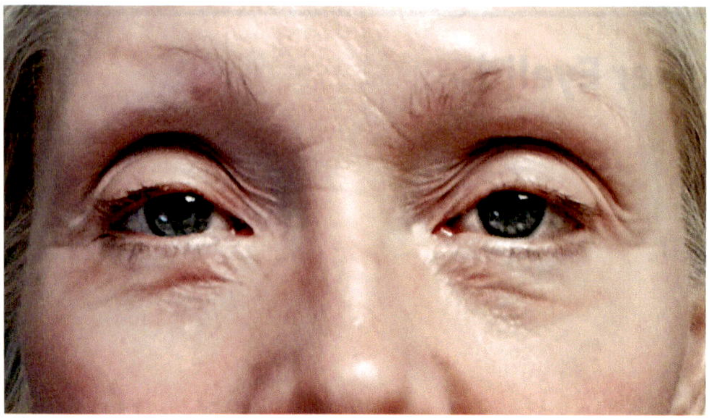

Fig. 27.1 Superior and inferior sulcus hollowing and shadows due to excessive fat removal and volume loss. (Image courtesy of Cat N. Burkat, MD FACS)

Understanding the anatomical structures involved in the aging lower eyelid for each individual patient is critical, as the surgical nuances will differ according to the preoperative assessment of these anatomic factors. Similar to the upper eyelid where dermatochalasis results in the loss of elasticity and support to the skin, lower eyelids can present with eyelid laxity, skin excess, and fat herniation. There are three fat pads in the inferior eyelid: the medial, central, and lateral fat pads (Fig. 27.1). The lower eyelid fat is most prominent on upgaze and less in downgaze [4]. The displacement of the orbital rim in relation to the cornea and lower eyelid margin can also be useful in preoperative assessment, and patients with a negative vector may have less optimal results without additional concurrent procedures [4]. With respect to the lower eyelid itself, lower eyelid laxity may impact whether horizontal eyelid shortening procedures are warranted. Location of the excess skin, orbicularis hypertrophy, orbital fat pseudoherniation, malar bags, or festoons should also be considered in relation to the eyelid anatomy.

General Complications

Although generally considered safe, numerous complications have been reported relating to lower eyelid blepharoplasty. These include but are not limited to globe perforation, fire, skin burns, eyelash injuries, dry eyes, corneal abrasion, prolonged chemosis, edema, hemorrhage, infection, lagophthalmos, diplopia, eyelid retraction, ectropion, or entropion.

Globe Perforation

Globe perforation is a feared complication in any eyelid procedure, including lower blepharoplasty, but can be avoided with careful surgical technique. The use of lidocaine with epinephrine is an effective and common way to anesthetize the eyelid. However, inadvertent penetration of the globe with the needle may rarely occur and is devastating. The surgeon should confirm that the needle is securely attached to the syringe, directed away from the globe, and then injected slowly [1]. Stabilizing the head and having the patient appropriately sedated for the injection portion are also useful to avoid sudden head movements. During the blepharoplasty procedure, a corneal shield lubricated with ophthalmic ointment can help protect the globe from iatrogenic injury from needles, blades, and lasers commonly used during surgery [8]. The shield also minimizes the risk of corneal abrasions. If there are any concerns for globe injury, an immediate indirect ophthalmoscopic examination should be performed to identify any area of perforation.

Fire, Skin Burns, and Eyelash Injuries

Intraoperative fires are a serious concern with approximately 100 intraoperative fires annually [1]. 15% of cases are associated with serious injuries to the patient or provider [1]. The increase in use of electric cautery and disposable drapes has led to the increase of such incidences. To minimize the risk, the surgeon should ensure that the oxygen is turned off or minimized during cautery use. It is important to always communicate with the anesthesiology team to let them know when cautery is being performed. The patient face should be draped open such that the nasal cannula is above the drape to avoid the trapping of oxygen, and the surgical team should be aware of the flammable objects that are near the surgical field [1]. The eyelashes and brow cilia can also be moistened to minimize the risk of burn injuries [1].

Dry Eye

Similar to most eyelid surgeries, dry eyes associated with or independent of lagophthalmos is common with blepharoplasty. Patients may note ocular irritation and mild discomfort. This is usually transient and can be treated with lubricants while symptoms persist. However, some patients may have persistent dry eyes due to unmasking of latent dry eyes. Treatment with punctal plug or cautery may be indicated in refractory cases.

Prolonged Chemosis

Chemosis can be a normal postoperative finding in the immediate or intermediate postoperative period, exacerbated by incomplete eyelid closure, ocular allergy, and postsurgical edema [9]. Chemosis can occasionally lead to corneal injury as edematous conjunctiva can prevent the appropriate distribution of the tear film [9]. Initial management consists of aggressive lubrication with artificial tears and ointment [9]. At times, a mild topical steroid eye drop may be used if the intraocular pressure and cornea are regularly evaluated [9]. Rarely, a suture tarsorrhaphy may be necessary to minimize exposure from chemosis [9]. Persistent chemosis lasting over 2 months can occur and be highly frustrating to the patient and surgeon. Options, such as incision of the inferior conjunctiva for drainage of chemosis or thermal cautery of the chemotic tissue to minimize recollection of fluid, have also been suggested for prolonged chemosis, but recurrences or need for repeat treatments is not uncommon.

Peribulbar and Retrobulbar Hemorrhage

Patients should expect to have eyelid ecchymosis and edema after surgery, which improve over the next several weeks. General postoperative management includes elevation of the head and use of cold compresses for at least 48 hours. During the early postoperative period, good blood pressure control and avoidance of blood thinners (with the approval of the treating physician) will allow for normal healing. The patient should be informed that sudden Valsalva maneuvers, such as coughing, sneezing, straining, or exercise during this period, can cause sudden increases in blood pressure and subsequent hemorrhage. If there is decreased vision, severe pain, tenseness to the tissues, or inability to stop the blood flow, the patient should notify the office immediately.

A small peribulbar hemorrhage or hematoma that is not enlarging can be appropriately managed at home with ice packs, direct pressure, head elevation, and reassurance. Rapid expansion of the hematoma, especially if associated with visual changes, may necessitate drainage. However, if the hemorrhage is stable, close observation can be considered given the concern for recurrent bleeding with active attempts to evacuate [1]. As mentioned previously, the preoperative assessment should include documenting any use of anticoagulation or vitamin supplements, prior medical history that could predispose to excessive bleeding, and prior ocular history including a baseline ophthalmologic exam. There also exist differing opinions on postoperative occlusive dressings which may address postoperative edema but potentially lead to a delayed diagnosis of severe orbital hemorrhages [9]. Therefore, most surgeons do not place occlusive dressings on the eyelids after routine blepharoplasty.

Retrobulbar hemorrhage is a serious concern with any eyelid surgery. The incidence of post-blepharoplasty retrobulbar hemorrhage has been reported to be 0.055% (1 in 2000) with an incidence of associated permanent blindness of 0.0045% (1 in 10,000) [10]. Significant bleeding can result in a tense orbital compartment syndrome that may lead to compressive optic neuropathy or even a central retinal artery occlusion [11, 12]. The vast majority, 96%, of retrobulbar hemorrhages occur within the first 24 hours of surgery, with more than half occurring intraoperatively or within the first 6 hours after surgery [9]. Therefore, any acute symptoms occurring postoperatively should be promptly assessed, keeping in mind that pain and pressure are the most common symptoms associated with hemorrhage after blepharoplasty [10]. If indicated, a meticulous physical examination should be performed to assess for changes in skin color, decreased visual acuity, eyelid edema, proptosis, subconjunctival hemorrhage, limitation of extraocular motility, increased intraocular pressure, and an afferent pupillary defect [9].

Should concern for a retrobulbar hemorrhage exist, control of intraocular pressure and hemostasis is critical. Topical and systemic glaucoma medications should be considered for elevated intraocular pressures, and systemic corticosteroids can be considered for significant edema [9]. If active hemorrhage occurs and there is risk of vision loss, surgical intervention may be necessary [9]. The incision is opened urgently and the surgical site explored for areas of hemorrhage. Any active bleeding should be identified and controlled [9]. In severe, vision-threatening cases, an immediate lateral canthotomy and cantholysis are performed to rapidly evacuate the orbital bleeding [1, 9]. If there continues to be no improvement and computed tomography (CT) imaging had demonstrated a posterior orbital hemorrhage, bony decompression may be indicated to address orbital apex compression [9]. However, if vision is at risk with active hemorrhage, surgical evacuation should not be delayed to wait for neuroimaging.

Infection

Although infection may occur with blepharoplasty, this is infrequent given the extensive vascularity of the eyelid and periorbital areas. The infection rate after upper and lower blepharoplasty is estimated to be approximately 0.2% [13]. If left untreated, infections can spread quickly and result in significant morbidity, including permanent visual loss. Symptoms and signs are often consistent with other wound infections including violaceous bullae, necrotic tissue, erythema, swelling, pain, and calor. Similar to other skin and soft tissue infections, *Staphylococcus aureus* and group A ß-hemolytic *Streptococcus* have been most commonly reported [14, 15]. Rarely, mycobacterial infections have also been reported following lower eyelid surgery and are more common than after upper eyelid surgery [16]. Broad-spectrum oral antibiotics can be considered for preseptal cellulitis or local infections without evidence of abscess formation [1]. Intravenous antibiotics and hospital admission must be considered for severe or progressive infections, in addition to careful monitoring of vision and clinical progression [1]. If there is no improvement despite appropriate medical therapy or if there are any signs of orbital involvement, neuroimaging is crucial to assess for orbital cellulitis or abscesses that may require surgical drainage and cultures [1]. Consultation with an infectious disease specialist to determine optimal organism-specific coverage may be warranted.

Volume Depletion from Excessive Fat Removal

Excessive fat removal during lower blepharoplasty can result in the appearance of shadowed or darkened lower eyelids, a more prominent tear trough deformity, a more tired appearance, and ultimately a dissatisfied patient (Fig. 27.1) [17]. Volume replacement with autologous fat grafting to the hollowed area, with or without a midface lift, are options for management.

Lagophthalmos

Lagophthalmos may occur after lower eyelid blepharoplasty. In the early postoperative period, lagophthalmos is usually caused by edema or orbicularis dysfunction from manipulation or anesthetic toxicity. It typically resolves without permanent sequela. Excessive lower eyelid tissue resection, however, may cause persistent lagophthalmos that may result in exposure keratopathy. Early mild postoperative lagophthalmos can be managed with frequent topical lubrication and reassurance. The management of persistent lagophthalmos is covered in the discussion of eyelid retraction and eyelid malposition.

Diplopia and Strabismus

Lower eyelid blepharoplasty carries the complication of diplopia and the causes are varied. It is important to determine if the patient symptoms are monocular or binocular. Monocular diplopia may be related to tear film disruption from dry eye or an irregular tear film following surgery [1]. Additionally, chemosis and eyelid edema can also contribute to monocular diplopia in the immediate postoperative period.

Binocular diplopia is more concerning but fortunately is typically transient. Persistent, binocular diplopia following blepharoplasty has been reported to be approximately 0.2% [18]. It may be secondary to injury to the inferior oblique or inferior rectus muscles [18–22]. Inadvertent infiltration of local anesthetic into either of these muscles often results in diplopia that resolves without intervention. However, the inferior oblique can be directly injured in lower blepharoplasty due to its position between the medial and central fat pads in the lower eyelid (Fig. 27.2). To minimize the risk of injury, the surgeon should avoid deep forniceal incisions, identify the oblique muscle when possible, and minimize excessive manipulation of the fat adjacent to the muscle. If the diplopia does not resolve, referral to a strabismus specialist is recommended [3].

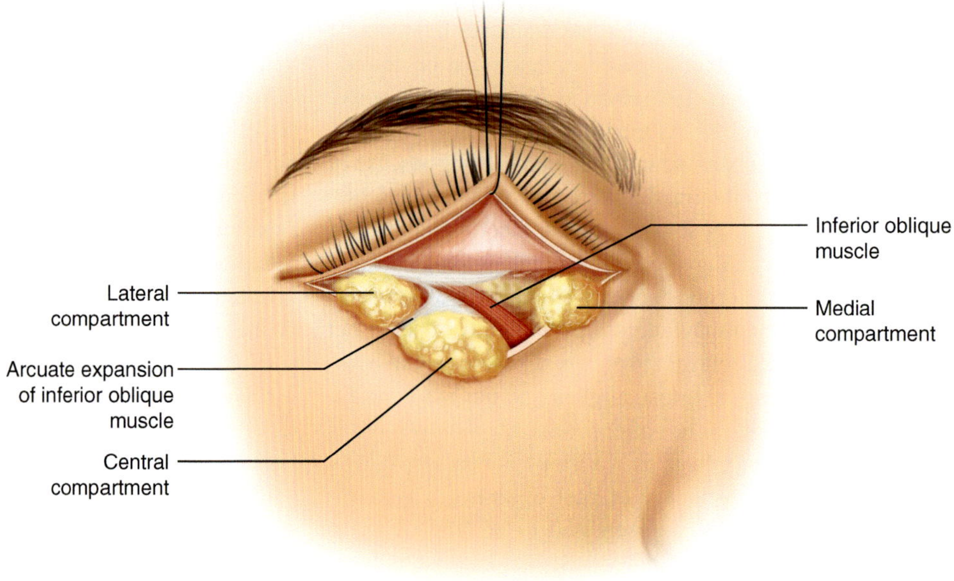

Fig. 27.2 Schematic diagram of the lower eyelid fat pads encountered during lower blepharoplasty. The relative position of the inferior oblique muscle is shown between the medial and central fat pads, and the arcuate expansion of the inferior oblique runs between the lateral and central fat pads

Eyelid Retraction and Eyelid Malposition

One of the most common long-term complications to lower blepharoplasty is eyelid malposition. Patients with untreated lower eyelid laxity, inferior rim hypoplasia, malar fat atrophy, and globe positions that are significantly more anterior than the maxilla (negative vector orbit) are at the greatest risk. Intraoperative bleeding, hematoma formation, and aggressive fat removal also increase the risk of complication. The transconjunctival incision and dissection should minimize the use of excessive cautery that could result in increased scarring and retraction of the posterior eyelid lamella. After lower eyelid surgery, the formation of cicatricial changes within the eyelid can lead to lower eyelid retraction and ectropion [23].

The severity of lower eyelid malposition can range from minimal inferior scleral show to severe cicatricial ectropion or retraction [9, 24]. It is important to note that eyelid retraction and cicatricial ectropion can occur simultaneously [25]. Cicatricial entropion may also occur due to significant cicatrization of the conjunctival layer. A transconjunctival approach that avoids disruption of the orbital septum has been reported to have a lower incidence of retraction [17, 21]. It has been suggested that when the septum is opened, there can be an increased risk of scarring of the middle and posterior lamellae, resulting in inferior eyelid displacement. Alternative sources have also suggested that transconjunctival lower eyelid blepharoplasty may actually carry the risk of elevation of the lower eyelid, particularly if the inferior retractor layer is not reattached to the tarsus [26].

Eyelid retraction can also occur in the setting of fat repositioning to augment the deep tear trough deformities. If the fat pedicle has not been well-released around the entire 360° base of the fat, the fine septal attachments to the fat will pull the eyelid inferiorly when the fat is transposed over the inferior orbital rim. This complication can be minimized by adequate dissection of the fat pedicles and full release of any circumferential septal connections.

Aggressive skin removal, especially in the setting of unresolved lower eyelid laxity, may lead to cicatricial ectropion. Avoidance of this complication is achieved by conservative skin excision during lower eyelid blepharoplasty. Typically, a few millimeters are removed, and the patient can undergo laser resurfacing to further tighten the skin postoperatively, if needed. Prior to excising the proposed amount of the skin, the patient can be asked to open and close his or her mouth. If this movement pulls on the pinched skin and lower eyelid, then the skin amount should be decreased.

A proper understanding of how to manage patients with eyelid malposition after lower blepharoplasty is essential. Cases of mild eyelid retraction or ectropion can initially be managed conservatively with upward massage for several months, with or without topical steroid therapy. Additionally, injections of steroid or fluorouracil 50 mg/mL have been shown to improve the cicatricial changes in the postoperative eyelid [17].

For cases of persistent, and symptomatic, eyelid malposition that are unresponsive to conservative measures, surgical intervention is often necessary. Regardless of the technique used to treat the malposition, stabilization of the eyelid is of the utmost importance. Any degree of eyelid laxity needs to be addressed. Beyond that, the type of malposition and the underlying cause dictate the specific treatment. Cicatricial ectropion secondary to anterior lamellar deficiency requires replacement of the skin. Skin grafting is generally considered the treatment of choice, although skin flaps can be utilized if appropriate for the patient. Eyelid retraction caused by middle and posterior lamellar scarring is treated by releasing areas of cicatrix and placement of a spacer graft (Fig. 27.3). Release of scar should be performed with scissors as much as possible, in order to minimize thermal cauterization that would potentially instigate more inflammation and scarring. The cicatrix is fully released once the eyelid is freely mobile and can be elevated into the proper position with any tethering. There are a variety of graft options that include, but are not limited to, hard palate, tarsus, nasal septum, ear cartilage, acellular dermal matrix, and other commercially available grafts. The recessed conjunctiva and retractor layers are sutured to the inferior graft edge with 6-0 chromic or polyglactin suture. Other options include suturing the conjunctiva over the graft edges. It is important to consult the patient about the risk of recurrence, the need for additional surgery, and the possibility of a suboptimal outcome [17, 25].

Entropion

While ectropion is an often discussed complication following lower eyelid blepharoplasty, cicatricial entropion is a rare complication. It is associated with the transconjunctival approach that can result in posterior lamellar scarring and deficiency (Fig. 27.4) [9, 27]. The lower eyelid may be scarred inferiorly toward the orbital rim (retraction) but can also demonstrate cicatricial entropion with inward directed lashes. Repair involves releasing of the cicatrix and placement of a graft such as hard palate, tarsus, ear cartilage, or one of the various alloplastic materials available [9].

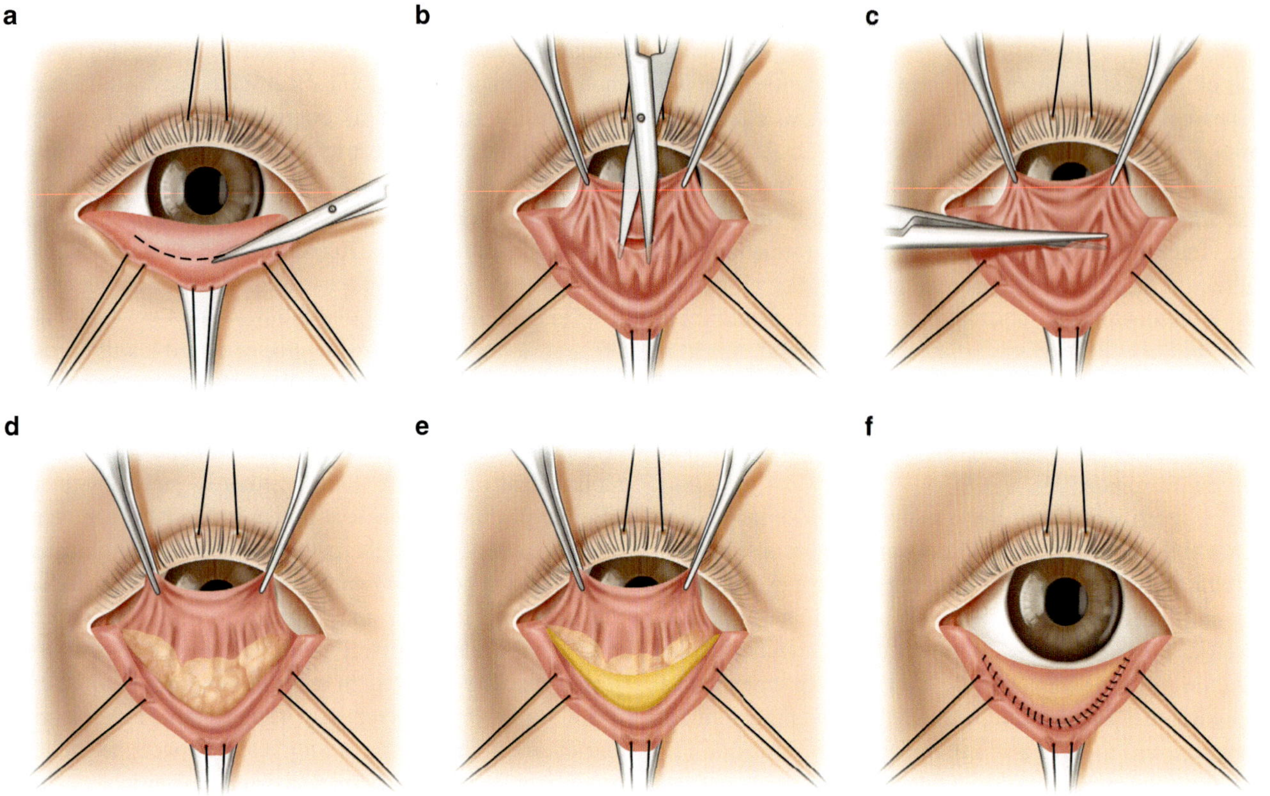

Fig. 27.3 Surgical steps for correction of lower eyelid retraction repair. (**a**) The lower eyelid is everted over a Desmarres retractor or with traction sutures, and the posterior conjunctiva and lower eyelid retractors are incised 3–4 mm inferior to the inferior edge of tarsus with a 15 blade scalpel; (**b**) the inferior retractor layer is incised horizontally to release it from the inferior tarsal border; (**c**) dissection is carried inferiorly into the fornix to completely release the retractors, conjunctiva, and areas of cicatrix, thus releasing the retraction pull on the lower eyelid; (**d**) a posterior lamellar defect results as the released conjunctiva, retractors, and cicatrix are allowed to recess into the fornix; (**e**) a rectangular tarsal-free graft with angled corners is trimmed to fit the posterior lamellar defect and sutured to the inferior recipient tarsus with the mucosal side facing the globe; (**f**) the recessed conjunctiva and retractor layers are sutured to the inferior tarsal graft edge with 6-0 chromic suture. Other options include suturing the conjunctiva over the graft edges

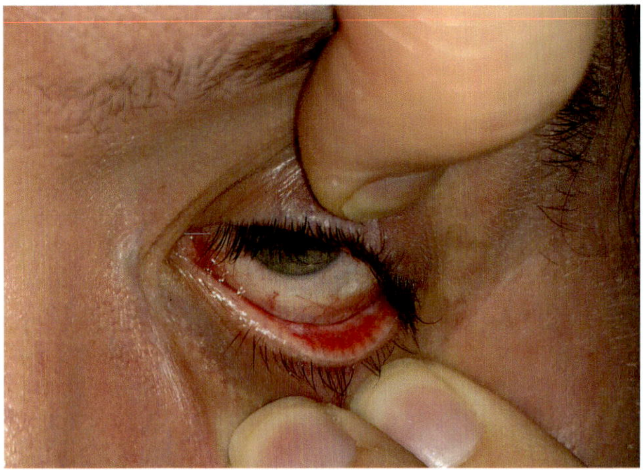

Fig. 27.4 Clinical photo demonstrating lower eyelid entropion secondary to posterior lamellar scarring and deficiency following prior transconjunctival surgery, as evidenced by the horizontal linear white scarring. (Image courtesy of Cat N. Burkat, MD FACS)

Conclusion

Complications associated with lower eyelid blepharoplasty can often be minimized with meticulous surgical technique. However, complications and suboptimal outcomes can still arise and require appropriate management. Many surgeons advocate for a more integrated approach to lower blepharoplasty, involving variations of fat excision, fat transposition, skin excision, trichloroacetic acid skin peels or laser resurfacing, temporary tarsorrhaphy, and lateral canthopexy tailored to each individual patient. Regardless of the surgical approach, it is important for the surgeon to be aware of the common and rare complications associated with each approach and be comfortable with addressing them should they arise.

References

1. Whipple KM, Korn BS, Kikkawa DO. Recognizing and managing complications in blepharoplasty. Facial Plast Surg Clin North Am. 2013;21(4):625–37.
2. Rizk SS, Matarasso A. Lower eyelid blepharoplasty: analysis of indications and the treatment of 100 patients. Plast Reconstr Surg. 2003;111(3):1299–306.
3. Klapper SR, Patrinely JR. Management of cosmetic eyelid surgery complications. Semin Plast Surg. 2007;21(1):80–93.
4. Naik MN, Honavar SG, Das S, Desai S, Dhepe N. Blepharoplasty: an overview. J Cutan Aesthet Surg. 2009;2(1):6–11.
5. Oestreicher J, Mehta S. Complications of blepharoplasty: prevention and management. Plast Surg Int. 2012;2012:1–10.
6. Bartley GB, Warndahl RA. Surgical bleeding associated with aspirin and nonsteroidal anti-inflammatory agents. Mayo Clin Proc. 1992;67(4):402–3.
7. Holck DE, Dutton JJ, Wehrly SR. Changes in astigmatism after ptosis surgery measured by corneal topography. Ophthalmic Plast Reconstr Surg. 1998;14(3):151–8.
8. Chen WP, Khan JA. Color atlas of cosmetic oculofacial surgery. Philadelphia: Saunders Elsevier; 2010. Print.
9. Lelli GJ, Lisman RD. Blepharoplasty complications. Plast Reconstr Surg. 2010;125(3):1007–17.
10. Hass AN, Penne RB, Stefanyszyn MA, Flanagan JC. Incidence of postblepharoplasty orbital hemorrhage and associated visual loss. Ophthalmic Plast Reconstr Surg. 2004;20(6):426–32.
11. Kelly PW, May DR. Central retinal artery occlusion following cosmetic blepharoplasty. Br J Ophthalmol. 1980;64:918–22.
12. Anderson RL, Edwards JJ. Bilateral visual loss after blepharoplasty. Ann Plast Surg. 1980;5:288–92.
13. Carter SR, Stewart JM, Khan J, et al. Infection after blepharoplasty with and without carbon dioxide laser resurfacing. Ophthalmology. 2003;110(7):1430–2.
14. Jordan DR, Mawn L, Marshall DH. Necrotizing fasciitis caused by group A streptococcus infection after laser blepharoplasty. Am J Ophthalmol. 1998;125(2):265–6.
15. Goldberg RA, Li TG. Postoperative infection with group A beta-hemolytic Streptococcus after blepharoplasty. Am J Ophthalmol. 2002;134:908–10.
16. Mauriello JA Jr, Atypical Mycobacterial Study Group. Atypical mycobacterial infection of the periocular region after periocular and facial surgery. Ophthal Plast Reconstr Surg. 2003;19:182–8.
17. Schwarcz RM, Kotlus B. Complications of lower blepharoplasty and midface lifting. Clin Plast Surg. 2014;42(1):63–71.
18. Hayworth RS, Lisman RD, Muchnick RS, Smith B. Diplopia following blepharoplasty. Ann Ophthalmol. 1984;16:448–51.
19. Alfonso E, Levada AJ, Flynn JT. Inferior rectus paresis after secondary blepharoplasty. Br J Ophthalmol. 1984;68:535–7.
20. Harley RD, Nelson LB, Flanagan JC, Calhoun JH. Ocular motility disturbances following cosmetic blepharoplasty. Arch Ophthalmol. 1986;104:542–4.
21. Baylis HI, Long JA, Groth MJ. Transconjunctival lower eyelid blepharoplasty: technique and complications. Ophthalmology. 1989;96:1027–32.
22. Syniuta LA, Goldberg RA, Thacker NM, Rosenbaum AL. Acquired strabismus following cosmetic blepharoplasty. Plast Reconstr Surg. 2003;111:2053–9.
23. Schwarcz R, Fezza JP, Jacono A, Massry GG. Stop blaming the septum. Ophthalmic Plast Reconstr Surg. 2016;32(1):49–52.
24. McCord CD Jr, Ellis DS. The correction of lower lid malposition following lower lid blepharoplasty. Plast Reconstr Surg. 1993;92:1068–72.
25. Patel BCK, Patipa M, Anderson RL, McLeish W. Management of postblepharoplasty lower eyelid retraction with hard palate grafts and lateral tarsal strip. Plast Reconstr Surg. 1997;99:1251–60.
26. Segal KL, Patel P, Levine B, Lisman RD, Lelli GJ. The effect of Transconjunctival blepharoplasty on margin reflex distance 2. Aesthet Plast Surg. 2016;40(1):13–8.
27. Korchia D, Braccini F, Paris J, Thomassin J. Transconjunctival approach in lower eyelid blepharoplasty. Can J Plast Surg. 2003;11(3):166–70.

Lateral Canthal Surgery

28

Seanna R. Grob, Jordan R. Conger, and Jeremiah Tao

Anatomy of the Lateral Canthal Angle and Surrounding Structures

The lateral canthus can be appreciated as the angle at which the upper and lower eyelids unite on the temporal aspect of the globe and orbit. Although significant variability exists between ethnicity, age, and sex, the lateral canthus sits slightly higher, on average, than its medial counterpart. This configuration is referred to as a positive canthal tilt. An abnormal negative canthal tilt is present when the lateral canthus sits lower than the medial canthus. This may be seen in euryblepharon or iatrogenic following lower eyelid surgery. The eyelashes extend to the lateral canthus. The gray line, or the most superficial portion of the orbicularis muscle, called the muscle of Riolan, of the upper and lower eyelid converge at the lateral canthus. During canthoplasty, the gray lines of the upper and lower eyelids are carefully re-approximated to form a sharp and distinct lateral canthal angle, and to forestall eyelid override or mild ectropion.

The exposed sclera on either side of the cornea form the medial and lateral scleral triangles. The lateral scleral triangle is defined by the upper and lower lids that join at the lateral canthus, and the corneoscleral limbus. The medial scleral triangle sits nasal to the cornea. The perception of the size of the palpebral fissure is related to the amount of scleral show. Whereas the medial scleral triangle size and shape remains fairly constant, the size and shape of the lateral scleral triangle varies more with eyelid malposition or surgery involving the lateral canthus [1]. Lateral canthal angle rounding, phimosis (commonly due to dehiscence of the lateral canthal tendon), canthal dystopia, or canthal webbing can distort the appearance of the eye shape.

S. R. Grob · J. R. Conger · J. Tao (✉)
Division of Oculofacial Plastic and Orbital Surgery, Gavin Herbert Eye Institute, Irvine, CA, USA

Department of Ophthalmology, University of California, Irvine, School of Medicine, Irvine, CA, USA
e-mail: jeremiat@uci.edu

The tarsoligamentous sling that supports the eyelids includes the tarsus of the upper and lower eyelids and the medial and lateral canthal tendons that attach to periosteum. The superior and inferior crura extend laterally from the superior and inferior tarsal plates and merge to form the lateral canthal tendon (LCT). The LCT is thought to contain both anterior and posterior divisions separated by adipose tissue [2, 3]. Although debated, the anterior portion of the LCT is thought to insert on the anterior surface of the lateral orbital rim [4–12]. The posterior portion extends deep to the septum on Whitnall's tubercle (orbital tubercle), found approximately 1.5 mm (SD, ±0.3 mm) posterior to the orbital rim, as the lateral orbital raphe [2]. The LCT is contiguous with the lateral horn of the levator aponeurosis superiorly [2, 4]. Anteriorly, the LCT merges with fibers from the preseptal and pretarsal orbicularis oculi muscles, and posteriorly, the LCT is continuous with the lateral rectus capsulopalpebral fascia (lrCPF), including the lateral cheek ligament [2, 4]. Inferiorly, the LCT receives fibrous connections from Lockwood's suspensory ligament. All of these structures together are collectively referred to as the lateral retinaculum.

The anterior component of the LCT is thought to provide some support to the lateral canthus, while the posterior component, with its connection to the lrCPF and lateral cheek ligament, provides the majority of the support to the eyelids and allows them to follow the curvature of the globe. The posterior component may also provide lateral movement of the canthal angle during temporal gaze to increase the temporal visual field via its connection to the lateral cheek ligament [4, 13–15]. However, other evidence suggests the canthal angle may actually move medially during temporal gaze, hypothesized to protect the globe in extreme versions [16].

Lastly, there has long existed a debate whether the LCT is a ligament or tendon [2, 4–12, 17]. This debate is beyond the scope of this chapter. For the sake of clarity, we will hereafter refer to it as the LCT.

A. J. Cohen, C. N. Burkat (eds.), *Oculofacial, Orbital, and Lacrimal Surgery*, https://doi.org/10.1007/978-3-030-14092-2_28

Preoperative Exam and Important Concepts to Consider

History

Patients requiring lateral canthal angle surgery present with a wide range of complaints and conditions, both functional and cosmetic. Appearance and function are intimately intertwined. Those requiring functional lower eyelid or canthal procedures may also be concerned about how the shape of their eyes may change. Conversely, many patients solely seeking lower eyelid aesthetic surgery may require surgical reinforcement at the lateral canthus to prevent lower eyelid malposition postoperatively.

Patients may present for many different reasons, ranging from dry eyes to bags or excess skin. Patient complaints often flow to diagnosing specific pathologic conditions that have specific treatment plans. For example, tearing can be secondary to lower eyelid laxity or ectropion or increased ocular surface exposure from eyelid retraction (Fig. 28.1). Once other possibilities such as ocular surface disease or tear outflow obstruction are ruled out, a horizontal tightening procedure such as the lateral tarsal strip may be appropriate. For patients seeking cosmetic surgery for periorbital and facial rejuvenation, patients may complain about "bags" under the eyes or "tired eyes" and lateral canthal surgery can be performed in combination with other interventions, such as lower eyelid blepharoplasty or midface lift. Importantly, lower eyelid malposition may be related to skin conditions or cancer, previous surgery (Fig. 28.2), or ocular pathology.

Lastly, non-oculofacial considerations such as coagulopathies or the use of anticoagulants must be discussed since bleeding may be associated with disastrous complications of surgical intervention. Smoking also negatively impacts results and can prolong postoperative healing [18].

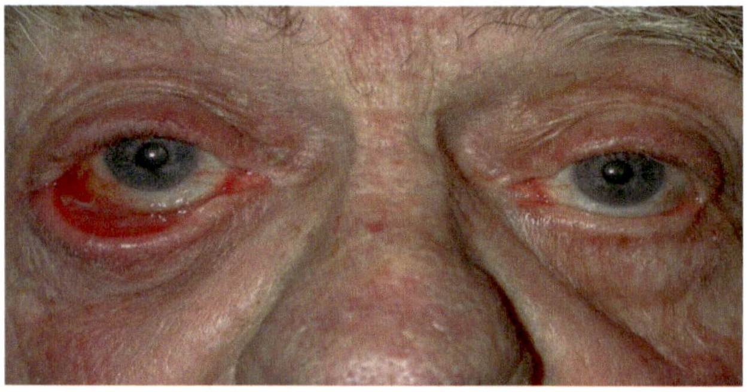

Fig. 28.1 Patient with ectropion and lower eyelid laxity on the right greater than the left lower eyelid with some lower eyelid retraction noted on the left

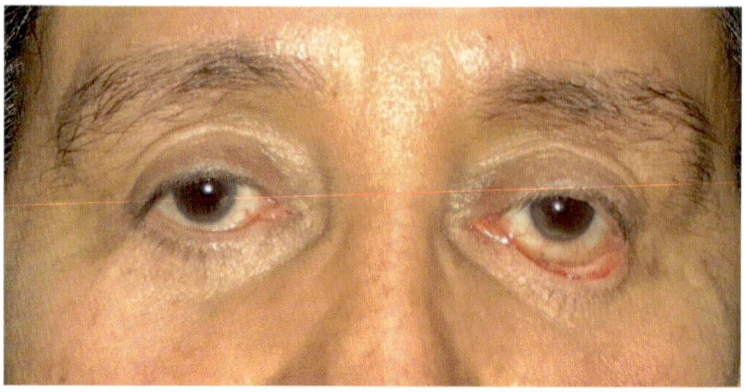

Fig. 28.2 Patient with cicatricial ectropion after a lower eyelid blepharoplasty

Examination

The whole face and eyes should be assessed prior to lateral canthal surgery. Examination should include an assessment of features associated with age, such as lower eyelid laxity. Lower eyelid malposition is one of the most common complications after lower eyelid blepharoplasty, midface rhytidectomy, and even lower facelift surgeries. In these cases, skin shortage induces a cicatricial downward vector on the eyelid (Fig. 28.2). Along with altered appearance post-blepharoplasty or facial cosmetic surgery, eyelid malposition commonly causes eye surface exposure that may manifest as redness, corneal dryness, reflex excess tears, or some combination of these [19].

Normal aging is associated with loss of elasticity and strength of the tarsoligamentous sling that, in turn affect tone, position, and movement of the lower eyelid. These aging changes can cause frank lower eyelid retraction or ectropion.

In many instances, eyelid laxity or pathology is not obvious with inspection alone, and laxity must be assessed with digital manipulation. In the snap back test, the eyelid is pulled down and away from the globe and then released and allowed to recoil back into position (Fig. 28.3a, b). A prolonged snap back test may suggest the need for lateral canthal support. A related test is the eyelid distraction test, in which the distance the lower eyelid can be pulled away from the globe is measured. More than 6 mm away from the globe suggests significant tarsoligamentous laxity and an abnormal eyelid distraction test, and a possible indication for lateral canthoplasty. Floppy eyelid syndrome is another condition in which these tests are abnormal. Additional correlates in this syndrome may be a papillary reaction on the palpebral conjunctiva and a history of sleep apnea.

Another test is the finger repositioning test to demonstrate the intended effects of surgery on the lateral canthus and midface (Fig. 28.4). By placing one finger at the lateral can-

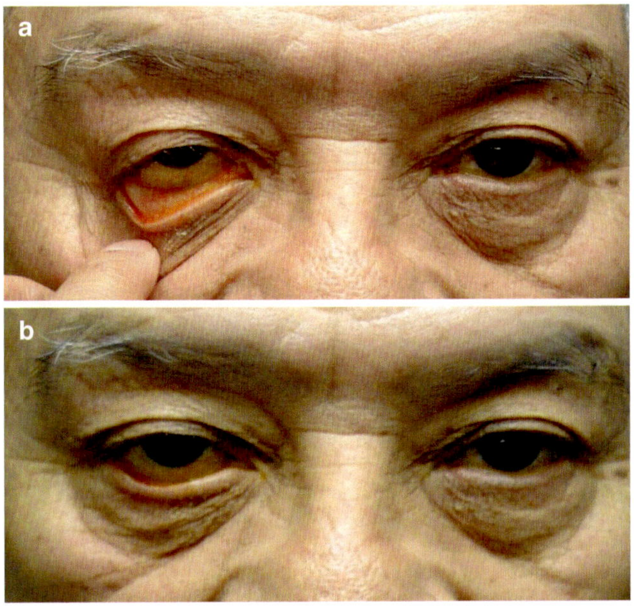

Fig. 28.3 Snap back test. Showing (**a**) the eyelid easily distracted away from the globe and with (**b**) poor apposition of the eyelid to the globe after release of the lower eyelid

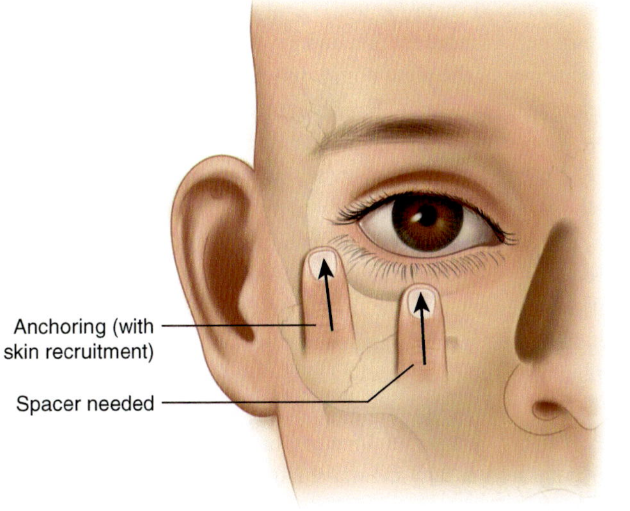

Fig. 28.4 A single finger is placed at the lateral canthus and the lower eyelid is pushed laterally and superiorly. If the lower eyelid assumes its normal position, then a lateral canthoplasty without the need of a spacer graft can be used. If a second finger is required at the medial lower eyelid to reposition the lower eyelid, then a spacer graft must be included as part of the surgery

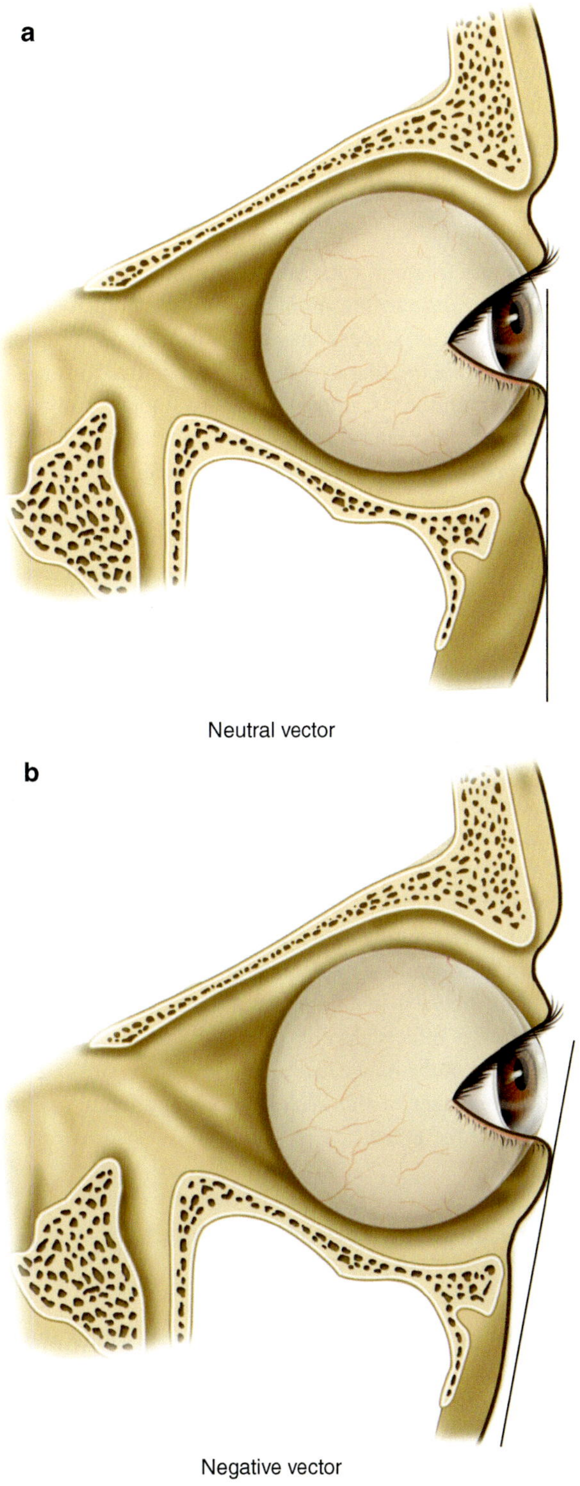

Fig. 28.5 (**a**) Neutral vector globe and maxilla in alignment. (**b**) Prominent eye with a negative vector showing the globe positioned anterior to the maxilla

thal angle, the effects of canthal anchoring such as a lateral tarsal strip can be predicted. If eyelid malposition remains with a single finger at the canthus, additional procedures may be necessary. For example, the need for additional finger elevation of the central eyelid or at the malar eminence may predict a need for other interventions including, but not limited to, spacer grafts or midface lifting [20]. In addition to laxity, these digital manipulation tests also assess for scar or stiffness in any layer of the eyelids or midface, commonly seen post trauma or after prior surgery.

Watching the patient blink involuntarily, volitionally, and forcefully determines orbicularis oculi muscle function. Patients with a seventh nerve palsy or paresis may present with lower eyelid malposition or an incomplete blink. Paretic vectors may demand additional treatments, such as eyelid weight loading or tarsorrhaphy, that are beyond lateral canthal surgery alone; these procedures are beyond the scope of this chapter.

Abnormal lateral canthus shape in the absence of symptoms or eyelid closure problems may be bothersome. Age, trauma, or prior surgery may cause canthal dystopia or phimosis or webbing that may be aesthetic indications for surgical intervention. Canthal angle dystopia may also be iatrogenic if the lateral tarsal strip is not secured back to the appropriate position 1–2 mm higher than the angle of the medial canthal angle.

Finally, the position of the globe is important. Prominent eyes cause a negative vector, which is seen on lateral view with the globe positioned anterior to the maxilla in the midline sagittal plane (Fig. 28.5). A positive vector indicates a deep set eye and is present when the globe is posterior to the maxilla in the midline sagittal plane. A Hertel exophthalmometer is not absolutely necessary but can be used to objectively measure the position of the globe. The standard eye position is approximately 15–18 mm with deep set eyes being less than 15 mm and prominent eyes being over 18 mm. Patients with prominent eyes or a negative vector are at an increased risk of lid malposition after lower eyelid surgery. Lower eyelid surgery should be approached with caution in these patients since lateral canthal procedures alone may not only be insufficient but also actually can lead to paradoxical effects. Eyelid tightening in the presence of a prominent globe may cause a "clotheslining, or sling, effect" with movement of the eyelid margin retracting toward the equator of the globe.

Tear Pump Dysfunction and Blink Lag with Poor Canthal Fixation

The tear pump system of the eye is an additional important component of lateral canthal physiology. The architecture of the periocular structures guides tears from the tear producing glands of the eyelids toward the medial canthus and into the lacrimal outflow system. A positive canthal tilt, the medial and lateral canthal tendons, and the orbicularis oculi muscle together function to pump tears in the inferonasal direction. Without proper canthal fixation to the orbital wall, the orbicularis cannot generate sufficient tension to generate a complete blink, resulting in impaired lacrimal pump functionality [21, 22].

Surgical Techniques of the Lateral Canthal Angle

Many surgeries have been developed to repair pathologic changes of the lateral canthal angle, or to enhance the area for cosmetic reasons [23–27]. Canthoplasty and canthopexy are two categories of horizontal tightening procedures that are used alone or in conjunction with other surgeries, such as blepharoplasty and midface lift. Lateral canthal anchoring is performed in many patients undergoing lower eyelid blepharoplasty to help provide lid support and prevent postoperative eyelid malposition. A canthoplasty refers to a tightening procedure that involves a canthotomy and cantholysis before reattaching the LCT to the orbital tubercle, whereas a canthopexy is a less invasive procedure that involves tightening of the LCT without cutting or removing lateral canthal tendon tissue. Both of these procedures have many different variations.

Canthoplasty with lower eyelid tightening by the lateral tarsal strip

First described in 1979, the lateral tarsal strip (LTS) procedure targets canthal tendon and eyelid laxity. This procedure remains one of the most commonly performed lateral canthal tightening procedures. Eyelid laxity or ectropion or entropion are common indications for this surgical procedure.

The procedure begins by making a lateral canthotomy and cantholysis (Fig. 28.6a–c). For correction of lower eyelid laxity, an inferior cantholysis is fashioned with sharp dissection. After cantholysis, the lower eyelid should be freed from lateral canthal attachments (Fig. 28.6d). The lower eyelid can then be pulled laterally and the amount of laxity and eyelid to tighten measured and marked along the lid margin. The eyelid is then split into anterior and posterior lamellae along the gray line of the eyelid, to the location of the marking. The palpebral conjunctiva may be shaved from the tarsal strip with a #15 blade. The strip can be pulled laterally to measure the amount of tissue resection and the tarsal strip can be trimmed (Fig. 28.7a). The tarsal strip is sutured directly to the periosteum near Whitnall's tubercle, just on the inner aspect of the lateral orbital rim (Fig. 28.7b–d). In the presence of a prominent eye, the fixation point may be more external. The tarsus can be secured to the lateral orbital rim with a single- or double-armed 4-0 or 5-0 polyglactin, polyester fiber, polydioxanone, or polypropylene suture depending on surgeon preference. As mentioned previously, the periosteal fixation should be slightly higher than the level of the medial canthal angle in order to avoid lateral canthal angle inferior dystopia. The lateral canthal angle is then re-approximated with a 6-0

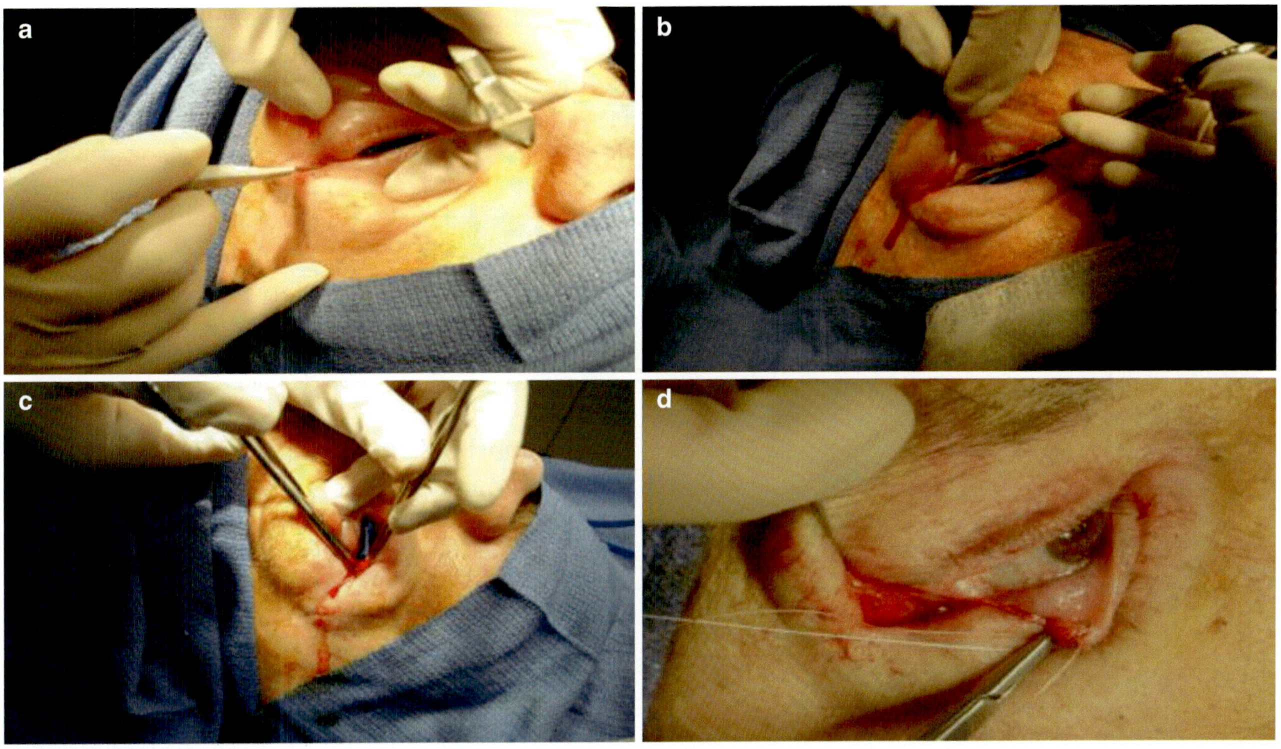

Fig. 28.6 Lateral tarsal strip canthotomy and cantholysis. (**a**) A #15 blade is used to incise the lateral canthal angle. (**b**) Straight iris scissors are used to complete a lateral canthotomy followed by (**c**) cantholysis. (**d**) The eyelid should be easily distracted away from the globe and free from any lateral canthal attachments

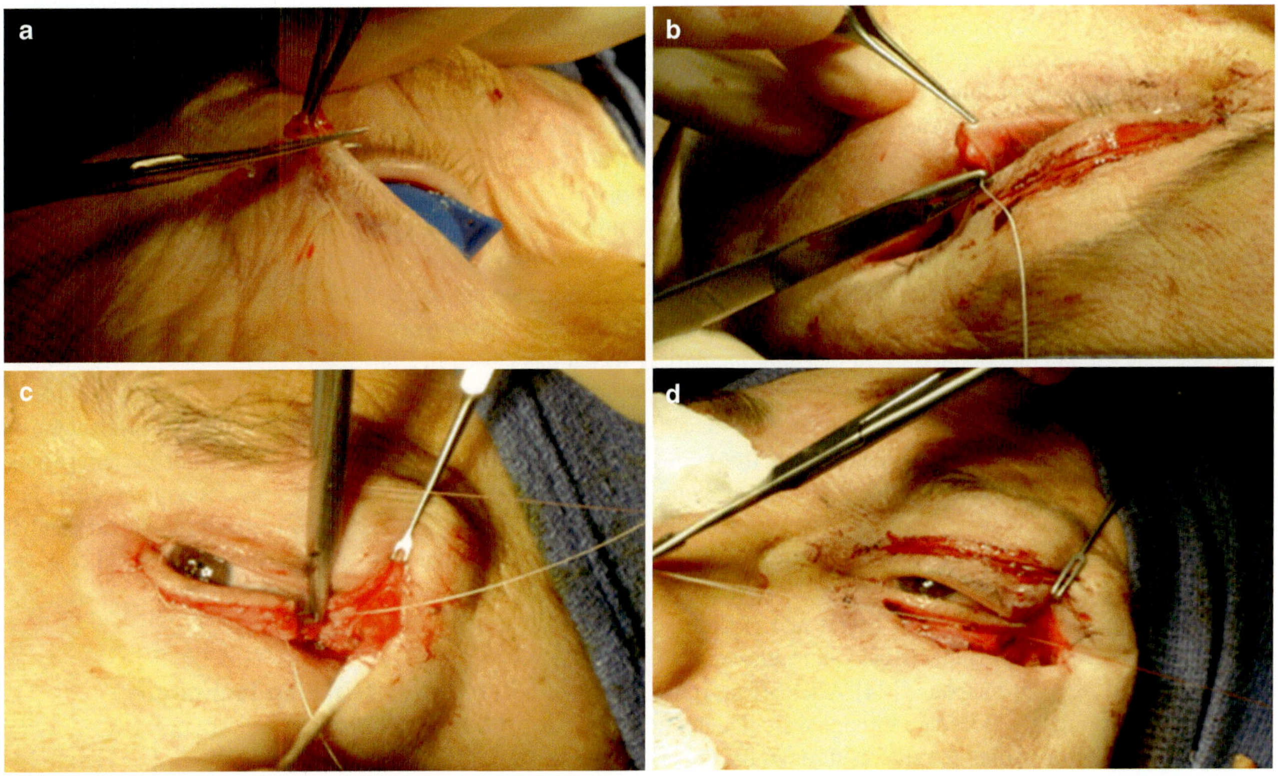

Fig. 28.7 Lateral tarsal strip. (**a**) Once the tarsal strip is formed, it can be trimmed based on the amount of tightening desired. (**b**) The tarsal strip is then secured with a 4-0 Vicryl suture (or other preferred suture). (**c**) The needle is then passed just inside the lateral orbital rim engaging periosteum to secure the strip to its near normal fixation location. (**d**) Once the suture is tied down, the lower eyelid positioning showed be checked

plain gut or polyglactin suture with a buried suture that reapproximates the gray line of the upper and lower eyelid. This prevents lateral canthal angle blunting or webbing, to create a sharp eyelid angle. The eyelid follicles present on the anterior lamella anterior to the repositioned tarsus are then removed and the excess skin can be trimmed and the lateral canthal skin incision is then closed [23].

A theoretical concern of this surgery is that the excision of LCT tissue and attachment of tarsus to the lateral orbital wall, replaces an elastic tissue with a rigid tissue [16]. This can lead to undesirable cosmetic effects, such as reduction in scleral show and/or loss of the normal lower eyelid contour. The LCT also has connections to the lateral cheek ligament thought to provide lateral canthal angle movement with temporal gaze [4, 13–15]. The lateral tarsal strip potentially decreases the dynamic aspects of the lateral canthus; however, in the authors' experience, these effects are mild or insignificant.

Canthopexy

A canthopexy is an option if the amount of eyelid laxity is mild and tucking the edge of the lower eyelid against the orbital rim is sufficient. More significant laxity requires lower eyelid resection procedures. Canthopexy can be conducted alone or in conjunction with other eyelid and midface surgeries. Commonly, the procedure is used to achieve subtle repositioning or tightening at the lateral canthus, or as adjunct support in cosmetic lower eyelid surgery.

If performed in isolation, the surgery utilizes one or two small incisions: a small (1 cm) incision in the lateral upper eyelid and a separate small (3 mm) lateral, subciliary incision. A double-armed 4-0 or 5-0 polypropylene or polyester fiber suture with large, half-circle needles is directed through the subciliary incision and passed through the proximal retinaculum and lateral canthal tendon. One of the needles is guided beyond the lateral commissure in the suborbicularis plane while Whitnall's tubercle is palpated through the lateral upper eyelid incision. The needle is then advanced through the periosteum at the level of the tubercle from posterior to anterior, and then pulled through the upper eyelid incision. This suture can then be reinforced at the level of the lateral canthal tendon using an additional suture. The original, double-armed suture can be secured at the upper eyelid wound site once the desired canthal height and tension is obtained. Finally, the two small incisions can be closed if no other procedures are to be completed [24]. Alternatively, others prefer performing this procedure through a single lateral raphe incision only, or pulling the sutures through the upper blepharoplasty incision if performed concurrently.

If performed in combination with other lower eyelid surgeries, then no additional incisions are necessary. A double-armed suture as above is passed through the lateral lower eyelid and then is introduced at the desired position inside the lateral orbital rim periosteum. The same pass is completed for the upper eyelid. For surgeons who prefer to use dissolvable sutures, a 4-0 or 5-0 polyglactin or polydiaxanone suture can be used in a similar fashion.

This surgery provides the advantage of being much less invasive than others described in this chapter, since lateral canthotomy and cantholysis are avoided. However, the primary limitation is its reduced longevity, where the lower eyelid slowly reassumes the preoperative position over time [16].

Lateral Canthoplasty or Canthopexy with Drill Hole

A drill hole lateral canthoplasty or canthopexy can be performed if a more powerful lower eyelid and midface suspension is required to help lift and suspend the lower eyelid and midface. It is an option if previous lateral canthoplasty with attachment to periosteum was unsuccessful or in cases with significant lower eyelid retraction or malposition after lower eyelid blepharoplasty. In some cases of multiple prior surgeries, intraoperative findings may demonstrate attenuated periosteum replaced with scar that is an ineffective anchor.

Through a lateral canthotomy incision, dissection is carried down to the lateral orbital rim. The periosteum is bluntly dissected from the lateral orbital rim bone. A high-speed drill is used to create a single hole just inside the lateral orbital rim at a level about 2 mm above the level of the lateral canthal angle [28]. A suture of choice such as a 4-0 polyester fiber or polyglactin on a small half-circle needle is then passed through the exposed lateral tarsus (i.e., lateral tarsal strip canthoplasty) or uncut canthal tendon (canthopexy) and secured through the drill hole. The suture is then passed through deep periosteal tissue just lateral to the drill hole or temporalis fascia more laterally and tied. Finally, the skin incision is closed in a layered fashion.

Other devices have been used to help anchor the lateral canthus and lower eyelid in settings of severe eyelid malposition or trauma. The Mitek Micro G2 Anchor System (Mitek Surgical Products, DePuy Mitek Inc., Raynham, MA) has been used as a suture anchor to reattach the lateral canthal tendon to the orbital wall, although availability and cost can be an issue [29].

A Tarsal Strip-Periosteal Flap Technique for Lateral Canthal Fixation

A tarsal strip-periosteal flap technique may be used in the setting of a prominent eye or in cases requiring tissue recruitment reconstruction such as after eyelid tumor

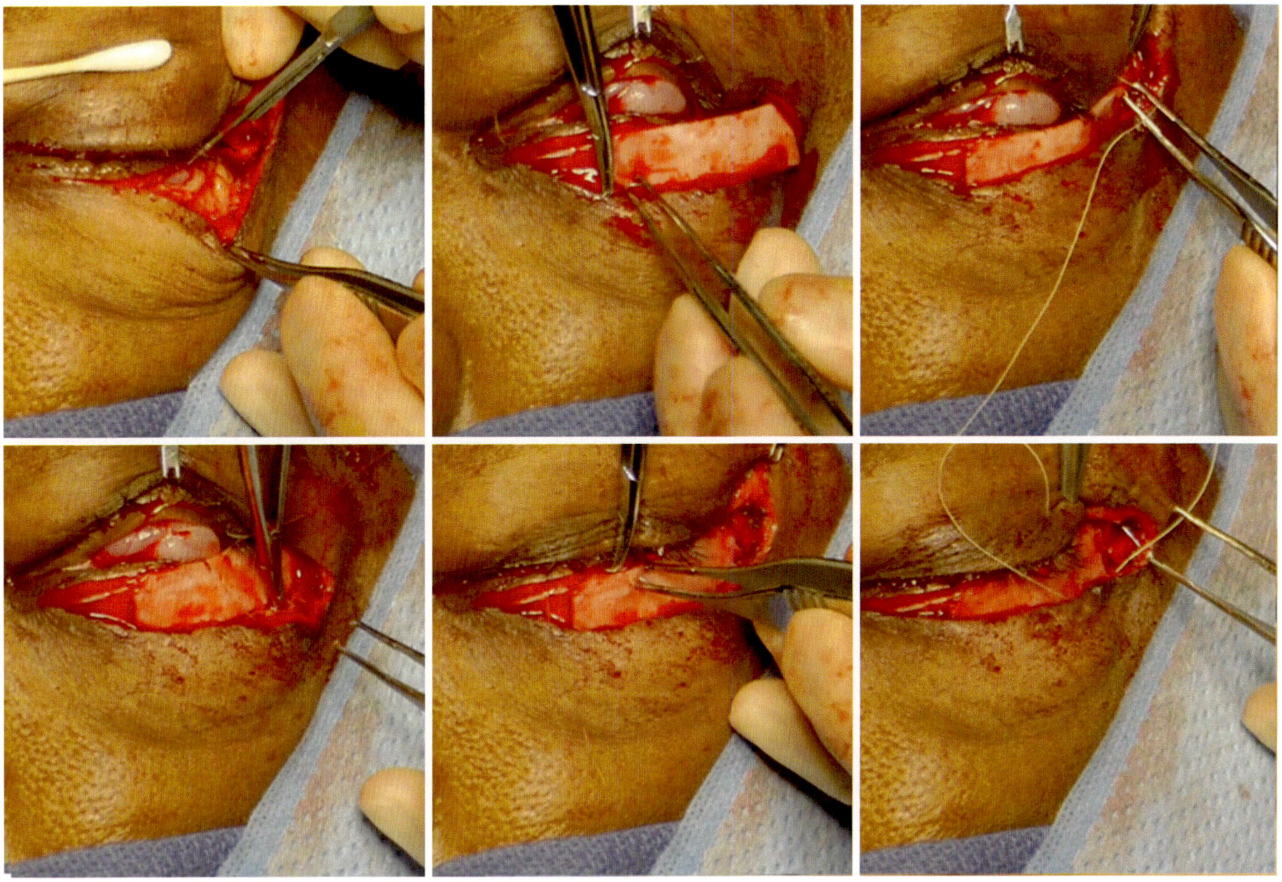

Fig. 28.8 Free tissue graft for lateral canthal fixation. A subciliary incision is made laterally in the lower eyelid and dissection is continued inferiorly (upper left). An Enduragen graft is positioned in the lower eyelid (upper middle) and should span to the lateral orbital rim (upper right). The graft can be secured into position with a running plain gut suture (lower left and middle) and is sewn from the middle lamella to the lateral orbital rim (lower right). The subciliary incision can then be closed with a running fast gut suture

excision. This can also be useful in prior eyelid surgeries in which the tarsal strip was excessively shortened, as the creation of the periosteal flap allows for posterior eyelid lengthening. Through a lateral canthotomy, dissection is carried down to the lateral orbital rim [30]. The periosteum along the lateral aspect of the rim is exposed. A surgical marking pen or methylene blue is used to draw the location of the planned periosteal flap in the desired configuration, keeping the width of the flap at least 10 mm [31]. The flap is incised with a #15 blade and gently elevated with a freer or Cottle elevator and remains attached just at the lateral orbital rim. The periosteal flap is then flipped horizontally, with its base attached at the orbital rim, and the free flap end sutured to the lateral aspect of the lower eyelid.

A Graft Patch Technique for Lateral Canthal Fixation

In rare instances, a free tissue graft may be indicated to provide additional lateral canthal support. Autologous tissues include temporalis fascia or fascia lata; allografts include sclera, dermis, and fascia; xenografts include bioengineered porcine and bovine collagen. The tissue graft is sewn from the middle lamella of the lateral eyelid to the lateral orbital rim periosteum to provide additional support in recalcitrant eyelid and canthal malposition [32]. The authors have found the patch graft useful in severe floppy eyelid syndrome owing to its elevating effect and also the stiffening effect on the eyelid (Fig. 28.8).

Complications

Complications unique and not uncommon to lateral canthal surgery include pyogenic granulomas, scarring, and canthal and eyelid malposition. All types of sutures are associated with a potential for reactivity with granuloma formation. Many of these suture reactions can be managed expectantly or with topical corticosteroids. In cases that persist for months or lead to frank abscess formation, excision of the inflammatory tissue and the inciting suture is indicated. Scarring is usually mild and inconspicuous if cutaneous incisions follow the relaxed skin tension lines. However, injections of corticosteroid or chemotherapeutic agents (e.g., 5-fluorouracil) are nonsurgical options. Anterior displacement of the canthus and ectropion can arise if the tarsus is not sutured to the inner aspect of the lateral orbital wall (at Whitnall's tubercle) and/or eyelid imbrication if shortening of the lower eyelid is too excessive [33–35]. Lid length disparity between the upper and lower eyelids can result in abnormalities during eyelid closure. Vertical descent of the lower eyelid can lead to rounding of the lateral canthal angle and deformity of the lateral lower eyelid [16]. Excess exposure of the ocular surface can cause significant ocular irritation and redness along with an unwanted appearance [19]. Additionally, surgery in the area can lead to problems with lymphatic drainage, predisposing the area to recalcitrant postoperative edema [16]. Damage to distal facial nerve fibers can potentially result in orbicularis weakness [36].

In some canthoplasty techniques, it may take several weeks for the eyelids to take final position, and patients may have an initial overcorrected appearance. Additionally, although both functional and cosmetic aspects of eyelid surgery should be considered, there are some instances, such as in reconstruction after cancer removal, where functionality may be held in higher regard. Additional surgery may be necessary in some cases.

Conclusion

The lateral canthus and its surrounding structures are quite complex. Proper function of all these structures is vital for normal ocular and orbital heath. Aging, prior surgery, infection, neoplasm, and trauma are just some of the ways in which the lateral canthus can be altered, and repair of the area requires extensive skill and knowledge. Over the last several decades, multiple approaches to lateral canthal surgery have been described. There have been few controlled studies comparing specific interventions, and surgeon experience combined with patient goals remains key.

Disclosures Authors have no relevant financial disclosures.

References

1. Gray H, Standring S, Ellis H, Berkovitz BKB. Gray's anatomy: The anatomical basis of clinical practice. 39th ed; New York, NY: Elsevier; 2005.
2. Gioia VM, Linberg JV, McCormick SA. The anatomy of the lateral canthal tendon. Arch Ophthalmol. 1987;105:529–32.
3. Bartley GB, Gerber TC. Eisler and his pocket. Am J Ophthalmol. 2006;141:417–8.
4. Kang H, Takahashi Y, Ichinose A, et al. Lateral canthal anatomy: A review. Orbit. 2012;31:279–85.
5. Whitnall SE. Anatomy of the human orbit and accessory organs of vision. 2nd ed. New York: Oxford University Press; 1932. p. 148–63, 295–8.
6. Duke-Elder S. System of ophthalmology, vol. 2. St Louis: C.V. Mosby Co; 1961. p. 522.
7. Kestenbaum A. Applied anatomy of the eye. New York: Grune & Stratton; 1963. p. 264.
8. Beard C, Quickert MH. Anatomy of the orbit. New York: Aesculapius Publishers; 1969. p. 2, 4, 9–10, 49.
9. Fox SA. Ophthalmic plastic surgery. 5th ed. New York: Grune & Stratton; 1976. p. 6, 10–2, 18–9.
10. Stewart WB. Ophthalmic plastic and reconstructive surgery. San Francisco: American Academy of Ophthalmology; 1984. p. 72–3, 78.
11. Rosenstein T, Talebzadeh N, Pogrel MA. Anatomy of the lateral canthal tendon. Oral Surg Oral Med Oral Pathol Oral Radiol Endod. 2000;89:24–8.
12. Jones LT, Boyden JLT. Duke-Elder S. System of ophthalmology, vol. 2. St Louis: C.V. Mosby Co.; 1961. p. 523.
13. Doxanas MT, Anderson RL. Clinical orbital anatomy. Baltimore: Williams & Wilkins; 1984. p. 68, 108–15.
14. Kakizaki H, Zako M, Nakano T, et al. Microscopic findings of lateral tarsal fixation in Asians. Ophthal Plast Reconstr Surg. 2008;24:131–5.
15. Kakizaki H, Athanasiov P, Selva D, Leibovitch I. Lateral tarsal fixation in Caucasians. Ophthal Plast Reconstr Surg. 2010;26:431–3.
16. Shorr N, Goldberg RA, Eshaghian B, Cook T. Lateral canthoplasty. Ophthal Plast Reconstr Surg. 2003;19:345–52.
17. Couly G, Hureau J, Tessier P. The anatomy of the external palpebral ligament in man. J Maxillofac Surg. 1976;4:195–7.
18. Lassig ADD, Bechtold JE, Lindgren BR, et al. Tobacco exposure and wound healing in head and neck surgical wounds. Laryngoscope. 2018;128(3):618–25.
19. Dortzbach RK. Lower eyelid blepharoplasty by the anterior approach. Prevention of complications. Ophthalmology. 1983;90(3):223–9.
20. Patipa M. Transblepharoplasty lower eyelid and midface rejuvenation: part I. Avoiding complications by utilizing lessons learned from the treatment of complications. Plast Reconstr Surg. 2004;113:1459–68; discussion 1475–7.
21. Shriver EM, Erickson BP, Kossler AL, Tse DT. Lateral canthal tendon disinsertion: clinical characteristics and anatomical correlates. Ophthal Plast Reconstr Surg. 2016;32(5):378–85.
22. Tse DT, Erickson BP, Tse BC. The BLICK mnemonic for clinical-anatomical assessment of patients with epiphora. Ophthal Plast Reconstr Surg. 2014;30:450–8.
23. Anderson RL, Gordy DD. The tarsal strip procedure. Arch Ophthalmol. 1979;97:2192–6.
24. Fagien S. Algorithm for canthoplasty: the lateral retinacular suspension: a simplified suture canthopexy. Plast Reconstr Surg. 1999;103:2042–53.
25. Jelks GW, Jelks EB. Repair of lower lid deformities. Clin Plast Surg. 1993;20:417–25.
26. Jelks GW, Glat PM, Jelks EB, et al. The inferior retinacular lateral canthoplasty: a new technique. Plast Reconstr Surg. 1997;100:1262–75.
27. Glat PM, Jelks GW, Jelks EB, Longaker M. Evolution of the lateral canthoplasty: techniques and indications. Plast Reconstr Surg. 1997;100:1396.
28. Oh SR, Korn BS, Kikkawa DO. Orbitomalar suspension with combined single drill hole canthoplasty. Ophthal Plast Reconstr Surg. 2013;29(5):357–60.
29. Alfano C, Chiummariello S, Monarca C, Scuderi N, Scuderi G. Lateral canthoplasty by the Micro-Mitek Anchor System. J Oral Maxillofac Surg. 2011;69(6):1745–9.
30. Lemke BN, Sires BS, Dortzbach RK. A tarsal strip-periosteal flap technique for lateral canthal fixation. Ophthalmic Surg Lasers. 1999;30(3):232–6.

31. Game J, Morlet N. Lateral canthal fixation using an oblique vertically oriented asymmetric periosteal transposition flap. Clin Exp Ophthalmol. 2007;35(3):204–7.
32. McCord C, Nahai FR, Codner MA, et al. Use of porcine acellular dermal matrix (Enduragen) grafts in eyelids: a review of 69 patients and 129 eyelids. Plast Reconstr Surg. 2008;122(4):1206–13.
33. Olver JM. Surgical tips on the lateral tarsal strip. Eye (Lond). 1998;12:1007–12.
34. Karesh JW, Nirankari VS, Hameroff SB. Eyelid imbrication. An unrecognized cause of chronic ocular irritation. Ophthalmology. 1993;100:883–9.
35. Donnenfeld ED, Perry HD, Schrier A, et al. Lid imbrication syndrome. Diagnosis with rose bengal staining. Ophthalmology. 1994;101:763–6.
36. Chong KK, Goldberg RA. Lateral canthal surgery. Facial Plast Surg. 2010;26(3):193–200.

The Subperiosteal, Drill-Hole, Midface Lift

29

Richard C. Allen

Various techniques to elevate the midface have been described [1–13]. In general, techniques differ depending on incision placement, desired vector, plane of dissection, and method of fixation. Incision placement can be through the eyelid (transcutaneous or transconjunctival) or from the temporal region. Access from each of these incisions can be augmented with a separate gingival incision. Depending on the placement of the incision, the vector invoked can be more vertical (through the eyelid) or diagonal (as with temporal incisions). The plane of dissection can be subperiosteal or preperiosteal. And, lastly, the method of fixation can be to strong connective tissue (temporalis fascia or periosteum) or to the bone.

Determining the choice of incision placement will depend upon whether other procedures will be performed concurrently and what the desired vector of pull is. In patients undergoing a browlifting procedure, adjunctive midface lifting through the temporal incision allows support with a diagonal vector. In those patients undergoing lower lid procedures, access through the transcutaneous or transconjunctival incision allows establishment of a vertical vector. The desired vector will depend upon the preoperative state. Cicatricial changes to the midface which cause lower eyelid malposition will respond more favorably to a vertical vector.

Determining the plane of dissection is usually dependent on the quantity of elevation desired. A subperiosteal lift will allow greater mobilization of the midface and thus, a more favorable lift. In addition, a subperiosteal dissection allows direct visualization of the neurovascular structures, in particular in the infraorbital neurovascular bundle. This visualization of the neurovascular bundle allows the midface to be fully mobilized. Lastly, the visualization is safer in regard to causing less damage to the neurovascular structures with less post-operative hypoesthesia.

R. C. Allen (✉)
Section of Ophthalmology, Department of Head and Neck Surgery, The University of Texas MD Anderson Cancer Center, Houston, TX, USA

Once mobilized, the midface will need to be fixated to a rigid structure in order develop scar in the post-operative period and have a lasting effect. For a trans-temporal lift, the fixation can be to the deep temporalis fascia or bone. For a trans-eyelid lift, the fixation can be to the periosteum or directly to the bone.

The purpose of this chapter is to describe a trans-eyelid, subperiosteal midface lift in which drill holes through the inferior orbital rim are used for fixation. This midface lift has the advantages of allowing the establishment of a strong vertical vector, full mobilization of the midface, and strong fixation to a rigid structure. It is most useful in cases of cicatricial lower lid retraction and ectropion.

Description of Technique [14]

The procedure can be safely performed under general anesthesia or monitored anesthesia care. The area of the midface, lower eyelid, and lateral canthus are anesthetized with 1% lidocaine and 0.375% bupivacaine with epinephrine. The patient is then prepped and draped in the normal sterile fashion. This midface lift is usually going to be performed for patients with cicatrical anterior lamellar and/or middle lamellar changes; therefore, a transconjunctival approach will almost always be used.

A 4-0 Silk suture is placed through the lower eyelid at the level of the Meibomian gland orifices to provide traction during the case. A lateral canthotomy and inferior cantholysis are then performed; this can be performed with a 15 blade and scissors, or with the monopolar, needle tip cautery. A transconjunctival incision is then made inferior to the inferior border of the tarsus, extending from the level of the punctum medially to the lateral canthotomy incision laterally. Dissection is then carried out between the orbicularis muscle and the orbital septum to identify the inferior orbital rim. This dissection is usually performed with the needle tip cautery. A 4-0 Silk suture is then placed through the cut end

A. J. Cohen, C. N. Burkat (eds.), *Oculofacial, Orbital, and Lacrimal Surgery*, https://doi.org/10.1007/978-3-030-14092-2_29

of the confluence of the conjunctiva, lower lid retractors, and orbital septum and fixated to the drape at the patient's forehead with a hemostat. The periosteum is identified. The needle tip cautery is then used to incise the periosteum at the inferior orbital rim. The Freer periosteal elevator is then used to elevate the periosteum from the midface. This is performed by retracting the eyelid with a Desmarres retractor and using a malleable retractor to displace the orbital septum from the view of the surgeon. The periosteum is elevated initially laterally and often the zygomaticofacial neurovascular bundle is identified. This can be cauterized and transected if needed, or preserved if possible. The periosteum is then elevated along the surface of the zygoma and dissection proceeds medially toward the maxilla. At the maxilla, the periosteum should be elevated superior to the infraorbital neurovascular bundle. There is often a ridge in this area that demarcates the insertion of the zygomaticus major and minor muscles. These muscles can be detached with the periosteum from the bone with no untoward post-operative effects.

The infraorbital neurovascular bundle should then be identified and gentle dissection is performed to mobilize the midface around the neurovascular bundle. Usually one can carefully dissect around it until it is visualized. Dissection then proceeds laterally, medially, and inferiorly to the infraorbital neurovascular bundle to the level of the gingival buccal sulcus.

At this point, a transgingival incision can be made to aid in release of the midface. If that is not desired, then the Freer periosteal elevator can be used to make an incision through the periosteum inferiorly in the dissection so that the periosteum is released from the bone to allow maximum mobilization of the midface. The midface is now fully mobilized.

To fixate the midface into the desired position, three drill holes will be made through the inferior orbital rim. These drill holes are made at a level medial to the neurovascular bundle, centrally, and laterally. The holes are made with a 1 mm drill bit (Stryker, Kalamazoo, MI). The periosteum of the inferior orbital rim should be elevated about 1 cm intraorbitally and the drill is then used to make the three holes at the edge of the rim. The malleable retractor should be used as a "backstop" so that the drill bit does not engage the soft tissue. The holes should traverse the edge of the inferior orbital rim so that a suture can be placed through them. This can at times be difficult because of the anatomy of the patient. Sometimes a hole needs to be begun anteriorly and finished from the posterior side of the rim. A 0 Bowman probe is useful to confirm the patency of the hole.

Attention is then turned to the cheek. Three stab incisions are made corresponding to the horizontal level of the drill holes. Vertically, the stab incision should be at least 1–2 cm inferior to the level of the inferior orbital rim. The stab incision should not be full thickness, but rather just enter the subcutaneous fat plane.

A 3-0 Nylon suture on an FS-1 needle is then placed in the subperiosteal dissection plane and the needle is placed full thickness through the cheek to exit out the stab incision. Usually it is best to start medial first. The needle is then turned around and placed back through the same stab incision, entering perpendicular to the surface of the skin and staying perpendicular until bone is felt. The needle is then retrieved from the subperiosteal plane. Thus, the suture has engaged the cheek and both ends of the suture exit out the dissection plane. Pulling on the sutures should demonstrate the vector of lift. A dimple in the cheek may be noted on the cutaneous side, which should be expected and is probably preferred.

The end of the suture without the needle is then threaded through the corresponding hole through the inferior orbital rim. The needle is too big to be placed through the hole. After the suture is retrieved from the hole, the suture is left untied and the excess suture is cut, and a clamp is placed around the sutures until they are tied later.

The steps for the 3-0 nylon suture are then repeated for the central and lateral stab incisions and drill holes. The medial suture is then tied and a dimple will usually be noted on the cheek. The same is performed for the central and lateral sutures. The skin of the stab incisions can be closed with a 6-0 prolene suture, but often these incisions will heal well without the need for suturing.

Attention is then directed to the transconjunctival incision which is closed with interrupted or running 7-0 Vicryl suture. If adjunctive procedures such as placement of inverting sutures or placement of a spacer, these procedures are then performed at this time prior to closing the transconjunctival incision. The lateral cantholysis is repaired usually with a lateral tarsal strip procedure: the strip is fashioned by dissecting between the anterior and posterior lamella laterally. The mucocutaneous junction of the posterior lamella is excised with Westcott scissors. The posterior surface of the strip is scraped with a 15 blade. The strip is then shortened to the appropriate amount depending on the tension desired. The strip is then sutured to the lateral orbital rim at the level of Whitnall's tubercle with a double armed 4-0 mersilene suture on an S-2 needle. The lateral canthotomy incision can then be closed with the 7-0 Vicryl suture used earlier on the transconjunctival closure.

Post-operatively, the patient is instructed to keep the head of the bed elevated for 2 days. Ice packs should be placed over the area of the repair for 2 days. Antibiotic ointment should be applied three times per day. There is no indication for systemic antibiotics.

Discussion

Indications for the subperiosteal drill-hole midface lift include the following: cicatricial lower lid retraction or ectropion, paralytic lower lid malposition, and severe involutional changes. Adjunctive procedures often performed with the midface lift will depend on the underlying condition. Cicatricial ectropion will usually also be treated with inverting sutures. Cicatricial retraction will usually have a spacer placed between the confluence of the orbital septum/lower lid retractors/conjunctiva and the inferior border of the tarsus. There are multiple types of spacers available including commercially available ones (porcine acellular dermal matrix), auricular cartilage, and hard palate.

The following are the advantages of this procedure: (1) complete subperiosteal dissection, (2) ability to elevate the midface medial to the infraorbital neurovascular bundle, and (3) full thickness engagement of the midface with the nylon sutures.

A subperiosteal dissection is advantageous for a number of reasons. Subperiosteal dissection allows complete dissection of the midface from the maxilla and zygoma with visualization of the neurovascular structures. Release of the periosteum at the level of the gingival buccal sulcus allows vertical movement of the soft tissue without significant tethering. Reestablishment of the periosteum to the bone results in a long lasting elevation.

Dissection medial to the neurovascular bundle is especially useful in cases which involve retraction or ectropion medially. In a preperiosteal dissection, the confidence of the medial dissection is less due to the inability to visualize the neurovascular structures. In addition, the currently available commercial, subperiosteal devices (e.g., Endotine Midface B, MicroAire, Charlottesville, VA) are designed to be placed lateral to the infraorbital neurovascular bundle.

Placement of the nylon sutures full thickness through the stab incisions insures adequate engagement of the soft tissue by the sutures. Although some early post-operative "dimpling" of the skin is noted in these areas of the sutures, the dimpling uniformly resolves with time.

In conclusion, the subperiosteal drill-hole cheek lift is an effective vertical midface lift which allows medial elevation and strong fixation to the bone and does not require a commercial device for the fixation.

References

1. Sclafani AP. Comprehensive periorbital rejuvenation with resorbable endotine implants for trans-lid brow and midface elevation. Facial Plast Surg Clin North Am. 2007;15:255–64.
2. Ramirez OM. Treatment of the aging midface. Plast Reconstr Surg. 2000;106:1653–6.
3. Codner M. Modifying the subperiosteal cheek lift. Aesthet Surg J/Am Soc Aesthet Plast Surg. 2003;23:203–4.
4. Albrecht P. Trans-inferior orbital rim anchorage and fascia roll multi-loop temporal anchorage in midface rejuvenation. Aesthet Surg J/Am Soc Aesthet Plast Surg. 2006;26:404–12.
5. DeFatta RJ, Williams EF 3rd. Evolution of midface rejuvenation. Arch Facial Plast Surg. 2009;11:6–12.
6. Finger ER. A 5-year study of the transmalar subperiosteal midface lift with minimal skin and superficial musculoaponeurotic system dissection: a durable, natural-appearing lift with less surgery and recovery time. Plast Reconstr Surg. 2001;107:1273–83; discussion 84.
7. Pontius AT, Williams EF 3rd. The extended minimal incision approach to midface rejuvenation. Facial Plast Surg Clin North Am. 2005;13:411–9.
8. Psillakis JM, Rumley TO, Camargos A. Subperiosteal approach as an improved concept for correction of the aging face. Plast Reconstr Surg. 1988;82:383–94.
9. Ben Simon GJ, Lee S, Schwarcz RM, McCann JD, Goldberg RA. Subperiosteal midface lift with or without a hard palate mucosal graft for correction of lower eyelid retraction. Ophthalmology. 2006;113:1869–73.
10. Sullivan SA, Dailey RA. Endoscopic subperiosteal midface lift: surgical technique with indications and outcomes. Ophthal Plast Reconstr Surg. 2002;18:319–30; discussion 29–30.
11. Chung JE, Yen MT. Midface lifting as an adjunct procedure in ectropion repair. Ann Plast Surg. 2007;59:635–40.
12. Jacono AA, Stong BC. Combined transconjunctival release and midface-lift for postblepharoplasty ectropion repair. Arch Facial Plast Surg. 2010;12:206–8.
13. Marshak H, Morrow DM, Dresner SC. Small incision preperiosteal midface lift for correction of lower eyelid retraction. Ophthal Plast Reconstr Surg. 2010;26:176–81.
14. Allen RC. Drill hole midface lift. 2015. http://www.eyerounds.org/video/plastics/2/Drill-hole-midface-lift.htm. Accessed 24 Jan 2016.

Transtemporal Midface Lift

30

Vito Quatela and Catherine Weng

Background

History

The philosophy of facial rejuvenation surgery evolved through the course of the twentieth century. Initially surgeons focused their efforts on reversing the effects of gravity developing rhytidectomy techniques to lift and remove excess skin. With time the focus of facial rejuvenation shifted more toward three-dimensional evaluation of facial aging. The importance of volume particularly in the midface was recognized as an important aspect of a youthful appearance. This led to the development and evolution of various surgical procedures for rejuvenation of the middle third of the face. The history of the transtemporal midface lift, as we know it, traces back to the development of the subperiosteal forehead lift. This was first reported by Tessier in 1979 when he presented his results on subperiosteal frontal rhytidectomy [1]. Following this, in the early 1980s Tessier, Psillakis, and Santana went on to describe midface lifting in the subperiosteal plane [2]. Hinderer described a subperiosteal elevation of the periorbital region from an open pretrichial approach. He demonstrated an improvement in the forehead periorbital tissues [3]. Psillakis also described success in midfacial lifting from a coronal approach with subperiosteal dissection in the periorbital and midface regions [4]. Their techniques all faced a similar challenge in the high risk of injury to the frontal branch of the facial nerve. They described rates of frontal branch injury of up to 20% [2]. These frontal branch injuries led some surgeons to limit their dissection to the anterior third of the zygoma; however this resulted in a less optimal lift. Ramirez later found that elevating the anterior 2/3 of the zygomatic periosteum could allow for more a favorable redraping of the midfacial tissues [5]. Then in the 1990s with the advent and application of the endoscope, surgeons were able to effectively elevate the forehead, temporal regions, and eventually midfacial tissues with smaller incisions and fewer frontal branch complications owning to the benefit of direct visualization of the dissection planes [2]. During this time, Ramirez described a combined endoscopic and transoral route for elevating the midfacial tissues with minimal complications compared previous reports [5].

V. Quatela (✉) · C. Weng
Quatela Center for Plastic Surgery, Rochester, NY, USA
e-mail: vquatela@quatela.com; cweng@quatela.com

Justification for Transtemporal Midface Lifting

Numerous techniques and approaches have been reported for lifting the midfacial tissues including transtemporal, transpalpebral, transoral, endoscopic, or combinations of all of the above [5]. The goals of all these procedures are all the same: to efface the nasolabial fold (NLF) and resuspend the descended malar and suborbicularis fat pads with their associated soft tissue and skin. When the endoscopic technique is applied, the midface is typically lifted in combination with an endoscopic forehead or temporal lift [5]. Our favored approach is through the transtemporal endoscopic method, which will be described in detail. We have found that with endoscopic guidance, curved dissectors, and appropriate technique, the midfacial tissues can be elevated effectively transtemporally without an intraoral incision. Additionally, the transtemporal approach to the midface lift imparts a more favorable vector of pull (more superolaterally) as compared to the preauricular or deep plane facelift approach [6].

There has also been variety in the proposed dissection planes for the midface lift. We prefer elevating the midface in the subperiosteal plane [7]. In the subperiosteal plane, we believe we can achieve an even elevation and resuspension of the tissues. Also, in this plane, we avoid risk of injury to the zygomatic and buccal branches of the facial nerve, which lie several layers superficial to this plane. Our technique for midface lifting produces benefit in several midfacial aesthetics: correction of midface ptosis and infraorbital hollowing,

A. J. Cohen, C. N. Burkat (eds.), *Oculofacial, Orbital, and Lacrimal Surgery*, https://doi.org/10.1007/978-3-030-14092-2_30

improvement in the depth of the nasolabial fold and even a degree of improvement in the of lower face jowling [8].

Anatomy

Perhaps more than in any other area in facial plastic surgery, a thorough and precise knowledge of the anatomy is essential to successful completion of endoscopic transtemporal midface lift without complication. Mastery of the fascial layers and understanding the location and depth of critical nerves and vascular structures can ensure safety during this surgery particularly in avoiding injury to the frontal branch of the facial nerve.

Scalp and Forehead

The scalp is comprised of five layers some of which extend into and continue into fascial structures in the temporal and midfacial regions. From most superficial to deep, the scalp comprises the skin, a dense subcutaneous layer of connective tissue, the aponeurosis also called the galea, loose areolar tissue, and the pericranium, which acts as the periosteum of the skull. The galea is made up of an inelastic tendinous sheet, which connects the frontalis muscle to the occipitalis muscle. The galea is continuous with the superficial muscular aponeurotic system (SMAS) and the temporoparietal fascia also called the superficial temporal fascia [7]. The frontalis muscle is located superficial to the periosteum of the forehead. Because the dissection in this region is subperiosteal, the frontalis is not encountered during the endoscopic forehead lift [7]. The depressor muscles of the brow include the corrugator supercilii, orbicularis oculi, and procerus which also lie above the periosteum but deep to the frontalis and can be dissected from beneath endoscopically [7].

Temple

In the temporal region, the fascial layers and locations are of great importance (Fig. 30.1). Just deep to the skin and subcutaneous fat is the temporal parietal fascia (TPF). The TPF is also sometimes referred to as the superficial temporal fascia [9]. The TPF is in a continuous layer that corresponds with the galea in the scalp and the SMAS in the face below the zygomatic arch [9]. The frontal branch of the facial nerve travels in this layer as it crosses the zygomatic arch. Some

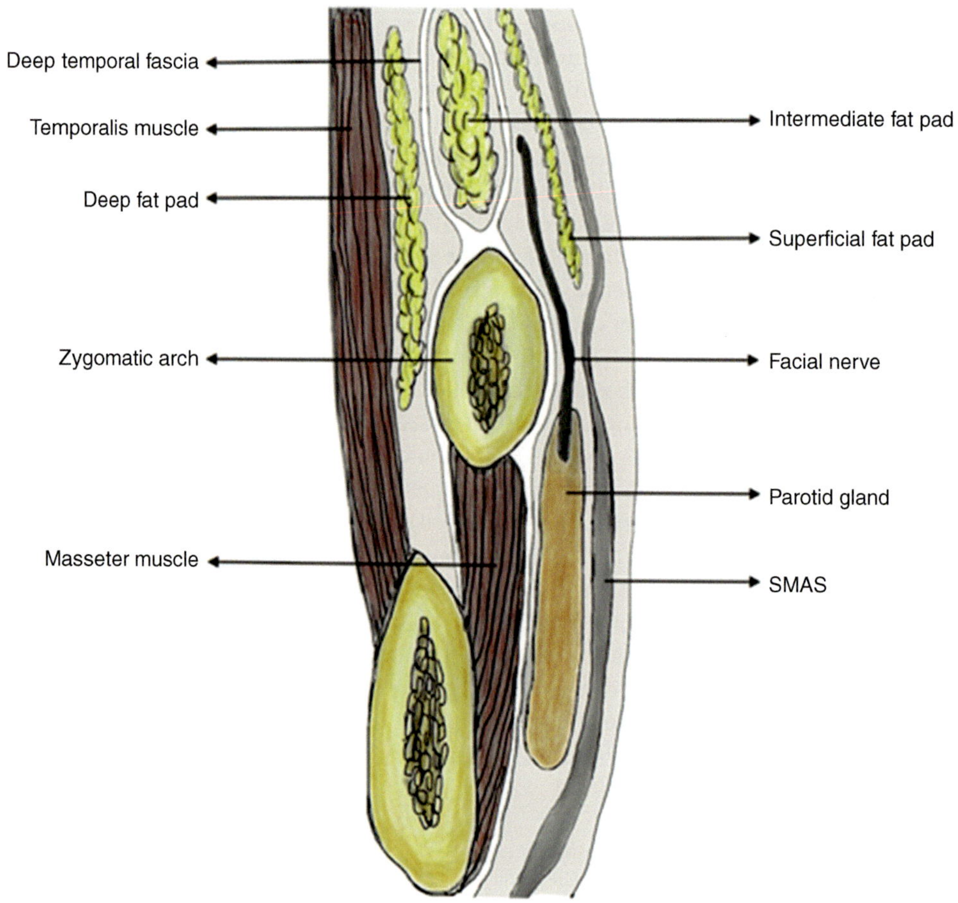

Fig. 30.1 The fascial planes through a coronal cut crossing the midportion of the zygomatic arch. One can observe the relationship between the facial nerve exiting the parotid gland and crossing superficially to the zygomatic arch and the intermediate temporal fat pad

surgeons argue that SMAS is not actually in continuation with the TPF but rather terminates within 1 cm of the zygomatic arch; however, both lie deep to the subcutaneous fat and superficial to the deeper layers [10]. Just deep to the TPF lies a thin superficial fat pad. Deep to the superficial fat pad is the deep temporal fascia complex. The deep temporal fascia, also called the temporalis fascia, exists as a single hearty fascial layer superiorly and then splits into two layers around the intermediate fat pad and zygomatic arch. The superficial layer of the deep temporal fascia attaches inferiorly to the lateral aspect of the zygomatic arch [9]. Between the superficial and deep layers of the deep temporal fascia sits the intermediate fat pad. The deep layer of the deep temporal fascia comprises the majority of the fascial fibers from the united single deep temporal fascia superiorly and attaches inferiorly to the medial aspect of the zygomatic arch [9]. Superiorly the deep temporal fascia directly overlies the temporalis muscle; inferiorly, after it splits into two layers, the deep temporal fat pad lies between the deep temporal fascia and the temporalis muscle fibers. The clinical significance of the deep temporal fat pad is that trauma to it can result in the appearance of temporal wasting.

The fascial layers have some variability in size and location at different levels from anterior to posterior in the coronal plane. One thing that remains constant is that the TPF, which contains the frontal branch of the facial nerve, remains superficial throughout this region and does not directly contact the bony zygomatic arch at any point. The size of the superficial fat pad between the TPF and the superficial layer of the deep temporal fascia can vary. The size of the intermediate fat pad between the superficial and deep players of the deep temporal fascia also varies; it decreases in size from anterior to posterior. Correspondingly, the location where the two layers coalesce into the single deep temporal fascia aka temporalis fascia lies more superior anteriorly and more inferior posteriorly [11].

Sensory and Motor Nerves

The sensory nerves of the forehead and scalp are the supraorbital and supratrochlear nerves and vessels exit the supraorbital notch in the forehead [7]. They can be seen endoscopically in the subperiosteal dissection of the forehead.

The frontal or temporal branch of the facial nerve is the main motor nerve that can be encountered in the dissection field in the transtemporal midface lift. Pitanguy originally described the course of the frontal branch. Pitanguy's line can be drawn as follows: First a line joining the lateral canthus to the superior portion of the tragus is identified and measured. The midpoint of this line is connected with the inferior aspect of the ear lobe, and this line bisecting the first line extending through the temple marks Pitanguy's line [9, 12] (Fig. 30.2). The frontal branch of the facial nerve crosses in the middle third of zygomatic arch and continues its course superomedially [9, 13]. This location approximately corresponds to halfway between the lateral canthus and the root of the helix [7]. The frontal branch is at greatest risk for injury as it courses over the zygomatic arch because there it has the least soft tissue thickness to protect the nerve from injury during dissection. Frequently, the frontal branch of the facial nerve exists not just as one branch but splits off into at least two smaller (sometimes up to four branches) in the temporal region as found in several cadaver studies [11–13]. In an anatomic study with fresh cadavers, Gosain et al. demonstrated that multiple rami of the frontal branch of the facial nerve cross the zygomatic arch [13]. They noted that the area of this crossing occupies less than half the length of the arch and the inferior aspect of the arch, greater than half the length of the arch on the superior aspect. These branches are centered around the midportion of the zygomatic arch [8, 13]. In the deep fascial layers between the TPF and deep temporal fascia, several veins can be seen crossing between the layers during surgical dissection. Sabini et al. performed a cadaver study that identified a series of bridging vessels crossing from the deep temporal fascia to the superficial temporal fascia [12]. The most robust among these veins, the sentinel vein, crosses between the deep temporal fascia and the TPF within 2 mm of temporal branch of the facial nerve [12].

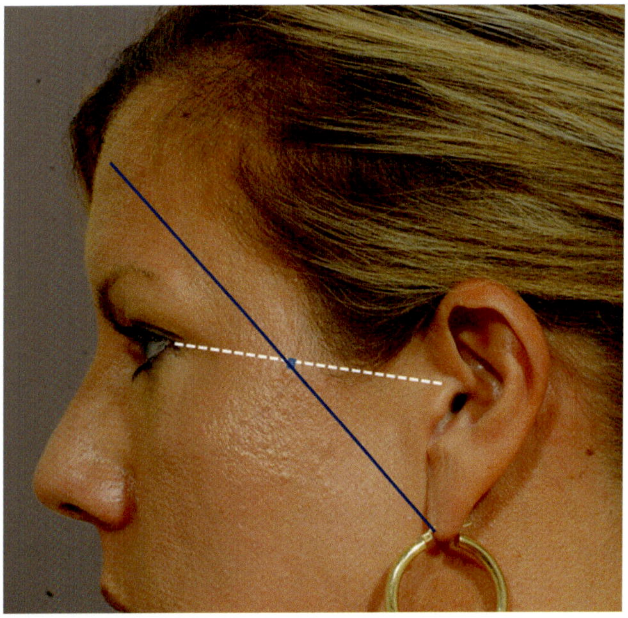

Fig. 30.2 Preoperative marking. Pitanguy's line is drawn as demonstrated. Dotted white line connects lateral canthus and root of helix. The midpoint of this line is connected with the inferior aspect of the ear lobe; extending this line creates Pitanguy's line approximating the path of the frontal branch of the facial nerve

Midface

The midface has been described as the area between the level of the mid-horizontal orbit and the mandibular margin [8]. In this region reside the lower eyelid, the bony orbital rim, the maxilla, and the malar and suborbicularis oculi fat (SOOF) pads and muscles of facial expression including the orbicularis oculi superiorly, the levator labii superioris, the zygomaticus major and minor, and the masseter deep. The lower eyelid-cheek junction can be seen as a curved line that runs slightly inferior and parallel to the infraorbital rim. The medial portion of the lower eyelid-cheek junction is sometimes referred to as the tear trough [9]. The lower eyelid-cheek junction marks the transition between the palpebral and orbital aspects of the orbicularis oculi muscle [9].

There are differences in the skin and subcutaneous tissues on either side of the lower eyelid-cheek junction. In the lower eyelid superiorly, the skin is extremely thin and lies directly over the orbicularis oculi. In contrast inferior to this junction, the skin is thicker and is separated from the orbicularis muscle by the malar fat pad [9]. Along this line in the medial portion, the orbicularis attaches firmly to the bone. Laterally, starting between the medial limbus and midpupillary line in the area of the SOOF, the orbicularis muscle attaches to the orbicularis retaining ligament, which then attaches to the bony orbital rim [9]. The SOOF contains two compartments: the medial compartment extends from the medial limbus to the lateral canthus and the lateral compartment extends from the lateral canthus to the temporal fat pad [9]. The malar fat pad comprises a triangular thickening of the subcutaneous fat in the cheek overlying the maxilla. It sits superficial to the SMAS and makes up most of the volume of the midface [9]. The zygomaticus major and minor, covered by the SMAS, lie deep to the SOOF and malar fat pads. The zygomatic branch of the facial nerve innervates the midfacial muscles of facial expression, which travel along the deep surface of these muscles. Thus, the dissection in the midface lift when carried out in a subperiosteal layer avoids these nerve branches entirely [9].

Midfacial Aging

The youthful midface contour is comprised of one continuous single smooth convexity. A number of changes can be observed during aging in the midface. The lower eyelids may develop palpebral bags. These palpebral bags can appear at an early age and are the result of pseudoherniation of orbital fat against a weak or lax orbital septum [14]. In addition, the orbicularis oculi muscle and its attachments can become lax and allow further deepening of this pseudoherniation. As aging progresses, the orbital septum weakens allowing protrusion of orbital fat and the midface descends [15].

Inferior to the orbital rim, malar mounds can develop and descend accentuating the nasolabial folds. The malar mounds are comprised of soft tissue that bulges directly from the malar prominence [14]. The appearance of these can worsen with smiling [14]. While the orbital septum protrudes, and the malar mounds descend, the arcus marginalis (which is the attachment of the orbital septum to the bony orbital rim) remains tightly adherent [15]. When the midface structures descend, the orbital rim is exposed, and the prolapsed orbital fat in the lower eyelid complex and ptotic SOOF create a double contour [7] like a beer belly over a tight belt [6, 8].

Hamra proposed that this attachment is a large contributor to the aged appearance of the lower eyelid and midface [15]. Hamra demonstrated that this convexity can be restored by release of the arcus marginalis [15]. This explains why fat removal or malar augmentation may be unsuccessful in restoring a youthful appearance. In fact, resection of the prolapsed fat without lifting the midface can even create an undesirable hollowed look [7].

There are several anatomic structures that contribute to midfacial aging. Proper release and elevation of these structures significantly contribute to midface rejuvenation. Gamboa et al. identified several of these in a cadaver study [16]. The orbicularis retaining ligament attaches to the orbicularis muscle medially near the lacrimal crest and laterally attaches to the lateral orbital thickening. The lateral orbital thickening is in continuity with the SMAS and the TPF. The prezygotic space overlies the zygoma, and dissection of this is required for proper repositioning of the midface. The zygomatic ligaments attach malar eminence soft tissues to the zygomatic periosteum [16].

Preoperative Assessment

As mentioned earlier, the ideal midfacial contour is that of a single uninterrupted convexity. In this situation, the inferior and lateral orbital rim should be padded with malar fat and SOOF [7]. The goal of the midface lift is to redrape the descended malar and SOOF fat pads over the orbital rim to eliminate the double convexity contour that emerges with the aging process. The postoperative appearance after the transtemporal midface lift can be simulated with finger elevation of the malar fat complex when describing and demonstrating the procedure to potential patients [9].

It is critical to document any preexisting anatomic conditions with photo documentation and discuss them thoroughly with the patient. Some important characteristics to take note preoperatively include the lower eyelid position, whether and to what degree is the inferior orbital rim exposed, the eyelid-cheek junction length, the presence of lower eyelid fat pseudoherniation, the estimated volume and size of the SOOF and malar fat pads, and the depth of the nasolabial fold [9]. Preexisting asymmetries such as brow asymmetries and eyelid ptosis should be carefully observed, noted, and pointed out to the patient preoperatively.

Patient education particularly appropriate postoperative expectations should be emphasized. Patients may experience initial tightness can have significant headache nausea in the immediate postoperative period [9]. The patient should be counseled and warned of this ahead of time. Particularly in the case of the transtemporal endoscopic midface lift, patients can expect prolonged postoperative edema 4–6 weeks as a result of the subperiosteal dissection [7]. Another important aspect of patient education prior to midface lifting is that often, midfacial descent is accompanied by volume loss. Therefore, midface lifting candidates may also benefit from midfacial volume augmentation. Patients should be made aware that in some cases lifting alone cannot comprehensively treat midfacial aging and they may need volume augmentation as well. This can be accomplished by fat grafting or filler injection [9].

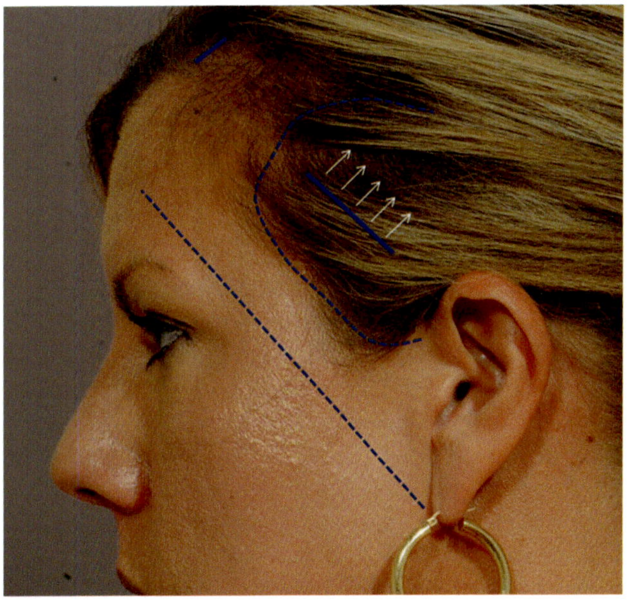

Fig. 30.3 Pitanguy's line is drawn as dotted blue line. The edge of the temporalis is mapped out as dotted blue line. The temporal incision is placed perpendicular to the direction of lifting setback from the hairline and at least 1.5 cm below the superior insertion of the temporalis. The frontal scalp incision (solid blue) is marked behind the hairline aligned with the lateral canthus

Surgical Technique

In order to optimize preoperative conditions, it is helpful to treat the glabella with botulinum toxin preoperatively. This allows easier reattachment of periosteum by obviating the downward pull of the depressor muscles on the brow during the initial postoperative healing process [7].

Preoperative Marking

Preoperatively, the patient should be marked while in upright position [9] (Fig. 30.3). Important anatomic markers are drawn out including the temporalis muscle boundaries and Pitanguy's line. The patient is instructed to clench her/his jaw, and the anterior and superior border of the temporalis muscle is marked with a marking pen. Pitanguy's line, which approximates the path of the frontal branch of the facial nerve, is drawn as described above. The bilateral supraorbital notches and glabellar frown lines should be marked [9].

The planned temporal and medial scalp incisions are marked out bilaterally. The temporal incision should begin 1 cm posterolateral to the temporal hairline at a level 1.5 cm inferior to the superior edge of the temporalis. This incision continues for 3 cm posteroinferiorly remaining at least 1 cm behind the hairline. This incision should be oriented with the direction of desired pull for lateral brow [7]. The medial scalp incisions are marked 1 cm behind the frontal hairline in line with the lateral canthus. These incisions are drawn 1–2 cm back from their anterior limit.

Assessment of the eyebrow position and the plan for any changes to it should be made preoperatively in the upright position [9]. In most patients 2–4 mm of brow elevation is all that is needed to bring the lateral brow to the ideal position (for women just above the orbital rim, for men at the orbital rim). The medial brow position is maintained as elevation can result in a surprised look. The preoperative medial brow position should be noted, and patients should be counseled that dissection of the corrugators can result in widening of the medial brow [9].

With elevation of the midfacial soft tissues, this often produces bunching of excess skin at the lower eyelid. In most cases this will require a skin pinch excision of the lower eyelid. This makes for an ideal opportunity to perform lower eyelid blepharoplasty in conjunction with transtemporal midface lift. If it is determined, transconjunctival fat removal will be necessary; the fat from the medial, middle, and lateral fat compartments should be assessed preoperatively in the upright position to identify the regions with excess orbital fat.

Incisions

A mixture of lidocaine and bupivacaine with epinephrine is injected at the marked incision sites and areas of dissection. The temporal incision is taken through the skin and TPF fascia down to but preserving the deep temporalis fascia. It is important to angle the bevel of the scalpel parallel to the hair follicles to preserve hair at the incision site [7, 9]. Up to about 5% of patients can experience telogen effluvium characterized by an area of alopecia 1 cm around the incision sites [9]. It is also important to keep the entire incision at least 1.5 cm below the superior extent of the temporalis muscle insertion so that the temporal soft tissue can be secured superiorly to the temporalis fascia in this location. The medial incisions are aligned with the lateral canthus and are used for endoscope entry sites and for forehead periosteal fixation [9].

After the temporal incision is taken through skin subcutaneous fat and the TPF, blunt dissection proceeds along the deep temporal fascia. Blunt dissection proceeds with a blunt endoscopic dissector: Ramirez EndoForhead "T" Dissector #4, (Black and Black Surgical, Tucker, Ga) [9] with gentle but firm pushing motion at a 30–40° angle to the surface of the deep temporal fascia [9]. Once the dissection plane is established and confirmed at the temporalis muscle fascia, a lighted Aufricht retractor is used for better visualization. Superomedially, blunt dissection transitions to the subperiosteal plane after passing the tenacious temporal line. The dissection continues to the level of the occiput posteriorly and connects across the midline to the contralateral subperiosteal dissection in the forehead. By extending the subperiosteal dissection posteriorly to the occiput, we are able to ensure the temporal tissues will redrape properly and avoid bunching near the temples once the temporal suspension is completed [9].

The dissection is carried inferiorly directly on the frontal bone in a subperiosteal plane. After releasing the periosteum from the frontal bar, a curved Ramirez Endoforehead Arcus Marginalis Dissector #6, (Black and Black Surgical, Tucker, GA) is used to release the arcus marginalis from its lateral end to within 1 cm from the marked supraorbital neurovascular bundle [9]. We use a bimanual technique in releasing the arcus marginalis with one hand placed on the skin at the orbital rim to prevent injury to the orbit with inferior dissection [9].

Endoscopic Forehead

The two medial incisions made behind the hairline at the level of the lateral canthus are taken down to the bone. A blunt dissector can be used to complete elevation of the periosteum circumferentially around these incisions. A bunt dissector is used to extend the subperiosteal forehead pocket to within 1 cm from the supraorbital notch. A downbiting subperiosteal elevator is used to elevate the medial attachments over the glabella and radix [8]. As mentioned earlier the arcus marginalis is released from the orbital rim with bimanual technique. In order to adequately elevate and resuspend the brows, it is critical to achieve full periosteal separation from the orbital rim at the arcus marginalis [7]. At the lateral canthus 1 cm region of periosteal attachment is maintained and not elevated. This helps to ensure the eye position and shape will not change in the long term after acute postoperative edema resolves.

A 30° endoscope with a protective cover is inserted through the medial incision to directly visualize the supraorbital neurovascular bundle [9]. Using a curved protected endoscopic grasper directed under endoscopic guidance, the corrugator supercilii muscles are cauterized and resected bilaterally. This step eliminates the vertical glabellar lines [9]. Resection and cauterization of the corrugators muscles can result in slight widening of the medial brows, which is desirable in some cases.

Midface

For the midface, our technique employs a subperiosteal release of the midface from the infraorbital rim to the inferior aspect of the maxilla and laterally over the entire zygomatic arch to the angle beneath the masseter aponeurosis [8]. There are several benefits to dissection of the midface in the subperiosteal plane: it can be elevated quickly and efficiently with minimal bleeding, and it is a safe plane for dissection with respect to the facial nerve [6].

Following complete elevation of the forehead and superior orbital rim, the dissection proceeds inferiorly with the lighted Aufricht retractor to optimize visualization and provide tension in the fascial planes [9]. We continue dissection inferiorly to the superior aspect of the zygomatic arch over deep layer of temporalis fascia deep to intermediate fat pad. This depth of dissection is carried anteriorly where the frontal branch of the facial nerve is protected by a layer of fascia and the intermediate fat pad [7]. As the plane of dissection from the superior and inferior pockets are connected on top of the deep temporalis fascia, several bridging veins are encountered which can be carefully cauterized with bipolar cautery close to the deep temporal fascia. The sentinel vein is encountered where Pitanguy's line crosses over the lateral orbital rim. This vein should be carefully preserved to protect the frontal branch and serve as a landmark for its. Sabini et al. performed a cadaver study that identified a series of bridging vessels crossing from the deep temporal fascia to the superficial temporal fascia. Among these is the sentinel vein, which enters the superficial temporal fascia within 2 mm of the frontal branch of the facial nerve [12] (Fig. 30.4).

While some surgeons prefer to dissect in the intermediate fat pad, we prefer to be deep to it on top of deep layer of deep temporal fascia as it provides the frontal branch of the facial nerve an extra layer of protection from traction and thermal injury during dissection [7, 8]. In this region care must also be taken to stay on top of the deep temporalis fascia. Penetration through the deep temporal fascia can lead to exposure the infratemporal fat pad. Even minimal trauma in this region can result in temporal wasting postoperatively [9].

Once the superior edge of zygomatic arch is reached, the periosteum of the zygomatic arch is entered anteriorly to ensure safety of frontal nerve [8]. A downcurved dissector is used to incise the periosteum over the arch exposing the periosteum over the entire superior aspect of the zygomatic arch [7, 9]. Posteriorly, the subperiosteal dissection is carried to within 1 cm anterior to the external auditory canal [9]. The masseteric aponeurosis attachments to the inferior aspect of the zygomatic arch are released with blunt dissection [7]. The endoforehead Arcus Marginalis Dissector #6 is used to release the periosteum over the anterior face of the zygoma. The zygomaticofacial foramen may be encountered, and the neurovascular structures should be kept intact if possible. This is an important landmark for suspension of the midface [9]. However, there is generally little consequence to this as bleeding is minimal and stops with packing pressure, and temporary postoperative numbness in the area usually resolves (Fig. 30.5).

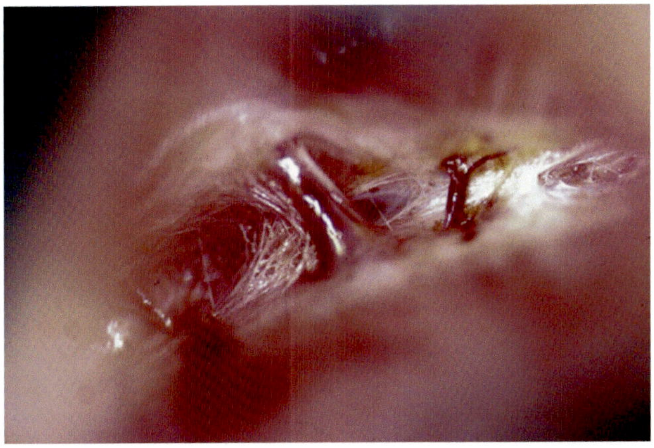

Fig. 30.4 The endoscopic surgical view of the sentinel vein

Subperiosteal dissection continues anteriorly and inferiorly along temporal line to orbital rim maintaining a 1 cm cuff of attached periosteum around the lateral cantus to avoid postoperative distortion of the eye [7–9]. "Dissection continues anteromedially over the anterior wall of the maxilla with a superior sweeping motion of the finger" [9].

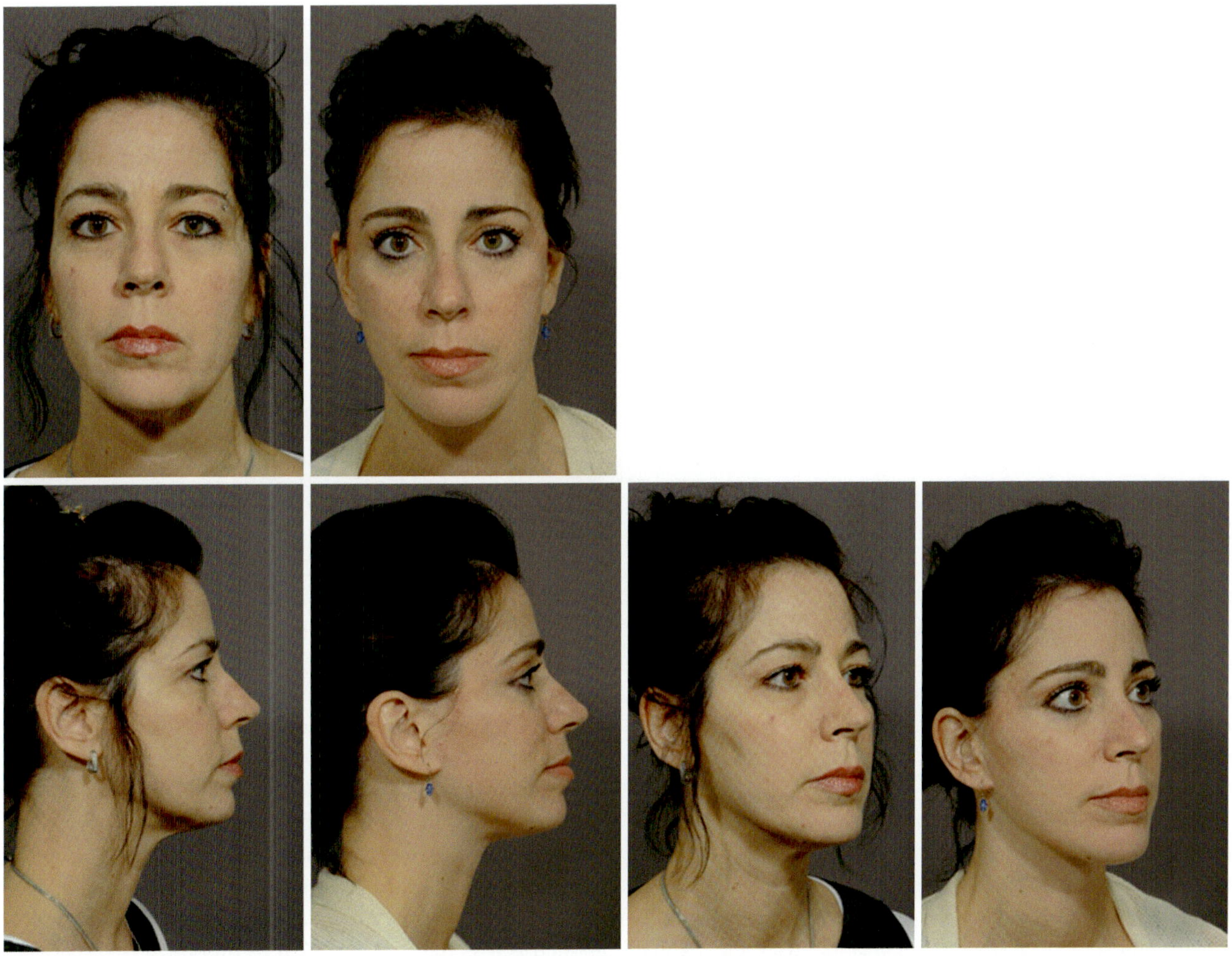

Fig. 30.5 A 45-year-old woman who underwent endoscopic forehead lift, transtemporal midface lift, upper and lower blepharoplasty, and facelift. Note significant improvement in midface volume and suspension

A finger is kept on the orbital rim as subperiosteal elevation is performed to protect the globe [7]. A thumb positioned over the infraorbital notch protects the neurovascular bundle. This continues toward the nose and ends at the pyriform aperture releasing all the tissue inferior to the infraorbital nerve taking care to avoid entering the oral mucosa [9].

A lateral pocket is made as the dissection proceeds inferiorly. Using the lighted Aufricht retractor, the tendinous attachments at the lateral aspect of the maxilla are lysed with the endoforehead Arcus Marginalis Dissector [8, 9]. The masseteric tendon is cut with a downward motion inferior to the inferior aspect of the zygomatic arch [8, 9]. The dissection continues inferiorly below the masseteric aponeurosis on top of the belly of the masseter muscle until reaching a position 1 cm superior to the gonial angle [8, 9]. The medial subperiosteal midface dissection pocket is connected to the lateral masseteric aponeurosis pocket with a sweeping finger dissection which is also used to confirm adequate release of midfacial tissues [9]. At this point a complete midface release is achieved. Once this point is reached, a complete release of the midfacial tissues is accomplished ensuring free mobility of the midface, malar fat pad, and SOOF [8, 9].

Lower Blepharoplasty

If fat excision is necessary to create an aesthetic lower eyelid contour, this should be performed transconjunctivally prior to suspension of the midface as the tension created from the suspension sutures will hinder access to the conjunctiva. If necessary, transconjunctival lower eyelid blepharoplasty should be performed at this point prior to suture fixation of the midface periosteum [7]. Fat removal or cauterization should be conservative [9]. Lower eyelid excess skin is addressed after midface suspension with a skin pinch excision [7].

Suture Fixation Midface and Temple

After complete subperiosteal elevation of the forehead and midface, a 10 French Jackson Pratt drain is placed through the hair bearing skin above the ear and tunneled subperiosteally across the supraorbital region with the tip of the drain beneath the contralateral brow. Care should be taken to avoid passing the trocar through the superficial temporal vessels during placement [7, 9].

A total of five sutures are used to suspend the midface and temple. We prefer using 0-Vicryl on UR6 needle (Ethicon, Sommerville, NJ) for these sutures as the curvature of the UR6 needle is particularly suitable for placement of the deeper midfacial sutures. Under direct visualization with the lighted Aufricht retractor, a 0-Vicryl is passed through periosteum just lateral to zygomaticofacial foramen back to temporalis fascia [7]. This stitch should exert a superior and slightly lateral vector of pull on the midfacial tissues attached to the periosteum including the malar fat pad and the SOOF [6, 9]. A second suture is placed proximal/superior to the frontal branch of the facial nerve just posterior to Pitanguy's line and is secured to the temporalis fascia superolaterally [6, 9]. Three additional sutures are placed in the superficial temporal fascia or galea layer of anterior skin edge and secured to the deep temporalis fascia [9]. These three sutures should suspend the skin posterior superiorly in the region of the temporal line [9]. By suspending the soft tissues around the temples, this prevents an unnatural appearing bunching of tissue in the temporal area.

Forehead Fixation

Many have proposed various approaches to fixation of the forehead including permanent micro screws left under the scalp, cortical tunnels to fix galea and pericranium, and temporary fixation screws [7]. We prefer temporary fixation as studies have shown that periosteal reattachment occurs rapidly and permanent fixation is unnecessary. With a preset hand drill guide holes are made toward the superior aspect of the medial incisions and a 14 mm removable screw is secured in place at each drill site. The scalp is retracted superiorly so that the leading edge of the incision rests against the screw and a staple is placed just behind the screw to maintain the forehead scalp in the lifted position hooked behind the screw. This fixation method prevents the forehead flap from gravitating inferiorly [9]. We have found that elevation of the medial endoscopic incision 8 mm from its starting point results in maintenance of preoperative brow height, while elevation of 10–12 mm will result in a 2–4 mm elevation of the brow [8]. In most cases 2–4 mm of elevation is all that is needed to bring the brow back into its ideal position.

Lower Eyelid Skin Pinch Blepharoplasty and Closure

After the midfacial soft tissue is suspended into its new position, there may be noticeable bunching of excess lower eyelid skin that requires a lower eyelid skin pinch to allow better redraping of the lower eyelid skin [9]. The lateral temporal incisions are closed with 5–0 nylon sutures in an interrupted vertical mattress fashion. Additionally if there are any gaps in the medial scalp incisions between the staples and the fixation screws, they are reinforced with 5–0 nylon vertical mattress sutures. The skin pinch incision is closed with 6–0 nylon interrupted sutures laterally and 7–0 silk running locking sutures below the lash margin. Half-inch paper tape is applied across the forehead skin to minimize postoperative edema. Then a light pressure dressing with cotton padding and Kerlix gauze is applied for gentle compression for the first postoperative night [7].

Postoperative Care

The postoperative care routine includes several office visits within the first 1–2 weeks after surgery. On postoperative day 1, the pressure dressing and drain are removed. The patient may experience significant nausea and tightness/headache in the immediate postoperative period. Often this discomfort is significantly relieved once the drain across the forehead is removed and typically resolves by 48 hours [9]. The paper tapes on the forehead are left in place for 1 week. On postoperative day 7, the tape, forehead screws and staples, as well as the temporal sutures are removed. While some authors prefer permanent fixation, we find that it is not necessary. By 1 week the periosteum of the forehead tissues has adhered sufficiently to obviate the need for long-term suspension with screws or other foreign materials. Kim et al. demonstrated in animal studies that by postoperative days 8–12, the shear stiffness and strength approach the preoperative stiffness and strength at the bone periosteum interface [17]. Functionally, stable fixation can be established in even less time. For these reasons, we prefer temporary fixation screws.

Periorbital bruising and edema are expected. Patients are allowed to cover any persistent edema with makeup at 1–2 weeks after surgery.

Patients can also expect mild temporary distortion of the lateral canthus and puckering of the skin above incision [7]. The superior lateral pull of the midface lift creates an unavoidable temporary pulling at the pericanthal skin in the same direction resulting in an elevated appearance of the lateral canthus [9]. Patients often need to be reassured in the postoperative period that this distortion is in fact temporary. By maintaining a 1 cm cuff of periosteal attachment around the lateral canthus attached in the surgical dissection, we ensure return of the lateral canthus position with time [9]. Lateral canthal massage can be performed to relax the pull on the pericanthal skin to help the patient regain their preoperative appearance [9].

Numbness of the forehead is expected as a result of the subperiosteal dissection which may last up to 6–12 months. Reinnervation begins proximally near the supraorbital nerve starting around 4 weeks and continues for up to a year at the occiput [9].

Lessons Learned

Additional Benefits

A number of lessons have been learned in the course of 1200 cases in the experience of the senior author. We have seen several additional benefits with our technique of transtemporal midface lift. One example is the shortened lower eyelid [18] (Fig. 30.6). The lower eyelid aesthetic was better with the combination of transtemporal endoscopic midface with lower blepharoplasty lift than after lower blepharoplasty alone [19]. This was shown by Marotta et al. when they compared two groups, and the lower eyelid height was similar in both groups preoperatively, but postoperatively there was an

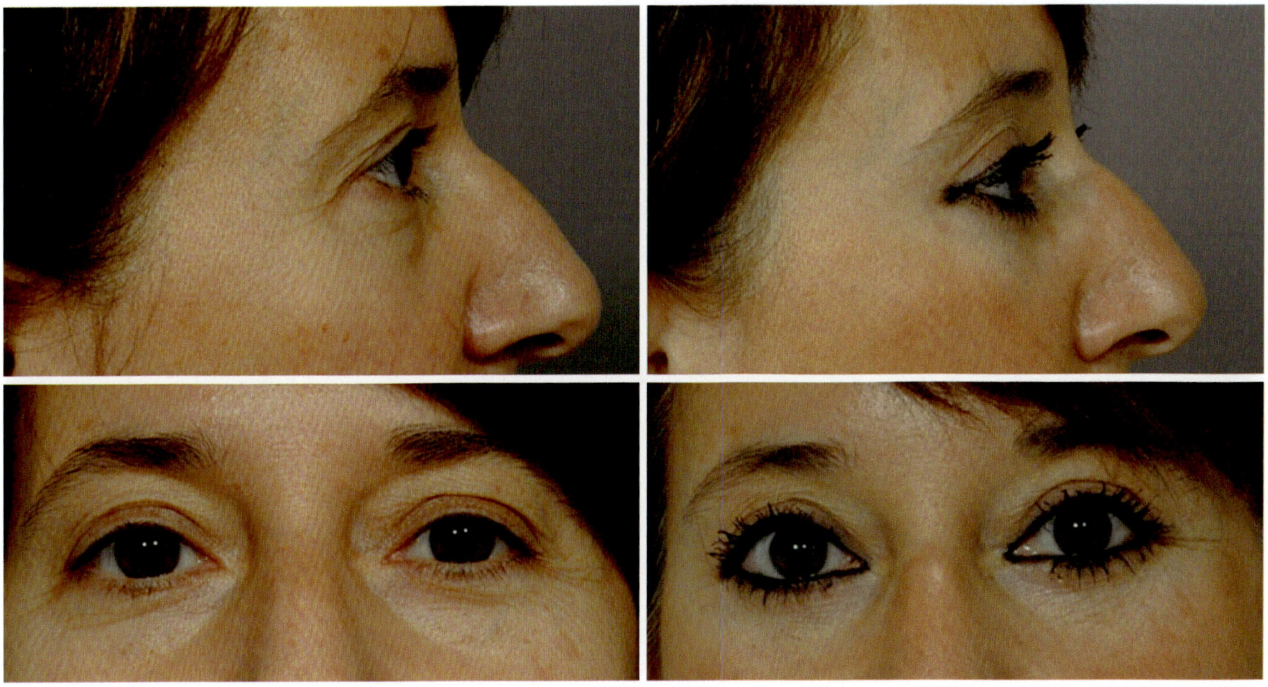

Fig. 30.6 A 48-year-old woman who underwent endoscopic forehead lift, transtemporal midface lift, and lower blepharoplasty. Note the periocular improvement and the appearance of shortened vertical height of the lower eyelids

average of 5.1 mm reduction in lower eyelid height with midface compared to 0 mm reduction with lower blepharoplasty alone including patients who underwent transconjunctival and skin pinch as well as those who underwent skin muscle flap methods [19]. In addition to reducing the vertical height of the lower eyelid, this technique also resulted in reduction of infraorbital hollowing and improved the double contour deformity more effectively than by lower eyelid blepharoplasty alone. This improvement was achieved by padding the infraorbital rim and excising pseudoherniated orbital fat transconjunctivally [19]. Also because of the vertical vector of lift, the ptotic midfacial soft tissues exert less downward stretch on the lower eyelid skin allowing for more aggressive skin resection with the lower blepharoplasty (up to 7 mm) [19].

Another benefit of transtemporal midface lifting is the increased tension of the lower eyelid [20]. This increased tension is long lasting – at least 12 months – and can help to combat lower eyelid laxity and avoid ectropion [20]. Scleral show can result from excessive excision from lower eyelid blepharoplasty. Midface suspension can raise the lower eyelid position and reduce sclera show from previous blepharoplasty and prevent scleral show when combined with lower blepharoplasty [7]. However, this increased lower eyelid tightness can also cause patients to experience postoperative dry eye. This may occur as a result of tension across the lower eyelid resulting in inadequate circulation of tear film [9].

By combining the midface lift with a temporal lift, we are able to avoid bunching of the temporal skin after lifting the midface [6] as can sometimes be seen with elevation of the midfacial soft tissues through other approaches (Fig. 30.7).

The vertical vector of pull on the midfacial tissues has several specific and unique benefits. It has a favorable effect on nasolabial fold. In a comparison with deep plane facelift, the transtemporal zygomaticofacial sutures result in more improvement than deep plane face lift on the nasolabial fold [18]. This is presumably because of the vertical rather than lateral vector of tension of the midfacial suspension sutures. Festoons and malar mounds are improved by vertical subperiosteal midface lift [14].

Although it was initially not expected when this technique first came into use, there is improvement in the appearance of the lower third of the face after transtemporal midface

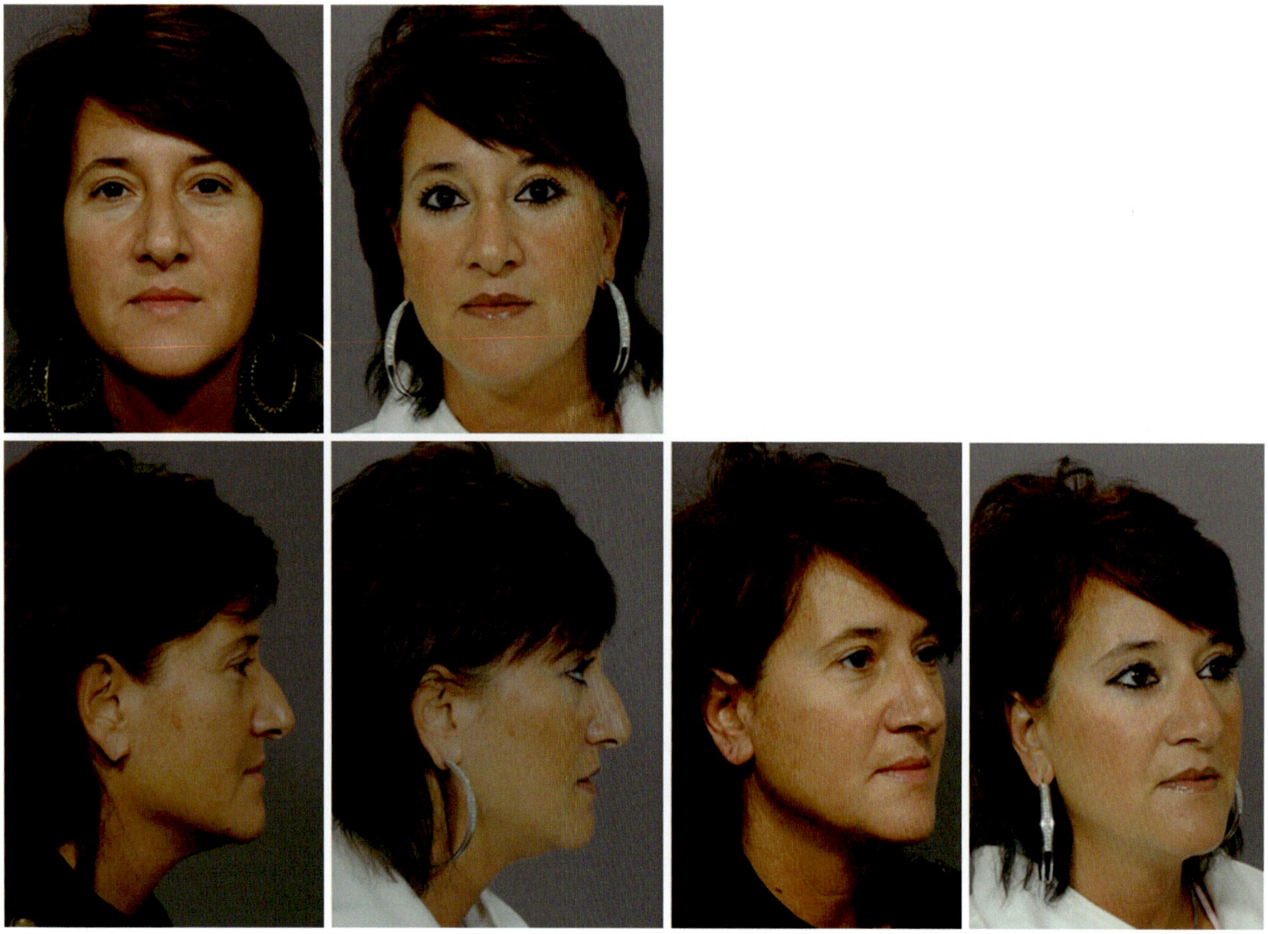

Fig. 30.7 A 48-year-old woman who underwent endoscopic forehead lift, transtemporal midface lift, and upper and lower blepharoplasty

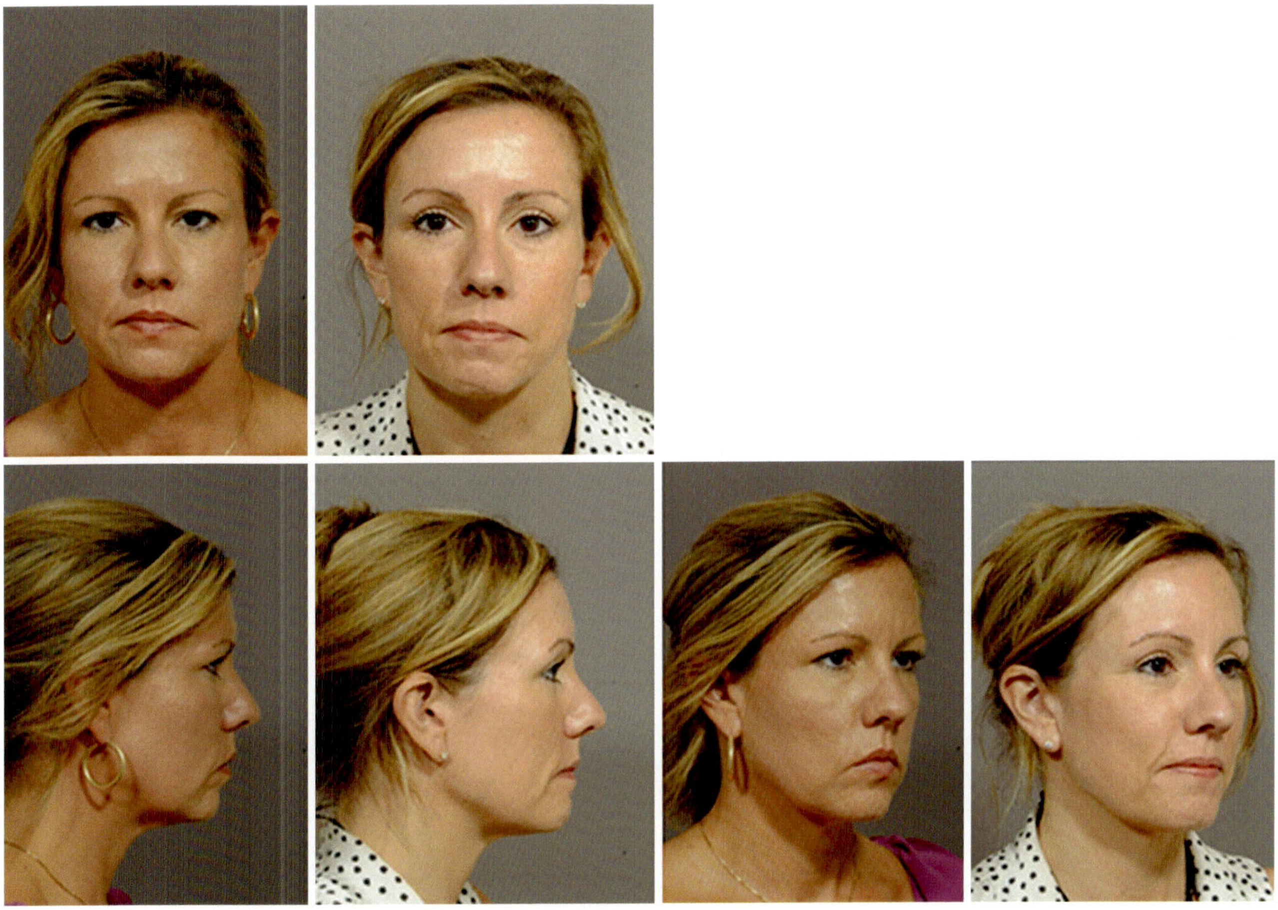

Fig. 30.8 A 42-year-old woman who underwent endoscopic forehead lift, midface lift, and upper and lower blepharoplasty. This patient did not have a lower facelift. Note pre- and postoperative photos demonstrate improvement in lower face jawline and jowling as a result of midface lift

lifting even with any direct surgical intervention on the lower face. The zygomatic periosteal suture typically imparts a 1–1.5 cm elevation of the skin overlying the angle of the mandible resulting in a significant improvement in jowling and rejuvenation for the lower face [21] (Fig. 30.8).

Another important lesson in midfacial rejuvenation is identifying preoperative overall volume deficit. While lifting the midfacial soft tissues can restore some of the volume loss due to midfacial descent, it may not be sufficient to restore a youthful appearance. It is said that the maxilla recedes 1.5 cm as we age. Midfacial resuspension may not be sufficient to compensate for this process, and additional valorization may be necessary such as fat injection or facial fillers.

Pitfalls/Complications

A number of lessons regarding postoperative complications and inconvenient consequences have been learned as well. Patients may experience masticatory tenderness as a result of the suspension sutures in the deep temporalis fascia and dissection over the masticator aponeurosis. This can be treated with muscle relaxants in the first week and NSAIDS thereafter [9]. This is expected to resolve within 2–8 weeks [7].

Chemosis is also relatively common postoperatively occurring in about 30% of patients [9]. Blurry vision and a change in refraction may occur if chemosis is present and usually resolves in 3–6 weeks [9]. If chemosis occurs, a regimen of hypertonic saline and prednisolone eye drops is initiated. Some patients may also experience photosensitivity and dry eye; these symptoms usually resolve within 3–6 weeks as well.

Hematoma is a rare complication after the transtemporal midface lift occurring in 1% or fewer cases. The major reason for this is that the subperiosteal plane is relatively avascular [9]. Potential sources of bleeding include bridging vessels near frontal branch or sentinel vein or the superficial temporal vessels being punctured or traumatized during drain placement. If a hematoma occurs, it may be difficult to identify as a certain amount of swelling is expected and much of the dissection is in the subperiosteal plain, it would be difficult to palpate. A hematoma in the midface can easily be drained transorally through a small mucosal incision.

Postoperative infection is a rare complication after transtemporal midface lift. Serious wound infections leading to abscess formation are exceedingly rare, estimated to occur at a rate of 1/1000 [9]. Although we have not seen any in our experience of over 1200 cases, we have seen stitch abscesses. These can form around a deep buried suture that can be treated with simple incision and drainage and removal of the retained stitch [9, 21].

Facial nerve injury is perhaps the most feared complication of this surgery. However with a thorough understanding of the anatomy and proper technique as detailed above, it is unlikely to be encountered. Temporary neuropraxia in the frontal branch of the facial nerve can occur in around 1% of cases. This is often secondary to traction of nerve or thermal injury form cautery of bridging veins. The temporary asymmetry that results can easily be treated by injecting botulinum toxin in the contralateral (functioning) brow, and most patients recover by 6 months [9]. Permanent frontal nerve injury is much less common. The senior author has only had 1 permanent paresis in 1200 cases in a patient with scarring from previous surgeries in the temporal region [9].

Hair loss may occur near the incision sites despite the surgeon's best effort to preserve hair follicles in incision planning. An estimated 5% of patients experience telogen effluvium or shock loss resulting in a 1 cm region of alopecia around incision sites [9]. Hair growth in this region almost always returns in 3–9 months. Patients should be reassured that hair growth will return in this region.

Irregularity over glabellar area such as localized depressions can occur due to corrugator resection [21]. These irregularities are less likely to occur if the periosteum is fully elevated over the orbital rim from the nasion medially to the arcus marginalis laterally. Another method to minimize these irregularities is by completely resecting the corrugators rather than merely performing a myotomy.

Superior oblique palsy has been described but is also rare and can be avoided with careful dissection technique [21].

Forehead and scalp paresthesias are not a complication but part of the expected postoperative experience. The paresthesias can be particularly distressing to some patients with itching and discomfort that is difficult to relieve. This can be expected to last 2–6 months but in some cases may continue for up to a year. Reinnervation begins at the supraorbital notch and proceeds superiorly reaching the crown by 9–12 months. Patients often need frequent reassurance in this regard.

Finally brow asymmetries can occur that are not due to temporary frontal nerve palsy or irregularities in the subcutaneous soft tissues. In evaluating such asymmetries, one must first carefully and critically study the patient's preoperative photos. Occasionally, there are preexisting asymmetries that the patient did not pay attention to before surgery. For example, a patient may have stronger brow elevation on one side that is long standing. If this asymmetry is identified preoperatively, it can be treated intraoperatively by performing lateral orbicularis oculi myotomy on the more active side [9]. If there were no preexisting asymmetries, a postoperative brow asymmetry may be the result of asymmetric placement of the medial incisions or screw fixation [9].

Summary

Midfacial rejuvenation evolved as the facial plastic surgery community developed a sophisticated understanding of the effects of aging in a three-dimensional perspective of the midface. With the transtemporal midface lift, we are able to reliably provide a lasting resuspension of the brow and restoration of a youthful midfacial appearance by restoring volume of the soft tissues in their original suspended position. With this surgery, several key maneuvers must be accomplished to achieve forehead and midface rejuvenation: (1) a subperiosteal dissection of the scalp to the level of the orbital rims and zygomatic arch, (2) release of the orbital periosteum, (3) selective myectomies of the glabella muscles, (4) subperiosteal dissection of the midface, and (5) suspension and reposition of the malar fat pad, SOOF, and soft tissue overlying the angle of the mandible [8].

References

1. Ramirez OM, Pozner JN. Subperiosteal endoscopic techniques in secondary rhytidectomy. Aesthet Surg J. 1997;17(1):22–6.
2. Ramirez OM. The subperiosteal rhytidectomy: the third-generation face-lift. Ann Plast Surg. 1992;28(3):218–32; discussion 233–4.
3. Hinderer UT, Urriolagoitia F, Vildosola R. The blepharo-periorbitoplasty: anatomical basis. Ann Plast Surg. 1987;18(5):437–53.
4. Psillakis JM, Rumley TO, Camargos A. Subperiosteal approach as an improved concept for correction of the aging face. Plast Reconstr Surg. 1988;82(3):383–94.
5. Ramirez OM. Three-dimensional endoscopic midface enhancement: a personal quest for the ideal cheek rejuvenation. Plast Reconstr Surg. 2002;109(1):329–40; discussion 341–9.
6. Keller G, Quatela VC, Antunes MB, Sykes JM, Magill CK, Seth R. Midface lift: panel discussion. *Facial Plast Surg Clin North Am.* 2014;22(1):119–37.
7. Graham H, Quatela V, Sabini P. Chapter 20: Endoscopic Approach to the Brow and Midface. In: Papel I, editor. Facial Plastic and Reconstructive Surgery. 3rd ed; 2008. p. 227–42.
8. Quatela VC, Jacono AA. The extended centrolateral endoscopic midface lift. Facial Plast Surg. 2003;19(2):199–208.
9. Quatela VC, Antunes MB. Transtemporal midface lifting to blend the lower eyelid-cheek junction. Clin Plast Surg. 2015;42(1):103–14.
10. Gosain AK, Yousif NJ, Madiedo G, Larson DL, Matloub HS, Sanger JR. Surgical anatomy of the SMAS: a reinvestigation. Plast Reconstr Surg. 1993;92(7):1254–63; discussion 1264–5.
11. Babakurban ST, Cakmak O, Kendir S, Elhan A, Quatela VC. Temporal branch of the facial nerve and its relationship to fascial layers. Arch Facial Plast Surg. 2010;12(1):16–23.

12. Sabini P, Wayne I, Quatela VC. Anatomical guides to precisely localize the frontal branch of the facial nerve. Arch Facial Plast Surg. 2003;5(2):150–2.
13. Gosain AK, Sewall SR, Yousif NJ. The temporal branch of the facial nerve: how reliably can we predict its path? Plast Reconstr Surg. 1997;99(5):1224–33; discussion 1234–6.
14. Hoenig JF, Knutti D, de la Fuente A. Vertical subperiosteal midface-lift for treatment of malar festoons. Aesthet Plast Surg. 2011;35(4):522–9.
15. Hamra ST. Arcus marginalis release and orbital fat preservation in midface rejuvenation. Plast Reconstr Surg. 1995;96(2):354–62.
16. Gamboa GM, de La Torre JI, Vasconez LO. Surgical anatomy of the midface as applied to facial rejuvenation. Ann Plast Surg. 2004;52(3):240–5.
17. Kim JC, Crawford Downs J, Azuola ME, Devon Graham H 3rd. Time scale for periosteal readhesion after brow lift. Laryngoscope. 2004;114(1):50–5.
18. Jacono AA, Stong BC. Anatomic comparison of the deep-plane face-lift and the transtemporal midface-lift. Arch Facial Plast Surg. 2010;12(5):339–41.
19. Marotta JC, Quatela VC. Lower eyelid aesthetics after endoscopic forehead midface-lift. Arch Facial Plast Surg. 2008;10(4):267–72.
20. Villano ME, Leake DS, Jacono AD, Quatela VC. Effects of endoscopic forehead/midface-lift on lower eyelid tension. Arch Facial Plast Surg. 2005;7(4):227–30.
21. Quatela VC, Choe KS. Endobrow-midface lift. Facial Plast Surg. 2004;20(3):199–206.

Evaluation of the Facelift Patient

31

Katherine Rose and John Siebert

In the public's view, there is no procedure more synonymous with plastic surgery than the facelift. The ultimate goal of a facelift is to provide patients with a natural, unoperated appearance that results in a younger, refreshed version of himself or herself. While individuals vary in the onset and rate at which they age, there is a fundamental pattern and sequence to changes in facial appearance that occurs throughout the decades of life. The surgeon must appreciate the anatomic pathogenesis of facial aging in order to address the signs of aging in a natural way.

This chapter summarizes the senior author's personal approach to the analysis of the facelift patient. The components and approaches to the procedure will be discussed elsewhere. Overall, the one principle of overriding importance in facelift is to restore harmony among the areas of the face with smooth transitions from the brow to the periorbital region to the midface to the jaw and to the neck. In consultation, it is important in the assessment to identify what areas need to be addressed and to understand the underlying pathogenesis that occurs with aging in order to restore this harmony.

Pathogenesis of the Aging Face

Bone

The bony skeleton of the face acts as a scaffolding for the overlying soft tissue. Changes in the bony structure with age will alter the appearance of the face. It was initially believed that the facial skeleton continued to expand with age. However, it is now accepted that there are specific areas of facial skeletal absorption that attribute to the appearance of the aging face. Bony resorption tends to occur in the fifth to sixth decade of life and leads to a loss of structural support of the soft tissue causing much of the aging stigmata that are observed (Fig. 31.1). In the periorbital region, there is resorption of the inferolateral and superomedial orbital rims with the changes in the inferolateral rim occurring earlier

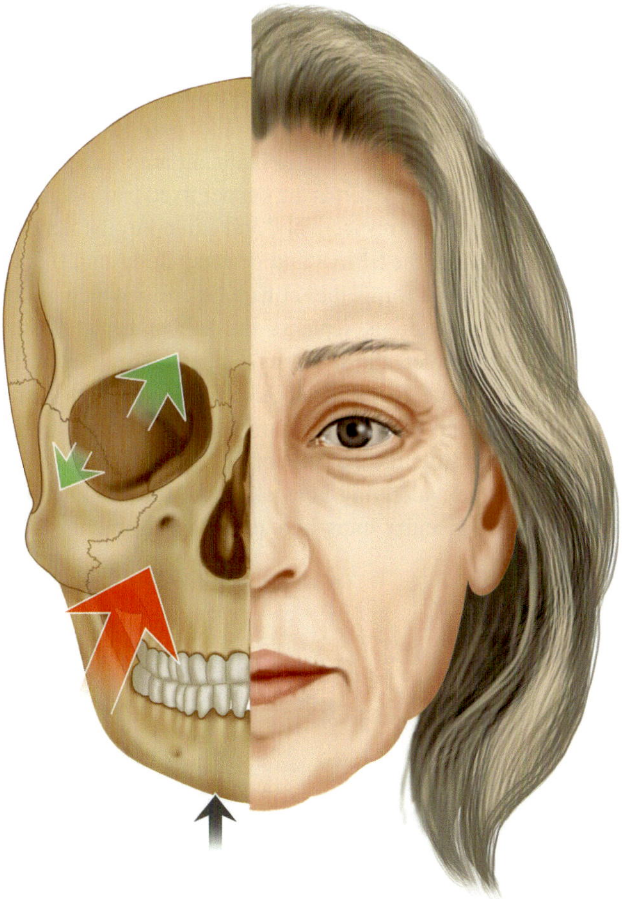

Fig. 31.1 Skeletal changes in the facial aging. The highlighted regions indicate areas of bone volume loss with age. The color corresponds with amount of bony resorption: the maxilla (red) has the greatest amount of bony resorption, followed by the orbit (green), and then the alveolus (black)

K. Rose · J. Siebert (✉)
Division of Plastic and Reconstructive Surgery, University of Wisconsin-Madison, Madison, WI, USA
e-mail: siebert@surg.wisc.edu

A. J. Cohen, C. N. Burkat (eds.), *Oculofacial, Orbital, and Lacrimal Surgery*, https://doi.org/10.1007/978-3-030-14092-2_31

than those in the superomedial rim. This bony resorption leads to lateralization of the orbit and an increased orbital area [1]. In the midface, there is predominantly resorption of the maxilla. Maxillary bone loss leads to midface retrusion, causing the tear trough deformity and a negative vector between the anterior globe and soft tissue cheek mass [2]. Resorption also occurs in the area of the pyriform aperture resulting in less support of the nasal base and an increased appearance of nasolabial folds [3]. In the lower face, there is a loss of alveolar bone resulting in decrease facial height [2].

Retaining Ligaments

The soft tissue of the face is supported over the bony structure with fibrous structures called retaining ligaments. The retaining ligaments extend perpendicularly either from the periosteum or deep fixed facial structures up to the dermis, penetrating through all the layers of the face. The orbitomalar (or orbital retaining ligament), zygomatic ligament, and mandibular ligaments are examples of osteocutaneous retaining ligaments that extend from the periosteum to the dermis. Of these ligaments, the zygomatic ligament is the most robust and stiff, followed by the orbital retaining ligament and the mandibular ligament [4]. The parotid ligament (Lore's fascia) and the masseteric ligament are examples of retaining ligaments that start at the deeper fixed parotid gland and masseter muscle, respectively, and extend to the dermis [5]. Once reaching the SMAS and dermis, the fascial thickening arborizes and forms the retinacular cutis, which leads to a complex of fibrous septa in the subcutaneous tissue (Fig. 31.2). Together, the retaining ligaments and the retinacular cutis create zones of adhesion in the face that form the superficial and deep fat compartments, providing the fat in the face with structure and support [6]. With aging and the alteration of the underlying bony skeleton, there is attenuation of the retinacular cutis and retaining ligaments. The ligaments bend along its course and form a hammock-shaped structure, decreasing the structural support of the respective fat compartment allowing the fat to descend, resulting in the sagging appearance associated with facial aging (Fig. 31.3) [4].

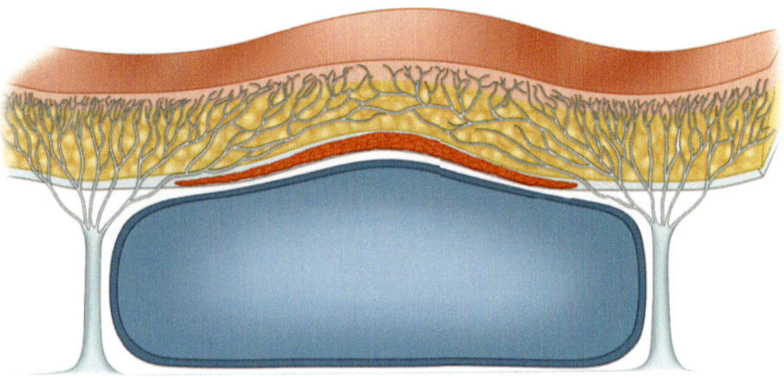

Fig. 31.2 Facial ligaments. The retaining ligaments of the face are dense fibrous adhesions between the periosteum or deeper fixed structures and the dermis. Once reaching the SMAS and dermal layer, the fascial structure divides and forms a complex network of fibrous septa in the subcutaneous tissue called the retinacular cutis. The combination of the retinacular cutis and retaining ligaments form the superficial and deep fat compartments of the face

Facial Muscles

The loss of mass and proper function of muscles with age is called sarcopenia. However, MRI studies have shown that the mimetic muscles are relatively resistant to atrophy, perhaps due to their constant use for facial expression [7]. As one ages, facial expression and mimetic motion diminish due to a change in muscle fiber orientation and resting tone. In youth, the facial muscles bow anteriorly due to the underlying fat pads. This convex shape results in more anteriorly projected facial expressions. Additionally, there is a greater amplitude in the muscle contractions, leading to more dynamic expressions [8]. In the older patient, the underlying fat has atrophied and been displaced, resulting in straighter and shorter muscle fibers, thus increasing the resting tone in the muscles. The relative hypertonicity of these muscles leads to shorter amplitudes with contraction and thus diminished facial expressions [3, 8].

Facial Fat

Facial fat is divided into superficial fat and deep fat, which are separated by the SMAS, with slightly more fat being in the superficial plane. Both the superficial fat and deep fat are divided into compartments by the retinacular cutis septa, retaining ligaments, and muscles of facial expression [2]. There are morphological differences in the fat between these two compartments with fat lobules in the superficial compartment being larger in size [3]. Recent anatomic studies have highlighted that there are approximately 22 superficial fat compartments in the face (Fig. 31.4a) [9].

In youth, there is a harmonious transition between each of the fat compartments leading to an overall smooth, rejuvenated appearance of the face. With aging, the superficial fat compartments atrophy at different stages and at different rates (Fig. 31.4b) [9]. This results in an abrupt contour change between the fat compartments, resulting in a less smooth transition across the face (Fig. 31.5). Volume loss in superficial fat compartments leads to temporal hollowing, ear lobe elongation, perioral thinning, and jowling. There are four deep fat compartments in the face: the medial and lateral sub-orbicularis oculi fat (SOOF), the deep medial cheek fat, and the buccal fat. These fat compartments are believed to allow for smooth muscle gliding during facial expression and mastication. (Fig. 31.6) [3]

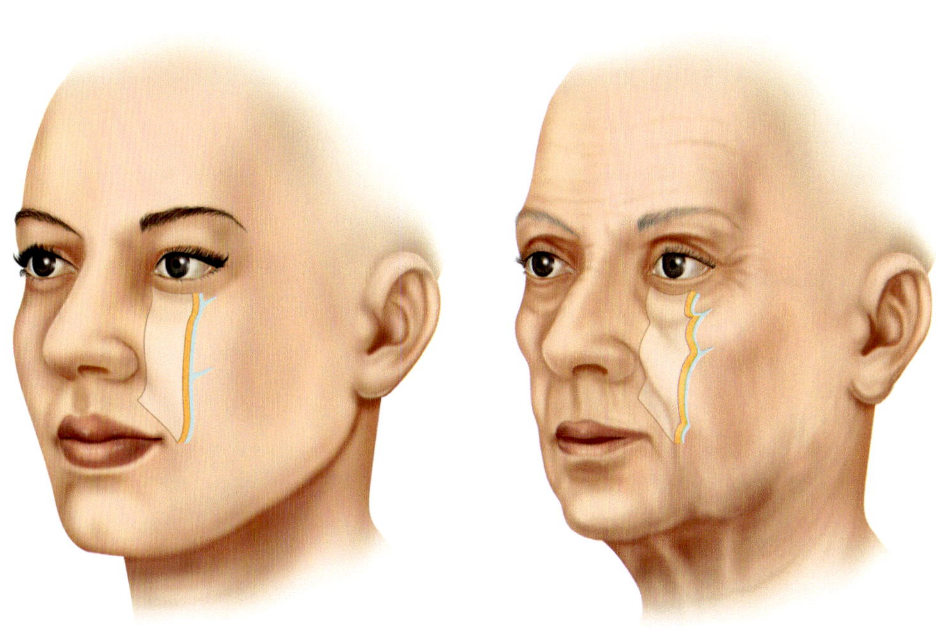

Fig. 31.3 Attenuation of facial retaining ligaments. With aging, the retaining ligaments begin to bow allowing bulging of the respective fat compartment. This contributes to the typical sagging appearance appreciated with facial aging

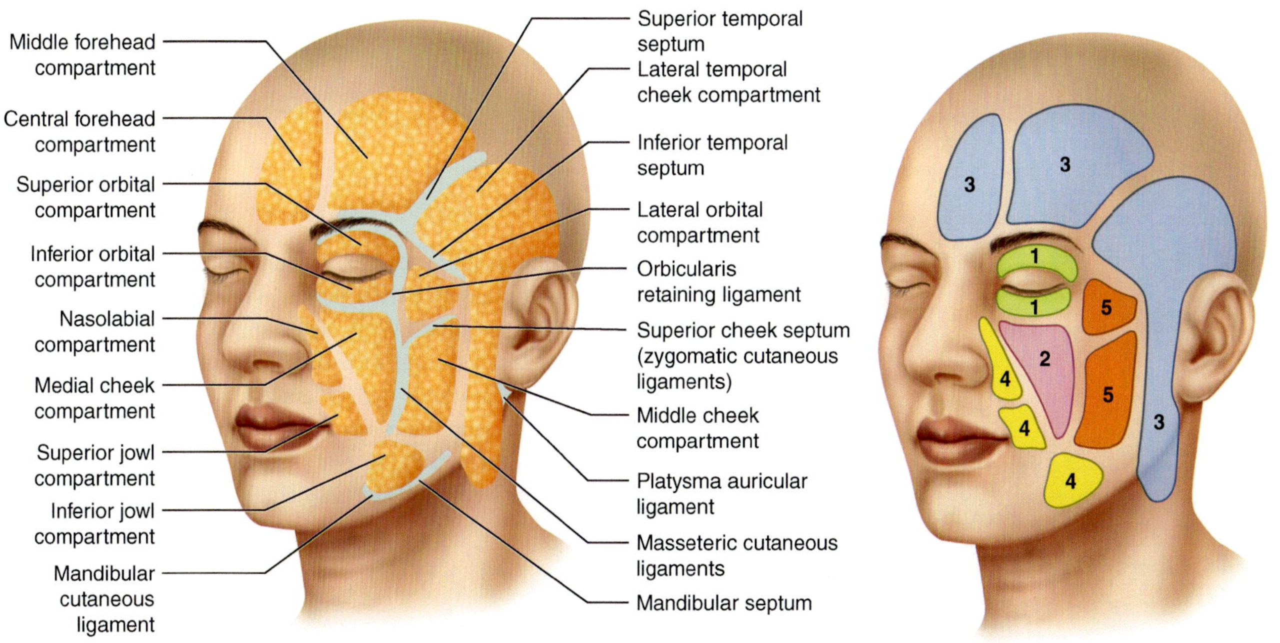

Fig. 31.4 (**a**) Superficial fat compartments of the face and (**b**) numbers correspond to the timing of the start of atrophy

Skin

Skin changes are some of the most recognized and bothersome aging changes for the patient. There is a loss of elasticity due to dermal elastosis, a reduction in the number of skin appendages, thinning of the dermis, and the development of rhytids from the traction forces that occur with muscle movements [2, 10]. These epidermal and dermal manifestations can be improved with chemical peels, topical agents, and laser procedures.

Facial Analysis

The clinical evaluation of the facelift patient is imperative to identify the signs of aging that need to be specifically addressed in facelifting surgery. A systematic analysis should be performed on all patients so that no area is overlooked. Additionally, all layers of the face (skin, fat, and structural support) should be assessed in each region. Assess for previous incisions and telltale signs of prior facial rejuvenation

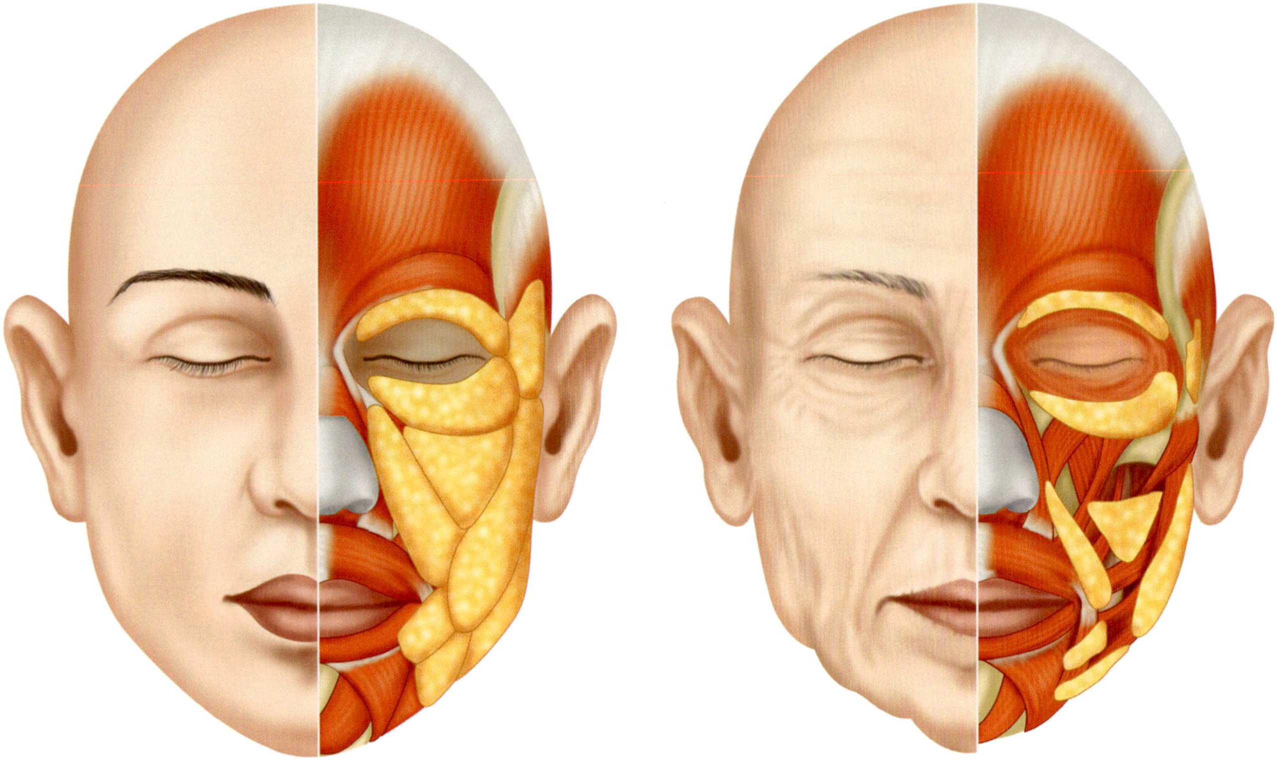

Fig. 31.5 Volume loss in the superficial fat compartments. Fat atrophy in the superficial fat compartments occurs at different times in life and at different rates. The varying atrophy leads to abrupt contour changes between the fat pads as opposed to the smooth transitions seen in the youthful face

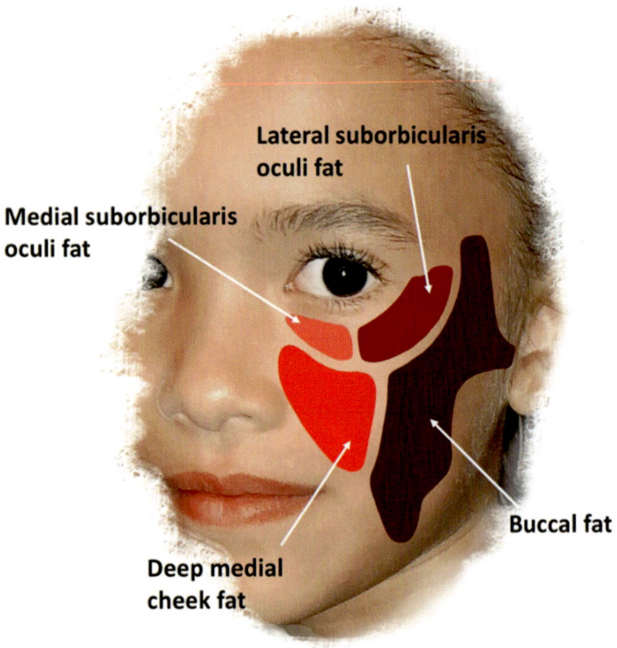

Fig. 31.6 Deep fat compartments of the face

procedures as these need to be addressed in the surgical plan. As aging is unique in each person, it is important to individualize treatment plans. While some surgeons may prefer more objective analysis and measurements, others may prefer to rely on their aesthetic eye. Overall, the most important principle is to restore harmony to the face with smooth transitions from the top to the bottom. We present a method for comprehensive facial analysis using a top-down approach.

Hairline

Starting at the top of the face, assess the patient's hairline. This is particularly important when the incision will influence the hairline. Examine whether the hairline is high or receding and whether the hair is thin in that region. Measure the distance between the top of the eyebrow and the start of the hairline to gain an appreciation of the forehead height. The distance between the hairline and the eyebrow should be approximately 1/3 the length of the total face for a harmonious appearance [11]. In a female, this will be approximately 5–6 cm in length, and in a male, it should measure approximately 6–7 cm [12]. Appreciate whether the hairline is distorted from previous surgeries and will need additional revision with the facelift.

Ears

Examine around the ears for previous incisions, which can be a sign of previous facial surgeries. In particular, look for preauricular, auricular, or retroauricular scars. If these scars are visible or unfavorable, it is important to revise these in the facelift procedure. Next, assess the position of the ear and the tragus. The characteristics of pre-tragal skin onto the face must be noted. This is important in the choice of incision placement since blunting of the natural pre-tragal convex contour needs to be maintained for a natural unoperated result. Similarly, heavy beard hair over the tragus should be avoided. Lastly, look to see whether the earlobes are attached or unattached. Changing an attached earlobe to an unattached one is preferred to hide scars, but this change to the ear should be discussed with the patient preoperatively.

Eyebrows

The ideal eyebrow position is unique for each person and differs based on gender and ethnicity. Additionally, the aesthetic preference in eyebrow fullness has changed with time – previously, thin eyebrows were considered more aesthetically appealing, and more recently, full eyebrows are more desired. In a woman, the eyebrow begins medially at the orbital rim in line with the alar base and the medial canthus. It gently slopes superiorly with a peak point approximately 2/3 of the way to the lateral end above the lateral limbus. Laterally, the eyebrow ends at the axis connecting the alar base and lateral canthus. The lateral eyebrow should be no more than 3 mm above the medial eyebrow. In a male, the eyebrow is lower, located at the level of the orbital rim, and is flatter in contour without a significant arch or peak [11, 13, 14]. The effect of aging on eyebrow position is controversial; however, it is clinically observed that the lateral eyebrow descends first with aging compared to the medial eyebrow, due to absence of frontalis muscle extension to the lateral eyebrow [15].

The position of the eyebrow is first assessed in relation to the orbital rim to determine whether there is eyebrow ptosis. Next, assess symmetry between the two sides, and note whether the eyebrow position or shape is asymmetric or flat. Eyebrow asymmetry can be caused by an underlying skeletal or soft tissue asymmetry, unilateral eyelid ptosis with compensation on that side, asymmetric frontalis muscle strength, unilateral facial nerve palsy, and/or previous surgical procedures that may have caused scarring in the temporal region (facial fractures, craniotomy, etc.). Eyebrow ptosis can be a common presenting symptom of facial nerve palsy; therefore, it is important to assess eyebrow mobility and test the frontal branch of the facial nerve.

Palpebral Aperture

The palpebral aperture, or fissure, is the elliptical shape opening between the medial and lateral canthi and the upper and eyelid margins of the eye (Fig. 31.7). The overall shape of the aperture should be evaluated; in particular, paying attention to blunting of the lateral canthal angle that may be apparent. Normally the upper and lower eyelid margins should join at the lateral canthus in a sharp angle, but rounding of the angle may be seen due to aging changes or prior lower eyelid or cosmetic surgery. The intercanthal horizontal distance, the distance between the medial and lateral canthal

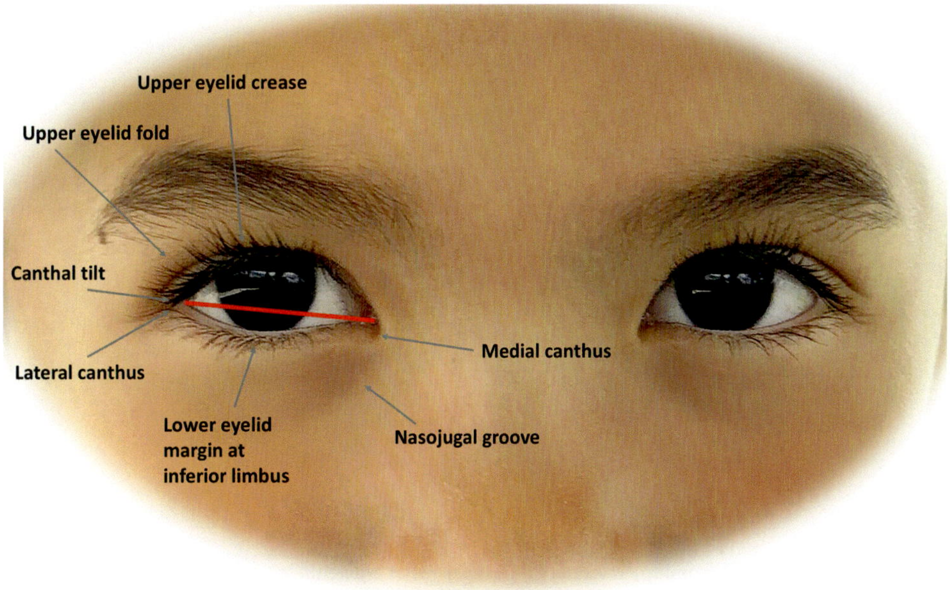

Fig. 31.7 Topographical landmarks of the palpebral aperture

angles, is typically 28–30 mm. The vertical distance between the upper and lower eyelid margins is 8–10 mm, on average [16]. The vertical interpalpebral fissure can be decreased if upper eyelid ptosis is present, or exaggerated with upper eyelid retraction, such as in thyroid eye disease, or lower eyelid retraction.

The relationship of the upper eyelid margin relative to the iris and pupil should be noted, both for unrecognized subtle ptosis and to restore symmetry between the two eyes. The lower eyelid margin should be evaluated for retraction, ectropion, or horizontal laxity. The lower eyelid margin typically rests at the level of the inferior limbus or slightly above or below the limbus. Inferior scleral show, if present, must be addressed to restore a youthful eye shape.

Next, assess the orientation or axis of the eyelid aperture. Ideally, there should be an upward canthal tilt where the lateral commissure is approximately 2 mm superior to the medial canthal angle [16, 17]. A negative canthal tilt may suggest lateral canthal laxity or dehiscence. Lower eyelid canthal attenuation can cause a rounded lateral canthus appearance with lower lid sag [17]. Normal involutional canthal dystopia and horizontal laxity can be addressed through a lateral canthoplasty or canthopexy, in addition to suborbicularis oculi lift, skin grafting, or bone tunnels, if needed.

Appropriate ocular history and examination are also important to minimize complications. Preoperative assessment of dry eye is imperative prior to any periorbital rejuvenation procedure as patients are at increased risk for worsened dry eyes after surgery. The Schirmer test, in which tear production is measured in a 5-minute period, or measuring the tear meniscus height using slit-lamp biomicroscopy can be useful to ascertain those patients at risk.

It is also important to assess the globe position relative to the orbital rim and malar eminence (Fig. 31.8). The preferred anatomic position is a positive vector, defined as when the globe does not project beyond the inferior orbital rim and malar eminence. A negative vector is when the globe projects more anteriorly than the lower lid margin and malar eminence, suggesting a lack of lower eyelid support from the inferior orbital rim. Hertel exophthalmometry is commonly used to measure globe prominence in relation to the lateral orbital rim. Typical measurements in Caucasians are between 16 and 18 mm with <16 mm suggesting enophthalmos and >18 mm suggesting exophthalmos, although a wide range of variations exist [17]. Racial differences are also significant, with some races having measurements over 20 mm normally. In patients with a negative vector orbit, performing a horizontal tightening procedure, such as a lateral tarsal strip, on the lower eyelid could result in lower lid retraction with the eyelid pulling down along the globe.

Upper Eyelid

In a youthful upper eye, there should be a well-defined upper lid crease lying above the eyelid margin called the eyelid, or supratarsal, crease. The crease has a gradual arch with the highest point positioned superior to the pupil. With aging, there is hollowing of the upper eyelid making this crease more defined. The eyelid fold is the skin that rests and hangs just over the crease. Symmetry should be assessed in the upper eyelid crease and fold. If there is asymmetry, it is important to assess the cause. Asymmetry can be caused by eyelid ptosis, eyelid retraction, asymmetry in tissue excess or laxity, and eyebrow ptosis. Greater dermatochalasis will result in a more significant eyelid fold that covers more of the pretarsal space and approaches the eyelash line.

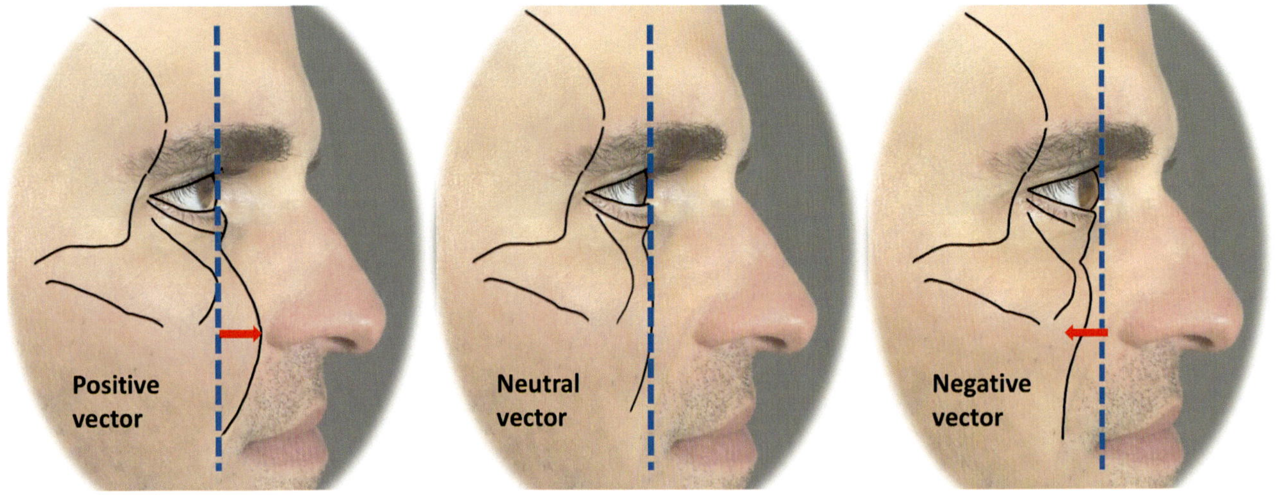

Fig. 31.8 Globe to malar prominence vector. (a) Positive vector where the anterior portion of the globe is positioned posterior to the infraorbital rim and malar eminence. (b) Neutral vector and (c) negative vector suggesting lack of lower lid support

A superiorly displaced eyelid crease is most commonly caused by dehiscence of the levator aponeurosis and should be addressed. The position of the eyelid margin may still be normal in early cases of levator aponeurosis attenuation. Additionally, it is important to assess the lateral eyebrow for excess or herniated supraorbital fat that would need to be removed to restore the aesthetic appearance of the eyelid.

Next, assess the eyelid margin relative to the pupil. In primary gaze, the superior margin is positioned 1–3 mm inferior to the superior limbus of the cornea but should not cover any of the pupil [17]. The margin should form a smooth contour with a slight peak between the medial limbus and the pupil. With age, this point shifts laterally as the tarsal plate migrates laterally [16, 17]. If there is a decrease in the distance between the eyelid margin and pupil, ptosis is present. Ptosis can be congenital, myogenic, neurogenic, and aponeurotic. If ptosis exists, assess levator function by immobilizing the head and measuring the distance the upper lid moves from downgaze to upgaze. A normal levator excursion is 10–15 mm. Detailed discussion of ptosis is covered in other chapters of this text.

The distance from the eyelid margin to the eyelid crease is called the pretarsal space, or pretarsal platform. The pretarsal space varies in individuals and in different ethnicities. On relaxed primary gaze, there should be approximately 3–6 mm pretarsal space in Caucasian patients, 1–4 mm in Indo-European and African patients, and 0–3 mm in Asian patients [16, 18]. With age, there is frequently a loss of pretarsal show secondary to eyebrow ptosis, supraorbital fat herniation, and dermatochalasis [16, 18]. Examine the patient for amount of pretarsal show and symmetry between the two eyes. While evaluating pretarsal show, look at skin laxity and excess. It is also important to assess for previous incisions to suggest a history of eyelid surgery or trauma.

Lastly, evaluate the amount of scleral show, which is the amount of sclera visible around the circumference of the cornea. There should be minimal scleral show at rest. An increase in inferior or superior scleral show suggests eyelid retraction, which could be a sign of thyroid eye disease or cicatricial changes to the eyelid.

Lower Eyelid

The lower eyelid should be assessed for excess skin, orbital fat herniation, malar bags, lower eyelid laxity, and positioning. The lower lid should be positioned at the inferior limbus with an upward canthal tilt [17]. An inferior position of the lower eyelid can be indicated by scleral show and can be caused by horizontal/tarsal laxity or lateral canthal attenuation. Excess eyelid skin is secondary to loss of skin laxity and support.

Horizontal eyelid laxity can be tested with the "snap-back" test where the inferior eyelid is retracted down and allowed to snap back. The eyelid should return to its normal apposition to the globe in less than 1 second. A slow return indicates eyelid/tarsal laxity and poor skin tone [16]. In some patients, the eyelid stays ectropic or only returns to the globe with a blink. The distraction test can also be used to assess laxity. In this test, the eyelid is distracted anteriorly from the globe and measured from the corneal surface. An eyelid distraction greater than 5–6 mm indicates significant laxity that will likely require horizontal tightening [16].

The appearance of excess skin is accentuated by orbicularis oculi laxity and attenuation of its ligamentous attachments, which results in bulging of the muscle. These changes are usually accompanied by orbital fat herniation due to attenuation of the retaining ligaments around the eye and the orbital septum [16]. There are three lower lid fat pads – medial, central, and lateral. The amount of fat and positioning of the fat in each of these compartments should be evaluated to determine if fat debulking or repositioning over the inferior orbital rim to minimize the tear trough deformity is most appropriate.

Midface

Aging of the midface results from skin laxity, atrophy and descent of the soft tissue mass of the cheek, and bony retrusion of the infraorbital rim and maxilla. Start by assessing the skin quality, thinness, and laxity. Next, focus on the fat quantity and distribution. The malar fat pad lies along the orbital rim and extends laterally to the zygoma. It is located superficial to the SMAS. As with other areas of the face discussed, there is atrophy and descent of the fat in the malar region causing volume loss and changes in fat distribution. The malar fat pad descents inferiorly and medially, leading to flattening of the malar prominence [5, 19]. The ptosis of the soft tissue mound of the midface uncovers the anatomy of the orbit, making the inferior fat pads and orbital rim more prominent. This creates a more defined groove at the orbitomalar ligament, called the tear trough, and at the lid-cheek junction (Fig. 31.9) [19, 20]. Look at the lid-cheek junction and note if the smoothness of this transition is disrupted by a prominent tear trough deformity. If a tear trough is present, note the severity on both sides and whether orbital fat is present to reposition into these areas.

The nasolabial folds should be evaluated carefully. As descent of the soft tissue continues, the displaced volume accumulates in the infrazygomatic part of the cheek and bulges over the nasolabial retaining ligament, making the nasolabial folds deeper and more noticeable [5, 20]. Additionally, due to constant muscle use of the mouth with mastication and facial expression, the soft tissue of the lower face is pushed laterally. This causes the face to expand radially and prolapse from the facial skeleton, attributing to the

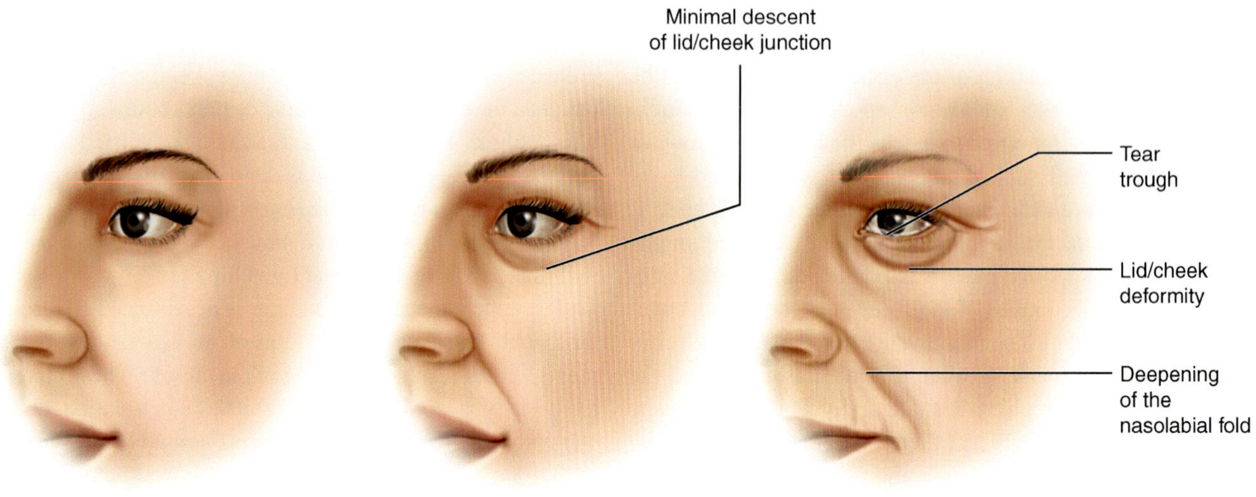

Fig. 31.9 Aging changes of the midface. Atrophy and descent of the malar fat and soft tissue pad causes descent of the lid-cheek junction with resulting deformity, tear trough deformity, and deepening of the nasolabial fold

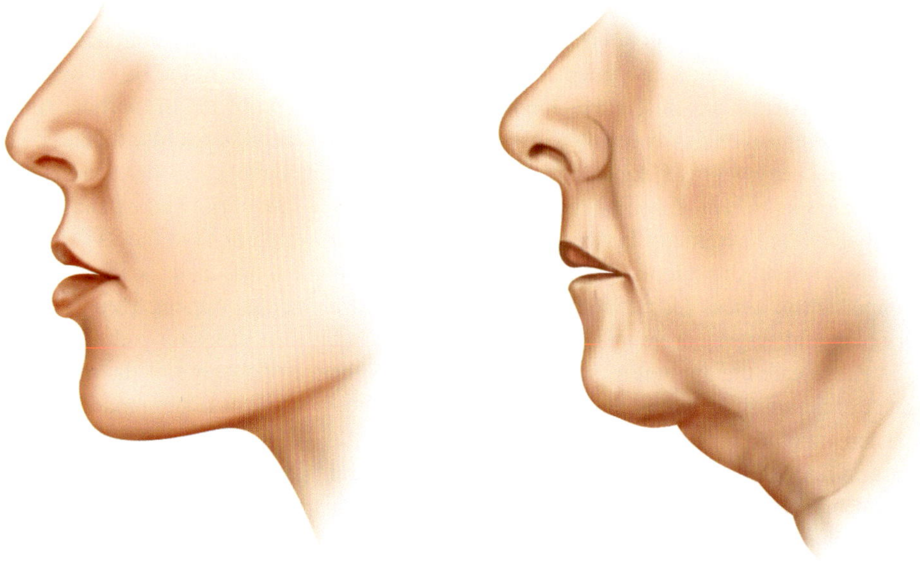

Fig. 31.10 Characteristic changes in the perioral region with aging: perioral rhytids, decreased lip volume, lengthening of the upper lip, loss of upper tooth show with lips in repose, thinning of the vermillion border, loss of vermillion border definition, and downward orientation of the oral commissure

prominence of the nasolabial fold in the aging face [5]. A midface lift and facelift, or 3D volume augmentation with dermal fillers or fat, can reposition the tissues to minimize the nasolabial folds.

Perioral Region

The perioral region is an area with significant aging manifestations and can be a large reason a patient is seeking facial rejuvenation. The perioral area is defined as the region from the subnasale to the mentum. The key landmarks include the philtrum, cupid's bow, vermillion border, oral commissure, nasolabial folds, marionette lines, and the lips. Aging will result in changes in all of these areas in very specific ways (Fig. 31.10). While a facelift will not address many of the changes seen in the perioral region, these areas should still be assessed in evaluation so that adjuvant treatments, such as soft tissue fillers, laser resurfacing, chemical peels, or botulinum toxin, can be discussed.

Facial analysis of the perioral region should start with assessment for overall symmetry, proportion, and harmony. On profile, the upper lip should occupy approximately one third of the lower third of the face, and the lower lip and chin should occupy the other two thirds [21]. Significant underlying skeletal changes occur with aging in the maxilla and mandible that affect the appearance of the perioral soft tissue. With atrophy of the maxilla, there is a relative lengthening in the upper lip length. While the youthful mouth has approximately 2–3 mm of incisor show with the lips in repose, the relative lip lengthening that occurs with aging results in less incisor show in the older patient [21].

In the youthful face, the upper lip is full and projects more anteriorly than the lower lip. With age, there is a loss in lip volume leading to a thinner and rolled lip appearance. With these changes, there is a loss of vermillion border definition, especially laterally near the commissure. Additionally, there will be flattening of the philtrum columns and cupid's bow [21, 22]. As these changes occur mainly due to a loss in volume, they can be addressed with volume augmentation with fillers or fat at the time of facelift.

The mouth is an area with significant animation during facial expression and mastication. Over time, the frequent, repeated animation causes the formation of perioral rhytids, which are further accentuated by thinning of the skin, loss of skin elasticity, and loss of fat volume that occurs with aging [21]. Many patients will present with complaints of perioral rhytids, which are frequently treated with different modalities of nonsurgical rejuvenation (chemical peels, lasers, botulinum toxin, and fillers), although maintenance treatments are necessary. Repetitive muscle activation, skin thinning, and the loss of elasticity also result in a downturn of the oral commissures that is characteristic of an older mouth. In younger patients, the oral commissure is on a transverse line through the occlusal plane. However, in an older patient, the oral commissures will turn inferiorly and form folds that lead into marionette lines and contribute to the appearance of jowling [21, 22]. Marionette lines, or labiomental folds, are a result of the laxity of the masseteric ligaments, allowing bulging of adjacent fat pads and deepening the fold [20]. Marionette lines are difficult to fully address with facelift; therefore, it is important to highlight this area to patients, discuss the limitations of facelift, and offer adjunctive procedures if this is an area of concern.

Jaw Line

A young face is characterized by a defined jaw line with a sharp cervicomental angle. The cervicomental angle should be 105–120° and approximately 3 mm posterior to the nose-lip-chin plane [23]. As we age, we lose definition in this area. The first physical finding to assess is jowling. The appearance of jowling is caused by attenuation of the masseteric cutaneous retaining ligament, which allows the descent and herniation of the fat pads below the mandible and into the submandibular fat compartment [2, 23]. Anteriorly, there is tethering of the mandibular ligaments leading to the prejowl sulcus. Radial expansion of the lower face also contributes to the appearance of jowls in the older face [5].

Next, it is important to analyze the chin structure, particularly in profile. Because of skin changes, fat atrophy, muscle atrophy, and mandible atrophy, the chin can become ptotic. Assess the projection of the chin. The maximal point of projection should be at the level of the pogonion, which is the most anterior point on the symphysis of the mandible on the midsagittal plane.

The width of the chin should be examined, with the chin point projection ideally in the midline. Assess for symmetry in the width of the chin from midline.

Neck

The last area of evaluation during facial analysis is the neck. Examine the neck for skin laxity and skin excess. Assess the platysma muscle for laxity and midline dehiscence. Excess laxity or dehiscence of the platysma can create platysmal banding, where two vertical bands extend from the submentum to the clavicle, and the appearance of a "turkey neck" deformity [20].

Fat quantity and distribution within the neck should be evaluated. There are two areas of fat deposition – supraplatysmal and subplatysmal. Examination should document whether there is excess fat in either of these compartments contributing to the aged appearance of the neck. With platysmal dehiscence, subplatysmal soft tissue, fat, and the submandibular gland descend into the submental and submandibular space creating a full appearance in the neck and loss of a sharp cervicomental angle.

References

1. Mendelson B, Wong C. Changes in the facial skeleton with aging: implications and clinical applications in facial rejuvenation. Aesthet Plast Surg. 2012;36:753–60.
2. Warren R, Aston S, Mendelson B. Face lift. Plast Reconstr Surg. 2011;128(6):747–64.
3. Cotofana, et al. The anatomy of the aging face: a review. Facial Plast Surg. 2016;32:253–60.
4. Brandt MG, Hassa A, Roth K, Wehrli B, Moore CC. Biomechanical properties of the facial retaining ligaments. Arch Facial Plast Surg. 2012;14(4):289–94.
5. Stuzin J. MOC-PSSM CME article: face lifting. Plast Reconstr Surg. 2008;121(1 Suppl):1–9.
6. Rohrich R, Pessa J. The retaining system of the face: histologic evaluation of the septal boundaries of the subcutaneous fat compartments. Plast Reconstr Surg. 2008;121(5):1804–9.

7. Fitzgerald R, et al. Update on facial aging. Aesthet Surg J. 2010;30(1 Suppl):11s–8s.
8. Le Louarn C, Buthiau D, Buis J. Structural aging: the facial recurve concept. Aesthet Plast Surg. 2007;31(3):213–8.
9. Rohrich RJ, Pessa JE. The fat compartments of the face: anatomy and clinical implications for cosmetic surgery. Plast Reconstr Surg. 2007;119:2219–27.
10. Bogle, et al. Evaluation of the aging face. In: *Atlas of cosmetic surgery*. Philadelphia: Saunders; 2009.
11. Guyuron B, Lee MA. Reappraisal of surgical techniques and efficacy in forehead rejuvenation. Plast Reconstr Surg. 2013;134(3):426–35.
12. Dhaliwal H. Analysis and diagnosis of upper facial region. Atlas Oral Maxillofac Surg Clin North Am. 2016;24(2):87–93.
13. Philips, et al. Forehead and brow rejuvenation. In: Grabb and Smith's plastic surgery. Philadelphia: Lippincott, Williams & Wilkins; 2013.
14. Codner, et al. Blepharoplasty and brow lift. Plast Reconstr Surg. 2010;126(1):1e–17e.
15. Matros E, Garcia JA, Yaremchuck MJ. Changes in eyebrow position and shape with aging. Plast Reconstr Surg. 2009;124(4):1296–301.
16. Codner M, Burke R. Blepharoplasty. In: Grabb and Smith's plastic surgery. Philadelphia: Lippincott, Williams & Wilkins; 2013.
17. Trussler A, Rohrich R. MOC-PSSM CME article: blepharoplasty. Plast Reconstr Surg. 2008;121(1 Suppl):1–10.
18. Drolet B and Sullivan P. Evidence-based medicine: blepharoplasty Plastic and reconstructive surgery, 2014; 133(5):1195–1205.
19. Heffelfinger R, et al. A simplified approach to midface aging. Arch Facial Plast Surg. 2007;9:48–55.
20. Coleman S, Grover R. The anatomy of the aging face: volume loss and changes in 3-dimensional topography. Aesthet Surg J. 2006;26(1 Suppl):S4–9.
21. Perenack J. Treatment options to optimize display of anterior dental esthetics in the patient with the aged lip. J Oral Maxillofac Surg. 2005;63(11):1634–41.
22. Austin HW, Weston GW. Rejuvenation of the aging mouth. Clin Plast Surg. 1992;19(2):511–24.
23. Narasimhan K, Stuzin J, Rohrich R. Five-step neck lift: integrating anatomy with clinical practice to optimize results. Plast Reconstr Surg. 2013;132(2):340–50.

Anatomy of Facelifting

32

Danny J. Soares and William E. Silver

Technical Terms and Abbreviations

BMI	Body mass index
MRL	Mandibular retaining ligament
RSTLs	Relaxed skin tension lines
SMAS	Superficial musculoaponeurotic system
TFA	Transverse facial artery
TPF	Temporoparietal fascia
UV	Ultraviolet
ZMM	Zygomaticus major muscle
ZRL	Zygomatic retaining ligament

Introduction

The human face is a marvel of functional and aesthetic engineering, enabling the key functions of static identity and dynamic expression of emotion; it is both a conduit for all the senses, and the emissary of language and speech while simultaneously housing the functions of mastication, deglutition, and respiratory airflow. The complexity of the human face is manifested in its aging process, and is highlighted by the history and evolution of the *cervicofacial rhytidectomy* procedure, or facelift, which has been punctuated by many technical successes and failures over its more than 110-year history. Part of the challenge of rhytidectomy has been that most faces are, by nature, unique, and thus require variations in surgical technique to achieve ideal outcomes. In addition, the surgeon must balance the desire to re-establish the contour of the lower facial skeleton against the critical need to ensure that the dynamic nature of facial soft tissue expressions remains "natural" and undisrupted. As a result, achieving a successful outcome in rhytidectomy requires, on the part of the surgeon, a nuanced understanding of (i) the underlying anatomy of the face and (ii) the natural aging process of the face. We shall review those two interrelated aspects of the face in detail in this chapter to promote a refined understanding of the process of facial rejuvenation through facelifting. A historical perspective on the procedure further complements a comprehensive look at this iconic surgery. It is only through re-living the challenges faced by surgeons over more than a century that one can truly appreciate the varied surgical rhytidectomy techniques that exist today.

Relevant Facial Anatomy

The complexity of the human face is underlined by the intricacy of its anatomy, which serves and supports its various functional needs. The structures that provide rigid identity and emotive expression to the human face can be roughly categorized into *static* and *dynamic* components (Fig. 32.1). The static component of the face consists of the facial skeleton, which forms a rigid framework upon which all facial soft tissues are suspended. The facial skeleton contributes to the overall facial identity by defining the shape and contour of the human visage but also by providing the structure against which all the moving soft tissue elements of the human face – collectively referred to in this chapter as the "mask of expression" – are fixed into position. The facial skeleton interfaces with the dynamic components of the face via its attachments to the mimetic and masticatory musculature as well as the retaining ligaments of the face.

D. J. Soares (✉)
Department of Otolaryngology, Head and Neck Surgery, University of Central Florida College of Medicine, Orlando, FL, USA

Mesos Plastic and Laser Surgery, Lady Lake, FL, USA
e-mail: Drsoares@mesoshealth.com

W. E. Silver
Department of Otolaryngology, Head and Neck Surgery, Emory University, Atlanta, GA, USA

Atlanta Institute for Facial Aesthetic Surgery, Atlanta, GA, USA

A. J. Cohen, C. N. Burkat (eds.), *Oculofacial, Orbital, and Lacrimal Surgery*, https://doi.org/10.1007/978-3-030-14092-2_32

Fig. 32.1 The static and dynamic components of the face. The facial skeleton forms the rigid base upon which the dynamic components rest, including the active dynamic components (musculature) and the passive dynamic components (overlying fat and skin)

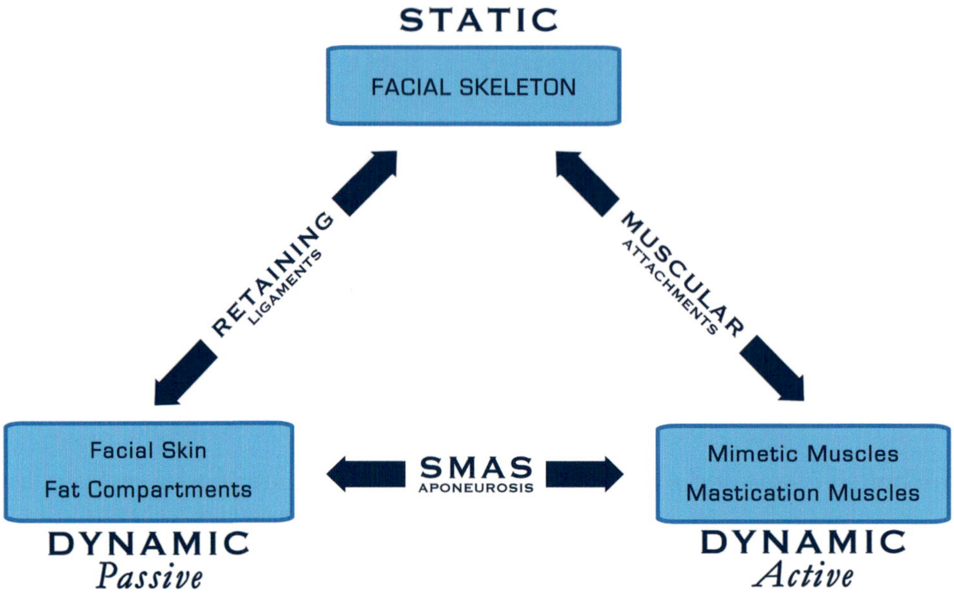

The *dynamic* components of the face subserve the function of expressiveness crucial to human communication and can be roughly divided into *active* and *passive*. The mimetic and masticatory muscles are the active dynamic elements of the face, serving as the "motor" that propels the motion of the facial soft tissues. The *passive* dynamic elements of the face move or are deformed in response to the action of the muscle movements and include the skin and adipose tissue compartments. The passive dynamic components are important to natural human expression and appearance because the facial movements that underlie facial expressions are transmitted from the muscles to the exterior via their actions on the overlying soft tissues.

The active and passive dynamic components of the face are interconnected via one unified fibrous aponeurotic layer, which together with the muscles of facial expression is known as the *superficial musculoaponeurotic system, or SMAS*. The SMAS serves as the intermediary through which facial expressions, rather than singular muscle movements, are created. This is accomplished via the numerous fibrous insertions arising from the SMAS that pierce through the superficial fat layer and insert onto the dermis. In effect, these insertions compartmentalize the adipose tissues and transmit minute movements to the facial skin, creating the large variety of possible human expressions. The skin and soft tissues of the face are additionally secured to the skeletal framework by the retaining ligaments of the face, thereby restricting their motion to fit within the facial skeletal frame. Finally, this dually static and dynamic facial framework is interlaced with a wide array of neural, vascular, and glandular structures, which direct its motion, perfuse its tissues, or serve other digestive and functional roles, respectively. We shall review each of these elements separately next.

Static Components of the Face

The Facial Skeleton

The bony skeletal framework of the face provides a rigid base upon which the soft tissue components of the face rest. From an aesthetic standpoint, the most important features imparted by the bony skeleton are the bony eminences and the external edges of the facial framework, as these provide shape to the face and segmental definition to the facial regions (Fig. 32.2). Thus, the *malar eminences*, the *zygomaticofrontal prominence*, the *mandibular angles*, the *nose*, and the *mentum* provide the key topographical landmarks upon which the facial structural identity rests. Furthermore, the *mandibular border*, *frontal bar*, and the *zygomaticofrontal* and *zygomaticotemporal processes*, together with the *cervicomental angle* of the neck, represent bony structural edges that impart shape to the face and neck. In addition, the relative projection and dimensions of these facial skeletal features is influenced by gender – granting either a masculine or feminine appearance to the face – as well as by one's genetic ancestry. Male faces typically demonstrate greater prominence of the frontal bars and projection of the chin compared to the average female face. Males also tend to have a wider mandibular width, or *intergonial distance*, relative to their respective maxillary width – known as the *intermalar distance* – with female faces having a greater relative intermalar distance than compared to males [1, 2]. These gender-specific differences occur along an entire spectrum that is normally distributed. *One of the most important goals of rhytidectomy is to reveal and showcase the underlying bony structural edges of the lower face and neck by re-suspending the ptotic tissues of the midface, lower face, and neck.* Re-establishing the mandibular border, as well as the cervicomental angle, yields a powerful form of facial rejuvenation.

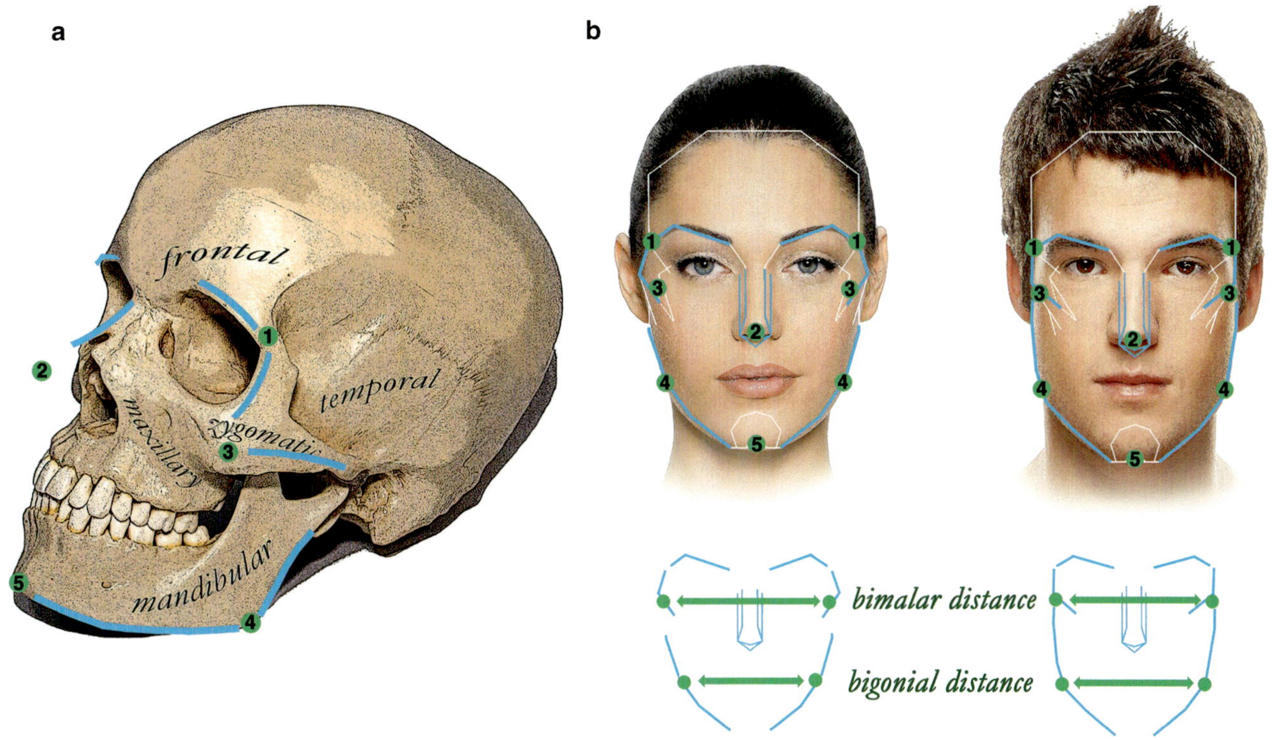

Fig. 32.2 Bony features of the facial skeleton. (**a**) The facial skeleton imparts shape to the face but also youthfulness when undisrupted by soft tissue laxity. From an aesthetic standpoint, the zygomaticofrontal prominence (1), nasal tip (2), malar eminences (3), mandibular angles (4), and the mentum are the most important facial prominences providing contour to the skeleton. The mandibular border, frontal bar, and the zygomaticofrontal and zygomaticotemporal processes also provide key bony structural edges that give shape to the face. (**b**) Differences in relative measurements of segments of bony skeletal framework are typically seen between male and female faces. The ratio of the bimalar to bigonial distances is one such example

The Facial Ligaments

The facial soft tissues are held in suspension from the bony skeleton via ligamentous attachments (Fig. 32.3). There are two major types of ligaments that anchor the skin and soft tissues of the face to the facial skeleton: *osteocutaneous ligaments* and *fasciocutaneous ligaments* [3, 4]. The osteocutaneous ligaments of the face provide a rigid attachment between the periosteum and the skin while fasciocutaneous ligaments typically originate from the SMAS or the fascia encasing the muscular and glandular elements of the face. *These ligaments are particularly important in facial aging and rhytidectomy as they form both an intrinsic barrier to facial aging and surgical rejuvenation alike*. The true osteocutaneous ligaments of the face include the zygomatic and mandibular retaining ligaments, as well as the *tear trough* ligament.

The *zygomatic retaining ligament* (ZRL) originates from the maxillary bone and inserts onto the skin overlying the superolateral malar eminence; it strongly resists the vertical descent of the midfacial soft tissues, delaying the aging of the midface relative to the lower face. The *mandibular retaining ligament* (MRL) originates from the mandibular parasymphysis; it provides a barrier to lower facial tissue descent beyond its position. While the ZRL truly opposes the gravitational descent of the midface, the MRL merely serves as an anteroinferior boundary to the aging soft tissues of the lower face, promoting instead the development of the marionette line as the jowl tissues advance over its position. This explains why significant midfacial ptosis tends to occur only later in life compared to aging of the lower face, which may begin as early as the third decade. As the face ages, the lower facial tissues are most susceptible to descent due to their lack of firm ligamentous support and their relative hypermobility due to their masticatory and mimetic functions. In turn, the midface remains more securely suspended against the zygoma and only begins to show descent in the fifth and sixth decades. The *tear trough ligament*, though not particularly relevant to rhytidectomy, forms an additional soft tissue attachment along the inferiomedial orbital rim that extends laterally as the *orbicularis retaining ligament* [5]. The tear trough ligament blocks the downward displacement of the orbital fat, forcing it to instead protrude outwardly and over the orbital rim. This creates the typical "lower lid bag" characteristic of steatoblepharon.

The osteocutaneous ligaments of the face are of critical importance in rhytidectomy, as they may need to be released in order to suspend the ptotic soft tissues of the face. Failure to release these ligaments may result in an inadequate suspension of the face, essentially guaranteeing the short-term failure of the procedure and potentially resulting in the

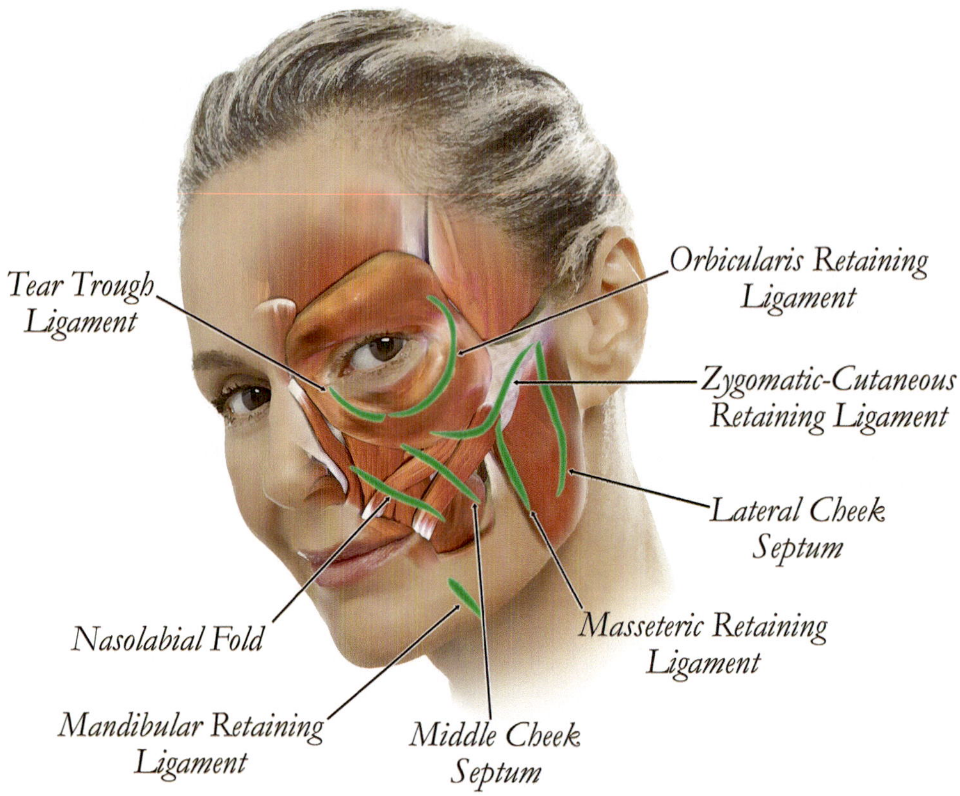

Fig. 32.3 The retaining ligaments of the human face

dynamic distortion of facial tissues due to uneven tension placed on the SMAS. In addition, improper release of the ligamentous attachments between the SMAS and the zygomaticus musculature may thwart the surgeon's efforts to correct the nasolabial fold, as we'll see later in our technical discussion of extended-SMAS lifts.

Fasciocutaneous ligaments originate from specific muscles and glandular structures and insert into the dermis, providing some additional degree of rigid anchoring of the facial soft tissues. The most significant fasciocutaneous ligaments pertaining to rhytidectomy are the *masseteric retaining ligament* and the *nasolabial fold*. The masseteric retaining ligament provides a rigid abutment of the SMAS to the masseter muscle. Together with the fibrous extensions from the parotid gland onto the skin (*lateral cheek septum*), the masseteric ligament serves to immobilize the submalar and pre-parotid midfacial soft tissues and resist age-related facial ptosis as well as its surgical suspension. Surgically, the masseteric and parotid fasciocutaneous ligaments may need to be released to allow for a uniform suspension of the SMAS with evenly distributed tension and a natural outcome. The nasolabial fold represents a condensation of fascial attachments originating at the insertion of the lip elevators onto the orbicularis oris muscle and into the overlying skin. The nasolabial fold resists descent, while the adjacent superficial fat pads gradually droop and hypertrophy, creating the increasingly prominent nasolabial fold that is characteristic of the aging face [6].

The remaining ligamentous structures of the mid- and lower facial regions represent *septal adhesions* that originate from the SMAS and insert into the skin [7]. These adhesions divide the superficial fat pads into distinct compartments, and include the *middle* and *lateral cheek septa*. Understanding how the aging process affects the adipose compartments of the face is key to understanding the volumetric component of facial aging, which will be discussed in further detail later in this chapter.

Dynamic Components of the Face

The dynamic nature of the face depends mostly upon the synchronized, coordinated activity of the approximately two-dozen individual muscles of facial expression. Although individual muscles can be easily identified, it is the conglomerate of facial muscles and their aponeurotic extensions, together forming the SMAS, that creates facial expressions. This conglomerate may be regarded as a living, moving mimetic syncytium that performs as the muscular motor of the "*mask of expression*." It is secured against the facial skeletal structure via the rigid ligamentous and muscular attachment points already described. Sitting atop this mask of expression lie the adipose tissue compartments, which are consistently partitioned by the ligaments and septal adhesions originating from the SMAS below and inserting onto the dermis above, which in turn act to transmit facial expressions into the external environment. As already described, the muscular and adiposal-dermal components of the face represent the active and passive dynamic elements, respectively, of facial expression.

Muscles of Facial Expression

At first glance, the facial mimetic musculature appears to comprise one uniform layer of muscles enveloped by fascial interconnections. However, with further scrutiny, it becomes clear that the muscles of facial expression are stratified into layers relative to the facial nerve and to each other. Excellent anatomical descriptions exist for the detail-oriented reader [8, 9]. The mimetic muscles can be broadly divided into *superficial* and *deep* layers according to whether they overlie or underlie the facial nerve, respectively. The layered organization of the facial muscles of expression is summarized in Table 32.1 and a simple review of the major mimetic muscles pertinent to rhytidectomy is shown in Fig. 32.4. Except for the *buccinator*, *levator anguli oris*, and *mentalis* muscles, all facial mimetic muscles lie superficial to the facial nerve and are innervated from their undersurface. Because those three muscles lying deep to the facial nerve are innervated from their surface, they are most susceptible to denervation injury, and the surgeon should be cautious when dissecting in their vicinity. The superficial mimetic muscles can themselves be divided into layers and a basic understanding of these layers assists the facelift surgeon in identifying key structures during facelifting, such as, for example, in distinguishing between the orbicularis oculi and zygomaticus major muscles at the level of the malar eminence.

Table 32.1 Anatomical layers of the distal branches of the facial nerve

Superficial (overlie facial nerve)	
Layer 1	Orbicularis oculi M. Zygomaticus minor M. Depressor anguli oris M.
Layer 2	Zygomaticus major M. Levator labii superioris alaeque nasi M. Depressor labii inferioris M. Risorius M. Platysma M.
Layer 3	Orbicularis oris M. Levator labii superioris M.
Deep (underlie facial nerve)	
Layer 1	Mentalis M. Levator anguli oris M. Buccinator M.

During rhytidectomy, two specific muscles bear special significance to the surgeon: the *zygomaticus major* and *platysma* muscles. The zygomaticus major muscle (ZMM) may be regarded as the most important muscle in rhytidectomy because it serves as a key landmark in facial dissection for the identification of the safe plane of midfacial dissection (Fig. 32.5). The zygomaticus major muscle originates superiorly from the malar eminence and inserts inferiorly into the commissural modiolus, blending with the fibers of the levator anguli oris and the orbicularis oris muscles while delivering fasciocutaneous attachments to the nasolabial fold. The site of the bony insertion of the superolateral ZMM lies near, and possibly even contributes to, the bulk of the zygomatic retaining ligament [10]. The superolateral insertion of the ZMM represents a critical landmark that allows the facelift surgeon to release the midface while safeguarding the integrity of the distal branches of the facial nerve, as well as spare injury to the transverse facial artery and the parotid duct. The

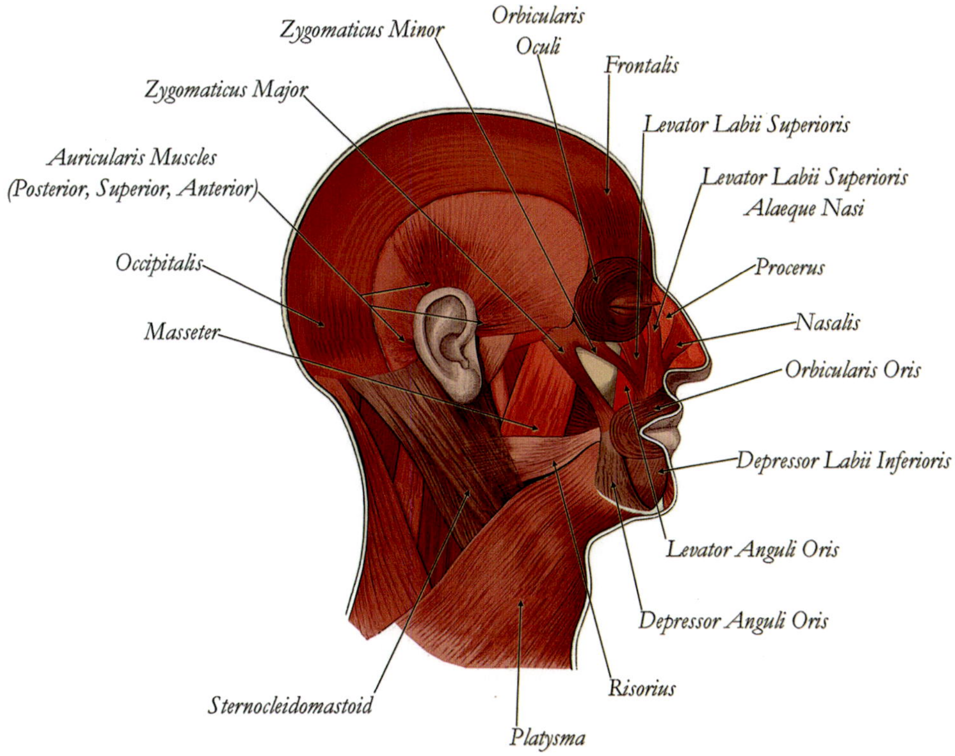

Fig. 32.4 The mimetic musculature of the human face

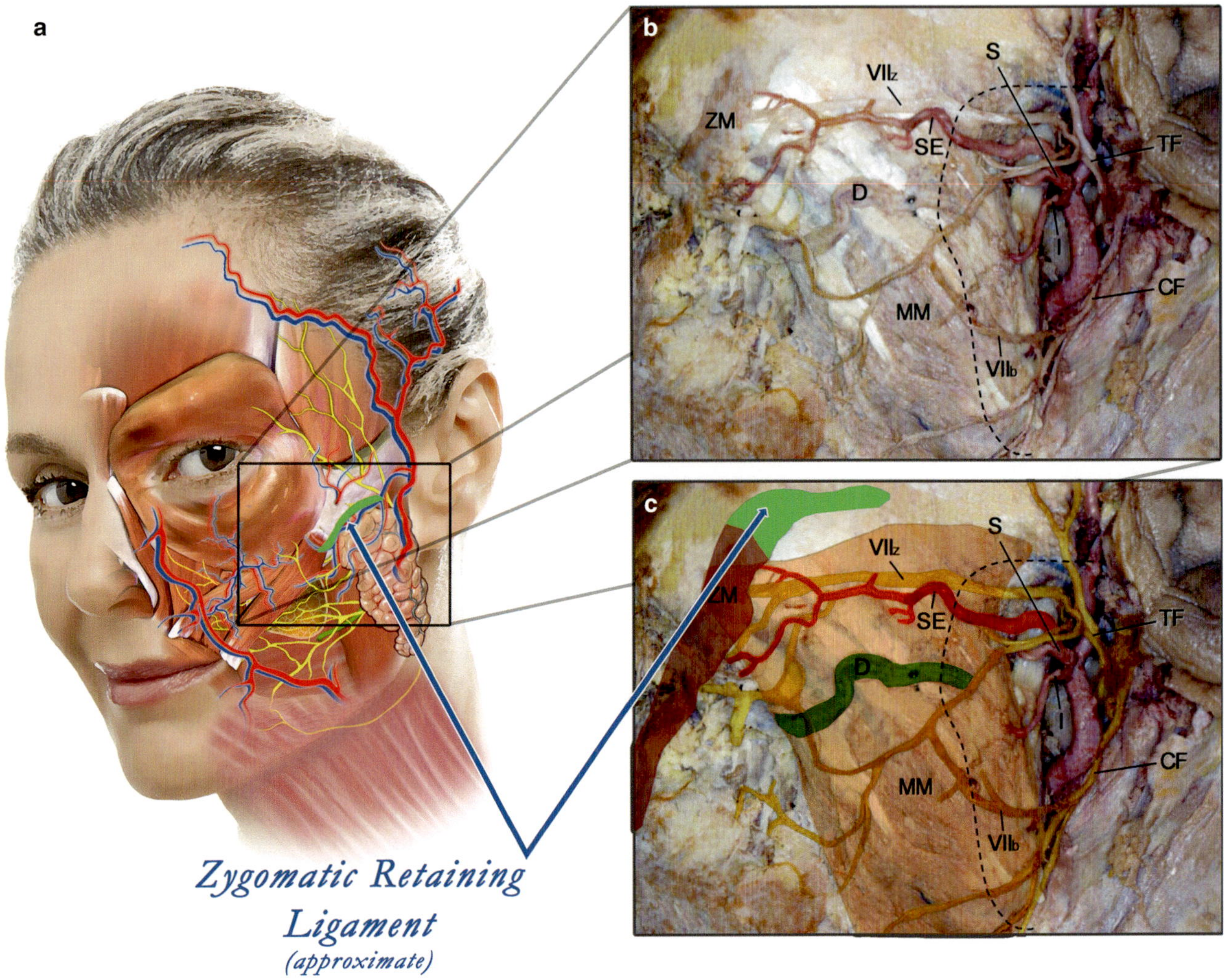

Fig. 32.5 The anatomy of the malar region. (**a**) The zygomaticus major muscle is closely associated with the *zygomatic retaining ligament* (in green) and the zygomatic (VIIz) and buccal (VIIb) branches of the facial nerve. (**b**) A close-up view of the parotidomasseteric region. *MM* masseter muscle, *ZM* zygomaticus major muscle, *D* parotid duct, *SE* superior emerging branch of transverse facial artery (TFA), *S* superior emerging branch of TFA, *I* inferior trunk of TFA, *VIIz* zygomatic branch of the facial nerve, *VIIb* buccal branch of the facial nerve, *CF* cervicofacial trunk of the facial nerve, *TF* temporofacial trunk of the facial nerve. Dotted line represents margin of removed parotid gland. (Used with permission from Yang et al. [30])

zygomatic branch is the division of the facial nerve that is most closely associated with the superolateral ZMM, traveling deep to the muscle, although the buccal branches also benefit from the clear identification of the ZMM during rhytidectomy as extending the dissection in a *supra-zygomaticus major muscle plane* into the buccal region ensures the safety of the buccal branches. In addition, the *transverse facial artery* (TFA) is closely associated with the ZMM, and it is a key vascular structure that must be preserved in rhytidectomy as it provides most of the blood supply to the facelift flap.

The *platysma muscle* represents the continuation of the SMAS into the neck, and it is the main target of suspension during the neck portion of the facelift procedure. The subplatysmal plane overlies the course of the marginal mandibular nerve, a fragile solitary facial nerve branch running underneath the platysma muscle on the surface of the superficial layer of the deep cervical fascia that is prone to injury with excessive manipulation. The importance of the platysma muscle in rhytidectomy will be further discussed later, along with the role of the SMAS in facial soft tissue suspension.

Fat Compartments

The adiposal tissues of the face play an important role in maintaining the youthful appearance of the face and contribute to the static and dynamic facial topography that is important to facial identity and expression. Rohrich et al. first described the organization of the fat pads of the face into specific compartments [11]. The facial fat compartments can be roughly divided into *superficial and deep* depending on

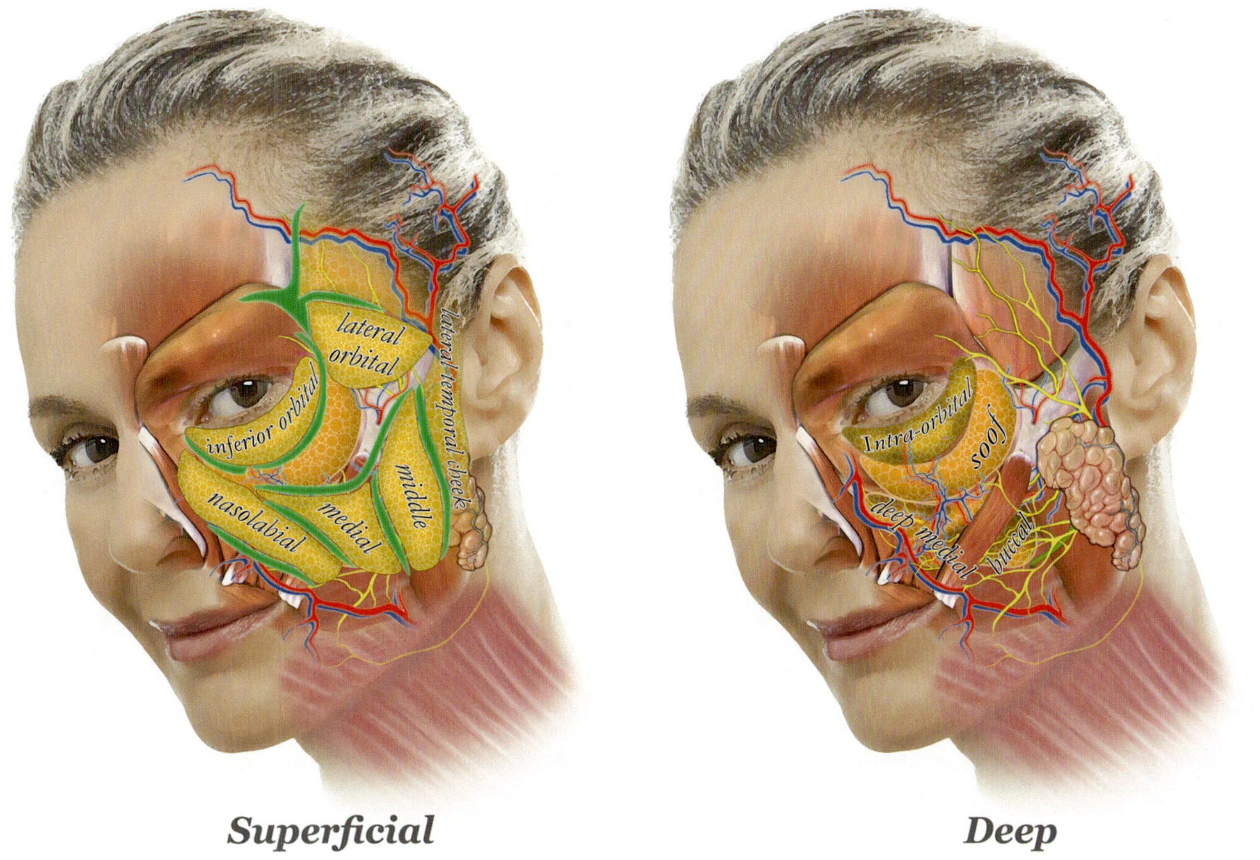

Fig. 32.6 The superficial and deep fat compartments of the human face

their location relative to the SMAS (Fig. 32.6). The compartmentalization of the superficial adipose tissues is the result of the retaining ligaments and septal adhesions originating from the underlying SMAS that pierce through the adipose tissue layers to insert into the skin. As a result, the superficial fat compartments are well preserved across individuals. As we will discuss further below, the volume of each compartment tends to change with aging, leading to a volumetric component of aging that must be addressed in order to maximize results in facial rejuvenation. Not all fat compartments become depleted of volume with aging; for instance, the nasolabial compartment tends to increase in volume with time, contributing to a deeper nasolabial fold [12, 13]. In contrast, the submalar region, which is bounded superficially by the medial and middle fat compartments and deeply by the buccal fat pad becomes depleted in old age and in individuals with extremely low BMI or lipodystrophy [14]. The superficial fat compartments sit atop the SMAS and are mobilized and distorted by each facial expression. The deep compartments sit deep to the SMAS and serve to create a soft gliding surface that decreases friction between mimetic muscles; in addition, they also provide youthful fullness to the face. The buccal fat compartment, known as Bichat's pad, is the largest facial fat compartment by volume and one of the most significant contributors to volumetric depletion of the face seen with aging [15, 16]. The volumetric loss of facial fat is not addressed by the rhytidectomy procedure, and many surgeons routinely perform simultaneous facial lipotransfer to maximize the outcomes of the procedure [17].

The Skin

The skin is perhaps the most-often ignored dynamic component of the face. While often seen merely as a protective encasing of the facial soft tissues, it is important to note that it is the specific insertion of fasciocutaneous ligaments onto the skin that allow the face to move in expression in the way that it does externally. The skin is essentially the outer border of the dynamic mask of expression of the face, creating the ultimate compartmentalization of the dynamic elements of the face. The skin of the face can be divided topographically into highly mobile and immobile regions, mimicking the mobility of the underlying SMAS below. The highly mobile regions of the face are adjacent to the perioral region and are easily moved because they are important for facial expression and less tethered to the facial skeleton, unlike the periorbital tissues. As a result, the perioral tissues are exposed to greater dynamic forces throughout an individual's life. This is evident in the more severe aging of the skin along these

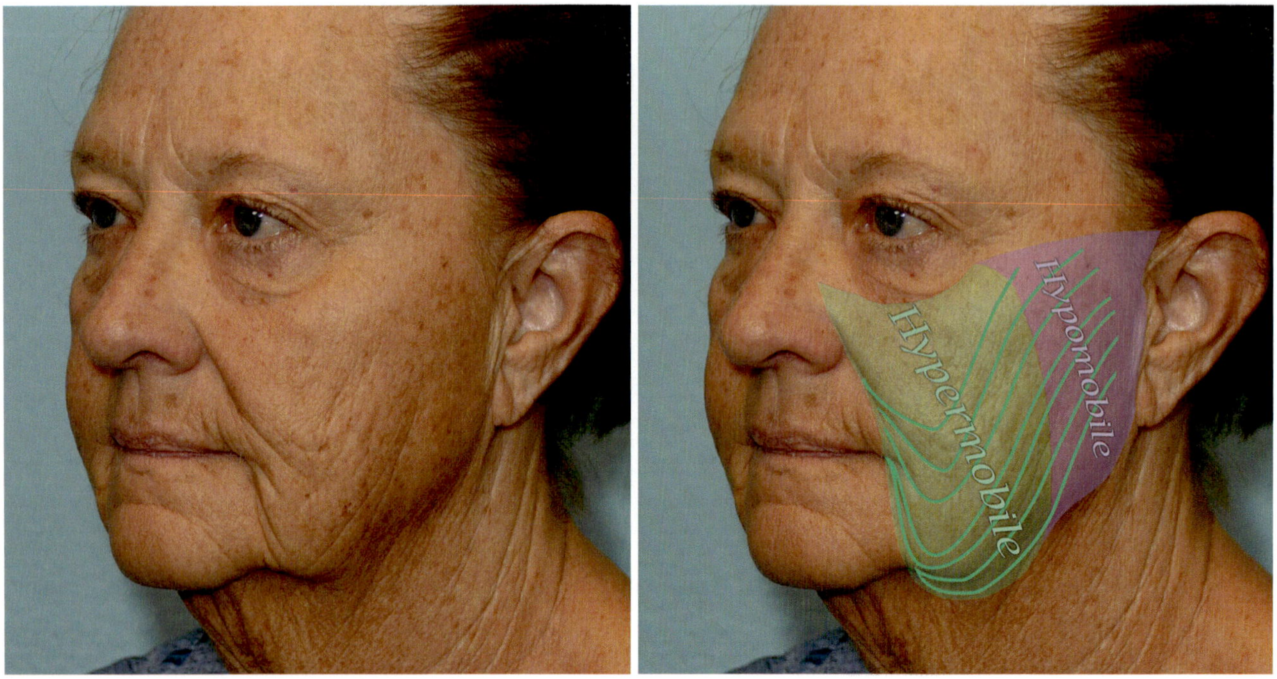

Fig. 32.7 Hyper- and hypomobile regions of the human face. Due to the expressive nature of the medial face, the tissues of the medial cheek and perioral regions demonstrate greater mobility compared to the fixed tissues of the lateral cheek and preauricular region. The rigidity of the hypomobile regions is secondary to the strong ligamentous support from the zygomatic and masseteric retaining ligaments and fibrous insertions from the parotid capsule

mobile areas (Fig. 32.7) compared to the less mobile facial regions of the preauricular and upper malar areas. Although the entire facial skin may be generally affected by external factors such as UV exposure and cigarette smoking, the more mobile areas of the face tend to age more aggressively over time. While rhytidectomy lifts the SMAS in a way that restores the firm suspension of the mobile face and simultaneously relieves the severity of rhytids, please note that the facelift procedure itself does very little to correct the intrinsic aging of the skin. As a result, many facelift surgeons typically routinely advocate for resurfacing of the facial skin simultaneously with – or staged following – rhytidectomy to maximize outcomes [18].

The Superficial Musculoaponeurotic System (SMAS)

The SMAS is a major component of the "mask of expression," providing a fluidity of motion that allows the overlying soft tissues to be dynamically altered during conventional expression while remaining restricted by bony ligamentous attachments to the bony skeleton. As a result, the SMAS acts as the link between the static skeletal framework of the face and the dynamic soft tissue mask of expression. As the name implies, the SMAS consists of *muscular* and fibrous *aponeurotic* components (Fig. 32.8). Laterally, the SMAS is mostly aponeurotic, existing as a continuous fibrous layer that is distinct from the parotid fascia and is continuous with the temporoparietal fascia (TPF) superiorly and the platysma muscle inferiorly. The aponeurotic SMAS is strongly pinned to the facial skeletal structure by the zygomatic, masseteric, mandibular, and orbicularis retaining ligaments. The aponeurosis serves both to allow the suspension of freestanding muscles of facial expression, such as the orbicularis oris and risorius, and to distribute tension from the mimetic muscles to the overlying skin in a way that can create a nearly infinite number of facial mimetic configurations [19].

As the aponeurotic SMAS is followed medially toward the central face, it splits to envelop the superficial muscles of facial expression (Fig. 32.9), most importantly the zygomaticus major muscle, which is a key facelift landmark. Medial to the zygomaticus major muscle, the SMAS then becomes mostly a thin membranous encasement of the mimetic musculature [20]. The muscular SMAS is thus used to describe the entirety of the mid- and lower facial mimetic musculature in its continuity with the SMAS aponeurosis; it is characterized by fibrous extensions from the musculature to the overlying dermis, allowing for precise manipulation of the skin during expression. Thus, the strong, firm aponeurotic SMAS largely disappears once the surgeon reaches the zygomaticus major muscle. If the surgeon performs a lamellar dissection and elevates the skin of the midface and then proceeds to elevate the SMAS separately, the surgeon would

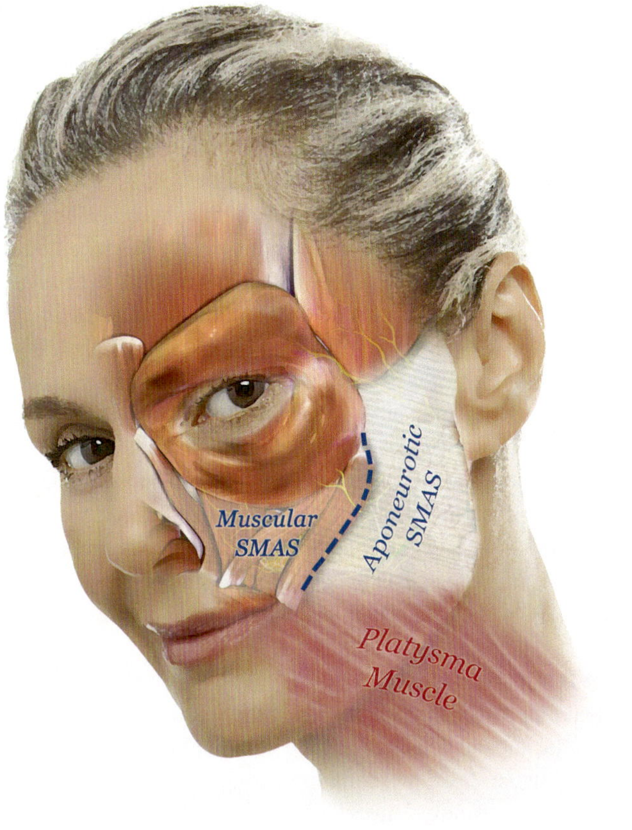

Fig. 32.8 The component regions of the superficial musculoaponeurotic system (SMAS). The SMAS is mostly aponeurotic in the lateral regions of the face. The SMAS gradually transitions to become a muscular layer medially, with the aponeurosis enveloping the mimetic musculature in a fascial covering. The aponeurotic SMAS is in continuity with the mimetic musculature medially, the temporoparietal fascia (TPF) superiorly, and the platysma muscle inferiorly

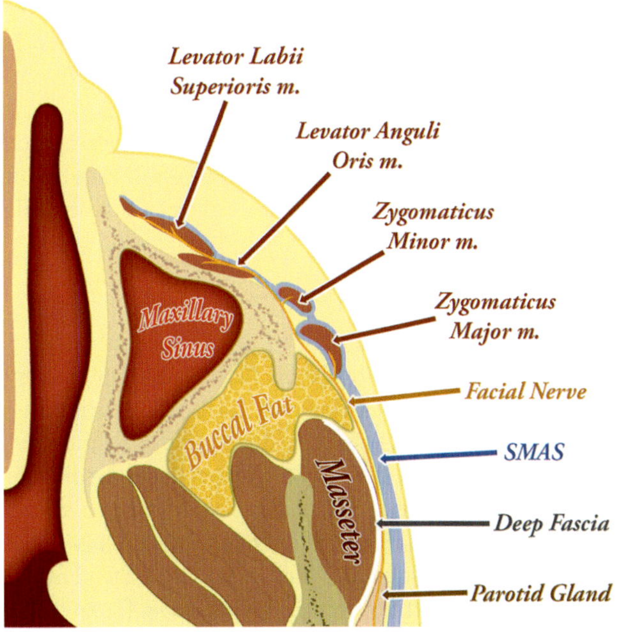

Fig. 32.9 The relationship between the aponeurotic SMAS and the mimetic musculature of the face. The SMAS exists mostly as an aponeurosis of variable thickness in the lateral aspect of the cheek and lower face. The aponeurosis envelops the mimetic musculature in a fascial covering, beginning with the zygomaticus major muscle. The zygomatic branch of the facial nerve courses under the aponeurotic SMAS to innervate the zygomaticus major and minor, and levator labii superioris muscles from their undersurface. The levator anguli oris muscle is innervated from its external surface, placing it at risk during aggressive sharp dissection in the medial cheek

find that the SMAS layer would be pierced upon reaching the zygomaticus major muscle as the SMAS splits at this point and becomes a thin facial encasement associated with the mimetic musculature. This is of significance in rhytidectomy because the SMAS can only be undermined as an independent fibrous layer laterally. Upon reaching the zygomaticus major muscle, if the surgeon chooses to continue in a supra-zygomaticus plane of dissection, the surgeon is now suddenly in the subcutaneous malar fat. The relevance of this key fact is central to avoiding the confusion generated by terms such as "the deep plane" which describes a deep subcutaneous dissection deep to the thick, superficial malar fat pads even though it is actually superficial to the SMAS (Fig. 32.10).

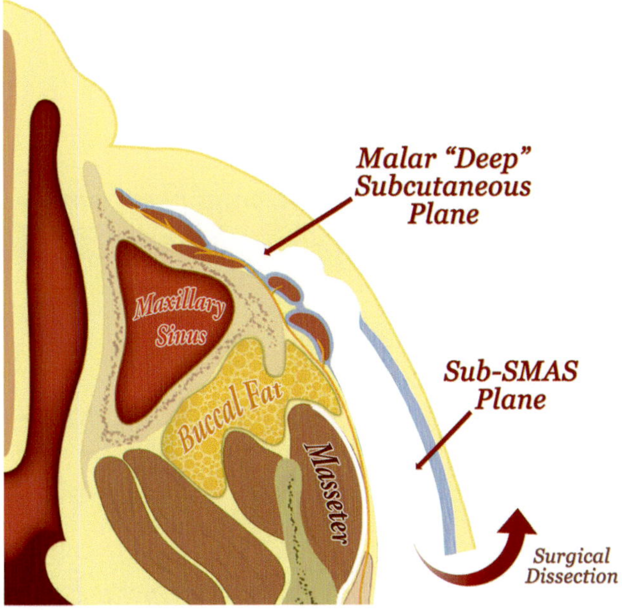

Fig. 32.10 The axial anatomy of the zygomatic region and the "deep plane." The deep plane of dissection starts in a sub-SMAS plane and gradually transitions to pierce through the SMAS at the level of the zygomaticus major muscle to then enter the deep subcutaneous plane of the cheek. While this plane is referred to as "the deep plane" it is actually superficial to the SMAS and mimetic musculature

Neurovascular and Glandular Structures

The many neural and vascular networks that sustain and direct the soft tissue mimetic mask add to the anatomical complexity of the face. The facial nerve is of critical importance to the facelift surgeon, as transection of motor nerves invariably leads to permanent paralysis unless early re-anastomosis can be performed. The vascular supply of the facial soft tissues is of importance as well because disruption of major nutrient vessels may compromise the viability of the skin and result in tissue necrosis, leading to unacceptable scarring.

The Facial Nerve

The facial nerve is of such critical importance in rhytidectomy that it has essentially shaped facelifting from the very beginning. Early on, surgeons abstained from performing any type of sub-SMAS dissection due to fear of injuring distal branches [21]. In time, with greater understanding of facial tissue planes and relationships, it became possible to approach even the midface from a lateral approach without significantly increasing the risk of injury to the facial nerve. The facial nerve emerges from the stylomastoid foramen and courses deep within the substance of the parotid gland, where it bifurcates into its two major divisions: the *temporofacial* and *cervicofacial* divisions. The temporofacial division further bifurcates into the *temporal* and *zygomatic* branches and variably contributes to the *buccal* branch, while the cervicofacial division bifurcates into the *marginal mandibular* and *cervical branches* and also variably contributes to the buccal branch (Fig. 32.11). Although the temporofacial division provides innervation to the upper and middle face and the cervicofacial division mostly innervates the lower face and neck, they are not exclusive in this arrangement. Many interconnecting branches network between the two divisions and between adjacent branches, meaning that specific innervation of any given muscle cannot consistently be traced back to only one facial nerve branch [22]. This redundant arrangement protects the innervation of the mimetic musculature of the face against severe paresis from single nerve branch injuries. However, because the facial nerve branches are fragile and run within the same plane of dissection along limited corridors, injury to one branch can often equate with injury to the remaining neighboring branches, causing devastating paralysis. This underlines the importance of having a solid understanding of the dissection planes of the face and the location of key landmarks in performing rhytidectomy safely, as explained further below.

The Temporal Branch

The temporal, or frontal, branch of the facial nerve originates from the substance of the parotid gland below the zygomatic arch as two to four intercommunicating branches that ascend in an increasingly superficial plane in a superomedial

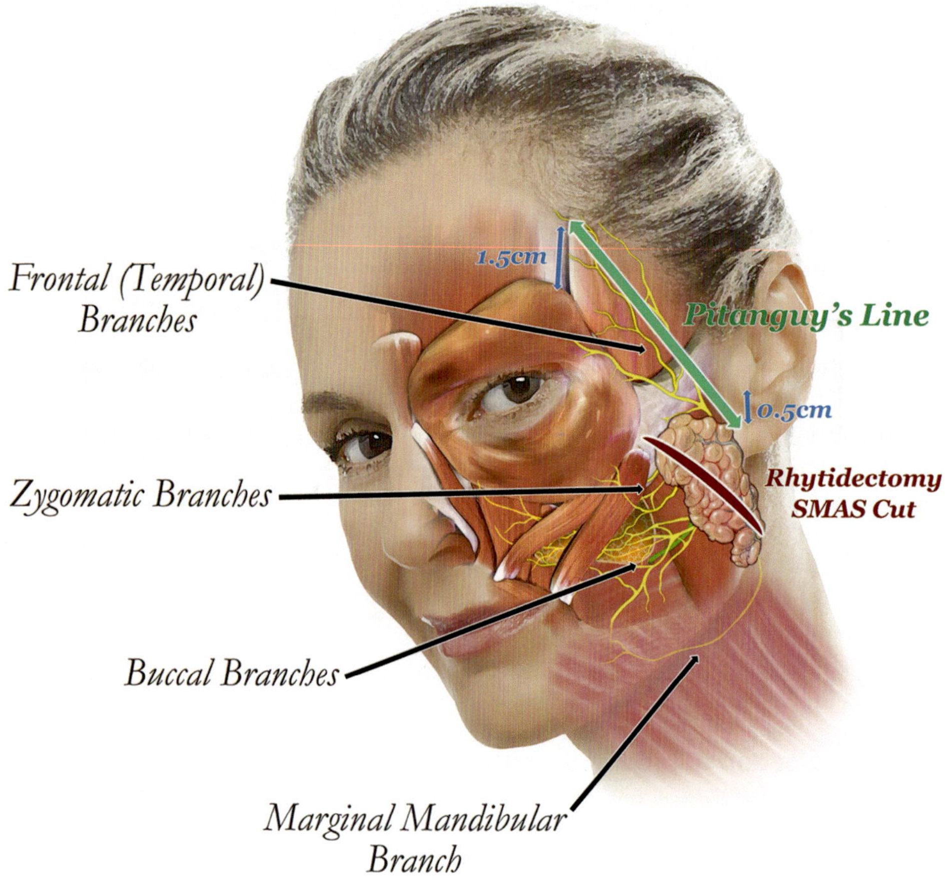

Fig. 32.11 The anatomy of the branches of the facial nerve. The temporal branch is typically found traveling above Pitanguy's line, drawn from 0.5 cm below the tragus to 1.5 cm above the brow

direction toward the lateral orbit and forehead (Fig. 32.11). At its exit from the parotid gland, the temporal nerve courses deep to the SMAS on top of the masseteric fascia – also known as the superficial layer of the deep fascia – that encases the masseter and temporalis muscles. The temporal branch continues underneath the SMAS, which becomes the *temporoparietal fascia* (TPF) above the zygomatic arch. At the level of the zygomatic arch, the frontal branch lies deep to the SMAS/TPF, sitting on top of the deep fascia, approximately 3 mm above the bone [23]. As it courses further superiorly, the temporal branch then gradually ascends to a more superficial course to travel within the temporoparietal fascia approximately 2 cm above the zygomatic arch [24]. The distal segments of the temporal nerve are the most superficial components of the entire facial nerve, lying largely unprotected as they travel through the temporal region. The nerve provides innervation to the upper orbicularis oculi muscle (with branches entering the muscle from underneath at approximately 3–4 mm from the lateral muscle edge), the frontalis (with branches entering at approximately 1.5–2 cm above the brow), and the corrugator and procerus muscles. Additionally, some communicating anastomoses are also sent to the zygomatic branches. Typically, the temporal branches cross over the zygomatic arch between approximately 3.8 cm and 6.0 cm from the bony lateral canthus along a line drawn over the arch [25]. During rhytidectomy, many surgeons rely on Pitanguy's line to quickly identify the approximate course of the temporal branch [26]. Pitanguy's line is drawn from a point 0.5 cm below the tragus to 1.5 cm above the brow (Fig. 32.11). With senescence, the brow may descend and fail to be useful as an external landmark, although an older patient with brow ptosis may still have a normal brow position when placed supine. In performing extended rhytidectomies, which release the midface, most surgeons will enter the sub-SMAS plane of dissection roughly along a line drawn from the malar eminence to the angle of the jaw. This entry cut essentially avoids the entire course of the temporal branch altogether, and, if the dissection is kept in an immediately sub-SMAS and supra-ZMM plane, the zygomatic and buccal branches should easily be kept out of harm's way as well. Of note, the SMAS cut performed in the high-SMAS technique, which will be discussed later, is often above the zygomatic arch; however, because the temporal branches usually remain deep to the temporoparietal fascia, this still remains safe, though closer to injury, relative to the frontal branch [24].

The Zygomatic Branch

The zygomatic branch of the facial nerve typically exits the parotid gland as two or three interconnected branches. These branches course medially over the masseteric fascia and then continue deep to the zygomaticus major muscle except for a small branch that courses *over* the upper third of the zygomaticus major to provide innervation to the inferior portion of the orbicularis oculi. This small nerve branch is at a higher risk of injury, and could lead to a weakening of lower eyelid closure that is typically temporary in nature. As the zygomatic branches travel under the zygomaticus major muscle, they innervate it from the undersurface of its inferior third before continuing further medially, deep to the levator labii superioris and superficial to the levator anguli oris, providing each of them with motor input. The zygomatic branch is most exposed to potential injury along a segment running between the anterior parotid border and the zygomaticus major muscle [27]. In this region, the zygomatic branch runs deep to the SMAS and on top of the masseteric fascia and is covered by a thin, wispy, and loose areolar tissue layer. Because the nerve courses on top of masseteric fascia, lifting the SMAS away from the face during sub-SMAS dissection allows the surgeon to dissect away from the facial nerve branch, as it will remain firmly adherent to the floor of the dissection plane. This becomes important in extended-SMAS facelift types employing a "deep plane" of dissection of the midface, as releasing the zygomatic retaining ligament is central to those techniques.

The Buccal Branch

The buccal branch of the facial nerve exits the parotid below the zygomatic branch and is often contributed by the temporofacial and cervicofacial divisions. The nerve travels medially over the masseteric fascia near the parotid duct and is covered by a characteristically thin, glistening areolar tissue layer. Occasionally, two branches traveling together, or even a plexus of nerves, may be encountered, with the most common arrangement being a single nerve traveling within 1 cm inferior to the parotid duct [28]. As the nerve continues further medially, it crosses over the buccal fat pad, which may be herniated in old age, and the buccinator muscle, largely unprotected. Furthermore, the course of the buccal branch is crisscrossed by the masseteric retaining ligament, which arises from the masseteric fascia along a vertical distribution and inserts onto the dermis above. *The safe dissection of the SMAS in the region of the masseteric ligament is critically endangered by failure to identify the proper dissection plane in the supra-zygomaticus major muscle plane in the buccal region*. The buccal branches are at greatest risk of injury during deep plane dissection. Surgeons dissecting along the sub-SMAS plane in the buccal region initially find a clean dissection plane along the surface of the parotid capsule and subsequently into the wispy areolar tissue overlying the masseteric fascia, near the parotid duct. If the surgeon attempts to extrapolate this cleavage plane into the deep plane of dissection in the upper buccal region, the surgeon will encounter the masseteric retaining ligament and will be likely to run directly into the buccal branch of the facial nerve, resulting in injury. This is especially true because the buccal region, in which the buccal nerve courses, is loose and mobile and outward traction of the SMAS during the dissection will fail to protect the buccal nerves, unlike with the zygomatic branches. *As a result, the supra-zygomaticus major muscle dissection plane should always be established prior to pursuing the release of the masseteric ligament and a sub-SMAS dissection in the buccal region.*

The Marginal Mandibular Branch

The marginal mandibular nerve is a long solitary branch that typically lacks the number of associated accompanying branches and anastomoses that would otherwise protect it from complete paresis following nerve injury. As a result, the marginal mandibular nerve is considered the most fragile motor nerve in facial plastic surgery. The marginal nerve has a curvilinear course; originating from the inferior portion of the parotid, it travels along the angle of the mandible in a plane deep to the platysma and on top of the superficial layer of the deep cervical fascia. The nerve tends to follow a course close to the mandibular border, extending no further than 2 cm away from the mandibular margin. The nerve then ascends gradually, crossing over the body of the mandible at a point posterior to the facial artery groove. It then courses over the facial artery and slowly gains a more superficial position as it ascends to branch and innervate the depressor anguli oris, depressor labii inferioris, orbicularis oris, and mentalis muscles. Anterior to the facial artery, the nerve is always found above the mandibular border, in contrast to its course posterior to the facial groove, where it tends to favor a position below the border of the mandible [29]. Because the SMAS and platysma are in continuity within the lower face, the subplatysmal plane of dissection from the lower face into the neck appears natural to most surgeons. However, this type of dissection can only be pursued safely posterior to the edge of the parotid and 2 cm below the mandible. Anterior to the parotid, it becomes important to use extreme caution, as the marginal mandibular nerve lies within and spans the subplatysmal dissection plane. As a result, most surgical techniques in rhytidectomy advocate for either a pre-platysmal dissection or a limited subplatysmal dissection that remains in the superolateral neck or below the mandible and avoids excessive manipulation anterior to the parotid border that could injure the marginal mandibular nerve.

Vascular Supply

The vascular anatomy of the face is pertinent to rhytidectomy because the major nutrient vessels to the facelift skin flap are near the dissection plane. Whetzel and Mathes demonstrated that the vasculature of the rhytidectomy skin flap depends heavily upon a limited number of arterial perforators arising from the *transverse facial artery* and *facial artery* [30, 31].

Transverse Facial Artery

The transverse facial artery (TFA) arises from the superficial temporal artery within the substance of the parotid gland. The TFA then courses anteriorly, following a path similar to the zygomatic branch of the facial nerve. The TFA gives rise to one or two perforators at a point located, on average, 3.1 cm lateral and 3.7 cm inferior to the lateral canthus, with a 95% confidence limit of 1.1 cm radius [32]. Hence, these important perforating vessels lie in close proximity to the zygomatic retaining ligament and zygomaticus major muscle. Facelift surgeons are typically cautious to avoid excessive skin undermining in the territory of the TFA if pursuing an aggressive skin flap, because inadvertent vessel ligation would devitalize the flap and increase the risk of skin necrosis. In rhytidectomy, the zygomatic retaining ligament can be properly released without requiring ligation of the TFA perforator(s), and a safe midfacial release can be performed without compromising flap vascularity (Fig. 32.12).

Facial Artery

The facial artery (FA) also provides significant vascular support to the facelift flap via *submental perforators*. The location of these perforators varies but are typically located on average 5.6 cm inferior and 3.1 cm lateral to the oral commissure, with a 95% tolerance limits at +/− 6 cm and +/− 3 cm, respectively [32]. Ligation of the submental perforator vessel can result in devascularization of the inferolateral (cervical) skin flap during rhytidectomy (Fig. 32.13). No large anastomotic connections between the TFA and FA exist and ligation of either perforator tends to diminish flap vascularity in the perioperative period. This is of importance to surgeons pursuing skin resurfacing simultaneously with rhytidectomy; although this practice has been shown to be safe and beneficial in maximizing facelift outcomes, the surgeon should be especially cautious to avoid inadvertent transection of these essential vessels if performing resurfacing simultaneously [18].

Parotid and Submandibular Glands

The parotid and submandibular glands are both important in rhytidectomy. The parotid gland acts as a natural protective encasement of the facial nerve that allows the surgeon to rapidly raise a skin and/or SMAS flap safely. This is incredibly helpful because establishing the sub-SMAS (supra-parotid capsule) plane in rhytidectomy facilitates further dissection and safeguards important structures. The parotid capsule extends fibrous attachments to the overlying skin, creating a thick adhesion that requires sharp dissection to elevate the skin flap in the preauricular region. Because of this, the substance of the parotid gland can be inadvertently entered, risking a sialocele, and care should be taken to preserve the integrity of the capsule at all times. The parotid duct, also known as Stensen's duct, exits the parotid approximately

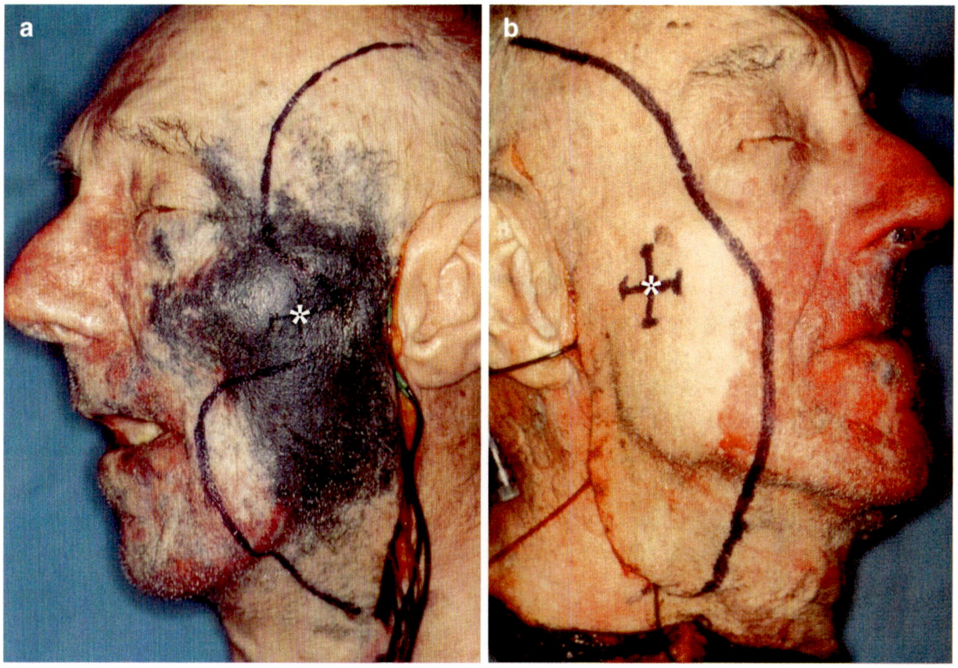

Fig. 32.12 The vascular supply of the facelift flap, before and after transection of TFA perforator(s). (**a**) Left facial cadaver dissection denoting the location of the transverse facial artery (TFA) perforator site (*) and its 95% confidence limits (cross). The dark line represents the extent of subcutaneous flap undermining; note that the TFA perforator site was not undermined. The dark blue ink represents the vascular territory of the TFA perforator while the red ink represents the vascular territory of the facial artery. (**b**) Right facial cadaver dissection denoting the site of the TFA perforator (*) and 95% confidence limits (cross). In this dissection, the entire area delineated by the dark blue line was undermined, including the site of the TFA perforator. No blue staining is seen in most of the flap due to transection of the perforator. In addition, the red staining from the facial artery perforator shows minimal overlap with the TFA territory. (Used with permission from Whetzel and Mathes [32])

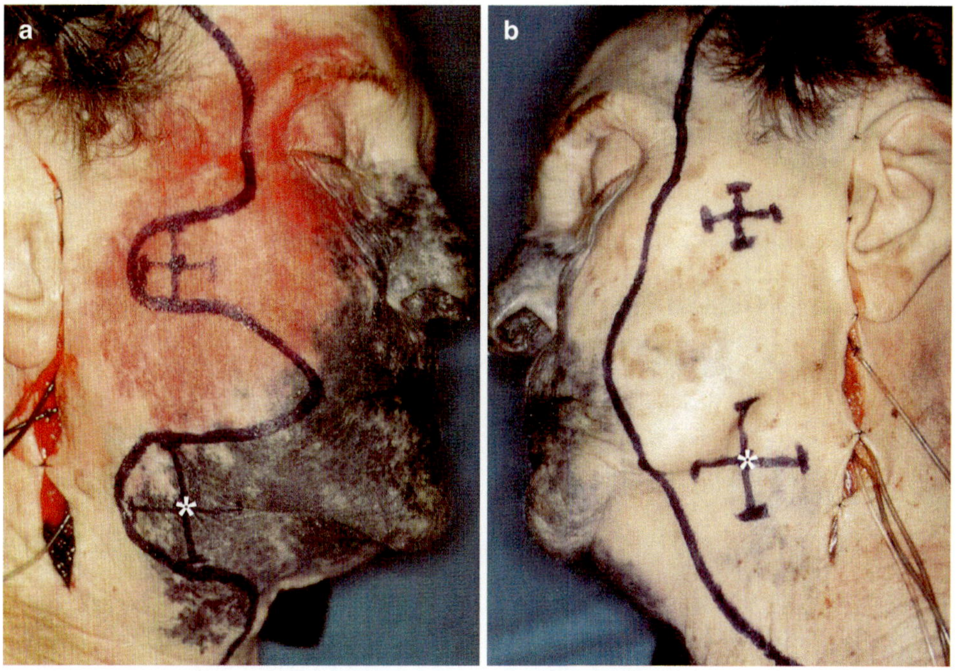

Fig. 32.13 The vascular supply of the facelift flap, before and after transection of submental perforator(s). (**a**) Right facial cadaver dissection denoting the location of the submental perforator site (*) and its 95% confidence limits (cross). The dark line represents the extent of subcutaneous flap undermining; note that neither the submental artery nor the transverse facial artery (TFA) perforator sites were undermined. The dark blue ink represents the vascular territory of the submental perforator while the red ink represents the vascular territory of the TFA perforator. (**b**) Left facial cadaver dissection denoting the site of the submental perforator (*) and its 95% confidence limits (cross). In this dissection, the entire area delineated by the dark blue line was undermined, including the sites of the submental and TFA perforators. No blue staining is seen in most of the flap due to transection of the submental perforator, and no red staining is seen due to transection of the TFA perforator. The red staining from the facial artery perforator shows only in the facial regions anterior to the submental artery branch. (Used with permission from Whetzel and Mathes [32])

halfway across the vertical length of the masseter muscle. The duct then courses anteriorly over the masseteric fascia, covered by the same wispy areolar tissue that overlies the branches of the facial nerve. The duct lies deep to the buccal branches of the facial nerve, and injury to the duct usually typically equates with injury to the buccal nerve branches as well [33]. Upon reaching the anterior edge of the masseter, the duct then turns deeply inwards and pierces the buccinator muscle to enter the oral cavity opposite the second maxillary molar.

The submandibular gland lies deep to the superficial layer of the deep cervical fascia and is often located below the plane of dissection during rhytidectomy. With the aging process, the submandibular glands become ptotic and their overlying fascia thinner; as a result, care should be taken to avoid inadvertent injury to the gland or its closely associated marginal branch during liposuction of the neck. In cases of significant contour issues relating to severe submandibular gland ptosis, the rhytidectomy surgeon may elect to perform a partial resection of the gland [34]. A detailed knowledge of the anatomy of the gland and its relationship to the facial vessels and marginal mandibular nerve is necessary for navigating this injury-prone region.

Relevant Cervical Anatomy

Dedo Classification of Cervical Deformities

Rejuvenation of the neck is a key goal of any successful cervicofacial rhytidectomy, and an understanding of cervical anatomy is central to determining which techniques should be employed to maximize the contour of the neck and jawline. This is especially true when considering the tremendous variation that exists in the shape and configuration of the neck across all individuals. Unlike the face, the anterior neck displays a less rigid arrangement – with the laryngeal framework varying in its position relative to the bony skeleton – and demonstrates greater variation in length and width as well as the distribution of subcutaneous and subplatysmal fat. In an attempt to categorize these anatomical variations into groups relative to their specific needs in surgical neck rejuvenation, rhytidectomy surgeons often employ the Dedo neck classification (Fig. 32.14), which can be summarized as follows [35]:

- *Dedo Class I* – Describes a youthful neck with smooth skin, without banding, and without adiposis. Class I necks have ideal projection of the mentum and a sharp cervicomental angle of 90–110° and are considered aesthetically ideal.
- *Dedo Class II* – Class II necks show excess skin laxity and thus rhytidosis of the anterior neck skin; with aging, all patients will develop at least this type of deformity.
- *Dedo Class III* – Dedo class III patients have excessive adipose tissue in the anterior neck. The fat can be in the subcutaneous or subplatysmal plane, and it is important to differentiate between the two, as conventional liposuction will not remove fat located under the platysmal muscle. Subplatysmal fat can be excised via an open lipectomy with anterior platysmal plication, as will be discussed later in this chapter.
- *Dedo Class IV* – These individuals demonstrate significant ptosis of the platysmal muscle, demonstrating vertical banding of the neck. Significant platysmal banding often requires partial excision and/or plication of the anterior muscle edges.
- *Dedo Class V* – Class V patients have receded chins. A receded chin shortens the hyo-mental distance, rendering a more obese or aged appearance to the individual. Augmentation genioplasty via implant placement or sliding genioplasty can successfully correct this deformity.
- *Dedo Class VI* – Class VI individuals may be the most challenging to treat and, in most instances, are less-than-ideal candidates for rejuvenation via a cervicofacial rhytidectomy. These patients have a more anteriorly and inferiorly positioned laryngeal framework and hyoid bone, which shortens the hyo-mental distance and blunts the cervicofacial angle to greater than 110 °. Dedo VI patients may still benefit from a rhytidectomy with a more aggressive open subplatysmal lipectomy with anterior plication of the platysma, though they should be provided limited expectations regarding the potential surgical outcome.

The Dedo classification can help organize the approach to neck rejuvenation during cervicofacial rhytidectomy, allowing the surgeon to maximize surgical outcomes by adding specific techniques in a customized approach that fits each patient's features. It is worth noting that the Dedo classes are not mutually exclusive, as often patients will present with multiple deformities; for example, an aging individual with rhytidosis and banding of the neck, a recessive chin, and subcutaneous adiposis would display Dedo class II, III, IV, and V features. However, because each feature requires its own specific procedure, maximal rejuvenation of a patient with Class II, III, IV, and V features would require a rhytidectomy, platysmal plication, liposuction and/or open lipectomy, and augmentation genioplasty, respectively.

De Castro Classification of Platysma Patterns

The platysma muscle also displays some variation in its configuration that may impact a surgeon's approach to neck rejuvenation during rhytidectomy. Figure 32.15 diagrams the three different platysmal patterns in the anterior neck

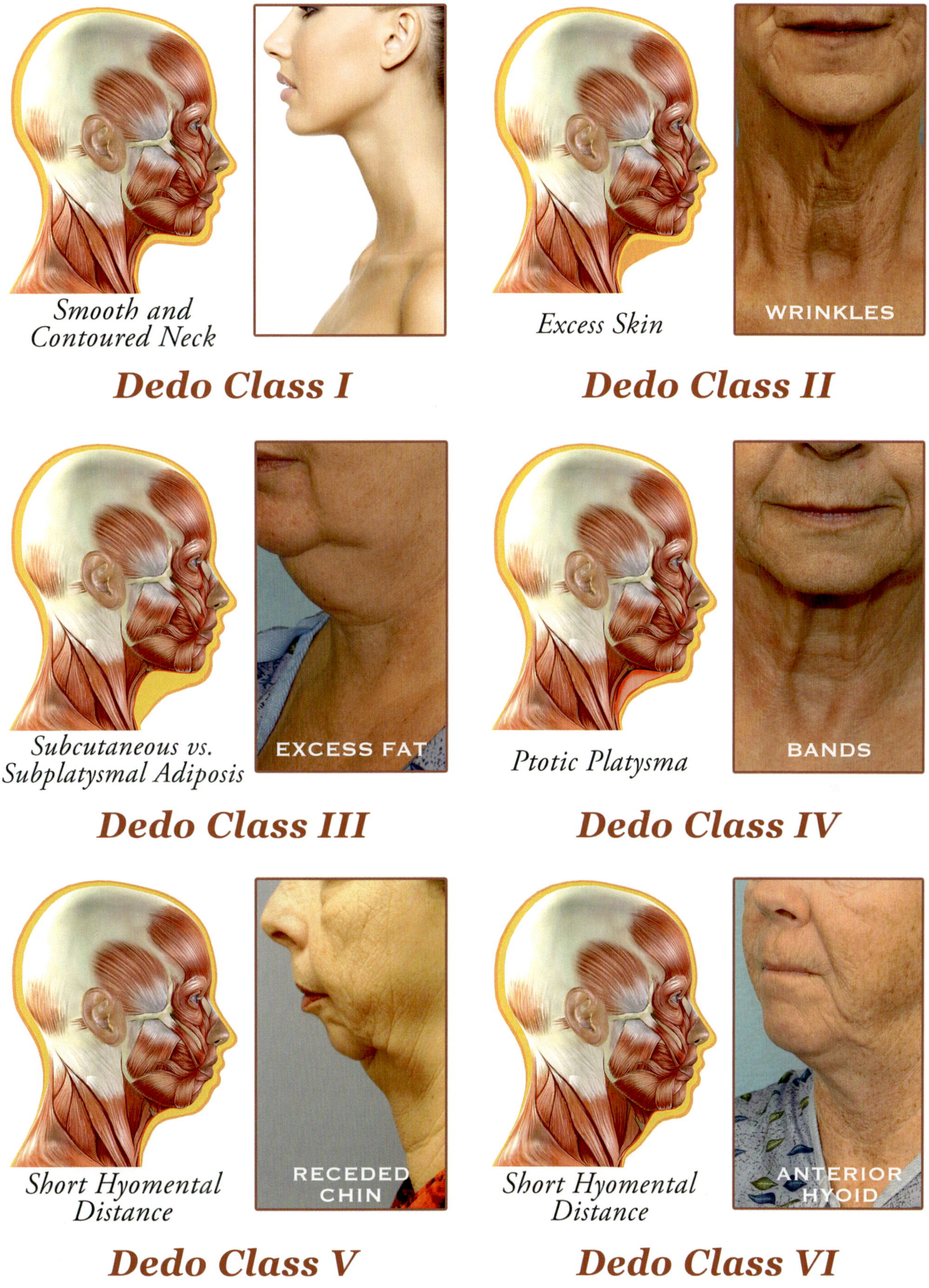

Fig. 32.14 The Dedo classification of cervical deformities

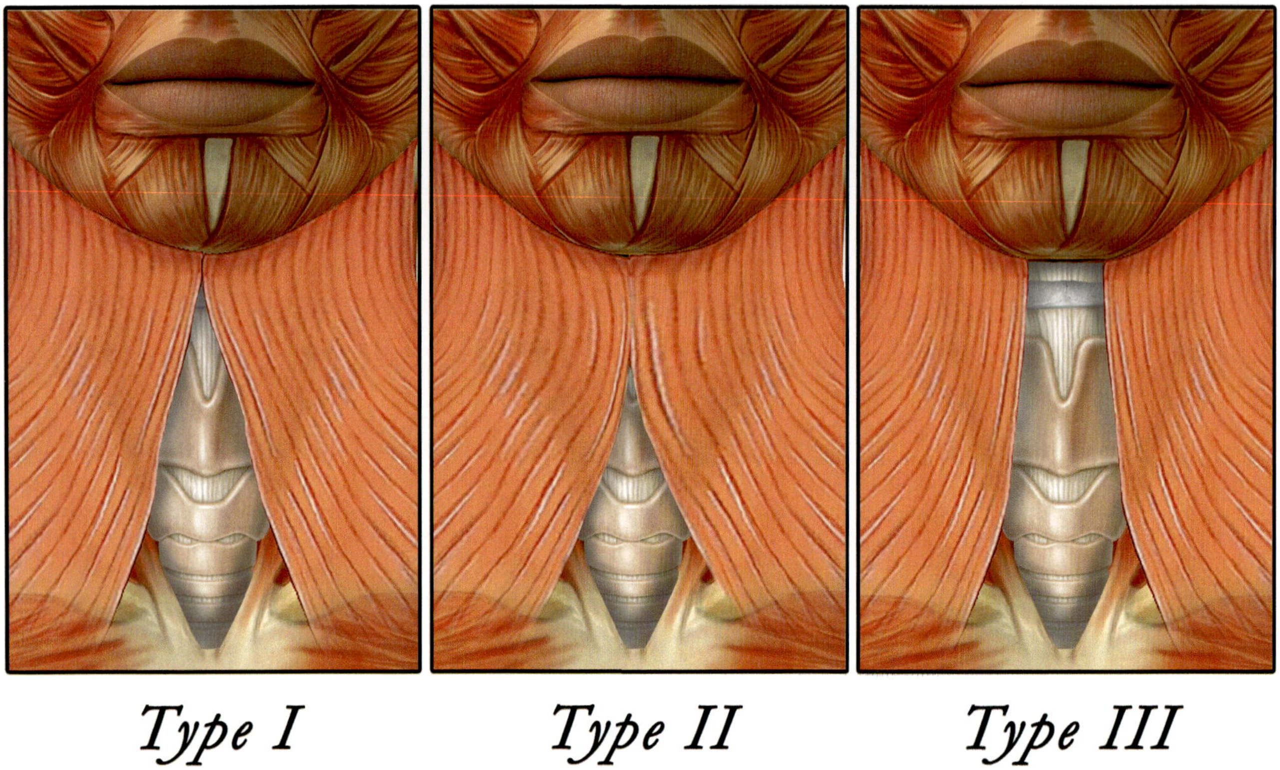

Fig. 32.15 The de Castro classification of the platysma muscle patterns

according to the de Castro classification [36]. The *type I pattern* is the most commonly encountered, with approximately 75% incidence across all individuals, and is characterized by a limited decussation of the platysmal fibers extending from the mentum to 1–2 cm below the mandibular symphysis. Individuals with the *type II pattern* show greater decussation, from the symphysis down to the thyroid cartilage, and make up 15% of all patients. Finally, the *type III pattern* is seen in 10% of individuals and shows no decussation along the entire length of the anterior platysma. The type of platysmal decussation can be useful to facelift surgeons, as those individuals with a type II platysma and minimal platysmal ptosis with a favorable cervicomental angle may do very well with a facelift without requiring any anterior (midline) platysmal work.

References

1. Farkas LG, Katic MJ, Forrest CR, Alt KW, Bagic I, Baltadjiev G, et al. International anthropometric study of facial morphology in various ethnic groups/races. J Craniofac Surg. 2005;16(4):615–46.
2. Le TT, Farkas LG, Ngim RC, Levin LS, Forrest CR. Proportionality in Asian and North American Caucasian faces using neoclassical facial canons as criteria. Aesthet Plast Surg. 2002;26(1):64–9.
3. Rossell-Perry P, Paredes-Leandro P. Anatomic study of the retaining ligaments of the face and applications for facial rejuvenation. Aesthet Plast Surg. 2013;37(3):504–12.
4. Rohrich RJ, Pessa JE. The retaining system of the face: histologic evaluation of the septal boundaries of the subcutaneous fat compartments. Plast Reconstr Surg. 2008;121(5):1804–9.
5. Wong CH, Hsieh MK, Mendelson B. The tear trough ligament: anatomical basis for the tear trough deformity. Plast Reconstr Surg. 2012;129(6):1392–402.
6. Yousif NJ, Gosain A, Matloub HS, Sanger JR, Madiedo G, Larson DL. The nasolabial fold: an anatomic and histologic reappraisal. Plast Reconstr Surg. 1994;93(1):60–9.
7. Alghoul M, Codner MA. Retaining ligaments of the face: review of anatomy and clinical applications. Aesthet Surg J. 2013;33(6):769–82.
8. Freilinger G, Gruber H, Happak W, Pechmann U. Surgical anatomy of the mimic muscle system and facial nerve: importance for reconstructive and aesthetic surgery. Plast Reconstr Surg. 1987;80(5):686–90.
9. Happak W, Burggasser G, Liu J, Gruber H, Freilinger G. Anatomy and histology of the mimic muscles and the supplying facial nerve. In: Stennert ER, Kreutzberg GW, Michel O, Jungehülsing M, editors. The facial nerve. Berlin/Heidelberg: Springer; 1994.
10. Furnas DW. The retaining ligaments of the cheek. Plast Reconstr Surg. 1989;83(1):11–6.
11. Rohrich RJ, Pessa JE. The fat compartments of the face: anatomy and clinical implications for cosmetic surgery. Plast Reconstr Surg. 2007;119(7):2219–27; discussion 2228–31.
12. Wan D, Amirlak B, Rohrich R, Davis K. The clinical importance of the fat compartments in midfacial aging. Plast Reconstr Surg Glob Open. 2013;1(9):e92.
13. Rohrich RJ, Pessa JE, Ristow B. The youthful cheek and the deep medial fat compartment. Plast Reconstr Surg. 2008;121(6):2107–12.

14. Tobias G, Binder W. The submalar triangle: its anatomy and clinical significance. Facial Plast Surg Clin North Am. 1994;2(3):255–64.
15. Zhang HM, Yan YP, Qi KM, Wang JQ, Liu ZF. Anatomical structure of the buccal fat pad and its clinical adaptations. Plast Reconstr Surg. 2002;109(7):2509–18; discussion 2519–20.
16. Yousuf S, Tubbs RS, Wartmann CT, Kapos T, Cohen-Gadol AA, Loukas M. A review of the gross anatomy, functions, pathology, and clinical uses of the buccal fat pad. Surg Radiol Anat. 2010;32(5):427–36.
17. Lam SM, Glasgold MJ, Glasgold RA. Complementary fat grafting. Philadelphia: Lippincott Williams & Wilkins; 2006.
18. Wright EJ, Struck SK. Facelift combined with simultaneous fractional laser resurfacing: outcomes and complications. J Plast Reconstr Aesthet Surg. 2015;68(10):1332–7.
19. Mitz V, Peyronie M. The superficial musculo aponeurotic system (SMAS) in the parotid and cheek area. Plast Reconstr Surg. 1976;58(1):80–8.
20. Broughton M, Fyfe GM. The superficial musculoaponeurotic system of the face: a model explored. Anat Res Int. 2013;2013:794682.
21. Barrett DM, Casanueva FJ, Wang T. Evolution of the rhytidectomy. World J Otorhinolaryngol Head Neck Surg. 2016;2(1):38–44.
22. Davies JC, Agur AMR, Fattah AY. Anatomic landmarks for localisation of the branches of the facial nerve. OA Anat. 2013;1(4):33.
23. Babakurban ST, Cakmak O, Kendir S, Elhan A, Quatela VC. Temporal branch of the facial nerve and its relationship to fascial layers. Arch Facial Plast Surg. 2010;12(1):16–23.
24. Trussler AP, Stephan P, Hatef D, Schaverien M, Meade R, Barton FE. The frontal branch of the facial nerve across the zygomatic arch: anatomical relevance of the high-SMAS technique. Plast Reconstr Surg. 2010;25(4):1221–30.
25. Ishikawa Y. An anatomical study on the distribution of the temporal branch of the facial nerve. J Craniomaxillofac Surg. 1990;18(7):287–2.
26. Pitanguy I, Ramos AS. The frontal branch of the facial nerve: the importance of its variations in face lifting. Plast Reconstr Surg. 1966;38(4):352–6.
27. Alghoul M, Bitik O, McBride JD, Zins JE. Relationship of the zygomatic facial nerve to the retaining ligaments of the face: the sub-SMAS danger zone. Plast Reconstr Surg. 2013;131(2):245e–52e.
28. Saylam C, Ucerler H, Orhan M, Ozek C. Anatomical landmarks of the buccal branches of the facial nerve. Surg Radiol Anat. 2006;28(5):462–7.
29. Batra APS, Mahajan A, Gupta K. Marginal mandibular branch of the facial nerve: an anatomical study. Indian J Plast Surg. 2010;43(1):60–4.
30. Yang H, Gil Y, Lee H. Topographical anatomy of the transverse facial artery. Clin Anat. 2010;23(2):168–78.
31. Whetzel TP, Mathes SJ. Arterial anatomy of the face: an analysis of vascular territories and perforating cutaneous vessels. Plast Reconstr Surg. 1992;89(4):591–603.
32. Whetzel TP, Mathes SJ. The arterial supply of the face lift flap. Plast Reconstr Surg. 1997;100(2):480–6.
33. Richards AT, Digges N, Norton NS, Quinn TH, Say P, Galer C, Lydiatt K. Surgical anatomy of the parotid duct with emphasis on the major tributaries forming the duct and the relationship of the facial nerve to the duct. Clin Anat. 2004;17(6):463–7.
34. Mendelson BC, Tutino R. Submandibular gland reduction in aesthetic surgery of the neck: review of 112 consecutive cases. Plast Reconstr Surg. 2015;136(3):463–71.
35. Dedo DD. "How I do it" practical suggestions on facial plastic surgery. A preoperative classification of the neck for cervicofacial rhytidectomy. Laryngoscope. 1980;90(11):1894–6.
36. de Castro CC. The anatomy of the platysma muscle. Plast Reconstr Surg. 1980;66(5):680–3.

Approaches to Facelifting

33

Danny J. Soares and William E. Silver

Technical Terms and Abbreviation

RSTLs Relaxed skin tension lines SMAS Superficial Musculoaponeurotic System

The Aging Process of the Face

The aging process of the face can be summarized objectively as *a gradual increase in complexity of the face*. It is a genetically pre-programmed insidious alteration of cellular tissues that results in the atrophy of the fibromuscular, bony, and adiposal components of the face along with the loss of elasticity and turgor of the facial skin. Although the severity of aging at a given age varies widely across individuals, it is generally accepted that a multitude of internal and external factors impact the rate of tissue decline, including but not limited to UV exposure, carcinogen exposure, stress, illness, hormonal and weight fluctuations, and prior surgical interventions. From an aesthetic standpoint, the process of facial aging can be regarded as primarily impacting three major facial characteristics: *contour*, *volume*, and *skin uniformity* (Fig. 33.1).

Loss of Contour

Contour loss is the clearest physical sign of facial aging; it can be defined as the loss of definition of the lower face and neck caused by the gradual ptosis of the lower facial and cervical soft tissues; it is abetted by the progressive distension of the SMAS and platysma muscles due to the chronic repetition of facial movements. Although the effects of gravity certainly assist in the process of facial aging, gravity itself likely acts more to reveal facial aging than to induce it. The soft tissues of the lower face, specifically the jowl and the anterior cervical region, see the most significant distension with advancing age because of the extreme mobility of the lower face and neck required for mimetic expression, speech, and mastication. Furthermore, the jowl tissues lack the ligamentous suspensory support that characterizes the mid and upper facial regions, resulting in the onset of visible senescence as early as the third decade of life. A validated grading scale for lower facial laxity helps to objectively quantify the degree of lower facial aging (Fig. 33.2) [1]. The descent of the jowl tissues distorts and conceals the linearity of the jawline and renders the facial shape squarer compared to the youthful countenance. Furthermore, bony remodeling is known to occur with facial aging, resulting in the inferolateral displacement of key support regions such as the malar and inferior orbital rim regions [2, 3]. In addition, the mandible also undergoes bony remodeling, with deepening of the pre-jowl sulcus and blunting of the mandibular angle [4].

The neck also undergoes dramatic contour loss during facial aging. Due to the descent of the lower facial tissues into the neck and the slow distension of the platysma muscle that often is associated with adiposal tissue hypertrophy in both the subcutaneous and the subplatysmal layers of the anterior neck and submental regions, the sharpness of the cervicofacial angle may become completely veiled by the ptotic and hypertrophied anterior cervical soft tissues. The Dedo classification previously described (Fig. 32.14) outlines the different classes of neck deformities, including all of those that relate to facial aging. Understanding this classification assists the rhytidectomy surgeon in determining the best surgical techniques necessary to achieve maximal rejuvenation in any patient.

D. J. Soares (✉)
Department of Otolaryngology, Head and Neck Surgery, University of Central Florida College of Medicine, Orlando, FL, USA

Mesos Plastic and Laser Surgery, Lady Lake, FL, USA
e-mail: Drsoares@mesoshealth.com

W. E. Silver
Department of Otolaryngology, Head and Neck Surgery, Emory University, Atlanta, GA, USA

Atlanta Institute for Facial Aesthetic Surgery, Atlanta, GA, USA

A. J. Cohen, C. N. Burkat (eds.), *Oculofacial, Orbital, and Lacrimal Surgery*, https://doi.org/10.1007/978-3-030-14092-2_33

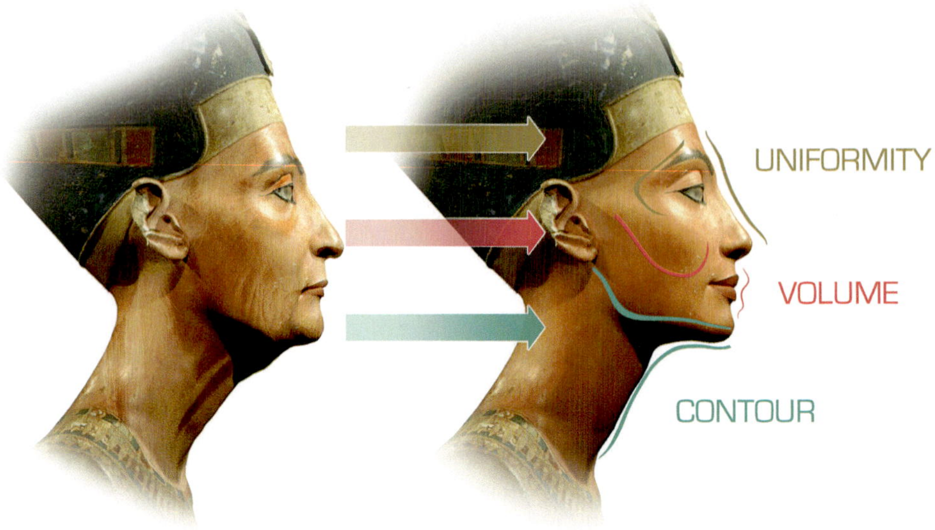

Fig. 33.1 The three major facial features affected by facial aging. Facial aging is characterized by a gradual increase in complexity of the face and can be described in terms of three separate features: loss of skeletal contour of the lower face, loss of volume, and loss of skin uniformity

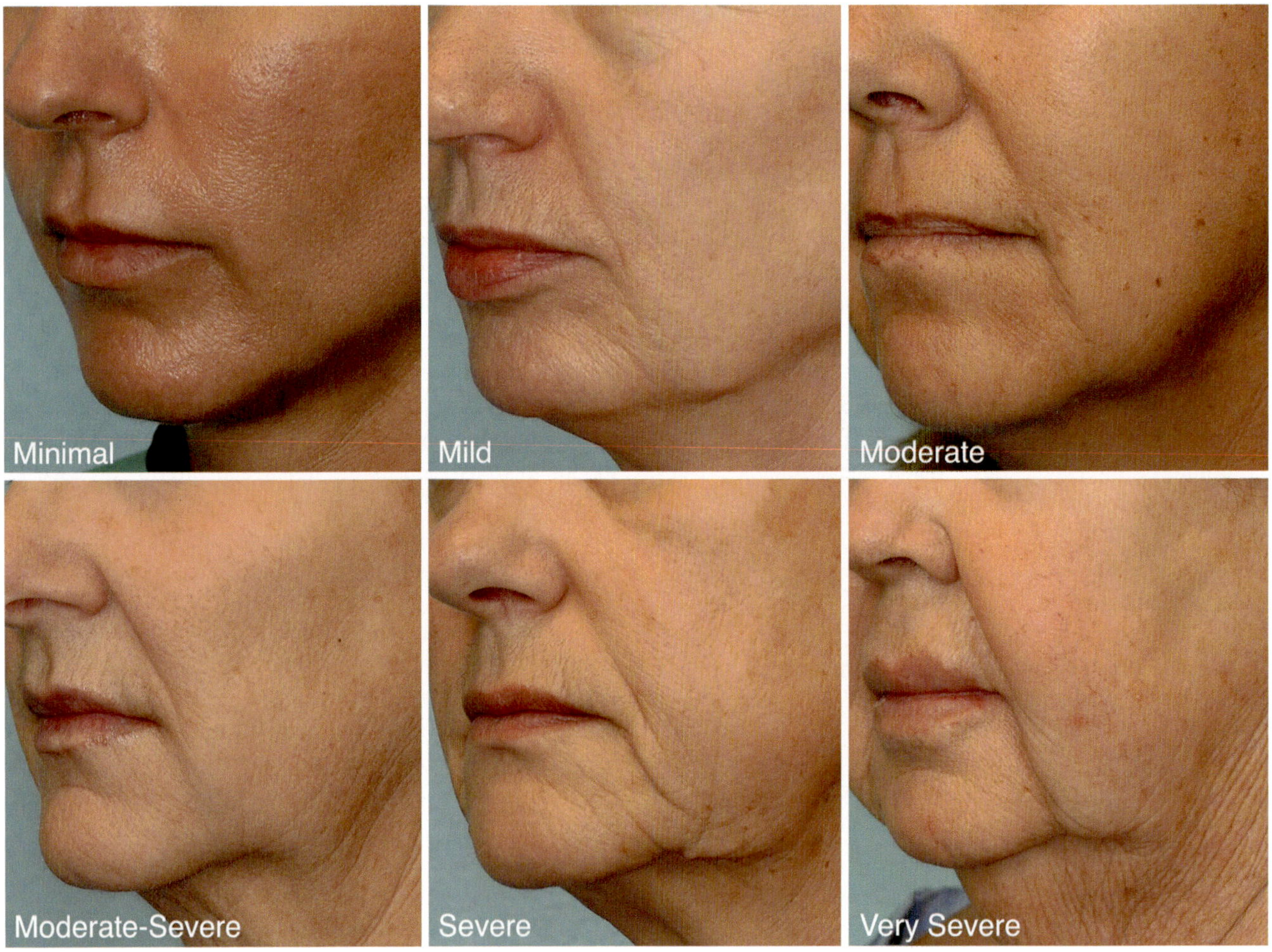

Fig. 33.2 Visual severity scale of lower facial tissue laxity

The midface can resist early malar soft tissue ptosis due to the suspensory function of the zygomatic and masseteric retaining ligaments, both of which directly counteract the repeated tension resulting from the upper lip elevators and the gravitational forces. Nonetheless, the midface eventually begins to descend due to the gradual elongation of the midfacial SMAS and the lytic bony remodeling associated with aging. These changes result in the loss of support of the malar fat pads, which simply ride atop the deeper fibromuscular tissues. Compounding the descent of the malar tissues, the volume of several fat compartments, such as the nasolabial and jowl fat pads, gradually increases, resulting in a *volumetric* component of aging that directly deepens the nasolabial folds [5]. The descent of the midfacial soft tissues results in the loss of contour of the midface as seen in the three-quarters facial view (Fig. 33.3). The malar descent causes the natural convexity of the cheek to flatten or even turn into a concave outline. Loss of midfacial support and malar descent are both of significance in rhytidectomy because ptotic midfacial tissues always compound and worsen the severity of aging of the lower face and neck, requiring a greater amount of lift to provide sufficient tissue excursion to restore the contour definition of the lower face and neck. This can only be achieved by a rhytidectomy technique that *(i) releases and re-suspends the midface* and *(ii) provides a powerful vertical vector of lifting*, as we'll see later in the chapter.

Loss of Volume

The volumetric nature of facial aging has been suspected and deliberated upon for decades, but has grown louder in recent years, now challenging the previous notion of gravitational tissue ptosis as the only force behind facial aging. In 2000, Donofrio first posited that "we have been conditioned for so long to accept 'sagging secondary to gravity' as a dictum that we have forgotten that it is only a supposition" [5]. Subsequently, in 2007, Lambros reintroduced the volumetric theory of aging in his photographic analysis of aging patients [6]. Although chronic fibromuscular distension due to repeated mimetic function, bony remodeling, dermal atrophy, and gravitational pull all contribute to facial aging, the apparent impact of volumetric alterations due to adiposal redistribution appears clear. Several studies have documented the gradual hypertrophy of specific facial fat compartments, directly leading to the development of deepened nasolabial and marionette folds. Lipoatrophy appears to coexist with adipose tissue hypertrophy in the aging face as well, with the latter seemingly impacting the submalar and suborbicularis oculi fat regions preferentially (Fig. 33.4) [7, 8]. The volumetric deflation of the midface secondary to lipoatrophy appears to compound and facilitate midfacial ptosis and aging. Our understanding of adipose tissue redistribution has helped rhytidectomy surgeons enhance their results through lipocontouring. Fat grafting is now often performed simultaneously, or in a staged fashion, with rhytidectomy [9]. Volume restoration to the submalar region and

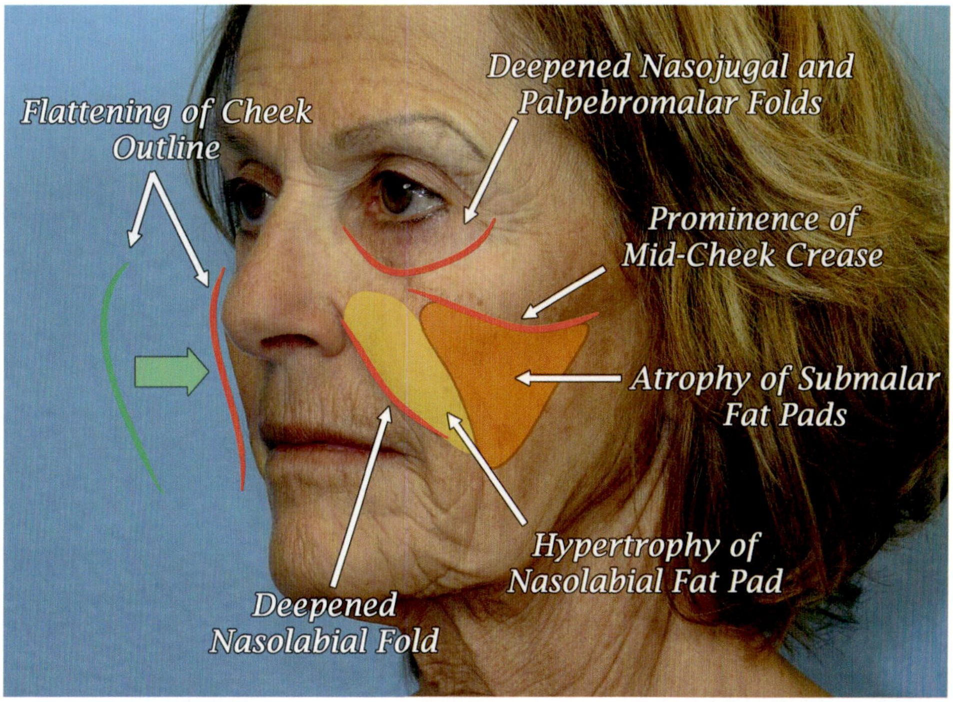

Fig. 33.3 The stigmata of midfacial aging. The process of aging is characterized by a gradual loss of volume in the submalar regions of the cheek along with ptosis of the midfacial soft tissues. In contrast, the nasolabial and jowl fat compartments witness an increase in adipose tissue volume. These changes result in a flattened midface, as seen in the three-quarter view, as well as a deepened nasolabial fold and pronounced nasojugal and palpebromalar folds. Volumetric depletion coupled with gradual ptosis of the midfacial tissues and bone loss in the orbitomalar region results in the development of the mid-cheek crease

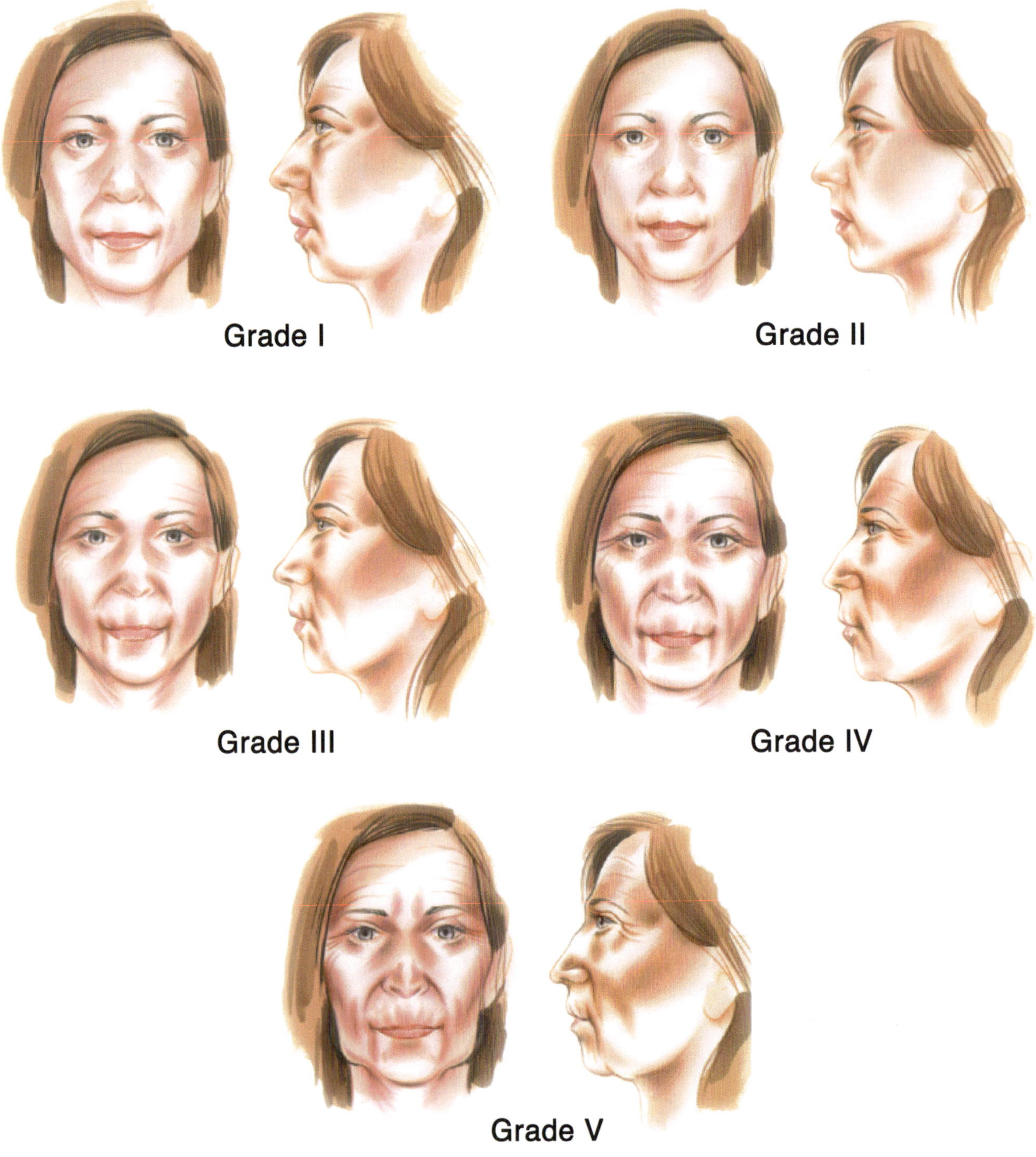

Fig. 33.4 Facial lipoatrophy scale. (Used with permission from Ascher et al. [8])

medial cheek is especially useful in re-contouring the cheek, restoring a natural fullness to the midface.

Loss of Skin Uniformity

The aging process impacts the uniformity of the skin more apparently than any other facial feature, and is objectively quantified by the Glogau scale (Fig. 33.5), summarized in Table 33.1 [10]. The gradual accumulation of genetic alterations, combined with the genetically driven dermal atrophy, aberrant collagen deposition, loss of elastic fiber content, and erroneous proliferation of dermal melanocytes, results in an extreme increase in the complexity of the skin surface. With aging, the dermis loses collagen, elastin, and glycosaminoglycan content, leading to the loss of the smooth texture and

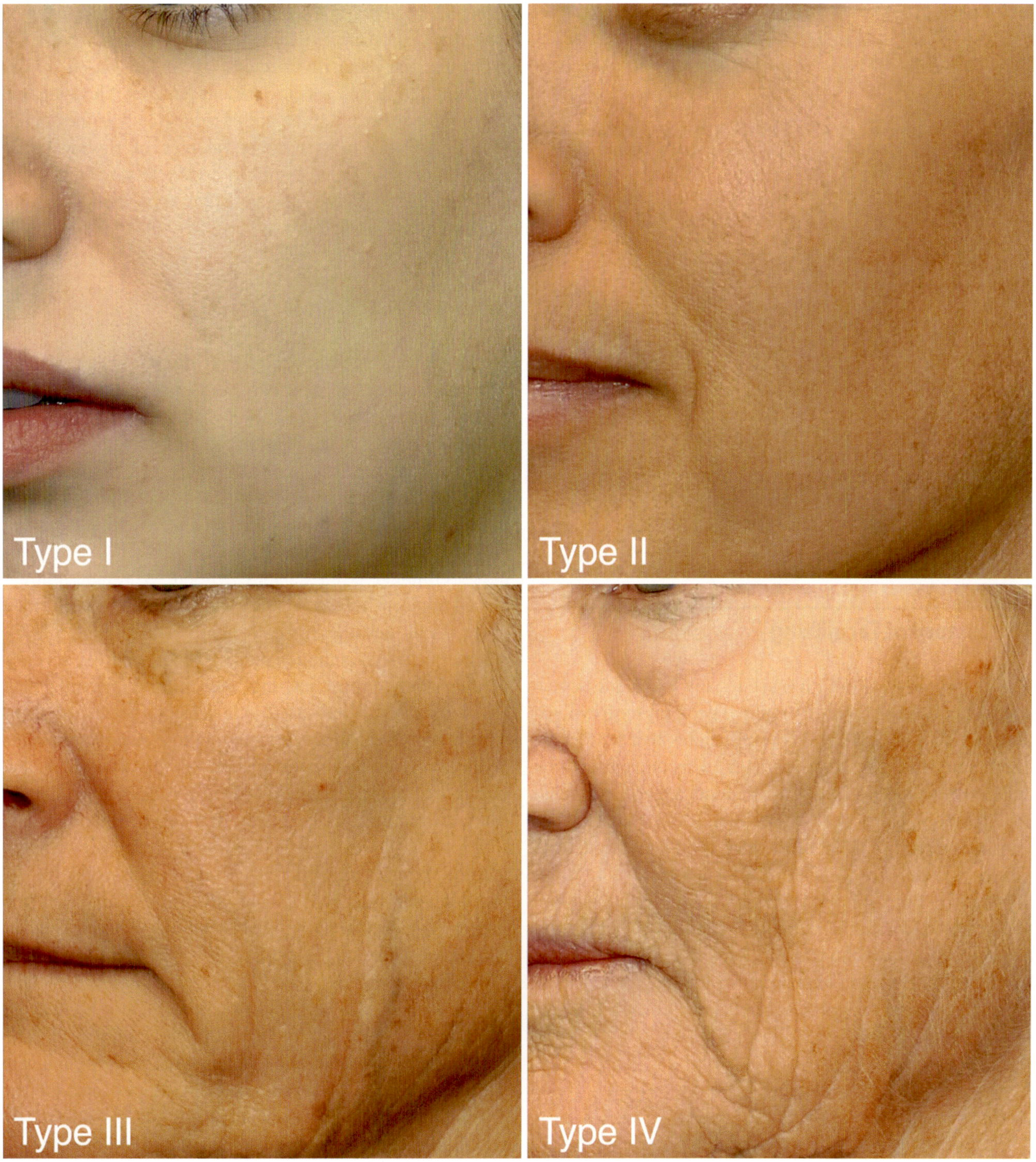

Fig. 33.5 A visual representation of the Glogau scale of photoaging of the facial skin

turgor that becomes evident as rhytidosis. The abnormal proliferation of melanocytes and endothelial cells promotes the development of solar lentigines, telangiectasias, and angiomas. Furthermore, the underlying ptosis of the fibromuscular layers of the face, compounded by the volumetric atrophy of facial fat pads, leads to the development of prominent folds and the exacerbation of facial rhytids. The rhytidectomy procedure is only capable of impacting one major factor influencing dermal aging, fibromuscular laxity. By suspending the ptotic facial SMAS, the surgeon can restore some degree of uniformity to the facial skin, improving the severity of rhytids. However, the procedure itself achieves no improvement in skin quality and provides no correction of age-associated dermal dyspigmentation. As a result, most modern rhytidectomy surgeons have incorporated skin resurfacing simultaneously with facelifting to maximize their surgical outcomes.

Table 33.1 Glogau photoaging classification[a]

Type I "No wrinkles"	*Patient age: 20–30s*	*Early photoaging* Mild pigmentary changes No keratoses Minimal wrinkles *Minimal or no makeup required*
Type II "Wrinkles in motion"	*Patient age: late 30–40s*	*Early-to-moderate photoaging* Early senile lentigines visible Keratoses palpable but not visible Parallel smile lines begin to appear *Usually wears some foundation*
Type III "Wrinkles at rest"	*Patient age: 50–60s*	*Advanced photoaging* Obvious dyschromia, telangiectasias Visible keratosis Wrinkles even when not moving *Always wears heavy foundation*
Type IV "Only wrinkles"	*Patient age: 60s +*	*Severe photoaging* Yellow-gray color of skin Prior skin malignancies Wrinkled throughout, no normal skin *Can't wear makeup, cakes, and cracks*

[a]From Glogau [10]

The History of Facelifting

The history of facelifting has seen many techniques come and go, but the central concepts of rhytidectomy have evolved to accumulate several rigid core principles that now guide the more-nuanced modern approach to facial rejuvenation that caters to the needs of each individual face. Although approximately half a dozen discernible rhytidectomy types exist today, each of them is especially suited to only handle specific patient-dependent degrees of aging. The apparent added complexity surrounding rhytidectomy today is more due to mere technicalities relating to how the SMAS should be suspended or which incision length or placement should be chosen than true advancements in the field of rhytidectomy. The rhytidectomy technique of choice could be thought of depending largely on the following factors:

1. *Severity of lower facial aging*
2. *Presence of significant midfacial ptosis*
3. *Presence of brow ptosis and periorbital aging*
4. *Dedo neck classification*

Identifying these factors objectively can help the surgeon determine the type of rhytidectomy procedure to pursue in order to achieve the best result. Please note that procedure cost, length of post-operative recovery, level of anesthesia, and duration of surgery are not primary factors used in determining the rhytidectomy technique of choice for a given patient cosmetically. Just as a surgical head and neck oncologist determines the most appropriate level of lymphadenectomy in the management of a specific stage of oropharyngeal cancer, the rhytidectomy surgeon must too determine the ideal rhytidectomy technique based on the degree of aging and specific patient features. The four factors outlined above will be discussed in detail as they apply to choosing the most appropriate type of rhytidectomy. First, however, it is necessary to briefly review the history of rhytidectomy and the genesis of the myriad of facelifting techniques available today.

History of Facelifting

1906–1976: The Skin-Only Rhytidectomy

The first facelift was reportedly performed in 1906 by Erich Lexer, a German surgeon, but only officially published as a procedure in 1912 by Eugen Van Höllander [11, 12]. Subsequently, several prominent surgeons of the time, including Joseph, Bourget, Passot, and Noël, published similar techniques in the first quarter of the twentieth century [13–16]. The earliest facelifts relied on strategically positioned elliptical skin excisions, without skin undermining, placed adjacent to the hairline and/or ears and performed under local anesthesia in a rapid fashion (Fig. 33.6). Although these techniques partially alleviated the severity of the facial rhytids, jowling, and neck skin laxity, they relied heavily on increased skin tension, predisposing to wide scarring and facial distortion. These issues were compounded by the fact that the skin was left attached to the underlying muscle and aponeurosis, rendering it significantly more unwieldy, especially at the level of the zygoma, which forced the surgeon to commit to exerting significant tension upon the skin. In 1927, Bames commented on the fact that such increased tension resulted in "stretching the surrounding skin so tightly that it gives an unnatural, harsh, and drawn appearance to the face" and thus better techniques were sought [17].

The second quarter of the twentieth century brought an increase in the popularity of the facelift, and with it the development of novel, though more invasive, techniques. Along with Bames, surgeons such as Burian and Seltzer promoted the wide subcutaneous undermining of the facial skin to facilitate the mobilization and suspension of the ptotic facial tissues (Fig. 33.7) [18, 19]. Such extensive skin undermining was not only thought necessary, but was regarded as crucial, as evidenced by the words of Burian in 1936:

> [When performing skin undermining during rhytidectomy] one must advance toward the cheekbone, where the skin is fixed to the periosteum through rather short and tight retinacula; this definitely must be separated, otherwise it will be impossible to correct the upper part of the [nasolabial] fold. One then continues down to the corner of the mouth, over the mandibular border, and then to the throat and the sternocleido-mastoideus muscle. [54]

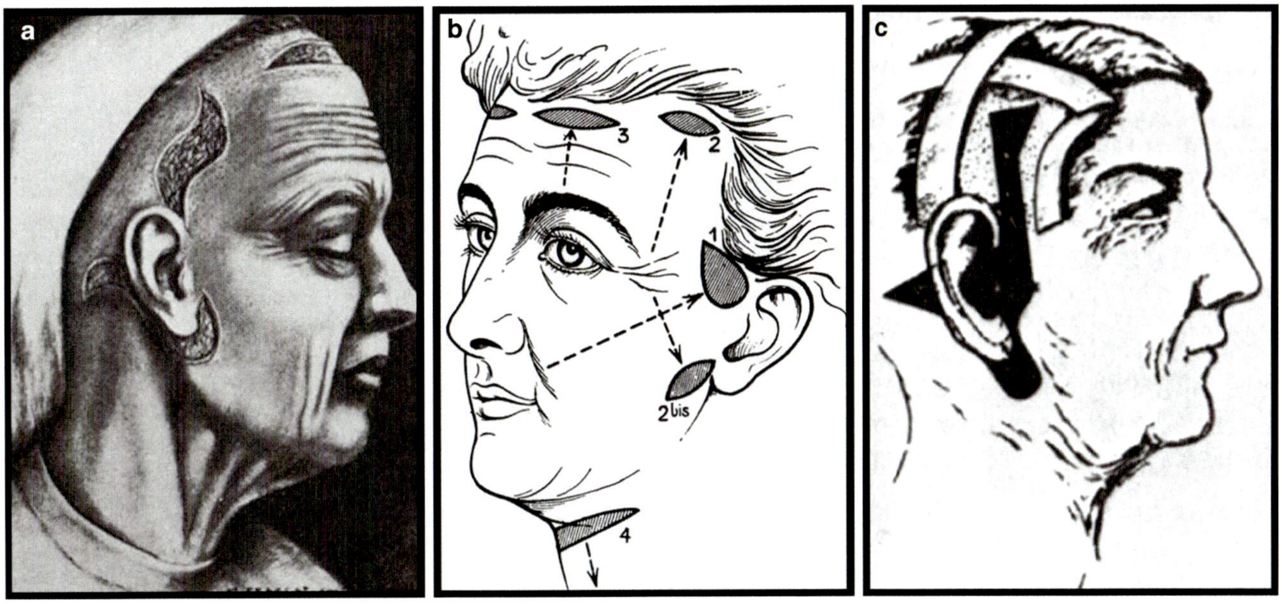

Fig. 33.6 Early rhytidectomy: Skin-only excisions without undermining. (**a**–**c**) Surgical technical illustrations published by Lexer (1931), Passot (1919), and Joseph (1928), respectively. (Used with permission from Gonzales-Ulloa [21, 70])

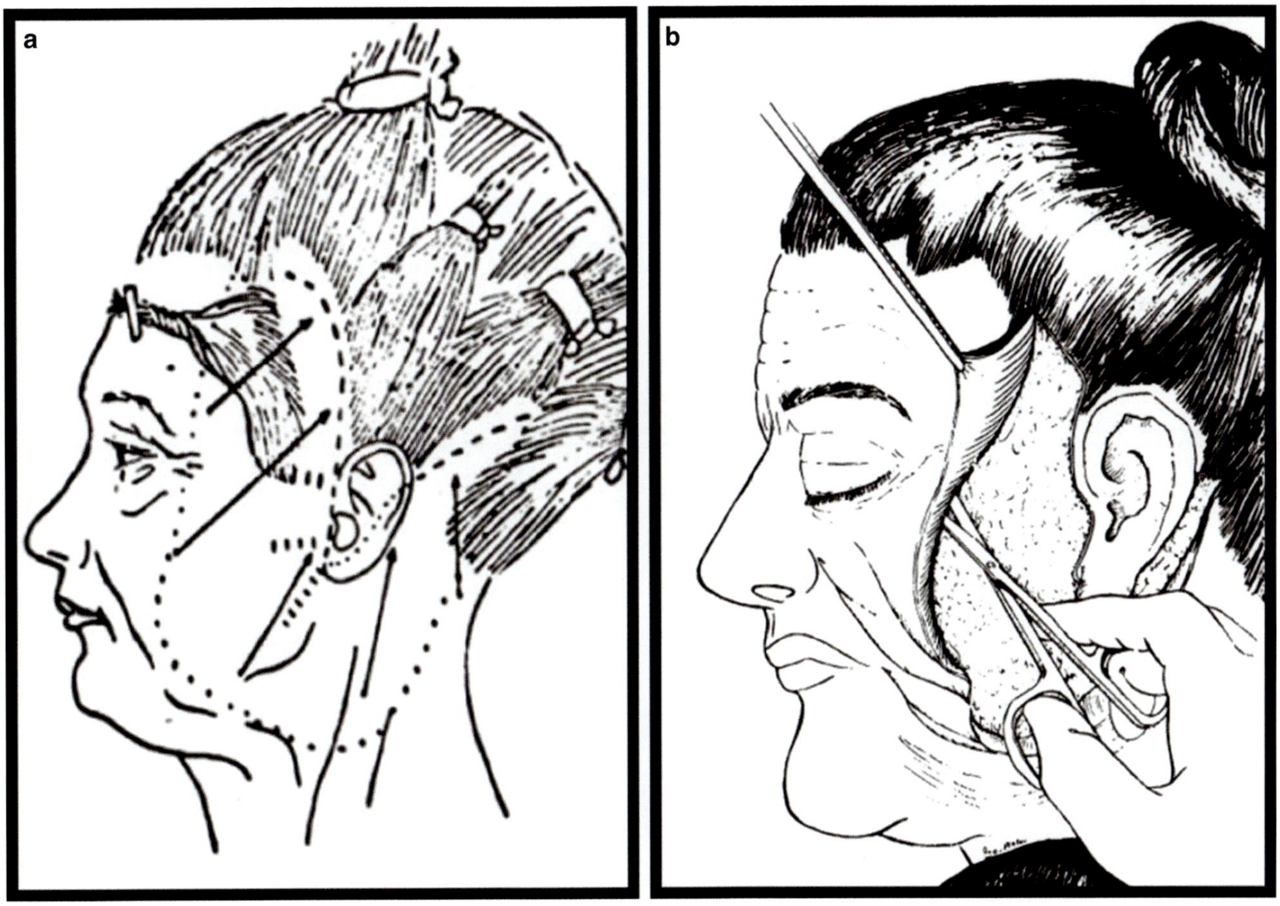

Fig. 33.7 Early rhytidectomy: Skin-only excision with subcutaneous undermining. (**a**, **b**) wide skin undermining was endorsed by Burian (**a**) in 1936 and Seltzer (**b**) in 1952. (Used with permission from Gonzales-Ulloa [70])

In describing these rigid areas of dermal attachments over the malar region, Burian was remarking on the dermal extension of the zygomatic retaining ligament, which restricts the motion of not only the skin but the SMAS and midface as well. The role of the zygomatic ligament and its restrictive nature preventing effective midfacial suspension and correction of the nasolabial fold would indeed receive the spotlight later in the evolution of the facelift.

In the 1950s, rhytidectomy techniques took on widely varying forms and degrees of invasiveness. While some surgeons experimented with modular combinations of rhytidectomy with brow/forehead lifting and upper and lower blepharoplasty, others, such as Gonzalez-Uloa in 1956, decidedly pursued ever more aggressive skin undermining (Fig. 33.8). However, with wide skin undermining, several problems also appeared, as illustrated by Johnson's comments in 1955:

> Slough of a portion of the flap may occur. This may possibly be due to a thin flap, a hematoma, or a combination of both. It may also occur from thrombosis of a vessel in the flap [20]

Furthermore, the high incidences of complications relating to heavy skin undermining, such as skin necrosis and hematoma, saw extraordinarily high numbers, with some large-scale studies revealing rates of 14% and 15.6%, respectively [21]. However, the most significant concern relating to skin-only lifting pertained to the limited longevity of skin-only lifts due to the skin's intrinsic elasticity, which precluded the long-term suspension of the ptotic soft tissues of the face. This was uniquely captured by Tord Skoog's remarks, prefacing the description of his rhytidectomy technique in 1974, which formed a watershed moment in the evolution of rhytidectomy:

> The facelift operation has recently gained wide-spread acceptance by the lay population and the medical profession at large. As in other aspects of plastic surgery, there has been a continuing search to improve techniques to achieve better and more lasting results, but surgical methods have remained basically unchanged and fairly routine. All the operations commonly employed share two principal features: (1) in undermining, the dissection is carried out almost exclusively within the subcutaneous tissue layer, close to the dermis, and

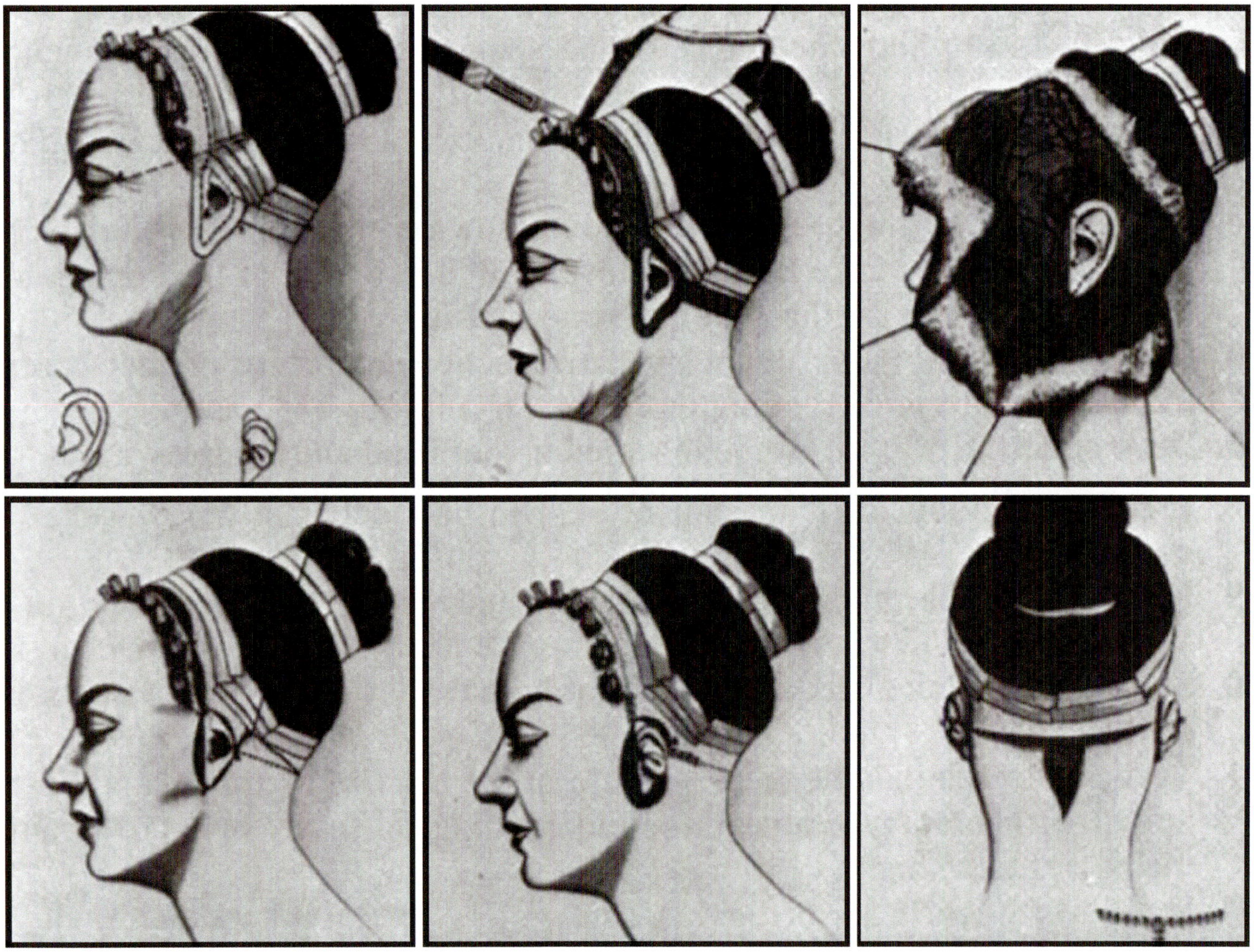

Fig. 33.8 Early rhytidectomy: Extended subcutaneous undermining. Gonzalez-Ulloa advocated for extended skin undermining of the face and neck in his "ear-island" technique published in 1956. (Used with permission from Gonzales-Ulloa [70])

> always external to the superficial fascia and the platysma; and (2) in closure, tension is placed mainly on the skin. This fails to consider an important relationship in the aging face. These deeper anatomic structures are in reality the foundation and architecture of the integument, and by deterioration in their position would automatically be reflected in facial form and expression. Yet, in spite of [this], nothing is done to readjust or reposition the deeper structures. When these basic anatomical changes are ignored and the surgical correction concerns itself with the skin alone, the result is compromised. [22]

The early contributions of Skoog, combined with the subsequent anatomical description of the SMAS, would form the core of the modern rhytidectomy.

1976–1990: The SMAS Rhytidectomy

The evolution of facelifting accelerated immensely with the description of the *superficial musculoaponeurotic system* by Mitz and Peyronie in 1976. Not only did they provide an anatomical and functional description of this important facial layer, but they also concluded their publication by surmising its potential use in facial cosmetic surgery:

> We have investigated the superficial musculo-aponeurotic system (SMAS) in the parotid and cheek areas by anatomical dissections, by radiographs, and by histological sections. The SMAS may be helpful in corrective surgery for facial palsy and during face lifting operations if a retrofascial approach is used.

With the birth of the SMAS rhytidectomy, surgeons saw an improvement in both the longevity and the contouring of the jawline and neck. The approach to the SMAS generated different techniques of suspension of the SMAS and platysma, ranging from simple folding (known as *plication*) to incising, undermining, and overlapping (known as *imbrication*) (Fig. 33.9). Still others performed a limited *SMASectomy*, in which a strip of SMAS was resected and re-approximated without undermining. Although facelifts employing a SMAS suspension yielded better and longer-lasting contouring of the lower face and neck, the method of SMAS suspension did not necessarily seem to matter [23]. Furthermore, surgeons noticed that SMAS mobilization appeared to have no beneficial impact upon the midface and nasolabial fold; in fact, it seemed to worsen the fold. This is showcased in Webster's commentary on SMAS techniques in 1982:

> We have heard some surgeons say that they are carrying out SMAS maneuvers to improve "nasolabial folds". There seems to be a misconception here as to what backward and upward pulls on the SMAS do to the [nasolabial] grooves. (…) By and large we found that the SMAS surgery did little to improve commissure position or depth of [nasolabial] grooving and, in fact, that it made the latter worse until the skin closures were performed. [23]

Furthermore, histological studies performed on the SMAS anatomy revealed that the SMAS itself was the reason why the nasolabial fold failed to improve with standard SMAS techniques. In 1990, Barton astutely noted:

> The superficial musculoaponeurotic system (SMAS) is seen to become the investing fascia of the zygomaticus major and minor muscles in the medial cheek. The pull on the cheek flap during rhytidectomy is diffused by the attachment of the SMAS to these muscles. I believe that this attachment accounts for the minimal change in the nasolabial crease after a Skoog-type sub-SMAS face lift. [24]

This notable finding exposed a limitation of SMAS lifts to that point, providing the impetus for further developments that ushered in the Golden Era of facelifting. In an attempt to correct the nasolabial fold without compromising the benefits of the SMAS rhytidectomy, Hamra developed the *deep plane* of dissection, leading to another critical evolutionary period in facelifting, as discussed next.

1990–2005: The Extended SMAS Rhytidectomy

The resistance of the nasolabial folds to rejuvenation via SMAS techniques fueled the technical breakthroughs of the 1990s. Surgeons had noticed that, although tightening of the SMAS created a significant improvement in the contour of the lower face and neck, SMAS techniques failed to provide significant improvement in the severity of the nasolabial fold. This was because the SMAS suspension was also directly pulling on the fold itself. The aponeurotic SMAS that exists in the lateral face splits to envelop the zygomaticus muscles, and they in turn insert onto the nasolabial fold skin. Thus, in essence, when surgeons suspended the SMAS in a superolateral vector, they found that the nasolabial fold actually worsened (Fig. 33.10). In fact, the nasolabial fold would improve only upon subsequent re-draping of the skin under tension [23]. This is because the pull on the skin forced the subcutaneous fat, which remained attached to the skin and sits above the SMAS, to roll outward and flatten the fold. However, surgeons found themselves once again relying on a high-tension closure of the skin to attain improvement of the nasolabial fold, which predisposed to wide scarring, dermal failure, poor longevity, and disruption of the face due to excessive, unnatural tension.

The Deep Plane Rhytidectomy

In 1990, Hamra published his seminal work on the first technique designed to tackle the nasolabial fold without compromising the benefits of SMAS suspension and without placing undue tension on the skin; he labeled it the *Deep Plane Rhytidectomy* (Fig. 33.11) [25]. This technique created a composite skin-SMAS flap that was undermined from lateral to medial; however, it introduced three important components previously absent in SMAS rhytidectomies:

(i) *It performed a heavy undermining of the SMAS over the zygoma and buccal regions.* This allowed for the complete release of the midfacial SMAS via lysis of the zygomatic retaining ligament and the masseteric

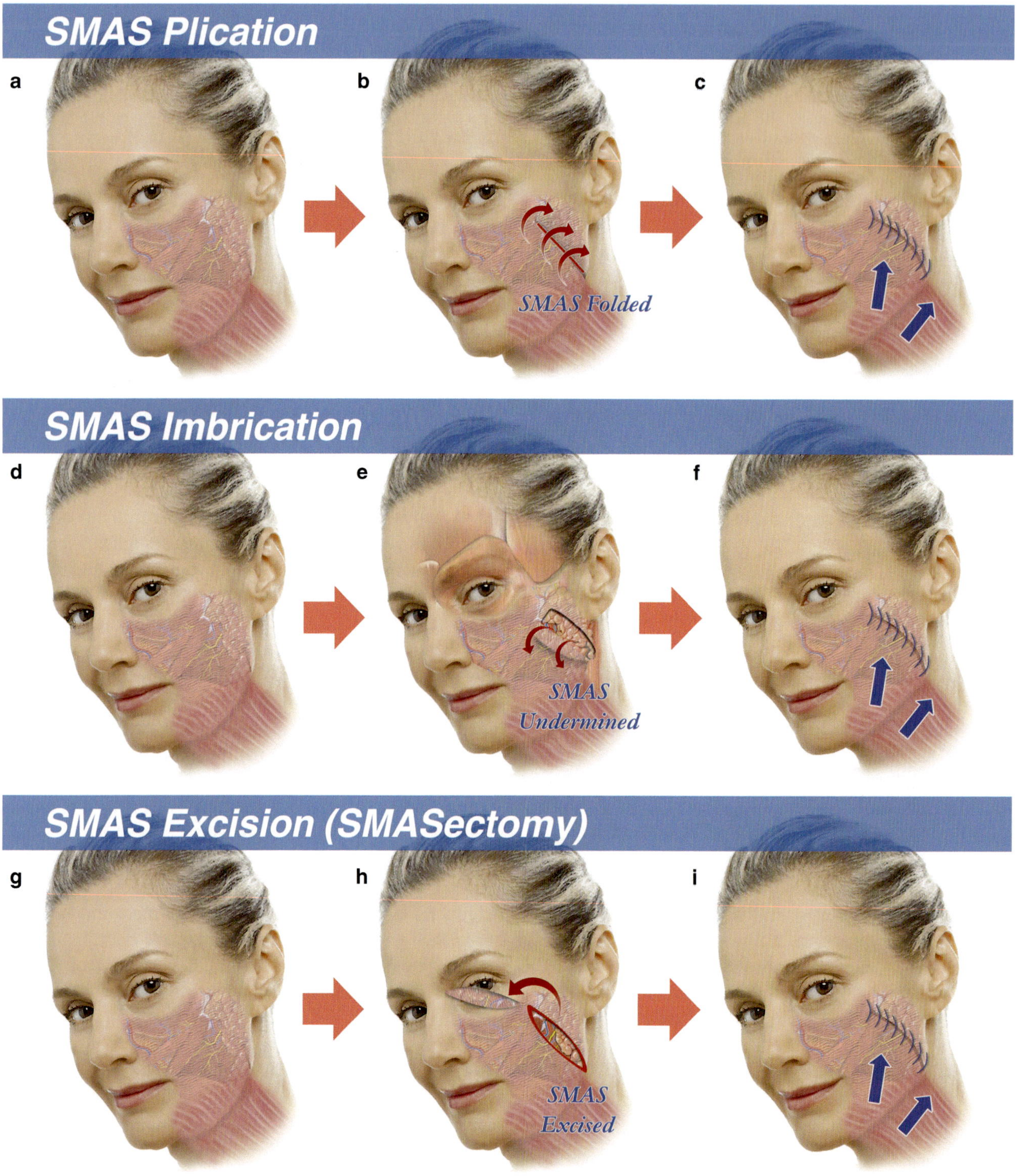

Fig. 33.9 SMAS suspension techniques. (**a–c**) SMAS plication: the SMAS is folded upon itself without need for SMAS cuts. (**d–f**) SMAS imbrication: the SMAS is incised, undermined, and then advanced posterosuperiorly. (**g–i**) SMASectomy: the SMAS is excised without undermining and then re-approximated

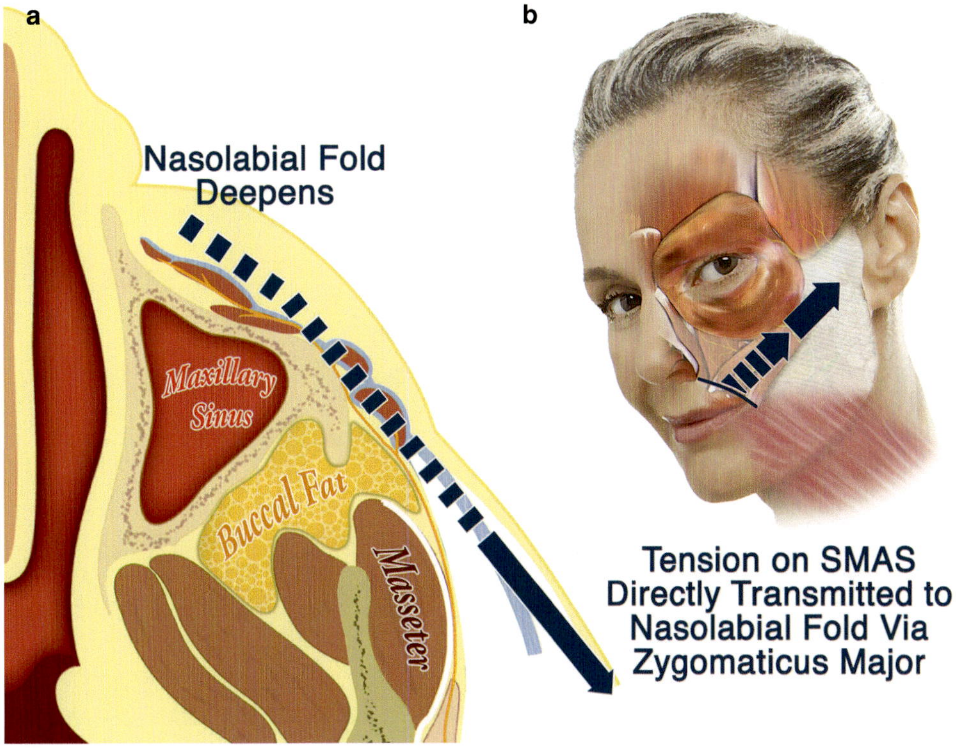

Fig. 33.10 The effect of SMAS tension on the nasolabial fold. (**a**) The aponeurotic SMAS envelops the zygomaticus musculature, which allows tension placed on the SMAS (dotted arrow) during rhytidectomy to be transmitted directly to the nasolabial fold. (**b**) Typical Skoog-type facelift techniques do not decouple the aponeurotic SMAS from the zygomaticus muscle, resulting in no improvement and possible worsening in the severity of the nasolabial fold due to the direct pull from the SMAS upon the nasolabial fold

retaining ligament, and for complete mobility of the midface. This expanded manipulation and undermining of the SMAs gave rise to the term *extended SMAS* rhytidectomies.

(ii) *It decoupled the midfacial SMAS from the zygomaticus musculature*. This had a dual effect: (1) it meant that the SMAS could now be suspended without directly pulling on, and worsening, the nasolabial fold, and (2) the suspension of the composite flap retained the ability to directly flatten the nasolabial fold due to it still being connected to the cheek subcutaneous fat.

(iii) *It relied on a composite flap of skin and SMAS*. This thick flap meant that extraordinarily high levels of tension could be placed on the suspension to allow for maximal correction of the nasolabial fold. Furthermore, because the SMAS was left attached to the skin, it also meant that the SMAS bore most of the tension, allowing the skin to be re-approximated with minimal dermal stress, thereby minimizing the risk of scarring and skin necrosis.

The term *deep plane* was coined by Hamra to differentiate from his previously published *tri-planar technique* (really an extended Skoog-type rhytidectomy) and to describe the dissection plane that allowed the surgeon to separate the midfacial SMAS from the zygomaticus musculature (Fig. 32.10) [26, 27]. If a surgeon extends a sub-SMAS dissection into the cheek, the dissection plane will naturally drive the surgeon directly underneath the zygomaticus major muscle because the SMAS splits to envelop the zygomaticus major muscle. The successful rhytidectomy surgeon will always avoid such a submuscular dissection as it carries a high risk of injury to the distal branches of the facial nerve. However, if the surgeon decided to pierce through the SMAS as it merges with the zygomaticus major muscle, the surgeon would then enter a new plane superficial to the zygomaticus muscle. This plane is Hamra's deep plane, which ironically is situated superficial to the muscular SMAS and sits immediately below the subcutaneous fat of the cheek. If the surgeon extends that plane bluntly, the entire cheek's soft tissue mass can be released from the underling musculature. The ultimate effect is one in which the lateral SMAS of the midface remains directly attached to the lower facial SMAS/platysma and the malar fat pads, but is decoupled from the zygomaticus major muscle, preventing the flap from directly pulling on the nasolabial fold upon suspension. The vector of pull in a deep plane rhytidectomy is intentionally superolateral in orientation, designed to be orthogonal to the nasolabial fold for maximum correction. Hamra's technique ushered a revolution in facelifting, gaining broad adoption, acceptance, and becoming a core technique used by surgeons today.

The High-SMAS Rhytidectomy

During the same period of expansive SMAS lifts, Barton himself developed and promoted his own perspective on a technique that closely mirrored that of the deep plane lift. Having himself understood and unearthed the importance of releasing the aponeurotic SMAS from the zygomaticus musculature, Barton constructed his own application of these

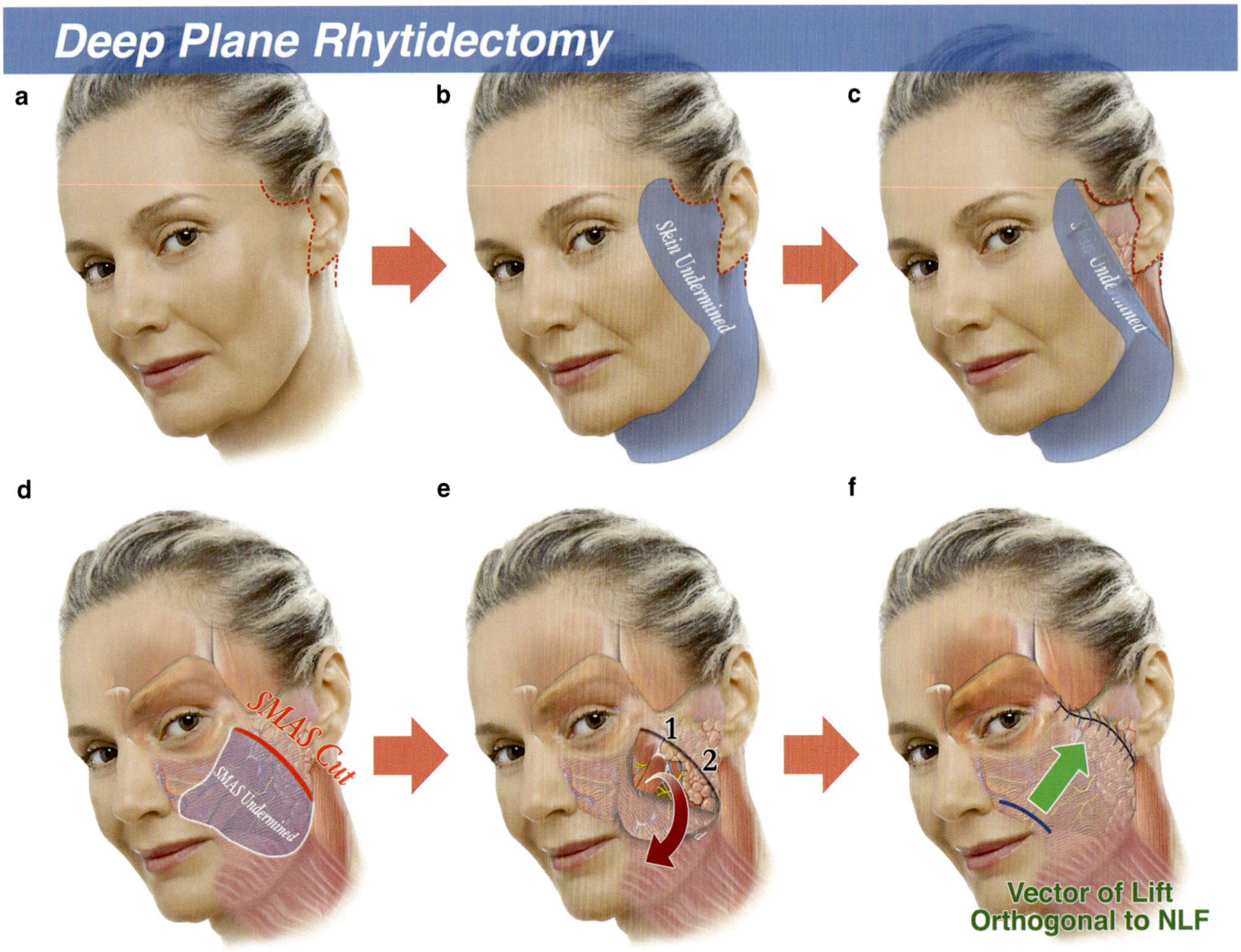

Fig. 33.11 Extended SMAS rhytidectomy: The deep plane technique. The deep plane technique as initially described by Hamra is defined by an extended sub-SMAS dissection that releases the malar soft tissues and decouples the SMAS from the zygomaticus major musculature, thereby allowing for greater correction of the nasolabial fold. (**a**) The skin incision for a deep plane facelift is typically placed in a trichophytic fashion along the temporal hairline due to the significant displacement of the midfacial soft tissues along the vertical vector. (**b**, **c**) The skin is undermined in the subcutaneous plane conservatively in the face but broadly in the neck due to the simultaneous anterior platysmal plication performed with this technique. (**d**) The SMAS is entered roughly along a line drawn from the malar eminence to the mandibular angle (red line). The SMAS is undermined sharply as a composite flap laterally and then bluntly along the deep plane of dissection between the zygomaticus muscles and the malar fat pads and into the buccal area (shaded region). (**e**) The sub-SMAS dissection effectively transects the zygomatic retaining ligament (1) and the masseteric retaining ligament (2), thereby freeing the midface and allowing for the suspension of the cheek soft tissues. (**f**) The cheek is suspended along a posterosuperior vector orthogonal to the nasolabial fold (green arrow). The procedure would later also incorporate an undermining of the medial zygomaticus-orbicularis (zygorbicular release) and a subciliary lower blepharoplasty with fat repositioning and septal reset, as described by Hamra

concepts in his *high-SMAS rhytidectomy*. [28]. Although similar in design to the deep plane facelift, employing a composite skin-muscle flap and releasing the SMAS aponeurosis from the zygomaticus musculature and the zygomatic ligament, the technique instead provided a more vertical vector of lifting (Fig. 33.12). The vertical vector of lift merged well with the vector of lift for the lower face, lending itself to improved tissue excursion and therefore a powerful rejuvenation of the lower face and neck in what is viewed as a more natural vector of suspension. However, because the midface had also been mobilized, the inferior component of the nasolabial fold also improved with this technique. The high-SMAS lift typically also combined an upper and lower blepharoplasty with lower orbicularis suspension, as well as an endoscopic forehead lift and a suprahyoid platysma plication.

The Subperiosteal Rhytidectomy

Although SMAS lifts dominated the evolution of rhytidectomy since their inception in 1974 with Tord Skoog, another major camp began to gain traction with the work of Tessier, first presented in 1979. Tessier advocated the use of an extended subperiosteal frontal rhytidectomy, which allowed for the repositioning of the entire upper facial soft tissues,

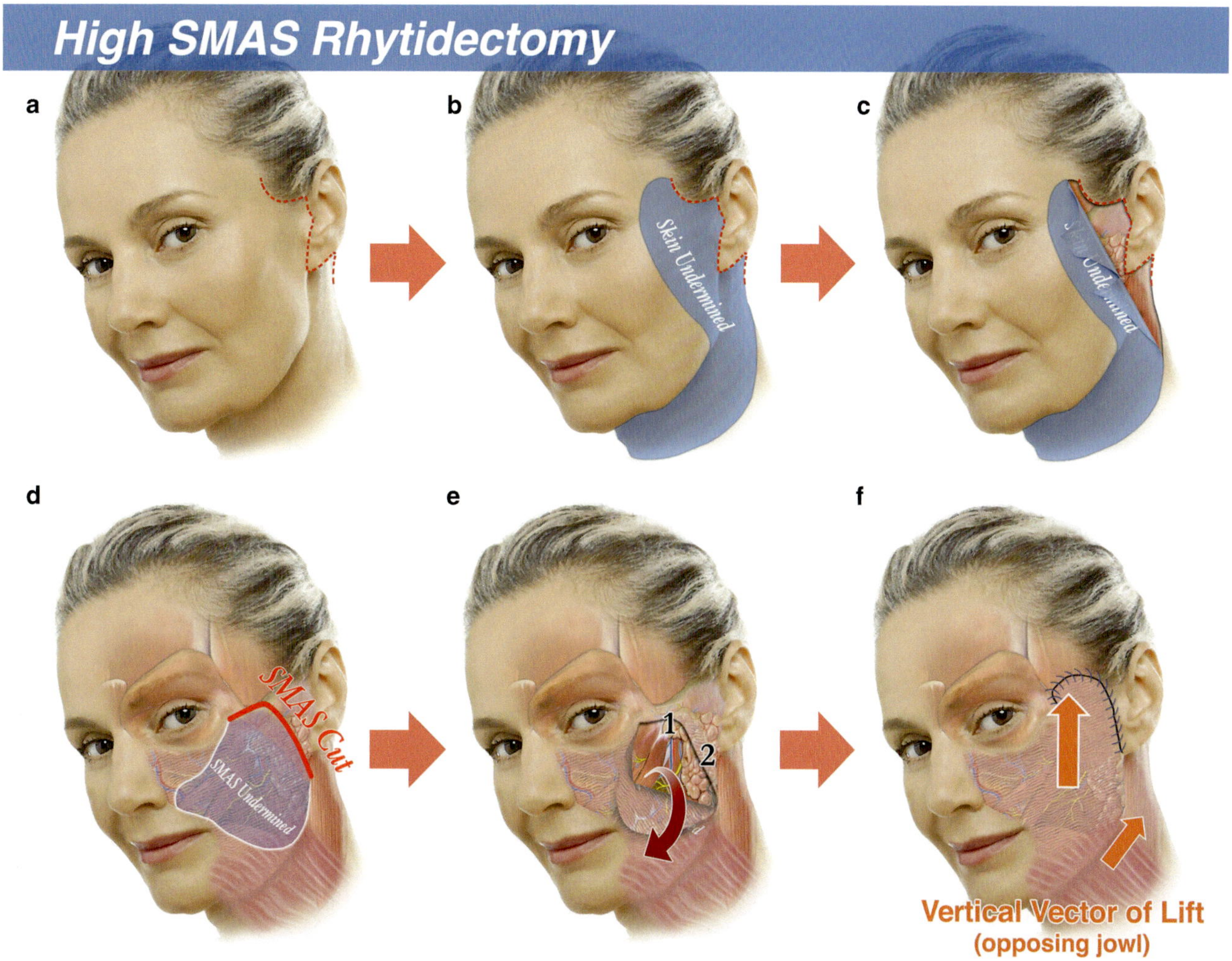

Fig. 33.12 Extended SMAS rhytidectomy: The high-SMAS technique. The high-SMAS technique, initially described by Barton, mirrors that of Hamra's deep plane and is also defined by an extended sub-SMAS dissection that releases the malar soft tissues and decouples the SMAS from the zygomaticus major musculature, thereby allowing for a greater correction of the nasolabial fold. (**a**) The skin incision for a high-SMAS facelift is typically placed in a trichophytic path along the temporal hairline due to the significant displacement of the midface along the vertical vector. (**b**, **c**) The skin is undermined in the subcutaneous plane conservatively in the face but broadly in the neck. (**d**) The SMAS is entered roughly along the zygomatic arch curving down toward the mandibular angle (red line). The SMAS is initially sharply undermined laterally as a composite flap and then dissected bluntly along the deep plane of dissection between the zygomaticus muscles and the malar fat pads and into the buccal area (shaded region). (**e**) The sub-SMAS dissection effectively transects the zygomatic retaining ligament (1) and the masseteric retaining ligament (2), thereby freeing the midface and allowing for the suspension of the cheek soft tissues. (**f**) The cheek is suspended along a largely superior vector (orange arrow) for maximal correction of lower facial aging and midfacial ptosis

including the brow and eyelid tissues, thereby preserving important anatomical relationships between periorbital structures [29]. In essence, the procedure represented an expanded subperiosteal brow lift that released the soft tissue attachments from the lateral orbital rim, superior zygoma, and anterior zygomatic arch. Gradually, with the work of Santana, Psillakis, and the seminal work by Ramirez in the 1990s, the procedure evolved to incorporate the release of the entire midface as well, through a subperiosteal/submuscular dissection plane [30, 31]. Ramirez's work modernized the procedure by adopting modifications that vastly reduced the incidence of temporal motor palsy (previously as high as 11%), and completely released the entire midface by joining the medial and lateral cheek/periorbital dissections (Fig. 33.13) [32, 33].

The subperiosteal rhytidectomy is unmatched in rejuvenation of the upper and middle face, and remains a core procedure to date. Despite its effectiveness in managing the aging of the upper face and middle face, the technique fails to address the aging of the lower face and neck, meaning that a concomitant standard SMAS rhytidectomy is still required for correction of the jowl and anterior neck laxity. For this reason, the subperiosteal rhytidectomy is regarded as a modular adjunct to facial rejuvenation rather than an alternative to the extended-SMAS techniques. The subperiosteal lift may be adopted in lieu of an extended SMAS technique such

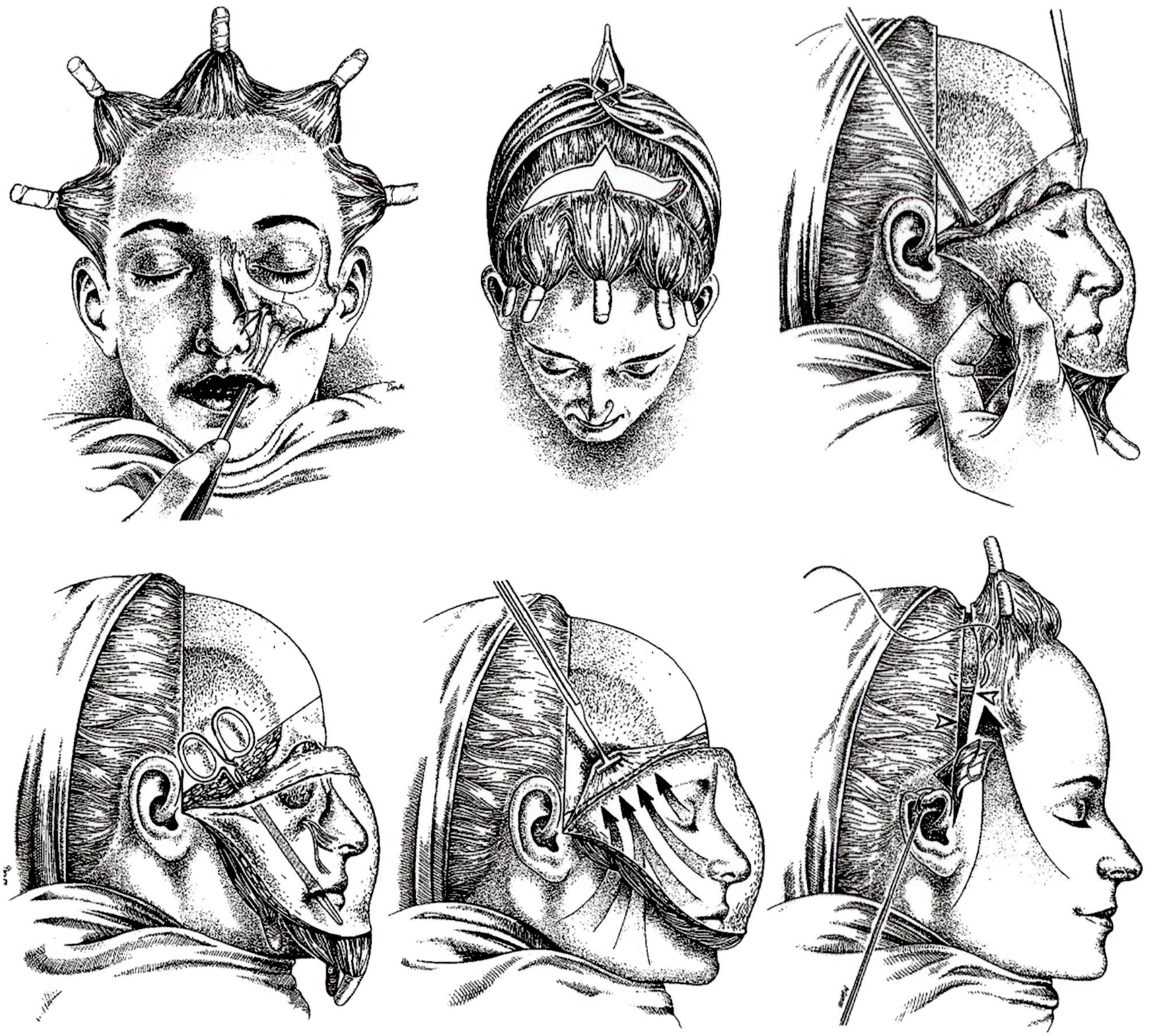

Fig. 33.13 The subperiosteal facelift. The subperiosteal rhytidectomy technique, initially described by Tessier, expanded on the frontal rhytidectomy and subperiosteal brow lift to incorporate a subperiosteal dissection of the entire midface and periorbital soft tissues. Despite its effectiveness in addressing the upper and *middle face*, it still required a conventional SMAS rhytidectomy to rejuvenate the lower face and neck. (Used with permission from de Saint Cyr et al. [33])

as the deep plane or high-SMAS rhytidectomies for the management of a ptotic midface and nasolabial fold.

With the advent of endoscopic techniques in the late 1990s, many surgeons switched to performing extended subperiosteal lifts endoscopically [34]. The subperiosteal lift is ideal for patients with upper and middle facial ptosis, and can be easily combined with other surgical procedures. This modularization of facial rejuvenation allowed surgeons to incorporate different surgical components into their surgical plan in an individualized approach. Nevertheless, some surgeons pursued *combo procedures* wherein whole-face rejuvenation of all aspects of facial aging was pursued; Hamra's *Composite Rhytidectomy*, published in 1992, served as the flagship technique.

The Composite Rhytidectomy

In an attempt to address the multiple aspects of upper, middle, and lower facial aging, Hamra introduced the composite rhytidectomy [35]. The procedure built on the standard deep plane technique but expanded the dissection to include the orbicularis oculi muscle into the composite flap and incorporated a coronal subgaleal brow lift, a subciliary lower blepharoplasty with fat repositioning, septal reset, and orbicularis suspension, and an upper blepharoplasty. The combined approach capably addressed aging in all aspects of the face, but proved to be an extensive (and more costly) undertaking not suitable for every surgeon and not immediately accessible to every patient. Although the

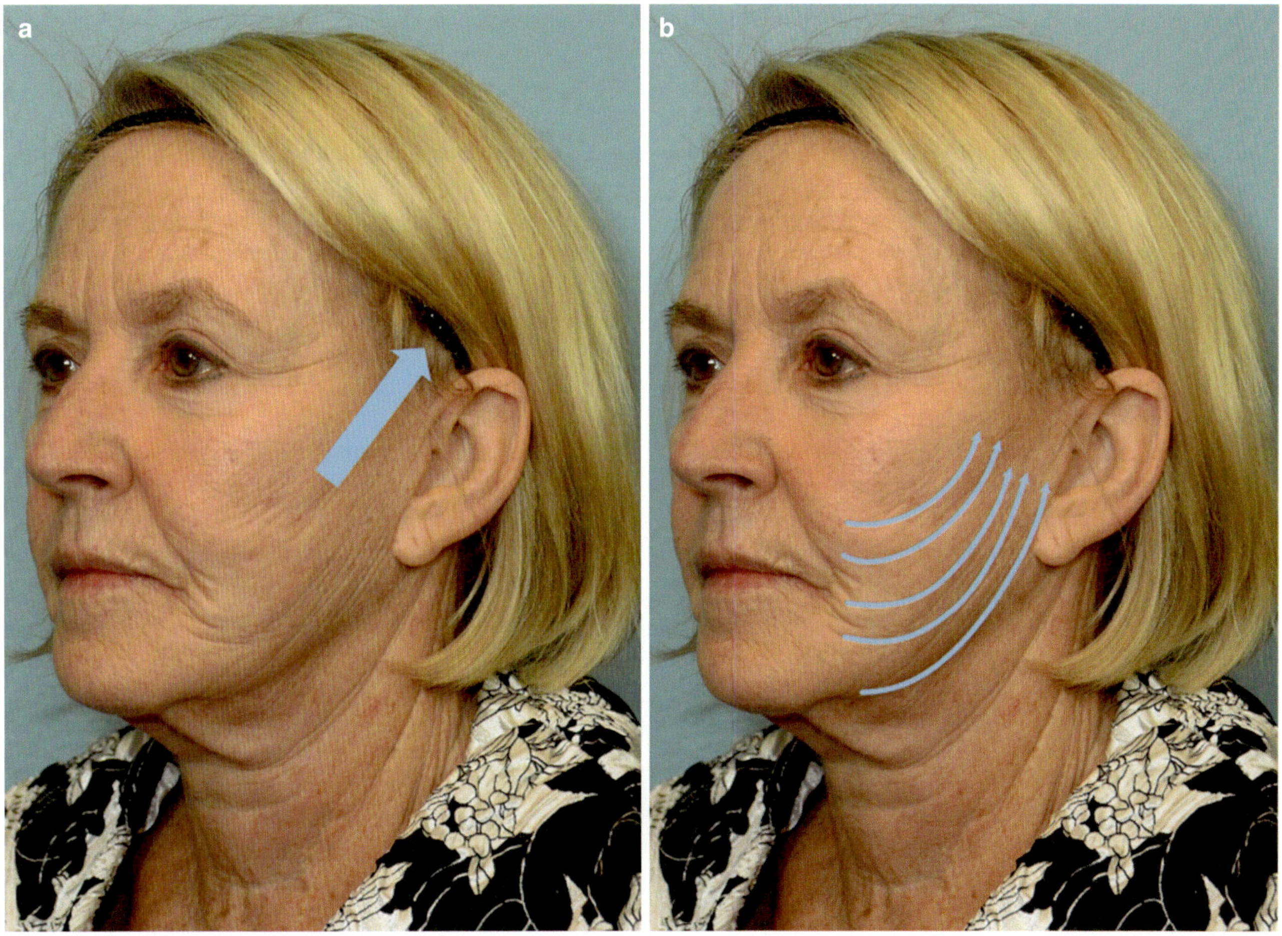

Fig. 33.14 Distorted facial RSTLs following a rhytidectomy technique employing a skin-SMAS composite flap. This patient had previously undergone a deep plane rhytidectomy, employing the traditional skin-SMAS composite flap. (**a**) The primary vector of lift for the SMAS is in the superomedial direction (orthogonal to the nasolabial fold) with the skin forcefully mobilized in the same direction and to the same extent as the SMAS. (**b**) Due to transmission of the SMAS tension onto the skin, this SMAS vector of tension distorts the facial relaxed skin tension lines (RSTLs), resulting in an unnatural appearance

composite rhytidectomy poignantly addresses the entirety of facial aging, it mostly reaffirms the modular nature of surgical facial rejuvenation, wherein individual procedures are combined to address each individual face maximally.

2005–Present: The Lamellar Extended-SMAS Rhytidectomy

The evolution of rhytidectomy continued into the new millennium with extended-SMAS rhytidectomies already established as the gold standard of rejuvenation of the midface, lower face, and neck. The modularization of facial rejuvenation continued to grow, incorporating endoscopic approaches to the brow and midface, as well as fractionated laser skin resurfacing methods. However, one challenge remained pertaining to the fact that a composite skin-SMAS flap forced the skin and SMAS to be repositioned in the same directional vector and to the same degree. The problematic nature of this issue became clear in patients with moderate-to-severe aging of the skin, in whom a tight suspension of the SMAS, required to counteract the severe ptosis of the face, still failed to correct all the laxity of the skin and instead forced the suspended SMAS to transmit its tension onto the skin, resulting in the distortion of the facial relaxed skin tension lines (RSTLs) (Fig. 33.14). Marten, who wrote about this issue in 2008, best documented its etiology:

> Composite-type dissections have the potential advantage that they can be performed more quickly and result in a comparatively thicker, arguably more durable flap composed of both skin and SMAS. These dissections have the distinct disadvantage, however, that skin and SMAS must be advanced by the same amount, in the same direction, and suspended under more or less the same amount of tension. Because skin and SMAS age at different rates and along somewhat different vectors however, optimal treatment of each layer is generally not possible when these techniques are used, and skin overshifting, skin overtightening, temporal hairline displacement, wrinkle shift from the neck to the cheek, and other objectionable occurrences and unnatural appearances can result. [36]

The need to specifically address excessive skin laxity in the moderate-to-severely aged face led to the *lamellar high-SMAS rhytidectomy* first described by Marten in 2005 [37]. In this technique, the skin and SMAS are both undermined, though the SMAS is kept in continuity with the platysma and the soft tissue mass of the cheek (Fig. 33.15). The SMAS undermining is pursued to the zygomaticus major muscle, releasing the zygomatic retaining ligament, and then proceeds to also separate the aponeurotic SMAS from the zygomaticus major muscle. However, special precautions should be taken when performing a lamellar high-SMAS rhytidectomy:

(i) *The skin undermining should not extend beyond the level of the zygomaticus muscle*—If the skin is undermined beyond this point, the surgeon may accidentally encounter the sub-SMAS plane, piercing the SMAS flap at the point where the dissection switches to a supra-zygomaticus major muscle plane, and disconnecting it from the midfacial soft tissue attachments as the two planes would merge. In such instance, the attachment of the SMAS flap to the cheek soft tissues would be disrupted, compromising the surgeon's ability to suspend the midface by pulling on the SMAS flap.

(ii) *An aggressive lamellar dissection theoretically carries a greater risk of injury to the transverse facial artery (TFA) perforators*—If the skin undermining and the sub-SMAS dissection is carried extensively into the submalar/buccal region, the perforating branches of the TFA may be harmed, significantly impeding the vascular supply to the majority of the flap.

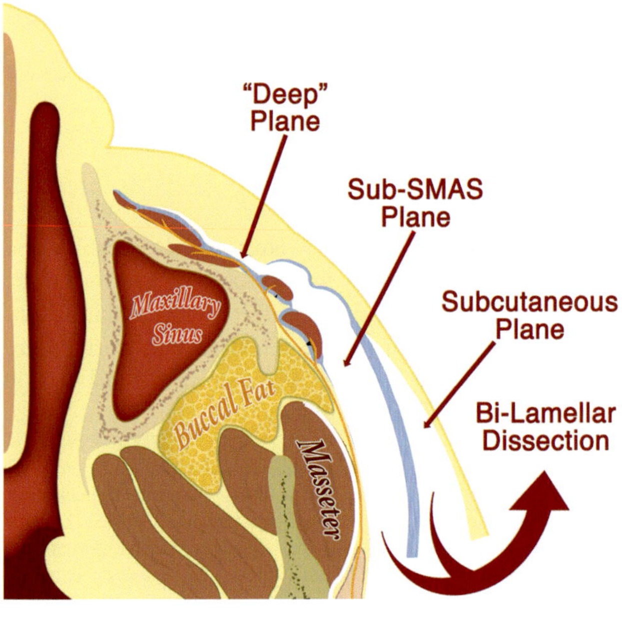

Fig. 33.15 Axial anatomy of a lamellar high-SMAS dissection. The lamellar high-SMAS rhytidectomy technique creates a bi-lamellar dissection of the skin and SMAS. The SMAS is separated from the zygomaticus major muscle and therefore decoupled from the nasolabial fold, just as it would with a high-SMAS or deep plane technique. In addition, the SMAS is still left partially attached to the midfacial soft tissues, allowing it to pull and suspend the cheek without worsening the nasolabial fold. The bi-lamellar dissection allows the skin and SMAS to be mobilized to different degrees and in different vectors, if necessary, thereby maximizing outcomes in patients with severe skin laxity and dermal elastosis

Though more time-consuming and demanding of a precise surgical technique, the lamellar dissection manages to re-drape the skin excess in a tension-free manner that maximally effaces facial rhytids without distorting the orientation of relaxed skin tension lines. However, the repositioning of the SMAS still allows the suspension of the face and neck tissues without requiring that any degree of tension be committed to the skin.

The Neck in Facelifting: A Brief History

From the very beginning, surgeons understood that a successful rhytidectomy, by default, also had to improve the contour of the lower face and cervicomental angle. The aging of the face and neck occurs together, and this is evidenced anatomically by the continuity of the SMAS into the platysma of the neck. The cervical platysma appears to elongate over time much in the same fashion as the SMAS, and distinguishing where the facial soft tissues end and the neck begins in the aged face can be quite difficult. Just like the SMAS, the platysma muscle has areas of firm attachments to the neck structure. The most significant attachment points occur laterally along the infra-lobular region (forming the platysma-auricular ligament) and along the anterior margin of the superior portion of the sternocleidomastoid muscle, as described by Furnas in 1989 (Fig. 33.16). The mandibular ligament also serves as a retention ligament for the platysma in the face. The platysma muscle, however, lacks any significant rigid attachments along the central neck, which allows the laryngeal framework to glide underneath during speech, mastication, and deglutition. For this reason, the laxity of the

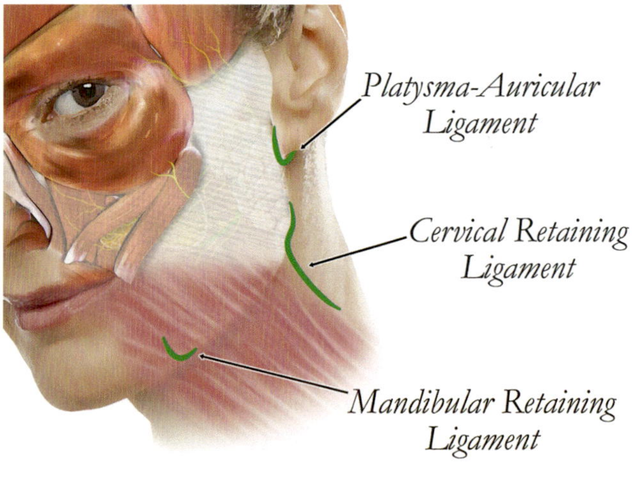

Fig. 33.16 The retaining ligaments of the platysma muscle. The platysma is affixed at several points within the cervical region. Mobilization of the platysma may be facilitated by the release of these ligaments

soft tissues of the neck is greatest in the central neck, while the resistance to lifting is greatest along the lateral neck.

The extent of cervical rejuvenation during the skin-only rhytidectomies of the early twentieth century centered around periauricular skin excisions, which pulled the skin laterally, stretching the skin into a sling that forced the neck tissues to be suspended. More courageous surgeons, such as Passot in 1919, would also excise central neck skin at the level of the hyoid bone [15]. Other surgeons, such as Maliniak in 1932, and later Millard, advocated for removal of excess subcutaneous fat from the submentum to improve the neck profile [38, 39]. In 1974, Tord Skoog began advocating for the suspension of the platysma muscle laterally against the mastoid periosteum in his rhytidectomy technique in order to achieve a longer-lasting rejuvenation of the neck. That same year, Guerrero-Santos published an elegant description of a laterally based platysma suspension [40]. The lateral suspension of the platysma muscle was thus born, serving as an immediate adjunct to the SMAS rhytidectomy.

In the ensuing years, surgeons began adopting techniques to remove soft tissue bulk from the central neck and plicate the anterior platysmal bands. In 1977, Connell and Aston both described their approach to neck rejuvenation via a combination of both a lateral and medial platysma suspension [41, 42]. Connel's approach also incorporated variable sectioning of the platysma muscle to achieve maximal correction of anterior laxity of the neck (Fig. 33.17) [43]. The evolution of the management of the neck thus reached a level of direct management that no longer relied simply on the rhytidectomy technique to improve neck contour.

With the development of extended-SMAS techniques in the 1990s, surgeons realized that the midface could be more easily repositioned, leading to greater vertical tissue excursion of the lower face. Incidentally, this enhanced ability to re-suspend the midface also heavily impacted the neck, as it generated a significant reduction in the bulk of tissue laxity in the cervical portion of the jowl and submental region. In 1990, Feldman also introduced his *corset platysmaplasty* in

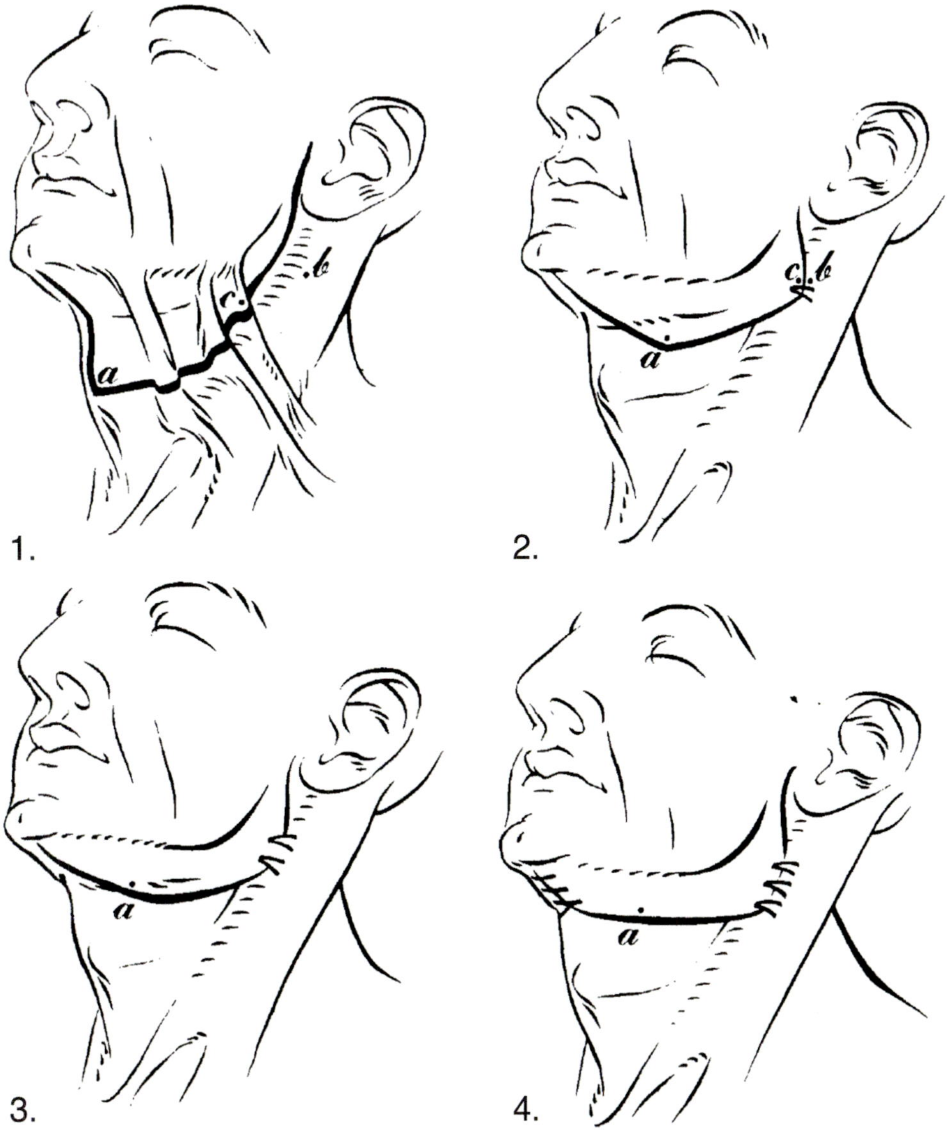

Fig. 33.17 Connell's lateral platysmal suspension with medial plication in 1978. (Used with permission from Connell [43])

an effort to completely eradicate platysmal banding along the entire length of the neck [44]. This procedure approximated the platysmal bands from the submentum to just above the sternal notch via a multi-pass running suture plication.

The development of these auxiliary surgical techniques helped the facelift surgeon maximize the rejuvenation of the neck in all patients. In addition to platysmal suspension, surgeons also began employing bony contouring of the mandible to correct microgenia or a pre-jowl sulcus [45]. Thus, modern surgeons have more surgical techniques and maneuvers available at their disposal than at any other point in the history of rhytidectomy. The challenge of the twenty-first century, nearly 115 years since the first rhytidectomy in 1906, now remains creating an algorithm-based modular approach to surgical facial rejuvenation that is custom-made to each individual face.

A Surgical Algorithm for Rhytidectomy

Every human has its own distinctive features, from their unique underlying bone structure to the intrinsic properties that govern the rate, configuration, and severity of aging unique to each face. As such, the combination of surgical procedures that offers near-ideal rejuvenation with the least invasive approach varies from person to person. Though the right procedure will always depend upon surgeon preference, training, and degree of familiarity, it is incumbent upon the surgeon to explore and gather an understanding of all the available techniques at his/her disposal. Ultimately, the priority of any surgeon is to "do no harm" well before it is to achieve maximal rejuvenation of the face. With that in mind, the surgeon should primarily assess the severity of aging of the neck and face, determine the existence of concurrent deformities, and formulate the least invasive plan that achieves the intended goal. The surgeon should consider the patient's intrinsic risk factors, including overall health, tolerance of anesthesia, and possible presence of tissue distortion from prior surgeries.

Choosing a Rhytidectomy Technique

Figure 33.18 summarizes the major techniques currently available to rhytidectomy surgeons already discussed in this

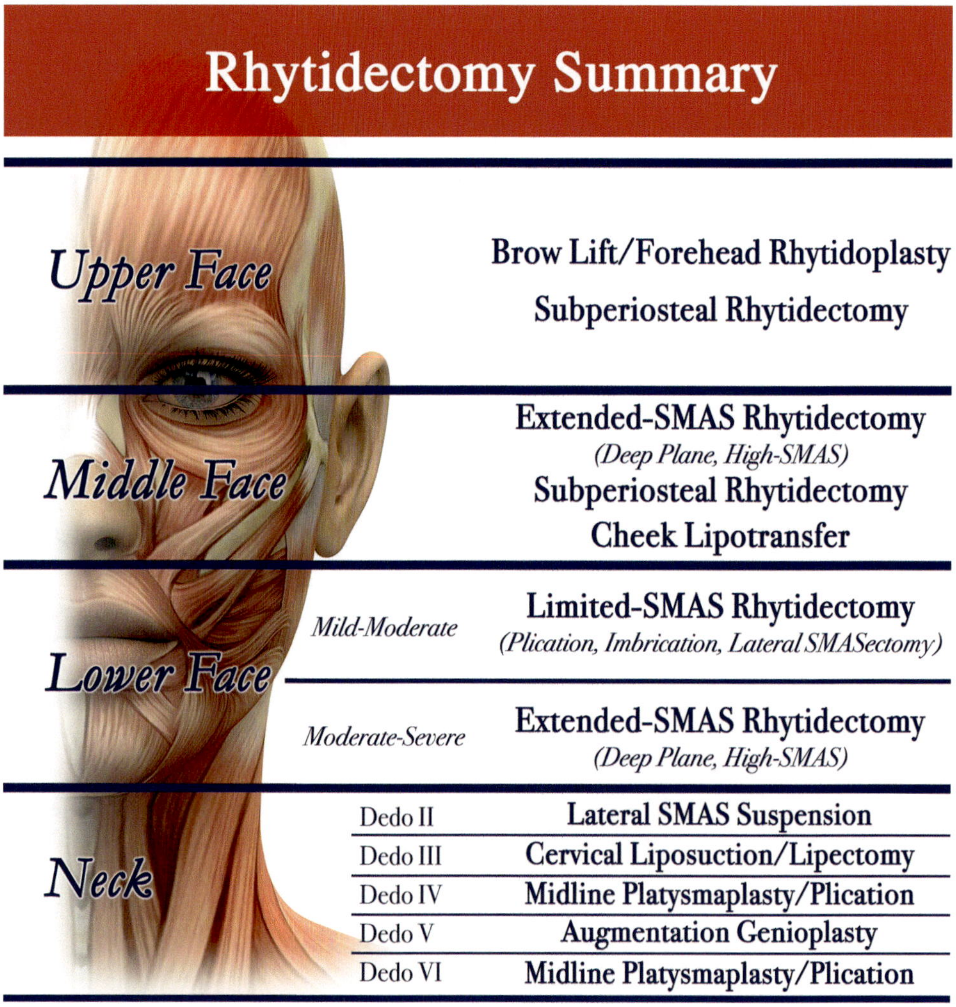

Fig. 33.18 The major rhytidectomy surgical techniques available to surgeons. The evolution of cosmetic surgery has resulted in the modularization of facial rejuvenation, which allows for the combination of multiple procedures to achieve maximal rejuvenation

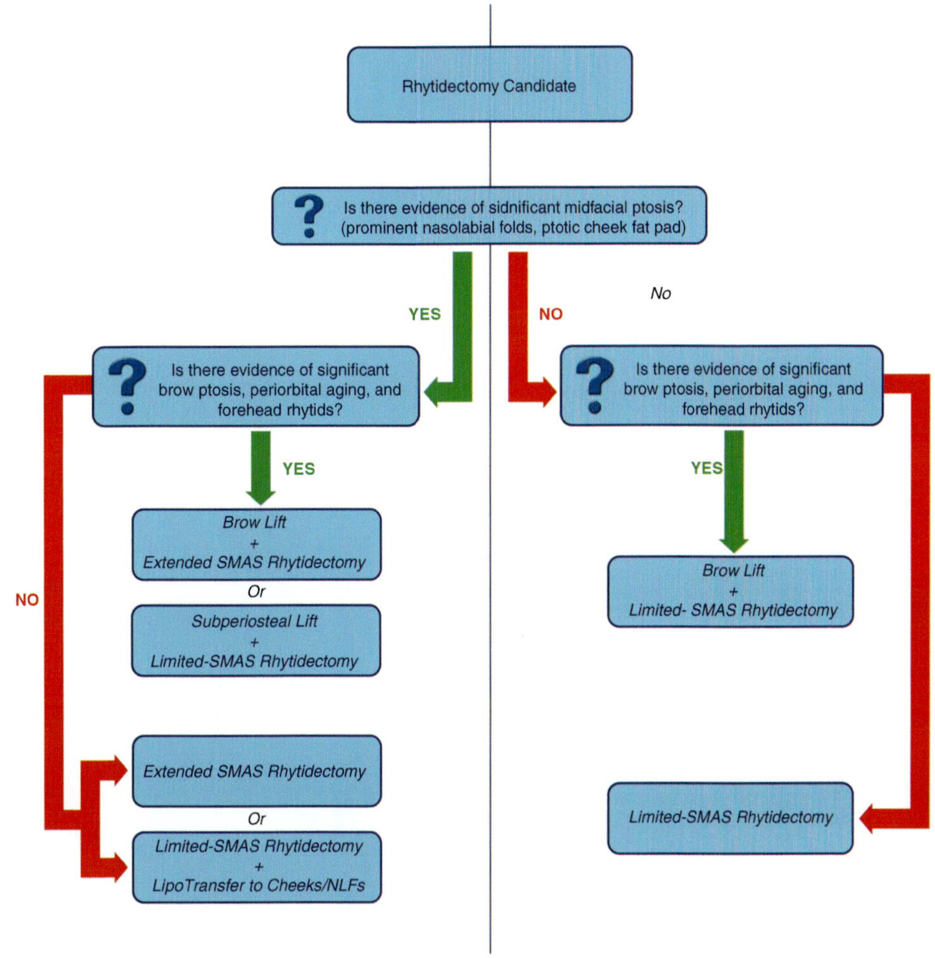

Fig. 33.19 Rhytidectomy surgical algorithm

chapter. Each technique is best suited for the management of a specific type, region, and severity of aging of the face. Although more aggressive techniques will undoubtedly still achieve successful outcomes in patients with mild aging, they are not often in the best interest of the patient given their longer anesthesia requirements and more prolonged recovery, as well as possibly increased risk of surgical complictions. Figure 33.19 outlines a brief algorithm that may be useful in guiding an approach to the rhytidectomy patient. In this algorithm, the first and most pertinent questions that surgeon must answer are:

1. *Is there evidence of significant midfacial ptosis?* Although it is incumbent upon the surgeon to determine what, in his/her view, should be regarded as significant midfacial ptosis, this author argues that severe midfacial ptosis is characterized by midfacial aging not completely overcome by isolated facial lipotransfer. Although lipotransfer can partially correct prominent nasolabial folds and midfacial ptosis, it is wholesomely inadequate in patients with moderate-to-severe midfacial ptosis. Significant midfacial ptosis can only be addressed via a procedure that releases and adequately suspends the midface, such as an extended-SMAS or subperiosteal lift.
2. *Is there evidence of significant brow ptosis, periorbital aging, and forehead rhytids?* The presence of brow ptosis and periorbital aging determines the need for rejuvenation of the upper face with brow/forehead suspension. If there is sufficient ptosis warranting surgical rejuvenation, the surgeon has the option of choosing between a subperiosteal lift—combined with a limited-SMAS rhytidectomy for lower face and neck aging—and a limited brow lift and an extended-SMAS rhytidectomy. Both combinations may be regarded as similar in the scope of effect and comprehensiveness of the lift.

Individuals with mild-to-moderate lower facial aging lacking any substantial midfacial or brow ptosis can be well served via a limited-SMAS rhytidectomy alone (Fig. 33.20). On the other hand, individuals with significant midfacial ptosis and/or brow descent will benefit from a more invasive combination of surgical procedures (Fig. 33.21). In essence, older patients may require more invasive procedures due to the presence of more advanced facial aging, although the medical status and health of the older patient deserves even greater scrutiny prior to contemplating any elective cosmetic surgery.

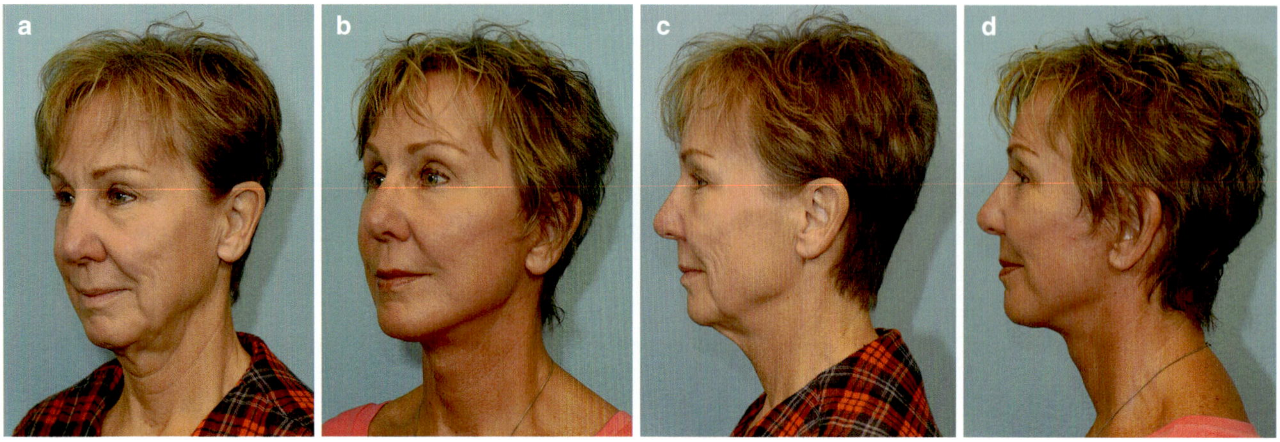

Fig. 33.20 Patient before (**a**, **c**) and 3 months following (**b**, **d**) lateral SMASectomy. The lateral SMASectomy allows for the suspension of the lower face and neck, without extended SMAS techniques and without anterior platysmal work

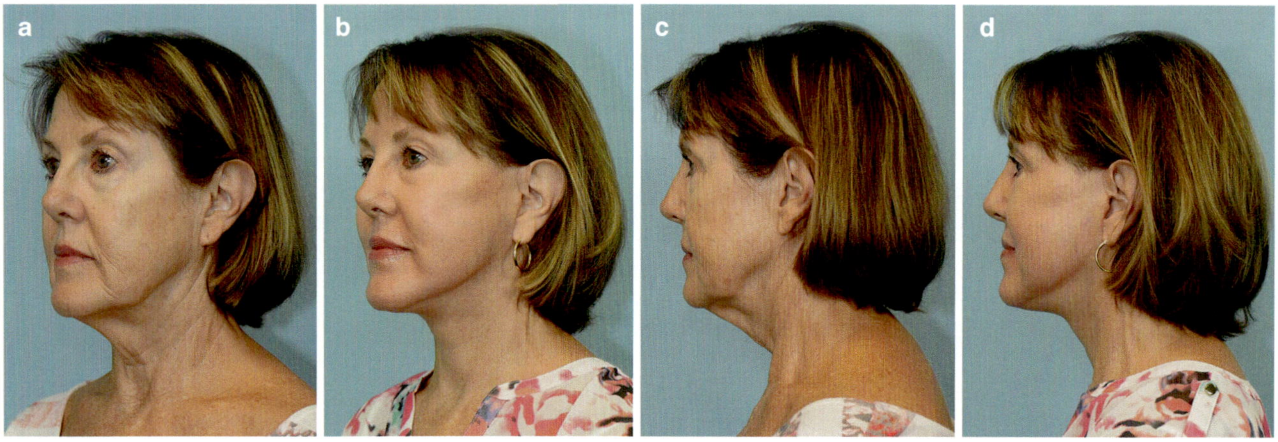

Fig. 33.21 Patient before (**a**, **c**) and 3 months following (**b**, **d**) a lamellar high-SMAS rhytidectomy with anterior platysmal plication and simultaneous fractional CO_2 laser skin resurfacing of the face. This patient demonstrated moderate ptosis of the midface with minimal brow ptosis; as a result, an extended-SMAS rhytidectomy was recommended. Due to the severity of anterior platysmal laxity, a simultaneous anterior platysmal plication was recommended

Individuals unable to undergo anesthesia or prolonged surgery should not be considered for rhytidectomy. It is also worth noting that "mini" procedures that aim to limit operative time by restricting the extent of skin undermining and SMAS/platysma suspension are not beneficial to individuals with advanced aging. Exposing an individual with advanced aging to a minimalistic rhytidectomy is harmful to their appearance, as the incongruence between the procedure and the degree of aging will often result in the lack of longterm improvement at best and facial distortion at worst. The surgeon should keep the following dictum in mind: *any aging not fully corrected by an incomplete rhytidectomy will get distorted by such rhytidectomy*. The surgeon should establish the most reasonable, least-invasive surgical plan for a patient's face, and then determine whether the patient is a medical candidate for the procedure. If the patient is not a candidate for medical reasons, then the conversation should be shifted toward non-surgical techniques that simply work to conceal aging, such as, for example, with the use of dermal fillers, skin resurfacing, and botulinum.

Choosing an Auxiliary Neck Procedure

Despite the variety of adjunctive neck procedures available today, all procedures rely on a concurrent rhytidectomy to deliver their rejuvenating effect. As such, the rhytidectomy surgeon should rarely ever rely on an isolated cervical procedure as the primary means of achieving neck rejuvenation. Regardless of the neck type and the severity of aging, all neck types benefit greatly from a rhytidectomy. Nonetheless, incorporating adjunctive neck procedures can enhance the outcome of rhytidectomy by improving the contour of the lower face and neck. The Dedo classification, already useful in describing the different types of cervical deformities, also serves well to guide the surgeon's approach to the neck during rhytidectomy, as outlined below:

- *Dedo Class II*—Dedo class II patients often require no significant adjunctive procedures because they have a sharp cervicomental angle and only mild laxity of the platysma and skin. Therefore, a simple lateral platysma suspension and a superior SMAS lift can achieve maximal correction of the neck (Fig. 33.22).
- *Dedo Class III*—Class III individuals benefit from fat removal from the neck at the same time as rhytidectomy. Class III individuals can be subcategorized into IIIa and IIIb subclasses (Fig. 33.23):
  - *Subclass IIIa*—These patients are characterized by primarily *subcutaneous* adiposis. They benefit significantly from a simple liposuction of the neck. Liposuction in rhytidectomy patients should always preserve a uniform layer of subdermal fat to minimize the chance of skin irregularities and dimpling (Fig. 33.24).

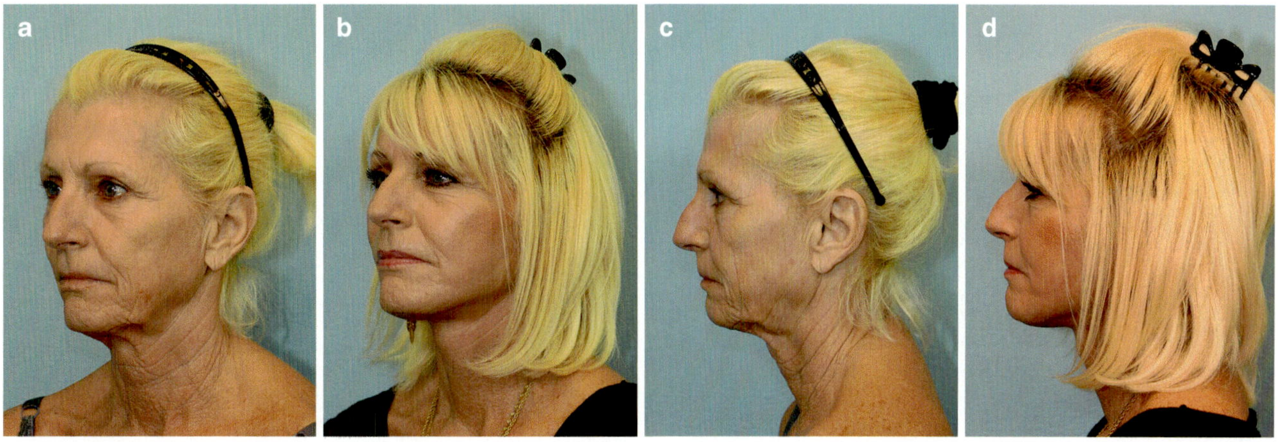

Fig. 33.22 A patient with a Dedo class II neck before (**a**, **c**) and 6 months following (**b**, **d**) a lateral SMASectomy. In this patient, due to the favorable neck structure and mild platysmal laxity, no anterior neck work was performed, relying solely on the lateral SMAS/platysma suspension for rejuvenation of the neck

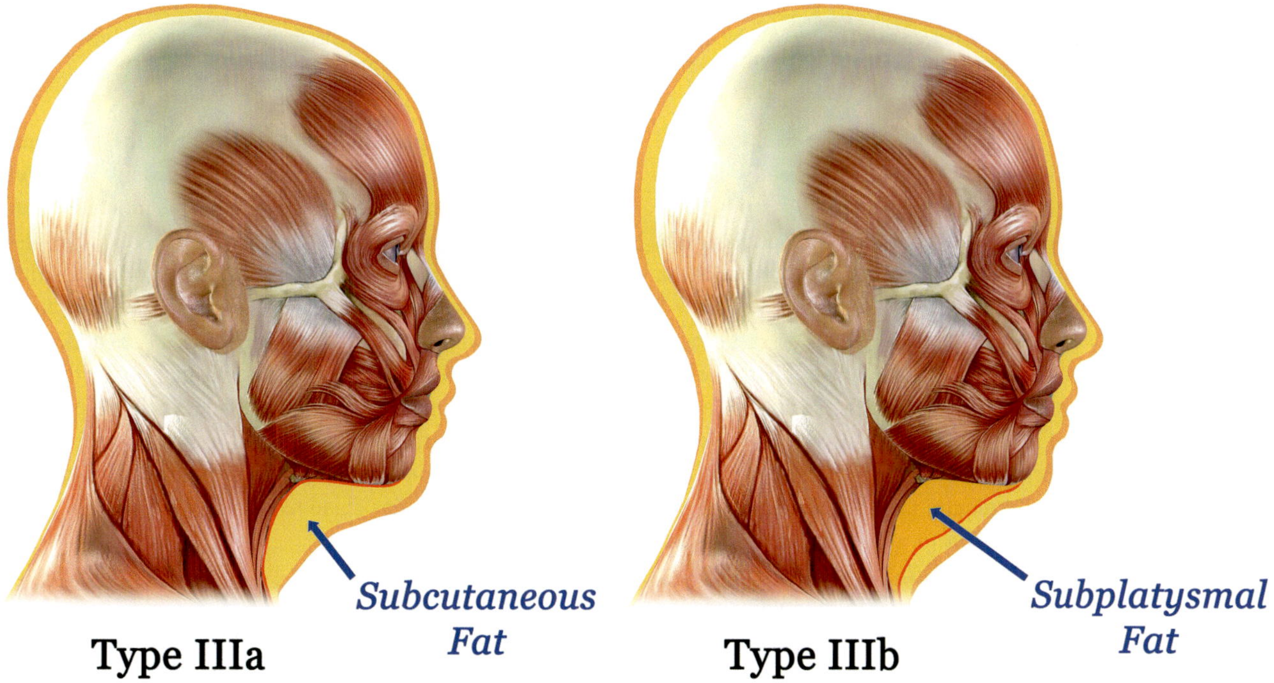

Fig. 33.23 Dedo class IIIa and IIIb neck types. Dedo class III patients are characterized by adiposis of the anterior neck. Class IIIa patients have mostly subcutaneous fat, amenable to simple liposuction. Class IIIb patients have moderate-to-severe adiposis of the subplatysmal compartment as well

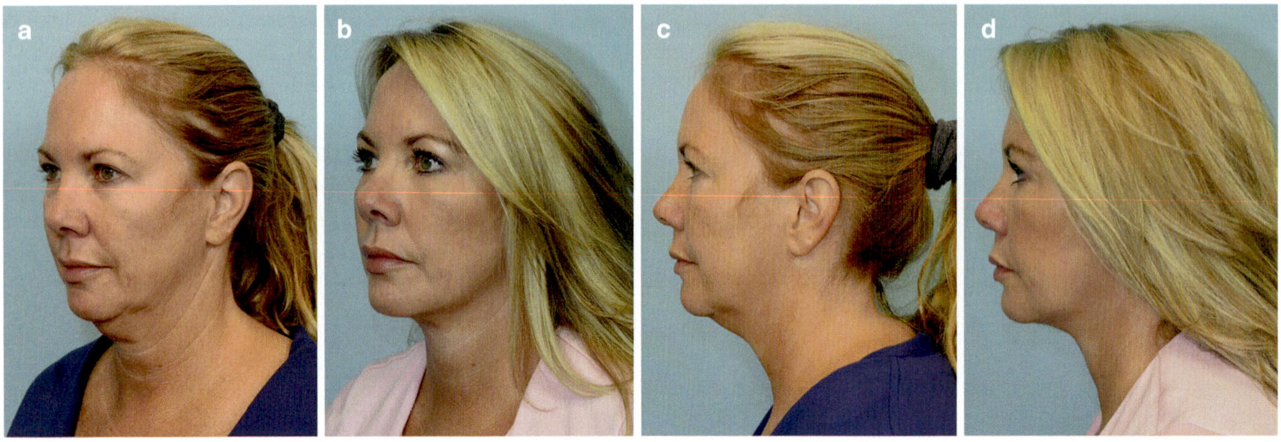

Fig. 33.24 Dedo class IIIa patient before (**a**, **c**) and 6 months following (**b**, **d**) lateral SMASectomy rhytidectomy and submental liposuction

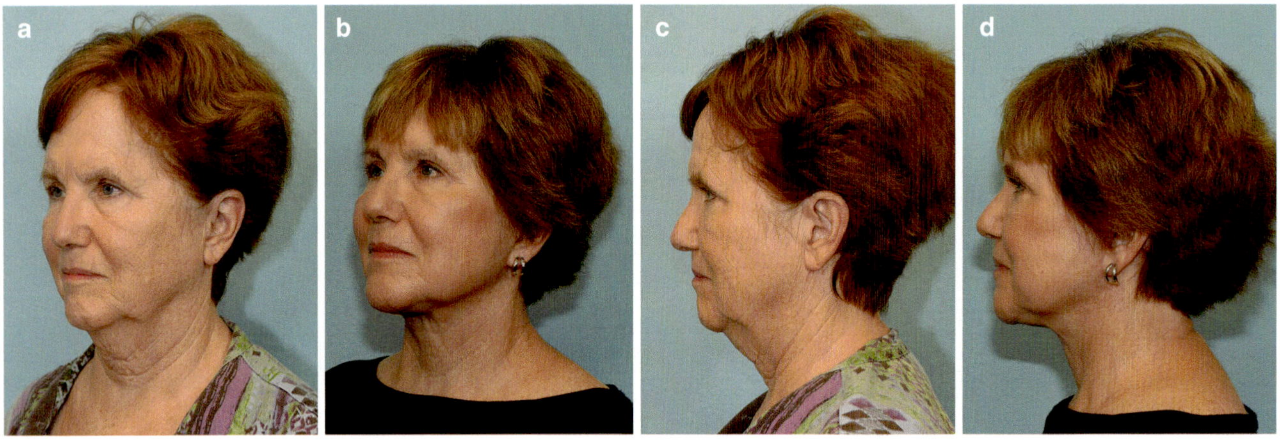

Fig. 33.25 Dedo class IIIb patient before (**a**, **c**) and 6 months following (**b**, **d**) lamellar high-SMAS rhytidectomy, submental liposuction, open submental subplatysmal lipectomy with anterior platysmal plication, and fractional CO_2 laser skin resurfacing of the face

  - *Subclass IIIb*—In IIIb patients, a large component of cervical adiposis lies within Level Ia, directly deep to the platysma, bounded by the anterior digastrics laterally and the mylohyoid muscle deeply. Subclass IIIb individuals benefit from an open lipectomy with an anterior platysma plication (Fig. 33.25).
- *Dedo Class IV*—Individuals with a Dedo class IV neck have moderate-to-severe platysmal aging characterized by significant banding. In these patients, due to the significant elongation of the platysma muscle, a simple lateral platysmal suspension is often insufficient; therefore, these patients typically require an anterior platysmal plication procedure in addition to a lateral suspension and SMAS rhytidectomy (Fig. 33.26).
- *Dedo Class V*—Class V patients benefit from an augmentation genioplasty either via the insertion of an alloplastic implant or advancement of the mandibular symphysis.
- *Dedo Class VI*—Although Class VI patients have been traditionally considered poor candidates for rhytidectomy, they still benefit from SMAS suspension for the eradication of the soft tissue ptosis of the mid and lower face. Most Dedo Class VI patients benefit from an open lipectomy with an anterior plication during rhytidectomy. However, the surgeon should be aware that, due to the more inferoanterior position of the hyoid bone, Class VI individuals also have more anteriorly positioned anterior digastrics. Lipectomy and platysmal plication will often unmask these prominent anterior digastric muscles, leading to noticeable submental paramedian bulges that also incorporate the submandibular triangle and salivary gland. In these patients, maximal contouring of the neck may require plication and/or partial resection of the digastric muscles with or without partial submandibular gland resection.

Surgical Technique: Lamellar High-SMAS Rhytidectomy

The lamellar high-SMAS technique borrows from Barton's high-SMAS rhytidectomy and pursues a bi-lamellar subcutaneous and sub-SMAS dissection [28, 37]. It extends the

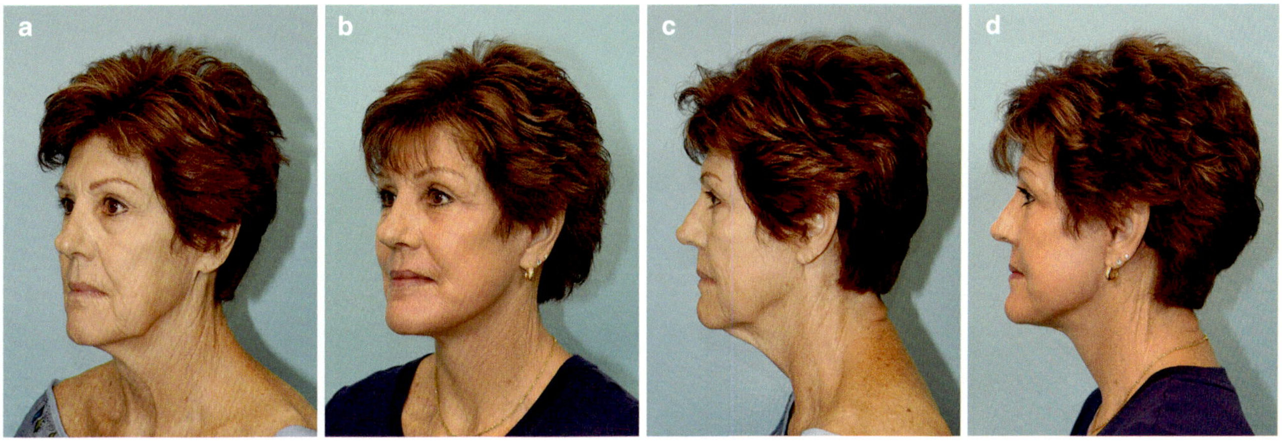

Fig. 33.26 Dedo class IV patient before (**a**, **c**) and 3 months following (**b**, **d**) lamellar high-SMAS rhytidectomy, anterior platysmal plication, and fractional CO_2 laser skin resurfacing of the face

sub-SMAS dissection into the malar region, releasing the zygomatic retaining ligament, and into the pre-parotid region to release the masseteric retaining ligament. The dissection further identifies and releases the SMAS attachments to the zygomaticus major musculature, decoupling the aponeurotic SMAS from the nasolabial fold. The lamellar dissection allows for the suspension of the aponeurosis in a largely superior vector, while the skin is allowed to re-drape in a tension-free, superolateral vector, ensuring that relaxed skin tension lines remain undistorted. The lamellar high-SMAS technique focuses on maximizing correction of moderate-to-severe jowling without distorting the relaxed skin tension lines of the face. The nasolabial fold is not the primary target of this technique, although it typically benefits in terms of both severity and length.

Technique Description

Preoperative Considerations

Prior to deciding whether to perform a lamellar high-SMAS rhytidectomy on any individual seeking surgical facial rejuvenation, the surgeon must thoroughly evaluate the patient and review all relevant medical history. Individuals with compromised cardiopulmonary function, or other medical contraindications to surgery and anesthesia, should not be deemed surgical candidates for rhytidectomy. In addition, individuals who are active tobacco smokers or users of any nicotine-containing products must completely cease all consumption for at least 1 month perioperatively. The ideal candidate for a lamellar high-SMAS facelift displays moderate-to-severe facial aging characterized by midfacial ptosis, prominent nasolabial folds, and moderate-to-severe jowling with variable degrees of neck skin laxity and platysmal ptosis; above all, however, the ideal candidate will also have significant elastosis of the skin, having prominent RSTLs that would be at risk for distortion with conventional skin-muscle flap techniques (Fig. 33.27). Incidentally, the ideal patients are typically in their mid-60s–70s and beyond.

Incisional Placement

The incisional placement in a high-SMAS rhytidectomy follows the standard periauricular configuration that is widely utilized in most rhytidectomy techniques, although with some notable variations that depend upon specific patient factors. The shape and location of the temporal portion of the incision is dependent upon the patient's hairline position and the degree of jowling present (Fig. 33.28). Despite the lamellar type of dissection in this technique, which allows for the skin to be re-draped in a more posterior vector than the SMAS, the lamellar high-SMAS technique still produces a significant vertical lift that is transmitted to the skin. In individuals with moderate-to-severe jowling in whom the temporal hairline is located at or above the level of the helical root, the temporal incision should be switched to a trichophytic design in order to prevent superolateral displacement of the hairline. In contrast, in individuals with lower temporal hairlines, in males, or in those with only limited jowling, the incision can be easily carried into the temporal hair tuft for maximal concealment.

The preauricular portion of the rhytidectomy incision is typically placed in a post-tragal configuration, which allows for maximal concealment. In males in whom there is an expectation of significant skin displacement, the flap can be easily ablated of its hair follicles with simple bipolar electrocautery of the follicular bulbs without harming the skin flap. A pre-tragal incision is justified in those with a prominent preauricular sulcus or crease. The remainder of the incision is placed in the postauricular sulcus with mild lateralization into the conchal cartilage to allow the incision to eventually displace into the sulcus during healing. Excessive lateral positioning of the postauricular incision can easily lead to obliteration of the postauricular sulcus, an often-frustrating sequela for patients. The occipital segment of the facelift

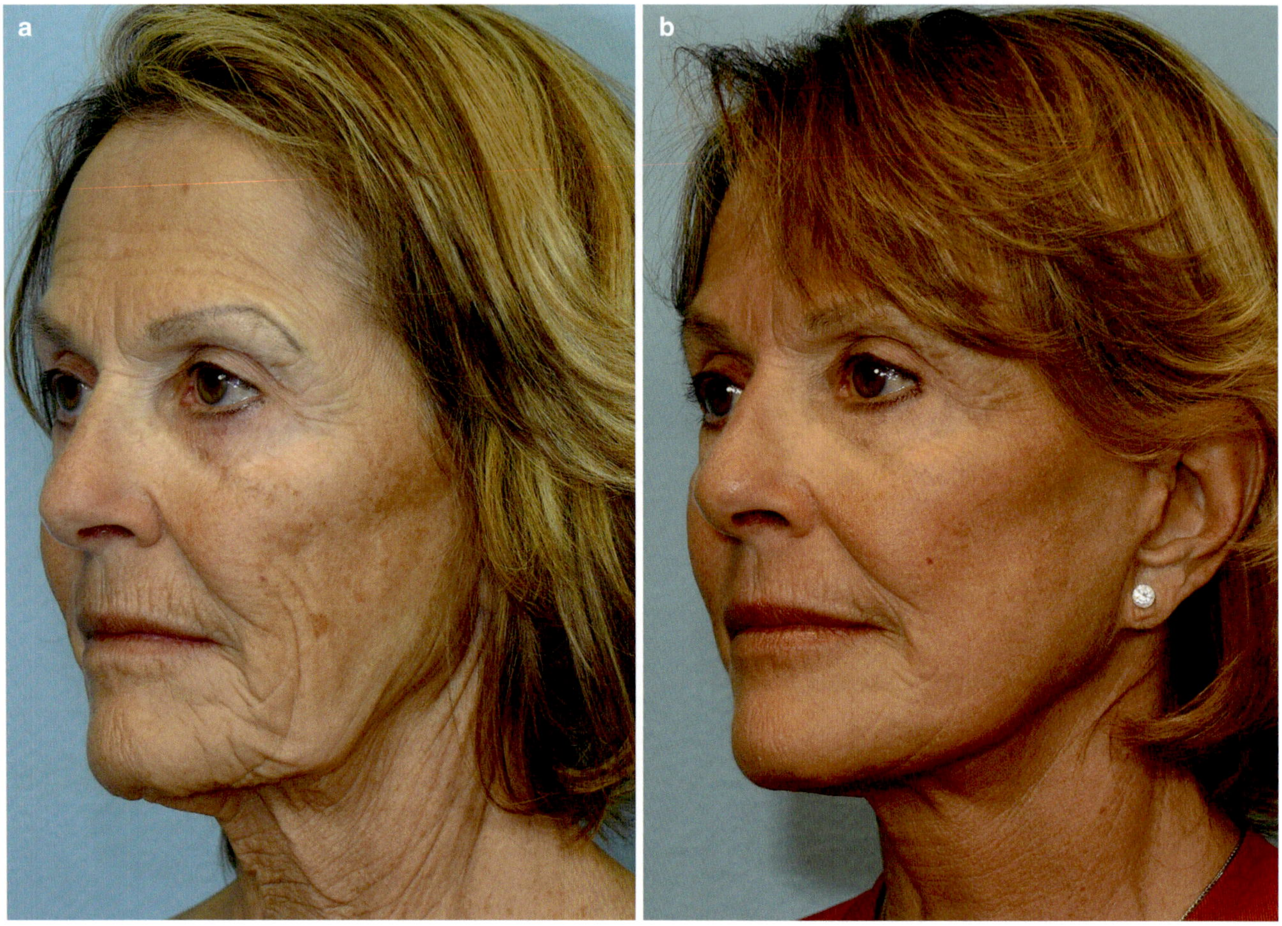

Fig. 33.27 Ideal candidate for a lamellar high-SMAS rhytidectomy. (**a**) This patient demonstrates moderate-to-severe aging of the lower face with ptosis of the midfacial soft tissues. In addition, there exists greater laxity of the skin than SMAS, evidenced by the deep jowl-complex rhytids. The prominent relaxed skin-tension lines (RSTLs) are maximally addressed by the lamellar high-SMAS procedure due to its separate undermining, mobilization, and excision of redundant skin independent of the SMAS. (**b**) Same patient 6 months following lamellar high-SMAS rhytidectomy with simultaneous fractional CO_2 laser skin resurfacing of the full face

incision is often necessary because lamellar-high SMAS patients often have significant cervical skin excess, despite the powerful vertical facial vector of lifting. The occipital incision is positioned in a lazy-S shape, initially following the occipital hairline before subsequently turning into the hair sharply. This configuration routinely allows for avoidance of step-offs or distortion of the occipital hairline.

Managing the Neck

The management of the neck is important during facelifting, especially in patients with moderate-to-severe aging in whom the lamellar high-SMAS technique is most beneficial. Individuals with moderate-to-severe facial aging typically have significant anterior neck laxity of the skin and platysma, as well as prominent platysmal banding. As such, these individuals typically benefit from the resection of excess midline platysma and cervical fascia, with possible simultaneous open removal of subplatysmal fat from level Ia. Excess subplatysmal fat can be identified pre-operatively by having the patient contract the platysma muscles. Subplatysmal fat is difficult to pinch with a contracted platysma, while subcutaneous fat remains easy to compress. Following subplatysmal lipectomy, the platysmal plication then ensures that platysma bands are eradicated and maximal contouring of the cervicomental angle can be achieved in any patient regardless of Dedo classification. The author's anterior neck technique closely mirrors that outlined in by Hamra in his *composite rhytidectomy* [35].

Operative Details

Once the patient is provided the selected level of anesthesia, the face and neck are infiltrated with a dilute mixture of 0.25% lidocaine with 1:400,000 epinephrine with sodium bicarbonate. A total of 70–120 cc is generally infiltrated, depending upon patient weight and size of the face and neck. The face is then carefully prepped with iodophore or chlorhexidine prep and allowed to dry for 15 minutes. The patient is draped in the standard sterile fashion, with the endotracheal tube and anesthesia circuit draped within a sterile sheath to allow for easy manipulation during the neck component of the surgery (Fig. 33.29).

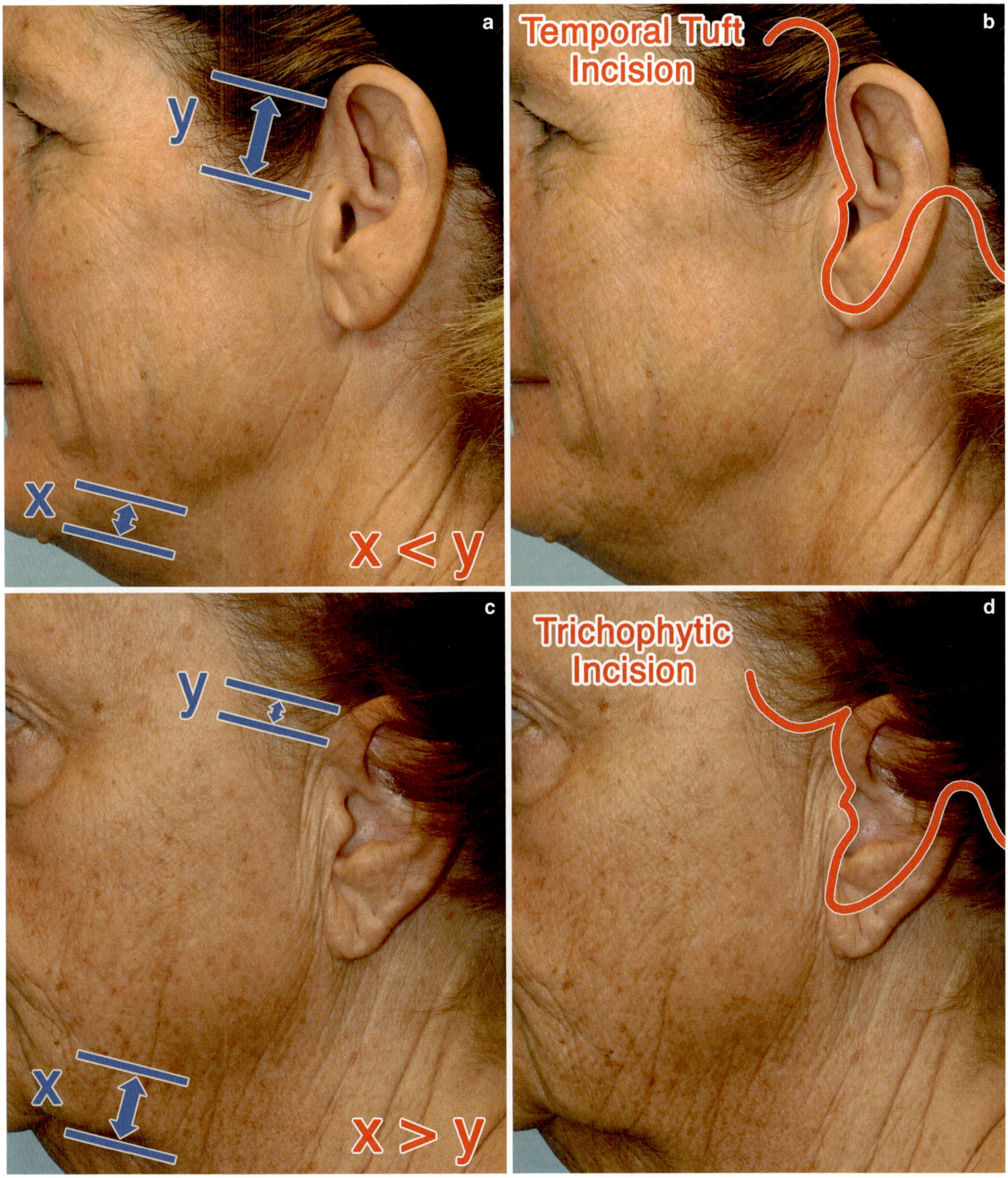

Fig. 33.28 Determining the ideal placement of the temporal segment of the rhytidectomy incision. Prior to deciding upon which incision to utilize, the surgeon should establish the severity of mid- and lower-facial aging and the position of the temporal hairline. In individuals requiring minimal vertical tissue mobilization (due to mild jowling only) and with a low temporal hairline (**a**), the ideal incision placement would be within the temporal hair tuft (**b**). Conversely, in individuals with severe mid- and lower-facial aging, in whom a powerful vertical vector of lift is expected to generate significant superior tissue excursion, and in whom the temporal hairline is high and sparse (**c**), the ideal incision would then follow the temporal trichophytic design (**d**)

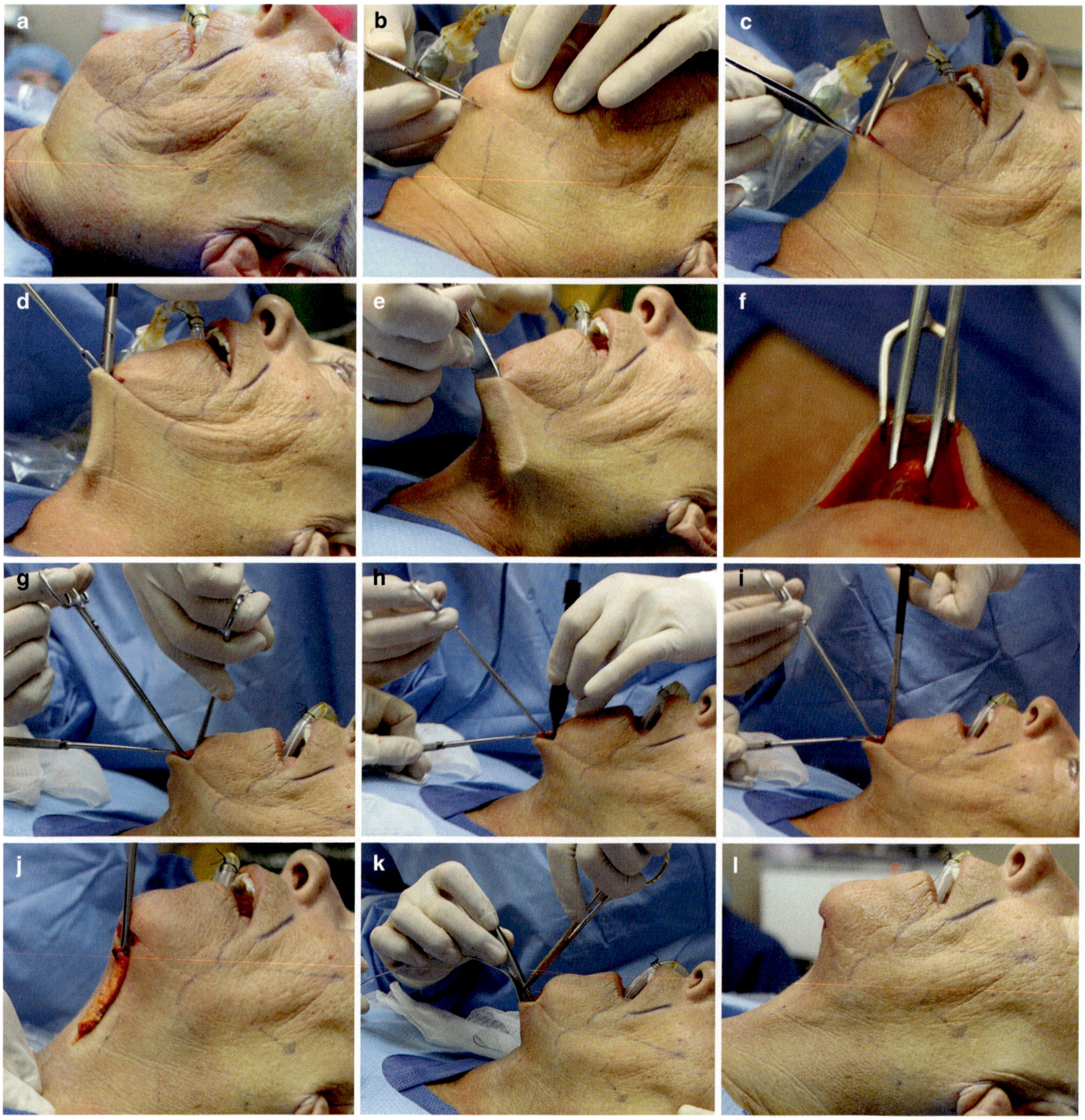

Fig. 33.29 Lamellar high-SMAS rhytidectomy: Cervical component. (**a**) Intraoperative, pre-procedural profile view of the neck. (**b**) An incision is made, measuring approximately 2.5 cm in length along the submental crease. (**c**) The skin of the submental region is undermined gently using fine dissecting blunt scissors subcutaneously. (**d**, **e**) The skin of the entire submental/midline neck and lateral neck is undermined along the subcutaneous plane. (**f–i**) The redundant midline cervical fascia and platysma is grasped with an Allis clamp (**f**) and them clamped with a curved Kelly clamp multiple times to crush the base of the excess tissue (**g**). The tissue base is then cauterized (**h**) and excised (**i**). (**j**) The excised midline tissue is displayed in its natural configuration prior to the surgery. (**k**) The platysmal muscle edges are then plicated with multiple inverted, interrupted 3-0 PDS sutures from the mentum to the thyroid notch. In the submental region, each bite of the platysma also grabs a portion of the ligamentous fascia connecting the platysma to digastric muscle. This allows for maximal rejuvenation of the cervicomental angle and minimizes the likelihood of developing submental paramedian bulges. (**l**) Intraoperative, post-platysmal plication profile view of the neck

Neck Component

A 2.5–3 cm incision is made along the submental crease centered on the midline. The incision is carried down to the subcutaneous fat. At this point, a standard subcutaneous liposuction is performed in the entire neck if indicated by the presence of significant cervical subcutaneous adiposis. Next, the skin of the neck is undermined, bordered by the mandibular edge superiorly, the cricoid-level inferiorly, and the anterior edges of the sternocleidomastoid muscles laterally. Subsequently, the midline platysma/cervical fascia is grasped with an Allis forceps at the anterior submental region, approximately 2 cm posterior to the inner symphyseal angle of the mandible. Next, a large Kelly clamp is used to repeatedly compress the excess midline platysma/fascial tissue. The line of compression is then cauterized with bipolar electrocautery and subsequently excised with curved facelift scissors down to the level of the thyroid notch, exposing subplatysmal level Ia fat and the platysma muscle edges. If excess subplatysmal fat is identified pre-operatively, a partial resection is performed, avoiding excess fat excision to prevent the *cobra neck deformity*. The platysma muscle edges are then plicated with interrupted 3-0 polydioxanone (PDS) sutures from the mentum down to at least the level of the hyoid bone. In individuals with more severe platysmal laxity, plication may need to be performed down to the level of the cricoid. Next, the surgeon ensures that the plication line is smooth without irregularities or prominent suture knots. The surgical site is usually sprayed with a fibrin sealant product (Artiss, Baxter Healthcare, Deerfield, IL, USA) and the incision re-approximated in a layered fashion utilizing interrupted 5-0 Monocryl sutures followed by a running interlocking low-tension 6-0 nylon suture. Surgical adhesive (Mastisol; Ferndale Laboratories, Ferndale, MI, USA) and half-inch iodophore-impregnated adhesive strips (Steristrips; 3 M Healthcare, St. Paul MN, USA) are applied to the anterior neck to help guide the skin during healing and ensure a smooth contour.

Facial Component: Skin Dissection

The facial component of the procedure is then performed (Fig. 33.30), by making the incision as previously described with a #15 scalpel. The skin is then undermined in the subcutaneous fat plane, leaving a 2 mm fat layer adherent to the skin flap to preserve topographic uniformity of the skin surface and to avoid disrupting the dermal vascular plexus. The skin is undermined to within 2 cm of the bony lateral canthus and extended inferiorly, in a radial configuration from the ear, into the lower face, superolateral neck, and postauricular region. The lateral neck dissection is connected to the central region of the neck subcutaneously to allow for maximal redraping of the skin, thereby minimizing any dimpling of the skin surface. Next. The SMAS is incised along a line roughly drawn from the mandibular angle to the inferior edge of the zygomatic eminence, being cautious to remain superficial to the parotid capsule and deep fascia. This portion of the procedure is best achieved in a safe manner by grasping and retracting the SMAS away from the face as it is incised. The SMAS can then begin to be gently undermined.

Facial Component: SMAS Dissection

The SMAS is initially undermined over the parotid gland as it can be easily and cleanly dissected off the parotid capsule thereby establishing a clear sub-SMAS plane of dissection (Fig. 33.31). This dissection is carried anteriorly in such a fashion until it reaches the anterior border of the parotid, at

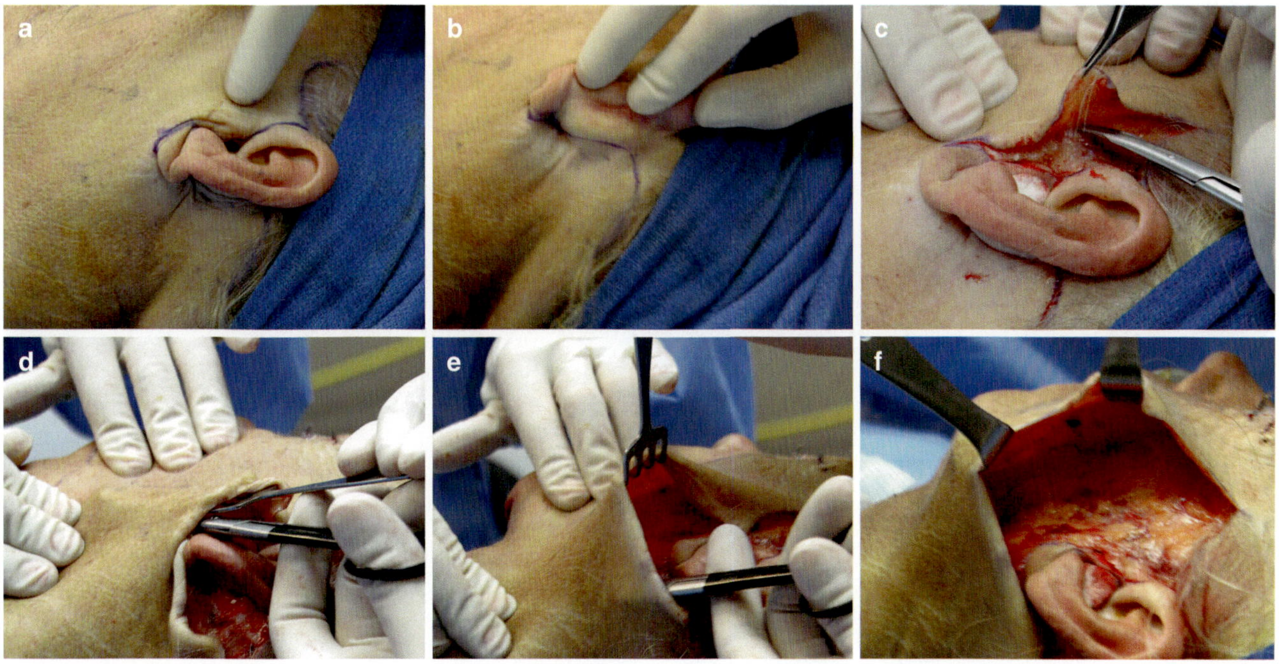

Fig. 33.30 Lamellar high-SMAS rhytidectomy: Facial subcutaneous dissection. (**a**, **b**) The skin incision is displayed. In this patient, due to the presence of severe lower facial and neck tissue laxity and the high temporal hairline, the rhytidectomy incision was designed with a temporal trichophytic incision. (**c**) The skin is carefully undermined utilizing fine blunt dissecting scissors. (**d**, **e**) Once the periauricular skin has been undermined, releasing the deeply attached skin from the parotid and perilobular regions, the dissection is then performed with the curved rhytidectomy scissors. The skin is undermined to approximately 1–2 cm from the lateral canthus and connected to the cervical dissection. (**f**) View of the tissue exposure upon completion of the skin undermining

which point we turn our attention to the malar region and the identification of the zygomaticus major muscle (ZMM). The sub-SMAS dissection is extended superiorly toward the zygomatic arch region with the SMAS under continuous tension away from the face; this helps keep any neighboring distal branches of the facial nerve safely down on the floor of the sub-SMAS dissection. As the dissection approaches the lateral aspect of the malar eminence, the zygomatic retaining ligament attachments become obvious and they are cautiously divided sharply. The dissection then continues bluntly toward the malar eminence until the superolateral segment of the ZMM is identified. Upon identification of the ZMM, the dissection is then extended inferomedially in a supra-muscular plane with the use of a Trepsat dissector along the zygomaticus major muscle into the medial cheek toward the nasolabial fold. *Please note, if the surgeon attempts to identify the ZMM below the malar eminence, the surgeon will inevitably be guided into the muscle's undersurface because the SMAS envelops the ZMM. Sub-ZMM dissection severely risks injury to the zygomatic and buccal branches of the facial nerve.* The surgeon should always aim to identify the ZMM superiorly, where it is attached to the bone and where blunt submuscular dissection is impossible. The dissection is then extended into the buccal region along the supra-ZMM plane, releasing the masseteric ligamentous attachments, which essentially allows the surgeon to release the attachments between the SMAS and the ZMM (Fig. 33.32).

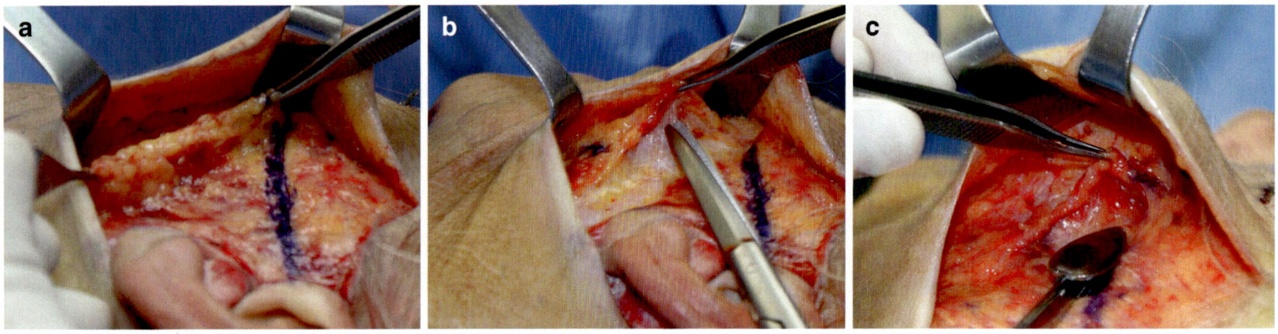

Fig. 33.31 Lamellar high-SMAS rhytidectomy: Upper SMAS work. (**a**) The SMAS is grasped and mobilized to determine its mobility. (**b**) The SMAS is then incised along a line from the angle of the mandible to the malar eminence and then carefully undermined under outward tension using blunt dissection. (**c**) Once the superolateral insertion of the zygomaticus major muscle (ZMM) is identified, the dissection is then carried in a supra-ZMM plane with the use of a Trepsat dissector

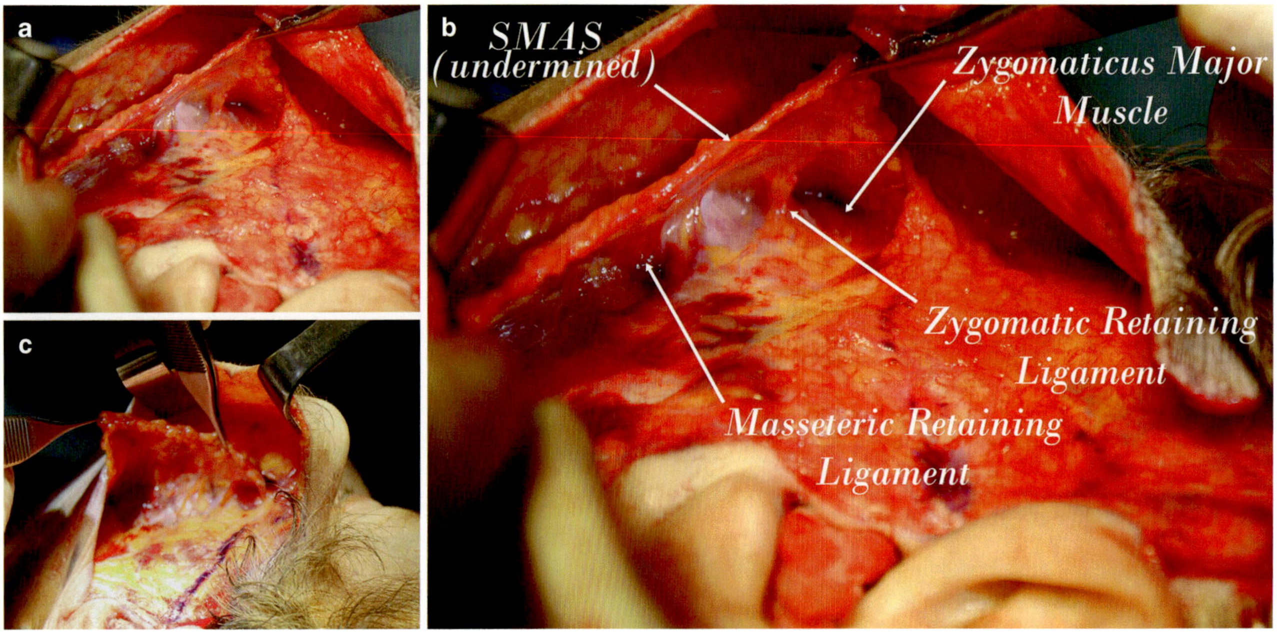

Fig. 33.32 Lamellar high-SMAS rhytidectomy: Lower SMAS work. (**a**) Upon completion of the upper SMAS work, the zygomaticus major muscle (ZMM) should be well identified. (**b**) Labeled view of (**a**). (**c**) The dissection is then carried into the buccal and mandibular regions of the lower face extrapolating from the supra-ZMM plane to ensure the safety of the distal branches of the facial nerve. Upon completion of the dissection, the skin and SMAS flaps should be easily mobilized to their respective degrees and vectors

The sub-SMAS dissection is extended into the subplatysmal plane of the inferolateral face and superolateral neck. The subplatysmal dissection at the angle of the neck reaches only as far anteriorly as the anterior edge of the parotid gland to preserve the integrity of the marginal mandibular branch of the facial nerve. However, the surgeon may choose to carry the subplatysmal dissection farther anteriorly if it is kept at least 2 cm below the mandibular border and performed carefully.

SMAS Suspension

Upon completion of the SMAS dissection, the SMAS is then imbricated with interrupted 2-0 PDS sutures, starting with the cheek SMAS, vertically upward against the temporalis fascia, and then proceeding diagonally downward toward the mandibular angle (Fig. 33.33). The imbrication is continued into the neck, where the platysma is imbricated and/or plicated against the mastoid periosteum with the use of interrupted 0 PDS sutures. If necessary, the SMAS flap may be divided at the mandibular angle, splitting the flap at the earlobe.

Skin Repositioning and Closure

The skin flap is then re-draped in a superolateral vector with only minor tension and without distortion of the RSTLs (Fig. 33.34). The excess skin is trimmed around the ear and complete hemostasis ensured with bipolar electrocautery. Next, fibrin sealant is sprayed on the surgical site, and the skin is once again re-draped and pressure applied for 3 minutes to allow the sealant to settle. The incision is typically closed with surgical staples for the hair-bearing portions of the temporal and occipital incisions. The preauricular incision is closed with 6-0 nylon sutures, while the post-tragal and postauricular incisions are closed with interrupted 5-0 fast gut and plain gut sutures, respectively. The segment of the incision situated between the postauricular sulcus and the occipital hairline is closed with interrupted 5-0 Prolene sutures. A facelift gentle compression dressing is then applied in a standard fashion, and the patient is then given back to anesthesia for awakening and extubation.

Post-operative Care

The patient is seen the next day for a short-term follow-up and removal of the dressing and surgical drains, although drains are not typically inserted if fibrin sealant is utilized.

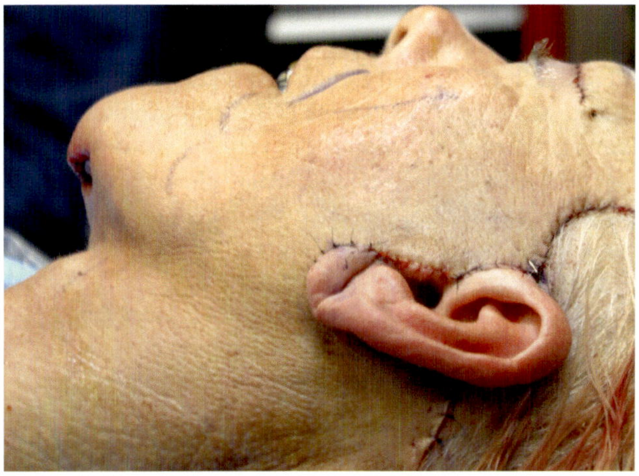

Fig. 33.34 Lamellar high-SMAS rhytidectomy: Skin closure. The skin incision is re-approximated under minimal tension. The trichophytic incision is closed with a running 5-0 fast gut suture. The preauricular incision is closed with a running 6-0 nylon followed by interrupted 6-0 nylon sutures for the perilobular incision. The post-tragal incision is closed with a running 5-0 fast gut suture. The postauricular incision is closed with a 5-0 plain gut suture. The occipital arm of the incision between the postauricular sulcus and the hairline is closed with interrupted 5-0 Prolene sutures, and the remainder of the incision is closed with surgical staples

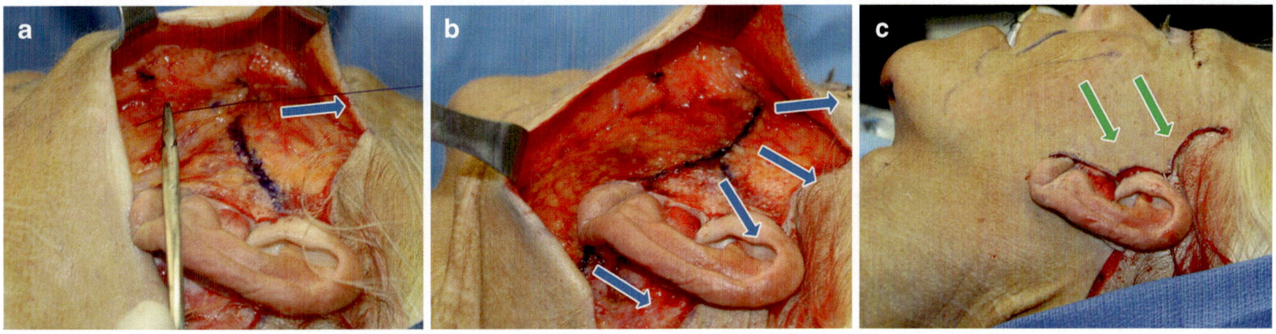

Fig. 33.33 Lamellar high-SMAS rhytidectomy: SMAS imbrication. (**a**) Once the SMAS flap has been undermined, it is then partially resected and imbricated against the temporal fascia with the use of interrupted 2-0 PDS sutures. The first suture provides a powerful vertical vector of lift to the mid- and lower-facial components (blue arrow). (**b**) The remainder of the SMAS is imbricated in a similar fashion utilizing interrupted 2-0 PDS sutures along a curved line down to the neck, providing for a multi-vector suspension (multiple blue arrows). The platysma muscle is imbricated against the mastoid periosteum with the use of interrupted 0 PDS sutures. (**c**) The skin is then re-draped and the excess is excised. Note that, other than at the helical root and the peak of postauricular sulcus incision, the entire skin incision is under no tension. The vector of mobilization of the skin differs from that of the SMAS, and is directed with a greater posterior component (green arrows)

The patient is then seen for two additional visits during the first 10 days for suture removal, monitoring, and guidance. Although lacking in sufficient supportive evidence, the authors routinely place rhytidectomy patients on post-operative antibiotic prophylaxis unless there is a known history of complications such as *Clostridium difficile* colitis, multiple severe allergies, etc. Patients are also routinely placed on a post-operative oral methylprednisolone taper to assist with post-operative edema. Patients are instructed to ambulate early and may be placed on venous thromboembolism chemoprophylaxis if their modified Caprini score is elevated. Garments are not routinely offered to the patient for post-operative use. Patients are additionally instructed to keep their head elevated for the first week, use gentle cold compresses on the face for 72 hours, and avoid any neck turning, wide mouth opening, or excessive chewing for the first two weeks. Post-operative standard photography is typically pursued at 3, 6, and 12 months if there is adequate patient adherence to follow-up visits.

Complications of Rhytidectomy

Post-rhytidectomy complications can be categorized into post-operative *surgical* complications and adverse *cosmetic sequelae*, with the former emphasizing issues that compromise the surgical integrity of tissues, functional performance, or introduce problems that threaten the medical status of the patient. By definition, cosmetic sequelae relate specifically to an inadequate correction of the original cosmetic issue or the introduction of additional issues that disrupt the cosmesis or natural appearance of the face.

Surgical Complications

Hematoma

Post-operative hematoma represents the most common serious complication following rhytidectomy largely owing to the degree of surgical dissection within the well-vascularized tissues of the face. Hematoma rates reported in the literature range between 2% and 15% of cases in the literature and can be roughly characterized into major and minor [46–48]. *Major hematomas* are high in volume, rapidly expanding, and distributed over 50% or more of the rhytidectomy flap territory. *Minor hematomas* are usually low-pressure, low volume, and restricted to small regions of the flap (e.g. post-auricular, infra-lobular, etc.). Major hematomas present a much more urgent challenge to the surgeon, due to the greater risk of devitalization of the skin flap.

Most hematomas present within the first 12 hours following surgery with asymmetric pain of a severity that is beyond that which is normally expected for the procedure, as well as asymmetric swelling and deep ecchymosis. The most common presentation of a post-rhytidectomy hematoma is that of a patient calling after-hours with significant pain on one side of the face that is poorly responsive to opioid narcotics. Even patients with only minor hematomas can present with intractable pain. Patients with suspected hematoma should be seen as soon as possible and their surgical sites evaluated thoroughly. If a major hematoma is identified, the patient should be brought back to an operating suite under safe and sterile conditions for immediate evacuation of the hematoma, identification of the bleeding vessel(s), and appropriate hemostasis followed by drain insertion and the placement of a compression dressing.

Minor hematomas present a lesser challenge to the facelift flap and, due to their typical low-caliber venous culprits, often result in self-tamponade early, thus affecting only a limited area of the flap. Nevertheless, minor hematomas will still lower the threshold for flap necrosis or infection and should be drained instead of simply monitored. Minor hematomas are often easily evacuated via needle drainage once liquefied. If a thick coagulum has formed, the incision should be opened along a short segment and the clot suctioned. Compression dressings should be reinstated and the patient seen within 24 hours to ensure that no re-accumulation of the hematoma has taken place. If evacuation of a minor hematoma required incisional re-opening, a small flexible rubber drain should also be placed.

Despite the varying degrees of invasiveness of different facelift techniques, no one technique appears to be significantly more prone to hematoma formation than others. In fact, even intraoperative blood loss fails to significantly correlate with a higher risk of post-operative hematoma. Instead, perioperative hypertension presents the most significant risk factor, with a reported 2.6-fold increase in risk [49]. Additional risk factors have also been well documented, such as smoking, male sex, and non-steroidal anti-inflammatory drug use, as well as exposure to vitamin E, fish oil, and various other herbal supplements. Patients who are maintained on anticoagulant therapy for medical reasons should be transitioned off anticoagulation prior to the surgery under the guidance of their prescribing physician. Such patients may require short-term transition with a low-molecular-weight heparin to minimize the length of time without anticoagulation. Most patients can safely restart their anticoagulation after 3–5 days following rhytidectomy. Individuals with a hereditary form of a blood-clotting disorder, such as von Willebrand disease (VWD), should be evaluated, undergo a coagulation profile, and be cleared by a hematologist or treating physician prior to considering rhytidectomy. In patients with mild VWD, preoperative desmopressin may be able to restore normal coagulation and minimize any bleeding risk. Individuals with an elevated risk of hematoma due to poor intraoperative blood pressure control and hereditary coagulopathies should be strongly considered for drain placement. The use of fibrin sealants also serves to significantly lower the risk of post-operative hematoma following rhytidectomy [50].

Skin Necrosis

Skin necrosis is a complication that is inherent to rhytidectomy due to the moderately aggressive degree of skin undermining and tendency for increased skin tension that is characteristic of facelifting (Fig. 33.35). The incidence of flap necrosis following rhytidectomy varies between 0% and 3% and is dependent upon both the surgical technique utilized and the surgeon's strict adherence to surgical principles of flap design and closing tension [51]. Facelift techniques employing a composite skin-muscle flap, such as that employed in deep plane and high-SMAS techniques, tend to create a more robust flap that is less susceptible to necrosis. However, excessive flap tension can result in necrosis even in such composite flaps, and the surgeon should adhere to the time-tested principles of minimizing unnecessary skin undermining, keeping flap tension to a minimum, and avoiding performing rhytidectomy in patients with an elevated risk of skin-flap failure.

Cigarette smoking results in an overall 12.6 increase in risk of skin necrosis, and individuals considering rhytidectomy should cease all nicotine intake for a minimum of 2 weeks before and 2 weeks after the surgery [52]. Additional risk factors also appear to predispose to flap necrosis, including diabetes mellitus, peripheral vascular disease, connective tissue disorders, and prior history of irradiation. Individuals deemed to be at a higher risk should not be exposed to aggressive skin undermining, exposure of the flap to significant tension, or concurrent skin resurfacing, meaning that the surgeon may need to alter his/her surgical technique to limit these risk factors or elect not to perform any surgery.

Skin necrosis typically presents within the first 5 days following surgery, with the skin quite possibly still managing to appear inconspicuously normal within the first 24 hours. However, with passing time, the flap begins to appear congested, dusky, and with varying degrees of superficial epidermolysis, ultimately hardening into a dark eschar in a gradual fashion. Typically, by five days the likely region of skin

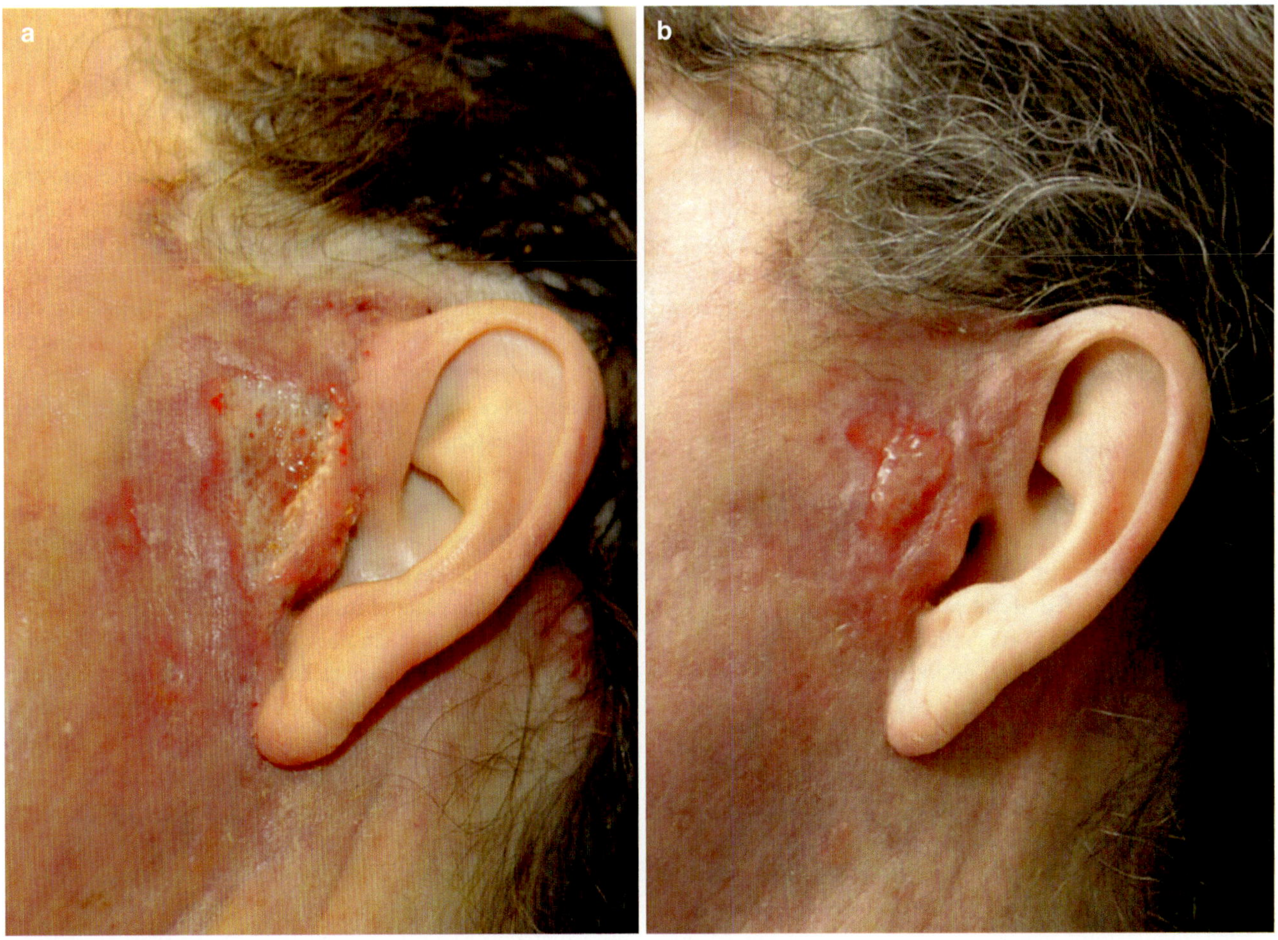

Fig. 33.35 Post-rhytidectomy skin-flap necrosis. (**a**) 1 week post-operatively, post-debridement. (**b**) 2 weeks post-operatively. Defect ultimately healed with minimal scarring

necrosis has started to demarcate, allowing the surgeon to establish the exact area of tissue devitalization.

The management of skin necrosis is typically conservative but work-intensive, as affected patients require regular follow-ups for wound care and reassurance. Fortunately, in most instances, post-rhytidectomy skin necrosis heals with minimal to no permanent scarring. The facelift surgeon now has at his/her disposal more resources than ever before in the management of flap necrosis, relying primarily on (1) serial debridement, (2) proper wound care, and (3) early adjunctive risk-modifying therapies. Nonetheless, the ideal approach to skin necrosis is one of prevention, and individuals with an elevated risk should not undergo rhytidectomy.

The mainstay of management of a necrotic area of tissue centers on serial debridements starting as soon as tissue demarcation has neared completion, typically by ten days. The removal of the eschar assists in encouraging a faster healing response, as the eschar and necrotic tissue act to suppress and slow down tissue recovery and re-epithelialization. A well-developed eschar provides a protective encasement of the region of dermal failure, but also poses a significant roadblock that delays the rapidity of re-epithelialization of the skin. In the presence of an eschar, re-epithelialization relies solely on peripheral healing against the dry and firm nature of the eschar, which is slowly degraded enzymatically. When performed, debridement of the eschar should be done conservatively to avoid injury to any remaining deep dermal and subcutaneous tissues. Following debridement, the surgeon should institute a thorough antimicrobial wound care regimen that retains moisture and provides a protective layer over the affected region. Silver- and chlorhexidine-impregnated clear silicone adhesive dressings (SurgiClear, Covalon Technologies, Ontario, Canada) provide a powerful antimicrobial environment that is shielded from external elements and dehydration by an adhesive silicone barrier. In addition, biological dressings consisting of naturally derived extracellular matrix xenografts provide a natural tissue scaffold that assists in rapid healing with maximum preservation of dermal integrity. Although the ideal type of dressing for post-rhytidectomy flap necrosis has not been objectively studied or documented, these new formulations have shown great promise [53, 54]. Treatments that modify the risk of necrosis in the early post-op period may also play a significant role in minimizing the severity of tissue failure, although sufficient supportive evidence is still lacking. Topical nitroglycerin may possibly serve as an adjuvant therapy in flaps prone to necrosis in the early period [55]. Similarly, the early use of hyperbaric oxygen therapy may assist in minimizing the area of flap tissue failure in patients with skin necrosis [56]. The healing period for full-thickness skin necrosis following rhytidectomy may require months to reach an acceptable appearance, and the surgeon should follow these patients more closely for management, guidance, and reassurance.

Facial Nerve Palsy

Facial paralysis presents a devastating complication to the rhytidectomy patient, resulting in an immediately noticeable cosmetic and functional deficit. The incidence of motor nerve injury following rhytidectomy is estimated to be between 0.5% and 2.6%, although the risk level may also be related to the type of procedure used and the surgeon's degree of familiarity with the technique [57, 58]. In general, the temporal and marginal mandibular nerve branches are most commonly injured in facelifting. The temporal branch travels superficially and is susceptible to inadvertent injury during simple hemostasis or suture suspension of the SMAS. Staying anterior and inferior to Pitanguy's line may help to avoid running directly into the territory of the temporal nerve branches. Techniques that may endanger the temporal branch include the high-SMAS and subperiosteal rhytidectomy technique. The high-SMAS technique typically calls for a high dissection of the SMAS/TPF up to 2 cm above the zygomatic arch. Barton showed that this dissection reliably avoids injury to the frontal branch, although the technique works in closer proximity to the nerve. The periosteal lift has classically been heavily associated with a high incidence of temporal nerve palsy as high as 11% [32]. However, since modifications by Ramirez, the incidence of palsy has been reduced dramatically [33].

The marginal mandibular nerve is also at risk during conventional rhytidectomy due to the long, fragile, and solitary nature of this single nerve branch. Marginal nerve injury is easily avoided by keeping the tissue dissection in the subcutaneous region as the nerve travels deep to the platysma. However, if the surgeon chooses to undermine the platysma, the dissection should be kept mostly over the parotid capsule and 2 cm or more below the angle of the mandible. Buccal and zygomatic nerve injuries are rare with limited-SMAS techniques but become naturally greater in theory when performing an extended-SMAS technique. In skilled hands, the incidence of buccal and zygomatic nerve injuries is still much lower than the rates seen with the temporal and mandibular nerves. As previously described, when performing an extended-SMAS rhytidectomy, the surgeon should always identify the superolateral insertion of the zygomaticus major muscle into the malar eminence and then maintain a supramuscular plane of dissection. Doing so will ensure that the zygomatic and buccal nerve branches will remain out of harm's way. Proper dissection technique and sufficient SMAS retraction, as previously described, are critical in protecting the facial nerve branches from injury during SMAS dissection in the midface.

The management of post-operative facial nerve palsy centers on an astute watchful waiting approach. Greater than 99% of facial nerve palsies in the first 12 hours following rhytidectomy are simply due to the local anesthetic. Motor nerve palsies persisting after 24 hours are likely due to nerve injury. Of those, approximately 85% of them result from neuropraxia and spontaneously recover over a period of weeks to months, depending on the extent of injury and presence of cross-innervation by neighboring branches [59]. Only a small percentage of facial nerve injuries involve an irreversible injury to the facial nerve. Because it is impossible to distinguish between severe neurotmesis and neuropraxia/axonotmesis within the first week from surgery, the surgeon must rely on their surgical instinct to determine the likelihood of serious injury to the nerve. In instances where the surgeon recalls a specific maneuver or unusual instance whereupon the paralyzed branch may have been accidentally injured, then return to the operative suite with exploration and primary nerve reanastomosis may be a reasonable option. However, in most instances, no such clear evidence exists, and surgical exploration may risk further nerve injury or fail to identify and repair the affected nerve. As a result, close monitoring and reassurance are usually the most appropriate course of management. Individuals should be followed closely for both guidance and reassurance. In instances where temporary nerve palsy poses a cosmetically significant asymmetry, contralateral botulinum therapy may be helpful in establishing a more natural appearance [60]. If a permanent injury is suspected beyond 6–12 months, then restorative surgery to address the specific deficit, when applicable, should be considered.

Infection

Infection is rare following rhytidectomy, with an overall risk that is less than 1% when appropriate aseptic technique is utilized and perioperative antibiotic therapy is instituted [61]. Infectious sequelae typically manifest as peri-incisional cellulitis with a propensity toward abscess formation. The most common early sign of infection is a seemingly inexplicable development of a unilateral focus of pain at approximately 5–7 days post-operatively. Patients subsequently begin to show visible signs at the affected portion of the incision, with erythema, dehiscence, discharge, and possibly fluctuance. Patients should be followed closely whenever an infection is suspected, and broad-spectrum empirical antibiotic therapy instituted that targets common staphylococcal and streptococcal species.

Given the rise of *community-acquired methicillin-resistant Staphylococcus aureus*, surgeons should consider instituting coverage with agents such as sulfamethoxazole/trimethoprim, clindamycin, or ciprofloxacin, depending on the local antibiogram, in patients with suspected post-operative infection. *Pseudomonas aeruginosa* is also a possible infectious agent in post-surgical incisional infections. The surgeon should institute broad-spectrum therapy early on and immediately seek to obtain a culture with sensitivity testing from the infection site to specifically tailor the treatment regimen against the causative organism. If an abscess is suspected, the surgeon should proceed with opening of the surgical site and drainage of purulence. A wick or surgical packing should be inserted to prevent re-accumulation, and consideration toward intravenous antibiotics given if no response is seen within 48 hours.

Seroma

A seromatous fluid collection is relatively rare in rhytidectomy due to the superficial nature of the procedure. Serous fluid accumulations usually present as low-tension, low-volume accumulations of fluid in the postauricular area diagnosed via aspiration of clear non-hematogenous fluid. Simple needle aspiration, sometimes requiring repeated management over the first 1–3 days, is often curative. Compression dressing, aided by a facial garment, assists in preventing recurrence until sufficient healing conclusively terminates the source of serous accumulation. Seromas should be differentiated from sialoceles, which tend to be much more resistant to simple needle evacuation.

Sialocele

Post-operative sialocele is another rare complication of rhytidectomy and is typically brought on by violation of the parotid capsule with injury to the glandular parenchyma. Sialoceles present much in the same way as seromas, although they tend to be located over, or immediately adjacent to, the parotid gland (e.g. preauricular or infra-lobular locations). Needle-tip fluid aspiration typically produces a yellowish, clear fluid that may be cloudy in appearance. The presence of elevated amylase levels typically clinches the diagnosis. Depending on the degree of injury, the volume of the sialocele may be minimal to very large. Large sialoceles imply a more significant parotid injury, possibly even to Stensen's duct, and often require significantly longer periods of time, and even operative intervention, to dissipate.

Management of sialoceles centers on repeated aspiration and/or evacuation, followed by placement of a compression garment. Unfortunately, large volume sialoceles often fail to respond significantly to such conservative approaches, requiring incisional opening and insertion of a Jackson–Pratt drain for simple care and monitoring of output by the patient. Patients should avoid sialagogues and be placed on anticholinergic agents, such as transcutaneous scopolamine. Finally, targeting of the affected parotid parenchyma with botulinum neurotoxin may aid in suppressing saliva production until the injury is able to heal.

Adverse Cosmetic Sequelae

Poor Scarring

Conspicuous scars following rhytidectomy present a disruptive problem to patients who seek the procedure without

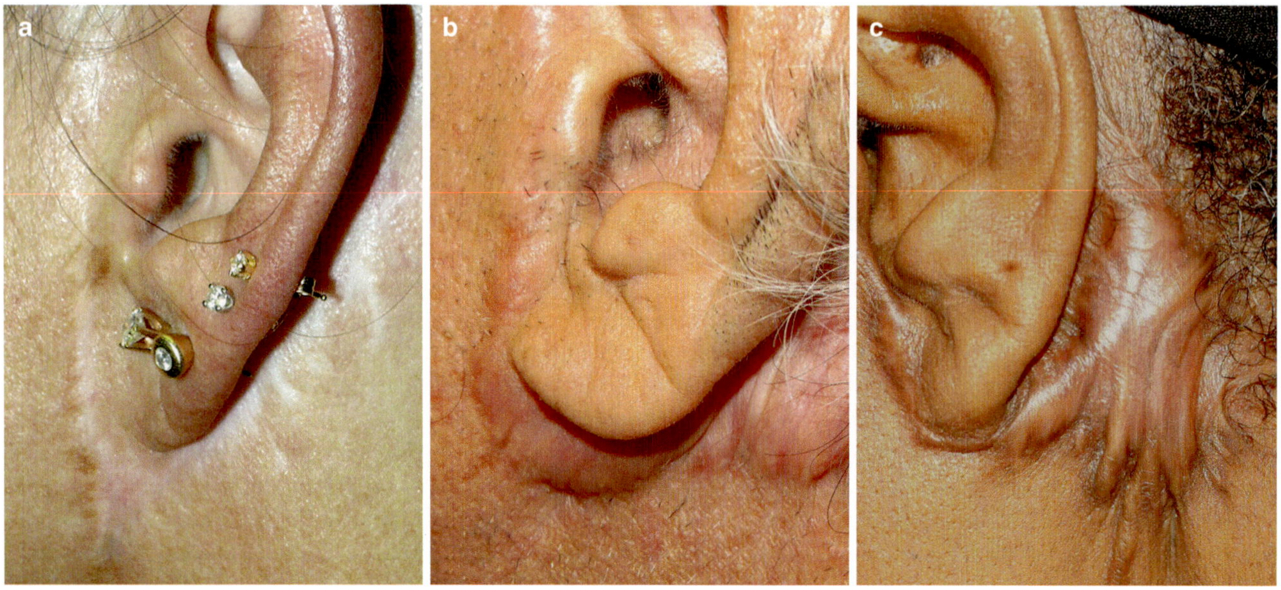

Fig. 33.36 Examples of poor scarring post-rhytidectomy. (**a**) Atrophic. (**b**) Hypertrophic. (**c**) Keloidal

stigmata of facelifting. As a result, maximal scar concealment is critical to achieving a successful outcome. Abnormal scarring, although rare, may present as *atrophic* or *hypertrophic* (Fig. 33.36). Prominent scarring following rhytidectomy is unusual given the favorable concealment afforded by the irregular shape of the auricle. The development of abnormal scarring typically points to excessive tension on the skin flap. Even in individuals predisposed to hypertrophic scarring, a well-designed, low-tension flap closure that abides by standard norms of tissue handling in plastic surgery will most often heal imperceptibly. Deep sutures are useful in strengthening the skin closure and should be used whenever mild tension is placed on the flap. Moderate-to-severe tension should never be placed on a rhytidectomy flap unless it is a composite skin-muscle flap capable of withstanding significant tension. Atrophic scarring typically develops in areas of tissue failure, or necrosis, of the skin adjacent to the incision, or in overly aggressive management of hypertrophic scarring with intralesional corticosteroids or antineoplastic agents.

Individuals prone to keloidal or hypertrophic scarring should have minimal skin resected to ensure that no undue tension is placed on the skin closure. The rhytidectomy surgeon should understand that increased skin tension fails to achieve any significant cosmetic benefit or longevity in rhytidectomy, as the SMAS layer of the face should be the target of the tissue suspension. If excessive skin tension is inadvertently placed on the skin and cannot be minimized, then the surgeon should ensure that deep sutures are placed. Furthermore, the use of surgical adhesive and dermal tape may be of benefit in re-distributing skin tension over a broader region. Patients prone to abnormal scarring should be monitored closely and, if necessary, undergo intralesional injection with triamcinolone and/or 5-fluorouracil [62]. Post-operative management with pulsed-dye laser therapy may also assist in the treatment of hypertrophic and keloidal scars [63, 64]. Atrophic scars are more easily concealed with cosmetics due to their smooth surface topography, but may still be noticeable due to the lack of normal pigmentation; cosmetic tattooing may be of benefit in some patients [65].

Displaced Hairline

A distorted and displaced hairline is another sign of rhytidectomy that most patients wish to avoid. Incisional placement should be carefully considered before surgery with objective measurements and appropriate planning essential to achieving ideal scar concealment. Individuals with moderate-to-severe aging are prone to more significant hairline distortion both due to the greater extent of skin excursion and resection, as well as the higher incidence of alopecia and receded hairlines. As previously outlined in this chapter, female patients with moderate-to-severe aging who are undergoing rhytidectomy, especially in whom a strong vertical vector of lift is expected, should have the temporal segment of the incision designed along the temporal hairline. Trichophytic incisions allow for resection of excess skin without displacing the hairline but are more prone to visible scarring. The incision should be carefully beveled to allow for hair growth through the incision, which can easily conceal the scar (Fig. 33.37). Male patients, due to the fusion of the sideburn into the beard, have essentially a limitless degree of tissue excursion vertically, although there are limitations relating to the posterior displacement of the hairline.

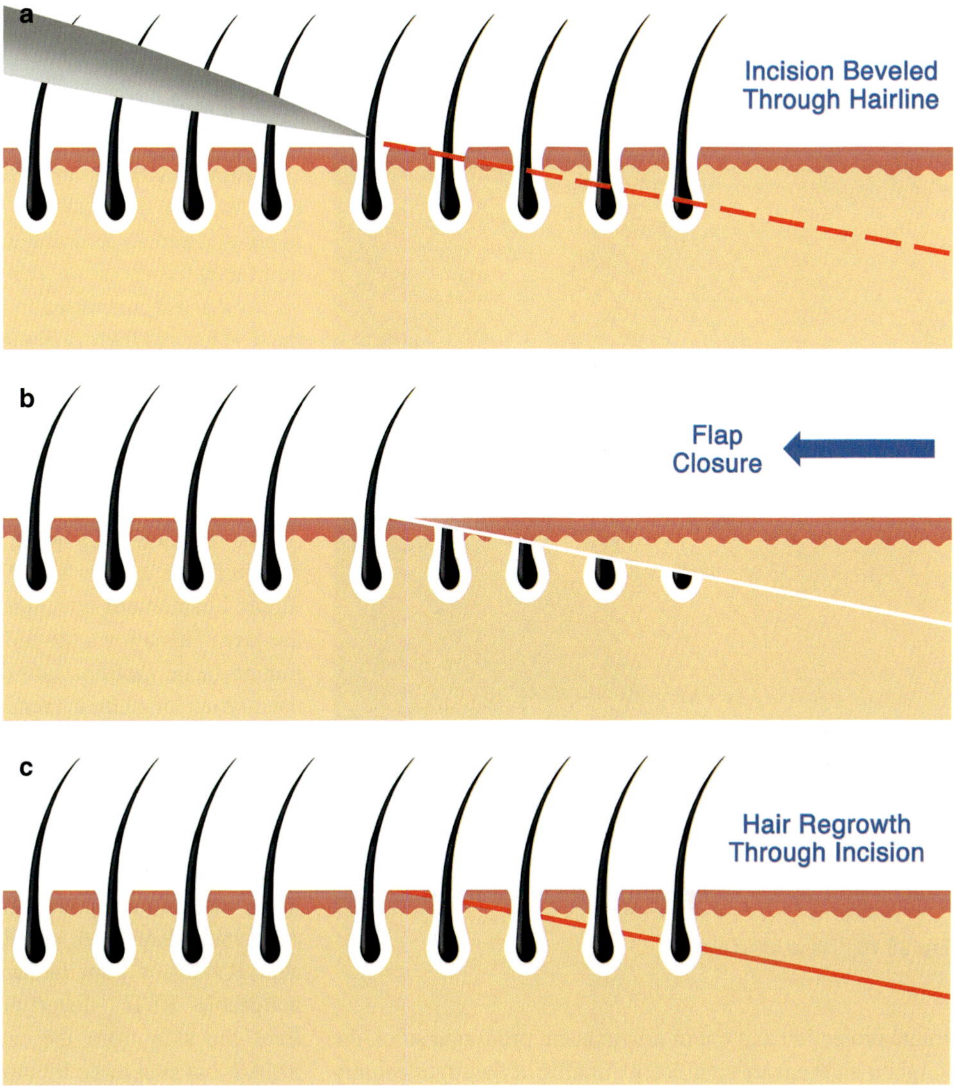

Fig. 33.37 Scalpel beveling in a trichophytic incision. Beveling of the incision is useful whenever a trichophytic incision is utilized. (**a**) The bevel is angled down toward the flap side, transecting the hair follicles in the process but preserving the follicular root. (**b**) When the skin flap is re-draped, trimmed, and then the skin closed, the hair follicles remain deep to the flap skin at the level of the incision. (**c**) As the hairs grow, they pierce through the skin into the exterior. The growth of the hair at the level of the incision helps to conceal the scar

The occipital incision should also be planned carefully. Typically, a lazy-S shape to the incision affords the surgeon the ability to use the occipital skin flap as an advancement-rotational flap, which typically lets the occipital hairline be re-aligned, minimizing post-operative step-offs of the incision, while still allowing the surgeon to hide the occipital incision within the hair. If a step-off is unfortunately created, scar revision via z-plasty can help realign the hairline. Transient hair loss in the temporal and occipital regions may occur due to *telogen effluvium*, a temporary shock loss of hair due to accelerated, concerted shedding of terminal scalp hairs. Topical minoxidil can help to accelerate hair re-growth. If permanent hair loss occurs, follicular unit transplantation can restore hair density to the affected area.

Tragal Effacement

Tragal effacement occurs when the displacement of the rhytidectomy flap over the tragal cartilage results in the loss of its topography (Fig. 33.38). Although the shape and prominence of the tragus vary widely among individuals, it is nonetheless always defined by a sharp protuberance that borders the anterior auditory canal wall. The tragus is a defining feature of a natural-looking auricle, and tragal effacement therefore results in yet another "facelift sign." Tragal effacement is almost always seen with post-tragal incisions, where the overlying skin is dissected off the cartilaginous base. If the surgeon neglects to thin the new tragal skin to the degree that characterized the original skin, the tragus may become less prominent, especially in individuals with already flattened tragi. Tragal effacement is especially common in patients undergoing skin-muscle flap elevation due to the much greater thickness of the flap. In composite-flap patients, even with significant thinning of the flap, the robustness of the skin-muscle flap may still obliterate the pre-tragal sulcus.

Prevention of tragal effacement can be easily achieved by appropriate pre-surgical planning. In patients with minimal

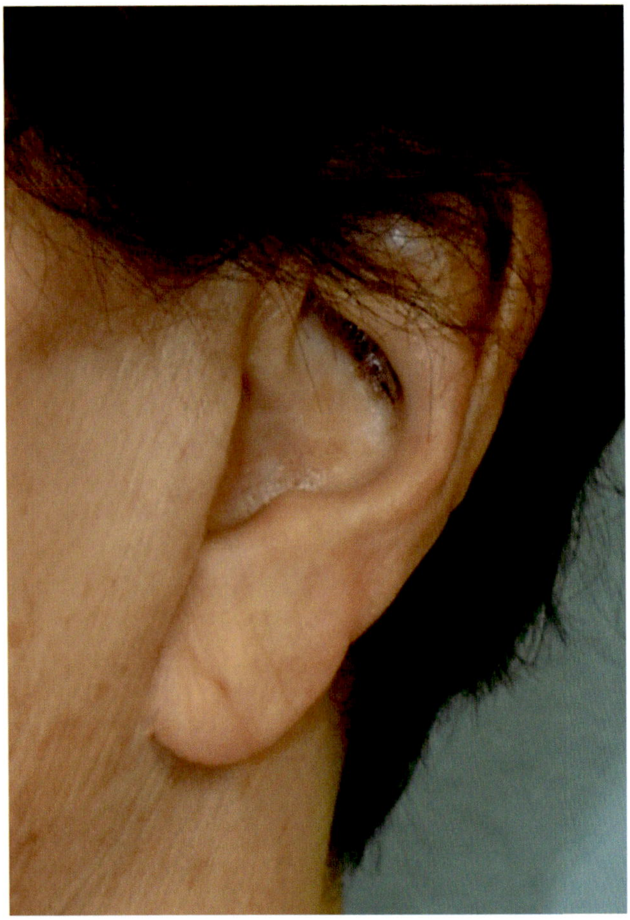

Fig. 33.38 Tragal effacement

tragal projection and flat or non-existent pre-tragal sulci, the surgeon must ensure significant thinning of the rhytidectomy flap from the tragal margin down to the level of the sulcus. If flap thinning still doesn't adequately prevent effacement, the surgeon may opt to place a deep subcutaneous suture from the flap to the fascia. In patients with severe post-surgical tragal effacement, secondary thinning of the soft tissue over the pre-tragal sulcus, with or without placement of quilting suture, may be all that is necessary. If tragal projection is lacking, auricular or nasal septal cartilage grafting may be beneficial [66]. Alternatively, hyaluronic acid or calcium hydroxylapatite filler augmentation of the tragal prominence may provide adequate correction of the problem.

Distorted RSTLs

In the youthful face, relaxed skin tension lines are barely visible, and serve only to assist the surgeon in planning surgical incisions that heal with minimal scarring. However, in the aged face, the RSTLs become quite prominent, even in patients with only mild solar elastosis. The RSTLs represent the natural grain of the facial lines, almost as a universal facial fingerprint that is consistent and well-preserved across individuals. Although these skin tension lines go mostly overlooked, once disrupted, they impart an artificial, unnatural appearance to the face. It is therefore important that the surgeon avoid disrupting this natural pattern of relaxed skin tension lines.

Distorted RSTLs are prone to occur whenever there is excessive pull of the skin in one direction, in which the skin is not allowed to re-drape uniformly, but is instead used to pull facial tissues along a predetermined vector. Any tension vector that is transmitted to the face will, by default, distort the RSTLs, and therein lies the critical nature of the problem. Although few modern rhytidectomy surgeons perform skin-only lifts, the composite skin-muscle flaps of several extended-SMAS techniques, namely the deep plane and high-SMAS techniques, may still result in the transmission of tension vectors onto the skin.

The role of SMAS in the natural configuration of RSTLs is significant, as the SMAS layer sends numerous microscopic ligamentous attachments into the dermis, throughout the face. This allows the SMAS to effectively transmit even minute facial motions into the overlying skin, allowing for the myriad of human facial expressions. Extended SMAS lifts tend to rely on a composite SMAS-skin flap that is more robust and better able to handle the higher tension required for suspension of the midfacial tissues. However, given that the SMAS is capable of transmitting tension onto the skin, these rhytidectomy techniques are inherently apt to result in RSTL distortion (Fig. 33.14).

In individuals with significant aging resulting in prominent RSTLs, a lamellar dissection is necessary to avoid noticeable RSTL distortion. Subcutaneous undermining frees the skin from the underlying SMAS, allowing the SMAS and skin to be mobilized along different vectors that better cater to their different individual degrees of laxity and aging. In most cases, fractional laser skin resurfacing will aid in improving skin uniformity and alleviate the severity of distorted facial rhytids. However, once done, the distortion of RSTLs cannot be undone until a repeat rhytidectomy is performed that re-orients the tension lines back into a normal configuration. The astute surgeon will therefore modify the technique in patients with at-risk features, in whom a lamellar dissection may help prevent or minimize RSTL distortion.

Lateral Sweep Deformity

Hamra first described the lateral sweep deformity in 1998 as the distortion of the lower facial tissues due to the incongruence between a tight lower face and a persistently ptotic midface that developed when limited-SMAS techniques were applied to moderate-to-severely aged faces (Fig. 33.39) [67]. Without the release of midfacial ligaments and the vertical suspension of the midface, Hamra argued the ptotic midfacial tissues will droop and sit atop the suspended lower facial

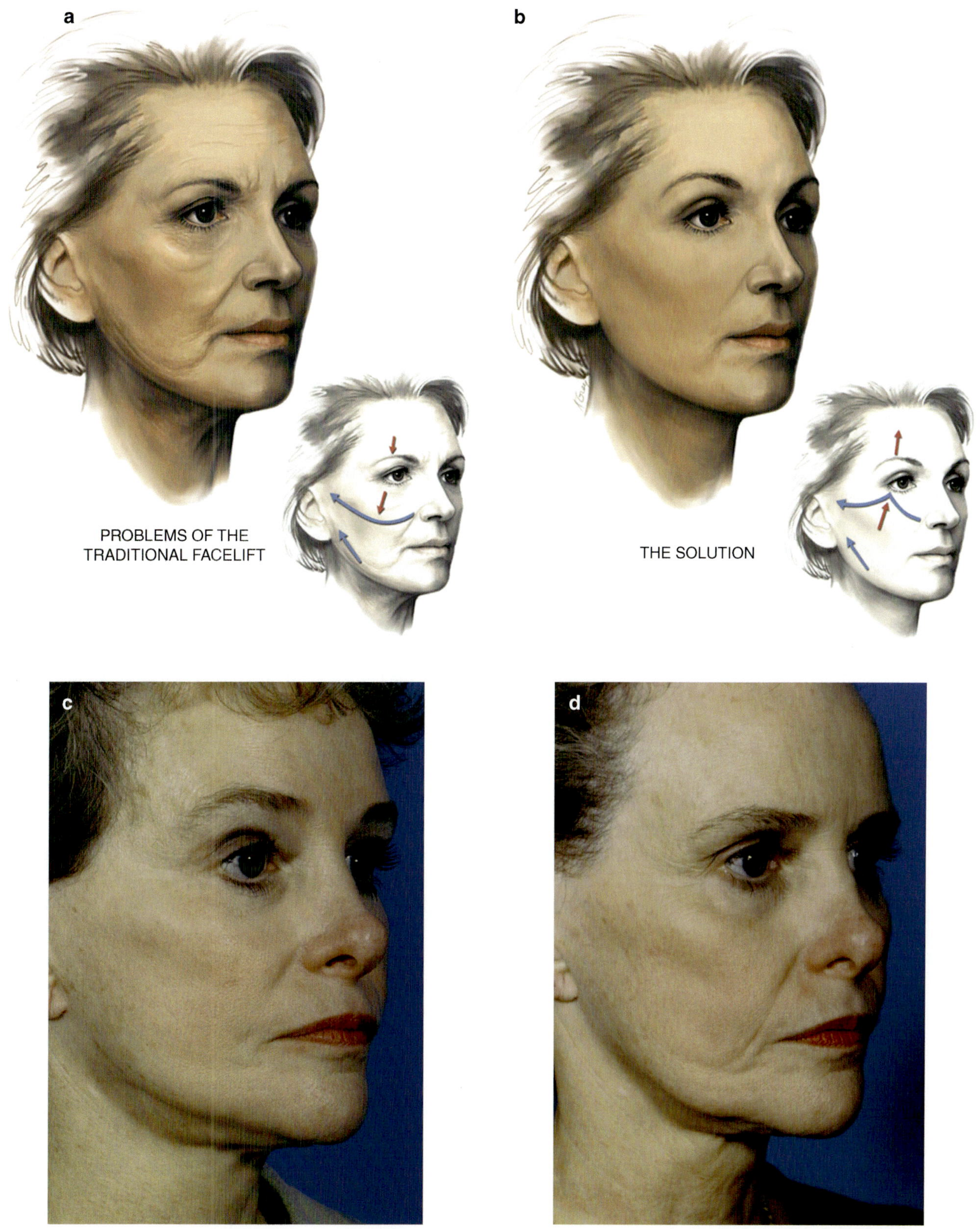

Fig. 33.39 The lateral sweep deformity. As initially described by Hamra, this deformity is reminiscent of a "Nike swoosh," ascending from medial to lateral. The lateral sweep occurs when a surgeon fails to adequately suspend the midface in a patient with moderate-to-severe facial aging. (**a**) The traditional limited-SMAS techniques do not reposition the midface; as a result, whenever a patient with moderate-to-severe facial aging is treated with such limited techniques, the lower face and neck are tightened, leaving the midface ptotic and resting on the lower facial tissues, reminiscent of a hammock. (**b**) Prevention of the lateral sweep deformity centers on providing a powerful vertical vector of lift to the midface. In individuals undergoing a deep plane technique (where a powerful superolateral vector is applied), the surgeon should consider adding a strong superomedial vector of lift to the midface, which is described by Hamra in his *composite rhytidectomy* technique. (Used with permission from Choucair and Hamra [67])

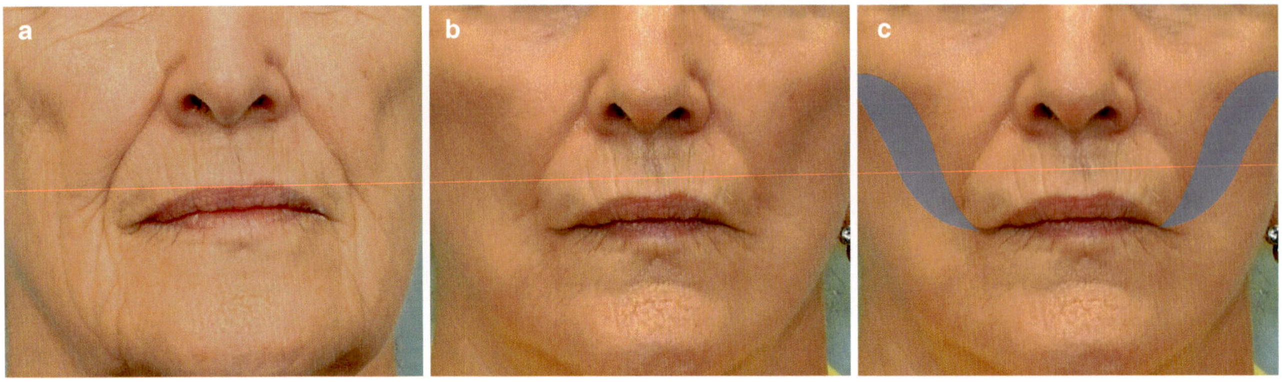

Fig. 33.40 The cross-cheek depression deformity. Known as the joker deformity, the cross-cheek depression, as originally defined by Lambros and Stuzin, describes a buccal depression that appears to "sweep" laterally along the inferior edge of the maxilla. This deformity should not be confused with the "lateral sweep" deformity described by Hamra. The joker deformity is common in individuals with high cheekbones, long faces, and buccal fat atrophy. The correction of this deformity relies mostly on simple volume correction via fat grafting, if the patient so wishes. (**a**) Preoperative view. (**b**) Post-operative view. (**c**) Labeled post-operative view highlighting the depression underlying the joker deformity

tissues, creating a "hammock effect"; this results in a distorted tension vector being transmitted to the skin, creating the "lateral sweep." Hamra's insight into this issue led to the development of his *composite rhytidectomy*, in which the cheek mass and orbicularis oculi muscle are suspended in a superomedial direction. This superomedial mobilization of the cheek creates an orthogonal vector of suspension that obliterates a lateral sweep line. The release of the orbicularis ligament, combined with a septal reset in which the lower eyelid fat pads were repositioned and in which the zygomaticus and orbicularis muscles were partially released from their midfacial attachments—termed the "zygorbicular release" by Hamra—was necessary for complete mobilization of the lid–cheek junction. Due to the need for exposure and the mobilization of periorbital tissues upward, the procedure, by default, necessitated a simultaneous subciliary lower blepharoplasty and coronal brow lift, leading to Hamra's coining of the term *composite* rhytidectomy.

Cross-Cheek Depression

The cross-cheek depression, or "Joker deformity," was described by Lambros and Stuzin in 2008 as a unique form of facial distortion that occurred in patients with a specific type of facial structure [68]. In their 2008 description, the authors described the issue as follows:

> Despite plastic surgeons' best efforts, deformities can be seen following a face lift. One of the most obvious signs of face-lift surgery is the cross-cheek depression or "joker line," which begins as an indentation in the region of the oral commissure and extends laterally and superiorly toward the ear. When this depression develops postoperatively, the face can appear harsh, pulled, and abnormal, creating a visual illusion that the corner of the mouth extends laterally onto the cheek. [68]

The *cross-cheek depression* is not a line and should not be confused with Hamra's *lateral sweep*. Instead, as the name suggests, the cross-cheek depression is a region of volume loss in the buccal segment of the face that is prone to distortion and accentuation in a way that appears to merge as an extension of the curvature of the commissure, thus creating the "joker" appearance (Fig. 33.40). As astutely noted by Lambros and Stuzin, this type of deformity is usually seen in patients with a long face, elevated cheekbones, and a paucity of adipose tissue in the buccal region. When these features coexist, the patient is prone to an accentuation of the buccal volume loss as the SMAS suspension lifts against the maxillary contour. Management of the cross-cheek depression relies on volume correction, typically via lipotransfer to the buccal region.

Pixie-Earlobe Deformity

The pixie or "satyr's" ear deformity represents an elongation and inferior displacement of the earlobe following rhytidectomy (Fig. 33.41d). This common deformity is regarded as a classic sign of facelifting, one which most patients wish to avoid. Although all patients are at risk for a pixie deformity following an overly aggressive rhytidectomy with excessive skin tension on the perilobular incision, patients with a non-cleft earlobe are at greatest risk. Cleft earlobes are characterized by an attachment point located above the inferior margin of the earlobe, which creates a cleft between the earlobe and the face (Fig. 33.41a–b). Non-cleft earlobes feature an earlobe that attach to the face along their entire length (Fig. 33.41c). Because of their configuration, cleft earlobes are naturally resistant against the development of a pixie earlobe because the distance that the earlobe attachment point needs to travel before it creates the appearance of a distended earlobe is significantly greater. Nonetheless, surgeons should still ensure that the skin flap is adequately tucked under the earlobe, providing sufficient support and resistance against the inevitable downward pulling that reflexively follows rhytidectomy.

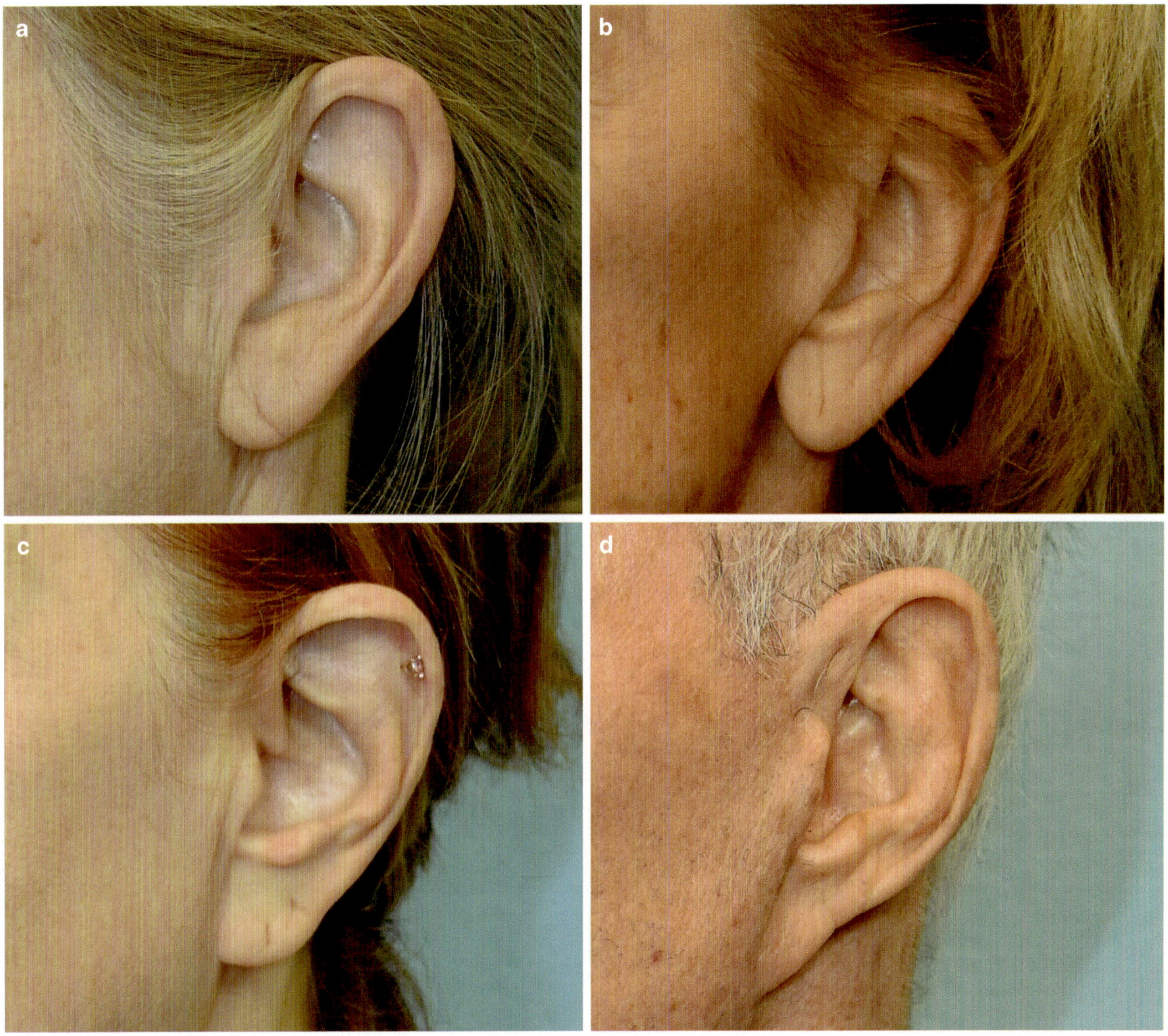

Fig. 33.41 Different earlobe types and the pixie earlobe deformity. Earlobes may be roughly divided into cleft or non-cleft, but they exist along a spectrum of earlobe insertion shapes. (**a**) Cleft earlobe, low insertion point. (**b**) Cleft earlobe, high insertion point. (**c**) Non-cleft earlobe. (**d**) Pixie earlobe deformity post-rhytidectomy; note the extension of the earlobe attachment point well below the inferior margin of the earlobe

The non-cleft earlobe lacks a cleft, and therefore even 2 mm of inferior excursion of the earlobe attachment point can result in a stretched earlobe. In individuals with a non-cleft lobe, it is of paramount importance to avoid placing any tension on the perilobular incision. In addition, deep subcutaneous sutures anchoring the earlobe to the platysma-auricular ligament may provide long-term resistance against any downward pull.

Several methods of repair exist for the management of the pixie earlobe deformity. Classically, a V-Y advancement flap may be utilized, pushing the earlobe insertion point upward. However, this approach can create a vertical incision that can be conspicuous. In patients with laxity of the lower face and neck skin, a revision facelift can be attempted, in which the perilobular tissues are once again lifted superolaterally and the excess skin is advanced superiorly to prop up the earlobe attachment point and limit skin tension. Finally, a conservative transcutaneous suture technique has been described by Hoefflin, in which a suture is looped subcutaneously around the earlobe via a stab incision at the base of the earlobe that is then anchored deeply to the periosteum of the auricular cartilage [69].

Conclusion

Throughout its more than 110-year history, the facelift procedure has seen great successes and failures, punctuated by several defining moments at key points in its existence. The evolution of the rhytidectomy has continued unimpeded into modern times, now invigorated by new advances in technology that have brought minimally invasive endoscopic approaches, and fractionated laser skin resurfacing into the forefront of this generation of surgical acumen. Despite all the new developments in this exciting, ever-changing field, the success of rhytidectomy still rests wholly upon a central understanding of facial anatomy and the challenges and limitations that it imposes upon the surgeon. The evolution of facelifting has taken this surgery from a skin-only excision through the development of limited-SMAS suspension techniques and then eventually to the extended-SMAS procedures that we see today. Only through understanding the challenges faced by past surgeons, in their attempts to modify and perfect the technique to yield the most natural results, can the modern surgeon be fully prepared to deliver optimal results and avoid complications.

References

1. Leal Silva HG. Facial laxity rating scale validation study. Dermatol Sure. 2016;42(12):1370–9.
2. Pessa JE, Zadoo VP, Yuan C, Ayedelotte JD, Cuellar FJ, Cochran CS, et al. Concertina effect and facial aging: nonlinear aspects of youthfulness and skeletal remodeling, and why, perhaps. Infants Have Jowls Plast Reconstr Surg. 1999;103(2):635–44.
3. Mendelson B, Wong C-H. Changes in the facial skeleton with aging: implications and clinical applications in facial rejuvenation. Aesthet Plast Surg. 2012;36(4):753–60.
4. Shaw RB Jr, Katzel EB, Koltz PF, Kahn DM, Girotto JA, Langstein HN. Aging of the mandible and its aesthetic implications. Plast Reconstr Surg. 2010;125(1):332–42.
5. Donofrio LM. Fat distribution: a morphologic study of the aging face. Dermatol Surg. 2000;26(12):1107–12.
6. Lambros V. Observations on periorbital and midface aging. Plast Reconstr Surg. 2007;120(5):1367–76.
7. Rohrich RJ, Pessa JE. The fat compartments of the face: anatomy and clinical implications for cosmetic surgery. Plast Reconstr Surg. 2007;119(7):2219–27.
8. Ascher B, Coleman S, Alster T, Bauer U, Burgess C, Butterwick K, et al. Full scope of effect of facial lipoatrophy: a framework of disease understanding. Dermatol Surg. 2006;32(8):1058–69.
9. Pallua N, Wolter T. The Lipo-facelift: merging the face-lift and Liposculpture: eight years experience and a preliminary observational study. Aesthet Plast Surg. 2013;37(6):1107–13.
10. Glogau RG. Aesthetic and anatomic analysis of the aging skin. Semin Cutan Med Surg. 1996;15(3):134–8.
11. Lexer E. In: Barth JA, editor. Die gesamte Wiederherslellung schiurgie, vol. 2. Leipzig; 1931. p. 548.
12. Hollander E. Cosmetic surgery. In: Joseph M, editor. Handbuch der Kosmetik. Leipzig: Veriag von Velt; 1912. p. 688.
13. Joseph J. Hangewangenplastik (melomioplastik). Dtsch Med Wochenschr. 1921;47:287.
14. Bourget J. La disparitionchiurgicale des rides etplis du visage. Bull Acad Med Paris. 1919;82:183.
15. Passot R. La chirurgieesthetique des rides du visages. Presse Med. 1919;27:258.
16. Noel A. La Chirurgieesthetique: Son Role Social. Paris: Masson et Cite; 1926.
17. Bames OH. Truth and fallacies of face peeling and face lifting. Med J Rec. 1927:126–86.
18. Burian F. Zur Technik der Gesichtshautspannung. Med Welt. 1936;10:930.
19. Seltzer AP. Reconstructive surgery for the elderly. Geriatrics. 1952;7(3):185–8.
20. Johnson JB. The problem of the aging face. Plast Reconstr Surg. 1955;15(2):117–21.
21. Gonzales-Ulloa M. The creation of aesthetic plastic surgery [book on the internet]. New York: Springer; 1985. Chapter 3: The history of rhytidectomy; p. 46–90. Available from: SpringerLink.
22. Skoog T. "Chapter XIII: The Aging Face". Plastic surgery: new methods. Saunders: Philadelphia; 1974. p. 328–9.
23. Webster RC, Smith RC, Papsidero MJ, Karolow WW, Smith KF. Comparison of SMAS plication with smas imbrication in face lifting. Laryngoscope. 1982;92(8 Pt 1):901–12.
24. Barton FE Jr. The SMAS and the nasolabial fold. Plast Reconstr Surg. 1992;89(6):1054–7; discussion 1058–9.
25. Hamra ST. The deep-plane Rhytidectomy. Plast Reconstr Surg. 1990;86(1):53–61; discussion 62–3.
26. Hamra ST. The tri-plane face lift dissection. Ann Plast Surg. 1984;12(3):268–74.
27. Hamra ST. Commentary on: total composite flap facelift and the deep-plane transition zone: a critical consideration in SMAS-release midface lifting. Aesthet Surg J. 2016;36(5):546–9.
28. Barton FE. The "high SMAS" facelift technique. Aesthet Surg J. 2002;22(5):481–6.
29. Tessier P. Le lifting facial sous-perioste. Ann Chir Plast Esthet. 1989;34(3):193–7. French.
30. Psillakis JM, Rumley TO, Camargos A. Subperiosteal approach on an improved concept for correction of the aging face. Plast Reconstr Surg. 1988;82(3):383–92.
31. Santana PM. Craniofacial methods in rhytidectomy. Cir Plast Iberolatinoamer. 1984;10:322–8.
32. Ramirez OM, Maillard GF, Musolas A. The extended subperiosteal face lift: a definitive soft tissue remodeling for facial rejuvenation. Plast Reconstr Surg. 1991;88(2):227–36.
33. de Saint Cyr BC, Maillard GC, Scheflan M, Ramirez O. The subperiosteal lift. Aesth Plast Surg. 1993;17(2):151–5.
34. Quatela VC, Jacono AA. The extended centrolateral endoscopic midface lift. Facial Plast Surg. 2003;19(2):199–208.
35. Hamra ST. Composite Rhytidectomy. St. Louis: Quality Medical Publishing; 1993.
36. Marten TJ. High SMAS facelift: combined single flap lifting of the jawline, cheek, and midface. Clin Plast Surg. 2008;35(4):569–603.
37. Marten TJ. Lamellar high SMAS face and mid-face lift. In: Nahai F, editor. The art of aesthetic surgery. St. Louis: Quality Medical Publishing; 2005. p. 1110–93.
38. Maliniak JW. Is the surgical restoration of the aged face justified? Med J Rec. 1932;135:321–4.
39. Millard DR, Garst WP, Beck RL. Submental and submandibular lipectomy in conjunction with a face-lift in the female and male. Plast Reconstr Surg. 1972;49(4):385–91.
40. Guerrero-Santos J, Espaillat L, Morales F. Muscular lift in cervical rhytidoplasty. Plast Reconstr Surg. 1974;54(2):127–30.
41. Connell BF. Contouring the neck in rhytidectomy by lipectomy and muscle sling. Plast Reconstr Surg. 1978;61(3):376–83.
42. Aston SJ. Platysma muscle in rhytidoplasty. Annals Plast Surg. 1979;3(6):529–39.
43. Connell BC. Cervical lifts: the value of platysma muscle flaps. Ann Plast Surg. 1978;1(1):32–43.
44. Feldman JJ. Corset platysmaplasty. Plast Reconstr Surg. 1990;85(3):333–43.
45. Mittelman H, Spencer JR, Chrzanowski DS. Chin region: management of grooves & mandibular hypoplasia with alloplastic implant. Facial Plast Surg Clin North Am. 2007;15(4):445–60.
46. Grover R, Jones BM, Waterhouse N. The prevention of haematoma following rhytidectomy: a review of 1078 consecutive facelifts. Br J Plast Surg. 2001;54(6):481–6.

47. Baker DC, Stefani WA, Chiu ES. Reducing the incidence of hematoma requiring surgical evacuation following male rhytidectomy: a 30-year review of 985 cases. Plast Reconstr Surg. 2005;116(7):1973–85; discussion 1986–7.
48. Kamer FM, Song AU. Hematoma formation in deep plane rhytidectomy. Arch Facial Plast Surg. 2000;2(4):240–2.
49. Berner RE, Morain WD, Noe JM. Postoperative hypertension as an etiological factor in hematoma after rhytidectomy. Prevention with chlorpromazine. Plast Reconstr Surg. 1976;57(3):314–9.
50. Spotnitz WD. Efficacy and safety of fibrin sealant for tissue adherence in facial rhytidectomy. Clin Cosmet Investig Dermatol. 2012;5:43–51.
51. Weissman O, Farber N, Remer E, Tessone A, Trivizki O, Bank J, et al. Post-facelift flap necrosis treatment using charged polystyrene microspheres. Can J Plast Surg. 2013;21(1):45–7.
52. Rees A, Aston SJ. Complications of rhytidectomy. Clin Plast Surg. 1978;5(1):109–19.
53. Kruper GJ, VandeGriend ZP, Lin H-S, Zuliani GF. Salvage of failed local and regional flaps with porcine urinary bladder extracellular matrix aided tissue regeneration. Case Rep Otolaryngol. 2013;2013:917183.
54. Kimmel H, Rahn M, Gilbert TW. The clinical effectiveness in wound healing with extracellular matrix derived from porcine urinary bladder matrix: a case series on severe chronic wounds. J Am Col Certif Wound Spec. 2010;2(3):55–9.
55. Robertson SA, Jeevaratnam JA, Agrawal A, Cutress RI. Mastectomy skin flap necrosis: challenges and solutions. Breast Cancer (Dove Med Press). 2017;9:141–52.
56. Francis A, Baynosa RC. Hyperbaric oxygen therapy for the compromised graft or flap. Adv Wound Care (New Rochelle). 2017;6(1):23–32.
57. Payne DL. Facial nerve deficits following face lift surgery. Am J Otol. 1992;13(1):91–2.
58. Liebman EP, Webster RC, Gaul JR, Griffin T. The marginal mandibular nerve in rhytidectomy and liposuction surgery. Arch Otolaryngol Head Neck Surg. 1988;114(2):179–81.
59. Kamer FM. One hundred consecutive deep plane face lifts. Arch Otol Head Neck Surg. 1996;122(1):17–22.
60. Clark RP, Berris CE. Botulinum toxin: a treatment for facial asymmetry caused by facial nerve paralysis. Plast Reconstr Surg. 1989;84(2):353–5.
61. LeRoy JL Jr, Rees TD, Nolan WB III. Infections requiring hospital readmission following face lift surgery: incidence, treatment, and sequelae. Plast Reconstr Surg. 1994;93(3):533–6.
62. Shah VV, Aldahan AS, Mlacker S, Alsaidan M, Samarkandy S, Nouri K. 5-fluorouracil in the treatment of keloids and hypertrophic scars: a comprehensive review of the literature. Dermatol Ther (Heidelb). 2016;6(2):169–83.
63. Tholen RH. Pulsed dye laser treatment of hypertrophic scars. Aesthetic Surgery Journal. 1996;16(2):92.
64. Kono T, Erçöçen A, Nakazawa H, Nozaki M. Treatment of hypertrophic scars using a long-pulsed dye laser with cryogen-spray cooling. Ann Plast Surg. 2005;54(5):487–93.
65. Drost BH, van de Langenberg R, Manusama OR, Janssens AS, Sikorska K, Zuur CL, et al. Dermatography (medical tattooing) for scars and skin grafts in head and neck patients to improve appearance and quality of life. JAMA Facial Plast Surg. 2017;19(1):16–22.
66. Perez CF, Gaball CW. Functional and aesthetic tragal reconstruction in the age of mobile electronic devices. Case Rep Otolaryngol. 2016;2016:2591705.
67. Choucair RJ, Hamra ST. Extended superficial musculaponeurotic system dissection and composite rhytidectomy. Clin Plastics Surg. 2008;35(4):607–22.
68. Lambros V, Stuzin JM. The cross-cheek depression: surgical cause and effect in the development of the "joker line" and its treatment. Plast Reconstr Surg. 2008;122(5):1543–52.
69. Hoefflin SM. Simple repair of pixie earlobe. Plast Reconstr Surg. 2001;107(6):1623–4.
70. Gonzales-Ulloa M. The history of rhytidectomy. Aesthet Plast Surg. 1980;4(1):1–45.

Alloplastic Contouring of the Orbital, Maxillary, and Zygomatic Regions

34

Danny J. Soares and William E. Silver

Technical Terms and Abbreviations

BMI	Body mass index
NJF	Nasojugal fold
ORL	Orbicularis retaining ligament
PMF	Palpebromalar fold
PTFE	Polytetrafluoroethylene
SMAS	Superficial musculoaponeurotic system
SOOF	Suborbicularis oculi fat
ZRL	Zygomatic retaining ligament

Introduction

The midface is a unifying component of the facial countenance, bringing together the complex regions of the orbit, nose, and mouth. Structurally, the cheek represents a keystone region of the face, serving as the rigid abutment into which the ligamentous and muscular attachments of the mimetic, masticatory, and orbital facial components insert. Aesthetically, the midface plays a central role in shaping facial identity – imparting gender and ethnic specificity to the human face – as well as influencing the perceived age of an individual. Due to its broad interfaced nature, the cheek demonstrates substantial anatomical complexity that must be understood to address its various types of facial deformities. Midfacial soft-tissue and bony deficiencies often underlie many common facial deformities, including malar under-projection, prominent nasojugal and palpebromalar folds, and deep temporal hollows. In this chapter, we review the pertinent anatomy of the midface and outline an algorithm for the management of common midfacial deformities.

D. J. Soares (✉)
Department of Otolaryngology, Head and Neck Surgery, University of Central Florida College of Medicine, Orlando, FL, USA

Mesos Plastic and Laser Surgery, Lady Lake, FL, USA
e-mail: Drsoares@mesoshealth.com

W. E. Silver
Department of Otolaryngology, Head and Neck Surgery, Emory University, Atlanta, GA, USA

Atlanta Institute for Facial Aesthetic Surgery, Atlanta, GA, USA

Midface Anatomy

Skeletal

The skeletal structure underlying the midface is comprised primarily of the *zygomatic* and *maxillary* bones (Fig. 34.1) and can be topographically partitioned into distinct regions of aesthetic importance. The *malar eminence* forms the most visible landmark of the midface, projecting outwardly as a three-dimensional domal protuberance that imparts shape to an individual's face. The malar eminence varies greatly in degree of projection relative to the orbit and maxilla, and can be defined spatially in terms of its anterior and lateral projection, as well as its vertical height relative to the facial length. Gender- and ethnicity-specific variations exist but are diffuse enough in distribution and spectrum of intensity such that no specific size, shape, or projection of the midface should be regarded as a defining characteristic of any group of individuals [1, 2]. An under-projected malar eminence creates the appearance of a flat face devoid of vitality and appears to predispose to more midfacial ptosis with aging.

Medially, the malar eminence seamlessly blends into the maxillary bone across the zygomaticomaxillary suture line into the *medial cheek*. This region of the midface is often flat and smooth, serving as the attachment for the lip elevators. The anterior projection of the bony medial cheek can play a critical role in the appearance of the face, as an under-projected maxilla results in an under-projected nose and receded orbital rim. Aesthetically, a deficient maxilla is characterized by a *negative vector* of the orbit, in which the globe projects farther anteriorly than the inferior orbital rim. Individuals with this type of bony insufficiency are

A. J. Cohen, C. N. Burkat (eds.), *Oculofacial, Orbital, and Lacrimal Surgery*, https://doi.org/10.1007/978-3-030-14092-2_34

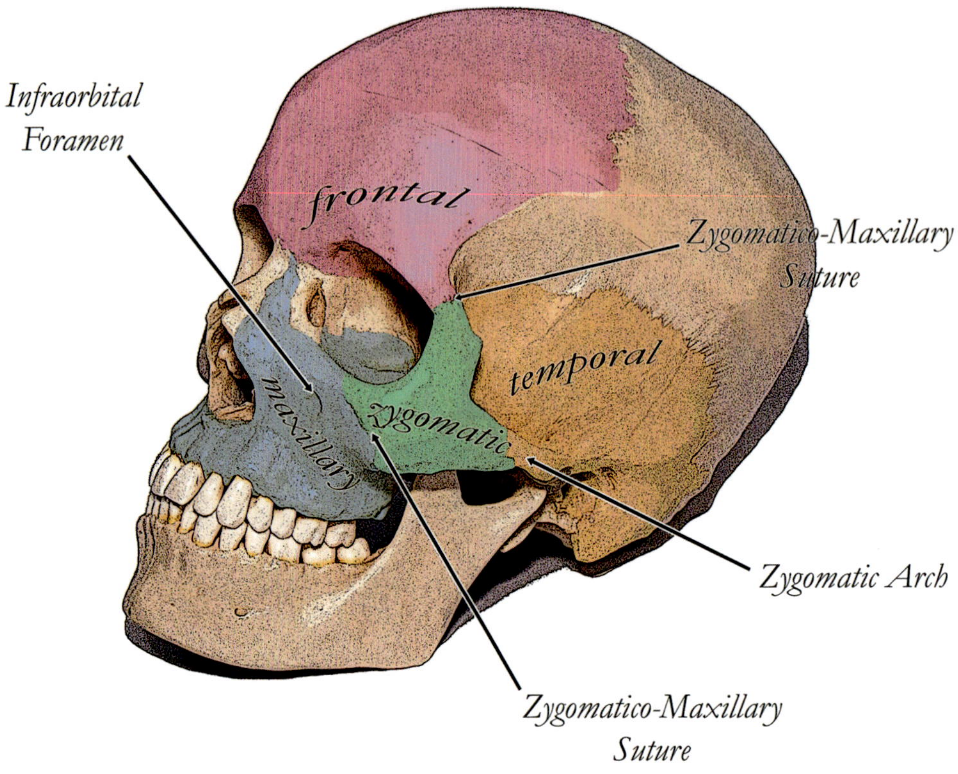

Fig. 34.1 The skeletal framework of the midface

prone to prominent tear trough deformities, including prominent nasojugal folds (NJFs) (Fig. 34.2), and are higher-risk candidates during external transcutaneous lower blepharoplasty due to a higher incidence of ectropion [3]. Maxillary deficiency also impacts dental projection and normal occlusion, with individuals often having poor lip projection and a type II malocclusion as defined by Angle's classification [4].

Superiorly, the malar eminence extends a process upward to meet the frontal bone across the *zygomaticofrontal suture line*, forming the *lateral orbital rim*. This superior extension of the malar bone demonstrates the same level of projection as the eminence itself such that individuals with under-projected eminences will also demonstrate a deficiency in the projection of the inferolateral orbital rim. This deficiency results in a greater tendency to develop prominent palpebromalar folds (PMFs) early due to the accentuation of any herniated lateral fat (Fig. 34.3).

Inferiorly, the surface of the bony midface drops off precipitously into the *submalar region*, a segment of the cheek largely dominated by soft tissue rather than bone. The submalar region is full in the healthy, youthful individual with normal body mass index (BMI) but sunken and gaunt in individuals with extremely low BMIs or in those with lipodystrophy (Fig. 34.4). The submalar region undergoes visible changes with aging as well, witnessing significant volume loss and soft tissue ptosis, which impart a "droopy" appearance to the aged face. The submalar region is roughly defined

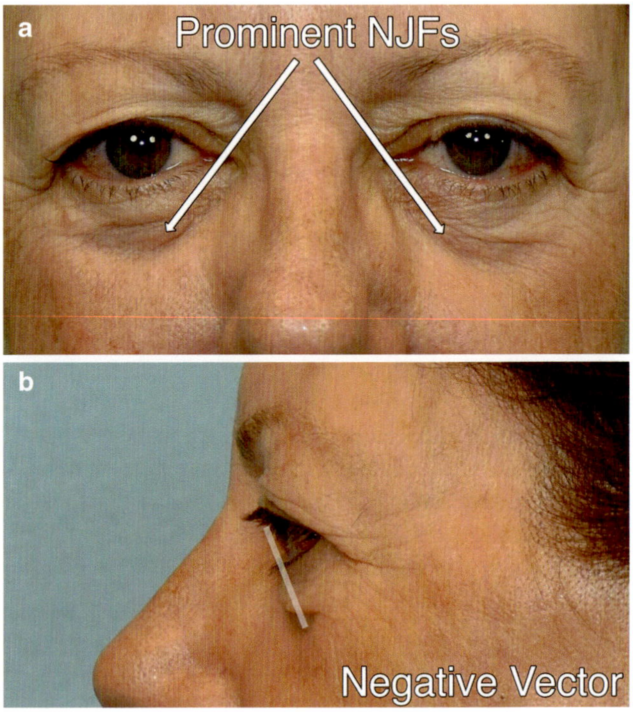

Fig. 34.2 Medial maxillary skeletal insufficiency. (**a**) Frontal view of a patient with maxillary insufficiency characterized by prominent nasojugal folds (NJFs). (**b**) Individuals with an under-projected midfacial skeleton typically display a "negative vector" configuration of the inferior orbital rim relative to the globe, wherein the globe projects farther anteriorly than the rim. Individuals with this type of configuration are particularly prone to cicatricial ectropion due to outer lamellar scarring following an external blepharoplasty

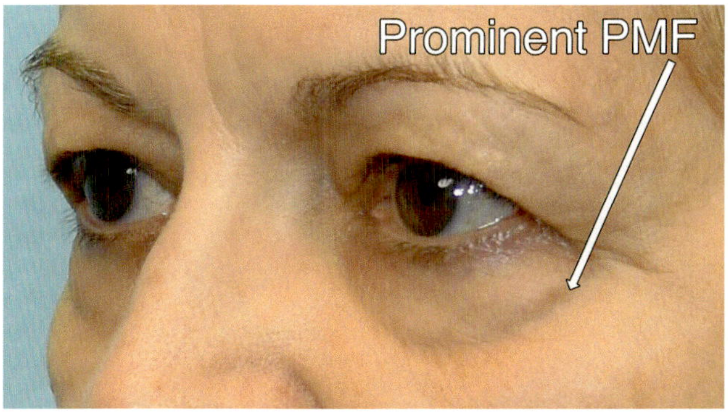

Fig. 34.3 Prominent palpebromalar folds (PMFs). Prominent palpebromalar fold in an individual with maxillary insufficiency

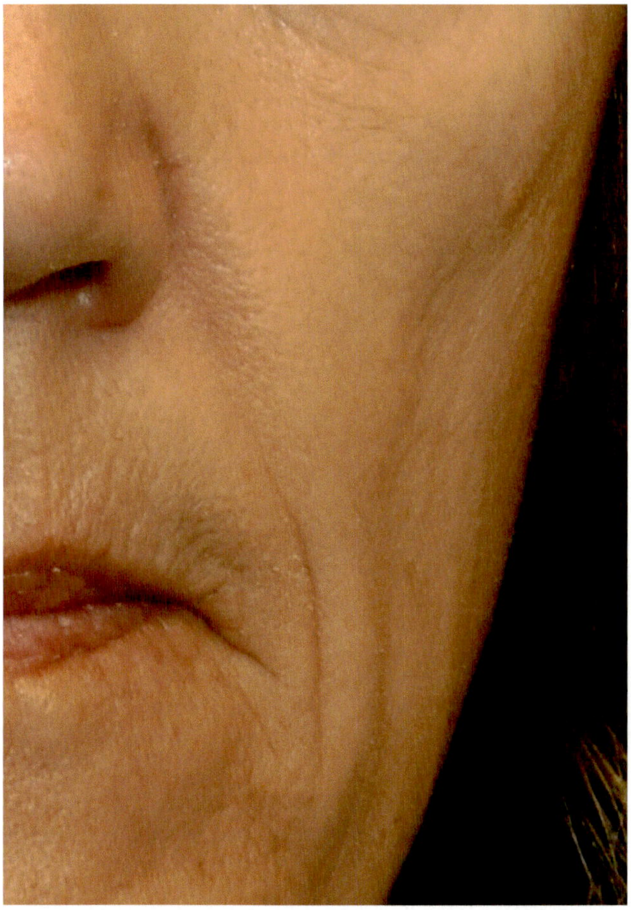

Fig. 34.4 Submalar lipoatrophy in an individual with a low body mass index (BMI)

as the triangular area located inferior to the malar eminence, bordered by the nasolabial compartment medially and the masseter muscle laterally [5].

Laterally, the zygoma extends another process toward the auricle, meeting the temporal bone across the *zygomaticotemporal suture line* and forming the *zygomatic arch* in the process. The zygomatic arch is associated with the temporalis muscle and thus also the temporal fat pads. The loss of volume in the superficial and deep temporal fat pads results in an increased prominence of the zygomatic arch and lateral orbital rim, deepening the temporal fossa (Fig. 34.5).

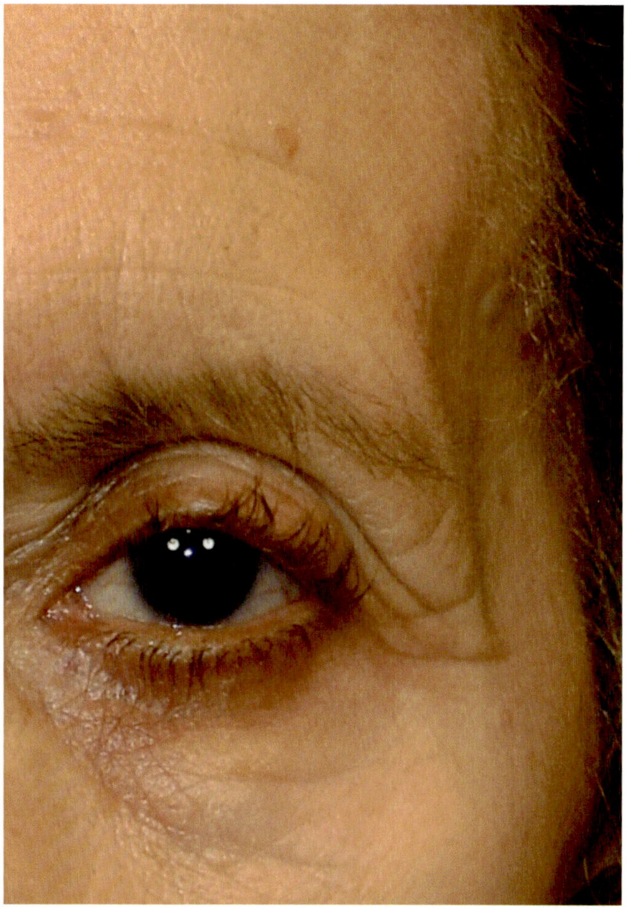

Fig. 34.5 Temporal lipoatrophy in individual with a low BMI

Muscular

The *masseter muscle* is the largest muscle originating from the midface, bridging the zygomatic arch and the mandibular angle (Fig. 34.6) and playing a powerful role in mastication. The masseter muscle contributes significant bulk to the lateral face and therefore influences the overall shape of the face. Individuals with significant masseter muscle hypertrophy tend to have relatively more square-shaped faces than those with less muscular volume, rendering the face more masculine. Treatment of masseter hypertrophy can be easily achieved via simple botulinum toxin type A injection therapy [6].

Multiple mimetic muscles also insert into the midfacial skeleton, including all the upper lip elevators. The zygomaticus major and minor muscles, as well as the quadratus levator labii superioris (i.e., levator anguli oris, levator labii

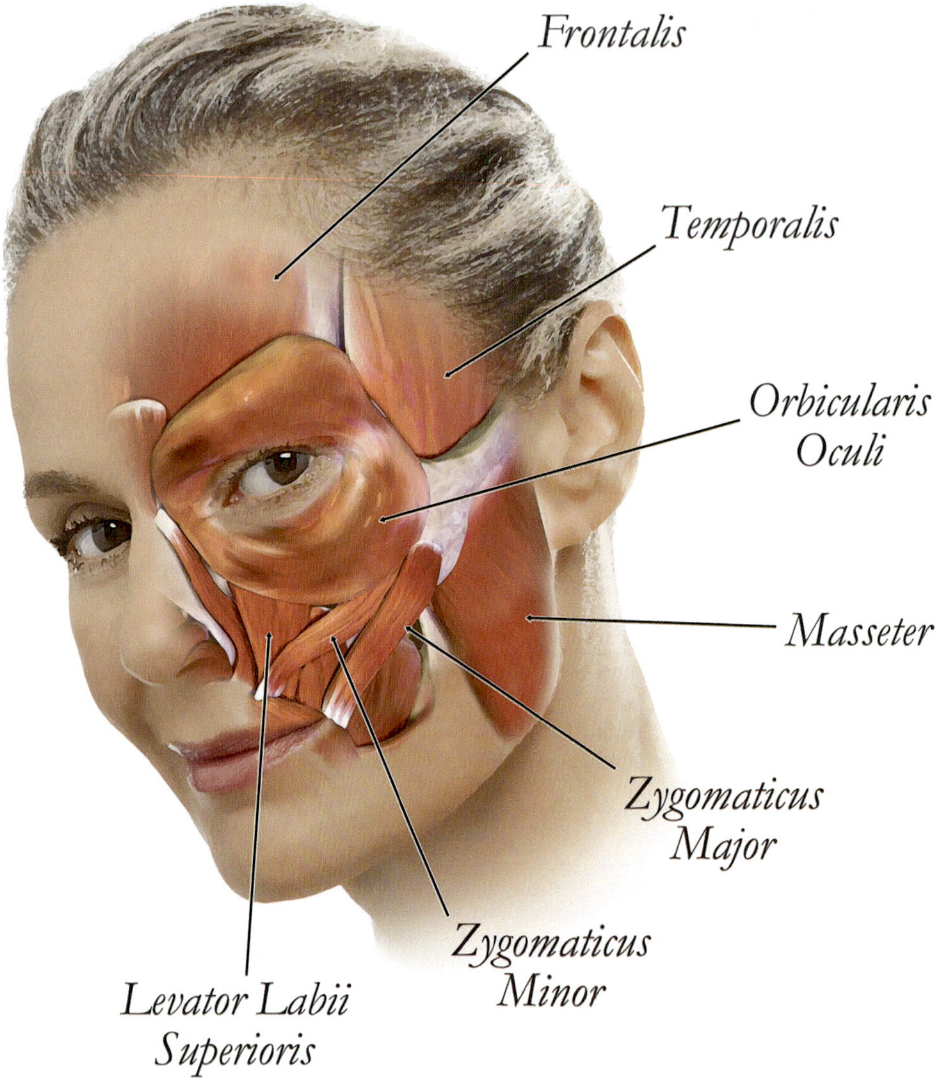

Fig. 34.6 Muscular anatomy of the midface. (Used with permission from Silver and Soares [33])

superioris, and levator labii superioris alaeque nasi), all insert onto the zygomaticomaxillary skeleton. Multiple retaining ligaments and fascial adhesions are associated with these midfacial muscles, forming important ligamentous attachments that support the midface and partition the fat compartments.

Ligamentous

Midfacial ligaments play a critical role in the suspension and organization of the midface, and underlie many of the stigmata of midfacial and periorbital aging [7, 8]. The midface features several important retaining ligaments, including the *zygomatic retaining ligament* (ZRL) and *orbicularis retaining ligament* (ORL) (Fig. 34.7). The ZRL arises from the lateral zygomatic region and inserts directly onto the skin, pinning the midfacial soft tissues firmly in place. Surgically, the ZRL forms a broad region of adhesion known as *McGregor's patch* that is often encountered in flap elevation during rhytidectomy. Superficially, the ZRL contributes to the diagonal *midcheek crease* that is often seen in the aged midface (Fig. 34.8).

The ORL serves as a rigid attachment point connecting the skin and the orbicularis muscle to the inferior orbital rim. This strong ligament precludes the descent of any intraorbital fat, resulting in the gradual outward herniation of the orbital fat that leads to the formation of lower eyelid steatoblepharon. The ORL forces the development of a superficial fold along the semicircular outline of the inferior orbital rim. Medially, this fold is referred to as the nasojugal fold; laterally, it is called the palpebromalar fold. Although the ORL and its associated displacement of orbital fat outwardly are responsible for the development of

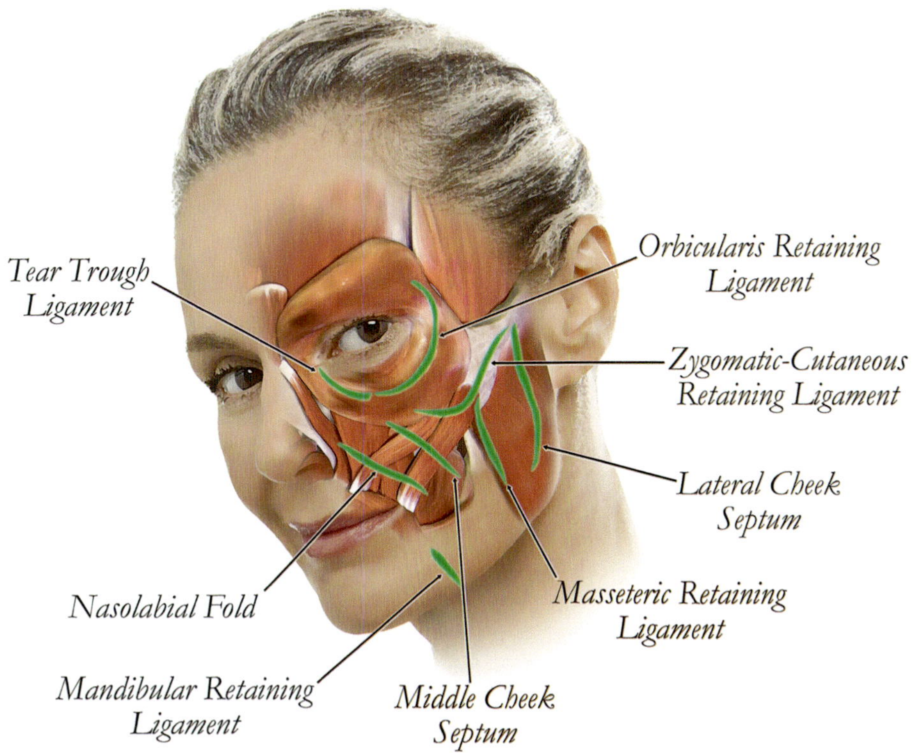

Fig. 34.7 The retaining ligaments of the face. (Used with permission from Silver and Soares [33])

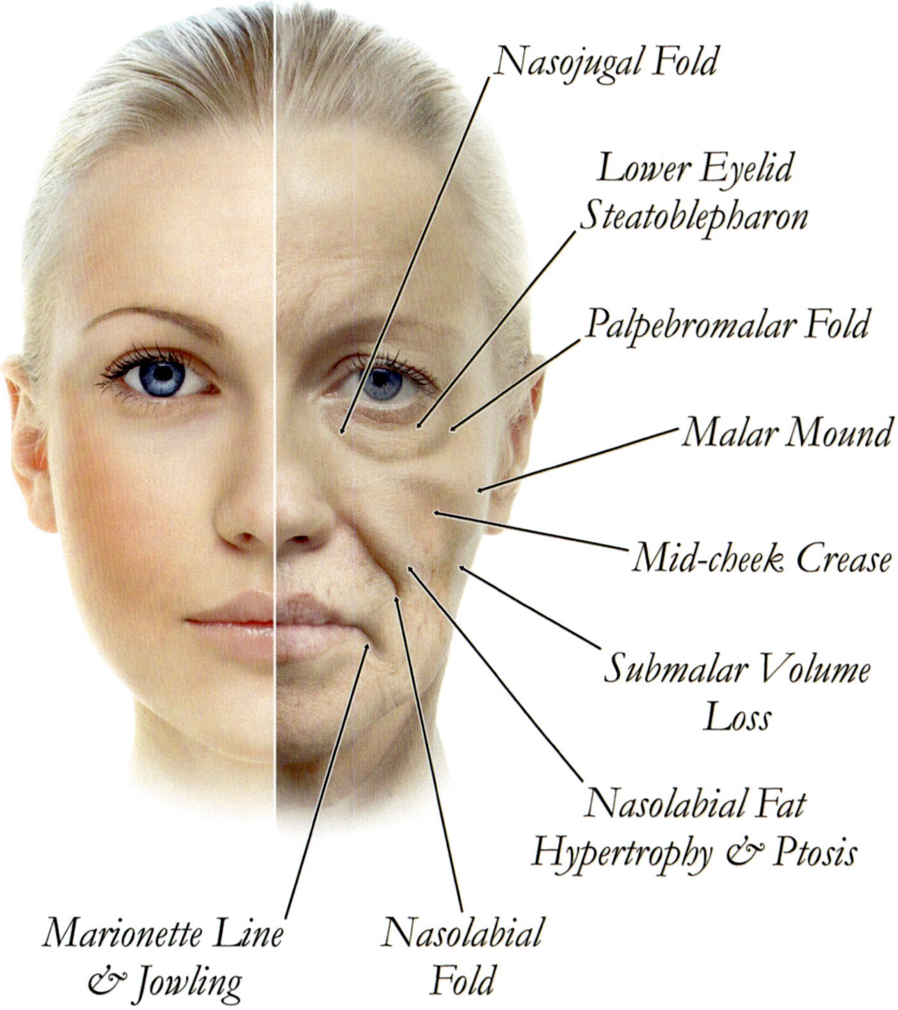

Fig. 34.8 Stigmata of facial aging. (Used with permission from Silver and Soares [33])

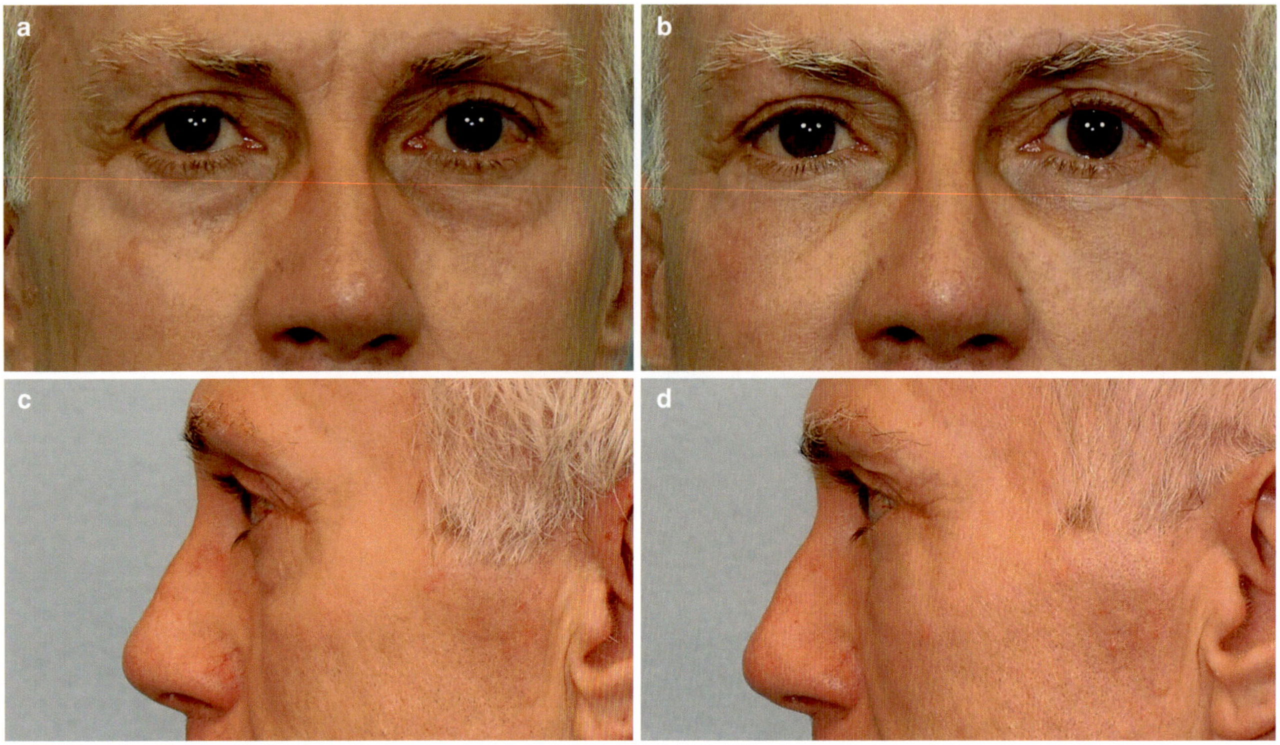

Fig. 34.9 Persistent tear trough deformity following lower blepharoplasty. (**a**, **c**) Frontal and lateral views of a patient who had previously undergone a lower blepharoplasty 5 years prior, displaying persistent bilateral tear trough deformities. (**b**, **d**) Frontal and lateral views of same patient 6 months following tear trough augmentation with a Flowers' silastic implant

the nasojugal fold, it is important to note that the degree of projection of the inferior orbital rim is also of critical importance in the cause of prominent tear troughs. An under-projected orbital rim is a common cause of persistent nasojugal folds following lower blepharoplasty with fat repositioning because this bony deficiency cannot be completely corrected using orbital fat alone; individuals with this type of bony insufficiency benefit greatly from alloplastic augmentation of the orbital rim and adjacent medial maxilla (Fig. 34.9) [9].

The remaining ligamentous structures of the midface represent septal adhesions originating from the deeper tissues of the face and serve to compartmentalize the superficial fat pads discussed next.

Adiposal

The human midface depends strongly upon having adequate adipose tissue volume for the smooth contour and shape of the cheek that defines youthfulness. The adipose tissue of the face is heavily partitioned into different compartments, which can be further subdivided into *superficial* and *deep* depending on whether they are located superficial or deep to the superficial musculoaponeurotic system (SMAS), respectively (Fig. 34.10) [10, 11].

Superficial Compartments

The superficial compartments of the midface include the *nasolabial, medial cheek, middle cheek, lateral temporal-cheek, inferior orbital, and lateral orbital* pads. Topographically, the nasolabial fat compartment contributes to the prominence of the *nasolabial fold* with aging due to a relative increase in volume as well as age-related ptosis [12]. The medial and middle cheek superficial fat compartments contribute subcutaneous adipose volume to the submalar region. Although these superficial fat pads are important in maintaining a smooth surface contour of the midface, they contribute a limited amount of volume when considering the volumetric depletion that is seen in the aged or lipodystrophic malar and temporal regions. Instead, it appears that the deep fat compartments of the face contribute a great deal more to the volumetric fullness of the cheek.

Deep Compartments

The deep fat compartments of the face lie deep to the SMAS and serve to provide bulky volume and a smooth gliding surface to the mimetic and masticatory musculature; they include the *buccal fat pad, deep medial cheek* compartment, and the *suborbicularis oculi fat* (Fig. 34.10).

The most significant deep fat compartment of the midface is the *buccal fat pad*, also known as *Bichat's pad,* which earned its name due to its prominent location within

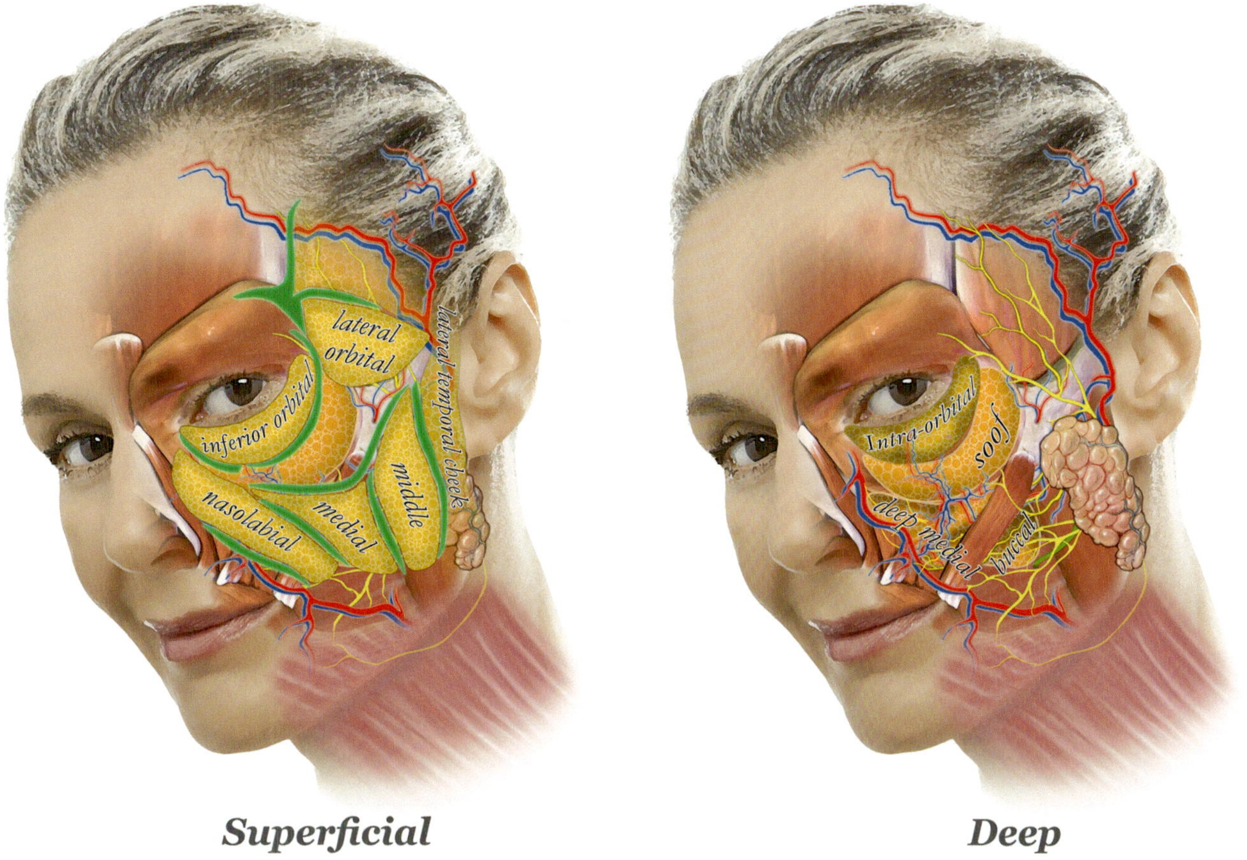

Fig. 34.10 The superficial and deep fat compartments of the midface. (Used with permission from Silver and Soares [33])

the buccal region. The buccal fat pad is a large amorphous fat conglomerate that is multilobulated in nature, containing additional extensions into the temporal region, pterygopalatine compartment, and the masticator space. However, aesthetically, the largest component of the buccal fat pad is the buccal segment, bounded medially by the buccinator muscle and laterally by the masseter muscle, SMAS, and facial nerve branches [13, 14]. The buccal fat contributes the bulk of soft tissue volume in the submalar region and appears to show significant atrophy with aging and facial lipodystrophy.

The deep medial cheek fat compartment lies deep to the zygomaticus muscles but superficial to the levator labii superioris muscle. The deep medial fat compartment significantly impacts the youthfulness of the medial cheek, and has thus become a common target of midfacial volume restoration via filler or fat injections [15].

The suborbicularis oculi fat (SOOF), as its name implies, is located deep to the orbicularis oculi muscle and bound superiorly by the ORL and inferiorly by the ZRL [16]. The SOOF should be distinguished from the intraorbital fat pads, which lie within the orbit and deep to the orbital septum and are compartmentalized into medial, central, and lateral.

Neurovascular

The blood supply to the midfacial soft tissues originates primarily from branches of the external carotid artery. Major branches, such as the facial, superficial temporal, and internal maxillary arteries, supply both the superficial and deep compartments. Distal branches, such as the *infraorbital*, *transverse facial*, and *zygomaticofacial* vessels, provide a redundant supply to the cheek tissues, and injury to one does not create a major disruption of tissue nourishment (Fig. 34.11). However, because most foraminal vessels supplying the midface travel with an accompanying sensory nerve, preservation of their afferent input is necessary to minimize disruption of facial sensation. Fortunately, these foramina can often be found consistently with knowledge of their typical locations. The infraorbital foramen is usually located approximately 1 cm below the inferior orbital rim at the midpupillary line and transmits important sensory nerve fibers for the central cheek via the infraorbital nerve [17]. The zygomaticofacial foramen lies approximately 1 cm diagonally from the inferio-lateral orbital angle and carries a sensory nerve by the same name supplying the lateral cheek [18].

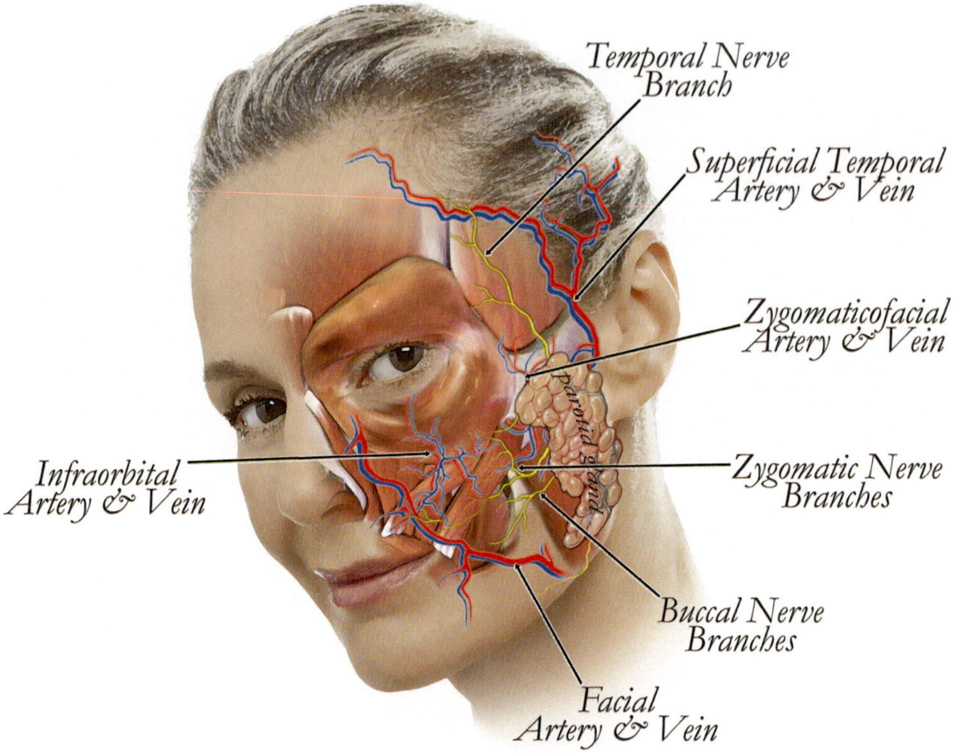

Fig. 34.11 Neurovascular anatomy of the midface. (Used with permission from Silver and Soares [33])

Evaluation of Midfacial Deformities

The treatment of midfacial deformities via alloplastic augmentation employs an objective approach that specifically targets each component of the midface. The cosmetic surgeon should understand when an alloplastic implant is both indicated and contraindicated in any given face. Alloplastic implants are designed to primarily correct bony deformities, and their lack of pliability, softness, and elasticity bars them from serving in the correction of soft tissue deficits. Because a unique balance between soft tissue and skeletal deformities characterizes each aesthetic region of the midface, the surgeon should seek to understand these regions thoroughly.

The midfacial/periorbital region can be subdivided into key areas (Fig. 34.12): the *malar eminence*, the *submalar region*, the *medial cheek*, and the *temporal fossa*, as well as the zygomatic arch and the lateral cheek (not pertinent in this chapter). Each of these regions demonstrates its own unique deformities and can benefit from targeted corrective procedures.

The Malar Eminence

Clinical Assessment

The malar eminence may be defined in terms of its anterolateral projection. An under-projected eminence renders the face flat on

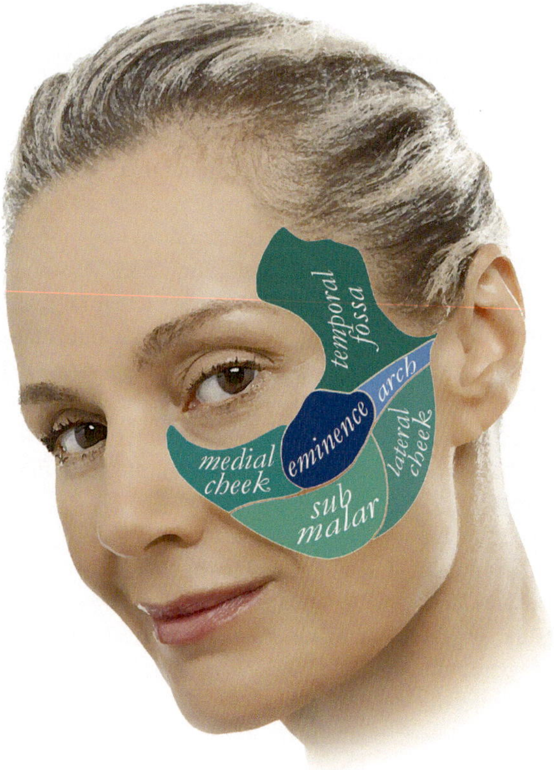

Fig. 34.12 Aesthetic areas of the midface

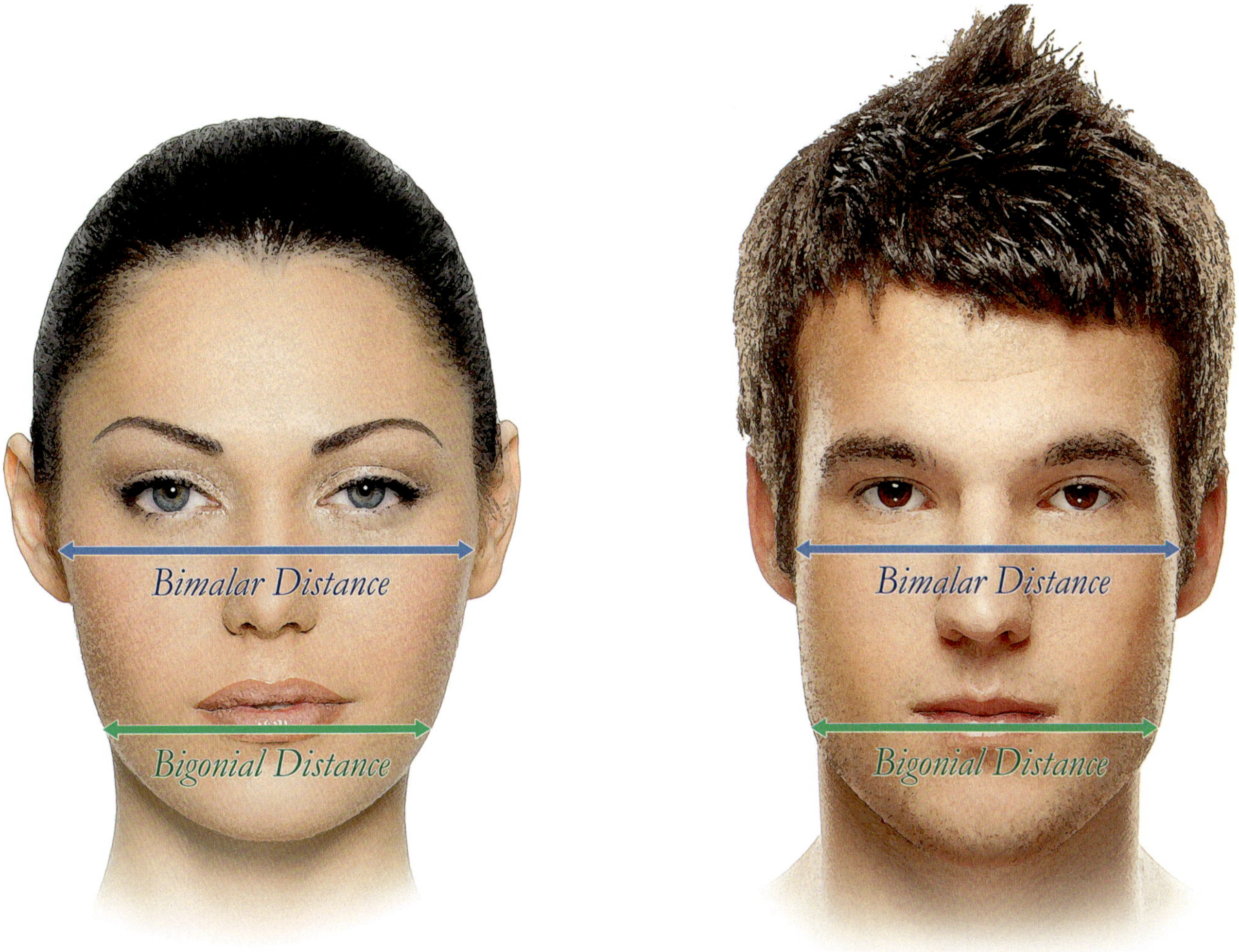

Fig. 34.13 Example of gender-dependent variations in bimalar: bigonial distances between female and male faces. (Used with permission from Silver and Soares [33])

frontal and three-quarters view and creates disharmonious facial shape. On lateral view, the malar crescent should reach within 5 mm of the nasolabial fold [19]. On frontal view, the malar eminence should project laterally farther than the mandibular (gonial) angle. This is particularly true in females, where, ideally, the bimalar distance is approximately 25% greater than the bigonial width (Fig. 34.13). In contrast, in males, this ratio tends to approach 1, rendering a squarer shape to the face [20].

Augmentation of the cheek eminence requires that the surgeon identify the ideal position of the malar promontory even in individuals lacking projection. Several techniques have been reliably used to establish the approximate location of the malar eminence: Hinderer's method, Wilkinson's method, and Silver's malar prominence triangle (Fig. 34.14).

Hinderer's Method

Hinderer's method uses simple approach to determine the approximate region of the eminence (Fig. 34.14a). The cheek is divided into quarters by intersecting two lines, one drawn from the ipsilateral nasal ala to the tragus, and the other marked from the ipsilateral oral commissure to the bony lateral canthus [21]. The region designated by the superolateral quadrant represents the area of the malar eminence.

Wilkinson's Method

Wilkinson's method drops a vertical line from the lateral canthus (Fig. 34.14b). The location of the malar promontory can reliably be located by dividing this line into thirds. The malar promontory is located one third of the way down from the canthus [22]. This method is also useful in enhancement of the cheekbone prominence with fillers (Fig. 34.15).

Silver's Prominence Triangle

Silver's prominence triangle utilizes multiple key topographical landmarks to objectively identify the area of cheek augmentation (Fig. 34.14c). This method is especially useful in

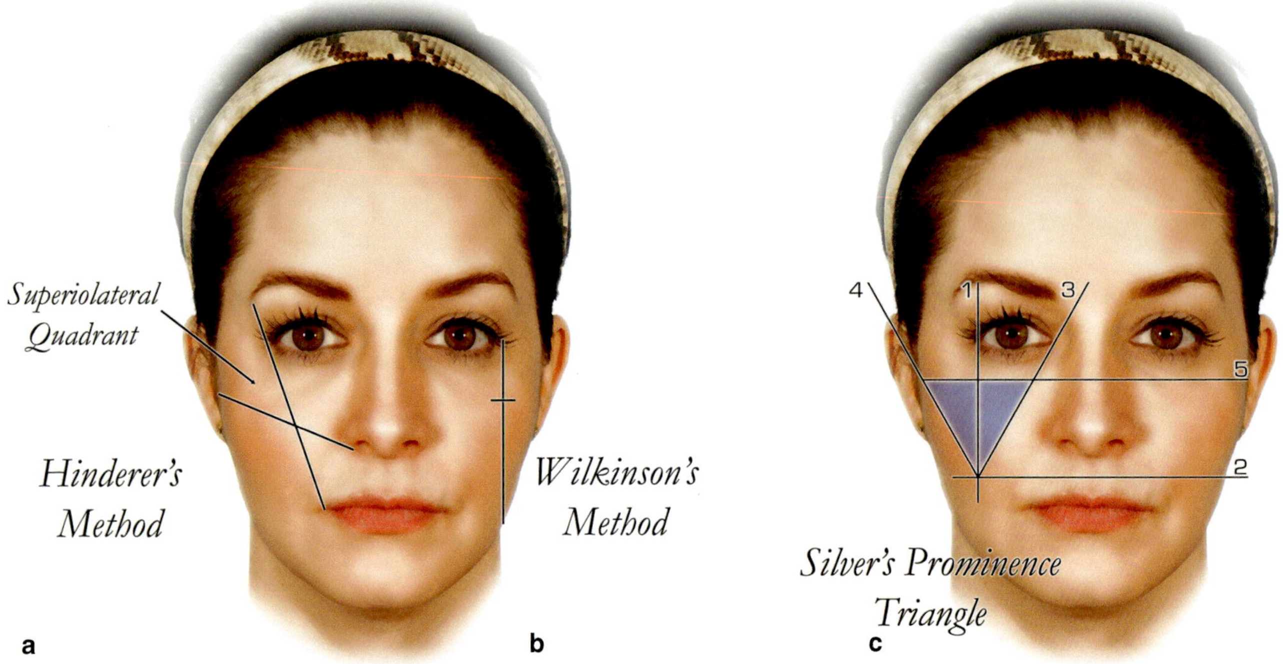

Fig. 34.14 Different methods commonly used in the identification of the malar prominence. (**a**) Hinderer's method. (**b**) Wilkinson's method. (**c**) Silver's method. (Used with permission from Silver and Soares [33])

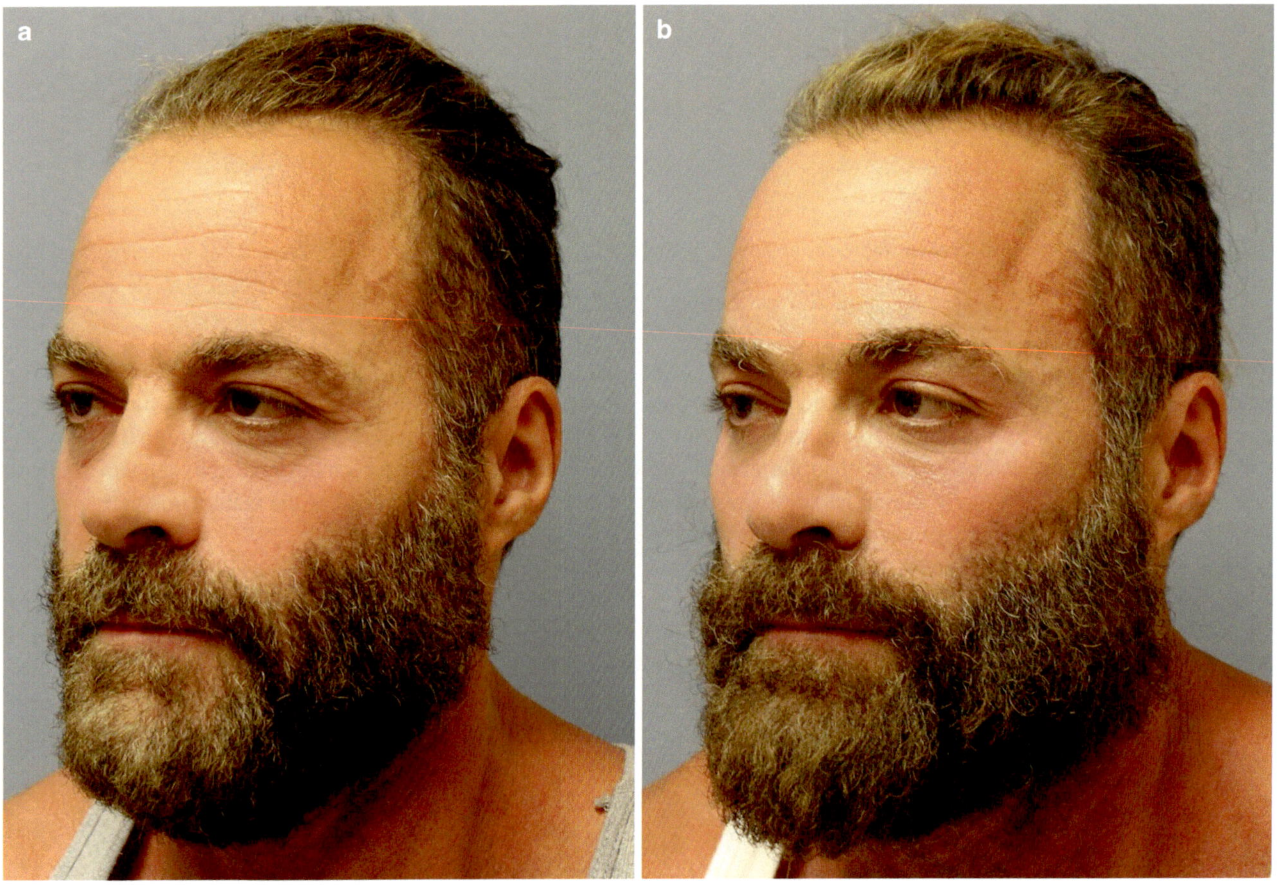

Fig. 34.15 Augmentation of the malar eminence with filler in a 46-year-old male. (**a**) Before and (**b**) 2 weeks following malar augmentation with supra-periosteal deposition of calcium hydroxyapatite filler

alloplastic augmentation of the cheeks due to its precise measurements, which help to ensure that the implant pockets are symmetrically created [23]. The triangle is constructed by drawing a vertical line (1) through the lateral canthus and then another line (2) perpendicular to line (1) located midway between the subnasale and the upper lip vermillion border. Next, a third line (3) is drawn from the medial canthus to the intersection point of the first two lines. Finally, line (3) is then reflected across the original vertical line (1) creating line (4). Lastly, the Frankfort horizontal line (5) is drawn; the triangle is outlined by lines (3), (4), and (5).

Grading System of Severity

The Binder classification of midfacial deformities (Fig. 34.16) is commonly referenced when discussing malar augmentation [24]. In this classification, both the malar and submalar regions are considered, ultimately allowing the surgeon to determine the ideal shape of implant to be used. Individuals with *Type I* deformities are characterized by a lack of bony projection of the malar eminence. *Type II* patients demonstrate normal malar bony projection but have significant aging-related volume loss and midfacial ptosis, featuring gaunt cheeks and sunken submalar regions. Finally, *Type III* patients display a combination of type I and type II deformities. The Binder classification was primarily designed to help aid the surgeon in determining the best implant shape for each Binder type (Fig. 34.17). However, because the submalar region is primarily defined by soft tissue volume, correction of submalar deficits is now preferentially corrected with soft tissue fillers such as autologous adipose tissue grafts and gels such as recombinant hyaluronic acid and calcium hydroxyapatite.

The Submalar Region

Clinical Assessment

The submalar region is triangle-shaped and bounded by the malar eminence superiorly, the masseter muscle laterally, and the nasolabial fold medially (Fig. 34.12) [5]. The submalar region consists mostly of soft tissue volume and is filled largely by the buccal fat pad. The submalar region experiences significant volumetric contraction with the aging process or in individuals with lipodystrophy such as those undergoing anti-retroviral therapy. In young, healthy individuals, submalar hollowing can also be encountered in extremely fit individuals with unusually low body fat percentage.

Clinically, the submalar region can be outlined easily by drawing a horizontal line at the subnasale, another diagonal line parallel to the nasolabial fold, and a line along the anterior edge of the masseter muscle. On palpation, this region should feel soft and pliable, without significant bony content.

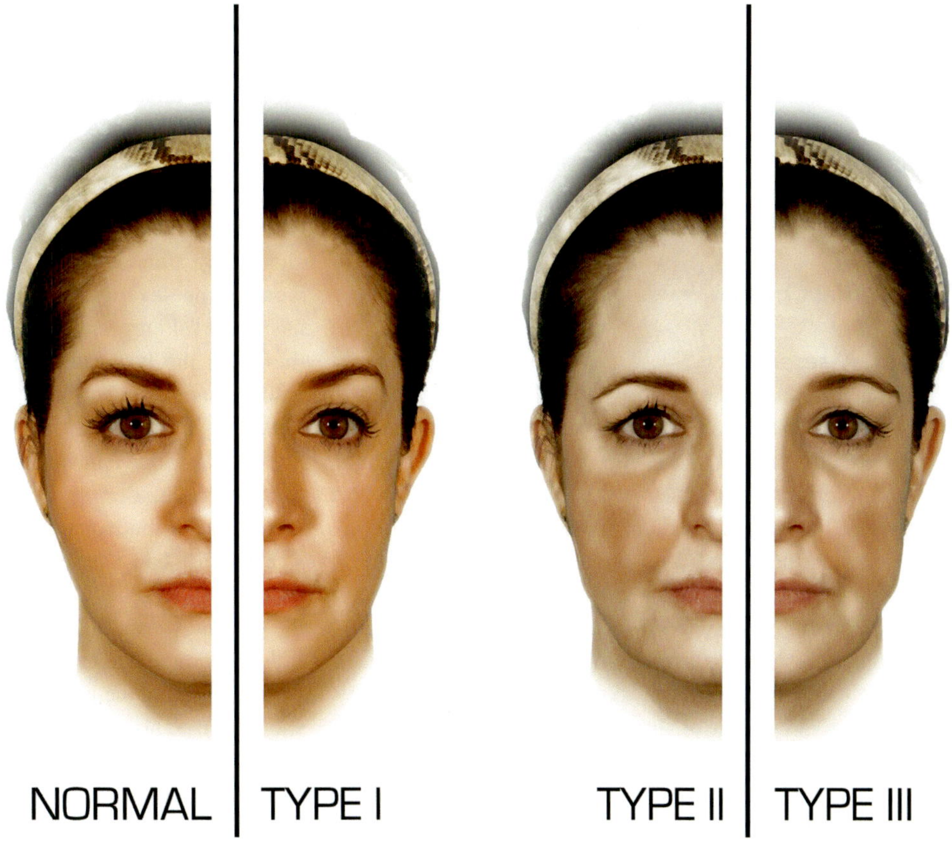

Fig. 34.16 Binder classification of midfacial deformities. Type I patients demonstrate mostly malar bony hypoplasia with otherwise normal submalar soft tissue pad. Individuals with type II cheeks have normal bony eminences but loss of submalar soft tissue volume due to aging-related volume loss and ptosis or secondary adipose tissue loss from lipodystrophy. Type III patients have a combination of bony hypoplasia and submalar soft tissue volume loss. (Used with permission from Silver and Soares [28])

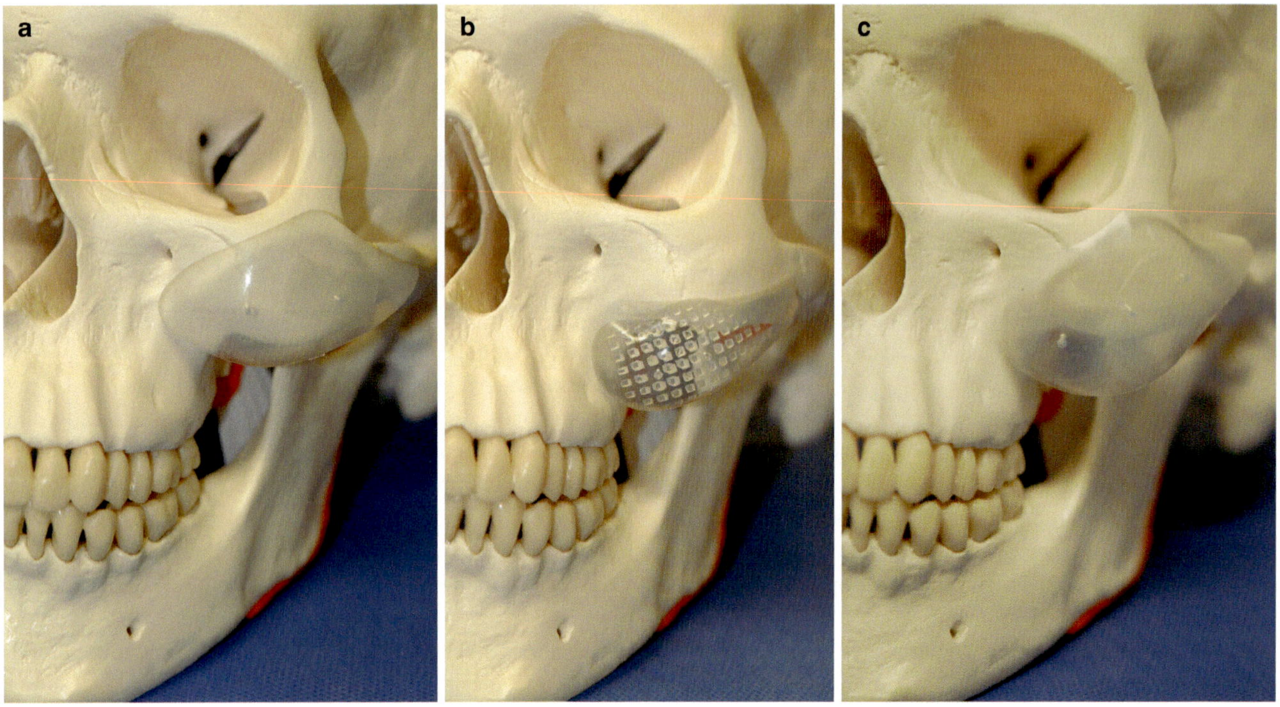

Fig. 34.17 Types of preformed malar implants from Implantech. (**a**) Malar. (**b**) Submalar. (**c**) Combined malar-submalar. (Used with permission from Silver and Soares [28])

Grading System of Severity

Several grading systems exist that allow clinicians to rate the degree of severity of submalar hollowing, as shown in Fig. 34.18 [25]. Grading the severity of submalar hollowing may be useful in determining the likely volume of autologous fat necessary for correction. Individuals with minimal volume loss may be candidates for simple soft tissue filler injections with hyaluronic acid or calcium hydroxyapatite.

The Medial Cheek

Clinical Assessment

The medial cheek can be roughly defined as the area situated between the pyriform aperture medially and the malar eminence laterally. It is bounded superiorly by the infraorbital rim and inferiorly by the nasolabial fold. The medial cheek consists of the medial maxillary bone, the upper lip elevators, and superficial and deep fat compartments. The most important feature of the medial cheek is the lower lid-cheek junction, otherwise known as the nasojugal fold. The nasojugal fold represents the insertion of the orbicularis retaining ligament, or ORL, into the skin. The ORL effectively restricts the movement or displacement of the soft tissues overlying the infraorbital rim and is responsible for the increasing prominence of the nasojugal fold with aging. In many, if not most, patients, the combination of orbital bone loss, pseudoherniation of orbital fat, and distension and elongation of the orbital septum and orbicularis muscle lead to the common “lower eyelid bags.” However, it is of critical importance that surgeons evaluate not just the soft tissues of the eyelid, but also the adequacy of projection of the underlying maxillary bone.

In 1969, Flowers coined the term *tear trough deformity* to describe a prominent *bony insufficiency* of the infraorbital rim and medial maxilla that often present with a deep depression along the lower lid and may coexist with, and thus worsen, the severity of the nasojugal fold [26]. While the nasojugal fold represents the attachment of the soft tissues to the bone, the tear trough deformity is regarded as a bony insufficiency due to midfacial skeletal hypoplasia. Individuals with tear trough deformities often have poorly projected midfaces and may have a prominent negative vector of the lower eyelid, under-projection of the nasal structure, and flat facies due to inadequate projection of the malar eminence. The lack of bony support in these individuals also predisposes them to accentuated lower eyelid bags with aging, as the gradual ptosis of the midfacial and lower eyelids meets little resistance due to the lack of a supportive bony “shelf.”

In evaluating the lower eyelid-cheek junction, the surgeon should differentiate between the following: medial maxillary under-projection due to bony hypoplasia (negative vector patients), true steatoblepharon of the lower eyelid due to excess orbital fat, and relative steatoblepharon due to lower

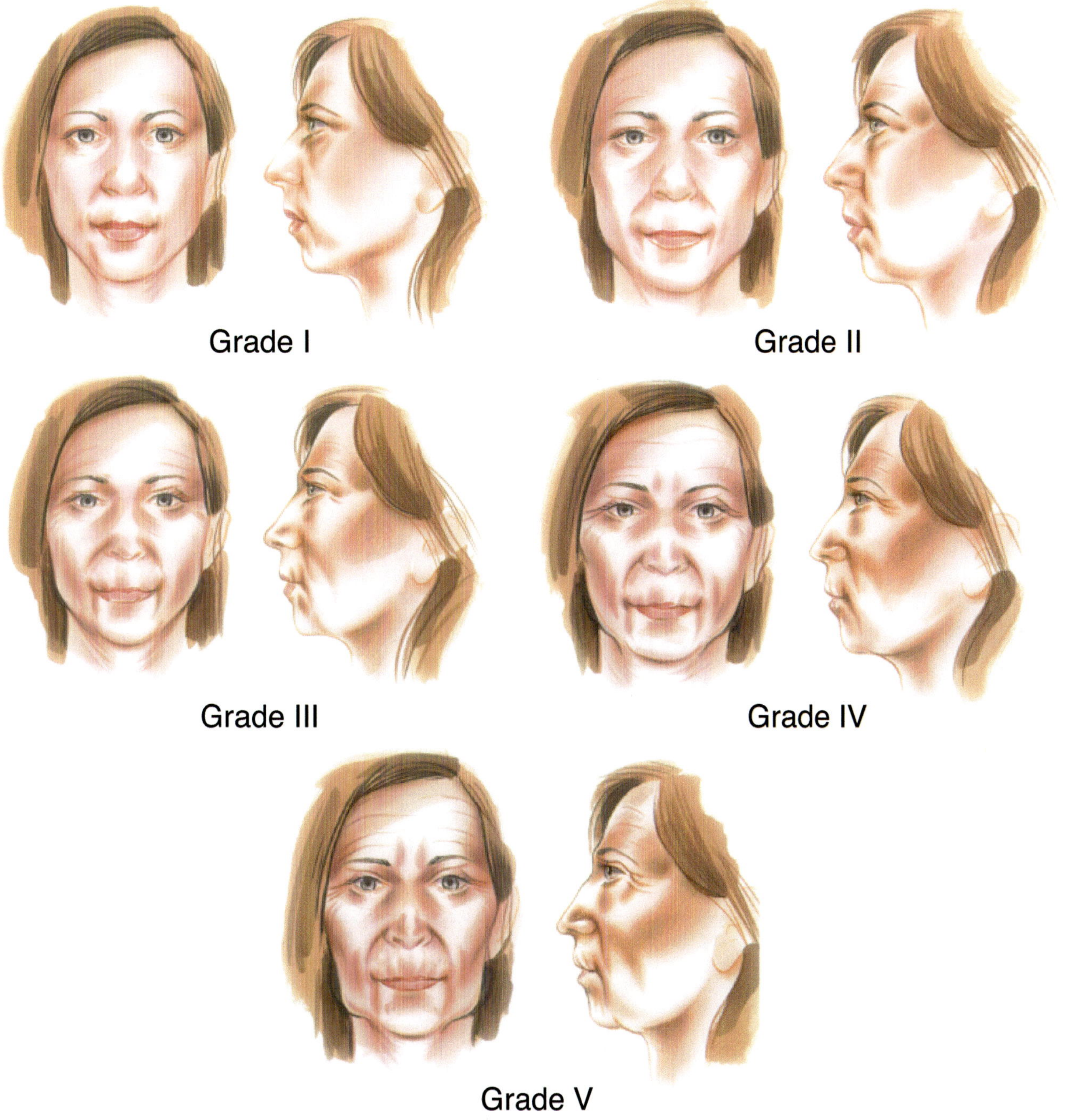

Fig. 34.18 Facial lipoatrophy grading scale. (Used with permission from Ascher et al. [25])

eyelid aging and ptosis (Fig. 34.19). In examining the patient, the surgeon must therefore determine whether there is a true lack of bony projection, and a true excess of orbital fat. Defining those two aspects will allow the surgeon to formulate the best method for correction of the prominent lid-cheek junction. Palpation of the lower eyelid allows the surgeon to easily determine the existence of maxillary insufficiency, as the globe sits anterior to the rim; a deep bony groove is easily formed by compression of the soft tissues of this region. Excess orbital fat in need of resection can be identified on close examination of the lateral view of the lower eyelid. In patients with normal maxillary projection, the lower eyelid should sit flush with the cheek, if true excess fat exists, the lower eyelid "bulges outward" past the anterior margin of the cheek. While fat resection is appropriate in patients with true fat excess, it is contraindicated in those without fat excess and in those with maxillary insufficiency, as they need all volume available for correction of the lower

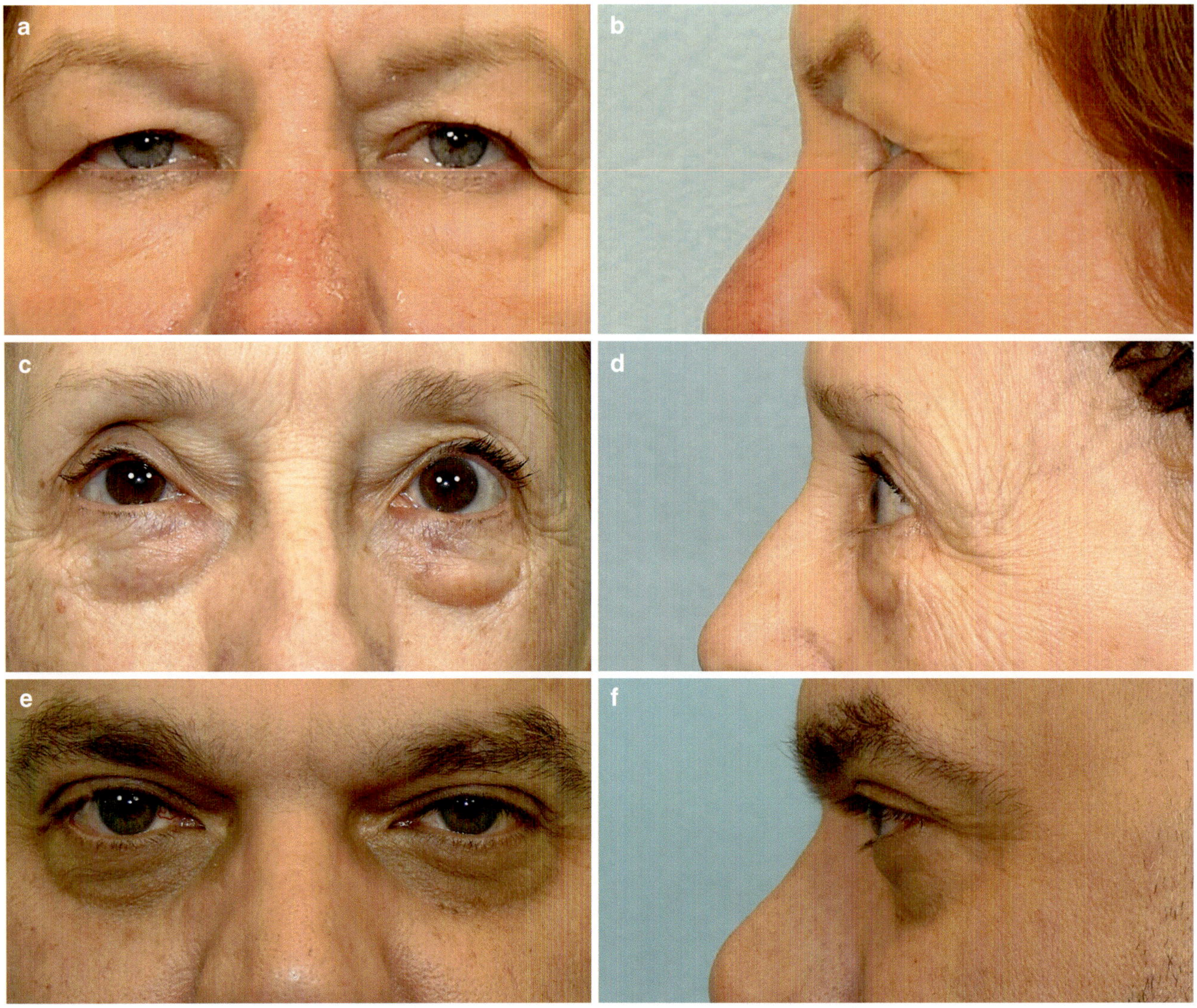

Fig. 34.19 Variations in lower eyelid-cheek junction defects presenting with prominent nasojugal folds. (**a**, **b**) Frontal and lateral views of individual with pseudoherniation of orbital fat with true fat excess. The steatoblepharon projects farther out than the midface characterized by normal soft tissue volume and normal bony projection of the midface/orbital rim. (**c**, **d**) Frontal and lateral views of an individual with pseudoherniation of fat in whom the orbital rim is adequately projected but in whom there exists midfacial soft tissue volume loss. In this patient, there is no true fat excess, and fat repositioning is likely to yield the best results. (**e**, **f**) Frontal and lateral views of an individual with midfacial/orbital rim deficiency. In this patient, there is no true excess or pseudoherniation of orbital fat; instead, there is significant under-projection of the orbital rim, characterized by a negative vector visible on the lateral views. This type of deformity responds well to alloplastic tear trough augmentation

lid-cheek junction. In those without excess fat, fat repositioning allows for correction of the pseudoherniation of fat and simultaneous partial filling of the nasojugal fold.

The Temporal Fossa

Clinical Assessment

The temporal fossa is smooth and full in youthfulness and in health, but develops into a prominent concavity with volume loss and aging (Fig. 34.5). Such volume loss can be seen naturally with the aging process of the face, severe weight loss, or secondary to lipodystrophy due to fitness and medication side effects. In addition, post-surgical atrophy of the temporal fat pads following cosmetic procedures such as brow and midface lifting, temporal craniotomies, or temporal trauma is also routinely seen. Due to its rigid nature, the temporal fossa presents a unique opportunity for alloplastic solid implant augmentation even though it represents mostly a soft tissue deficiency.

The temporal fossa is bounded anteriorly by the frontozygomatic process, inferiorly by the zygomatic arch, superiorly by the temporal crest, and posteriorly by the temporal bone topography and/or temporal hairline. The temporal fossa is largely occupied by the temporalis muscle and its associated superficial and deep fat compartments. Correction of temporal hollowing can be performed via implant placement deep to the temporalis muscle or superficial to the temporalis muscle, below the fascia [27].

Alloplastic Correction of Midfacial Deformities

Alloplastic Implants in Facial Contouring

Our knowledge of the physical attributes and biocompatibility of a large variety of alloplastic implant materials has evolved over centuries of use. As early as 3000 BC, silver and gold implants were utilized by the Incas in Peru for repair of trephination defects. However, historically, the wide adoption of alloplastic implantation had been hindered by the inherent risk of postsurgical infection, implant rejection, and implant extrusion. With the advent of the sterile surgical technique and antibiotics in the late nineteenth and early twentieth centuries, the widespread use of alloplastic implants in facial surgery became possible.

The ideal implant material should mimic the exact physical characteristics of the tissue it is attempting to replace. For alloplastic implants, due to their solid nature, their most immediate application presented in the form of bony augmentation. Nonetheless, material elasticity and tensile strength became important characteristics allowing for implant carving, contouring, and molding as needed to fit the region of interest. Furthermore, implant material characteristics that allowed for implant stabilization and biocompatibility, such as implant porosity, chemical inertness, resistance to enzymatic biodegradation, and lack of carcinogenicity became priorities in the modern era of facial plastic surgery. Following decades of trial and error, intense research, and extensive intraoperative utilization, several implant materials have solidified their preferred status as the choice materials for alloplastic augmentation [28].

Dimethylsiloxane (Silicone)

Solid silicone implants gained immediate acceptance in the 1950's due to their inertness and tissue biocompatibility. At the molecular level, silicone is a synthetic polymer of dimethylsiloxane monomers, and can exist in multiple physical states, ranging from liquid to solid, depending upon the degree of cross-linking between polymer chains. When dimethylsiloxane polymers are vulcanized along with silica particles, the resulting material is a solid silicone rubber material (*Silastic*, Dow Corning, Midland, MI) (Fig. 34.20). Silicone rubber is pliable and easily carved, with significant chemical inertness and bioenzymatic resistance. Furthermore, silicone rubber can withstand autoclave sterilization unchanged [29, 30]. Solid silicone is completely non-porous, displaying a smooth and hydrophobic surface. As a result,

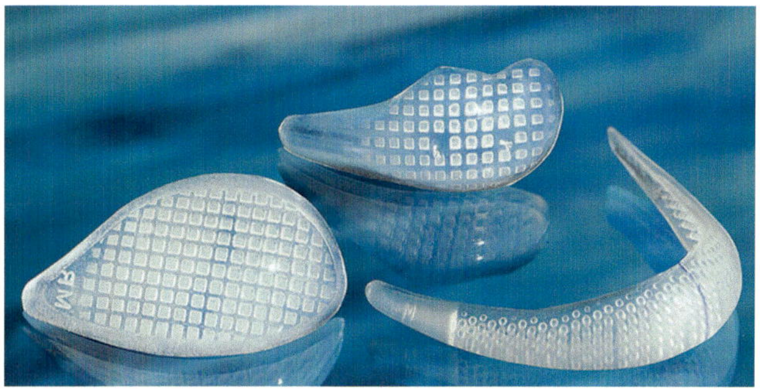

Fig. 34.20 Preformed silicone facial implants. (Courtesy of Implantech Associates, Inc., used with permission)

silicone implants heal by capsular formation, which typically further serves to stabilize the implant into position. The smooth surface of the implant, and its non-porous nature, allows for swift surgical removal if necessary though a tendency for implant mobility and displacement in the early post-operative period mean that some degree of fixation is necessary, especially if excessively large implant pockets have been created.

Polytetrafluoroethylene (PTFE)

Polytetrafluoroethylene (PTFE) was first introduced in 1975 and readily incorporated into medical prosthetics. PTFE is a synthetic polymer of ethylene bonded to fluorine, a covalent bond that is unable to be broken by natural human enzymatic activity. As a result, PTFE displays incredible tissue stability and is non-biodegradable. Solid PTFE implants are microporous in nature, featuring pore sizes ranging from 10 to 30 nanometers. This microporous nature allows for only limited tissue ingrowth, which facilitates tissue stabilization while still allowing for relative ease of implant removal. Current PTFE implants (*Gore-tex*, W.L. Gore and Associates, Flagstaff, AZ) are available in sheets or as preformed augmentation implants for the chin, cheek, and nose and have gained increased adoption over the last several decades over silicone (Fig. 34.21).

High-Density Polyethylene (HDPE)

High-density polyethylene was first introduced in the 1970's as a mesh for abdominal wall reconstructions because of its inertness and resistance to bioenzymatic degradation. High-density polyethylene implants (Medpor, Porex Surgical Inc. College Park, GA) are macro-porous in nature, displaying pore sizes of 125–250 nanometers, which allows for significant tissue ingrowth during healing. For this reason, HDPE implants feature the greatest implant stability post-surgically but are often difficult to remove, requiring that a cuff of normal tissue be excised simultaneously, which can be deleterious in areas with minimal tissue coverage. HDPE implants are available as blocks or preformed implants for midfacial, nasal, and mandibular augmentation (Fig. 34.22).

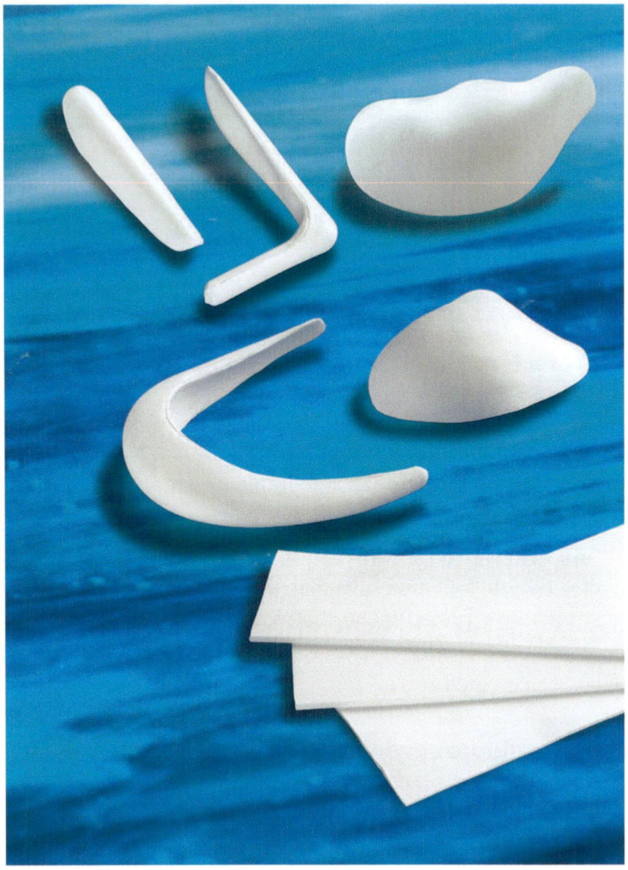

Fig. 34.21 Preformed polytetrafluoroethylene (PTFE) facial implants. (Courtesy of Implantech Associates, Inc., used with permission)

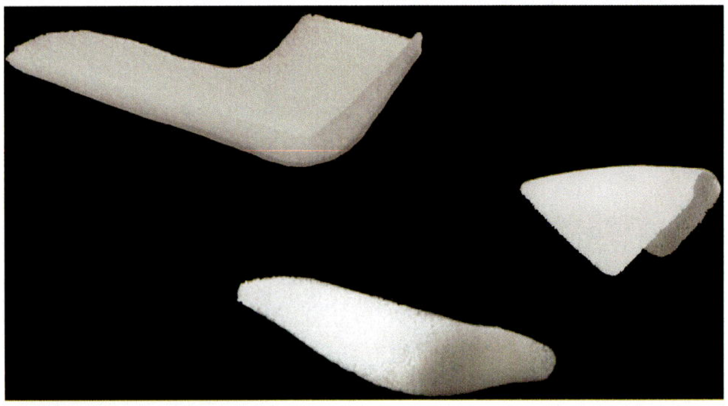

Fig. 34.22 Preformed polyethylene (HDPE) facial implants. (Courtesy of Stryker Inc., used with permission)

Cheek Augmentation

Surgical Technique

The surgical technique for transoral placement of malar implants is shown in Fig. 34.23. Preoperative inspection and evaluation of the regions to be augmented are of paramount importance in order to achieve an ideal result. The surgeon should carefully evaluate the malar eminences and the submalar regions to determine the best implant shape and size to be used. Preoperative facial asymmetries should be noted and if necessary addressed via insertion of different-sized implants or through custom implant carving. The risks and benefits of the procedure should be thoroughly discussed with the patient preoperatively, including the risk of infection, extrusion, displacement, and deformation, as well as the risk of motor or sensory nerve injury and reaction to anesthesia. Fortunately, alloplastic midfacial augmentation lends itself well to all anesthesia levels, allowing the surgeon to tailor the procedure to each patient's needs and tolerance.

The surgeon should begin by outlining the malar eminence through any one of a variety of methods discussed previously. In the authors' experience, constructing the Silver malar prominence triangle is a reliable method of ensuring that the implant site is symmetrically positioned. The implant shape is then marked inside the triangle, allowing the surgeon to create an implant pocket that is just large enough to fit the implant snuggly. The location of the infraorbital rim and foramen is also delineated, providing the surgeon awareness of these important landmarks that should not be breached. Appropriate preoperative antibiotic prophylaxis is established via standard intravenous antibiotic dosing, and the surgeon then proceeds to anesthetize the midface. Local anesthesia is established via injection of 1% lidocaine with 1:100,000 epinephrine, injected into the vicinity of the infraorbital foramen and the zygomaticofacial foramen. The substance of the cheek and the maxillary gingivobuccal sulcus are also infiltrated and at least 15 minutes allowed for maximal vasoconstriction of the tissues prior to the surgical incision. The face is prepped with iodophore or chlorhexidine solutions and draped in the usual sterile fashion.

The procedure begins with an intraoral incision made with needle-tipped electrocautery. The incision is made at the level of the canine fossa and at least 1 cm above the gingival margin to allow for easy closure of the incision at the completion of the procedure. Because the gingival mucosa stretches easily, a short 1 cm long incision is sufficient for placement of the implant. The incision is carried down to and through the maxillary periosteum. The surgeon then creates the implant pocket by carefully performing a subperiosteal elevation of the midfacial soft tissues while being aware, at all times, of the location of the infraorbital foramen and the infraorbital rim. Dissection over the superior portion of the masseter muscle is often necessary to create a sufficiently large implant pocket, especially if submalar augmentation is also being performed. Care should be taken to stay on the masseter muscle and avoid pressure on the overlying tissues to minimize the chance of facial paresis due to facial nerve injury.

Prior to insertion of the cheek implant, the surgeon should verify the size and shape of the implant by testing sizers of different shapes and dimensions. The surgeon should ensure, upon insertion of the sizers, that facial symmetry is preserved.

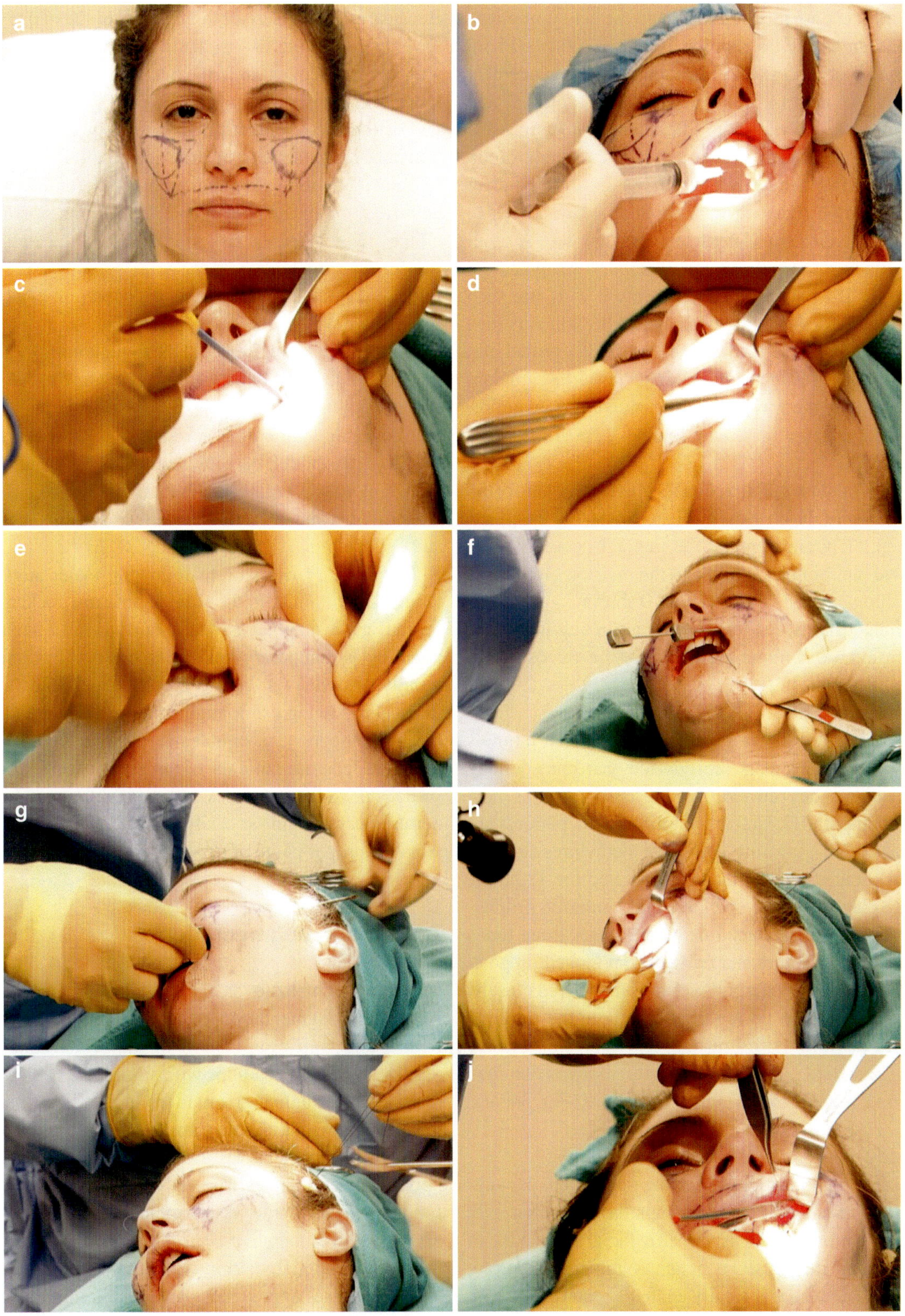

Fig. 34.23 Alloplastic malar augmentation operative sequence. (**a**) Appropriate cheek markings are placed with the patient in a sitting position. (**b**) Infiltration of local anesthetic into the cheek and incision site. (**c**) Gingivobuccal incision carried down to periosteum with electrocautery. (**d, e**) Adequately sized implant pocket created subperiosteally. (**f–h**) Implant is guided into position with a Stamey needle aimed at the superolateral corner of the pocket, exiting out of the temporal tuft. The Stamey needle carries in its tip a silk suture that was previously pierced through the superolateral corner of the cheek implant. The tip of the needle, along with the silk suture ends, is retrieved at the temporal exit site following stab incision overlying the needle tip. The implant is driven into position by pulling on the suture until resistance is met. (**i**) The implant is secured in position by tying the silk suture ends over a gauze bolster. (**j**) The gingivobuccal incision is closed in a layered fashion with chromic gut sutures. (Used with permission from Soares and Silver [23])

The implant sizers are then retrieved and the actual implants immersed in an antibiotic solution (such as 300 mg/15 ml clindamycin solution) prior to insertion. Implant placement is assisted via the use of a *Stamey needle.* The implant is tied to the Stamey needle via a 2-0 silk suture that pierces the implant at its superolateral corner and is fed through the tip of the needle. The needle is then driven into the implant pocket through the transoral incision and gently advanced subcutaneously into the ipsilateral temporal hair tuft. A small incision is made at the exit site in the temporal scalp and the needle tip pushed outward. The silk suture ends are then retrieved and released from the Stamey needle, which is then pulled out. The silk suture is then gradually pulled out through the temporal incision, guiding the cheek implant into position along the way. The suture is tied over an antibiotic-impregnated gauze bolster for immediate post-operative stabilization.

Once the implant is stabilized in its intended position, the external contour of the cheek is evaluated to ensure that it has been appropriately augmented. The implant pocket is then irrigated with antibiotic solution and the incision closed in a layered fashion, utilizing interrupted 3-0 chromic gut sutures for the submucosal tissues followed by a running interlocking low-tension 4-0 chromic gut suture for the mucosa.

Post-operative Care

Post-procedure care following malar augmentation requires minimal work, but patients are advised that considerable midfacial edema may develop for at least 2 weeks post implant placement [31]. Unless contraindicated, patients are usually started on a tapering course of methylprednisolone and are encouraged to keep the head elevated for 48 hours. Patients are placed on post-operative oral antibiotic prophylaxis and started on chlorhexidine mouth rinses three times daily. The retaining suture and bolster are removed on post-operative day 5 and the intraoral incisions monitored closely. Patients are asked to avoid repeated trauma to the gingivobuccal sulcus during tooth brushing and to avoid abrasive food items. Standard post-operative photography is obtained at 3, 6, and 12 months following the procedure (Fig. 34.24).

Complications

Post-procedure complications following transoral malar augmentation are rare. Commonly, patients have concern over mild facial asymmetry from asymmetric facial edema due to head positioning during sleep or an asymmetric swelling response. Reassurance is typically all that's required in these instances, as long as the surgeon feels confident that the intraoperative augmentation yielded a symmetric result. Implant displacement post-procedure is very rare and likely to result from post-operative facial trauma. Significant implant displacement would necessitate a repeat operation to reposition the implant in place prior to capsular formation. Because of the considerable thickness of the malar soft tissue envelope overlying the implant, even mild implant displacement is inconsequential to the overall success of the augmentation and likely remains insignificant.

Post-operative infection is always possible due to the transoral surgical route of insertion of a foreign body but is unusual. Patients are kept on perioperative antibiotic therapy, and irrigation of the pocket and implant intraoperatively has effectively negated the risk of infection in the authors' experience. Due to the robust vascular supply of the midface, infection remains an extremely rare occurrence [32]. If infection does develop, the early treatment varies depending on the implant material utilized. Due to their non-porous nature, silicone implants may be left in place while broad-spectrum empiric antibiotic therapy is trialed and tailored to bacterial culture results; if the infection fails to clear within 3–5 days, the implant should be removed. If reinsertion is contemplated, at least 3 months should be allowed to pass to allow for sufficient tissue healing, revascularization, and scar tissue remodeling.

Nerve injury is also rare following malar augmentation. Due to its proximity to the surgical implant pocket, the infraorbital nerve may occasionally sustain mild stretch injury, resulting in temporary midfacial sensory dysfunction that rapidly resolves within 3–6 months. Facial nerve injury is unusual following malar augmentation and would likely represent a temporary, reversible neuropraxia. Due to significant midfacial edema, patients often experience a "Mona Lisa smile" due to limited cheek excursion during smiling. Motor nerve injury should be easily avoided if the surgeon maintains the proper plane of dissection.

Tear Trough Augmentation

Surgical Technique

Alloplastic augmentation of the tear trough region begins with a thorough examination of the orbital and midfacial regions. Not all individuals with significant "lower lid bags" require tear trough augmentation. In fact, most patients can be managed with a simple transconjunctival lower blepharoplasty with orbital fat excision or repositioning, depending upon whether there is true fat excess or not, respectively. Individuals with true under-projection of the orbital rim often display a *negative vector*, which itself can contribute to lower eyelid malposition with outer lamellar scarring following external approaches. As a result, the transconjunctival approach is the preferred route of implant placement for most individuals. Occasionally, if the degree of under-projection is severe, the transconjunctival route may prove difficult, as the orbital rim may be challenging to dissect due to limited visibility secondary to its position deeper under the globe. In such instances, performing a simultaneous

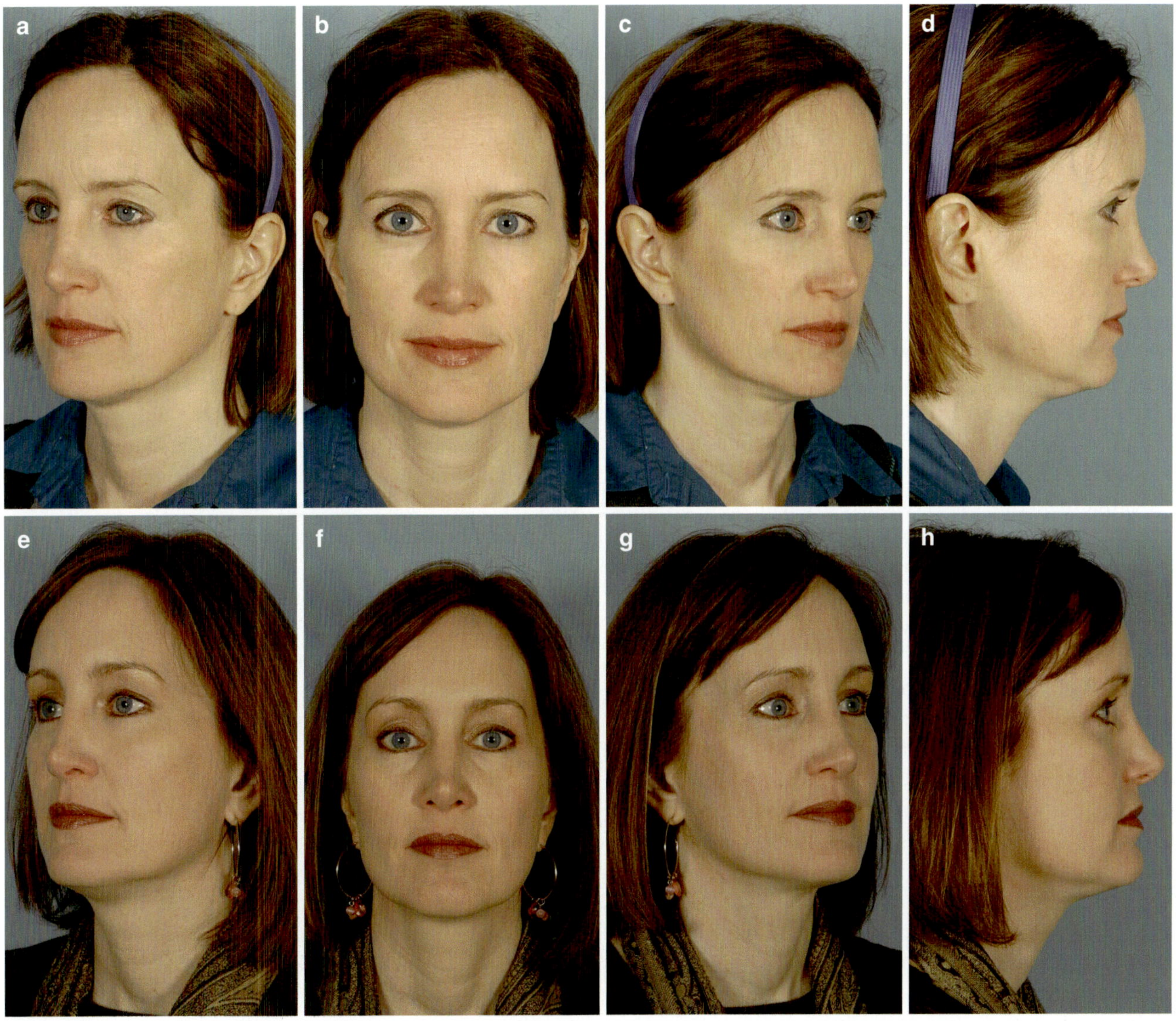

Fig. 34.24 Pre- and post-operative photos following malar augmentation. (**a–d**) Preoperative photos showing a patient with Binder type I deformity. (**e–h**) Post-operative photos 3 months after cheek augmentation with malar implants and endoscopic brow lift. (Used with permission from Silver and Soares [28])

transoral subperiosteal dissection may aid the surgeon in safely carrying out a subperiosteal dissection.

Individuals with bony under-projection of the orbital rim will also benefit from fat repositioning during implant placement, as the combination of procedures can completely eradicate the nasojugal fold. In fact, a common presentation for patients with bony insufficiency of the orbital rim is the persistence of "lower lid bags" following lower blepharoplasty. If a moderate to severe lack of bony deficiency is not corrected, a lower blepharoplasty is typically unable to completely correct the appearance of the "lower eyelid bags." Once the patient is identified as a surgical candidate, the risks and benefits of alloplastic tear trough augmentation should be discussed, including the risk of implant extrusion, infection, bleeding, motor and sensory nerve dysfunction, contour deformities, palpable implant edges, and, rarely, eyelid malposition. Individuals with lax lower eyelids typically benefit from canthopexy or canthoplasty depending on the severity of lower eyelid laxity. Although the transconjunctival placement of a midfacial implant typically does not aggravate lower eyelid laxity, it will do little to improve it.

The patient is marked in the preoperative setting, outlining the region to be augmented and the likely position of the infraorbital nerve. The transconjunctival placement of a midfacial implant typically requires deeper anesthesia but can be successfully performed in permissive awake patients. The midface is infiltrated with 1% lidocaine with 1:100,000 epinephrine, targeting the infraorbital region and the substance of the medial cheek. The palpebral conjunctiva is also infiltrated with the anesthetic mixture. If the patient is kept awake, the globe is anesthetized with topical tetracaine solution. A plastic corneal shield is placed in all instances to avoid accidental corneal injury. The face is then appropriately prepped with iodophore or chlorhexidine solutions and the patient draped in the usual sterile fashion.

The surgery begins with a standard transconjunctival incision through the palpebral conjunctiva approximately halfway between the inferior edge of the tarsus and the fornix or 2–3 mm below the inferior edge of the tarsal plate. The incision is then carried past the lower lid retractors and maintained in a pre-septal plane of dissection just deep to the orbicularis oculi muscle. Upon reaching the orbital rim, the orbicularis retaining ligament, evident as the fused ligamentous arcus marginalis, is incised down past the periosteum. The dissection is then continued in the subperiosteal plane, dissecting the soft tissues off the anterior wall of the maxilla and infraorbital rim. Care is taken to avoid injury to the infraorbital nerve by performing a 360° dissection around the foramen. It's important that the subperiosteal pocket be extended medially onto the ascending process of the maxilla and nasal bone and laterally into the medial aspect of the malar eminence.

Once the implant pocket has been created, standard sizers are inserted to determine the ideal implant size. Typically, if possible, the surgeon should trial one size up and one size down to determine the ideal dimensions of the implant. If all sizers appear to be inadequate, custom implant carving can be easily performed. A hole is placed through the implant via a 3 mm punch biopsy tool at the site of the infraorbital nerve and then the hole is connected to a vertical cut through the inferior edge of the implant to allow for the implant to be fit into position around the infraorbital nerve. A nerve hook can assist with gentle retraction and manipulation of the nerve during implant placement. It is critical that the implant not impinge upon the nerve, to avoid post-operative dysesthesia or chronic pain.

Once the implant is in position, it is secured against the infraorbital periosteum or arcus with interrupted 5-0 PDS sutures. The implant and pocket are irrigated with antibiotic solution. Any redundant orbital fat is then released and transposed over the implant and sutured to the SOOF via interrupted 5-0 PDS sutures. Prior to completion of the closure, a small butterfly drain is passed outward through the alar-facial junction as described by Flowers [9]. The palpebral conjunctiva and lower lid retractors are reapproximated with a running subcuticular 6-0 nylon suture exiting transcutaneously. The corneal protector is then removed, the eye is irrigated, and a forced duction test is then performed to ensure no gaze restriction.

Post-operative Care

The post-operative course is typically straightforward for most patients, although some pain can be expected due to the midfacial subperiosteal dissection. Early on, moderate edema is to be expected and a post-operative tapering course of methylprednisolone accelerates the clearance of the edematous phase. The butterfly drain is typically removed the following day unless significant output is noted. The patient is kept on standard post-operative oral antibiotic prophylaxis and frequent lubrication with artificial tears. The running nylon suture is removed on post-operative day 5. Standard post-operative photography is obtained at 3, 6, and 12 months following the procedure (Fig. 34.25).

Complications

Complications following transconjunctival alloplastic augmentation of the tear trough region are rare. As seen with cheek augmentation, post-operative infection is exceedingly rare owing to the excellent vascular supply of the orbital and cheek tissues and standard perioperative prophylaxis. Temporary neuropraxic injury to the infraorbital nerve may result in partial anesthesia of the midface that typically resolves within 6 months. Although temporary weakness of the orbicularis oculi is rare, the surgeon should avoid excessive or unnecessary lateral suborbicularis oculi dissection. Lower eyelid malposition is rarely encountered, mirroring the relative safety of the transconjunctival lower blepharoplasty procedure. Cicatricial entropion can be seen if the lower eyelid retractors are not properly approximated and scar against the exposed orbicularis oculi muscle tissue. Individuals with laxity of the lower eyelids may typically find improved lower eyelid position post-operatively due to the support afforded by the implant, though laxity will persist unless addressed independently. Because alloplastic augmentation of the medial cheek corrects only bony deficiency, patients may still require soft tissue volume correction via fat or soft tissue filler injections. Furthermore, due to the high incidence of overall maxillary insufficiency, these patients may also benefit from alloplastic malar augmentation. Combined augmentation can be performed simultaneously, although, if staged, it would be preferable to position the malar implant first to prevent the potential displacement of the tear trough implant during malar augmentation.

Temporal Fossa Augmentation

Surgical Technique

Alloplastic augmentation of the temporal fossa is a simple procedure that requires small, concealed incisions and minimal anesthesia. The procedure is well tolerated and offers a short recovery period. Specialized implants have been developed for augmentation of the depressed temporal fossa (Fig. 34.26). The operative sequence begins with a thorough examination of the region to be augmented, outlining the boundaries of the temporal fossa. A small incision is marked

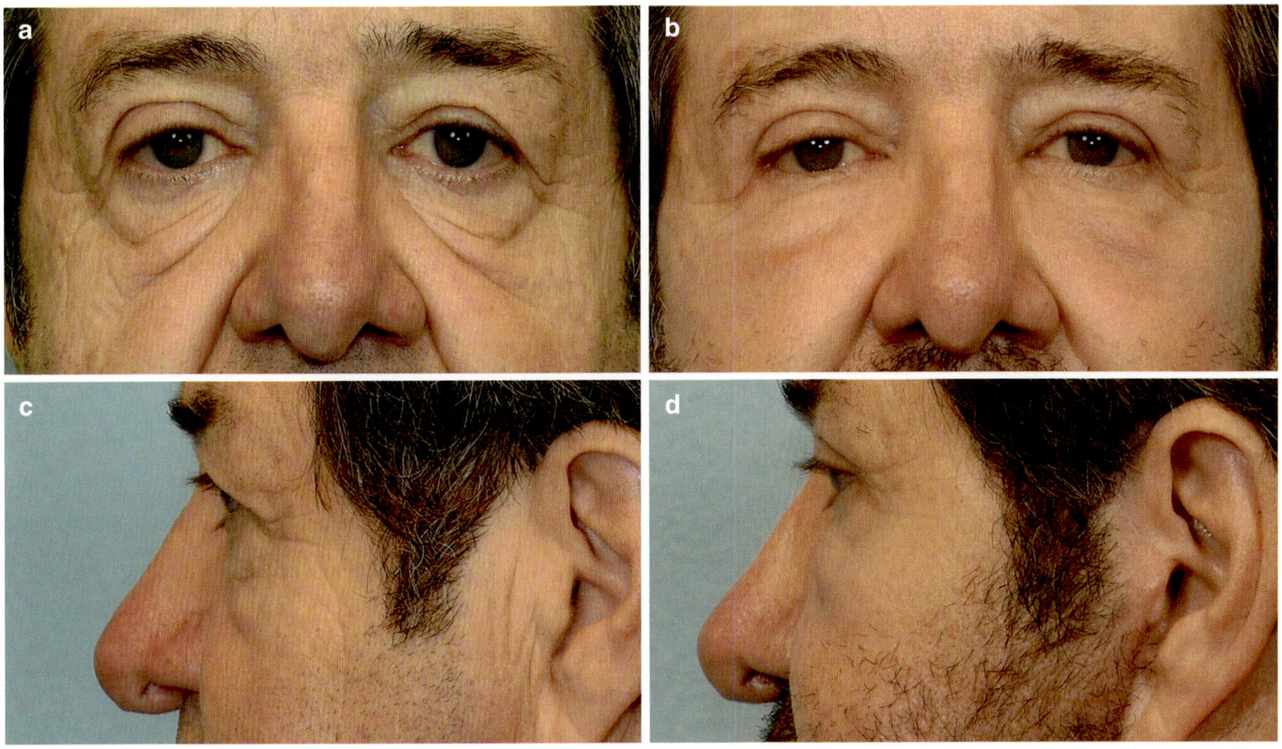

Fig. 34.25 Pre- and post-operative photos following midfacial augmentation. (**a**, **c**) Preoperative frontal and lateral views. (**b**, **d**) Post-operative frontal and lateral views of patient 3 months following alloplastic malar augmentation, transconjunctival alloplastic tear trough augmentation, midfacial lipotransfer, and upper blepharoplasty

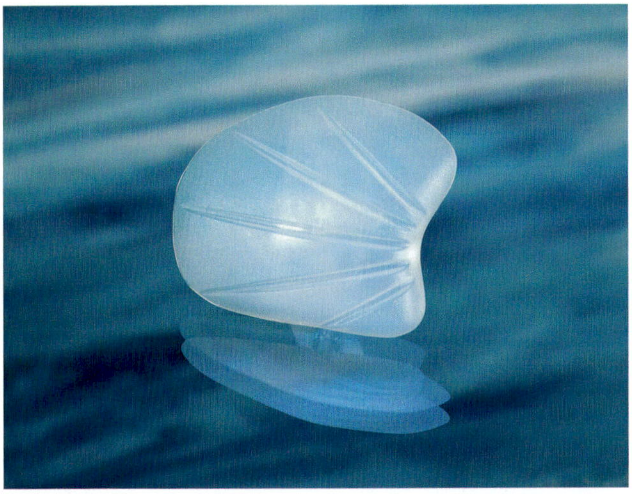

Fig. 34.26 Preformed silicone temporal fossa implant. (Courtesy of Implantech Associates, Inc., used with permission)

vertically within the temporal hair tuft, and the surgical region is infiltrated with 1% lidocaine with 1:100,000 epinephrine. The area is prepped with iodophore or chlorhexidine solutions and draped in the typical sterile fashion.

A #15 blade is used to make a beveled incision parallel to the hair follicles to avoid transection and subsequent hair loss. The incision is carried past the temporoparietal fascia down to the superficial layer of the deep temporal fascia. This fascia is then incised, and a subfascial pocket is created over the temporalis muscle similar to the well-known Gillies' approach to the zygoma used in trauma. Once the pocket has been created, the implant is sized and carved appropriately, ensuring tapering of the edges, and then placed in position. The implant can be affixed to the overlying temporal fascia along its periphery with interrupted 5-0 PDS sutures. The implant and pocket are irrigated with antibiotic solution prior to closure. The incision is then closed in a layered fashion, reapproximating the temporoparietal fascia with interrupted 5-0 monocryl sutures followed by surgical staples or Prolene sutures for the skin. The area is then stabilized via a traditional head wrap with clinging gauze.

Post-operative Care

Post-operatively, patients may experience mild to moderate headache and will notice some edema of the temporal region. Head elevation and a post-operative steroid course, if not contraindicated, may assist in speeding up clearance of the edematous phase. The head wrap is removed after 24 hours and the patient is encouraged to sleep supine, avoiding resting sideways on the temples. Mild bruising may occur, typically resolving within 1 week. Complications following this procedure are rare owing to the stability of the region and the excellent vascular supply of the tissues.

Alloplastic augmentation performed in this fashion helps correct prominent temporal fossae due to adipose tissue atrophy. If available, autologous fat grafting is well suited for this purpose as well, although individuals with significant temporal wasting due to low BMI will often have inadequate fat reserves. Individuals lacking bony projection of the frontotemporal region, either postsurgically or developmentally, may benefit from skeletal augmentation via placement of methyl methacrylate implants submuscularly [27].

Conclusion

Alloplastic augmentation of the midface and periorbital tissues serves a distinct role in the management of common midfacial deformities. Alloplastic implants, due to their rigid nature and tissue biocompatibility, remain the ideal material for correction of facial deformities originating from bony insufficiency. Soft tissue volume loss is best addressed with soft tissue fillers, especially fat grafting, whenever possible. Despite the foreign material of alloplastic implants, their use in facial augmentation is characterized by very low rates of extrusion, infection, or deformity. Surgeons should carefully examine the patient's facial features to determine whether a bony insufficiency exists, wherein alloplastic augmentation will typically provide the most natural results.

References

1. Farkas LG, Katic MJ, Forrest CR, Alt KW, Bagic I, Baltadjiev G, et al. International anthropometric study of facial morphology in various ethnic groups/races. J Craniofac Surg. 2005;16(4):615–46.
2. Le TT, Farkas LG, Ngim RC, Levin LS, Forrest CR. Proportionality in Asian and North American Caucasian faces using neoclassical facial canons as criteria. Aesthet Plast Surg. 2002;26(1):64–9.
3. Rajabi MT, Gholipour F, Ramezani K, Hosseini SS, Rajabi MB, Tabatabaie SZ. The influence of orbital vector on involutional entropion and ectropion. Orbit. 2018;37(1):53–8.
4. Angle E. Classification of malocclusion. Dental Cosmos. 1899;41:248–64.
5. Tobias G, Binder W. The submalar triangle: its anatomy and clinical significance. Facial Plast Surg Clins North Am. 1994;2(3):255–64.
6. Yu CC, Chen PK, Chen YR. Botulinum toxin a for lower facial contouring: a prospective study. Aesthet Plast Surg. 2007;31:445–51; discussion 452–3.
7. Alghoul M, Codner MA. Retaining ligaments of the face: review of anatomy and clinical applications. Aesthet Surg J. 2013;33(6):769–82.
8. Wong CH, Hsieh MK, Mendelson B. The tear trough ligament: anatomical basis for the tear trough deformity. Plast Reconstr Surg. 2012;129(6):1392–402.
9. Flowers RS. Tear trough implants for correction of tear trough deformity. Clin Plast Surg. 1993;20(2):403–15.
10. Rohrich RJ, Pessa JE. The fat compartments of the face: anatomy and clinical implications for cosmetic surgery. Plast Reconstr Surg. 2007;119(7):2219–27; discussion 2228–31.
11. Wan D, Amirlak B, Rohrich R, Davis K. The clinical importance of the fat compartments in midfacial aging. Plast Reconstr Surg Glob Open. 2013;1(9):e92.
12. Yousif NJ, Gosain A, Matloub HS, Sanger JR, Madiedo G, et al. The nasolabial fold: an anatomic and histologic reappraisal. Plast Reconstr Surg. 1994;93(1):60–9.
13. Zhang HM, Yan YP, Qi KM, Wang JQ, Liu ZF. Anatomical structure of the buccal fat pad and its clinical adaptations. Plast Reconstr Surg. 2002;109(7):2509–18; discussion 2519–20.
14. Yousuf S, Tubbs RS, Wartmann CT, Kapos T, Cohen-Gadol AA, Loukas M. A review of the gross anatomy, functions, pathology, and clinical uses of the buccal fat pad. Surg Radiol Anat. 2010;32(5):427–36.
15. Rohrich RJ, Pessa JE, Ristow B. The youthful cheek and the deep medial fat compartment. Plast Reconstr Surg. 2008;121(6):2107–12.
16. Hwang SH, Hwang K, Jin S, Kim DJ. Location and nature of retro-orbicularis oculus fat and suborbicularis oculi fat. J Craniofac Surg. 2007;18(2):387–90.
17. Aziz SR, Marchena JM, Puran A. Anatomic characteristics of the infraorbital foramen: a cadaver study. J Oral Maxillofac Surg. 2000;58(9):992–6.
18. Krishnamurthy A, Roshni S, Murlimanju BV, Nayak SR, Jiji PJ, et al. Foramina on the zygomatic bone: its clinical significance. Clin Ter. 2011;162(5):419–21.
19. Blyer SM. Facial implants in cosmetic surgery. In: Fonseca RJ, Turvey TA, editors. Oral and maxillofacial surgery. 2nd ed. St. Louis: Elsevier Saunders; 2009.
20. Powell N. Proportions of the aesthetic face. New York: Thieme Medical; 1984.
21. Hinderer UT. Malar implants for improvement of the facial appearance. Plast Reconstr Surg. 1975;56(2):157–65.
22. Wilkinson TS. Complications in aesthetic malar augmentation. Plast Reconstr Surg. 1983;71(5):643–9.
23. Soares DJ, Silver WE. Midface skeletal enhancement. Facial Plast Surg Clin North Am. 2015;23(2):185–93.
24. Binder WJ, Azizzadeh B. Malar and submalar augmentation. Facial Plast Surg Clin North Am. 2008;16(1):11–32.
25. Ascher B, Coleman S, Alster T, Bauer U, Burgess C, Butterwick K, et al. Full scope of effect of facial lipoatrophy: a framework of disease understanding. Dermatol Surg. 2006;32:1058–69.
26. Flowers RS. Correcting suborbital malar hypoplasia and related boney deficiencies. Aesthet Surg J. 2006;26(3):341–55.
27. Gordon CR, Yaremchuk MJ. Temporal augmentation with methyl methacrylate. Aesthet Surg J. 2011;31(7):827–33.
28. Silver W, Soares D. Facial contouring with implants. In: Sclafani A, editor. Sataloff's comprehensive textbook of otolaryngology head and neck surgery. Vol. 3, Facial plastic and reconstructive surgery. Philadelphia: JP Brothers Medical Publishers; 2014.
29. Eppley BL. Alloplastic implantation. Plast Reconstr Surg. 1999;104(6):1761–83.
30. Quatela VC, Chow J. Synthetic facial implants. Facial Plast Surg Clin North Am. 2008;16(1):1–10.
31. Hopping SB, Joshi AS, Tanna N, Janjanin S. Volumetric facelift: evaluation of rhytidectomy with alloplastic augmentation. Ann Otol Rhinol Laryngol. 2010;119(3):174–80.
32. Rubin JP, Yaremchuk MJ. Complications and toxicities of implantable biomaterials used in facial reconstructive and aesthetic surgery: a comprehensive review of the literature. Plast Reconstr Surg. 1997;100(5):1336–53.
33. Silver W, Soares D. Introduction to the midface anatomy. In: Cohen AJ, Ali MJ, editors. Compendium of oculofacial, orbital and lacrimal surgery. 1st ed. Switzerland: Springer International Publishing; 2015.

Autologous Fat Transfer to the Eyelids and Face

35

Robert Schwarcz

Volume depletion has become a vital hallmark of facial aging further unmasking gravitational changes. Using autologous fat as a facial augmentation tool has long been heralded as an accepted form of facial volumization [1, 2]. Unlike nonfat filler material, autologous fat can be readily available and easily accepted by the host injection sites. A known limitation of this procedure is grafted adipocyte viability resulting in contour inconsistency. Since these are live tissue grafts, a blood supply is vital to survival, and thus preparation and technique are important [1]. There are other beneficial reasons to utilize this technique. Facial fat grafting can be combined with other facial cosmetic surgical procedures to augment the aesthetic result. Some authors also have reported the differentiation of adipose-derived cells into chondrocytes, myocytes, osteoblasts, and, most recently, neural progenitor cells, thus demonstrating beneficial in reconstructive cases and those with profound asymmetry [3].

Surgical Technique

Harvesting Fat

Fat can be harvested from a plethora of donor sites. Most commonly it is harvested from the abdomen, hips, or thighs. The procedure begins with proper sterile technique and infiltration with tumescent solution which is employed to allow for anesthesia and hemostasis [4]. One technique is to utilize approximately 200cc of 0.1% lidocaine with 1:1,000,000 epinephrine with an infiltration cannula. After adequate time is allowed for infiltration of the tumescent anesthesia, a hand liposuction approach is administered to minimize adipocyte damage (Fig. 35.1). Microharvesting cannulas are typically used. Harvest sites are based on available fat from patient sites. Common harvest locations are abdomen, flanks, and outer thighs but can also include inner thighs/lower extremities if needed [2, 5].

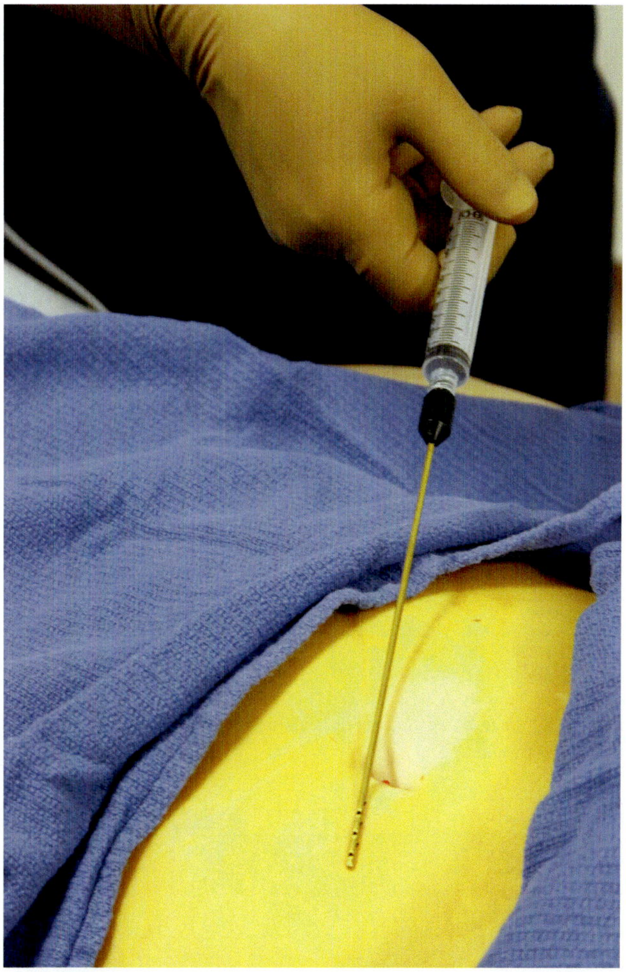

Fig. 35.1 After adequate time is allowed for infiltration of the tumescent anesthesia, a hand liposuction approach is administered to minimize adipocyte damage

R. Schwarcz (✉)
Ophthalmology, Division of Oculoplastic Surgery, Mount Sinai Hospital, ICAHN School of Medicine, New York, NY, USA

A. J. Cohen, C. N. Burkat (eds.), *Oculofacial, Orbital, and Lacrimal Surgery*, https://doi.org/10.1007/978-3-030-14092-2_35

Fat Handling

Once harvested, there is a slurry of fat, tumescent solution, and blood products (Fig. 35.2). The author's preference is to centrifuge this intermediate product (Fig. 35.3). It is customary for others to allow the fat to rest and decant in the harvesting syringe, with separation of the layers manually. Others have utilized a seize method, and there are closed disposable devices for this as well. The author prefers centrifuging for 3 minutes at 1500 rpm, but there are many suitable variations. Once the layers have separated using either method, the diluent is carefully poured off (Fig. 35.4). The remaining fat is then transferred to a more manageable 1 cc luer lock syringe (Fig. 35.5). There have been various methods described which involve straining the fat, transferring it to a Telfa pad, or adding protein-rich plasma. These methods involve an intermediary step or a portion in which the fat is exposed. It is speculated that keeping the technique closed cell without exposing the fat may decrease the chance for cross contamination.

Once transferred to the 1 cc syringe with a luer lock female to female adapter, the compact, yellow rich-looking fat is ready to be transferred to the host site. For periorbital areas it is preferable to use a smaller cannula such as a 0.7 mm (Fig. 35.6), while in other parts of the face a larger cannula such as a 0.9 or 1.2 mm or 19 gauge equivalent can be more efficient.

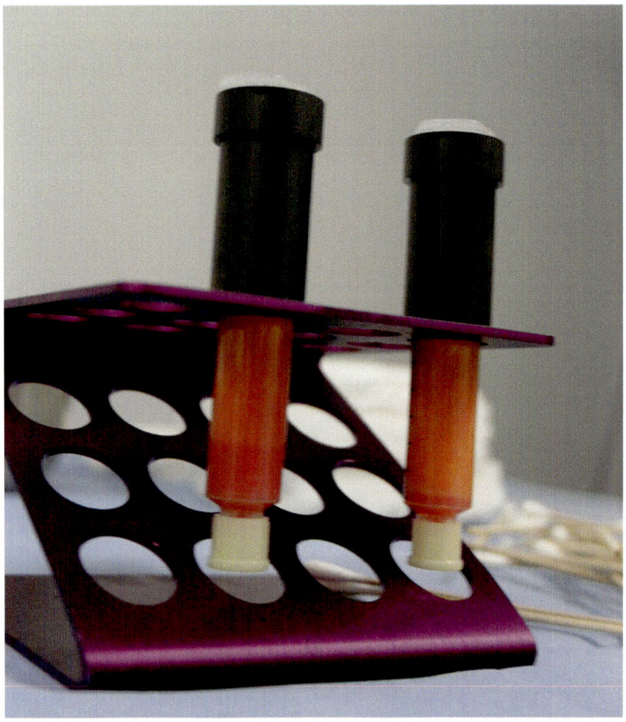

Fig. 35.2 Once harvested, there is a slurry of fat, tumescent solution, and blood products

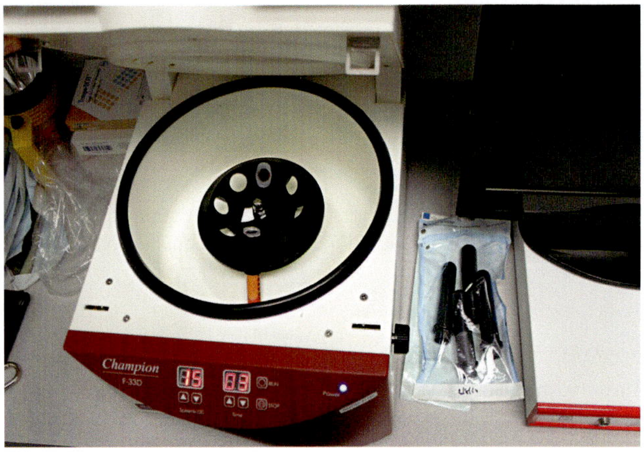

Fig. 35.3 This intermediate product is then centrifuged

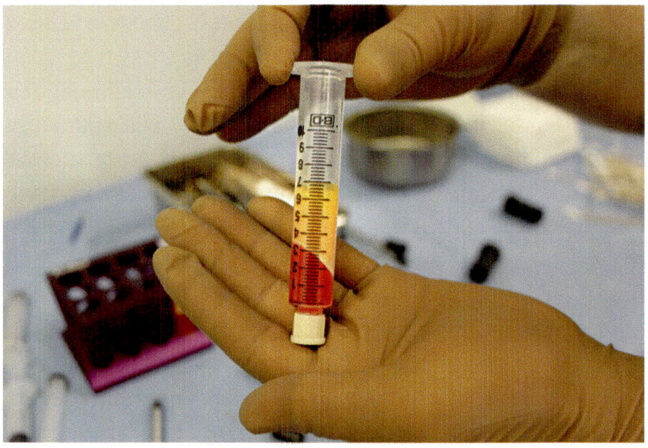

Fig. 35.4 Once the layers have separated using either method, the diluent is carefully poured off

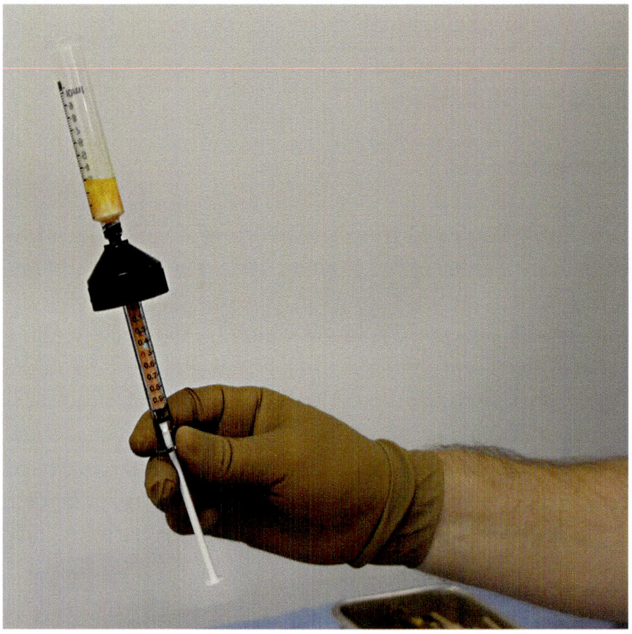

Fig. 35.5 The remaining fat is then transferred to a more manageable 1 cc luer lock syringe

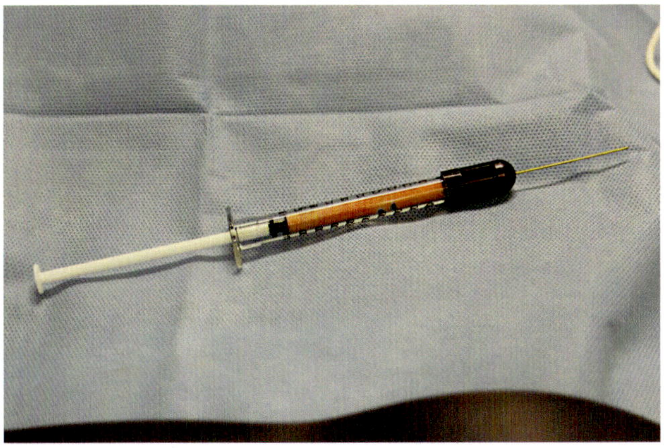

Fig. 35.6 For periorbital areas it is preferable to use a smaller cannula such as a 0.7 mm, while in other parts of the face a larger cannula can be more efficient

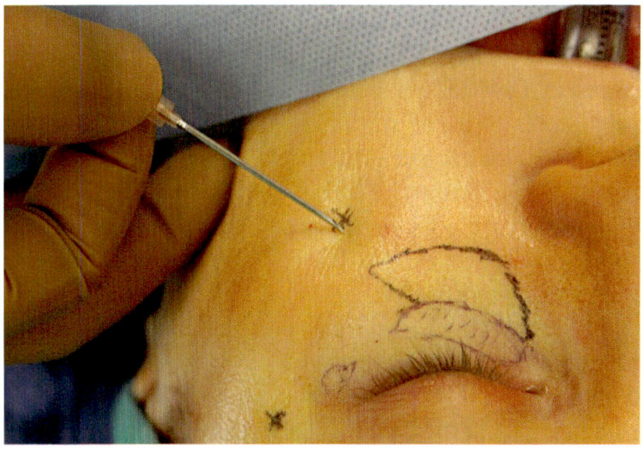

Fig. 35.7 An 18 g needle is pierced into skin in areas that the cannula can easily reach the targeted site

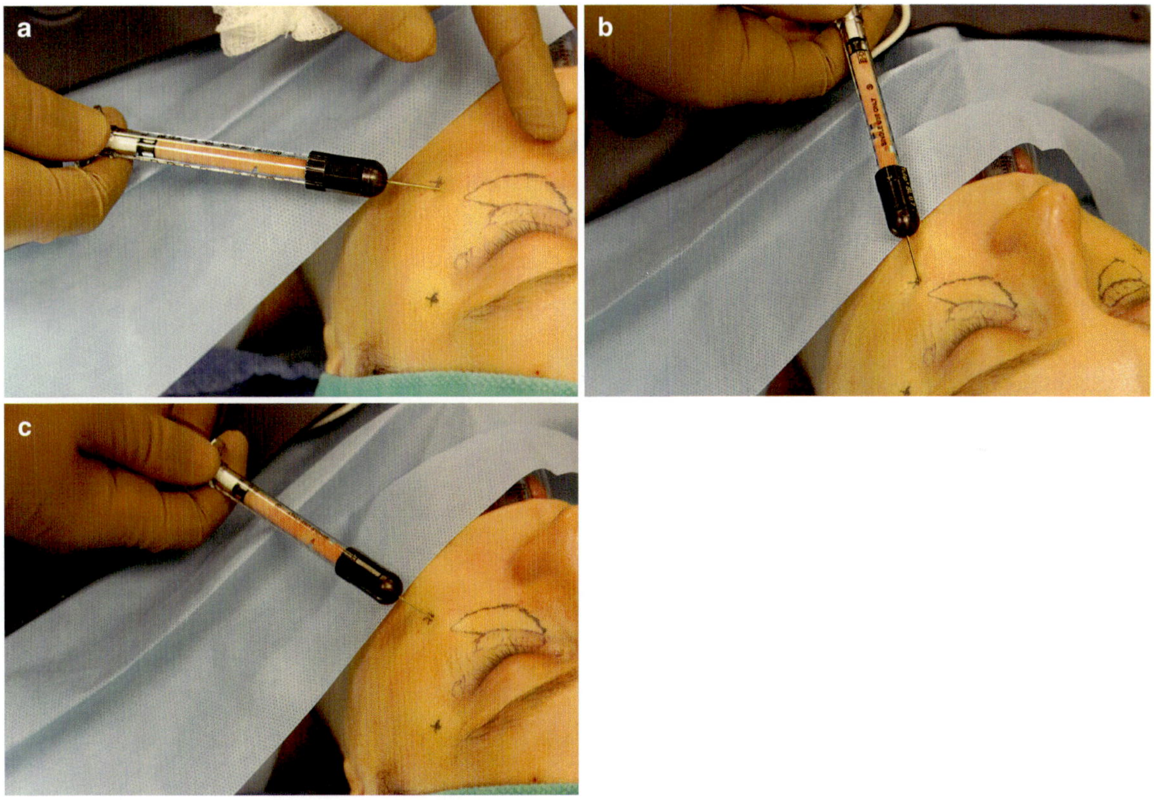

Fig. 35.8 Very small aliquots of fat are injected with each pass back and forth in a fanning technique in different angles directed upwards (**a**–**c**)

Transferring the Fat

Once ready in the 1 cc syringe with the appropriate cannula, the syringe is primed, and the first few fat globules are observed coming out to assure no blockage is noted. An 18 g needle is pierced into the skin in areas that the cannula can easily reach the targeted site (Fig. 35.7). The cannula enters the skin, and the depth is achieved by guiding the cannula perpendicular and then parallel. Optimal depth is to be intramuscular or submuscular to avoid superficial contour defects. The distal end of the cannula is felt with the "smart hand" (non-dominant hand). Very small aliquots of 0.1 cc of fat are injected with each pass back and forth in a fanning technique (Fig. 35.8a–c). For the periorbital region, a 0.7 mm (22 gauge) cannula is used to inject 1.5–3 cc per side into the infraorbital region with the entry port being in the upper cheek.

The fanning passes are directed upward. See Fig. 35.9 for typical entry port sites and volumes injected.

For supraorbital or superior sulcus defects, a 0.7 mm cannula is utilized in the suborbicularis muscle plane with fat averaging 1 cc per side. The entry port is at the suprabrow region fanning downward in the suborbicularis oculi muscle plane [2]. Ideally, the depth should be in the submuscular and intramuscular plane to allow for better integration and lessen the chance of visible contour irregularities.

For midface filling the entry port site can be at the mid nasolabial fold fanning upward in a multiplanar approach (both intramuscular and submuscular). A 0.7 or 0.9 mm cannula can be used, and typically 2–6 cc are transferred per side.

For perioral region filling, one can use a few entry ports depending on the location that requires the most volumization. Ports can be the same as for midface at the nasolabial fold with fanning downward, as well just lateral to the jowl at the mandibular border, thus filling medially toward the pre-jowl sulcus. Typically, 1–2 cc of fat per side are placed here, blending anterior to the sulcus. The lips can be filled as well with port of entry at the lateral commissure and filling with a 7 mm cannula. Fat is placed submucosal toward the midline with an average of 1 cc for the upper lip and 1.5 cc to the lower lip [2].

For posterior facial filling at the jawline, the entry port could be made at the inferior aspect of the nasolabial fold. Using a 1.2 mm cannula (18 gauge), fanning could be achieved laterally and superolaterally, with 2–5 cc typically placed per side. In this location fat should be placed preperiosteally so as not to disturb the masseter muscle or parotid gland.

Temporal filling is performed using a 0.7 or 0.9 mm cannula, with the port at the hairline edge. Fanning injections are performed inferiorly into the temporal region. Fat is placed subcutaneously in this region, using 3–5 cc per side (Fig. 35.9).

Complications

The most common complication with fat transfer is contour irregularities. This is usually secondary to superficial injection depth or possibly due to fat necrosis or graft inability to attain an adequate blood supply. Once edema is diminished and a blood supply to the grafted fat has been established, early recognition of any contour irregularity is important to note. At this point injectable therapy could be used in the form of 5-fluorouracil or kenalog (triamcinolone) given monthly (Fig. 35.10). If this does not adequately resolve the contour, the next alternative would be microliposuction with a 19 gauge cannula or similar equivalent. It is important to trap the offending fat mound with the surgeon's smart hand and actively liposuction the unwanted fat (Fig. 35.11). Only

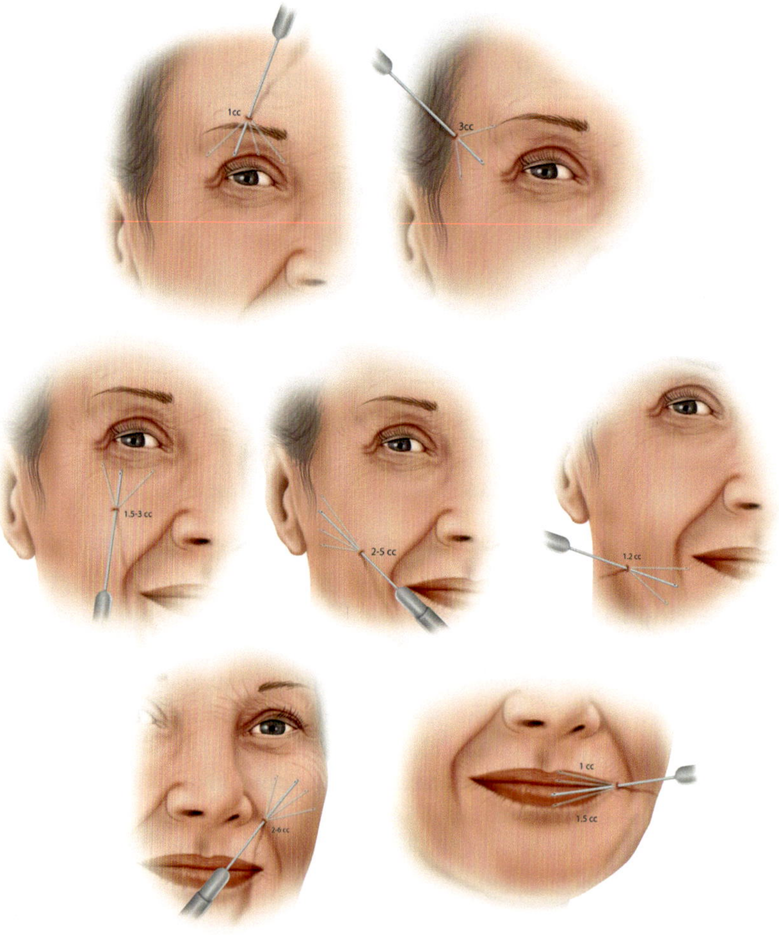

Fig. 35.9 Average port entry zones and fill volumes

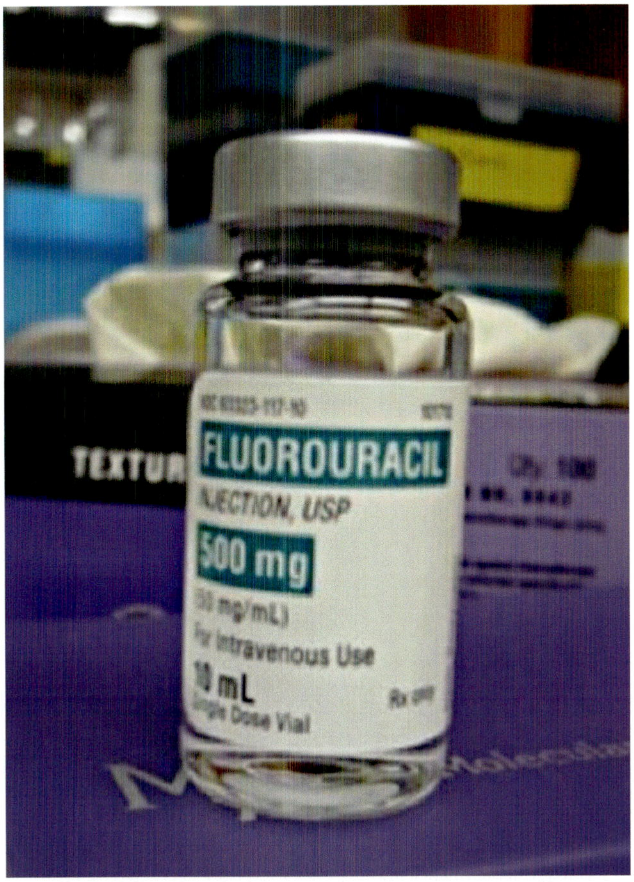

Fig. 35.10 Contour irregularity may be treated with injectable therapy, such as 5-fluorouracil or triamcinolone

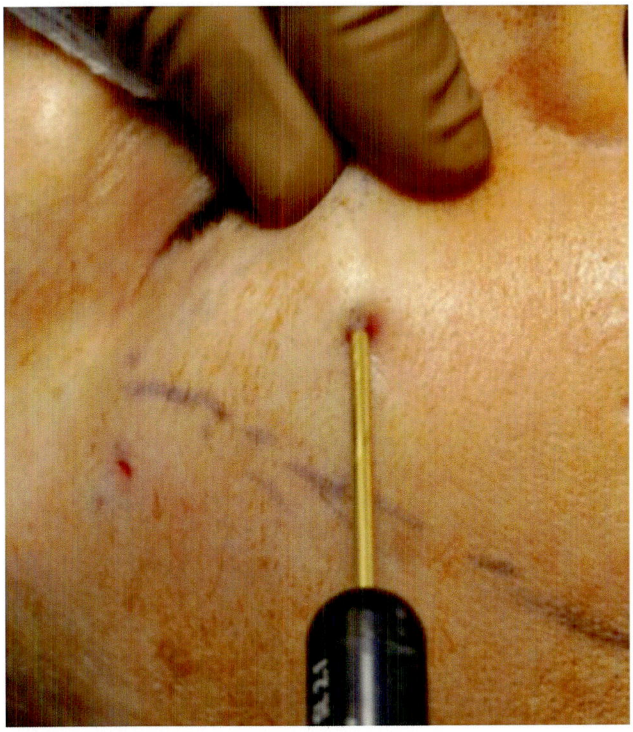

Fig. 35.11 The persistent fat mound should be palpated and isolated with the surgeon's smart hand, followed by active liposuction of the unwanted fat

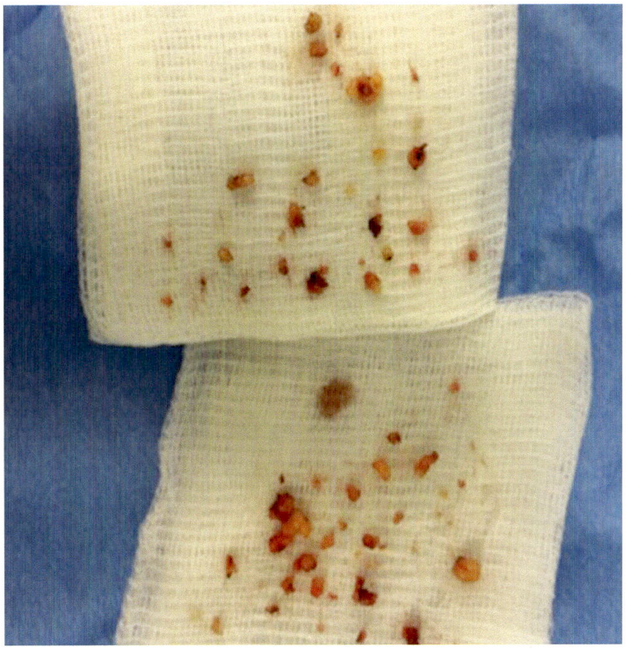

Fig. 35.12 Grafted fat is often encountered in small, fibrotic, very adherent globules

after swelling subsides and at least 3 months of healing have occurred, it may be appropriate to consider surgically removing residual unwanted fat. However, this may be difficult due to the multiplanar placement and fibrotic nature of grafted fat. The fat is often encountered in small, fibrotic, very adherent globules (Fig. 35.12) [5–7].

Another common complication includes atrophy or necrosis of the fat, and additional fat transfer procedures may be necessary to achieve optimal results. Very rarely, complications such as blindness or cerebral vascular insult have been reported [8, 9]. Grafted adipolysis can lead to oil droplets which can cause inflammation and result in cicatrization and calcification. This can be minimized by grafting smaller-sized fat particles. Once developed, oil cysts can be tender and inflamed for a prolonged period of time, and it is advisable to open the cyst with a large bore needle to allow drainage of material [9]. Other complications that could ensue include infection or hematoma. There can also be a risk of damage to underlying structures including muscle, tendons, blood vessels, or nerves. There could also be infection, hematoma, or, more commonly, contour irregularities noted at the harvest site [9].

Discussion

Facial fat transfer is a vital tool in a cosmetic surgical armamentarium. Aging is customarily accompanied with facial fat deflation, and often volumization is adequate without lifting procedures. When performing any necessary tightening and lifting procedures, the surgeon should always be aware of volume loss, and the potential benefit fat grafting could

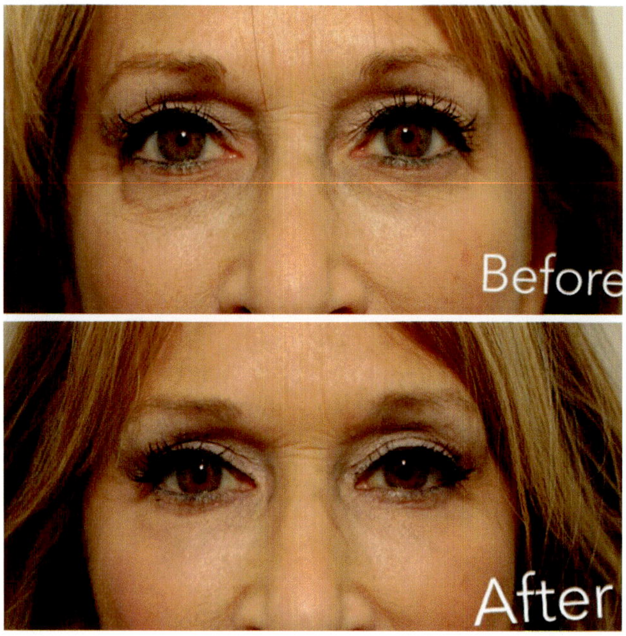

Fig. 35.13 Fat grafting to the eyelids, in combination with rhytidectomy procedures, can create a more three-dimensional rejuvenation of the face

provide in conjunction with these procedures. Adding fat grafting to eyelid (Fig. 35.13) and rhytidectomy procedures can add for a more three-dimensional enhancement with a natural appearing result. Fat transfer along the jawline, midface, temples, periorbital, and perioral region combined with standard rhytidectomy, eyelid, and midfacial procedures can be quite powerful. Facial fat grafting is valuable in softening and enhancing the periorbital area when volume depletion is noted. It can provide a smooth transition from the midface to the lower eyelid junction while performing lower eyelid rejuvenation procedures, and with careful technique it can enhance a hollow superior sulcus. Fat added to hollowing temples and perioral regions can enhance face- and brow-lifting procedures or can be provided as a stand-alone procedure. Recent advances have allowed finer instrumentation with smaller cannulas, thus leading to lower complication rates and enhanced outcomes [10]. Facial volumization with autologous fat transfer continues to be an area of growth, and is a vital tool in the cosmetic surgery armamentarium that can have a lasting impact on facial appearance.

References

1. Coleman SR. Structural fat grafts: the ideal filler? Clin Plast Surg. 2001;28:111–9.
2. Marten TJ, Elyassnia D. Fat grafting in facial rejuvenation. Clin Plast Surg. 2015;42(2):219–52.
3. Kokai L, Rubin P, Kacey G. The potential of adipose derived adult stem cells as a source of neuronal progenitor cells. Plast Reconstr Surg. 2005;116:1453–60.
4. Sykes JM, Tapias V, Pu LL. Autologous fat grafting viability: lower third of the face. Facial Plast Surg. 2010;26(5):376–84.
5. Coleman SR, Katzel EB. Fat grafting for facial filling and regeneration. Clin Plast Surg. 2015;42:289–300.
6. Duncan DI, Chabaty R. Clinical safety data and standards of practice for injection lipolysis: a retrospective study. Aesthet Surg J. 2006;26(5):575–85.
7. Coleman SR. Lower lid deformity secondary to autogenous fat transfer: a cautionary tale. Aesthet Plast Surg. 2008;32(3):415–7.
8. Lee DH, Yang HN, Kim JC, et al. Sudden unilateral visual loss and brain infarction after autologous fat injection into the nasolabial groove. Br J Ophthalmol. 1996;80:1026–7.
9. Yoshimura K, Coleman SR. Complications of fat grafting: how they occur and how to find, avoid and treat them. Clin Plast Surg. 2015;42:383–8.
10. Klein JA. The tumescent technique. Anesthesia and modified liposuction technique. Dermatol Clin. 1990;8(3):425–37.

36 Nonsurgical Periorbital and Facial Rejuvenation: A Paradigm Shift for Patients and Surgeons

Christopher C. Lo, Ashley Campbell, and Joseph A. Eviatar

While oculofacial surgery was once the primary option for facial rejuvenation, minimally invasive, nonsurgical treatments are now known to successfully restore a well-rested, youthful appearance to the well-selected patient. Although some patients may elect for a surgical correction expecting that they will only ever need one procedure to achieve the desired look, it must be understood that even surgical procedures also have a corrective timeline and will need maintenance and future corrections. Many techniques discussed in this chapter can be used as adjunctive therapy to surgical corrections; thus a thorough understanding of nonsurgical periorbital and facial rejuvenation strategies is crucial to every oculoplastic surgeon.

As with all facial enhancements, the goal should be to restore a healthy, youthful appearance in a subtle and natural manner. Historically, many surgeons focused on reversing laxity and descent of facial structures. With the understanding of panfacial volume loss came a shift to facial revolumization with fat [1–3]. Now with the advent of lasers and other devices with minimal healing time, skin tightening can be targeted after improvement of the underlying structures. Each patient's corrective requirements can be widely variable – tightening, volumization, and contouring can all be required to a certain extent, depending on patient age, gender, Fitzpatrick skin classification, ethnicity, and expectations. Understanding balance, shadows, and symmetry is crucial in reaching a tasteful and natural aesthetic endpoint.

The decision whether to perform an invasive or noninvasive procedure is based on a patient's desire and also the underlying components that contribute to an aged appearance. In most cases, revolumization and skin improvements are needed to some degree. There has also recently been a shift in the age of the patient population undergoing aesthetic procedures as many younger patients may seek "preventative" treatments. We believe this trend will continue as patients continue to become more educated on these less invasive techniques.

Evaluation of the Nonsurgical Patient

Prior to any treatments, an in-depth knowledge of facial anatomy and proportions is imperative to achieving the optimal aesthetic outcome. During facial analysis and pre- and peri-procedural planning, lateral, oblique, and "worm's-eye" views may be helpful vantage points. However, the frontal view must be constantly evaluated and revisited as this view allows for critical evaluation of volume, symmetry, balance, and shadows.

The patient's age, skin type, genetics, environmental exposures, and underlying soft tissue and bony architecture not only guide where treatments are needed, but also what level of improvement is attainable with nonsurgical techniques. Each individual patient's "foundation" must be established, and the areas to be addressed should be prioritized based on need, cost of treatment, and which treatments may serve as the base for subsequent treatments. Balance and harmony of the facial structures should be the goal – "youth" is elusive and may be unattainable except in the sense of soft tissue rejuvenation. Mimicking aesthetic fads may lead to a disharmonious appearance and not improve overall attractiveness. As with surgical patients, realistic expectations are crucial and should be established immediately. It is imperative that the physician and patient discuss these issues and agree on a treatment plan together.

C. C. Lo
Oculoplastic and Orbital Surgery, UCLA Doheny and Stein Eye Institutes, Los Angeles, CA, USA

A. Campbell
Division of Oculoplastics, John Hopkins Wilmer Eye Institute, Baltimore, MD, USA

J. A. Eviatar (✉)
Facial Aesthetics, Omni Aesthetic MD, New York, NY, USA
e-mail: JEviatarMD@OmniAestheticMD.com

A. J. Cohen, C. N. Burkat (eds.), *Oculofacial, Orbital, and Lacrimal Surgery*, https://doi.org/10.1007/978-3-030-14092-2_36

Varying degrees of facial asymmetry is the norm and needs to be recognized, documented, and communicated with the patient. In addition to involutional or age-related changes, the patient should be thoroughly evaluated for asymmetries caused by thyroid eye disease, Horner's syndrome, Bell's palsy, myasthenia gravis, trauma, and other etiologies. During treatments, symmetry can be approximated between the two sides of the face by treating each side of the face with varying amounts of product [4].

Digital photography and assessment of facial photos with the patient has been an invaluable tool to highlight subtle changes and clarify the goals of each treatment session. Without facial documentation, it is impossible for the patient and surgeon to accurately differentiate day-to-day changes from aging or treatments. While some of these procedures are considered short term or temporary, there is a subtle semipermanent effect that exists with each of these corrections that can only be documented with serial photographs. To this end, standardized lighting and camera angles are necessary to capture these nuanced volume and contour changes.

As with surgical enhancements, gender norms are essential considerations in nonsurgical treatments. While both male and female patients share the common goal of looking rejuvenated, healthy, and energetic, gender dimorphism dictates anatomical norms which differ in females and males. For example, stereotyped females may have a smaller forehead, convex brow with lateral flare, higher eyelid tarsal platform show, and a narrow nasal bridge, chin, and jaw. Alternatively, a stereotyped male often has a large forehead, flat brows, prominent orbital ridge and glabellar projection, lower eyelid tarsal platform show, and a wider chin and jaw [5]. Harmony is crucial; a male jaw aesthetically favors a larger volume, which could be enhanced with a structural filler. A similar injection in a female would create an unbalanced appearance. Alternatively, a female face favors full lips, strong cheekbones, and shaped eyebrows, which would be normally considered undesirable corrections for a male face. Furthermore, specific areas, such as forehead lines, may require more units of neurotoxin for adequate treatment in male patients [5]. Additional considerations should be made for ethnic norms, and procedures should enhance and optimize an individual's personal facial features with strategies that are specific to that ethnicity to ensure the best aesthetic outcomes and patient satisfaction [6, 7]. There is absolutely no single recipe for rejuvenation; each patient must be evaluated individually.

Enhancement, Rejuvenation, or Reconstruction

Following an integrated model of facial aging, it is understood that increasing skin laxity, subcutaneous fat atrophy, and repositioning of soft tissue due to loss of elasticity and gravity all are involved in facial aging [1–3, 8, 9]. MRI volumetric studies have further quantified that a dramatic volume loss in the temporal, infraorbital, lateral, and medial cheek areas occurs between young and middle-age women, which corroborates the importance of selective tissue augmentation and volume correction strategies in facial rejuvenation [10, 11].

Deflation and descent lead to accentuation of the periorbital hollows, which are stereotypic of the aged face [12]. The complex soft tissue layers in the face are interconnected and attach to the underlying facial skeleton with retaining ligaments [7]. Anatomic studies have been performed that have elucidated superficial and deep facial fat compartments surrounded by fibrous condensations [13, 14]. Understanding these discrete compartments allows us to fill and volumize precise locations of the face, including the deep medial cheek and nasolabial, superficial middle, and lateral cheek fat pads [15]. Furthermore, filling the deep medial cheek fat allows for scaffolding that can set the foundation for further manipulations of more superficial fat compartments and allow for lifting with filling. Targeted filling of the periorbital hollows, superior sulcus, and eyebrow region can enhance the three-dimensional contours and restore a rejuvenated appearance to the periorbital area [9, 16–20].

Dynamic changes to the skeletal morphology also play a large role in the appearance of the aged face. CT studies have documented facial bone ratio and angle changes, which can result in disharmony when the remodeling disrupts the balance between bone and soft tissue [8]. According to the Lambros theory of aging and skeletal remodeling, there is a clockwise rotation of the profile of the midface relative to the cranial base, which results in a change of profile and facial vectors; the pyriform and inferior maxilla move posteriorly, and the superior orbit and glabella move anteriorly [21, 22]. These changes have been confirmed with both two-dimensional and three-dimensional CT analysis [22, 23]. From a frontal view, the orbit width and height was not found to change with age; however, the superomedial upper orbit and the inferolateral orbit recede, further unmasking medial upper eyelid fat and accentuating lower eyelid lag [2, 23]. Mandible height and projection may recede with time and, with blunting of the mandibular angle, can result in loss of jaw definition and unmasking of jowls and neck laxity [2]. Overall, loss of bony architectural support and diminution of overlying facial volume create the visual impression of lines, shadows, and sagging. These changes reflect the reconstructive challenges that are addressed during both surgical and nonsurgical repair. Understanding which layers are affected allows for targeted treatment at the specific level.

Enhancement, rejuvenation, and reconstruction are three different strategies that are employed during nonsurgical plastic surgery. Enhancement focuses on improving symmetry, balance, and aesthetic appeal. Rejuvenation repairs and reverses the damage associated with aging, while reconstruction involves re-making defective parts, from age or disability, to recreate a desired appearance. While older patients, with atrophic changes to the skin, soft tissue structures, and bony morphology, may require reconstruction, rejuvenation, and enhancement, a more youthful patient may experience optimal result with only rejuvenation or enhancement.

Neurotoxins

Botulinum neurotoxin is a protein produced by *Clostridium botulinum* that inhibits the release of acetylcholine at the neuromuscular junctions, thus inducing flaccid muscle paralysis. While first studied to protect against botulism toxicity in the food canning industry, this chemical was further concentrated and weaponized during World War II. This agent was first injected clinically to treat strabismus, but its applications have extended beyond ophthalmic and neurologic indications to treat urologic, hypersecretory, gastrointestinal, and complex pain disorders [24–27]. After noting improvement of wrinkles in patients treated for blepharospasm, botulinum toxin type A (onabotulinumtoxinA) was approved in 2002 by the Food and Drug Administration (FDA) for temporary correction of moderate-to-severe glabellar lines. Since then, there have been many cosmetic applications for these neurotoxins, including injections in the mid and lower face to prevent the appearance of wrinkles by lessening the contraction of hyperdynamic muscles [28]. Botulinum toxin type A (onabotulinumtoxinA) was then FDA approved for the treatment of crow's feet in 2013, followed by being the first neurotoxin to be approved in 2017 for the amelioration of moderate to severe forehead lines caused by frontalis muscle hyperactivity.

Superficial, low-dose injections of botulinum toxin type A have also been used for hyperhidrosis, improving recalcitrant acne, rosacea, and psoriasis [29–32]. As with injectable filler implants, the "off-label" clinical uses of neurotoxins for aesthetic applications in the face are vast and powerful. Following the facial feedback hypothesis, there is evidence that neurotoxin injection can have a positive influence on patient mood by altering facial expressions [33]. These techniques may not all be FDA approved but have become the standard of care for advanced injectors.

There are currently three neurotoxins approved for use in the United States, Botox (onabotulinumtoxinA; Allergan), Dysport (abobotulinumtoxinA; Ipsen, Ltd.), and Xeomin (incobotulinumtoxinA; Merz Aesthetics, Merz Pharmaceuticals). Dysport and Xeomin were FDA approved based on noninferiority trials to Botox. Since then, various clinicians have identified nuanced variations to the properties of these medications, related to proprietary formulations [34]. A fourth formulation, RT002 (daxibotulinumtoxinA; Revance), is currently seeking FDA approval for glabellar lines. There are also new neurotoxins in the FDA pipeline that are formulated as topical, rather than injected, products. Further research and experience will be needed to direct the proper use of these new products.

Clinical onset for Botox is detected by 1 week following injection, and effects can last approximately 3–4 months. Some clinicians find that Dysport has more rapid onset of action with a similar duration of effect. Xeomin is produced without the additive proteins present in the other formulations that may or may not contribute to increased immunogenicity and therefore may prevent secondary treatment failure. It is unclear if this is truly significant in clinical practice. Xeomin does not require refrigeration and has also been shown to be stable in extreme heat. Xeomin also has a more rapid onset of action, but has recently been found to have shorter duration of effect when compared to that of Botox [35]. Various clinicians have tried alternating neurotoxins for varying results for patients that have "resistance" to the medications, although there is debate if these theoretical possibilities have any role in clinical practice. Clinical experience with each seems to be the best guide as all three have a similar mechanism of action and each plays a potential role in practice.

Studies have shown a high level of treatment satisfaction with long-term use of Botox. Treatments at a regular interval both maintain and improve outcomes [36]. Following this paradigm, gradual muscle atrophy is expected; as a result, the cumulative annual dose of neurotoxin tends to decrease over time, and fewer visits may be needed to maintain the desired result. Additionally, the location of injections may need to slightly change each visit to prevent the appearance of rhytids due to relative overaction of adjacent muscles in untreated areas.

While the FDA label may provide a standard for injection dose and location, a customized and tailored approach is preferable. There are a wide variety of injection techniques that take into account individual patient characteristics, with the goal of creating a natural, and not "frozen," look. Understanding the anatomy of the facial muscles can allow for a judicious approach toward injecting neurotoxin, which allows for softening of the fine dynamic rhytids, without removing all movement and expression.

Although generally well tolerated, injections of neuromodulators have known risks, such as bleeding, discomfort, bruising, soft tissue infection, undercorrection, and irreversible, albeit temporary, paralysis of muscles by inadvertent injection, which could lead to lagophthalmos, ptosis, diplopia, dysphagia, or respiratory distress. There is evidence that activating the injected muscle areas may increase stimulation to the muscles and lessen the duration of overcorrection. After the launch of Xeomin, the FDA required publishing a black box warning, where patients should be warned of the risk of systemic toxicity and even death. However, the low doses used for cosmetic medicine can be safely injected with proper technique without cause for concern.

Upper Face Injections

- *Glabella*: The glabellar region was the first FDA-approved region for neuromodulator injection [37]. The procerus muscle, corrugator and depressor supercilii, medial orbicularis oculi, and frontalis muscle form the glabellar complex and create vertical glabellar rhytids. Injection of this area is well tolerated with high patient satisfaction scores for up to 4 months after injection [38, 39].
- *Forehead*: The frontalis muscle is also a common neuromodulator treatment site for forehead rhytids [40, 41]. The muscle fibers are oriented vertically, and there are often two distinct muscle bodies. There is variation among depth of forehead rhytids and the orientation of the frontalis muscle fibers, requiring a nuanced approach to injection in this region [42]. The goal in treatment is to minimize the appearance of transverse lines, while avoiding a frozen, inexpressive appearance. Techniques include multiple injection sites with small amounts of neurotoxin or larger volumes of saline with dilute neurotoxin. Care should be taken to prevent inadvertent brow ptosis from overinjection of the lower frontalis brow elevators. Injecting semipermanent hyaluronic acid fillers to support the frontalis at the subgaleal area can improve the shape of the forehead, decrease unwanted shadowing, decrease the number and depth of lines, and decrease the total required neurotoxin to soften these lines.
- *Eyebrow*: Advanced injectors can use neurotoxins to improve the shape of the brow, without limiting animation of this expressive region. Understanding and manipulating the elevators and depressors of the brow allow for improvement of this aesthetically focal area. Injectors can raise and flatten the brow in men to create a masculine facial frame. In women, injectors can shape and arch the brow with approximately 2 units strategically placed under the desired arch of the eyebrow to weaken the orbital orbicularis oculi.

It has been historically taught that forehead injections should stay at least 1 cm above the supraorbital rim to avoid eyelid ptosis. However, most cases of eyelid ptosis are likely preexisting and become manifest after neurotoxin treatment because of weakening of the frontalis muscle, which has otherwise been compensating for underlying ptosis. Meticulous observation of the eyelid, eyebrow, and forehead complex position to rule out ptosis should be done prior to injection. Also, air bubbles should be carefully removed from the tip of the syringe prior to injection as infiltration of air may inadvertantly violate the soft tissue planes allowing the neurotoxin to travel to an undesired location. If ptosis does develop, the patient should be observed to see if the ptosis is related to the eyelid or due to overparalysis of the frontalis muscle. An induced eyelid ptosis can be temporarily improved with topical adrenergic agonists, such as apraclonidine (0.5%) and brimonidine (0.1% or 0.2%), or sympathomimetics, such as neosynephrine hydrochloride (2.5%) [43, 44].

- *Outer eyelids*: The lateral periorbital rhytids, commonly known as "crow's feet," are formed from age- and sun-related skin changes and forceful contraction of the lateral orbicularis oculi muscle. The orbital subdivision of the orbicularis oculi muscle should be targeted at multiple sites during injection with caution to avoid disrupting function [45]. Overzealous injection of this area can "freeze" periocular expression during a natural smile. Misplaced injection of the lower orbicularis fibers can inadvertently paralyze the zygomaticus mimetic muscles and distort the smile.
- *Lower eyelids*: Injecting 1–2 small amounts of 2–3 units of Botox can be used to relax the preseptal and pretarsal orbicularis and flatten the tarsal roll. This can be especially useful in Asian patients with high riding lower eyelid orbicularis. Overcorrection must be avoided to prevent lagophthalmos, ectropion, and other unwanted eyelid malpositions. Also, as the skin in this region is extremely thin, the lower eyelid can be gently distracted over the orbital rim for injection, to avoid inadvertent injury to the globe. Ecchymosis is more common in the lower eyelids as well. In some cultures, this lower eyelid orbicularis roll (or "love band") is considered youthful, welcoming, and attractive, and it is important to always maintain cultural considerations and patient preference.
- *Upper eyelids*: Some have also injected neurotoxin to temporarily improve a mild upper eyelid ptosis by weakening the pretarsal orbicularis of the upper lid. However, only experienced injectors should attempt these given the unpredictability of results and possible exacerbation of ptosis.
- *Nasal lines*: Contraction of the transverse portion of the nasalis muscle creates nasal dorsum lines or "bunny lines." Advanced injectors have developed multiple techniques to inject low doses of neurotoxin near the medial canthus to avoid distortion of the smile.

Lower Face Injections

- *Mouth*: The orbicularis oris, depressor anguli oris, and mentalis are commonly addressed with botulinum toxin. Excessive contraction of the orbicularis oris can create vertical upper lip lines, known as "smoker's lines," which can be minimized by careful, symmetric microinjections to the upper lip area. The depressor anguli oris muscle inserts from the jawline into the angle of the mouth, and injection to these points can elevate the "frowning" corners of the mouth.

- *Gummy smile*: Small (2.5 units) injections to the levator labii superioris alaeque nasi at the upper nasolabial fold, levator labii superioris, and/or zygomaticus major/minor can be used to reduce incisor and gingival show [46, 47]. In general, injections in the lower third of the face should be conservative as excessive paresis could cause drooling, dysarthria, and inability to drink from straws or purse the lips [48].
- *Chin*: An overactive mentalis muscle, paired with age-related subcutaneous fat loss, can create a diffuse dimpling of the chin, which can be improved with neuromodulators. This improvement can be further supplemented by dermal fillers to smooth the volume loss in the chin.
- *Jawline*: An overactive masseter muscle can create a square-shaped jawline that can be successfully contoured with botulinum toxin to create a rounder/more oval, feminine facial appearance, something particularly valued in certain Asian cultures [49–51]. The goal of treatment in this case is to induce muscle atrophy rather than limit muscle contraction to reduce wrinkles. Starting doses are much higher than other areas in the face, often requiring up to 40 units of Botox (approximately 15–20 units per masseter, unless there is asymmetric masseter size). Overparalysis of the masticatory muscles should be avoided as this can cause weakness in chewing in up to 30% of patients [52].
- *Neck*: The platysma is a broad, thin muscle overlying the anterior aspect of the neck that functions to lower the mandible and pull the lower lip inferolaterally. Although static rhytids and subcutaneous fat loss of the neck cannot be fully improved with botulinum neuromodulators, the appearance of platysmal bands can be softened with multiple direct injections into the bands [53–55]. In addition to relaxing the platysmal bands, delivery of small aliquots of Botox at approximately 1.5–2 cm intervals into the platysma can improve neck skin texture, color, and smoothness and accentuate the cervicomental contour [56]. Injection deep into the neck muscles, however, may cause dysphagia, dysarthria, or even respiratory distress.

Injectable Fillers in the Facial Region

As the understanding of facial aging and rejuvenation has changed, there has been a shift from surgical skin tightening procedures toward restoring subcutaneous and bony volume first. There are currently many options for FDA-approved fillers, each with distinct properties to formulate an optimal treatment plan based on perceived deficits. Properties that differentiate these products and their usage in the clinical setting include particle size and shape, cohesiveness and the degree of cross-linking, G-prime, flow characteristics, varying thickness, and the ability to lift rather than just spread.

Table 36.1 Commonly treated facial areas. (Many indications are off-label)

Location	Suggested injections or fillers
Forehead	Neurotoxins, structural hyaluronic acid (HA) fillers,[a] superficial HA fillers to target lines
Temples	HA fillers or customized deep fillers, calcium hydroxyapatite (CaHA), poly-L-lactic acid (PLLA) fillers[a]
Hair line (for lifting)	PLLA fillers,[a] CaHA fillers
Brows	HA fillers or customized deep fillers, PLLA fillers,[a] threadlifting[a]
Glabella	Neurotoxin, HA fillers,[a] CaHA fillers[a]
Lower periocular volume loss (tear trough)	HA fillers, CaHA fillers,[a] PLLA fillers[a]
Nose	Neurotoxin, HA fillers,[a] CaHA fillers[a]
Cheeks	HA fillers, CaHA fillers, PLLA fillers, threadlifting[a]
Canine Fossa/NLF	HA fillers, PLLA fillers, CaHA fillers
Lips	Neurotoxins, structural and nonstructural HA fillers depending on desired correction[a]
Jawline	CaHA fillers, HA fillers, neurotoxins
Masseter	Neurotoxins
Parotid hypertrophy	Neurotoxins
Neck	Neurotoxins, customized CaHA (dilute),[a] HA for fine lines, Kybella (fat melting and skin rejuvenation), cool sculpting, threadlifting[a]
Facial sweating	Neurotoxins
Acne scars	HA fillers, CaHA fillers,[a] PLLA fillers[a]
Ear lobes	HA fillers, CaHA fillers[a]

[a]Complicated techniques to be used only by advanced injectors

Injectable fillers and neuromodulators work exceptionally well together to rejuvenate various areas of the aging face (Table 36.1).

Injection Technique

While technique may vary with product and practitioner, there are general principles to administering cosmetic fillers. To lower periprocedural bleeding risk, cessation of nonessential anticoagulants or herbal medications is recommended. Topical antiseptic is often sufficient, but antiviral or antibiotic prophylaxis can be considered for specific at-risk populations. While neurotoxins are considered medications, these injectable fillers are semipermanent implantable devices that require greater attention to sepsis prevention as there is a risk of infection or biofilm.

Product viscosity, which can be customized with off-label saline or lidocaine reconstitution, often dictates needle size and surgeon preference. In general, smaller gauge needles prevent periprocedural pain and bleeding. Needle length is also an important consideration as longer needles can more easily access the mid or deep dermis. There is an ongoing debate regarding the role of cannulas in reducing the possibility of adverse events. Both needles and cannulas are acceptable methods of delivering the implants, although there are slight variations in the techniques required. The temples and upper eyelid/brow regions may be good locations for the use of cannulas, although other injectors find more versatility and facile use with needles. Knowledge of the anatomy and vascular supply is more critical in regard to avoiding complications.

Commonly used injection techniques include serial puncture, threading, fanning, and cross-hatching. Depth of injection, product viscosity, and desired effect must be collectively considered prior to injection. Serial puncture technique involves holding the skin taut while the needle is inserted directly in the area of defect. Once the intended injection depth has been achieved, the product should be delivered as the needle is being withdrawn in a small bolus. Threading technique requires a longer needle as the needle is tunneled through a larger area of defect at the appropriate depth. Product is delivered as the needle is withdrawn in a slow, continuous stream. Slow, small injections are critical as large boluses may acutely occlude a vessel if there is inadvertent intravascular injection. In the fanning technique, multiple threads are delivered through a single insertion point without removing the needle. For areas of more extensive volume loss, a cross-hatching technique can be used, where the fanning technique can be overlapped with multiple entry points.

Following treatment, the practitioner can provide gentle massage to assist with shaping of product and to avoid formation of nodules. Ice should be applied for the day, and exercise should be avoided for 24 hours. Patients should be instructed to refrain from aggressive facial movement or unnecessary manipulation until the product settles.

Injectable Facial Fillers (Table 36.2)

- Autologous fat transfer was first explored as a facial volumizer in the late 1800s and regained prominence in the 1970s with the advent of improved liposuction techniques to harvest fat tissue [57]. These injections are safe and have good result with deep tissue filling, though have variable longevity given high rates of resorption in certain locations [58]. There are ongoing attempts to make fat injection more predictable and longer lasting, though in reality patients seeking fat injection only have this done in conjunction with other surgeries as surgical downtime after harvesting and injection is considerable following these procedures. In addition, the surviving fat has the potential to hypertrophy after weight gain or after menopause and may be challenging to remove at this stage [59]. Fat transfer to the face is discussed in more detail in a separate chapter.
- Collagen, a naturally found component of the biological matrix, can be injected in varying concentrations to restore facial volume. The first FDA-approved product for injected facial augmentation, this product can be harvested from cadaveric or bovine sources, although it has gained more use after laboratory cultures of human fibroblast cells have further improved immunogenicity [60]. Bovine collagen was one of the first injectable implants used to define the lip line; however, now it has limited current usefulness. Other collagen products have since emerged but have generally lost favor due to quick, unpredictable absorption and the requirement of antigenic testing prior to injection.
- Nonpermanent hyaluronic acid fillers are the most widely used and marketed for facial implantation and have supplanted collagen as the "gold standard" for volumizing facial injection [60]. Hyaluronic acid is a naturally occurring scaffold for connective tissue and collagen development in the human dermis. This biomaterial has been modified to allow for more long-lasting space filling. One of the undeniable benefits of hyaluronic acid fillers are the ability to dissolve out the treatment with injectable hyaluronidase. Restylane/Restylane Fine/Restylane Silk/ Restylane Lyft (previously known as Perlane)/Restylane Refyne/Restylane Defyne (Galderma), Voluma/Juvederm/ Vollure/Volbella (Allergan), and Belotero (Merz Aesthetics) are FDA-approved, well tolerated, bacterial-cultured hyaluronic acids. These products have varying superficial and deep tissue applications based on the particle size, G-prime, thickness, and flow of each specific product [61].

For example, Galderma has tailored their products' rheology to fit various needs around the face. Restylane Refyne has high flexibility and can be used to lessen the appearance of fine nasolabial folds and marionette lines, without sacrificing movement in these areas. On the opposite side of the spectrum, Restylane and Restylane Lyft have a high G-prime and provide strong structural support and volume. Restylane Defyne lies in the middle of the spectrum and balances structural support with flexibility. Allergan has similarly developed Juvederm Ultra with increased flexibility. Voluma and Vollure have higher G-prime in comparison, while Ultra Plus has been engineered to provide moderate flexibility and support.

Various synthetic compounds have been developed that have potential for long-term cosmetic effect while maintaining limited immunogenicity. Paraffin and liquid silicone were initially attempted for cosmetic injections; unfortunately, patients developed nodules and severe granulomatous reactions to these injected materials [62, 63]. More recent and successful synthetics involve biostimulatory suspended microparticles. As the fluid volume of the injectable absorbs, the stimulatory nature of the product stimulates elastin and collagen deposition. In addition, fibrosis can induce lifting properties that complement volume improvements.

Table 36.2 Options for injectable fillers in the face

Filler type	Name	Indication	Advantages	Disadvantages
Autologous products	Fat	Deep defects	Skin improvement, fewer adverse or allergic events	Technique and technician dependent, reserved for patients undergoing surgery given long recovery time, requires availability from donor site, unpredictable resorption, not easily reversible
	Autologous collagen/ autolagen (collagenesis, Beverly, MA; Isolagen, Exton, PA)	Fine lines, lip definition	Natural product, less chance of immunogenicity	Short acting, costly
Fillers	Restylane Lyft (previously Perlane)/Restylane/ Restylane Fine Lines/ Restylane Silk/Restylane Refyne/Restylane Defyne (Galderma)	Deep to superficial rhytids/lines based on formulation and customization	Reliable, predictable, longer lasting than collagens depending (longevity based on product and placement), immediately reversible	Hydrophilic causing 24–48 hours edema, rare immunologic reactions, bruising, nodules, vascular occlusions, necrosis
	Voluma/Juvederm Ultra Plus/Juvederm Ultra/ Vollure/Volbella (Allergan)	Deep to superficial rhytids/lines based on formulation and customization	Reliable, predictable, less spread, possibly longer lasting	Hydrophilic causing 24–48 hours edema, rare immunologic reactions, bruising, nodules, vascular occlusions, necrosis, costly for significant volumizing
Volumizers/ fillers	Radiesse (calcium hydroxyapatite microspheres) and Belotero (Merz) with full line coming to the US pending FDA approval	Radiesse: deep to superficial rhytids/lines based on customization Belotero: fine lines, superficial corrections on the lips, neck, acne	Not hydrophilic, skin improvement, collagen synthesis, can be used with tightening and lifting devices	Not truly reversible, rare nodules or immune reactions, vascular occlusions, necrosis
Volumizers	Sculptra (poly-L-lactic acid microparticles) (Dermik Laboratories, Berwyn, PA)	Deep to superficial rhytids/lines based on customization	Long-term gradual results, skin improvement, can be used along with tightening and lifting devices	Nonreversible, nodule formation, rare immune reaction, vascular occlusion, necrosis
Permanent	Bellafill (PMMA, Suneva)	Moderate to severe rhytids and lines, acne	Long-term results but still needs maintenance therapy for correction	Requires skin test due to bovine product. Nonreversible except with surgical excision and generally avoided, lifetime possibility of complications, infection, or reactions for patient, use of other agents may incite an unpredictable reaction in the same location

Sculptra (Valeant Pharmaceuticals) is composed of poly-L-lactic acid microparticles with a biostimulatory mode of action. This treatment is FDA approved for both aesthetic treatments as well as for HIV-associated facial lipodystrophy. After refluxing the needle to prevent vascular occlusion, this substance can fill directly over the bone. This injectable can also be delivered subdermally and intradermally to improve collagen and volume overall, though this may require multiple treatments. Radiesse (Merz Aesthetics) is an admixture of calcium hydroxylapatite microscopheres suspended in a gel structure of sterile water, glycerin, and carboxymethylcellulose. The characteristically high G-prime of Radiesse, which is a measure of elasticity, makes it a suitable product for lifting and contouring [64]. This product can be customized through reconstitution with lidocaine to allow for more superficial filling.

Bellafill (previously Artefill) (Suneva) is a polymethyl methacrylate filler with improved product longevity. However, it has been noted to have erythema at the injection site and, like other synthetic compounds, should be injected deeply into tissue to avoid palpable nodules or other unwarranted side effects. There is a general consensus among many practitioners, however, that the use of nonreversible fillers, such as Bellafill, and the off-label use of silicone, is problematic as they are unable to be removed without surgical intervention. These products harbor the long-term potential for deep tissue infection. In addition, as aging continues to change the facial anatomy, these permanent products can become unwanted and are difficult and unpredictable to remove. Patients seeking "permanent" correction should be educated that no outcome, whether surgical or injectable, can be permanent on the impermanent human face. However, permanent dangers do exist. Excellent alternatives, such as long-lasting, cross-linked hyaluronic acid fillers, fat transfer, or other surgical interventions, should be discussed. (See Figs. 36.1, 36.2, 36.3, 36.4, and 36.5 for examples of patients with facial fillers).

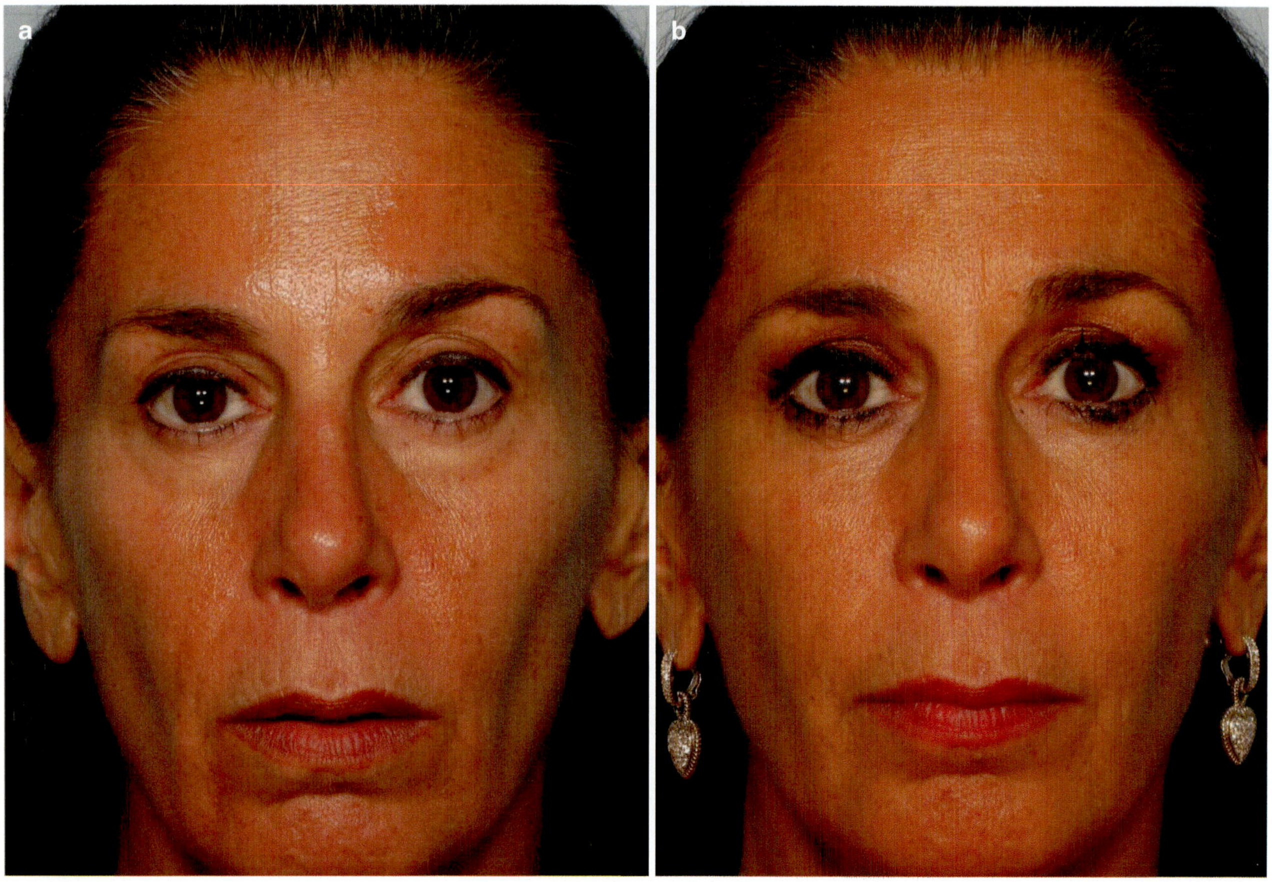

Fig. 36.1 (**a**) Before. A 50-year-old woman with panfacial volume loss and shadowing in the hollowed contours of the temples, tear trough, cheek, and midface. (**b**) After. Sculptra (PLLA) filler injected in the midface, cheek, and temple area to stimulate collagen formation and global volumization. After three treatments of two vials each, the patient had improved periorbital, midface, and lower face volume

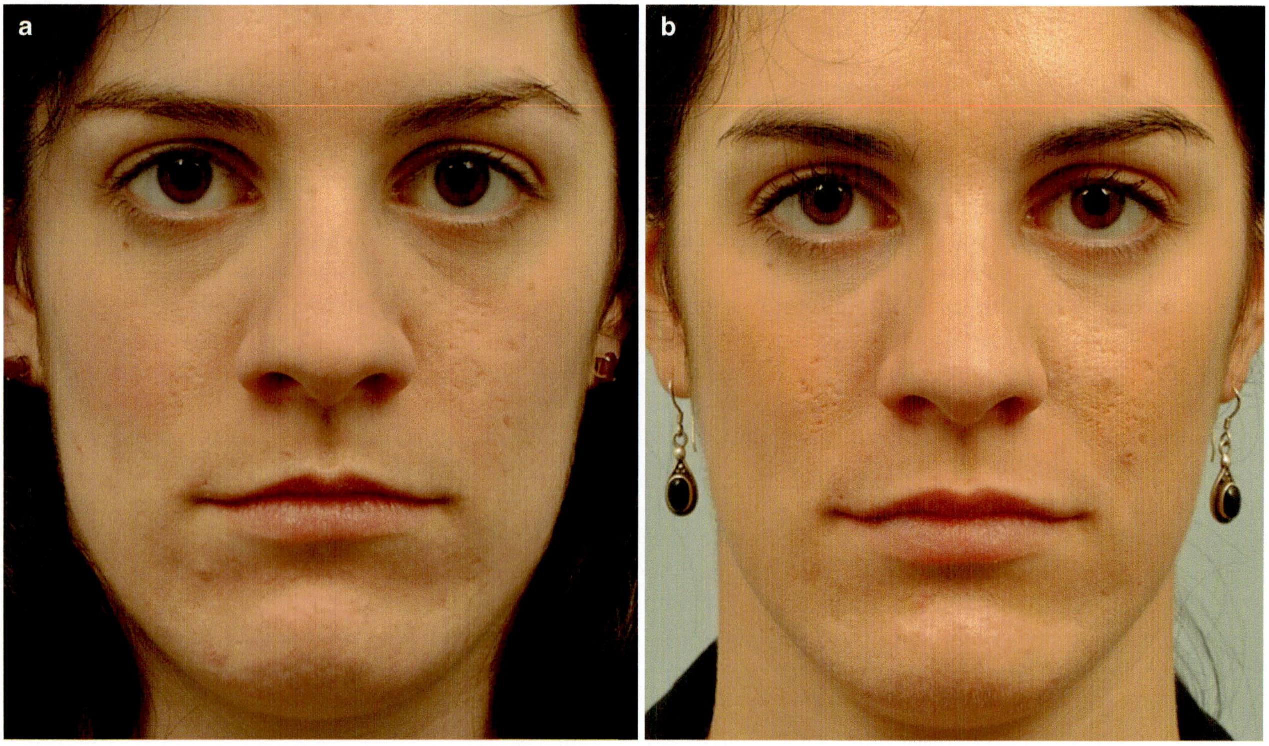

Fig. 36.2 (**a**) Before. A 27-year-old woman with prominent tear trough and thin lips. (**b**) After. The patient received one vial of hyaluronic acid (Restylane) to the tear trough and one vial of Juvederm Ultra Plus to the lips to improve coloration of the tear trough and restore balance and harmony to the facial proportions

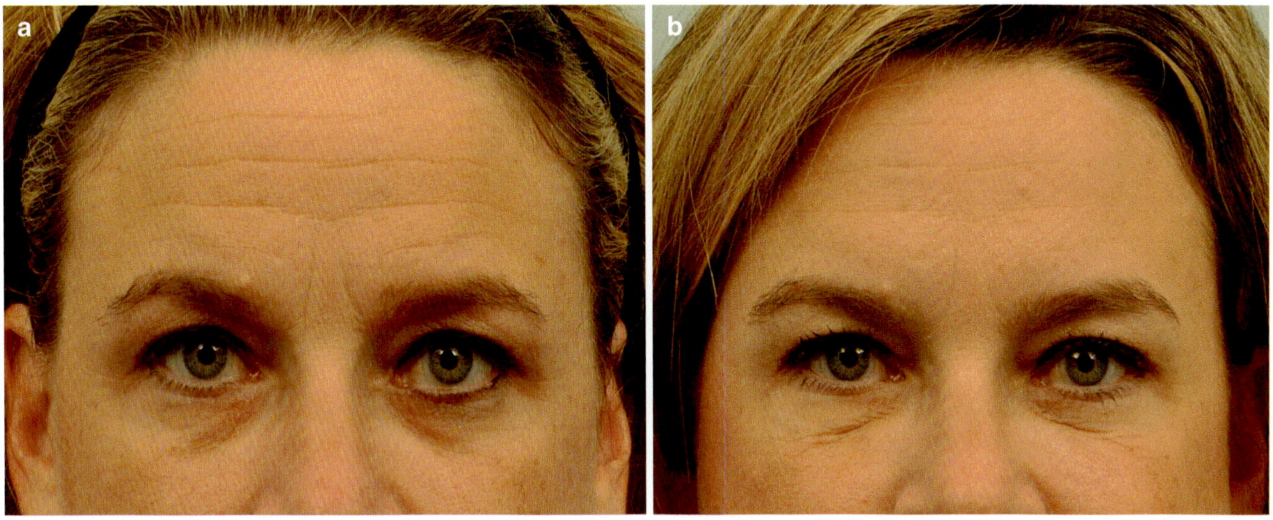

Fig. 36.3 (**a**) Before. A 44-year-old woman with prominent static and dynamic lines in the forehead, glabella, and crow's feet area due to skin changes and repetitive animation. (**b**) After. Neurotoxin (50 units) smoothens furrows in forehead and crow's feet. Injection of one syringe of Belotero further improves the under eye shadowing and fills the tear trough

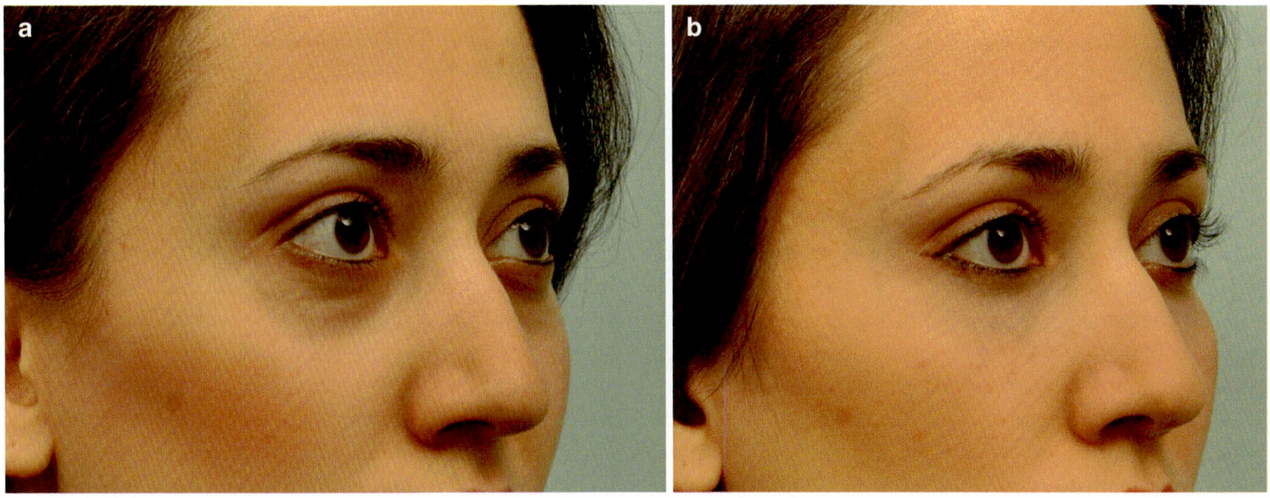

Fig. 36.4 (**a**) Before. A 28-year-old woman with volume loss and shadowing from prominent tear troughs. (**b**) One syringe of hyaluronic acid (Restylane) and one syringe of Perlane injected to periorbital region to restore a youthful under eye contour

Complications of Injectable Fillers

Formation of unsightly nodules is a feared complication of injectable facial treatments. Unlike with hyaluronic acid fillers, which can be dissolved with hyaluronidase, there is no "reversing agent" for other synthetic compounds. Smaller nodules that are generally not visible respond well to conservative treatment with digital massage.

Large nodules, which are rare in experienced hands, can be treated by breaking up the product overaccumulation with an injection of normal saline and lidocaine. Small amounts of 5-fluorouracil can be mixed with an equal amount of lidocaine or lidocaine with epinephrine to be injected directly into the nodules to reduce fibroblastic activity in these sites and break up the nodule. This technique induces a mechanical reduction in the collection of product and prevents further volume creation by inhibiting its biostimulatory properties. Anecdotally, serial injection of 5-fluorouracil and lidocaine has been able to reverse Sculptra and Radiesse contour issues in areas of overinjection.

Injection of steroid into these noninflammatory nodules has been largely abandoned due to the potential for permanent tissue thinning and skin depigmentation, which may result in a potentially worse problem for the patient. In select cases, however, small amounts of steroid can be added to 5-fluorouracil, saline, or lidocaine mixtures to decrease local inflammation, although excellent success can be achieved without the addition of steroid. In severe cases, surgical excision of permanent or semipermanent product may be required.

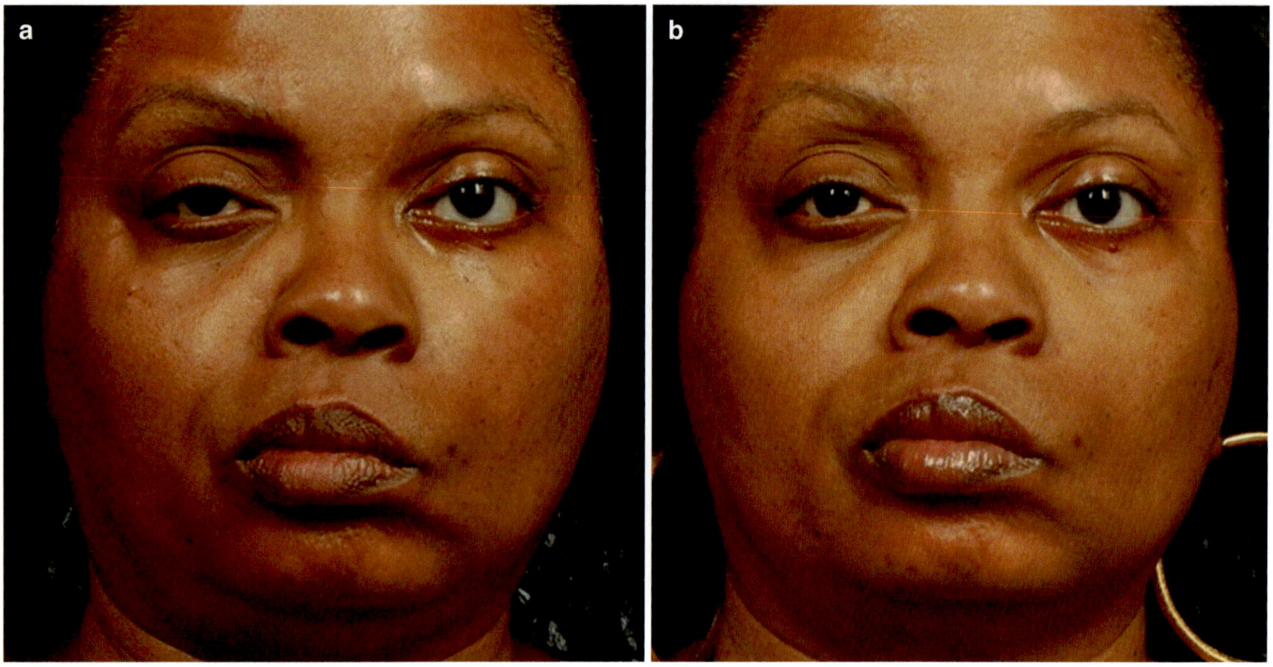

Fig. 36.5 (**a**) Before. A 53-year-old woman with marked facial asymmetry and hemifacial paralysis after a dental fracture. (**b**) While perfect symmetry is not possible in all cases, overall balance can be achieved. One syringe of Voluma and one syringe of Juvederm Ultra used to augment midface and periorbital region for improvement of overall harmony

Common side effects that patients can expect include mild bruising, tenderness, and swelling, which can be sometimes unpredictable. These may be mitigated with use of smaller gauge needles, avoidance of NSAIDS or other blood thinners, and strategic placement of needles. Swelling may require compresses or a short course of oral steroid, though close observation is necessary to rule out infection.

Serious complications from injectable fillers include infection, inflammatory or allergic response, anaphylaxis, or vascular occlusion that can lead to tissue necrosis, strabismus, ocular ischemia, retinal vascular occlusion, nerve damage, and permanent vision loss in one or both eyes [17, 63, 65–73]. The complex facial vascular system is full of anastomoses with potential for retrograde flow; intravascular filler emboli and peripheral compression of vasculature have been proposed mechanisms of vascular compromise, although animal models support intravascular injection as the leading cause of nonperfusion [74]. These catastrophic complications have been reported with all of the injectable fillers [68]. Although risk of inadvertent cannulization of facial vasculature with a larger gauge cannula is theoretically reduced, the risk still exists [68]. Particular areas of concern are the periocular and glabella region as well as the canine fossa and nose, although there are truly no "safe" sites [75]. Attention to the vascular anatomy in these regions, small bolus delivery, and slow retrograde injection techniques will minimize the possibility of these rare, but possible, events.

Vascular Occlusion Management for Injectable Fillers

Standardized protocols in the event of vascular occlusion have been suggested to prevent tissue necrosis and blindness, but no consensus has yet been found. The rarity of these events makes them difficult to study in a randomized, controlled fashion. In addition, there is stigma associated with presenting these complications, especially in an aesthetic practice. However, it is critical that anyone using injectable fillers should be cognizant of the subsequent steps should a complication occur.

At the onset of vascular compromise, oral aspirin 81 mg should be administered. Ischemia to the skin has been reported to abate after high-dose pulsed injection of hyaluronidase to the area, though there have not been reports comparing treatment with the natural course if left untreated [76–78]. As the skin may slough, antibiotic ointment or emollients can be recommended. Retrobulbar infiltration of orbit after blindness with high volumes of hyaluronidase (1500–3000 units) is a treatment that theoretically makes sense and can be considered, although this salvage treatment has not been reported to successfully reverse central retinal artery occlusion or posterior ischemic optic neuropathy in case reports or animal models [79–82]. Timing of infiltration with hyaluronidase likely plays a role and it is important to weigh this potential benefit against further truama and ocular injury. Hyperbaric oxygen has been used as an adjunct after ophthalmic artery obstruction, and recovery in vision has been reported in few cases, especially those with cilioretinal artery present [83, 84]. The use of nitroglycerin paste has been discussed, although a recent study showed that vasodilation could propagate intra-arterial particles and decrease potential collateral circulation and worsen end point ischemia [85]. Systemic prostaglandin E1 or other vasodilatory and antiplatelet aggregation medications may play a role in reversing these complications, but further studies and experience are needed to validate its use [86]. No "antidote" can be prescribed except for vigilance in diagnosis of this underreported event. Patients should be kept for observation and reexamined by the physician prior to discharge. The office staff should be on alert if a patient complains of pain, blanching, or any signs of possible occlusion, as these symptoms and signs can even present within hours to a few days after the injection procedure.

Cutaneous Lasers

Laser technology currently plays an important role in improving aging skin, reducing scar tissue, and improving the appearance of rhytids. Popular since the early 1990s for resurfacing, the CO_2 emits invisible infrared radiation at 10,600 nm, which is absorbed by intracellular and extracellular water.

Transferring thermal energy directly into these tissue layers induces fibrosis, collagen formation, and tightening. Fractionated CO_2 technology was developed in 2007 to allow this treatment to be interspersed among areas of nontreatment; this approach reduces pain, erythema, and scar formation [87–89]. Erbium:YAG cutaneous lasers function similarly to CO_2 lasers, though erbium laser has a more favorable thermal relaxation time and thus is better tolerated by patients. The erbium:YAG laser emits at 2940 nm and can successfully treat rhytids, actinic photodamage, and dyschromias. Fractionated erbium:YAG at 1550 nm further improves patient recovery time while still delivering improved results [90]. Combining laser therapy with peels or other agents can be very effective to decrease pigmentation and rosacea. This continues to be an area of great interest including the use of stem cells following laser treatment as a way to allow dermal penetration of stem cells with minimal injury.

As advancements in laser technology continue, there have been numerous ablative and nonablative products released on the market. Although they have improved tolerability, decreased recovery time, and decreased adverse events like depigmentation, these treatments have not superceded the original CO_2 lasers, which can effectively penetrate the deeper layers of the skin to induce dermal remodeling [91, 92]. A complete review and comparison of the available laser therapies, indications, safety profiles, and results are outside the scope of this chapter.

Prior to any laser treatment, however, thorough evaluation and counseling are necessary. Select laser treatments in pigmented patients (with Fitzpatrick scores above 3–4) should be approached with caution as post-inflammatory hyperpigmentation or depigmentation can occur. A test spot can be considered in patients prior to full treatment. Pre-treatment for herpetic infections and fungal infections is recommended. In addition, for ablative treatments, rigorous wound care and often a lengthy recovery period should be discussed as part of the pre-procedural evaluation.

Light-Based Therapy

Intense pulsed light (IPL), also known as photo rejuvenation or photofacial treatment, is a device that targets clinical signs of photoaging such as brown spots, sun damage, irregular skin pigmentation, as well as rosacea wrinkles, laxity, enlarged pores, telangiectasias, and spider veins. IPL devices emit polychromatic incoherent high-intensity pulsed light of a certain wavelength spectrum, fluence, and pulse duration. The wavelength and pulse duration can be adjusted based on the patient's skin type and skin condition and can be applied to a wide spectrum of skin conditions. The light then transfers energy to chromophores within the skin generating heat and leading to destruction of the targeted area [93]. In a study comparing histology of skin biopsies before and after IPL treatment, it was found that both type 1 and type 3 collagen increased after treatment and elastin fibers were more neatly arranged [94]. In randomized controlled split-face studies evaluating skin rejuvenation, most demonstrate improvement in telangiectasia and irregular pigmentation between treated and untreated sides, but there has not been shown to be a great improvement in rhytids [95].

Most people have some discomfort during the procedure, yet this is usually mediated by premedication with an NSAID, cold compresses, or topical anesthesia. Adverse events of IPL can include erythema, swelling, hypopigmentation, hyperpigmentation, atrophy, scarring, keloid formation, and infection. Blistering and crusting are from overtreatment. Patients with a history of herpes simplex should take appropriate antiviral prophylaxis. Patients taking medications that increase photosensitivity or patients with suntans are not good candidates. Often, a test shot at a nonvisible site is recommended so that the reaction can be evaluated 6 weeks after the shot. Patients must avoid significant light exposure after treatment for at least 8 weeks [93]. Topical daily sunscreen after treatment is important to minimize early recurrence. Otherwise, patients treated with IPL have virtually no downtime after treatment and the majority of patients appreciate an improvement in the effects of skin aging. Home IPL treatments have also been developed for patient self-administration.

Other superficial skin rejuvenating treatments, for example, Clear + Brilliant (Valeant), are designed like IPL to be used both in a physician office and a spa setting. Skilled technicians can increase the efficacy of the device with knowledge of a patient's skin type and pretreatment. Less experienced aestheticians or physicians need to use the light-based devices and superficial lasers with caution even though they are not as potentially dangerous as focused laser light sources. However, around the periocular region, light-based treatments are potentially more harmful to the uvea than other laser modalities and therefore should be used with appropriate globe protection at all times.

Devices

As interest in noninvasive and minimally invasive skin tightening procedures continues to rise, so too does the number of technologies available in the devices realm. These include radiofrequency and ultrasound devices. The goal behind these devices is to heat the targeted tissue to a point that causes disruption of the upper dermal collagen, deeper facial layers, and fibrous septum anchoring dermis to fascia, which are all thought to play a role in aging of the skin [96]. When this is done, collagen fibers become denatured and stimulate de novo collagen while avoiding damage to surrounding tissue. As with any procedure, appropriate patient selection is critical. The target audience for these devices are patients with mild to moderate skin laxity in the targeted area. While these devices are marketed separately and tested for efficacy by the FDA as stand-alone devices, frequently their efficacy has been more effective in conjunction with neurotoxin and fillers, especially in older patients, where collagen and elastin production is more limited.

Radiofrequency

Unipolar and bipolar radiofrequency have been used to tighten skin by delivering energy to different subcutaneous layers through various handpieces or microneedling cartridges. An example of a radiofrequency device is ThermiRF (ThermiAesthetics), where specific temperatures target stimulation to specific tissue layers. Approved in 2013 by the FDA, it uses a 10 cm 18-gauge cannula to directly target dermal and subdermal planes in the upper neck and jowl area. The surface probe has a temperature sensor at the end that initiates an automatic feedback loop to ensure that the temperature stays between 50 °C and 60 °C. The device also uses a forward-looking infrared camera (FLIR) that is able to capture the entire surface temperature in the field, including monitoring of the epidermis to avoid superficial burns which can happen above temperatures of 43 °C. Typically, three treatment zones are mapped out and sterile preheated tumescent solution is infiltrated through small entrance sites at the apex of each treatment area. Results from this technology can be seen in as little as 1 month and continue to show benefits for 6–8 months with minimal downtime. Usually, postprocedure pain is minimal and does not require analgesics. Adverse events include superficial burns, which occur less than 0.1% [97].

Thermage (Valeant Pharmaceuticals) is a device that delivers pulses of energy through various-sized tips to tighten skin, lift eyebrows, and stimulate collagen formation. Other devices such as Exilis (BTL Aesthetics) use continuous radiofrequency to attempt similar results as well as reduce subcutaneous fat. Two other developments have sprung from the ThermiRF technology – ThermiSmooth and ThermiRase. ThermiSmooth is used for areas around eye, including crow's feet, crepey skin under the eye, and upper eyelid tightening. A probe is applied flat to the skin surface to deliver the energy. Usually three to six treatments are required to achieve a significant amount of skin tightening. ThermiRase uses radiofrequency technology to ablate nerves helping to reduce frown lines. An external nerve stimulator is used initially to map out the nerves to target. Several treatment applications are then applied until patient is unable to frown. This has been seen to have immediate effects for up to 24 months.

While Radiesse and Sculptra can be used with radiofrequency tightening devices, extreme caution should be exercised if hyaluronic acid-based fillers were used in the past as they can melt the subcutaneous filler. Same-day treatment with both skin tightening and non-hyaluronic acid-based fillers can increase the efficacy and allow for a more rapid final result. Combining treatments for a synergistic effect is an area in need of further studies and exploration.

Ultrasound

Microfocused ultrasound (MFU) uses sound waves to produce areas of necrosis in the subcutaneous planes. The penetration depth depends on the frequency, with higher frequencies producing shallower degrees of injury. A commercially available device, Ulthera (Ulthera Inc.), also combines the use of high-resolution imaging to allow for visualization of tissue up to a depth of 8 mm. Initially Ulthera obtained FDA approval in 2009 for eyebrow lifts. Subsequently, it was granted FDA approval in 2012 for lifting submental and neck tissue. The facial superficial musculoaponeurotic tissue is targeted for tightening, with ultrasound energy targeted to temperatures over 65 °C, the point at which collagen starts to denature. Treatment lasts for 30–60 minutes. This technology is typically ideal for people with mild to moderate skin and soft tissue laxity [98]. In a study assessing the efficacy of Ulthera for facial and neck skin laxity, it was determined that 67% of subjects showed improvement at 180 days based on blinded reviewer assessments [98]. Another study demonstrated that efficacy improved when multiple treatments were used [99].

The most common symptom is discomfort during the treatment, usually obviated with pretreatment with oral acetaminophen or oral nonsteroidal anti-inflammatory drugs. Oral diazepam is also useful. Other side effects that have been reported are transient erythema, edema, and bruising. Other uncommon adverse events include post-inflammatory hyperpigmentation, muscle weakness, transient numbness, and striated linear skin patterns [98].

Chemical Peels

Medical grade chemical peels can improve melasma, improve skin tone, shrink pores, and also promote superficial collagen formation. Many variables such as agent, concentration, zone of treatment, skin thickness, and permeability make chemical peels an individualizable treatment. Superficial peels (alpha-hydroxy acids, glycolic acid, lactic acid, and salicylic acid) may improve fine lines and hydrate the skin; deeper peels (TCA 30–50%, Phenol, Baker-Gordon) can induce more lift, but may have more complications, such as depigmentation, scarring, prolonged healing, infection, and cardiac arrhythmia. Stronger peels may require anesthesia, while lighter peels can be safely and comfortably performed in the office setting. Pigmented individuals (Fitzpatrick 4–6) and patients with freckles are generally poor candidates for this treatment. Pregnancy and oral contraceptive pills are contraindications as increased circulating estrogens can cause hyperpigmentation. Prophylactic treatment of herpetic outbreak is recommended. Patients will need to use a bland emollient multiple times a day during the desquamation period, and patients should be counseled that an unsightly healing process, based on the depth of the peel, may occur. Skin texture changes and slight depigmentation are common side effects and should be discussed during the evaluation period.

Cold

Cryolipolysis is a nonsurgical alternative to liposuction. Currently, CoolSculpting (ZELTIQ Aesthetics) technology currently dominates the market with hand pieces devised for different parts of the body. This new technology targets and freezes fat cells, which are then naturally metabolized. The adipose tissue destruction is permanent as with liposuction but requires several months for the adipocytes to be eliminated from the body. Though long-term, randomized controlled trials are still needed, cryolipolysis has been found to be safe and improves the short-term appearance of subcutaneous lipid stores [100].

Results can be repeated with multiple treatments. Depending on the hand piece, approximately 20% of the fat in the targeted area can be permanently removed. Most patients are young enough where the overlying skin is able to remodel. Older patients may require subsequent skin tightening procedures.

Common adverse effects include temporary numbness to the treatment area; paradoxical lipid hyperplasia has also been reported in the literature but requires more study [101]. Cryolipolysis has been used throughout the body, as well as applied to the neck to decrease subcutaneous fat and improve the neck appearance.

Solutions, Cosmeceuticals, and Botanicals

Kybella (Kythera biopharmaceuticals) is made from deoxycholic acid, which is a substance produced in the body that helps absorb fat. This FDA-approved product has been injected into the fat pads below the chin, in a controlled grid pattern to the submental fat area, to tighten the chin area and sculpt the jaw. Several treatments are required to achieve full correction and this may be paired with other techniques, such as cold or radiofrequency. This is done over a several month period. Patients need to be warned that extreme swelling and a tight sensation may be a side effect lasting for weeks, particularly at the initial treatment. Otherwise, the product has a favorable side effect profile with short-term bleeding, bruising, pain, and numbness from injections. Dysphagia, thought to be secondary to pain and induration from submental injection, resolves spontaneously. There will likely be other applications of this technology as experience with the product grows.

Microdermabrasion and Microneedling

Microdermabrasion is a deep surface exfoliation of the skin with the use of crystals to smoothen and brighten coarse skin. The body replaces the superficial layer of the epidermis to improve skin texture, areas of discoloration, and fine lines. Microneedling, with or without chemical peel, can be a treatment option to stimulate collagen, tighten skin, reduce scars, and improve penetration of adjunctive topical agents. This technology creates small areas of dermal penetration similar to the technique used in tattoo removal, in which a chemical is also added to this area to dissolve the ink. Others have recommended following microneedling with application of topical antiaging skin care vitamin and serum products.

Nonsurgical Thread-Lifting

Previously, thread-lift sutures have been developed as a minimally invasive technique to lift sagging tissues as an alternative to a surgical face or neck lift. While these techniques were first introduced in the 1990s, there has recently been a resurgence of thread-lifting sutures by the cosmetic industry. While these products are minimally invasive, require little downtime, and can provide immediate perceived improvement, these treatments are not substitutes for skin strengthening and volumizing treatments. Patient selection is critical, as those with more tissue descent may not achieve adequate or lasting results with this technique. In addition, the literature has yet to demonstrate durability of the lifting effect in all the iterations of this product [102]. In the author's experience, the Silhouette InstaLift (Sinclair) can reposition soft tissue in the midface, lower face, neck, and brow after proper reinflation of the face and neuromodulation to rebalance facial contours. Patients with significant soft tissue laxity due to weight loss are better served with tissue resection with surgery.

Conclusions

It is truly an exciting time for the development of facial rejuvenation technologies. For the carefully selected patient, there are many nonsurgical options for facial enhancement, rejuvenation, and reconstruction. Optimal treatment is often achieved by considering each product and device as a unique tool to be used toward the creation of a desired result. The combination of treatments with fillers, toxins, and devices is the norm, rather than single product treatment as has traditionally been required for demonstrating safety and efficacy to the FDA. We are currently fortunate to have a plethora of approved treatment options, which will only continue to increase.

These treatments have been widely accepted by the public at large, drawing in many patients who would otherwise not consider surgical rejuvenation. It is our obligation to explain that it is not a question of "surgical" or "nonsurgical." Nonsurgical treatments can be disfiguring and dangerous with improper technique – as can surgical treatments. These treatments often best go hand in hand; and pre-treatment and maintenance with nonsurgical techniques can improve and prolong results. These procedures should be viewed as a useful tool in our armamentarium to refine and maintain the appearance of ageless attractiveness in both women and men.

References

1. Friedman O. Changes associated with the aging face. Facial Plast Surg Clin North Am. 2005;13(3):371–80.
2. Kahn DM, Shaw RB. Overview of current thoughts on facial volume and aging. Facial Plast Surg. 2010;26(5):350–5.
3. Zoumalan RA, Larrabee WF Jr. Anatomic considerations in the aging face. Facial Plast Surg. 2011;27(1):16–22.
4. Mancini R, Khadavi NM, Goldberg RA. Nonsurgical management of upper eyelid margin asymmetry using hyaluronic acid gel filler. Ophthal Plast Reconstr Surg. 2011;27(1):1–3.
5. Keaney TC, Anolik R, Braz A, et al. The male aesthetic patient: facial anatomy, concepts of attractiveness, and treatment patterns. J Drugs Dermatol. 2018;17(1):19–28.
6. Talakoub L, Wesley NO. Differences in perceptions of beauty and cosmetic procedures performed in ethnic patients. Semin Cutan Med Surg. 2009;28(2):115–29.
7. Wong C-H, Mendelson B. Facial soft-tissue spaces and retaining ligaments of the midcheek: defining the premaxillary space. Plast Reconstr Surg. 2013;132(1):49–56.
8. Pessa JE, Zadoo VP, Yuan C, et al. Concertina effect and facial aging: nonlinear aspects of youthfulness and skeletal remodeling, and why, perhaps, infants have jowls. Plast Reconstr Surg. 1999;103(2):635–44.
9. Gosain AK, Klein MH, Sudhakar PV, Prost RW. A volumetric analysis of soft-tissue changes in the aging midface using high-resolution MRI: implications for facial rejuvenation. Plast Reconstr Surg. 2005;115(4):1143–52; discussion 1153–55.
10. Wysong A, Kim D, Joseph T, MacFarlane DF, Tang JY, Gladstone HB. Quantifying soft tissue loss in the aging male face using magnetic resonance imaging. Dermatol Surg. 2014;40(7):786–93.
11. Wysong A, Joseph T, Kim D, Tang JY, Gladstone HB. Quantifying soft tissue loss in facial aging: a study in women using magnetic resonance imaging. Dermatol Surg. 2013;39(12):1895–902.
12. Goldberg RA. The three periorbital hollows: a paradigm for periorbital rejuvenation. Plast Reconstr Surg. 2005;116(6):1796–804.
13. Rohrich RJ, Pessa JE. The retaining system of the face: histologic evaluation of the septal boundaries of the subcutaneous fat compartments. Plast Reconstr Surg. 2008;121(5):1804–9.
14. Gierloff M, Stöhring C, Buder T, Gassling V, Açil Y, Wiltfang J. Aging changes of the midfacial fat compartments: a computed tomographic study. Plast Reconstr Surg. 2012;129(1):263–73.
15. Ramanadham SR, Rohrich RJ. Newer understanding of specific anatomic targets in the aging face as applied to injectables: superficial and deep facial fat compartments – an evolving target for site-specific facial augmentation. Plast Reconstr Surg. 2015;136(5 Suppl):49S–55S.
16. Lee S, Yen MT. Nonsurgical rejuvenation of the eyelids with hyaluronic acid gel injections. Semin Plast Surg. 2017;31(1):17–21.
17. Mustak H, Fiaschetti D, Goldberg RA. Filling the periorbital hollows with hyaluronic acid gel: long-term review of outcomes and complications. J Cosmet Dermatol. 2017; https://doi.org/10.1111/jocd.12452.
18. Morley AMS, Taban M, Malhotra R, Goldberg RA. Use of hyaluronic acid gel for upper eyelid filling and contouring. Ophthal Plast Reconstr Surg. 2009;25(6):440–4.
19. Mustak H, Fiaschetti D, Gupta A, Goldberg R. Eyebrow contouring with hyaluronic acid gel filler injections. J Clin Aesthet Derm. 2018;11(2):38–40.
20. Goldberg RA, Fiaschetti D. Filling the periorbital hollows with hyaluronic acid gel: initial experience with 244 injections. Ophthal Plast Reconstr Surg. 2006;22(5):335–41; discussion 341–43.
21. Pessa JE. An algorithm of facial aging: verification of Lambros's theory by three-dimensional stereolithography, with reference to the pathogenesis of midfacial aging, scleral show, and the lateral suborbital trough deformity. Plast Reconstr Surg. 2000;106(2):479–88; discussion 489–90.
22. Mendelson BC, Hartley W, Scott M, McNab A, Granzow JW. Age-related changes of the orbit and midcheek and the implications for facial rejuvenation. Aesthet Plast Surg. 2007;31(5):419–23.
23. Shaw RB Jr, Kahn DM. Aging of the midface bony elements: a three-dimensional computed tomographic study. Plast Reconstr Surg. 2007;119(2):675–81; discussion 682–83.

24. Scott AB. Botulinum toxin injection into extraocular muscles as an alternative to strabismus surgery. Ophthalmology. 1980;87(10):1044–9.
25. Jankovic J, Brin MF. Therapeutic uses of botulinum toxin. N Engl J Med. 1991;324(17):1186–94.
26. Felber ES. Botulinum toxin in primary care medicine. J Am Osteopath Assoc. 2006;106(10):609–14.
27. Binder WJ, Brin MF, Blitzer A, Schoenrock LD, Pogoda JM. Botulinum toxin type A (BOTOX) for treatment of migraine headaches: an open-label study. Otolaryngol Head Neck Surg. 2000;123(6):669–76.
28. Wu DC, Fabi SG, Goldman MP. Neurotoxins: current concepts in cosmetic use on the face and neck – lower face. Plast Reconstr Surg. 2015;136(5 Suppl):76S–9S.
29. Zanchi M, Favot F, Bizzarini M, Piai M, Donini M, Sedona P. Botulinum toxin type-A for the treatment of inverse psoriasis. J Eur Acad Dermatol Venereol. 2008;22(4):431–6.
30. Glaser DA, Pariser DM, Hebert AA, et al. A prospective, nonrandomized, open-label study of the efficacy and safety of onabotulinumtoxinA in adolescents with primary axillary hyperhidrosis. Pediatr Dermatol. 2015;32(5):609–17.
31. Min P, Xi W, Grassetti L, et al. Sebum production alteration after botulinum toxin type a injections for the treatment of forehead rhytides: a prospective randomized double-blind dose-comparative clinical investigation. Aesthet Surg J. 2015;35(5):600–10.
32. Shah AR. Use of intradermal botulinum toxin to reduce sebum production and facial pore size. J Drugs Dermatol. 2008;7(9):847–50.
33. Alam M, Barrett KC, Hodapp RM, Arndt KA. Botulinum toxin and the facial feedback hypothesis: can looking better make you feel happier? J Am Acad Dermatol. 2008;58(6):1061–72.
34. Rappl T, Parvizi D, Friedl H, et al. Onset and duration of effect of incobotulinumtoxinA, onabotulinumtoxinA, and abobotulinumtoxinA in the treatment of glabellar frown lines: a randomized, double-blind study. Clin Cosmet Investig Dermatol. 2013;6:211–9.
35. Jandhyala R. Relative potency of incobotulinumtoxinA vs onabotulinumtoxinA a meta-analysis of key evidence. J Drugs Dermatol. 2012;11(6):731–6.
36. Carruthers A, Sadick N, Brandt F, et al. Evolution of facial aesthetic treatment over five or more years: a retrospective cross-sectional analysis of continuous onabotulinumtoxinA treatment. Dermatol Surg. 2015;41(6):693–701.
37. Carruthers JD, Carruthers JA. Treatment of glabellar frown lines with C. botulinum-A exotoxin. J Dermatol Surg Oncol. 1992;18(1):17–21.
38. Molina B, Grangier Y, Mole B, et al. Patient satisfaction after the treatment of glabellar lines with Botulinum toxin type A (Speywood Unit): a multi-centre European observational study. J Eur Acad Dermatol Venereol. 2015;29(7):1382–8.
39. Carruthers JD, Lowe NJ, Menter MA, Gibson J, Eadie N, Botox Glabellar Lines II Study Group. Double-blind, placebo-controlled study of the safety and efficacy of botulinum toxin type A for patients with glabellar lines. Plast Reconstr Surg. 2003;112(4):1089–98.
40. Lizzul PF, Narurkar VA. The role of calcium hydroxylapatite (Radiesse) in nonsurgical aesthetic rejuvenation. J Drugs Dermatol. 2010;9(5):446–50.
41. Carruthers A, Carruthers J. A single-center, dose-comparison, pilot study of botulinum neurotoxin type A in female patients with upper facial rhytids: safety and efficacy. J Am Acad Dermatol. 2009;60(6):972–9.
42. Wieder JM, Moy RL. Understanding botulinum toxin. Surgical anatomy of the frown, forehead, and periocular region. Dermatol Surg. 1998;24(11):1172–4.
43. Steinsapir KD, Groth MJ, Boxrud CA. Persistence of upper blepharoptosis after cosmetic botulinum toxin type A. Dermatol Surg. 2015;41(7):833–40.
44. Scheinfeld N. The use of apraclonidine eyedrops to treat ptosis after the administration of botulinum toxin to the upper face. Dermatol Online J. 2005;11(1):9.
45. Ghalamkarpour F, Robati RM, Aryanejad F, Toossi P. Supraciliary wrinkles and botulinum toxin A. Clin Exp Dermatol. 2010;35(4):388–91.
46. Mazzuco R, Hexsel D. Gummy smile and botulinum toxin: a new approach based on the gingival exposure area. J Am Acad Dermatol. 2010;63(6):1042–51.
47. Polo M. Botulinum toxin type A in the treatment of excessive gingival display. Am J Orthod Dentofac Orthop. 2005;127(2):214–8; quiz 261.
48. Gart MS, Gutowski KA. Aesthetic uses of neuromodulators: current uses and future directions. Plast Reconstr Surg. 2015;136(5 Suppl):62S–71S.
49. Choe SW, Cho WI, Lee CK, Seo SJ. Effects of botulinum toxin type A on contouring of the lower face. Dermatol Surg. 2005;31(5):502–7; discussion 507–8.
50. Wu WTL. Botox facial slimming/facial sculpting: the role of botulinum toxin-A in the treatment of hypertrophic masseteric muscle and parotid enlargement to narrow the lower facial width. Facial Plast Surg Clin North Am. 2010;18(1):133–40.
51. Kim N-H, Chung J-H, Park R-H, Park J-B. The use of botulinum toxin type A in aesthetic mandibular contouring. Plast Reconstr Surg. 2005;115(3):919–30.
52. Peng H-LP, Peng J-H. Complications of botulinum toxin injection for masseter hypertrophy: incidence rate from 2036 treatments and summary of causes and preventions. J Cosmet Dermatol. 2018;17(1):33–8.
53. Matarasso A, Matarasso SL. Botulinum A exotoxin for the management of platysma bands. Plast Reconstr Surg. 2003;112(5 Suppl):138S–40S.
54. Rohrich RJ, Rios JL, Smith PD, Gutowski KA. Neck rejuvenation revisited. Plast Reconstr Surg. 2006;118(5):1251–63.
55. Kane MAC. Nonsurgical treatment of platysma bands with injection of botulinum toxin a revisited. Plast Reconstr Surg. 2003;112(5 Suppl):125S–6S.
56. Wu WTL. Microbotox of the lower face and neck: evolution of a personal technique and its clinical effects. Plast Reconstr Surg. 2015;136(5 Suppl):92S–100S.
57. Kaufman MR, Miller TA, Huang C, et al. Autologous fat transfer for facial recontouring: is there science behind the art? Plast Reconstr Surg. 2007;119(7):2287–96.
58. Buck DW 2nd, Alam M, Kim JYS. Injectable fillers for facial rejuvenation: a review. J Plast Reconstr Aesthet Surg. 2009;62(1):11–8.
59. Lambros V. Fat grafting: a growing problem? Plast Reconstr Surg. 2018;141(2):527–8.
60. Murray CA, Zloty D, Warshawski L. The evolution of soft tissue fillers in clinical practice. Dermatol Clin. 2005;23(2):343–63.
61. Center for Devices, Radiological Health. Dermal fillers (soft tissue fillers) – dermal dillers approved by the Center for Devices and Radiological Health. https://www.fda.gov/medicaldevices/productsandmedicalprocedures/cosmeticdevices/wrinklefillers/ucm227749.htm. Accessed 10 Aug 2018.
62. Narins RS, Beer K. Liquid injectable silicone: a review of its history, immunology, technical considerations, complications, and potential. Plast Reconstr Surg. 2006;118(3 Suppl):77S–84S.
63. Glicenstein J. The first "fillers", vaseline and paraffin. From miracle to disaster. Ann Chir Plast Esthet. 2007;52(2):157–61.
64. Eviatar J, Lo C, Kirszrot J. Radiesse: advanced techniques and applications for a unique and versatile implant. Plast Reconstr Surg. 2015;136(5 Suppl):164S–70S.

65. Andre P, Lowe NJ, Parc A, Clerici TH, Zimmermann U. Adverse reactions to dermal fillers: a review of European experiences. J Cosmet Laser Ther. 2005;7(3–4):171–6.
66. Lowe NJ, Maxwell CA, Patnaik R. Adverse reactions to dermal fillers: review. Dermatol Surg. 2005;31(11 Pt 2):1616–25.
67. Ramesh S, Fiaschetti D, Goldberg RA. Orbital and ocular ischemic syndrome with blindness after facial filler injection. Ophthal Plast Reconstr Surg. 2018;34(4):e108–10.
68. DeLorenzi C. Complications of injectable fillers, part 2: vascular complications. Aesthet Surg J. 2014;34(4):584–600.
69. DeLorenzi C. Complications of injectable fillers, part I. Aesthet Surg J. 2013;33(4):561–75.
70. Kim YJ, Kim SS, Song WK, Lee SY, Yoon JS. Ocular ischemia with hypotony after injection of hyaluronic acid gel. Ophthal Plast Reconstr Surg. 2011;27(6):e152–5.
71. Sung MS, Kim HG, Woo KI, Kim Y-D. Ocular ischemia and ischemic oculomotor nerve palsy after vascular embolization of injectable calcium hydroxylapatite filler. Ophthal Plast Reconstr Surg. 2010;26(4):289–91.
72. Sung W-I, Tsai S, Chen L-J. Ocular complications following cosmetic filler injection. JAMA Ophthalmol. 2018;136(5):e180716.
73. Myung Y, Yim S, Jeong JH, et al. The classification and prognosis of periocular complications related to blindness following cosmetic filler injection. Plast Reconstr Surg. 2017;140(1):61–4.
74. Chang S-H, Yousefi S, Qin J, et al. External compression versus intravascular injection: a mechanistic animal model of filler-induced tissue ischemia. Ophthal Plast Reconstr Surg. 2016;32(4):261–6.
75. Scheuer JF 3rd, Sieber DA, Pezeshk RA, Gassman AA, Campbell CF, Rohrich RJ. Facial danger zones: techniques to maximize safety during soft-tissue filler injections. Plast Reconstr Surg. 2017;139(5):1103–8.
76. Fang M, Rahman E, Kapoor KM. Managing complications of submental artery involvement after hyaluronic acid filler injection in Chin region. Plast Reconstr Surg Glob Open. 2018;6(5):e1789.
77. DeLorenzi C. New high dose pulsed hyaluronidase protocol for hyaluronic acid filler vascular adverse events. Aesthet Surg J. 2017;37(7):814–25.
78. Sun Z-S, Zhu G-Z, Wang H-B, et al. Clinical outcomes of impending nasal skin necrosis related to nose and nasolabial fold augmentation with hyaluronic acid fillers. Plast Reconstr Surg. 2015;136(4):434e–41e.
79. Zhu G-Z, Sun Z-S, Liao W-X, et al. Efficacy of retrobulbar hyaluronidase injection for vision loss resulting from hyaluronic acid filler embolization. Aesthet Surg J. 2017;38(1):12–22.
80. Hwang CJ, Mustak H, Gupta AA, Ramos RM, Goldberg RA, Duckwiler GR. Role of retrobulbar hyaluronidase in filler-associated blindness: evaluation of fundus perfusion and electroretinogram readings in an animal model. Ophthal Plast Reconstr Surg. 2018; https://doi.org/10.1097/IOP.0000000000001132.
81. Carruthers JDA, Fagien S, Rohrich RJ, Weinkle S, Carruthers A. Blindness caused by cosmetic filler injection: a review of cause and therapy. Plast Reconstr Surg. 2014;134(6):1197–201.
82. Carruthers J, Fagien S, Dolman P. Retro or peribulbar injection techniques to reverse visual loss after filler injections. Dermatol Surg. 2015;41(Suppl 1):S354–7.
83. Hwang K. Hyperbaric oxygen therapy to avoid blindness from filler injection. J Craniofac Surg. 2016;27(8):2154–5.
84. Henderson R, Reilly DA, Cooper JS. Hyperbaric oxygen for ischemia due to injection of cosmetic fillers: case report and issues. Plast Reconstr Surg Glob Open. 2018;6(1):e1618.
85. Hwang CJ, Morgan PV, Pimentel A, Sayre JW, Goldberg RA, Duckwiler G. Rethinking the role of nitroglycerin ointment in ischemic vascular filler complications: an animal model with ICG imaging. Ophthal Plast Reconstr Surg. 2016;32(2):118–22.
86. Takai Y, Tanito M, Matsuoka Y, Hara K, Ohira A. Systemic prostaglandin E1 to treat acute central retinal artery occlusion. Invest Ophthalmol Vis Sci. 2013;54(4):3065–71.
87. Lowe NJ, Lask G, Griffin ME, Maxwell A, Lowe P, Quilada F. Skin resurfacing with the ultrapulse carbon dioxide laser. Observations on 100 patients. Dermatol Surg. 1995;21(12):1025–9.
88. Goldman MP. Observations on the use of fractionated CO_2 laser resurfacing. J Drugs Dermatol. 2009;8(1):82–6.
89. Ortiz AE, Goldman MP, Fitzpatrick RE. Ablative CO_2 lasers for skin tightening: traditional versus fractional. Dermatol Surg. 2014;40(Suppl 12):S147–51.
90. Chiu RJ, Kridel RWH. Fractionated photothermolysis: the Fraxel 1550-nm glass fiber laser treatment. Facial Plast Surg Clin North Am. 2007;15(2):229–37, vii.
91. Doshi SN, Alster TS. 1,450 nm long-pulsed diode laser for nonablative skin rejuvenation. Dermatol Surg. 2005;31(9 Pt 2):1223–6; discussion 1226.
92. Ang P, Barlow RJ. Nonablative laser resurfacing: a systematic review of the literature. Clin Exp Dermatol. 2002;27(8):630–5.
93. Babilas P, Schreml S, Szeimies R-M, Landthaler M. Intense pulsed light (IPL): a review. Lasers Surg Med. 2010;42(2):93–104.
94. Feng Y, Zhao J, Gold MH. Skin rejuvenation in Asian skin: the analysis of clinical effects and basic mechanisms of intense pulsed light. J Drugs Dermatol. 2008;7(3):273–9.
95. Hedelund L, Due E, Bjerring P, Wulf HC, Haedersdal M. Skin rejuvenation using intense pulsed light: a randomized controlled split-face trial with blinded response evaluation. Arch Dermatol. 2006;142(8):985–90.
96. Tsukahara K, Tamatsu Y, Sugawara Y, Shimada K. Relationship between the depth of facial wrinkles and the density of the retinacula cutis. Arch Dermatol. 2012;148(1):39–46.
97. Pritzker RN, Robinson DM. Updates in noninvasive and minimally invasive skin tightening. Semin Cutan Med Surg. 2014;33(4):182–7.
98. Fabi SG. Noninvasive skin tightening: focus on new ultrasound techniques. Clin Cosmet Investig Dermatol. 2015;8:47–52.
99. Lee HS, Jang WS, Cha Y-J, et al. Multiple pass ultrasound tightening of skin laxity of the lower face and neck. Dermatol Surg. 2012;38(1):20–7.
100. Derrick CD, Shridharani SM, Broyles JM. The safety and efficacy of cryolipolysis: a systematic review of available literature. Aesthet Surg J. 2015;35(7):830–6.
101. Singh SM, Geddes ERC, Boutrous SG, Galiano RD, Friedman PM. Paradoxical adipose hyperplasia secondary to cryolipolysis: an underreported entity? Lasers Surg Med. 2015;47(6):476–8.
102. Gülbitti HA, Colebunders B, Pirayesh A, Bertossi D, van der Lei B. Thread-lift sutures: still in the lift? A systematic review of the literature. Plast Reconstr Surg. 2018;141(3):341e–7e.

Facial Feminization Surgery

37

Cat Nguyen Burkat and Scott R. Chaiet

Introduction

Facial Feminization Surgery

Facial plastic surgical procedures performed on the transgender patient to feminize the facial skeleton and soft tissue are collectively referred to as the field of facial feminization surgery, and may be offered as a part of the transition process for a transgender, or gender expansive, individual in the treatment of gender dysphoria. Gender dysphoria, a DSM-5 diagnosis, results in distress from the differences between one's experienced gender and sex-assigned gender at birth.

Facial feminization surgery was initially popularized in the 1980s by Douglas Ousterhout, with further description in his more recent book, *Facial Feminization Surgery: A Guide for the Transgendered Woman*. Although many of these procedures are commonly performed throughout the United States on cisgender patients (those whose gender identify is in agreement with sex assigned at birth), other techniques, such as shaping of the thyroid cartilage (laryngochondroplasty), may require specialized training and experience. This chapter will present a wide variety of procedures performed today in facial feminization surgery, outline a conceptual approach to facial analysis of a patient with male sex assigned at birth seeking surgical consultation for feminization, and describe technical pearls.

Prior to surgery, it is important to review if the patient has initiated hormone therapy, as hormonal supplementation with estrogen complements the surgical process of feminization by reducing facial hair, altering fat distribution, and changing skin appearance and texture [1]. Estrogen and testosterone blockers also suppress testosterone and reduce the rate of growth of male-pattern hair [2]. Any surgical therapy on the male to female transgender patient should also be performed in collaboration with a medical team. While the Standards of Care of the World Professional Association for Transgender Health (WPATH) does not require a mental health letter for facial surgery, it is required for chest and genital surgery. Rather, the guidelines state, *Mental health professionals can play an important role in helping patients choose the timing and implications of these procedures during the transition process.*

Facial feminization surgery alleviates gender dysphoria for many patients. Research demonstrates that facial feminization surgery positively affects the quality of life for transgender individuals, with patients scoring statistically higher on physical, mental, and social functioning outcome scales following facial feminization surgery compared to those without surgery [3].

As with any other surgery, proper preoperative understanding of goals and counseling is critical. Informed consent includes a discussion of risks, benefits, and alternates to the procedure. The transgender patient may often present with specific goals and photographs of a desired result, or have travelled long distances for expert care for surgeries that were researched on the internet. Therefore, a careful discussion together will provide a mutual understanding of realistic expectations of the perioperative process and expected outcomes [4].

Facial Analysis

Recognition of Facial Femininity

While some patients will identify precise facial attributes contributing to gender dysphoria, it may be overwhelming for other patients and/or surgeons to embark on facial

C. N. Burkat (✉)
Department of Ophthalmology and Visual Sciences, University of Wisconsin-Madison, Madison, WI, USA
e-mail: cburkat@wisc.edu

S. R. Chaiet
Division of Otolaryngology – Head and Neck Surgery, Department of Surgery, University of Wisconsin-Madison, Madison, WI, USA
e-mail: chaiet@surgery.wisc.edu

A. J. Cohen, C. N. Burkat (eds.), *Oculofacial, Orbital, and Lacrimal Surgery*, https://doi.org/10.1007/978-3-030-14092-2_37

feminization surgery. Thus, it is important to first understand the facial analysis of patients and which facial features, on average, will create the most feminine appearance for a transgender patient. Facial plastic surgeon, Jeffrey Spiegel, performed research to determine which facial aspects are most associated with femininity, by feminizing frontal and lateral photographs (using digital modification) of individuals with male sex assigned at birth in either the forehead, midface (nasal and lip modifications), or the jaw. Then, 100 adult research participants assessed the frontal and lateral photographs and ranked, in both views, that forehead modification resulted in the most stereotypically feminine appearance. Spiegel's research also showed that facial feminization procedures can result in recognition as a woman 6 out of 7 times, with the upper third of the face as a major determinant of femininity [5]. Therefore, this chapter discusses the surgical options starting from, and focusing on, the upper face, while balancing the natural aesthetic facial proportions [6]. Descriptions of facial characteristics typical for each "gender" will be in reference to biologic sex which are based on societal and historical publications. These characteristics may not necessarily apply to all cultures, races, or ethnicities but will provide a platform to describe differences between the masculine and feminine facial skeleton and soft tissue.

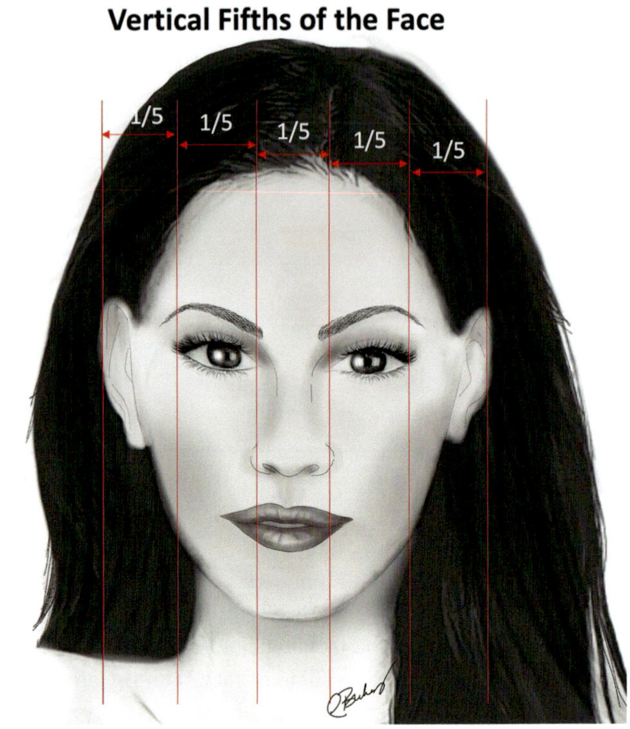

Fig. 37.1 Facial analysis with "vertical fifths" to assess symmetry and facial proportions

Facial Units

Studies by Powell and Humphreys (1984) are often considered a foundation for objective facial analysis of facial angles, proportions, widths, and heights for each sex [7]. In comparing the biologic male (masculine) and female face (feminine), the authors state that "the male's bone structure is sterner, bolder and more prominent. The dominance of the forehead, nose, and chin is more striking than the females. The zygoma and mandible produce much stronger contours in the male face." Further analysis by facial unit will assist the patient and/or surgeon focus on precise changes to remove or soften these masculine features.

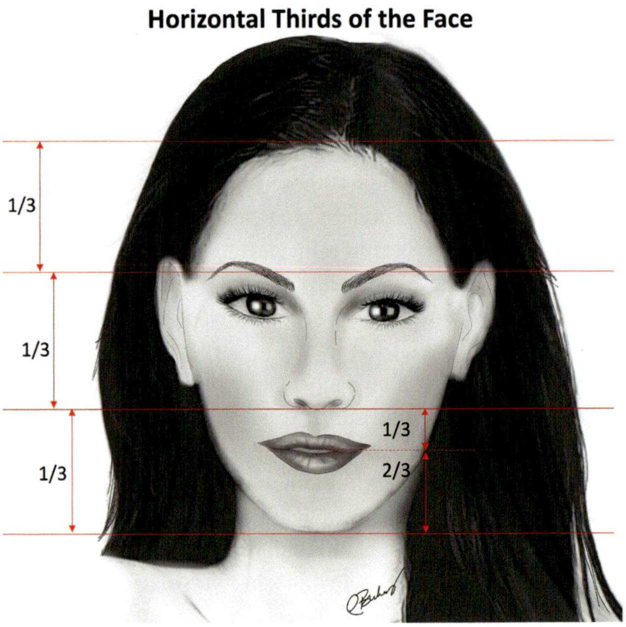

Fig. 37.2 Facial analysis with "horizontal thirds," including further division of the lower face demonstrating upper and lower lip relationship

Conceptually, the face is divided into five equal vertical segments and three equal horizontal segments: the "vertical fifths" and "horizontal thirds" (Figs. 37.1 and 37.2). The vertical portions are aligned with the medial and lateral canthal eyelid angles and the outer helical rims so that each fifth is equal to the width of one eye (Fig. 37.1). Practically, the vertical fifths analysis is used as a starting point to measure the width of the base of the nose, identify asymmetries within a face, and as guidance for facial feminization surgery.

The horizontal thirds are divided by the trichion (hairline), glabella, subnasale, and menton (chin) (Fig. 37.2) [8]. The masculine hairline is commonly higher [8] and displays an "M" shape with central downward peak, with or without male pattern baldness or a receding hairline, creating an elongated upper third of the face. The eyebrow position should be carefully measured and palpated, as the masculine eyebrow typically rests at or below the bony supraorbital rim, whereas the feminine brow rests up to 1 cm above the orbital rim. When evaluating the eyebrow position, it is important to keep in mind that the patient may pluck the eyebrows, which may give the appearance of falsely elevated eyebrow heights. In addition, the masculine eyebrow shape is flatter in contour, compared to an arching feminine eyebrow that peaks near the lateral limbus of the eye. Hairline and eyebrow position are intimately related in facial appearance and critical to facial aesthetic balance of the horizontal thirds, particularly in the transgender patient who has experienced the effects on hair loss by testosterone.

The masculine forehead may often reveal "frontal bossing," seen as a prominent bone shape across the glabella and prominent supraorbital ridges, that may be addressed by facial feminization. Bony forehead projection can be seen in both frontal and lateral views.

In general, the eyelid fissure measures 30 mm horizontally, on average, and has a slight upward canthal tilt, such that the lateral canthus measures 1–2 mm above the medial canthal angle. The upper eyelid should rest 1–1.5 mm below the superior corneal limbus centrally, whereas the lower eyelid margin is located just above or at the inferior limbus. The eyelid crease may be prominent or subtle, and represents the terminal attachments of the anterior fibers of the levator aponeurosis to the subcutaneous tissue and orbicularis muscle. Typically, the crease measures higher in the feminized eyelid, lower in masculine eyelids, and 3–5 mm in the eyelids of Asian patients. The feminine upper eyelid crease is often more curved, or semilunar, compared to a horizontal flatter line in the masculine eyelid. In the eyelids of Asian patients, the medial crease will blend into the epicanthal fold and medial canthus, which is a critical ethnic feature to retain. Upper eyelid skin should measure approximately 19–20 mm from the eyelid margin to the transition of eyebrow skin, in order to allow for adequate eyelid closure and ocular protection. In some patients, the eyelid crease may be asymmetric in height or demonstrate multiple creases. An abnormally elevated eyelid crease greater than 12 mm or more may often indicate an underlying levator aponeurosis dehiscence that may require repair to elevate the eyelid. The upper eyelids have two anatomic fat pads, the medial and preaponeurotic (or central) fat, that may be sculpted to provide a deeper, feminized superior sulcus. Any lateral fullness in the eyelid should suggest prolapse of the lacrimal gland.

Key Points: Facial Analysis

- Facial analysis using the "vertical fifths" and "horizontal thirds" provides a starting point to assess facial proportions.
- The upper third of the face contains many key landmarks in facial feminization surgery, such as hairline location, eyebrow position, and forehead projection.
- The feminine eyebrow typically rests higher above the orbital rim and is more arched in contour.
- Prominent supraorbital bones result in frontal bossing in the masculine upper face.
- The feminine upper eyelid often has a higher and curved eyelid crease, a deeper sulcus, and greater visibility of the tarsal region.
- A feminine nose tends to demonstrate concavity at the nasal dorsum, a slightly upturned nasal tip, and a smaller shape.
- The masculine mandible is wider with a square shape and greater masseter bulk.
- The masculine cheek bones are typically wider, but lack the prominence and height of the feminine midface.
- Anterior chin projection is often less in the feminine chin.

In the central face, the nasolabial angle on lateral view is formed between lines along the nasal columella and the upper lip. The angle defines nasal tip rotation and has been reported as 90–95 ° in the masculine nose, and more obtuse at 95–110 ° in the feminine nose [9]. In other words, the stereotypical feminine nasal tip looks turned slightly upward (Fig. 37.3).

From a side view, the upper nose is stereotypically straight in the masculine nasal dorsum, in contrast to the slight concavity of the female dorsum. The feminine nasofrontal angle measured between the nasal dorsum and forehead is also more obtuse as the glabellar region is less pronounced [10, 11] (Fig. 37.3). Patients often seek to reduce a dorsal convexity, or "hump," which is often performed in conjunction with nasal tip surgery to create a balanced feminine nose, called reductive rhinoplasty. The width of the lower nose, the alar base, should align with the vertical fifths, although may be wider in a non-Caucasian nose.

The lower horizontal third can be further divided into horizontal segments to analyze the ideal ratio of the upper lip (one-third) to the lower lip and chin (two-thirds) (Fig. 37.2). A long vertical chin height is more common in the masculine jaw. Lower facial and neck analysis should focus on the underlying bone structure of the jaw, particularly the prominence of the mandibular angles. The anterior chin shape and projection should be evaluated, as anthropologic studies show the chin is more pointed in a biologic female [11]. Although no standard bone measurements exist, the mandibular angles (posterior inferior corners of the jawbone) are typically wider and lower, creating a square shape in males.

This may be accompanied by upper lip deflation and elongation seen with aging. Shortening the length of the

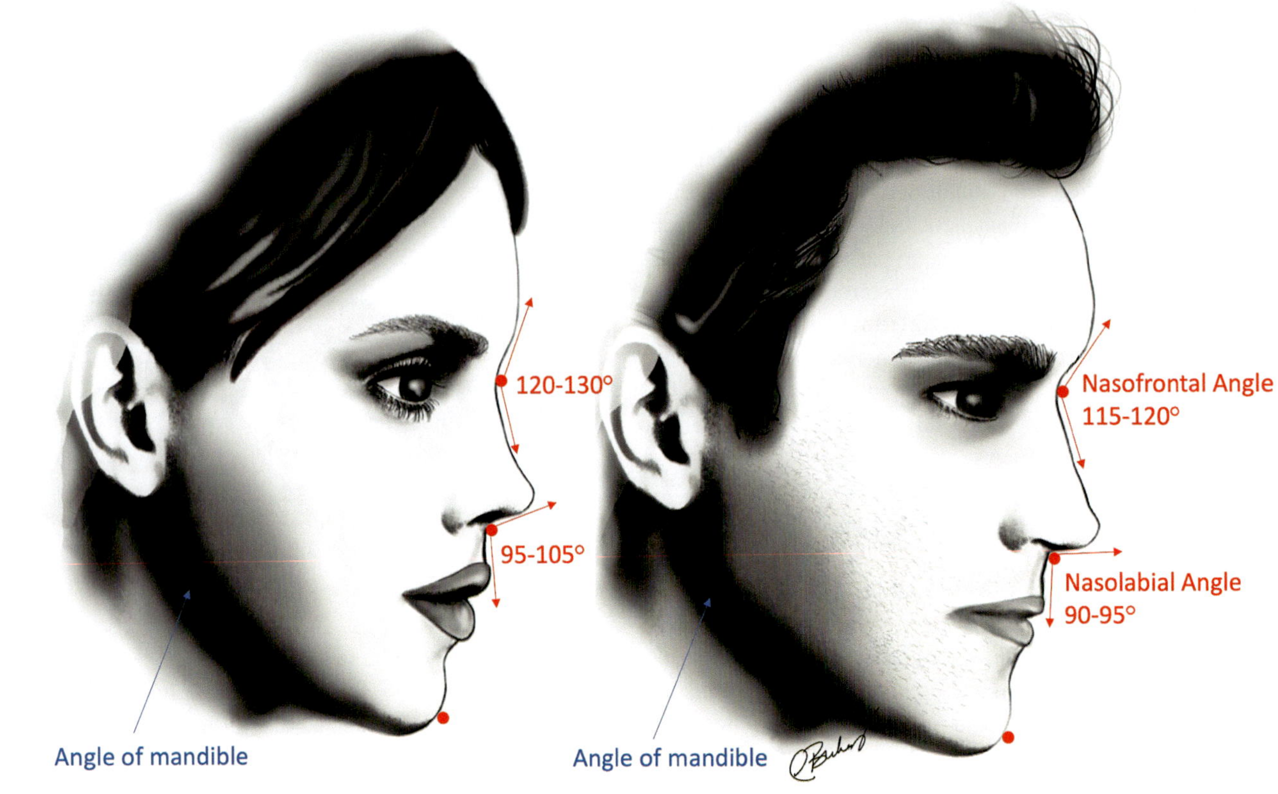

Fig. 37.3 The nasolabial angle on lateral view, formed between lines along the nasal columella and the upper lip, defines nasal tip rotation and is generally more obtuse in the feminized face. The masculine nasofrontal angle measured between the nasal dorsum and forehead is typically more acute due to greater glabellar and frontal bone prominence

lower lip and chin, in conjunction with adding volume to the upper lip, will therefore recreate the ideal balance of a feminized face.

Many methods are available in the literature that describe lower facial harmony by measuring the lip and chin projection. The Gonzalez-Ulloa assessment in the lateral view of the face is commonly used, where a tangential line extends downward from the nasion (soft tissue depression above the nose) perpendicular to the Frankfort horizontal plane. This line should transect the anterior soft tissue prominence of the chin (pogonion) and may indicate over-projection or under-projection of the chin [12]. Alternately, a line can be extended downward through the red-white vermillion lip borders of the upper and lower lips; anterior chin projection should rest behind this line in a feminine chin where the masculine chin extends to the line, or farther anterior.

Similarly, width of the midface is important for facial feminization, as the masculine zygomatic (cheek) bones have more bulk, but less prominence and height compared to the feminine female face [1]. Visualizing the lines of vertical fifths may help aid in analysis of chin shape, jaw and cheek width, and contour of the mandible. Upper and lower lip length and projection are then measured as the distance from each lip to a line from subnasale (soft tissue depression under nose) to the anterior chin prominence (Fig. 37.4).

Neck analysis, not included in the horizontal thirds, completes the facial analysis. A prominent thyroid cartilage, or "Adam's apple," develops with exposure to testosterone during puberty and is a marker of the masculine neck. The degree of jowls, tissue laxity, neck fullness, and neck skin redundancy should also be assessed.

Surgical Procedures for Facial Feminization

Surgery of the Forehead, Eyebrow, and Hairline

The upper face contains important features that contribute to a stereotypically feminine face, such as hairline position, forehead height as measured between the eyebrows and hairline, eyebrow location relative to the bony supraorbital rims, and glabellar and nasal dorsum prominence (Fig. 37.5).

Brow lifts are commonly performed in the United States and include various techniques that are performed through upper blepharoplasty incisions, with an endoscope via small incisions within the hairline, or through a long coronal incision [13]. These approaches, however, do not address the forehead distance between the hairline and brows and may actually cause an unwanted elevation of the hairline.

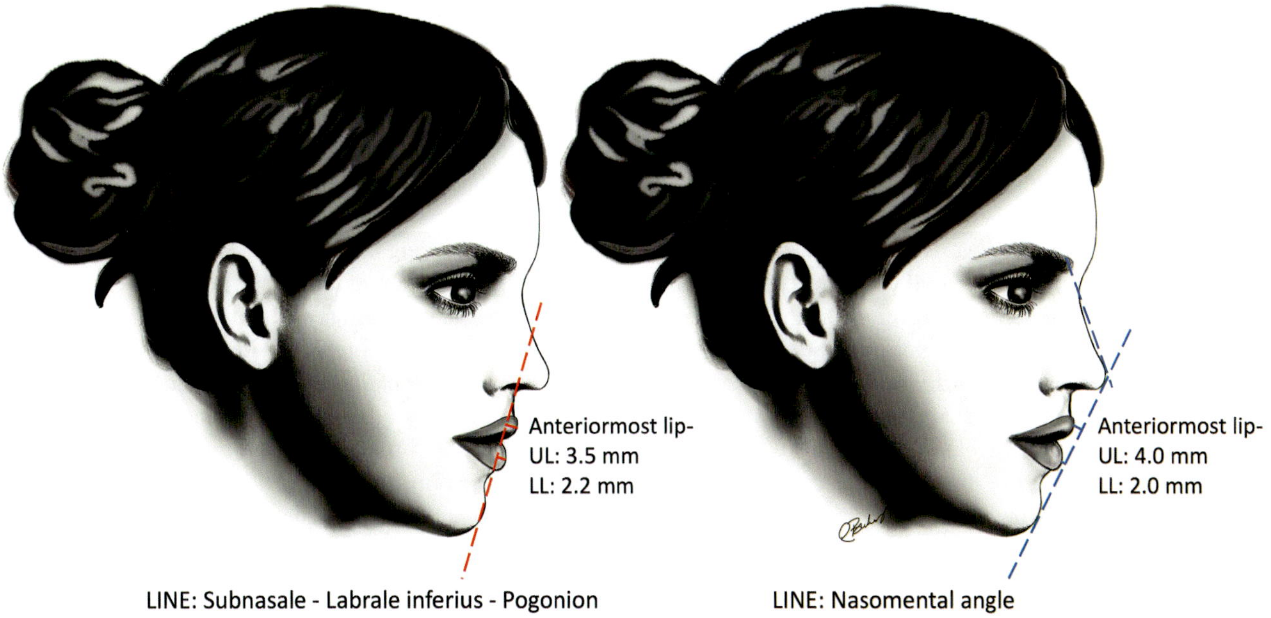

Fig. 37.4 Ideal lip projection can be measured in several ways
Left figure: A line is drawn from the subnasale through the labrale inferius to the pogonion of the chin; perpendicular lines from this to the anteriormost point of each lip define its horizontal position. The upper and lower lips project approximately 3.5 mm and 2.2 mm anterior to this line, respectively
Right figure: This measurement uses the nasomental angle to determine horizontal lip position, with the lips falling just 4.0 mm behind this line for the upper lip and 2.0 mm behind the line for the lower lip

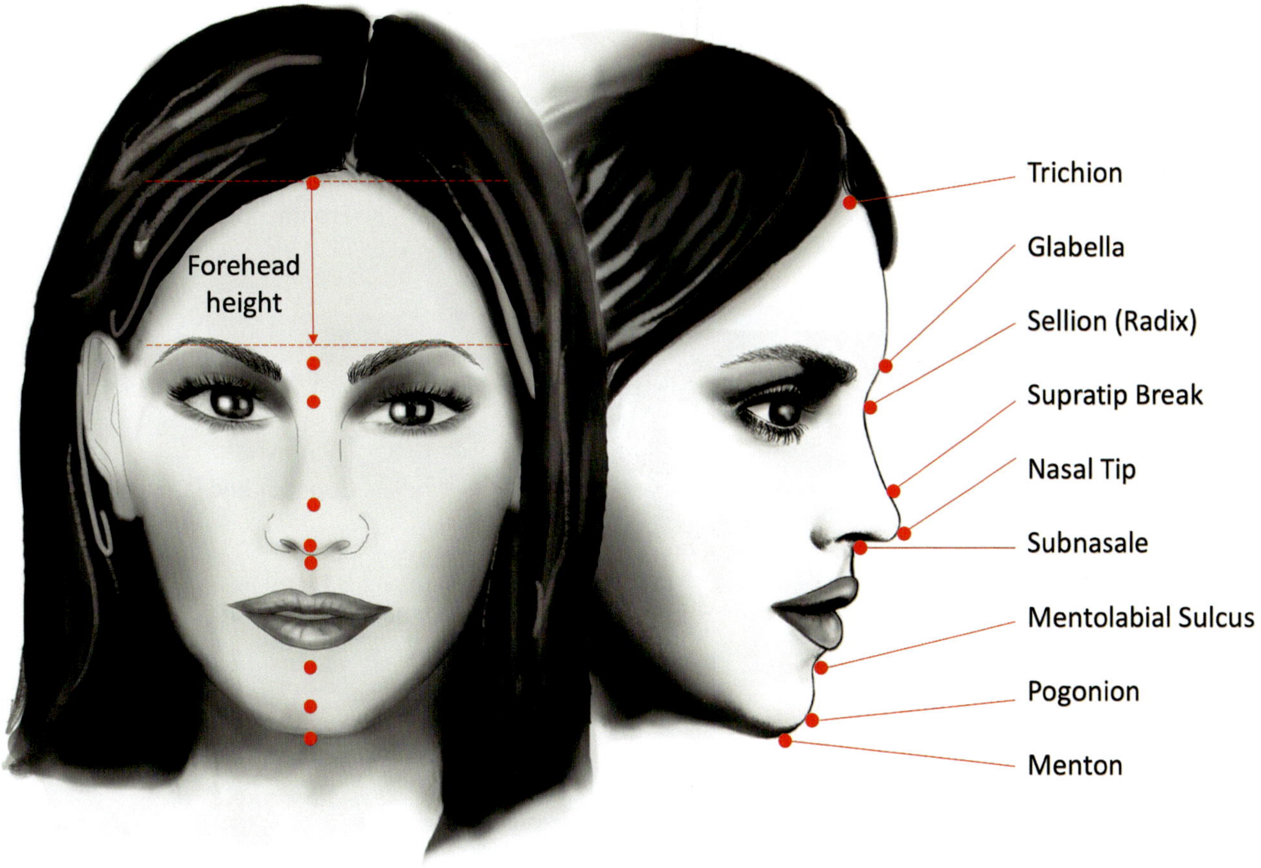

Fig. 37.5 Pertinent anatomic landmarks of the face to consider for optimal facial feminization

In facial feminization of the upper horizontal facial third, it is important to consider lowering the hairline position, also referred to as scalp advancement, while concurrently elevating the eyebrow height. Both of these procedures can often be approached through a trichophytic hairline incision. The feminized brow should ideally demonstrate an arched contour that peaks above the lateral limbus (lateral border of the iris), although one study suggests that the ideal peak is more lateral above the canthal angle [14]. A feminized brow tends to be higher above the supraorbital rim compared to the masculine brow that is typically positioned at the bony rim. These differences help optimize aesthetic results as compared to a masculine brow shape that is flatter in contour, low-lying, heavy, and thick-haired. Additional eyebrow contouring to further feminize the upper face can be done with careful epilation (eyebrow plucking) to thin the vertical brow and to taper the tail of the brow after the peak.

Once the eyebrow has been elevated to a more feminized location, excess non-hair-bearing forehead skin and soft tissue may be excised and advanced to create a rounded feminine shape. Relaxing incisions in the galea under the hair-bearing scalp can be helpful to advance the high hairline. Beveling the blade when creating the incision, as well as limited hair transplantation, can camouflage the scar and improve the aesthetic result along a new hairline [15, 16]. Hormone therapy with testosterone blockers may complement the surgical procedures by diminishing male-pattern hair growth [2]. However, a transgender patient with significant receding hairline may elect to defer scalp advancement completely. A hairpiece may be more practical and economical if limited donor hair exists.

An important aesthetic change in facial feminization surgery requires reducing the prominent supraorbital ridges and glabella, known as frontal bossing. Forehead cranioplasty surgery can reshape the forehead through either a trichophytic or coronal incision. A forehead with a thick anterior table (frontal bone anterior to the frontal sinus) can be reduced with a surgical burr to sculpt the forehead and orbital rims (Figs. 37.6 and 37.7). Alternately, a traditional osteoplastic flap can be performed to remove the anterior table with an oscillating saw, reshape the bone with burrs, and then secure it back in place with miniplates to the newly contoured glabella and supraorbital rims [17] (Fig. 37.8). Techniques that have replaced the bone flap without plating have been shown to have higher risks of nonunion and flap shifting. Ousterhout also described the adjunctive use of bone filler, methyl methacrylate, to fill in the concavity above the recontoured supraorbital rims [11]. However, due to rare infections with methyl methacrylate, it has been replaced by hydroxyapatite cement

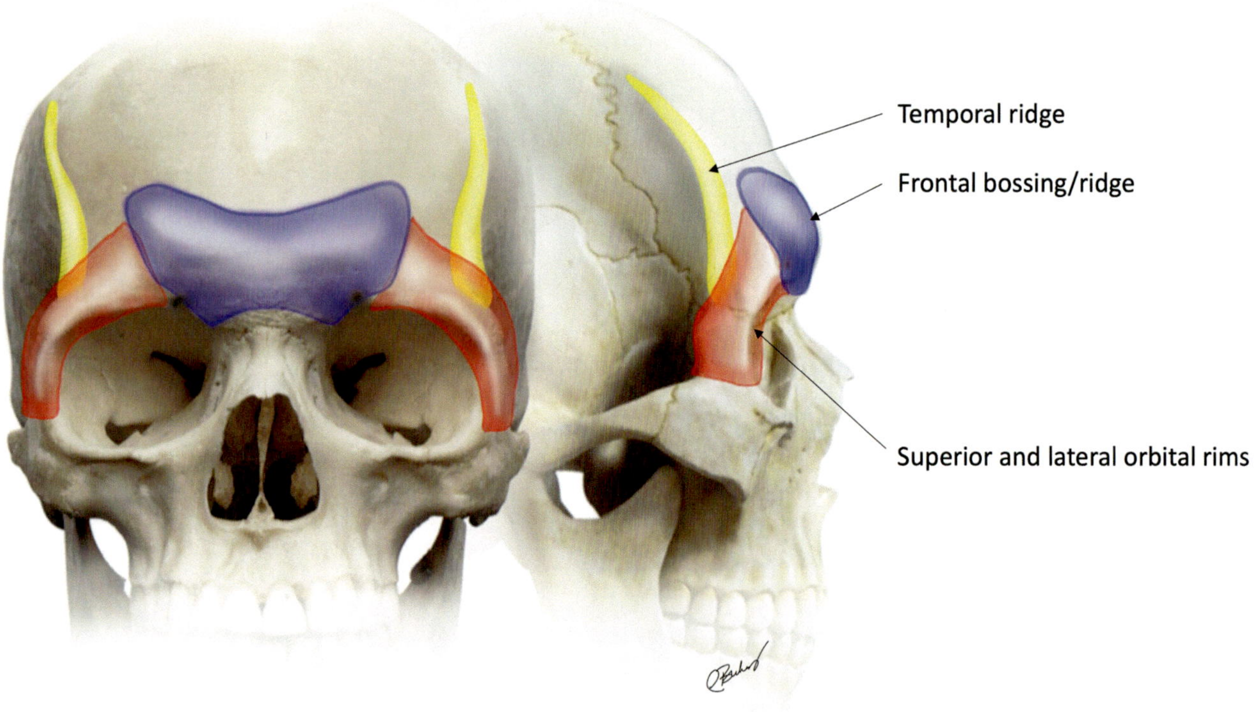

Fig. 37.6 Prominent frontal bossing can be reduced by high-speed burrs to shave down the excess projection of the frontal bone, glabella, and the supraorbital rims for upper facial feminization; a wide orbital rim and thick temporal ridge can also be sculpted

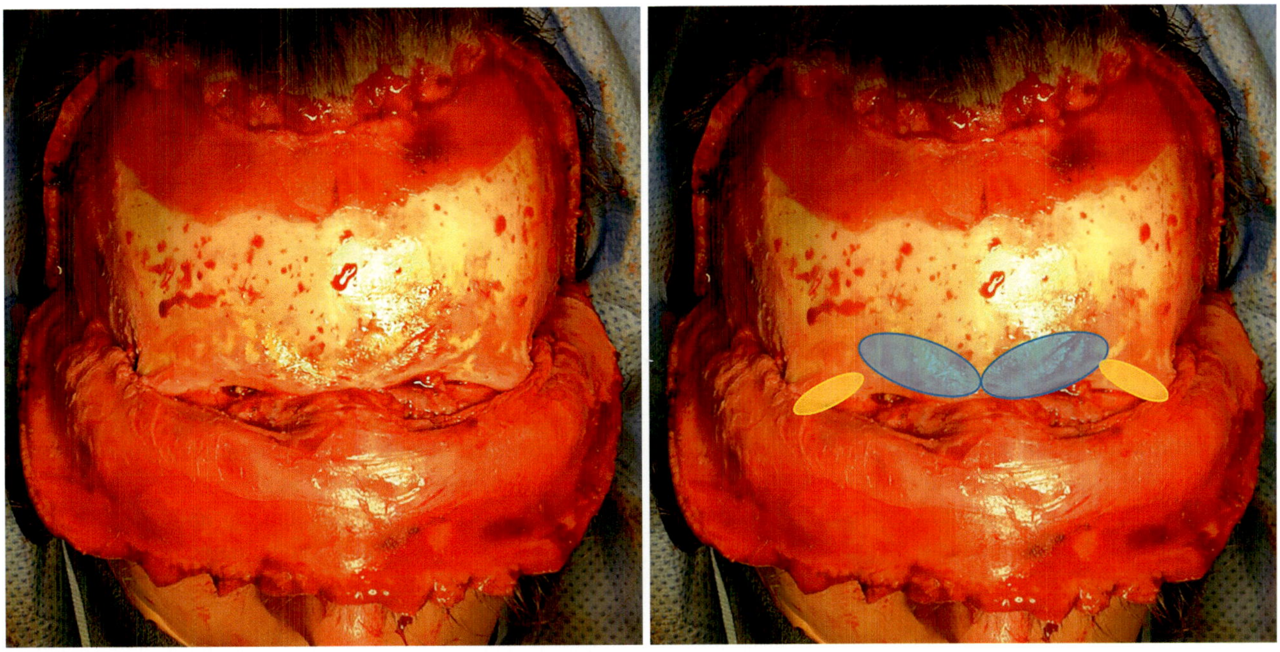

Fig. 37.7 Surgical view of the frontal bossing and prominent supraorbital ridges that are reduced

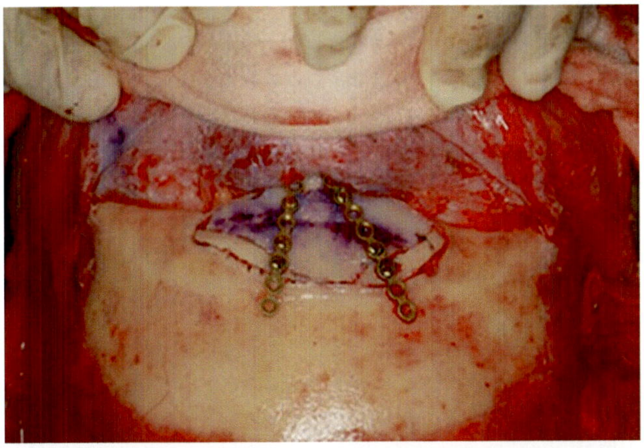

Fig. 37.8 Surgeon view of a reshaped frontal bone flap secured with miniplates to the newly contoured supraorbital rims (With permission from Springer Science + Business Media: Cho and Jin [17])

and less often performed than reductive techniques [18]. With any approach, care must be taken to avoid injury to the supratrochlear sensory nerve and frontal sinus.

Key Points: Surgical Concepts

- A trichophytic incision along the hairline can be used to simultaneously reduce the forehead height (scalp advancement) and elevate the eyebrows.
- Forehead cranioplasty surgery can reduce the prominent glabella and supraorbital ridges.
- The upper eyelids in a feminized face typically demonstrate a higher and semilunar eyelid crease, with greater visible area of the pretarsal skin.
- Cheek augmentation with implants, autologous fat, or injectable fillers helps create the feminine high cheekbones.
- The ideal "heart-shaped" female face is characterized by prominent, wide cheekbones and contrasting submalar concavities.
- Reducing the width and square shape of the mandible will result in a more stereotypical feminized appearance.
- Masseter muscle hypertrophy contributes to lower facial width and can be softened with neurotoxin injection.
- Occlusion of the teeth should be carefully examined when considering genioplasty surgery to alter the appearance of the chin.

Eyelid Surgery

In general, the basic steps of eyelid blepharoplasty or other eyelid surgeries will fundamentally be similar for facial feminization surgery. The main landmarks of the periorbital region that contribute to a feminine appearance include the eyebrows and the prominence of the glabellar bone and superior orbital rims. As mentioned in the previous section, frontal bossing and excessive projection of the orbital bones can be contoured and flattened, when present. Care should be taken to avoid injury to the globe, supraorbital neurovascular bundle, trochlea medially, and the lacrimal gland just below the superior orbital rims. Ideally, the eyebrow should be positioned higher, up to 1 cm above the orbital rim, and with a delicate or more pronounced arch, depending on personal preference.

The key defining features of the eyelid, in regard to feminization, are the eyelid crease and eyelid fold. The eyelid fold refers to the soft tissue skin and orbicularis muscle that are directly above the crease and hang over the crease. Although variations exist among ethnicities, in general, the masculine upper eyelid will typically have a more prominent eyelid fold that rests lower over the crease to cover most of the upper tarsal region. In contrast, a feminine eyelid fold will often be more compact and hang minimally over the eyelid crease. This allows more of the eyelid tarsal platform to be seen, or more "eyeshadow space." The superior sulcus may also be deeper and more accentuated in the feminine upper eyelid, compared to the fuller masculine superior sulcus that blends into the more prominent skin fold. This may involve conservatively debulking some medial and central preaponeurotic fat pads to create a gentle depression of the superior sulcus.

A shorter skin fold should be created in conjunction with a higher eyelid crease in the feminized eyelid, with biologic female creases located typically 8–12 mm above the eyelid margin. The eyelid crease is often lower at 6–8 mm above the eyelid margin in biologic men, and lower at 3–5 mm in eyelids of Asian descent. The crease should also be more rounded and curved, tapering toward both canthi, in contrast to the lower and flatter profile of the biologic male or Asian eyelid crease. The patient should bring in photos of their preferred eyelid appearance, in particular for eyelids of Asian descent, in order to properly discuss the possible outcomes of surgery in regard to eyelid crease height, skin fold, epicanthal fold, preaponeurotic fat, and crease definition and contour.

The lateral canthal angle should demonstrate a gentle upward slope and rest 1–2 mm above the level of the medial canthal angle in the feminine eye. The canthus should have a sharp angle so that the eyelids have an aesthetically appealing "almond" shape that can be further accentuated with eyeliner techniques. This canthal shaping can be formed with a buried 6-0 or 7-0 polyglactin suture to secure the gray line or posterior lamellar lines of the upper and lower lateral eyelid margins, with the knot rotated away from the ocular surface.

Nasal Surgery

Although a full discussion of rhinoplasty surgery is beyond the scope of this chapter, reductive rhinoplasty that yields a smaller feminized nose can result in a dramatic facial change for a transgender patient. When considering reductive rhinoplasty, there are several key items notable for facial feminization.

(a) The stereotypically female nasal dorsum has a slight concavity compared to the straight male dorsum.
(b) The nasofrontal angle is wider at the junction of the nose and forehead.
(c) The nasal tip is slightly upturned with a supratip break, corresponding to a more obtuse nasolabial angle (Figs. 37.3 and 37.5).
(d) Nasal size should be congruent to the rest of the facial proportions. Therefore, if a patient undergoes forehead reduction and mandibular angle contouring, reductive rhinoplasty to the nasal dorsum, tip, and reduction to the alar base width to create a more petite nose to maintain the aesthetic balance.

Various surgical techniques include nasal bone osteotomies, tip bulk reduction with suture techniques and cephalic trim of the lower lateral cartilages, and alar base reduction. In addition, rhinoplasty to create a nose in harmony with the feminized face should preserve nasal breathing function.

A recent study showed that facial feminization rhinoplasty increased the nasofrontal angle from 141.6 ° to 150.5 °, increased the nasolabial angle from 107.4 ° to 115.2 °, and created a supratip break [10].

Surgery of the Midface

Although the zygomatic bones (cheekbones) have more bulk in the biologic male face, they lack the prominence to create the stereotypical feminine appearance of "high cheekbones." A high cheekbone is ideally juxtaposed by a concavity below the malar eminence, which gives the appearance of the shadowed contour below the "blush" of the cheek. To contour the midface, autologous fat injection or alloplastic malar implants can be placed through oral incisions above the upper teeth, and secured to the underlying bone. Osteotomies and/or bone grafts to lateralize the zygoma are less commonly performed [1].

When lifting the midfacial soft tissues does not provide enough contrast between the cheekbones and the contour beneath, debulking buccal fat can provide the desired submalar concavity [16]. In the office, filler injection with hyaluronic acid (HA) can similarly achieve a feminizing change to the midface, by providing volume to the upper cheeks and lifting the malar soft tissue, albeit non-permanently. Nonsurgical interventions have dramatically increased in popularity across the world in recent years due to limited downtime and healing. Estrogen hormone therapy will change the soft tissue distribution to create a feminized cheek volume but may take 12 or more months on the therapy; therefore, filler injection can be an excellent starting point for facial feminization during these months. Whether by surgical or nonsurgical means, artistic sculpting to create prominent cheekbones with submalar hollowing will result in the ideal feminine-shaped face [16, 19]. Additional facial contouring can be achieved with cosmetic techniques to darken/shadow the submalar concavity while applying highlighter to the higher cheek prominence. Chin shape alterations can complete the feminized heart shape, and will be discussed in the next section.

Surgery of the Lower Face and Mandible

Rhytidectomy (facelift) is a commonly performed procedure in the United States to increase facial beauty by lifting and resuspending the soft tissue [13]. A unique aspect of lower facial surgery in facial feminization is the underlying mandible shape, particularly the prominence of the mandibular angles and the shape of the chin. The biologic male lower face is typically wider, contributed in part by larger masseter muscles overlying the bone. Therefore, both the bulk of the bone and masseter should be addressed in order to achieve a more feminized lower facial shape. Bone reduction through a posterior oral incision softens the prominence of both wide and square-shaped, mandibular angles. After wide subperiosteal dissection, bone is removed using high-speed burrs or by osteotomies using saws and curved osteotomes [16] (Fig. 37.9). Lower face and neck surgery is otherwise quite similar to aging face procedures for cisgender patients, but should be performed only after reductive bone work is completed to fully assess the position of the soft tissue.

Masseter muscle reduction can lessen the wide appearance of the jaw, and can be achieved through direct surgical debulking, as well as chemodenervation. Softening the masseter muscle is also common in Asian biologic female patients to create a desirable oval or heart-shaped jawline. Botulinum toxin injected into the masseter muscles results in muscle inactivity for 3–4 months, which softens the "strong" square shape of the mandibular angle, and often can reduce muscle bulk over time. Large volumes are typically required, and injections should be placed posteriorly and inferiorly to prevent diffusion into muscles of facial expression, such as the zygomatic smiling muscles [20].

The masculine "boxy" chin shape can be modified in the transgender patient to achieve a pointier shape, to complete the ideal feminine "heart-shaped" face. Genioplasty surgery can reposition bone pieces to create anterior projection and simultaneously reduce vertical height. Changes to chin shape may also be accomplished with an alloplastic implant, with care to avoid injury to the mental sensory nerves exiting the mandible. If preoperative teeth alignment reveals overbite or underbite, referral to an oral surgeon is recommended prior to surgery.

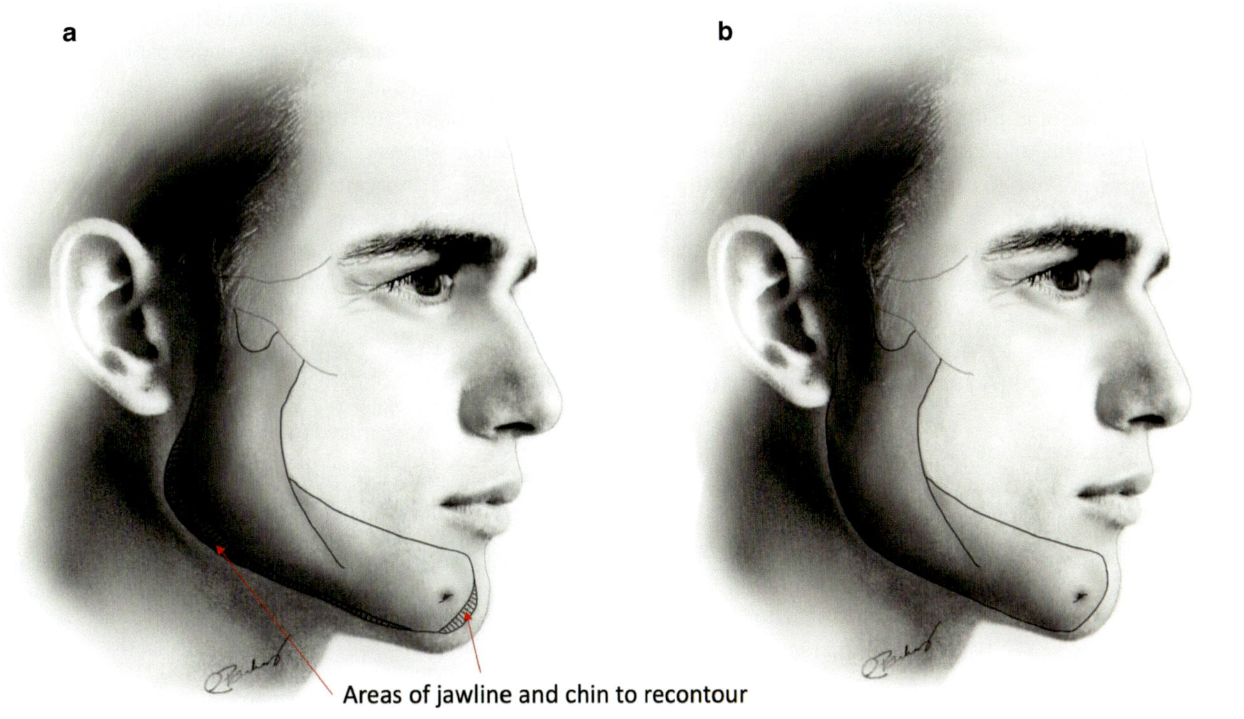

Fig. 37.9 Reduction of a wide prominent mandible angle (**a**) with a resultant decrease in mandibular vertical height and softening of the jawline angle (**b**). The anterior bony chin is similarly softened with surgical burrs or osteotomes

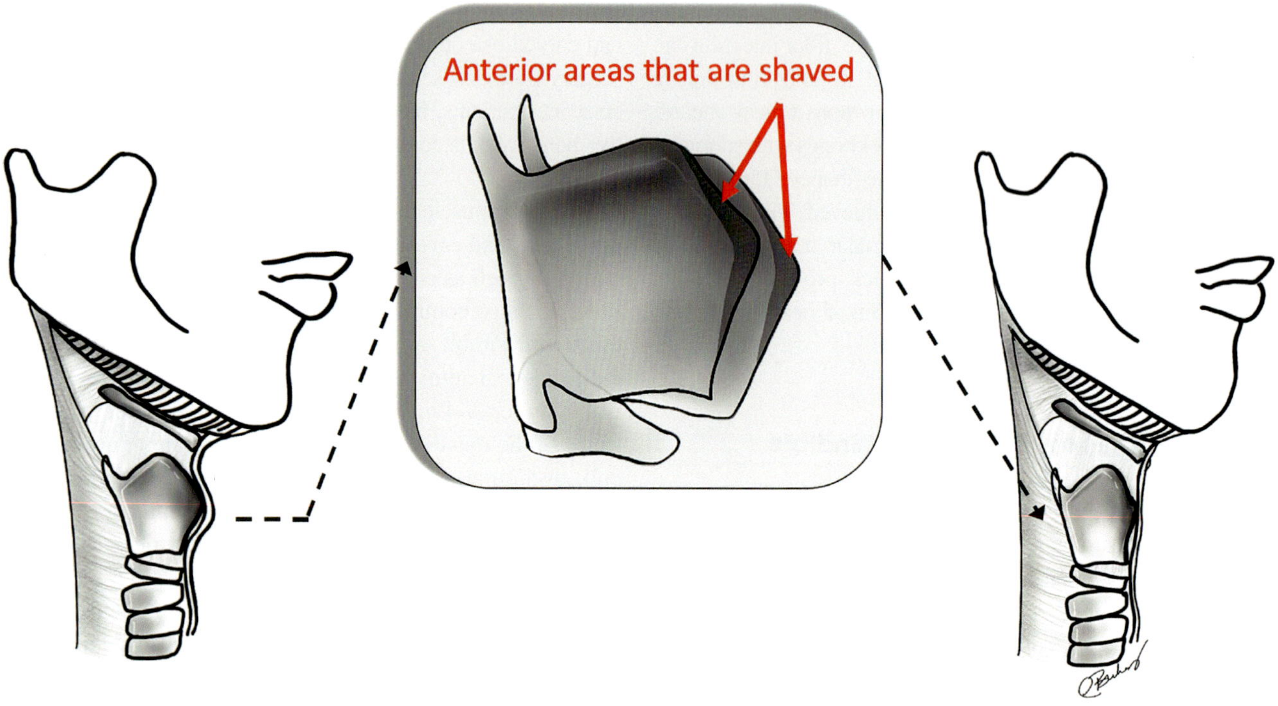

Fig. 37.10 Prominent thyroid cartilage “Adam’s apple” and a flattened, more feminine appearance after anterior tracheal shave

Finally, augmenting lip volume and reshaping the lips may complement other facial feminization surgical procedures. Usually, a hyaluronic acid filler optimally provides volume to the lips and can be performed in the office. The lips should be shaped to create fuller lips with increased projection and volume to the bodies (or “pillows”) of the lips and to outline a well-defined cupid’s bow and vermillion border. In some patients, dermal or fat grafts can add additional volume and longevity to the lips. The height of the visible upper red lip can be surgically lifted with a cheiloplasty (lip lift) which simultaneously shortens a long upper white lip (distance between the base of the nose and the upper vermillion border).

Thyroid Cartilage (Adam’s Apple) Alteration

Transgender patients may desire laryngochondroplasty or a “tracheal shave” to reduce and flatten the superior prominence of the thyroid cartilage (Adam’s apple). Those familiar with the complex anatomy of the larynx can safely remove excess cartilage with preservation of the vocal fold attachment through a small horizontal incision in the anterior neck (Fig. 37.10) [21]. Speech therapy can also be an important adjunct to change the voicing style and pitch of phonation.

Conclusion

Facial feminization surgery is an important part of treatment for transgender patients seeking to feminize the facial skeleton and soft tissue in the treatment of gender dysphoria. Alterations of the face help transgender patients achieve recognition as a woman, and can result in better physical, mental, and social functioning outcomes following facial feminization surgery. A meaningful patient and physician collaboration is necessary to achieve optimal outcomes and can be highly rewarding.

References

1. Becking AG, Tuinzing DB, Hage JJ, LJG G. Transgender feminization of the facial skeleton. Clin Plast Surg. 2007;34(3):557–64.
2. Spack NP. Management of transgenderism. JAMA. 2013;309(5):478–84.
3. Ainsworth T, Spiegel JH. Quality of life of individuals with and without facial feminization surgery or gender reassignment surgery. Qual Life Res. 2010;19(7):1019–24.
4. Spiegel JH. Challenges in care of the transgender patient seeking facial feminization surgery. Facial Plast Surg Clin North Am. 2008;16(2):233–8.
5. Spiegel JH. Facial determinants of female gender and feminizing forehead cranioplasty. Laryngoscope. 2011;121(2):250–61.
6. Ousterhout DK. Facial feminization surgery: a guide for the transgendered woman. Omaha: Addicus Books; 2009.

7. Powell N, Humphreys B. Proportions of the aesthetic face. New York: Thieme Medical Publishers; 1984.
8. Morgan JPI, Haug RH. Evaluation of the craniomaxillofacial deformity patient. In: Greenberg AM, Prein J, editors. Craniomaxillofacial reconstructive and corrective bone surgery. New York: Springer; 2002. p. 5–21.
9. Zimbler MS. Aesthetic facial analysis. In: Flint PW, Haughey BH, Lund VJ, Niparko JK, Richardson MA, Robbins KT, et al., editors. Cummings otolaryngology – head and neck surgery: head and neck surgery. 5th ed. Philadelphia: Mosby Elsevier; 2010. p. 272–3.
10. Noureai SAR, Randhawa P, Andrews PJ, Saleh HA. The role of nasal feminization rhinoplasty in male-to-female gender reassignment. Arch Facial Plast Surg. 2007;9(5):318–20.
11. Ousterhout DK. Feminization of the forehead: contour changing to improve female aesthetics. Plast Reconstr Surg. 1987;79(5):701–13.
12. Gonzalex-Ulloa M. Quantitative principles in cosmetic surgery of the face (profileplasty). Plast Reconstr Surg Transplant Bull. 1962;29:186–98.
13. The American Society for Aesthetic Plastic Surgery. Cosmetic Surgery National Data Bank [Internet]. 2013. Available from http://www.surgery.org/media/ statistics
14. Roth JM, Metzinger SE. Quantifying the arch position of the female eyebrow. Arch Facial Plast Surg. 2003;5(3):235–9.
15. Ramirez AL, Ende KH, Kabaker SS. Correction of the high female hairline. Arch Facial Plast Surg. 2011;11(2):84–90.
16. Altman K. Facial feminization surgery: current state of the art. Int J Oral Maxillofac Surg. 2012;41(8):885–94.
17. Cho S-W, Jin HR. Feminization of the forehead in a transgender: frontal sinus reshaping combined with brow lift and hairline lowering. Aesthet Plast Surg. 2012;36(5):1207–10.
18. Hoenig JF. Frontal bone remodeling for gender reassignment of the male forehead: a gender-reassignment surgery. Aesthet Plast Surg. 2011;35(6):1043–9.
19. Glasgold MJ, Glasgold RA, Lam SM. Volume restoration and facial aesthetics. Facial Plast Surg Clin North Am. 2008;16(4):435–42.
20. Bentsianov B, Francis A, Blitzer A. Botulinum toxin treatment of temporomandibular disorders, masseteric hypertrophy, and cosmetic masseter reduction. Oper Tech Otolaryngol Head Neck Surg. 2004;15(2):110–3.
21. Conrad K, Yoskovitch A. Endoscopically facilitated reduction laryngochondroplasty. Arch Facial Plast Surg. 2003;5(4): 345–8.

Part III

Lacrimal

38 Evaluation and Imaging of Lacrimal Drainage Disorders

Jonathan J. Dutton

The lacrimal drainage system is a mucous membrane-lined duct whose function results from a complex interplay of anatomy and physiology [1, 2]. Drainage of tears depends upon a variety of factors. These include the volume of tear production, eyelid position, orbicularis muscle pump mechanisms, anatomic status of the puncta and drainage passages, capillary attraction forces, gravity, and nasal air convection currents [3]. Any patient with symptomatic epiphora may have a normally patent anatomic system that is overwhelmed by excessive secretion of tears. On the other hand, the lacrimal drainage system can be compromised by stenosis or blockage and unable to handle normal or even reduced tear production. Patients may have a partial or complete blockage of the nasolacrimal drainage system, and yet experience no symptoms at all, or may even have symptoms of dry eye. This situation can be seen if tear production is significantly reduced. The clinical picture of epiphora depends on the total balance between tear production on the one hand and tear drainage on the other. It is not related exclusively to the absolute function of either production or drainage alone.

The causes of lacrimal drainage insufficiency can relate to anatomic abnormalities or to physiologic dysfunction. Anatomic obstruction refers to a structural blockage of the lacrimal drainage system. This can be a partial or complete obstruction. Complete blockage can result from closed puncta, canalicular occlusion, or nasolacrimal duct fibrosis. Partial obstruction is seen with punctal or canalicular stenosis, inflammatory narrowing of the nasolacrimal duct, or from a mechanical obstruction within the lacrimal sac or duct from tumors or from concretions. Nasal polyps or tumors also can rarely cause a partial obstruction to tear drainage.

Physiologic etiologies result from failure of functional pump mechanisms even in the face of normal drainage apparatus anatomy. Dysfunction results from punctal eversion or other eyelid malpositions or from lacrimal pump inadequacy from poor orbicularis muscle tone, paralysis, or significant horizontal eyelid laxity [4, 5]. In an interesting study on tear production and clearance, Yen et al. showed a reduction in tear production and in both conjunctival and corneal sensation following punctal occlusion, more so with both upper and lower occlusions [6]. These parameters returned to preocclusion levels 14–17 days after removal of the plugs. They concluded that an autoregulatory mechanism was responsible for altering these parameters.

Clinical Evaluation

The clinical evaluation of gross lacrimal function is usually not difficult, and the diagnosis of epiphora often is made on history alone. However, the determination of a specific etiology may be more difficult and usually requires one or more clinical diagnostic procedures. There is no single test that will localize the anatomic site or physiologic basis for the imbalance between tear production and tear drainage. Several clinical tests have been described, many of which are often used together to diagnose the specific disease processes in any particular case [7].

Clinical History

Clinical history is important in the evaluation of any patient with symptomatic epiphora. An adequate history will usually reduce the possible causes and in many cases will allow the surgeon to decide what further tests may be necessary. Epiphora in a child with a history of tearing since birth is typically the result of a developmental blockage at Hasner's membrane, whereas acquired epiphora in an adult will have a very different etiology such as canalicular or lacrimal duct obstruction. It is important to elicit any history of facial trauma, the use of some specific ophthalmic topical medications, certain systemic chemotherapeutic agents, or orbital irradiation.

J. J. Dutton (✉)
University of North Carolina, Durham, NC, USA
e-mail: Jonathan_dutton@med.unc.edu

A. J. Cohen, C. N. Burkat (eds.), *Oculofacial, Orbital, and Lacrimal Surgery*, https://doi.org/10.1007/978-3-030-14092-2_38

Previous sinus surgery, particularly intranasal antrostomy, polypectomy, or ethmoidectomy, might suggest potential direct lacrimal duct injury. History of a rapidly growing palpable medial canthal mass or bleeding from the puncta suggests the presence of malignancy. Intermittent epiphora can be seen with allergic rhinitis or sinusitis. Episodes of dacryocystitis suggest distal nasolacrimal duct (NLD) obstruction.

External Examination

Evaluation of epiphora begins with a careful examination of the ocular surface and eyelid structures for evidence of corneal keratitis, eyelid malpositions, or mechanical obstruction to tear drainage. Conjunctival or corneal irritation, either inflammatory or mechanical, may cause hypersecretion with resultant epiphora. Blepharitis and allergic conjunctivitis will often trigger increased lacrimation, as will trichiasis or conjunctival scarring.

Stenosis or occlusion of the puncta will slow or block tear drainage. A narrow medial palpebral angle can result in apposition of the upper and lower puncta, with mechanical occlusion even when the puncta are otherwise normal (Fig. 38.1). Conjunctivochalasis is seen with increasing frequency with advancing age and with contact lens use [8, 9]. In severe cases the redundant conjunctiva can mechanically overhang and occlude the inferior punctum [10] (Fig. 38.2). Mass lesions in the medial canthal region or conjunctival symblephara may also mechanically obstruct tear drainage. Careful palpation of the lacrimal sac will uncover distension suggestive of a sac mucocele (Fig. 38.3), and pressure on the lacrimal sac may produce reflux of mucopurulent material demonstrating some degree of lower nasolacrimal obstruction (Fig. 38.4). In some cases, periorbital cellulitis is seen as erythema and edema of the lower eyelid and medial canthus (Fig. 38.5).

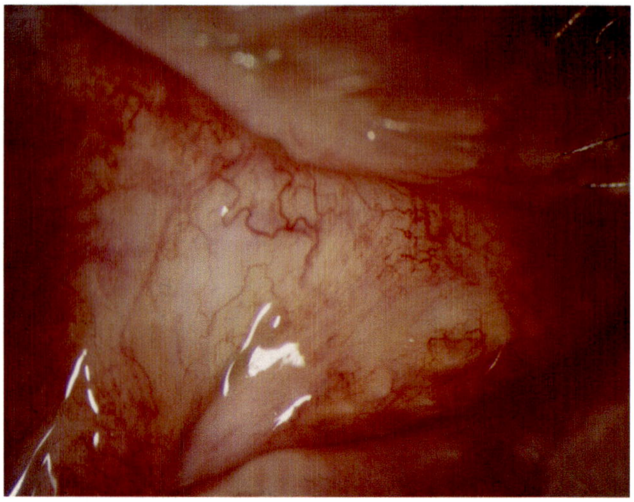

Fig. 38.2 Medial conjunctivochalasis overhanging and occluding the inferior punctum

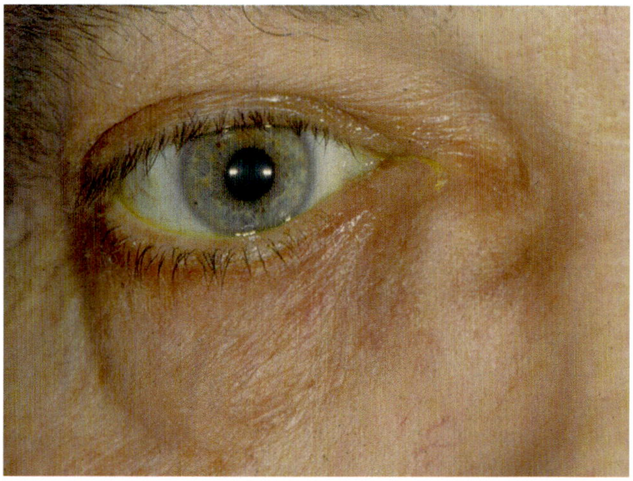

Fig. 38.3 Right dacryocystitis with a distended lacrimal sac

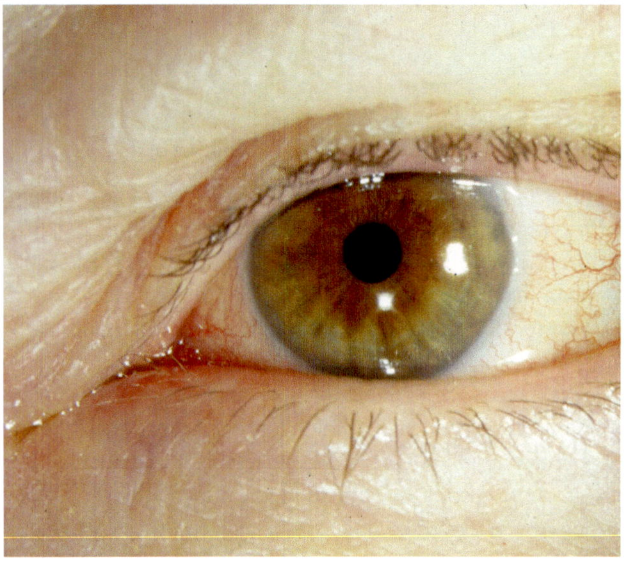

Fig. 38.1 Narrow medial canthal angle with kissing puncta and increased tear meniscus

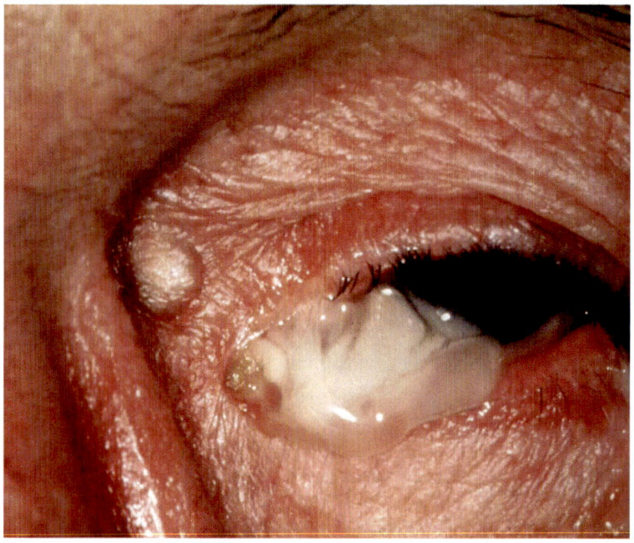

Fig. 38.4 Left dacryocystitis with copious reflux of mucopurulent discharge

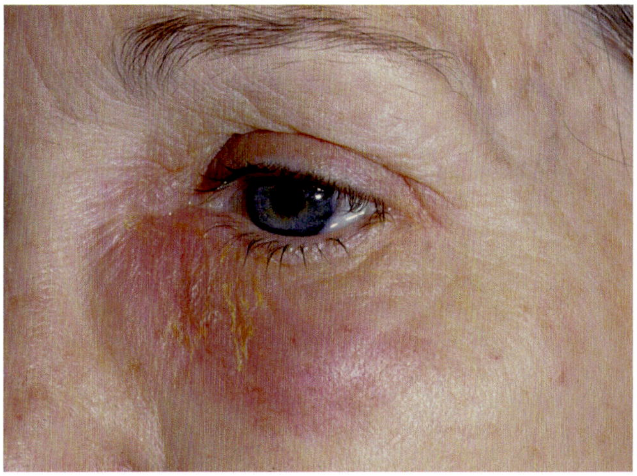

Fig. 38.5 Left dacryocystitis with lower eyelid cellulitis

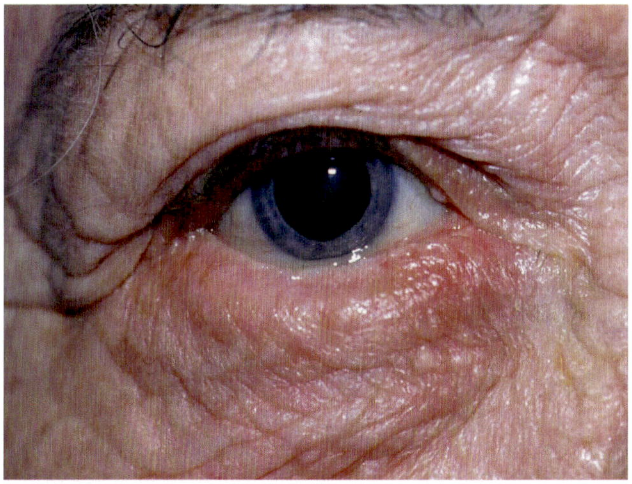

Fig. 38.6 Right lower eyelid involutional entropion with inversion and mechanical occlusion of the inferior punctum

Examination of the nasal vestibule is mandatory to uncover possible hypertrophic mucosa or nasal polyps that can obstruct the nasolacrimal ostium [11]. In children a narrow inferior meatus can often impede drainage even after successful probing. Although there is some controversy regarding the value of inferior turbinate infracturing [12–14], our experience suggests this is helpful in some cases, so that a careful nasal exam should be performed. Rarely, a nasal tumor can obstruct the nasolacrimal ostium.

Mild to moderate involutional eyelid laxity and decreased orbicularis muscle tone may result in functional epiphora from impaired pump mechanism [15–17]. There may be no evidence of punctal or canalicular stenosis or of eyelid malposition, and the NLD can be patent to irrigation without reflux. Eyelid laxity can also be associated with frank eyelid malpositions such as entropion that can produce corneal irritation and secondary reflex hypersecretion (Fig. 38.6). Ectropion from involutional eyelid laxity or from facial nerve palsy may lead to exposure keratopathy and reflex epiphora. Medial ectropion causes the punctum to rotate away from the tear lake, impairing tear drainage. When this is long-standing, the punctum may become stenotic or occluded.

Punctal stenosis is a common finding, reported in more than 50% of normal individuals and increases with advancing age [18]. The prevalence is increased with eyelid inflammatory diseases such as chronic blepharitis. Punctal and canalicular stenoses are also common complications of chemotherapy such as systemic 5-fluorouracil and docetaxel or with the use of topical mitomycin-C for conjunctival tumors [19–21]. Kashkouli et al. [22] showed a significantly higher rate of proximal lacrimal obstruction in patients using topical antiglaucoma medications (timolol, dorzolamide, pilocarpine), with 77% involving the canaliculi. Since punctal stenosis can be seen without accompanying eyelid laxity, any epiphora evaluation should specifically look for this condition. Agenesis of one or more puncta is not a common cause of epiphora (Fig. 38.7) but has been observed in 14% of patients with congenital nasolacrimal duct obstruction [23]. Multiple puncta may sometimes be seen, but these are more often associated with dry eye symptoms (Fig. 38.8).

Some cases of dacryocystitis may be associated with a cutaneous fistula from the lacrimal sac. There is usually a history of tearing or mucoid discharge from the skin at the medial canthus, and this should elicit a careful examination for a small opening in the skin over the lacrimal sac area. Irrigation through the punctum with fluorescein will usually demonstrate the fistula as dye-stained fluid egresses on the skin. Occasionally a fistulous tract may extend some distance from the medial canthus even down onto the mid cheek (Fig. 38.9).

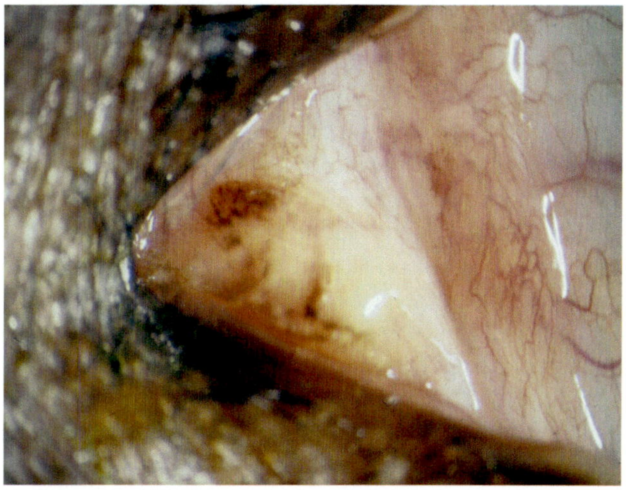

Fig. 38.7 Congenital absence of superior and inferior puncta

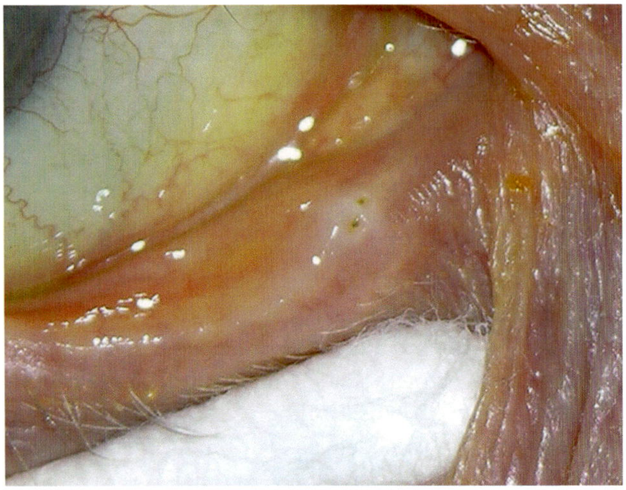

Fig. 38.8 Double inferior punctum

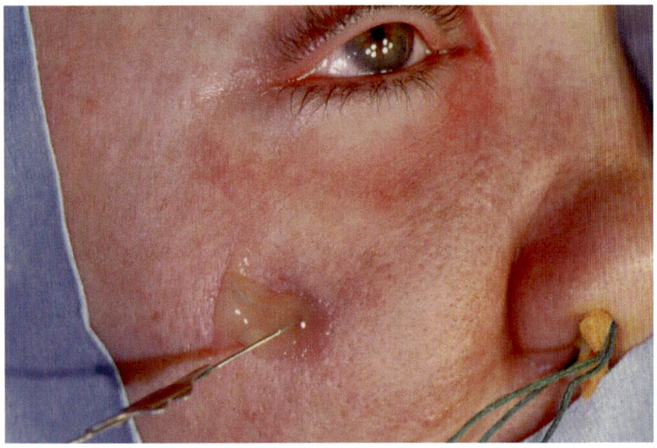

Fig. 38.9 Right dacryocystitis with a fistula from the lacrimal sac draining onto the cheek

Clinical Evaluation of Lacrimal Drainage

Like many diagnostic evaluations in medicine, most tests of lacrimal drainage require some subjective interpretation in order to determine the probable etiology of epiphora (Table 38.1). In most cases, careful clinical evaluation in the office will adequately demonstrate the cause of tearing and allow appropriate therapeutic decisions. Some cases, however, present a more difficult diagnostic challenge. This is especially true for those patients with proximal system anatomic stenosis and physiologic dysfunctions. Beigi et al. [24] evaluated 36 eyes originally diagnosed with nasolacrimal duct obstruction by syringing alone performed by non-lacrimal specialists and referred for DCR. Re-examination by an experienced observer used a more accurate methodological approach employing the dye disappearance test, Jones I test, detailed eyelid examination, and in appropriate cases canalicular probing and mini-endoscopic examination. They found that only 22% of the 36 patients carried the correct diagnosis. In the other 72%, canalicular or punctal stenosis was the correct diagnosis, and in 6%, ocular surface disease caused hypersecretion without NLD obstruction.

Table 38.1 Results of primary and secondary Jones tests and probable sites of lacrimal system obstruction

Jones I	Jones II	Probable site of obstruction
+	Not needed	Patent system, probably normal
–	+, dye in the nose	Partial NLD obstruction vs. functional
–	+, saline in the nose, no dye	Partial canalicular obstruction vs. functional
–	–, regurgitation of dye from opposite punctum	Complete lower NLD obstruction
–	–, regurgitation of saline from opposite punctum, no dye	Complete distal common canaliculus or upper sac obstruction
–	–, regurgitation of dye from same punctum only	Complete opposite canalicular obstruction with lower NLD obstruction
–	–, regurgitation of saline from the same punctum, no dye	Complete distal canalicular obstruction

NLD nasolacrimal duct; + positive, dye appearing in the nose; – negative, no dye in the nose

Tear Meniscus

Overflow tearing is a common symptom in patients with lacrimal drainage dysfunction. Increase in the tear lake height is often recognized as a clinical sign of NLD obstruction [17]. Burkat et al. quantitatively demonstrated an increase in the lower eyelid tear meniscus in patients with NLD obstruction [25]. The mean meniscus in normal control eyes was 0.2 mm compared with a meniscus mean height of 0.6 mm in eyes with NLD obstruction demonstrated by irrigation. The mean ratio difference between the normal side and the obstructed side was 2.5, but the authors concluded that a ratio of ≥1.5 was suggestive of obstruction.

Schirmer Tests

The Schirmer test is a clinical tool for the diagnosis of dry eye and hypersecretion syndromes. While there has been some controversy regarding the reliability and interpretation of this test, nevertheless, it is widely used in clinical practice. The Schirmer I test, performed without topical anesthetic, evaluates gross tear production, both basic and reflex. A strip of filter paper 35 mm long and 5 mm wide is folded 5 mm from one end, and the small folded portion is placed into the conjunctival fornix near the lateral third of the lower eyelid (Fig. 38.10). The amount of wetting on the filter paper is

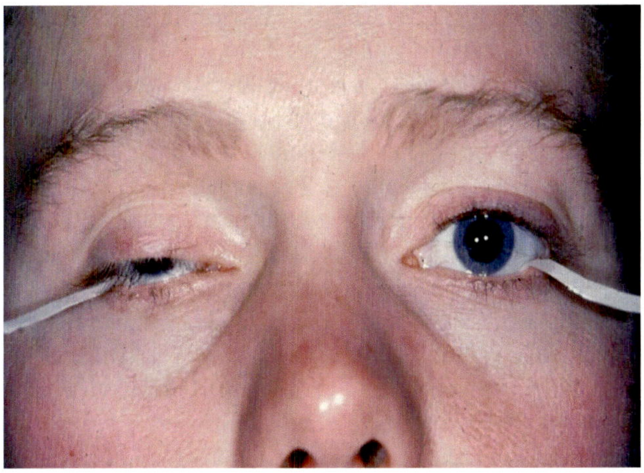

Fig. 38.10 Schirmer's tear volume test. The filter paper strips are placed in the conjunctival sac at the junctions of the middle and lateral lower eyelids

measured from the fold in millimeters at 5 minutes [54]. The test is performed in subdued lighting, and both eyes are tested simultaneously. This test measures the aqueous component of the tear film but does not distinguish between basic and reflex tear production. It gives only a very crude estimate of absolute tear flow, since the paper itself may stimulate some reflex lacrimation. It is important to blot any tears that are in the fornix prior to performing this test to prevent an excessive degree of wetting on the filter paper. If the tear drainage system is functioning, some volume of tear flow will pass into the puncta without being recorded on the paper strip. The fractional volume lost in this manner is in proportion to the adequacy of the drainage system and may be significantly more than the volume recorded on the strip. Normal values for the Schirmer I test range from 10 to 30 mm of wetting at 5 minutes, with values over 25 mm typical of patients under age 30 and values of 5–10 mm in those over age 60.

The 5-minute testing interval used in the standard Schirmer test can cause discomfort to some patients and may cause hypersecretion that can produce a falsely elevated test result. Karampatakis et al. [26] showed that a 2-minute test gave acceptable results that correlated well with the 5-minute results in 94.5% of cases, where most normal individuals show wetting equal to or greater than 10 mm.

When the Schirmer I test result is abnormally low, the Schirmer II test may give a better indication of stressed reflex capability by bypassing the normal conjunctiva-cornea to lacrimal reflex arc. Topical anesthetic is used in the eye, and the nasal mucosa is stimulated mechanically with a cotton swab or chemically with ammonium chloride. The amount by which the Schirmer II test exceeds basic production represents stressed reflex secretion. Clinically, this test is invasive, tends not to be very useful, and is rarely performed.

Tear Break-Up Time

Tear film stability depends in part upon its basal mucin layer which increases the hydrophilic quality of epithelial cells to allow uniform wetting of the corneal surface. With deficiency of this mucin component, the tear film will bead up on the relatively more hydrophobic corneal surface. The tear break-up time is a simple clinical test for evaluation of this component of tear function. One drop of fluorescein is placed in the eye, and the patient is instructed to blink once. The corneal surface is observed under slit-lamp magnification using cobalt blue illumination, and the observer notes how many seconds it takes for dry spots to appear in the tear film. Normal tear break-up time is between 15 and 30 seconds. A tear break-up time of less than 10 seconds indicates a probable mucin deficiency that may result not only in dry eye symptoms but also in reflex hypersecretion and epiphora.

Dye Disappearance Test

The dye disappearance test (DDT) was first described by Zappia and Milder in 1972 [27]. It is only a crude measure of the rate of tear flow out of the conjunctival sac. Nevertheless, it is a simple, effective, and reliable test for gross nasolacrimal duct obstruction in adults [28, 29]. One drop of 2% fluorescein is placed into the lower conjunctival fornix, and the amount of dye remaining after 5 minutes is graded on a subjective 0–4+ scale, where 0 represents no dye remaining and 4+ represents all the dye remaining. Little or no fluorescein remaining in the conjunctival sac (a positive test) indicates probable normal drainage outflow. Most or all of the dye remaining in the conjunctival sac (a negative test) suggests a partial or complete nasolacrimal drainage system obstruction or failure of the lacrimal pump mechanism. It is important to prevent loss of tears onto the cheek, and the patient is instructed not to blot the eyes with tissue during the test. The test cannot distinguish between physiologic and anatomic causes of drainage dysfunction, nor can it localize the site of any mechanical blockage. It only indicates whether tear flow out of the fornix is relatively normal or delayed and therefore correlates with the history of epiphora. The dye disappearance test has been shown to be positive (normal outflow) in 95% of asymptomatic normal individuals and may be more sensitive than the primary Jones test discussed below. Unlike the latter, however, it does not appear to be dependent upon gross tear flow as measured by the Schirmer test.

In the face of a normal Schirmer test of basic and reflex tear response, the dye disappearance test can be a sensitive, though subjective, indicator of gross drainage. With a normally draining system, fluorescein should be almost gone within 5 minutes. Epiphora due to physiologic dysfunction or partial anatomic obstruction will show prolonged presence of dye in the conjunctival sac, whereas epiphora resulting from hypersecretion syndrome with normal drainage should yield normal or even rapid disappearance of dye. It is important to realize that the rate of dye clearance through the lacrimal system is strongly influenced by the pressure head from above. Even in the presence of decreased drainage function, a large volume of fluorescein augmented by increased reflex tear secretion from conjunctival irritation may result in an artifactually rapid dye disappearance. It is therefore important to administer this test under conditions as nearly physiologic as possible, with the patient in an upright position, blinking normally, and receiving only one drop of fluorescein. Increased voluntary blinking during the test can significantly shorten the test time and can allow the use of a reduced fluorescein concentration of 0.25% [30].

Primary Jones Dye Test

In 1961, Jones described a simple test of lacrimal drainage function that has become one of the most used procedures in the evaluation of epiphora [31]. The primary Jones dye test (Jones I) is a functional test and should be carried out in as nearly physiologic conditions as possible. The patient is tested while sitting upright and is asked to blink normally. Topical anesthetic is not used, although the clinician may anesthetize the nasal mucosa for comfort. Two percent fluorescein solution is instilled into the conjunctival sac. After 2 minutes and again after 5 minutes, a fine cotton-tipped applicator is introduced beneath the inferior turbinate to the level of the nasolacrimal ostium to recover any dye that passed down the lacrimal duct. Alternatively, the patient can blow their nose onto a clean tissue.

There is some confusion in the literature regarding what constitutes a positive and negative result. Some authors use positive to refer to dye reaching the nose (this was the original usage by Jones), while others use this designation to mean dye does not reach the nose. Here, we refer to the former and recommend recording the actual result. The Jones I test is considered positive if dye is recovered in the nose, and this indicates patent NLD anatomy and adequate physiological pump function. However, the dye may be very difficult to retrieve resulting in a high false-negative rate. Transit time for the dye to reach the nose is quite variable and shows a significant correlation with the Schirmer test. Even in normal individuals, passage of dye into the nose may take considerably longer than the 5 minutes allowed for the test. A 10-minute interval will result in a greater number of positive tests. In addition, the testing conditions can alter the results since transit time is influenced by factors such as blink rate, head position, gravity, and fluorescein volume. Tucker and Codère showed that the volume of fluorescein greatly influenced the transit time. In their study 44% of normal volunteers showed a transit time of ≥10 minutes with one drop and only 8% ≥10 minutes with multiple drops [32]. Hagele et al. showed that patient age was a significant factor in transit time [33]. In patients younger than 45 years of age, 91% passed dye to the nose in ≤6 minutes. In patients 45 years of age or older, 84% passed in ≤12 minutes.

Experience in placing the dye (drops vs. strips) and techniques for recovering dye from the nose also will influence the recovery rate. A positive test strongly suggests a patent drainage duct, since the dye passed down the nasolacrimal system under physiologic conditions. However, this does not completely rule out some physiological dysfunction or mild anatomic obstruction. More importantly, a negative test alone does not necessarily indicate abnormal drainage. Even in asymptomatic normal patients, the overall positive recovery rate is typically only in the range of 80–85% [34].

The fluorescein appearance test, described by Flach, is a modification of the primary Jones dye test [35]. This test was designed to avoid the difficulty and variability involved in recovering dye from the inferior nasal meatus. Two percent fluorescein is placed in the conjunctival sac, and the oropharynx is examined with ultraviolet light, beginning at 5 minutes and continuing up to 1 hour if necessary. With this technique, 90% of normal individuals show oropharyngeal fluorescence within 30 minutes and 100% within 60 minutes. This procedure can be employed in the event of a negative primary Jones test and can be performed 20–30 minutes later. Because of the persistence of fluorescence in the oropharynx, only one eye can be tested by this technique during a single office visit.

In 1973, Hornblass [36] elaborated on a variation of the primary Jones dye test originally mentioned by Lipsius [37]. In this version, 0.4 ml of 1% sterile solution of sodium saccharin is instilled into the conjunctival sac, and the patient is asked to report when they taste the solution. Hornblass found a mean transit time to the nose of 3.5 minutes, with 65% of normal individuals reporting a positive test within 6 minutes and 90% within 15 minutes. Transit times in excess of 15 minutes suggest partial nasolacrimal duct obstruction. The test depends on a subjective response from the patient, and before the patient can taste the solution, it must pass into the pharynx where threshold taste sensitivity is quite variable. Lipsius noted that 3% of normal individuals were incapable of tasting saccharin [37].

Secondary Jones Dye Test

A negative primary Jones dye test suggests delayed transit time through the lacrimal drainage system. However, it does not differentiate physiologic pump dysfunction from anatomic obstruction. The secondary Jones dye test (Jones II) is used to evaluate anatomic patency of the system in such cases (see Table 38.1). Residual fluorescein left from the primary test is irrigated from the conjunctival sac, and topical anesthetic is instilled. The patient sits with the head tilted slightly forward while clear saline is irrigated into one canaliculus through a cannula. The patient is instructed to blow or spit out any fluid that passes into the nose or pharynx onto a clean tissue. The passage of any fluid into the nose indicates gross anatomic patency of the nasolacrimal system. In this situation, complete obstruction is not present since saline did traverse the system under increased hydrostatic pressure. Dye in the recovered fluid demonstrates normal punctal and canalicular anatomy, since the dye must have passed freely into the lacrimal sac during the previous Jones I test. However, such a result does not rule out a partial anatomic block at the level of the lower sac or duct.

If the secondary Jones test is positive, but there is resistance to irrigation and some dye-stained fluid regurgitates from the puncta, then there likely is a partial block in the distal system at the lower sac or duct. Remember that even in a normal system, retrograde flow out of the puncta may be seen with excessive injection pressures.

Recovery of clear saline in the nose without any fluorescein suggests punctal or canalicular stenosis or pump failure, where dye from the primary Jones test did not enter the lacrimal sac. If irrigated fluid does not reach the nose at all, but regurgitates from the puncta, a high-grade NLD obstruction is likely that cannot be overcome with increased hydrostatic pressure. Punctal regurgitation of dye-stained fluid suggests blockage at the level of the lower sac or duct, with residual dye in the sac being flushed out by the irrigation. Regurgitation of clear saline from the opposite punctum suggests obstruction at the level of the distal common canaliculus or upper sac with no residual dye from the primary Jones test. When clear saline regurgitates from the same punctum that is being irrigated, without flow from the opposite punctum, a proximal obstruction in that canaliculus is likely.

During the irrigation of saline, distension of the lacrimal sac may rarely be seen, suggestive of lower nasolacrimal duct obstruction. Under such conditions, a palpable sac without fluid passing into the nose suggests complete nasolacrimal duct blockage, whereas a palpable sac with fluid passing into the nose implies a partial obstruction. A sac that is contracted and fibrotic because of chronic inflammation will not dilate under these conditions.

Probing

If the secondary Jones test indicates canalicular obstruction, the canaliculus in question should be probed gently to the lacrimal sac with a small Bowman probe. First, the punctum is dilated if necessary by pulling the lid laterally to prevent canalicular kinking and inserting a dilator. The distance of the stenosis or blockage from the punctum is noted in millimeters by measuring directly on the probe. In most individuals, a short common canaliculus is present 6–9 mm from the puncta. Probing is more sensitive for canalicular stenosis or obstruction than any imaging technique, but the canalicular system should not be probed without prior indication of possible obstruction because of the risk of inadvertent injury and subsequent fibrosis.

Diagnostic Imaging

In most cases, the diagnosis and etiology of epiphora are relatively simple and straightforward with careful clinical examination and tests as discussed above.

Even with these tests, the status of the lacrimal drainage system and the precise location of any obstruction may not be obvious. In these cases, and where epiphora persists following appropriate surgery, imaging studies may be useful. In a 2010 survey of members of the American Society of Ophthalmic Plastic and Reconstructive Surgery, less than 5% of respondents used any form of lacrimal imaging for most patients with epiphora and relied upon the clinical evaluation alone [38]. When imaging was used, computed tomography (CT) and dacryocystography (DCG) were the most common.

While a number of imaging modalities and variations have been described, the major techniques in common usage are dacryocystography, dacryoscintigraphy, computed tomography, magnetic resonance imaging, and diagnostic ultrasound.

Contrast Dacryocystography

The first attempt to visualize the lacrimal drainage system radiographically was made by Ewing in 1909 [39]. He used bismuth paste for retrograde filling of the nasolacrimal duct, but such early attempts proved unsatisfactory. The technique was used infrequently until the introduction of better aqueous contrast media such as Sinografin and Angiografin and especially the low-viscosity iodized oils such as Pantopaque, Ethiodol, and ultrafluid Lipiodol. In a standard dacryocystography (DCG) study, the canaliculi are intubated with catheters. Contrast material is injected into the lower canaliculus on each side, and films are taken immediately in Caldwell's posteroanterior frontal projection and in both lateral projections. Repeat films are obtained at 5 minutes and again at 15 minutes. DCG can also be combined with CT or MR imaging to give further information on the nasolacrimal system.

In 1968, Iba and Hanafee described the technique of distension dacryocystography, first used by Barrie Jones in

1959 [40]. Here images are recorded during injection of 0.5–1.0 ml of contrast material so that the lacrimal system is seen in a distended state. Injection is accomplished through the placement of canalicular indwelling tapered Teflon catheters or IV catheter tubing, and both sides are studied simultaneously. This method provides maximum visualization of the anatomic structure of the system and, because of the back pressure, gives good filling of the canaliculi. It is the best technique for demonstration of fistulae, diverticula, supernumerary canaliculi, and the presence of concretions or lacrimal sac tumors. However, it does not reveal accurate sac and duct dimensions under normal physiologic conditions. This test also requires either an ophthalmologist or a skilled technician to be in the radiology suite to inject the contrast material.

Improved imaging was achieved with a technique adopted from subtraction angiography that eliminates confusing bony shadows (Fig. 38.11). A scout film is taken before injecting contrast material and is used to produce bone-free images of the dacryocystogram. More sophisticated computer-assisted digital subtraction images can be produced using fluoroscopically controlled angiographic equipment and an image intensifier [40, 41]. Saleh showed that DCG was comparable to syringing in the detection of NLD obstruction (88% vs. 84%) but that DCG was better in delineating details such as dacryoliths, fistulae, and malpositions at the sac-duct junction [42].

The dacryocystogram of a normal lacrimal drainage system will usually show the canaliculi when less viscous aqueous contrast media are used [43]. The lacrimal sac appears as a smooth narrow structure to the sac-duct junction. The duct widens at the level of the bony rim, and its inner surface becomes more irregular because of the presence of mucosal folds. Such folds may be exceptionally well developed in younger patients. Further constrictions are seen in the midportion of the duct, in the region of Hytle's and Taillefers' valves. Finally, in its lower third, the duct widens again.

Visualization of the nasolacrimal system by DCG reveals considerable variation in the structure of the sac and duct among normal individuals. Atypical areas of narrowing and widening, as well as unusual angulations and diverticula, may all be seen in the absence of clinical symptoms.

A combination of subtraction, distension, and macrodacryocystography provides the best visualization of the anatomic structure of the lacrimal drainage system. This approach will provide accurate localization of any anatomic obstruction in the majority of cases. Imaging of the canaliculi with dye failing to pass into the sac or duct implies obstruction at the common canaliculus. A blockage at the sac-duct junction usually results in a dilated sac with no contrast material reaching the duct or nose, even on late films (Fig. 38.12). Obstruction at the level of the lower nasolacrimal duct will show dilatation of the sac, and contrast material in the duct, but not reaching the nose. A patent dacryocystorhinostomy ostium is easily demonstrated by passage of contrast into the nose at the level of the middle meatus. Demonstration of patent lacrimal passages by DCG in the face of epiphora suggests physiological dysfunction or a mild incomplete anatomic block.

Although DCG, with or without dynamic phase extension or digital subtraction, remains important for diagnostic imaging of lacrimal obstruction, it still has not become a routine diagnostic test. In most cases, a careful clinical examination with dye disappearance and Jones tests will determine functional from anatomic abnormalities and will give precise localization of any obstruction. For cases where clinical

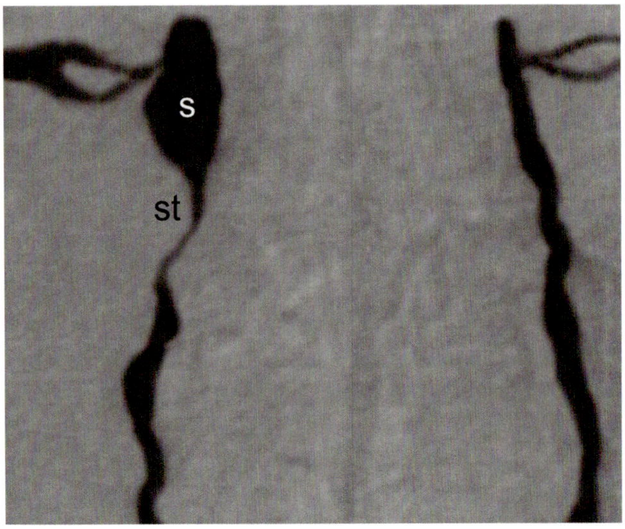

Fig. 38.11 Dacryocystography with normal drainage on the left, but stenosis (st) on the right with dilatation of the lacrimal sac (s)

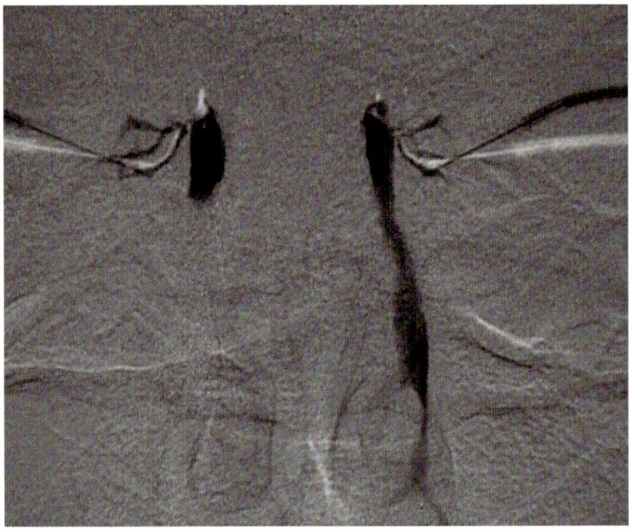

Fig. 38.12 Dacryocystography with complete blockage of the lower lacrimal sac on the right side

evaluation is equivocal, however, the DCG is considered the gold standard for imaging of the nasolacrimal system. It does not allow for imaging of the soft tissue or bony structures surrounding the nasolacrimal sac or duct, but it can be combined with CT or MR studies to get a complete picture of the nasolacrimal system and the surrounding anatomy.

In a recent study, Lee et al. used fluoroscopic dacryocystography to evaluate dynamic changes in lacrimal drainage system anatomy during the blink cycle [4]. This study showed that with eyelid closure the canaliculi contract while the lacrimal sac dilates, both contributing to the pump mechanism. This has expanded to our knowledge of lacrimal physiology under normal conditions and may add to an understanding of proximal system pathology.

Dacryoscintigraphy

The first use of radionuclide tracer to image the lacrimal drainage system was by Bozoky and Korchmaros, who used radioactive Au^{198} (gold) and measured the buildup of activity over the sac and duct [44]. Rossomondo et al. [45] introduced the first modern nuclear imaging technique for a more physiological assessment of the tear flow. They instilled a drop of saline with [99mTc] sodium pertechnetate and imaged the system with a gamma camera. In the first clinical evaluation of the technique, Carlton et al. [46] demonstrated its value in visualizing the lacrimal system and in measuring some physiological parameters of tear flow. In their study of 28 asymptomatic volunteers, they recorded a transit time of 4–43 seconds for tracer to reach the level of the lacrimal sac and 4–323 seconds to reach the nose. Since dacryoscintigraphy is a physiologic test, it is very sensitive in localizing the site of anatomic blockage as well as finding abnormalities in patients with physiologic pump dysfunction [47, 48]. A high correlation has been shown between symptomatic epiphora and quantitative lacrimal scintigraphic measures of tracer flow times [49].

Dacryoscintigraphy is not a first-line diagnostic test. The procedure is mostly indicated for patients with epiphora who, on clinical evaluation with Jones I and II tests, show patency of the lacrimal drainage system and no other obvious cause for their symptoms. Epiphora in the face of an apparently patent drainage system to irrigation is the result of either partial nasolacrimal system obstruction or to a physiologic delay in drainage from lacrimal pump failure.

The technique commonly employed today uses [99mTc] sodium pertechnetate in saline or technetium sulfur colloid delivered as a 10 μl drop placed into the lateral conjunctival sac by micropipette. The patient is positioned in front of the pinhole collimator of a gamma camera and is instructed to blink normally. The nasolacrimal system is imaged every 10 seconds for the first 2–3 minutes. Late images are obtained every 5 minutes thereafter for a total of 20 minutes (Fig. 38.13). The specific activity of this dose is in the range of 50–150 μCi and results in radiation exposure to the lens of less than 2% of that for a complete contrast dacryocystogram [45, 50].

Dacryoscintigraphy does not provide the same detailed anatomic visualization available with contrast DCG. In standard nuclear studies, the proximal canalicular system is poorly imaged unless dilated. The lacrimal sac and duct are usually nicely outlined [2]. Complete or partial obstructions of the drainage system are seen, with a sensitivity of better than 90% [51]. The precise site of obstruction is difficult to determine with scintigraphy alone, but the approximate level, such as presac, preduct, or intraduct, can often be determined [49]. Generation of dynamic activity curves for specific

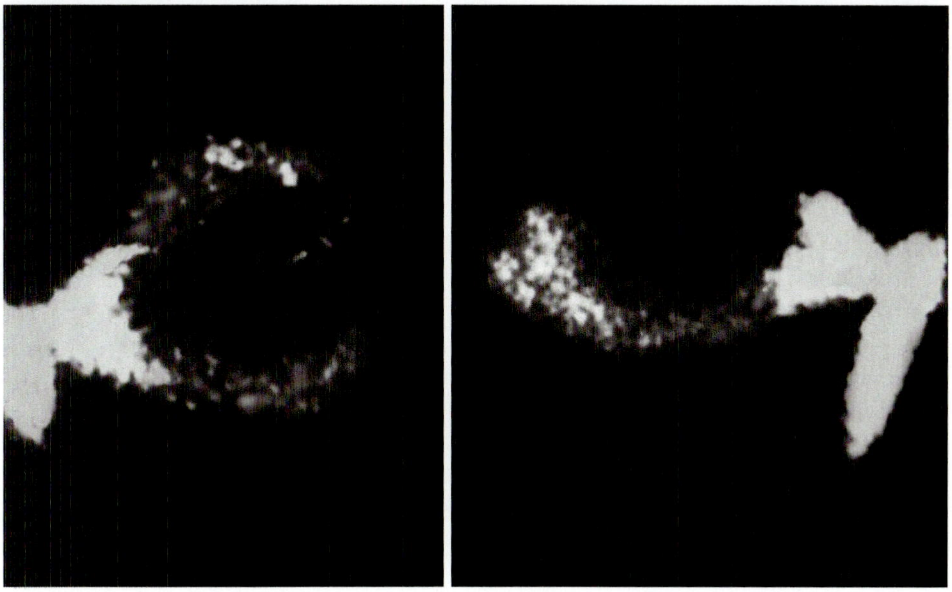

Fig. 38.13 Dacryoscintigraphy showing normal canalicular and upper lacrimal sac flow on the right side and superior canalicular obstruction on the left side

regions of interest will demonstrate incomplete anatomic obstructions as well as rather subtle degrees of functional impairment [50, 52]. This technique is the most accurate and reproducible for the lacrimal sac and upper duct.

In asymptomatic normal volunteers, dacryoscintigraphy may show abnormalities in up to 40% of individuals, with 25–32% showing no tracer reaching the nose [50, 52]. This correlates with the observation that 15–35% of asymptomatic individuals will be negative on the Jones I test. Presumably, these individuals have subclinical abnormalities that delay drainage.

In most cases, dacryoscintigraphy is evaluated by visual analysis based on the times taken for tracer to reach the lacrimal sac, duct, and nose. The site of obstruction is identified by gross inspection [53]. Wearne et al. identified three areas of obstruction: presac delay defined as blockage at the medial canthus, preduct delay where the sac fills with tracer but none passes to the duct, and intraduct delay where tracer gets into the upper duct but not beyond [48].

Transit times are measured as the time to attain maximum counts in regions of interest within the drainage system. Unfortunately, there is little agreement of normal and abnormal parameters for this test. Hurwitz et al. [54] gave mean values as 5.2 minutes to the lacrimal sac and 11.2 minutes to the lacrimal duct. Peter and Pearson, on the other hand, argued that transit time was delayed if it was ≥2 minutes to the sac, ≥3 minutes to the duct, and ≥6 minutes to the nose [55].

Quantitative dacryoscintigraphy attempts to provide better objective data on tear flow by using radioactive half-times and transit times [46, 54]. Following a standard instillation of tracer, dynamic time-activity curves are constructed for each area of interest. Transit times are calculated as the time at which maximal counts are present in the sac, duct, and nose. Numerous different techniques have been elaborated [47, 50, 52, 54], but in general these are rather complex and rarely used in routine clinical practice.

In addition to initial clinical evaluation of epiphora, dacryoscintigraphy can be useful in evaluating persistent epiphora following dacryocystorhinostomy surgery [56]. It can show the status of the surgical ostium and demonstrate partial or complete obstructions or decreased tear transit at the presac or sac level.

Computed Tomography

In selected cases computed tomography (CT) of the lacrimal system can be useful in the evaluation of epiphora [57]. This is especially helpful when patency of the lacrimal system is uncertain and when dacryolith or tumor is suspected [58]. This technique also allows evaluation of surrounding tissues in cases of trauma or anatomic variants that may complicate planned surgery [59].

Axial scans through the lower orbit will show the lacrimal sac fossa as a depression in the anteromedial orbital wall (Fig. 38.14a). In successively lower sections, the lacrimal duct appears as a round to oval defect in the frontal process of the maxillary bone at the anteromedial corner of the maxillary sinus (Fig. 38.14b). The duct may be filled with air or fluid. Traced inferiorly, the duct opens beneath the inferior nasal turbinate. Cross sections of the system are seen on coronal images since the line of section is oriented downward and obliquely

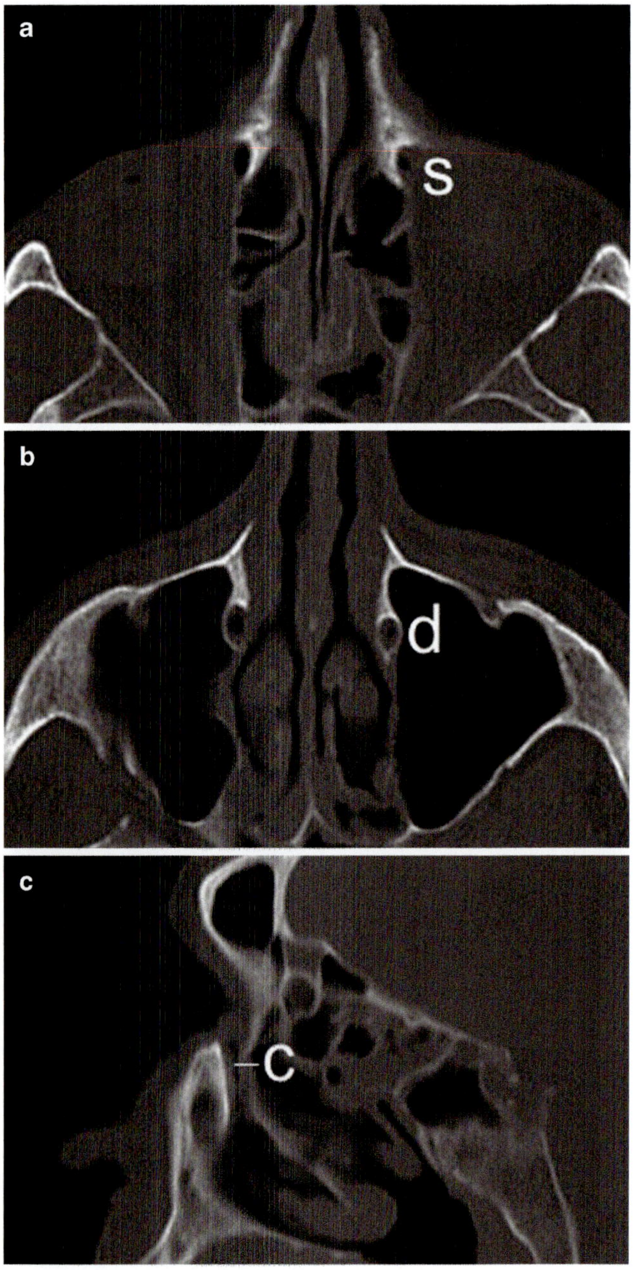

Fig. 38.14 Bone window CT. (**a**) Axial section through the lacrimal sac fossae (s), (**b**) axial section through the lacrimal ducts (d) as they approach the inferior meatus, (**c**) sagittal section showing the lacrimal canal (c) in longitudinal section

backward. Sagittal images can sometimes reveal the entire length of the system in longitudinal section (Fig. 38.14c).

Dilatation of the lacrimal sac from dacryocystitis can easily be seen on CT (Fig. 38.15). The modality is also useful in detecting lacrimal sac mucoceles and fistulae (Fig. 38.16) and can sometimes show concretions within the sac and duct. Extrinsic lesions such as tumors, sinusitis, and nasal polyps that can cause tear drainage dysfunction may also be visualized [60]. When epiphora follows trauma, and subsequent clinical studies indicate nasolacrimal duct obstruction, CT dacryocystography may reveal facial fractures compressing the sac or duct [61]. CT imaging can distinguish a dacryocystocele from sinonasal tumors [62]. In most cases of suspected malignancy, especially if there is a history of bloody epiphora or pain, CT may demonstrate a soft tissue mass in the sac or in the adjacent paranasal sinuses (Fig. 38.17). In cases of congenital lacrimal amniocele, CT will reveal the dilated sac and duct, often associated with bony changes (Fig. 38.18). It is essential to differentiate this soft, near-midline dilated lacrimal conduit from a meningocele. MRI is more sensitive for soft tissue abnormalities but does not image the bony structures well.

When combined with dacryocystography, three-dimensional CT (3-D CT-DCG) is excellent at identifying bony structures around the nasolacrimal system. Using modern spiral CT techniques with topical or injected contrast material, the surgeon can identify obstructions in the nasolacrimal system [58, 63, 64]. This can especially be useful in patients that have had facial trauma, prior sinus or lacrimal surgery, or tumors of the medial canthus [4]. Newer techniques utilizing spiral CT and 3D reconstruction technology

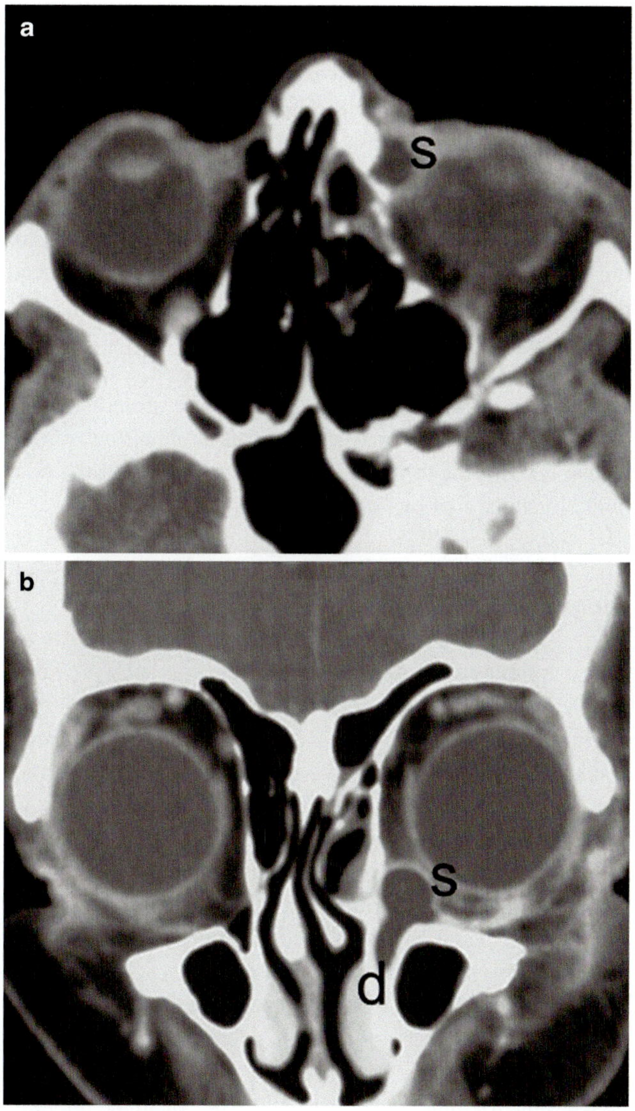

Fig. 38.15 Tissue window CT showing dacryocystitis. (**a**) Axial section through the dilated lacrimal sac (s), (**b**) coronal section showing the dilated sac (s) and upper duct (d)

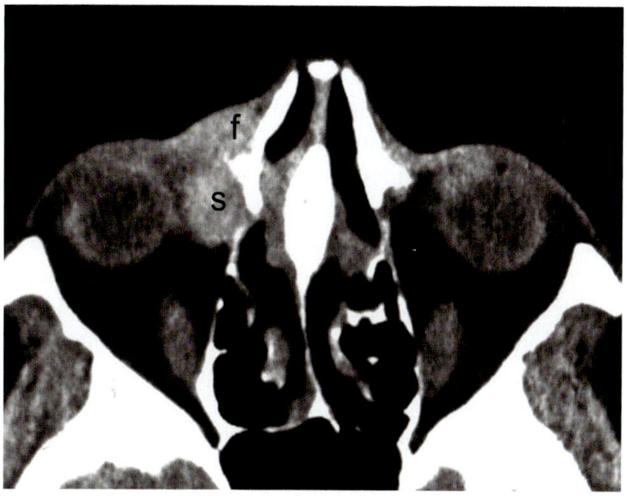

Fig. 38.16 Axial CT scan with dacryocystitis (s) and an anteriorly draining fistula (f)

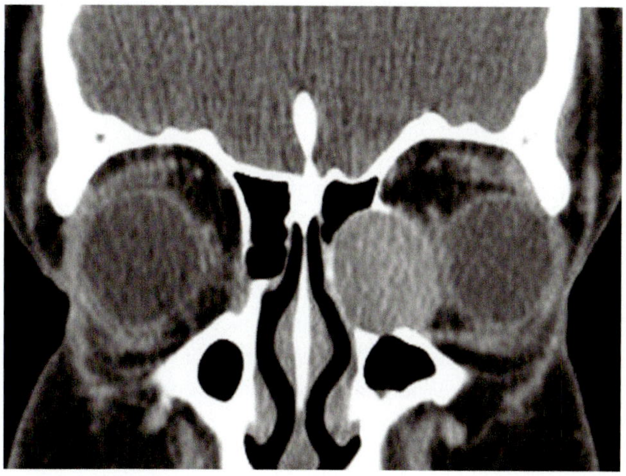

Fig. 38.17 Coronal tissue window CT showing a transitional cell carcinoma of the left lacrimal sac

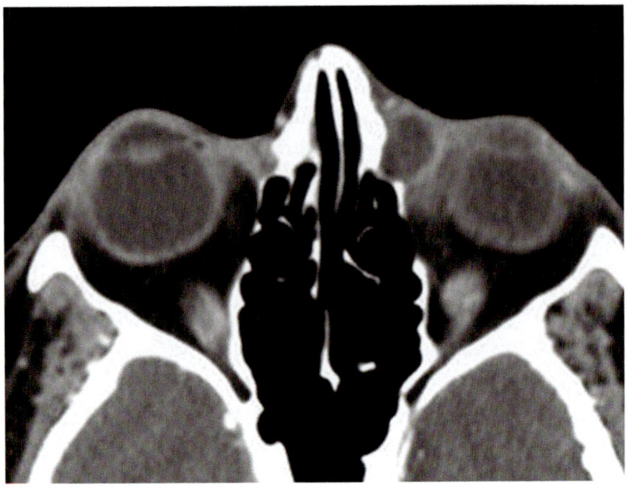

Fig. 38.18 Congenital lacrimal amniocele on the right side. (Courtesy of Dr. Rona Silkiss)

have improved the diagnostic accuracy in patients with partial obstructions of the nasolacrimal system by allowing the surgeon to view a 3D rotational image of the entire system from multiple projections [41].

Cone-beam computed tomography is a newer technology that utilizes a C-arm angiography system that rotates around the patient to produce high-resolution 3D images with computer reconstructions in axial, coronal, and sagittal planes. The technique allows the simultaneous assessment of the nasolacrimal duct together with its surrounding soft tissue and bony structures [59].

There are some disadvantages to CT scan. As mentioned previously it is not the best study for evaluating soft tissue masses of the nasolacrimal system. Also, in standard CT the sequences are presented as a series of axial images that make identification of small obstructions difficult. Longitudinal and oblique images can be created, but this reconstruction results in decreased spatial resolution in the reformatted images. The exposure to ionizing radiation is also more than for standard DCG and is less appropriate for young children.

Magnetic Resonance Imaging

Since 1990 dynamic magnetic resonance imaging dacryocystography (dMRI-DCG) has been used as an adjunctive diagnostic test in the evaluation of lacrimal system pathology that allows for excellent resolution of the nasolacrimal system [65–68]. When combined with a contrast agent, 3D MRI offers several advantages over other imaging techniques [67]. Gadolinium, given as a topical solution diluted from 1:10 to 1:100 with normal saline, is administered one drop to each eye per minute for 5 minutes. The patient stays in an upright position until just prior to image acquisition. Because the lacrimal system is not cannulated and therefore not under increased hydrostatic pressure, this study gives a picture of the functional status of the nasolacrimal system. There have been no reports of ocular complications from the administration of topical gadolinium, and this obviates the need to risk damage to puncta from the direct injection of contrast agents.

dMRI-DCG has a very high correlation with the gold-standard contrast DCG in detecting NLD obstruction. It has a sensitivity of 94% and a specificity of 100% in detecting a dilated sac [69]. MRI also allows high-resolution evaluation of soft tissue structures within and surrounding the nasolacrimal drainage system [69–73]. The superficial location of the drainage system facilitates imaging with small surface coils that can give a spatial resolution of $0.3 \times 0.3 \times 3$ mm or better [68]. Manipulation of signal intensities, repetition times, and tip angles, as well as the use of fat suppression algorithms, can often allow for differentiation of mucous or blood from solid neoplasms. Because of volumetric acquisition, MRI images can be viewed in any plane without degradation of the image quality. This is a key advantage over CT-DCG, which requires reformatting of out-of-plane images that results in degradation of image resolution. Coronal images are superior for determining the distal extent of contrast transit, and axial images are excellent for examining the lumen of the nasolacrimal duct and intraductal pathology.

Although MRI can be a useful diagnostic study, it is expensive and therefore is not routinely used. Other drawbacks include poor ability to image bony structures, and there can be artifact from the nearby ethmoid air cells. MRI is also susceptible to movement artifact because of the relatively long acquisition times required.

Diagnostic Ultrasonography

The techniques of A- and B-mode ultrasonography provide a simple and noninvasive method for evaluating the normal lacrimal sac and duct (Fig. 38.19) [74]. Using ultrasonic visualization Pavlidis was able to demonstrate the contributions of the medial orbicularis muscle, canaliculi, medial canthal tendon, and upper lacrimal sac to blinking and to the lacrimal pump mechanism [75]. Using ultrasound biomicroscopy (UBM), Al-Faky demonstrated high-resolution images of reduced or absent fluid turbulence in the lacrimal sac in patients with facial nerve palsy [76].

Echography has also proved useful in the evaluation of gross anatomic lacrimal system abnormalities [77–79]. Physiological dysfunction cannot be evaluated, nor can the precise site of anatomic obstruction be localized in most cases. However, a dilated lacrimal sac can easily be distinguished from one of normal dimensions (Fig. 38.20). It is also possible to differentiate air from mucus or solid masses, making the identification of lacrimal sac neoplasms possible [80]. Lacrimal sac concretions can be visualized with ultrasound (Fig. 38.21), and these may occur in 6–7% of patients with NLD obstruction [81].

With the B-mode probe placed in the medial canthus, oriented vertically and aimed toward the lacrimal sac fossa, an oblique longitudinal cross section of the lacrimal sac and upper duct is obtained. Although the canaliculi cannot typically be imaged, Tost et al. reported visualization of the canaliculi with intracanalicular injection of sodium hyaluronate [82]. The diameter of the sac and upper duct may be estimated and the thickness of the walls appreciated [83]. Diverticuli may also be identified (Fig. 38.22), and a variety of echogenic densities within the system such as inflammatory membranes and tumors can be detected. The position and size of a surgically created ostium may also be imaged with this technique (Fig. 38.23), although its patency cannot easily be evaluated [55].

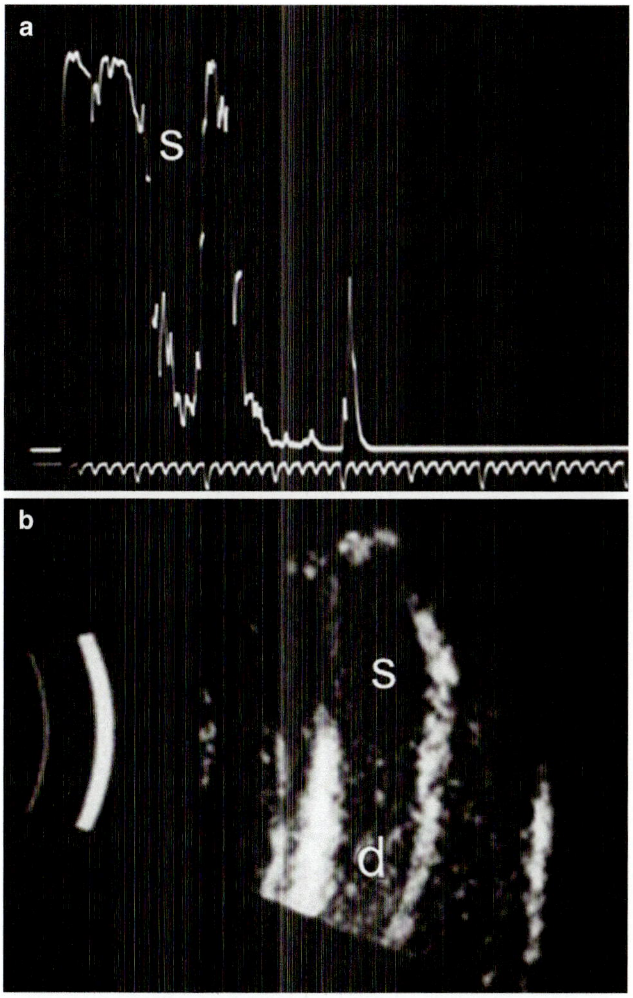

Fig. 38.19 Ultrasonography of the normal lacrimal drainage system. (**a**) Standardized A-scan showing the relatively echolucent lacrimal sac (s), (**b**) B-scan showing the lacrimal sac (s), and duct (d)

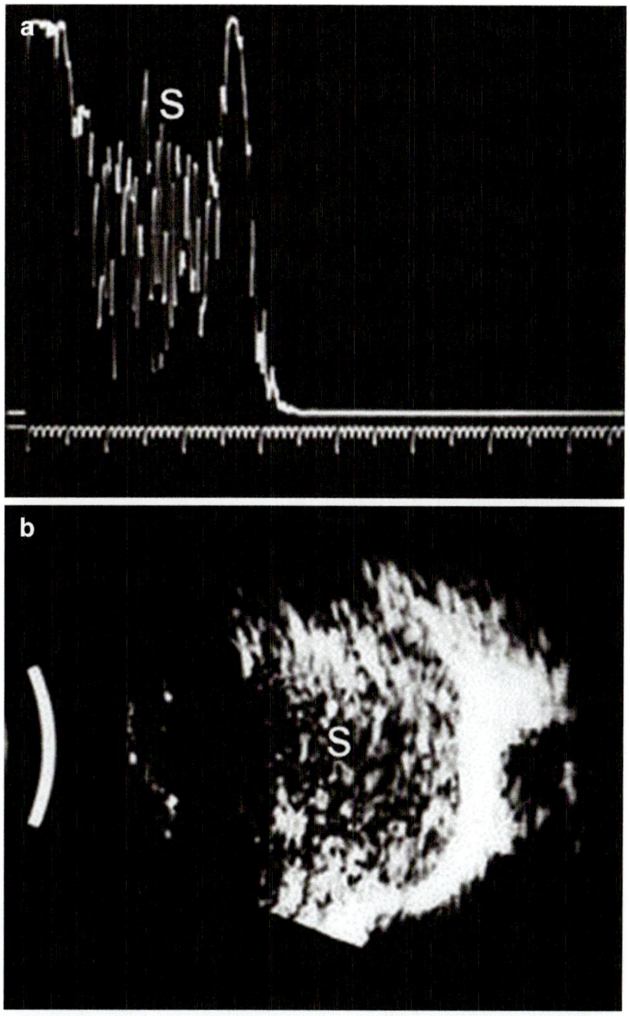

Fig. 38.20 Ultrasonography of dacryocystitis showing a dilated lacrimal sac with mucoid debris (s). (**a**) Standardized A-scan, (**b**) B-scan

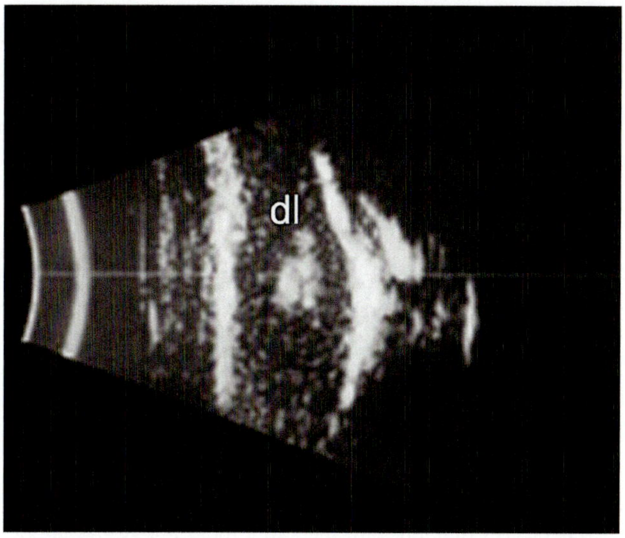

Fig. 38.21 B-scan echogram showing a slightly dilated lacrimal sac with a dense central echo representing a dacryolith (dl)

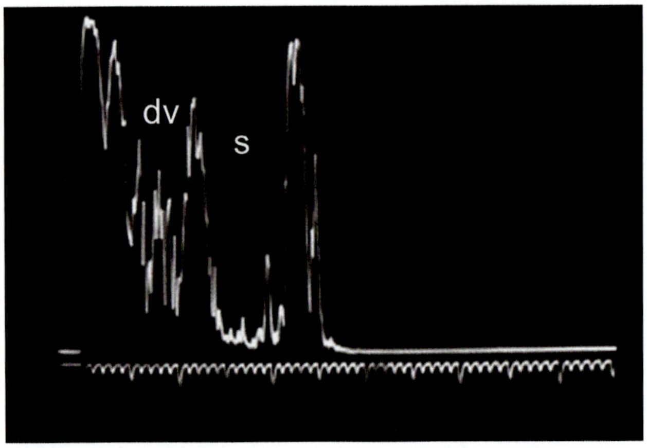

Fig. 38.22 A-scan echogram of dacryocystitis with a dilated lacrimal sac (s) and an anterior diverticulum (d)

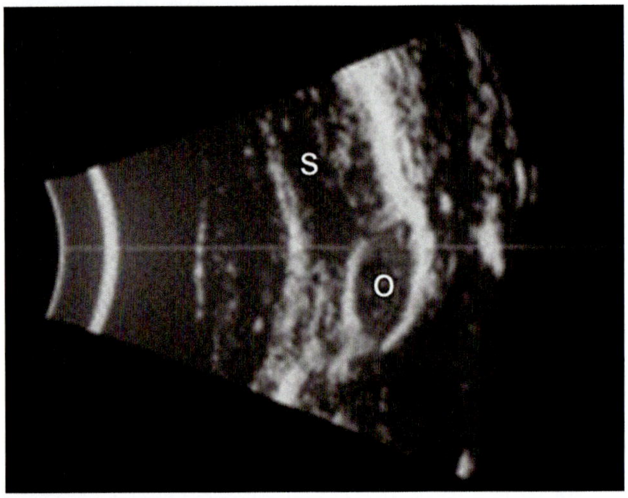

Fig. 38.23 B-scan echogram showing the lacrimal sac (s) and a postsurgically created DCR ostium (o)

For precise measurements of the sac and evaluation of the internal reflectivity of the sac contents, A-mode scanning is used. The A-probe is first oriented as for a paraocular orbital study but with the beam aimed just behind the anterior lacrimal crest toward the sac fossa so that an oblique anterolateral-posteromedial transit of the sac is obtained. If the sac is filled with air, it appears as an echolucent defect bounded by sharply defined vertical anterior and posterior sac walls [77]. Often, the presence of dilated diverticula can be detected. Mucus in the sac produces uniform, homogeneous, low-density internal echoes, and inflammatory exudates and membranes show higher, more irregular echoes. Multiple strongly echogenic irregular echoes with irregularity of the sac walls suggest a sac tumor. A transocular A-mode image of the sac is obtained with the probe held above the lateral canthus and directed toward the lacrimal sac fossa through the eye. This technique gives an approximate horizontal cross section of the sac. The average dimensions of the sac in normal individuals are 2.5 mm (SD = 0.95 mm) in horizontal diameter and 4.0 mm (SD = 1.49 mm) in anteroposterior extent. A sac more than 4.5 mm wide or 7.0 mm deep should be considered abnormally dilated.

References

1. Dutton JJ. Atlas of clinical and surgical orbital anatomy. London: Elsevier; 2011. p. 165–74.
2. Olver J. Colour atlas of lacrimal surgery. Oxford: Butterworth Heinemann; 2002. p. 1–28.
3. Dutton JJ. Diagnostic tests and imaging techniques. In: Linberg JV, editor. Lacrimal surgery. New York: Churchill Livingstone; 1988. p. 19–48.
4. Lee MJ, Kyung HS, Han MH, et al. Evaluation of lacrimal tear drainage mechanism using dynamic fluoroscopic dacryocystography. Ophthal Plast Reconstr Surg. 2011;27:164–7.
5. Becker BB. Tricompartment model of the lacrimal pump mechanism. Ophthalmology. 1992;99:1139–45.
6. Yen MT, Pflugfelder SC, Feuer WJ. The effect of punctal occlusion on tear production, tear clearance, and ocular surface sensation in normal subjects. Am J Ophthalmol. 2001;131:314–23.
7. Dutton JJ. Clinical evaluation and imaging of lacrimal drainage obstruction. In: Cohen AJ, Mercandetti M, Brazzo B, editors. The lacrimal system. 2nd ed. Heidelberg: Springer; 2015. p. 75–94.
8. Mimura T, Usul T, Yamamoto H, et al. Conjunctivochalasis and contact lenses. Am J Ophthalmol. 2009;148:20–2.
9. Mimura T, Yamagami S, Usul T, et al. Changes of conjunctivochalasis with age in a hospital-based study. Am J Ophthalmol. 2009;147:171–7.
10. Li QS, Zhang XR, Zou HD, et al. Epidemiologic study of conjunctivochalasis in populations equal or over 60 years old in Caoyangxincun community of Shanhai. Zhonghua Yan Ke Za Zhi. 2009;45:793–8.
11. Figueira EC, Boustred N, Wilcsek GA. Epiphora in the presence of a simulated mucocele secondary to nasal polyposis in a patient with samter triad. Ophthal Plast Reconstr Surg. 2008;24:160–2.
12. Wesley RE. Inferior turbinate fracture in the treatment of congenital nasolacrimal duct obstruction and congenital nasolacrimal duct anomaly. Ophthalmic Surg. 1985;16:368–71.
13. Migliori ME, Putterman AM. Silicone intubation for the treatment of congenital lacrimal duct obstruction: successful results removing the tubes after six weeks. Ophthalmology. 1988;95:792–5.
14. Attarzadeh A, Saijadi M, Owji N, et al. Inferior turbinate fracture and congenital nasolacrimal duct obstruction. Eur J Ophthalmol. 2006;16:520–4.
15. Knijnik D. Tearing and eyelid laxity with no ectropion: is tarsal strip always effective? Arq Bras Oftalmol. 2006;69:37–9.
16. Narayanan K, Barnes EA. Epiphora with eyelid laxity. Orbit. 2005;24:201–3.
17. Vick VL, Holds JB, Hartstein ME, Massry GG. Tarsal strip procedure for the correction of tearing. Ophthal Plast Reconstr Surg. 2004;20:37–9.
18. Bukhari A. Prevalence of punctal stenosis among ophthalmology patients. Middle East Afr J Ophthalmol. 2009;16:85–7.
19. Billing K, Karagiannis A, Selva D. Punctal-canalicular stenosis associated with mitomycin-C for corneal epithelial dysplasia. Am J Ophthalmol. 2003;136:746–7.
20. Eiseman AS, Flanagan JC, Brooks AB, et al. Ocular surface, ocular adnexal, and lacrimal complications associated with the use of systemic 5-fluorouracil. Ophthal Plast Reconstr Surg. 2003;19:216–24.

21. Esmaeli B, Valero V, Ahmani MA, Booser D. Canalicular stenosis secondary to docetaxel (taxotere): a newly recognized side effect. Ophthalmology. 2001;108:994–5.
22. Kashkouli MB, Pakdel F, Hashemi M, et al. Comparing anatomical pattern of topical anti-glaucoma medications associated lacrimal obstructions with a control group. Orbit. 2010;29:65–9.
23. Kamal S, Ali MJ, Gupta A, Naik MN. Lacrimal and nasal masquerades of congenital nasolacrimal duct obstructions: etiology, management, and outcomes. Int Ophthalmol. 2015;35:807–10.
24. Beigi B, Uddin JM, McMillan TF, Linardos E. Inaccuracy of diagnosis in a cohort of patients on the waiting list for dacryocystorhinostomy when the diagnosis was made by only syringing the lacrimal system. Eur J Ophthalmol. 2007;17:485–9.
25. Burkat CN, Lucarelli MJ. Tear meniscus level as an indicator of nasolacrimal obstruction. Ophthalmology. 2005;112:344–8.
26. Karampatakis V, Karamitsos A, Skriapa A, Pastiadis G. Comparison between normal values of 2- and 5-minutes Schirmer test without anesthesia. Cornea. 2010;29:497–501.
27. Zappia RJ, Milder B. Lacrimal drainage function. The fluorescein dye disappearance test. Am J Ophthalmol. 1972;74:160–2.
28. Roh JH, Chi MJ. Efficacy of dye disappearance test and tear meniscus height in diagnosis and postoperative assessment of nasolacrimal duct obstruction. Acta Ophthalmol. 2010;88:e73–7.
29. Kashkouli MB, Mirzajani H, Jamshidian-Tehrani M, et al. Reliability of fluorescein dye disappearance test in assessment of adults with nasolacrimal duct obstruction. Ophthal Plast Reconstr Surg. 2013;29:167–9.
30. Kim C, Lee MJ, Khwarg SI. Voluntary blinking and use of 0.25% dye on fluorescein dye disappearance test. Can J Ophthalmol. 2013;48:99–103.
31. Jones LT. An anatomical approach to problems of the eyelids and lacrimal apparatus. Arch Ophthalmol. 1961;66:111–24.
32. Tucker NA, Codère F. The effect of fluorescein volume on lacrimal outflow transit time. Ophthal Plast Reconstr Surg. 1994;10:256–9.
33. Hagele JE, Guzek JP, Shavlik GW. Lacrimal testing. Age as a factor in Jones testing. Ophthalmology. 1994;101:612–7.
34. Wright MM, Bersani TA, Frueh BR, Musch DC. Efficacy of the primary dye test. Ophthalmology. 1989;96:481–3.
35. Flach A. The fluorescein appearance test for lacrimal obstruction. Ann Ophthalmol. 1979;11:237–42.
36. Hornblass A. A simple taste test for lacrimal obstruction. Arch Ophthalmol. 1973;90:435–6.
37. Lipsius EI. Sodium saccharin for testing the patency of the lacrimal passages. Am J Ophthalmol. 1957;43:114–5.
38. Nagi KS, Meyer DR. Utilization patterns for diagnostic imaging in the evaluation of epiphora due to lacrimal obstruction: a national survey. Ophthal Plast Reconstr Surg. 2010;26:168–71.
39. Ewing AE. Roentgen ray demonstration of the lacrimal abscess cavity. Am J Ophthalmol. 1909;24:1.
40. Iba GB, Hanafee WN. Distention dacryocystography. Radiology. 1968;90:1020–2.
41. Galloway JE, Kavic TA, Raflo GT. Digital subtraction macrodacryocystography. Ophthalmology. 1984;91:956–62.
42. Saleh GM, Gauba V, Tsangaris P, Tharmaseelan K. Digital subtraction dacryocystography and syringing in the management of epiphora. Orbit. 2007;26:249–53.
43. Malik SRK, Gupta AK, Chaterjee S, et al. Dacryocystography of normal and pathological lacrimal passages. Br J Ophthalmol. 1969;53:174–9.
44. Bozoky L, Korchmaros I. Über die Untersuchung der Tranenableitung mittels radioaktiver Isotope. Zbl Ges Ophthalmol. 1967;87:185.
45. Rossomondo RM, Carlton WH, Trueblood JH, et al. A new method of evaluating lacrimal drainage. Arch Ophthalmol. 1972;88:523–5.
46. Carlton WH, Trueblood JH, Rossomondo RM. Clinical evaluation of microscintigraphy of the lacrimal drainage apparatus. J Nucl Med. 1973;14:89–92.
47. Jager PL, Mansour K, Vrakkink-de Zoete H, et al. Clinical value of dacryoscintigraphy using a simplified analysis. Graefes Arch Clin Exp Ophthalmol. 2005;243:1134–40.
48. Wearne MJ, Pitts J, Frank J, et al. Comparison of dacryocystography and lacrimal scintigraphy in the diagnosis of functional nasolacrimal duct obstruction. Br J Ophthalmol. 1999;83:1032–5.
49. Jabbour J, Van der Wall H, Katelaris L, et al. Quantitative lacrimal scintigraphy in the assessment of epiphora. Clin Nucl Med. 2008;33:535–41.
50. Amanat LA, Hilditch TE, Kwok CS, et al. Lacrimal scintigraphy II. Its role in the diagnosis of epiphora. Br J Ophthalmol. 1983;67:720–8.
51. Fard-Esfahani A, Tari AS, Saghari M, et al. Assessment of the accuracy of lacrimal scintigraphy based on a prospective analysis of patients' symptomatology. Orbit. 2008;27:237–41.
52. Hilditch TE, Kwok CS, Amanat LA. Lacrimal scintigraphy I. Compartmental analysis of data. Br J Ophthalmol. 1983;67:713–9.
53. Sagili S, Selva D, Malhotra R. Lacrimal scintigraphy: "interpretation more art than science". Orbit. 2012;31:77–85.
54. Hurwitz JJ, Maisey MN, Welham RA. Quantitative lacrimal scintillography. I. Method and physiological application. Br J Ophthalmol. 1975;59:308–12.
55. Peter NM, Pearson AR. Comparison of dacryocystorhinostomy and lacrimal scintigraphy in the investigation of epiphora in patients with patent but nonfunctioning lacrimal systems. Ophthal Plast Reconstr Surg. 2009;25:201–5.
56. Palaniswamy SS, Subramanyam P. Dacryoscintigraphy: an effective tool in the evaluation of postoperative epiphora. Nucl Med Commun. 2012;33:262–7.
57. Freitag S, Woog JJ, Kousoubris PD, Curtin HD. Helical computed tomography dacryocystography with three-dimensional reconstruction. Ophthal Plast Reconstr Surg. 2002;18:121–32.
58. Bonnet F, Ducasse A, Marcus C, Hoeffel C. CT dacryocystography: normal findings and pathology. J Radiol. 2009;90:1685–93.
59. Wilhelm KE, Rudorf H, Greschus S, et al. Cone-beam computed tomography (CBCT) dacryocystography for imaging of the nasolacrimal duct system. Clin Neuroradiol. 2009;19:283–91.
60. Frances IC, Kappagoda MB, Cole IE, Bank L, Dunn GD. Computed tomography of the lacrimal drainage system: retrospective study of 107 cases of dacryostenosis. Ophthal Plast Reconstr Surg. 1999;15:217–26.
61. Glatt HJ. Evaluation of lacrimal obstruction secondary to facial fractures using computed tomography or computed tomographic dacryocystography. Ophthal Plast Reconstr Surg. 1996;12:284–93.
62. Debnam JM, Esmaeli B, Ginsberg LE. Imaging characteristics of dacryocystocele diagnosed after surgery for sinonasal cancer. Am J Neuroradiol. 2007;28:1872–5.
63. Udhay P, Noronha OV, Mohan RE. Helical computed tomographic dacryocystography and its role in the diagnosis and management of lacrimal drainage system blocks and medial canthal masses. Indian J Ophthalmol. 2008;56:31–7.
64. Ashenhurst M, Jaffer N, Hurwitz JJ, et al. Combined computed tomography and dacryocystography for complex lacrimal problems. Can J Ophthalmol. 1991;26:27–31.
65. Amrith S, Goh PS, Wang SC. Tear flow dynamics in the human nasolacrimal ducts – a pilot study using dynamic magnetic resonance imaging. Graefes Arch Clin Exp Ophthalmol. 2005;243:127–31.
66. Goldberg RA, Heinz GW, Chiu L. Gadolinium magnetic resonance imaging dacryocystography. Am J Ophthalmol. 1993;115:738–41.
67. Karagulle T, Erden A, Erden I, et al. Nasolacrimal system: evaluation with gadolinium-enhanced MR dacryocystography with a three-dimensional fast spoiled gradient recalled technique. Eur Radiol. 2002;12:2343–8.

68. Rubin PA, Bilyk JR, Shore JW, et al. Magnetic resonance imaging of the lacrimal drainage system. Ophthalmology. 1994;101:235–43.
69. Cubuk R, Tasali N, Aydin S, Saydam B, Sengor T. Dynamic MR dacryocystography in patients with epiphora. Eur J Radiol. 2010;73:230–3.
70. Hoffmann KT, Anders N, Hosten N, et al. High resolution functional magnetic resonance tomography with Gd-DTPA eye drops in diagnosis of lacrimal apparatus diseases. Ophthalmologe. 1998;95:542–8.
71. Kirchhof K, Hähnel S, Jansen O, et al. Gadolinium-enhanced magnetic resonance dacryocystography in patients with epiphora. J Comput Assist Tomogr. 2000;24:327–31.
72. Manfrè L, de Maria M, Todaro E, et al. MR dacryocystography: comparison with dacryocystography and CT dacryocystography. Am J Neuroradiol. 2000;21:1145–50.
73. Weber AL, Rodrigues-De Velasquez A, Lucarelli MJ, Cheng HM. Normal anatomy of the lacrimal sac and duct: evaluated by dacryocystography, computed tomography and MR imaging. Neuroimaging Clin N Am. 1996;6:199–217.
74. Al-Faky YH. Anatomic utility of ultrasound biomicroscopy in the lacrimal drainage system. Br J Ophthalmol. 2011;95:1446–50.
75. Pavlidis M, Stupp T, Grenzebach U, et al. Ultrasonic visualization of the effect of blinking on the lacrimal pump mechanism. Graefes Arch Clin Exp Ophthalmol. 2005;243:228–34.
76. Al-Faky YH. Physiological utility of ultrasound biomicroscopy in the lacrimal drainage system. Br J Ophthalmol. 2013;97:1325–9.
77. Dutton JJ. Standardized echography in the diagnosis of lacrimal drainage dysfunction. Arch Ophthalmol. 1989;107:1010–2.
78. Rochels R, Lieb W, Nover A. Echographic diagnosis in diseases of the efferent tear ducts. Klin Monatsbl Augenheilkd. 1984;185:243–9.
79. Stupp T, Pavidis M, Busse H, Thanos S. Presurgical and postsurgical ultrasound assessment of lacrimal drainage dysfunction. Am J Ophthalmol. 2004;138:764–71.
80. Montanara A, Mannino G, Contestabile M. Macrodacryocystography and echography in diagnosis of disorders of the lacrimal pathways. Surv Ophthalmol. 1983;28:33–41.
81. Repp DJ, Burkat CN, Lucarelli MJ. Lacrimal excretory system concretions: canalicular and lacrimal sac. Ophthalmology. 2009;116:2230–5.
82. Tost F, Bruder R, Clemens S. 20-MHz ultrasound of presaccular lacrimal ducts. Ophthalmologe. 2002;99:25–8.
83. Tobias S, Pavlidis M, Busse H, Thanos S. Presurgical and postsurgical assessment of lacrimal drainage dysfunction. Am J Ophthalmol. 2004;138:764–71.

Punctal Disorders, Malpositions, and Management

39

Moisés Enghelberg and Cat Nguyen Burkat

The anatomical position of the lacrimal punctum is paramount for proper functioning of the lacrimal excretory system. The superior and inferior lacrimal puncta, although simple in appearance, do have a complex organization. A relatively avascular fibrous ring surrounds the opening and produces a mild elevation called the lacrimal papillae. The muscle of Riolan encircles the cuff of the puncta as well, aiding in the lacrimal pump mechanism [1]. The average in vivo external opening of the punctum approximates 646 μm. The inferior, or lower eyelid, punctum tends to be displaced more laterally than the superior, or upper eyelid, punctum from the medial canthus due to early facial growth. Proper apposition of the puncta to the globe and its corresponding tear lake is necessary for adequate tear drainage [2].

Patency of both puncta is required to provide optimal tear drainage. Studies that examined the relationship between tear drainage via occlusion of the upper or lower puncta demonstrated similar tear outflow behavior by occluding either the upper or lower punctum [3].

Evaluation

The proper position of the punctum is best examined using the slit-lamp biomicroscope, assessing adequate posterior rotation toward the globe so that the punctum is apposed to the tear lake, as well as to evaluate for patency, irregular slit configuration, or multiple puncta. Instillation of fluorescein dye and consequently its disappearance is an important step in determining the patency of the puncta and overall function of the lacrimal drainage system. The practitioner may also ask the patient to close their eyes to evaluate for proper movement of the punctum during the dynamic state. Examination should also include measurement of the tear lake under biomicroscopy, which is seen as the height of the tear fluid that rests above the lower lid margin, best measured with a straight short slit beam. The lower tear meniscus height tends be on average 0.1–0.2 mm in height. Measurements above 0.4 mm by the clinician may prompt a diagnosis of underdrainage (excretory system blockage) or tear oversecretion. The practitioner may also attempt to express the punctum to gauge resistance to flow and to evaluate for tear reflux [4, 5].

Punctal Disorders

Congenital Causes

Agenesis of the lacrimal puncta is a relatively rare condition in which the puncta do not develop in the newborn. Punctal agenesis is usually associated with the absence of underlying canalicular tissue. When both puncta are absent, careful exploration of the internal opening of the common canaliculus is to be performed during surgical dissection. If no canalicular tissue can be identified intraoperatively, a conjunctivodacryocystorhinostomy with insertion of a Jones tube is indicated [1, 6].

Congenital stenosis is a rare condition in which the puncta do not cannulate in their entirety, leading to stenosis. This condition can also be related to the exuberant development of the lacrimal ampullae surrounding the puncta. The condition tends to be benign with patent and well-developed lacrimal canaliculi and nasolacrimal ducts. Patients may present with epiphora. The affected punctum can be opened by using a punctal dilator, a snip punctoplasty, or in severe cases, a canalicular cutdown with temporary placement of a monoka monocanalicular stent [1, 7].

M. Enghelberg
Department of Ophthalmology, Larkin Community Hospital, South Miami, FL, USA

C. N. Burkat (✉)
Department of Ophthalmology and Visual Sciences, University of Wisconsin-Madison, Madison, WI, USA
e-mail: cburkat@wisc.edu

A. J. Cohen, C. N. Burkat (eds.), *Oculofacial, Orbital, and Lacrimal Surgery*, https://doi.org/10.1007/978-3-030-14092-2_39

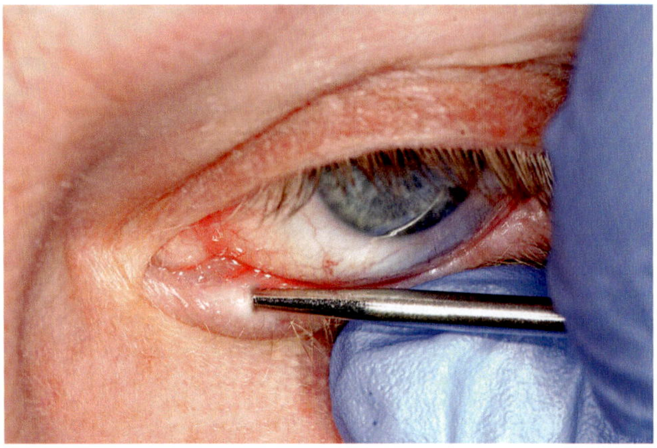

Fig. 39.1 Punctal dilator used to enlarge a stenosed or occluded punctum

Imperforate punctum or punctal atresia is a congenital condition in which a fine overlying membrane covers the punctum, secondary to failure of the epithelial bud to open at the punctum. The membranous cover tends to be comprised of fine orbicularis muscle, which typically covers the eyelids while in utero and aids during canalization of the lacrimal system. The membrane can also be due to conjunctival tissue that failed to perforate. Interestingly, the upper and lower puncta tend to not be imperforate at the same time given that the upper and lower eyelids have a separate embryological origin. The upper eyelid is derived from the frontal nasal process, while the lower eyelid is derived as an extension of the maxillary process. This condition is easily managed by canalizing the punctum with a fine punctal dilator (Fig. 39.1). Patients tend to respond well to treatment [8–10].

Supernumerary (or accessory) punctum is an underreported congenital anomaly, in which there is more than one lacrimal punctum. These anomalies are thought to arise from incomplete separation of the epithelial core or by failure of canalization between the conjunctival sac and the nasal cavity. Epiphora or excessive tearing has been documented in patients with accessory puncta, although some patients are asymptomatic. Accessory puncta are typically located on the lower eyelid medial to the normal punctum with a slit-like appearance (Fig. 39.2) [8–10].

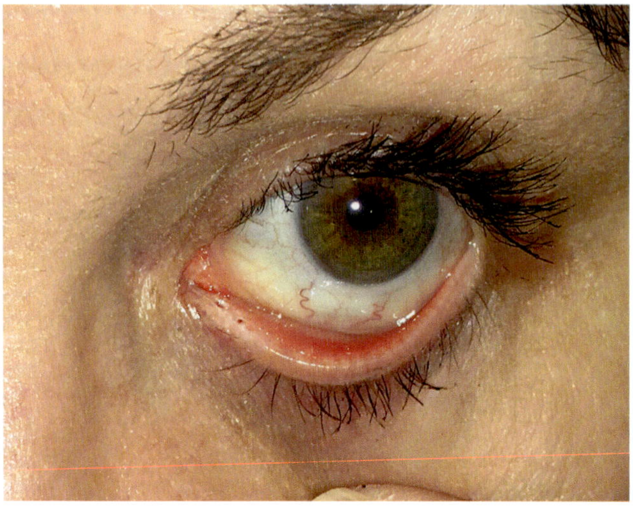

Fig. 39.2 Supernumerary, or accessory, puncta are typically located on the lower eyelid medial to the normal punctum (left lower eyelid)

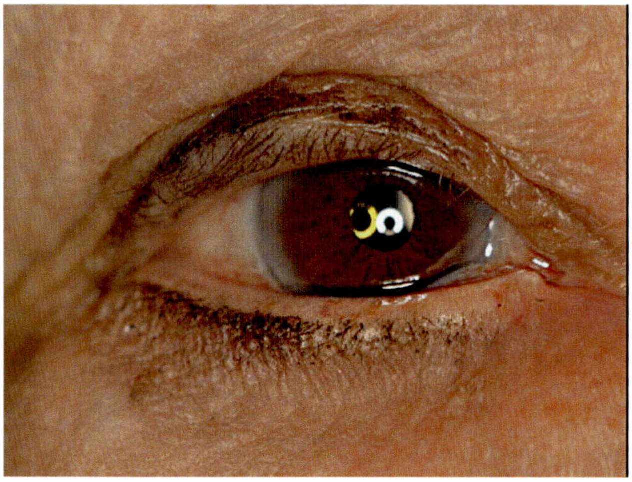

Fig. 39.3 Conjunctivochalasis resting over the punctum, right lower eyelid

Acquired Causes

Punctal stenosis tends to present in patients with chronic ocular dryness, environmental allergies, or patients on long-term ocular antihypertensive drops. It has also been reported in patients with chronic blepharitis, likely due to chronic inflammation. Elderly patients and females have been reported to have an increased incidence of this condition, and punctal stenosis has also been reported as a side effect after some chemotherapeutic agents that are excreted in the tear film. Changes in the composition of the tear film can alter the puncta by inducing an inflammatory state to the peri-punctal tissues. Pervasive ocular dryness can potentially also lead to atrophy of the puncta and subsequent stenosis. These patients often complain of tearing, however, due to increased reflex tear secretion. Punctal stenosis can be resolved by addressing the underlying dry eye state, and performing dilation with a punctal dilator, or a three-snip punctoplasty to create a greater opening for tear drainage [7]. Restenosis may occasionally recur and require repeat treatment.

Conjunctivochalasis can potentially impede appropriate tear drainage through the puncta, by essentially creating a mechanical valve that blocks the punctal opening. Elastotic degeneration of the conjunctiva increases its laxity, potentially making it redundant and floppy. The degenerated conjunctiva can interfere with the architecture of the tear meniscus and distort the tear film, making it difficult for tears to reach the puncta. Conjunctival prolapse can also mechanically obstruct the punctal orifice (Fig. 39.3), leading to symptoms of epiphora. If other causes of tearing have been explored and ruled out, and significant conjunctivochalasis has been identified as the source of tearing, patients can successfully undergo medial conjunctival resection or thermocautery of the redundant tissue [11].

Iatrogenic Causes

Punctal plugs and cautery can also lead to lacrimal outflow issues. Indwelling permanent silicone plugs tend to present a higher complication rate than collagen punctal plugs, which dissolve weeks to months after insertion. Epiphora, mattering, discharge, crusting eyelids, and canaliculitis are the most common complications of punctal plugs. Canaliculitis presents with pouting of the puncta, erythema of the punctum, and medial eyelid margin overlying the canaliculus, tenderness, and purulent discharge (Fig. 39.4). Purulence can often be expressed from the puncta. The characteristic focal swelling is located at the punctum and medial canalicular eyelid margin, in contrast to the inferonasal swelling in the medial canthus overlying the lacrimal sac in dacryocystitis. Definitive treatment of canaliculitis often entails canalicular curettage, canaliculotomy to remove retained plugs or dacryoliths, and consideration of silicone intubation or antibiotic drops or irrigation. If a retained punctal plug is suspected to be more distal in the lacrimal sac or duct, a dacryocystorhinostomy (DCR) with silicone intubation may be necessary to remove the plug and/or treat the obstruction.

Punctal cautery is another iatrogenic cause of punctal occlusion (Fig. 39.5a–c). This technique is commonly used to treat chronic dry eyes, such as in those not tolerant to punctal plugs. In some patients, the puncta may need to be re-dilated due to intolerance to the procedure with secondary epiphora, an inflammatory tear film, or tear oversecretion given deficiency in the mucinous or lipid layer of the tear film. The punctal opening can be reestablished though a three-snip punctoplasty technique or canaliculotomy in the office or operating room [11].

Slit punctum can also be an iatrogenic or congenital abnormality of the punctum. It often occurs in the setting of silicone bicanalicular intubation that may have been secured too tightly, such that the tube pulls through the canalicular eyelid margin and elongates the punctal opening into a slit configuration (Fig. 39.6). A slit-like punctum may also result from an overly aggressive snip punctoplasty. Tearing and lacrimal outflow issues may ensue, due to an excessively large opening that affects the lacrimal pump mechanism. In some cases, the slit punctum may need to be sutured smaller into a round orifice.

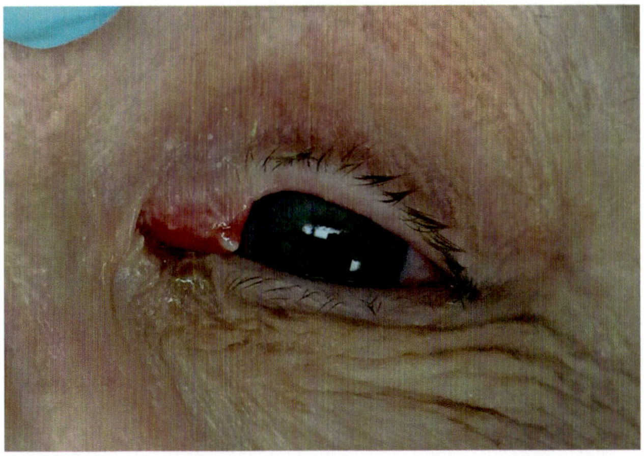

Fig. 39.4 Canaliculitis and pouting swollen punctum of the left upper eyelid

Punctal Malpositions

Congenital Causes

Centurion syndrome is an anomaly which consists of an anterior displacement of the anterior limb of the medial canthal tendon and a prominent nasal bridge. This results in punctal malposition away from the globe and displacement of the lacrimal punctum out of the tear lake. Centurion syndrome is one of the few causes of primary punctal malposition. Patients tend to present with symptoms consistent with epiphora, as well as an increased tear lake. Surgical correction may include medial spindle conjunctivoplasty to rotate the punctum toward the ocular surface, or posterior repositioning of the medial canthal tendon in severe cases [12].

Acquired Causes

Punctal ectropion most often occurs secondary to involutional changes of the tarsoligamentous attachments of the eyelid that become lax. Cicatricial punctal ectropion can also arise secondary to a shortening of the anterior lamella (skin and/or muscle layer), such as seen after eyelid thermal or chemical burns (Fig. 39.7), aggressive skin blepharoplasty, laser resurfacing, chronic dermatitis, ichthyosis (Fig. 39.8), or chronic solar changes. Paralysis or weakness of the orbicularis oculi muscle following a stroke or degenerative systemic condition, such as Guillain-Barre syndrome, Bell's palsy, or myasthenia gravis, may lead to paralytic ectropion of the punctum. Weakness of the orbicularis oculi muscle leaves the lower eyelid retractors unopposed in their action, thus increasing the eyelid eversion. Involutional punctal ectropion typically requires a medial spindle conjunctivo-

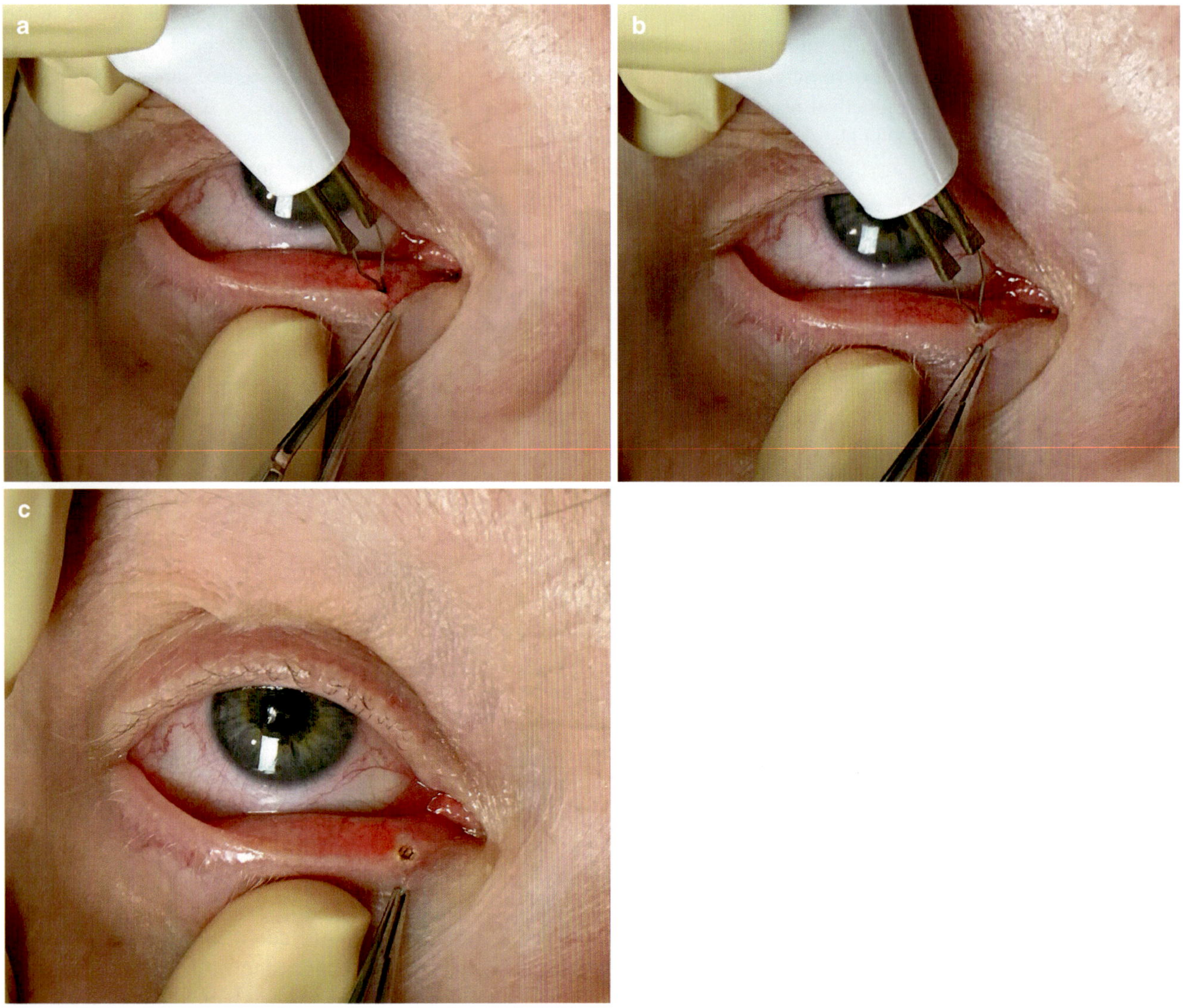

Fig. 39.5 Iatrogenic punctal occlusion by cauterization of the punctum: (**a**) low temperature cautery tip inserted into punctum, (**b**) short bursts to cauterize punctum, (**c**) punctum thermally occluded

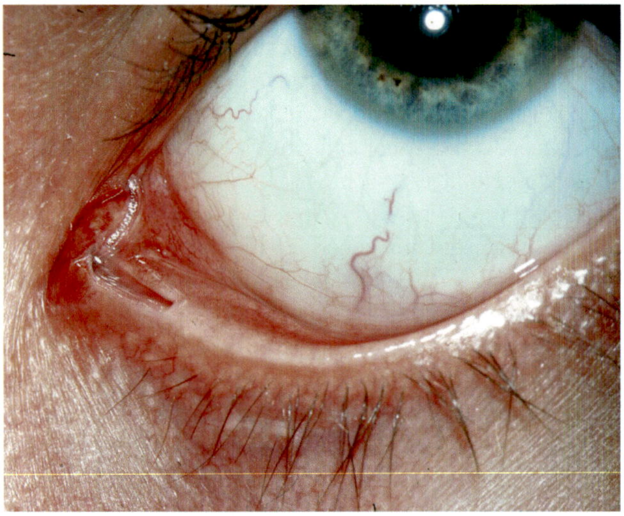

Fig. 39.6 Slit punctum, left lower eyelid, due to tight silicone intubation in the medial canthus

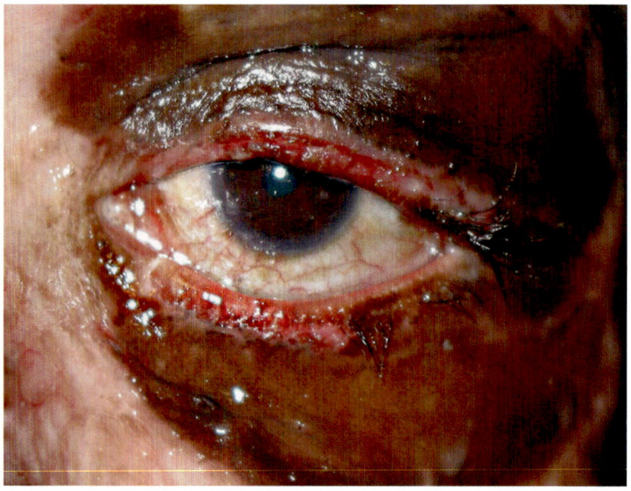

Fig. 39.7 Cicatricial punctal ectropion secondary to extensive thermal burn to the face

plasty procedure, but if significant horizontal eyelid laxity is present, a horizontal eyelid tightening procedure is necessary, such as a lateral tarsal strip procedure or wedge resection. Cicatricial punctal ectropion may often require release of anterior lamellar cicatrix, with placement of a full-thickness skin graft to elongate the skin surface for optimal punctal correction. Paralytic etiologies may require medial canthoplasty, tightening/repositioning of the medial canthal tendon, or even medial tarsorrhaphy [11].

Punctal apposition syndrome, also known as "kissing puncta," is a relatively underreported condition in which the puncta are in contact at any given time apart from the active blinking cycle. This contact acts as a mechanical obstruction to the puncta and thus the drainage system. Patients tend to present with epiphora or plerolacrima. It is important to evaluate the upper eyelid position, as some cases of "kissing puncta" are secondary to upper eyelid ptosis, with the droopy upper eyelid touching and blocking the inferior punctum (Fig. 39.9a). This condition is generally managed by either a levator resection/advancement surgery to elevate the upper eyelid if eyelid ptosis is present or by horizontal tightening of the lower eyelid, such as with a lateral tarsal strip procedure. Horizontal tightening can be simulated during the office evaluation, observing for correction of the kissing puncta when the lateral tension distracts the punctum away from the upper punctum (Fig. 39.9b).

Floppy eyelid syndrome, also regarded as upper eyelid ectropion, is a condition associated with a variety of comorbidities such as keratoconus, obesity, and sleep apnea, although patients can be of normal body habitus as well. Patients present with severely increased rubbery laxity of the upper eyelid which displaces the upper lacrimal punctum, as well as papillary conjunctivitis, eyelash ptosis, and eyelid mattering (Fig. 39.10a, b). The increased eyelid laxity may lead to corneal epithelial erosions, spontaneous nocturnal eyelid eversion, and tearing. While managing this condition, it is important to address the underlying comorbidities and prompt referral to an internist, and a sleep medi-

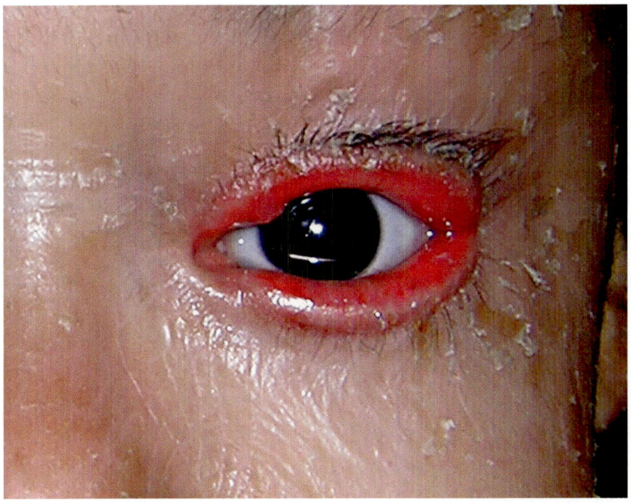

Fig. 39.8 Cicatricial eyelid and punctal ectropion due to ichthyosis causing anterior lamellar shortage

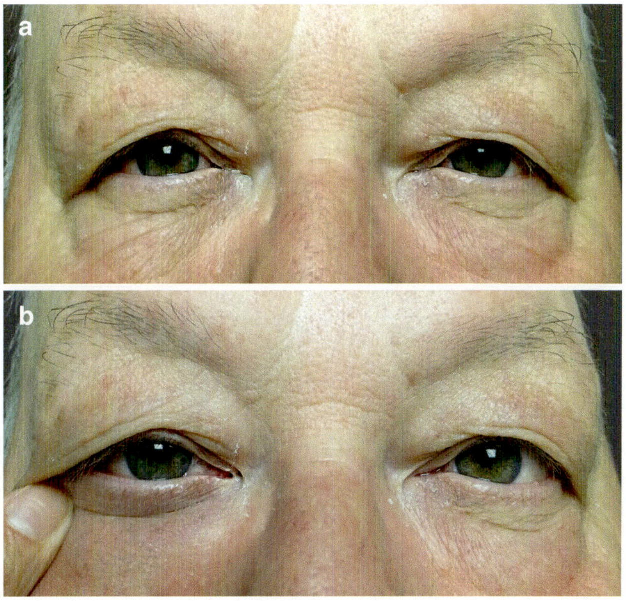

Fig. 39.9 Bilateral punctal apposition syndrome, or "kissing puncta," with upper eyelid ptosis (**a**). Simulated lateral tightening resolves the punctal apposition, indicating that a horizontal tightening procedure is necessary (**b**)

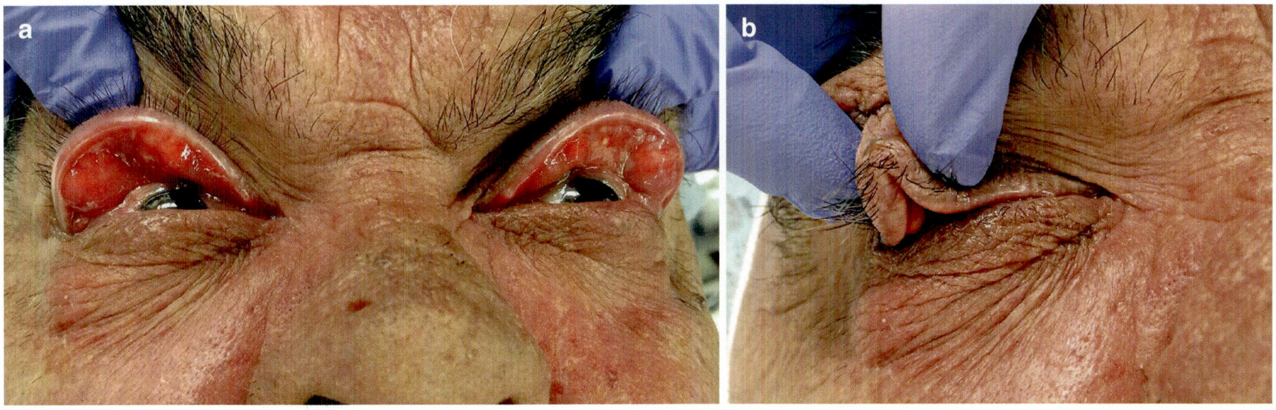

Fig. 39.10 Bilateral floppy eyelid syndrome with easily everted and horizontally lax upper eyelids (**a**, **b**)

cine specialist is recommended. When addressing this malposition, surgical management involves performing a tarsal strip procedure or full-thickness eyelid wedge resection, with many variations reported in the literature, and canthoplasty. This combination leads to reformation of the lateral canthal angle while fixing the upper eyelid and punctum into a more stable position in relation to the ocular surface (Fig. 39.11) [13, 14]. Recurrences are not uncommon and may require additional surgery. Patients should also be educated to avoid sleeping on the face and to consider wearing an eye shield at night to minimize rubbing or nocturnal eyelid eversion.

Surgical Management

Medial spindle conjunctivoplasty is performed to invert the punctum back toward the ocular surface and tear lake. If an ectropic punctum corrects with horizontal tightening, as evaluated in the office, then a lateral tarsal strip procedure may be sufficient (Fig. 39.12a, b). However, if the punctum remains ectropic despite horizontal pull, then a medial spindle conjunctivoplasty is indicated. Typically, sharp scissors are used to excise a diamond of conjunctiva and lower eyelid retractors just below the inferior border of tarsus at the level of the punctum. A small piece of the retractors must be included in this excision. The superior apex of the diamond should be immediately below the lacrimal ampulla, which is approximately 3–4 mm below the punctum at the eyelid margin. The incision is closed with chromic catgut or polyglactin 5-0 or 6-0 double-armed sutures. The cut edge of the white retractor band immediately anterior to the forniceal conjunctiva is first grasped with forceps and pulled superiorly (Fig. 39.13). Each arm of the suture is first passed through the white inferior retractor layer, passing posteriorly to anteriorly, with the two needle passes approximately 3 mm apart (Fig. 39.14a). Each arm is then passed through the inferior tarsal edge, exiting out on the tarsal conjunctival side (Fig. 39.14b). The sutures are then passed back through the conjunctival surface of the inferior incision edge (Fig. 39.14c) and directed anteriorly full-thickness through the retractors, septum, orbicularis muscle, and skin. Both arms of the suture exit the skin approximately 6 mm inferior to the punctum and approximately 2–4 mm apart from each other (Fig. 39.14d). The ends are tied on the skin, thus rotating the punctum inward (Fig. 39.15) [15]. Other variations of this technique have included using multiple buried sutures to reattach the inferior retractor band to the inferior tarsus, without passing externally through the skin.

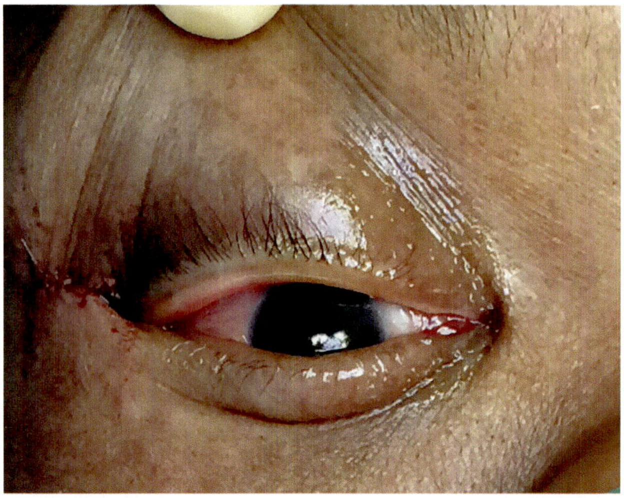

Fig. 39.11 Improved eyelid distraction after surgical resection of lateral redundant floppy upper eyelid and canthopexy

Lateral tarsal strip involves performing a canthotomy and inferior or superior cantholysis to release the appropriate lateral canthal tendon limb. The tarsal strip is created by dividing the lateral eyelid at the gray line, splitting the eyelids into the anterior and posterior lamella. The length

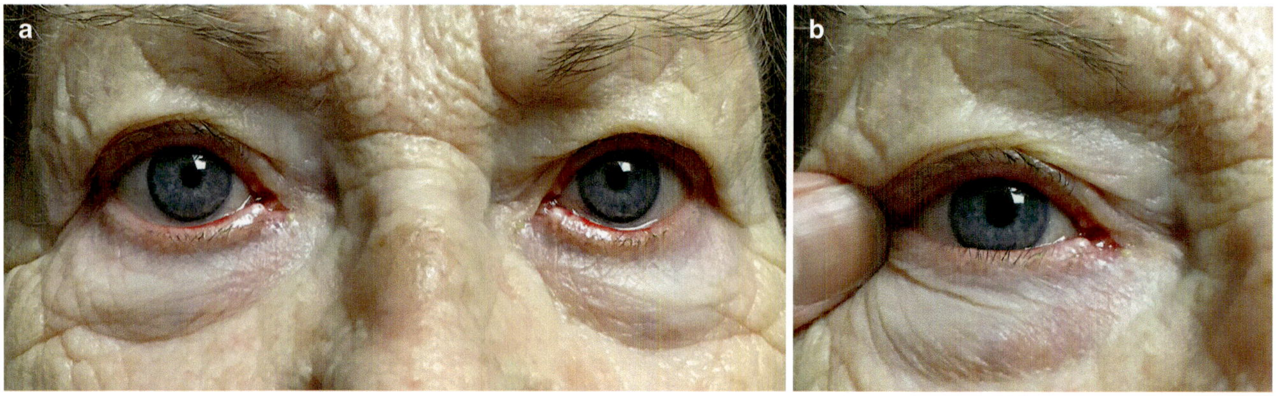

Fig. 39.12 Right lower eyelid punctal ectropion (**a**) corrects with lateral horizontal tightening on examination (**b**), suggesting that medial spindle conjunctivoplasty is not needed

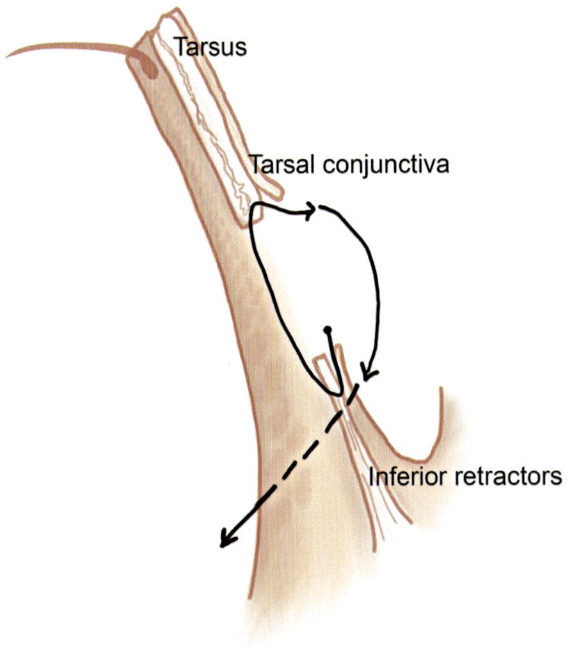

Fig. 39.13 Schematic of the medial spindle conjunctivoplasty technique to correct punctal ectropion. Double-armed sutures are typically passed several millimeters apart

of the tarsal strip created is dependent on the laxity of the eyelid, and thus how much the eyelid needs to be shortened. If significant eyelid laxity is present, a portion of the excess lateral eyelid and tarsus can be excised. Avoid aggressive shortening the tarsal strip as this may result in lower eyelid retraction once reattached to the lateral orbital

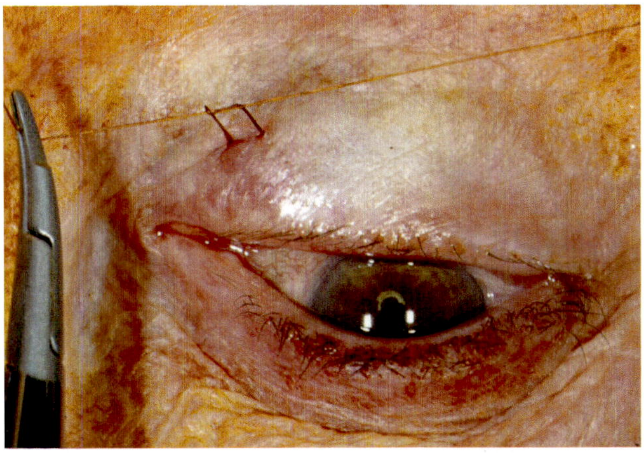

Fig. 39.15 Suture ends are tied on the skin, rotating the punctum inward

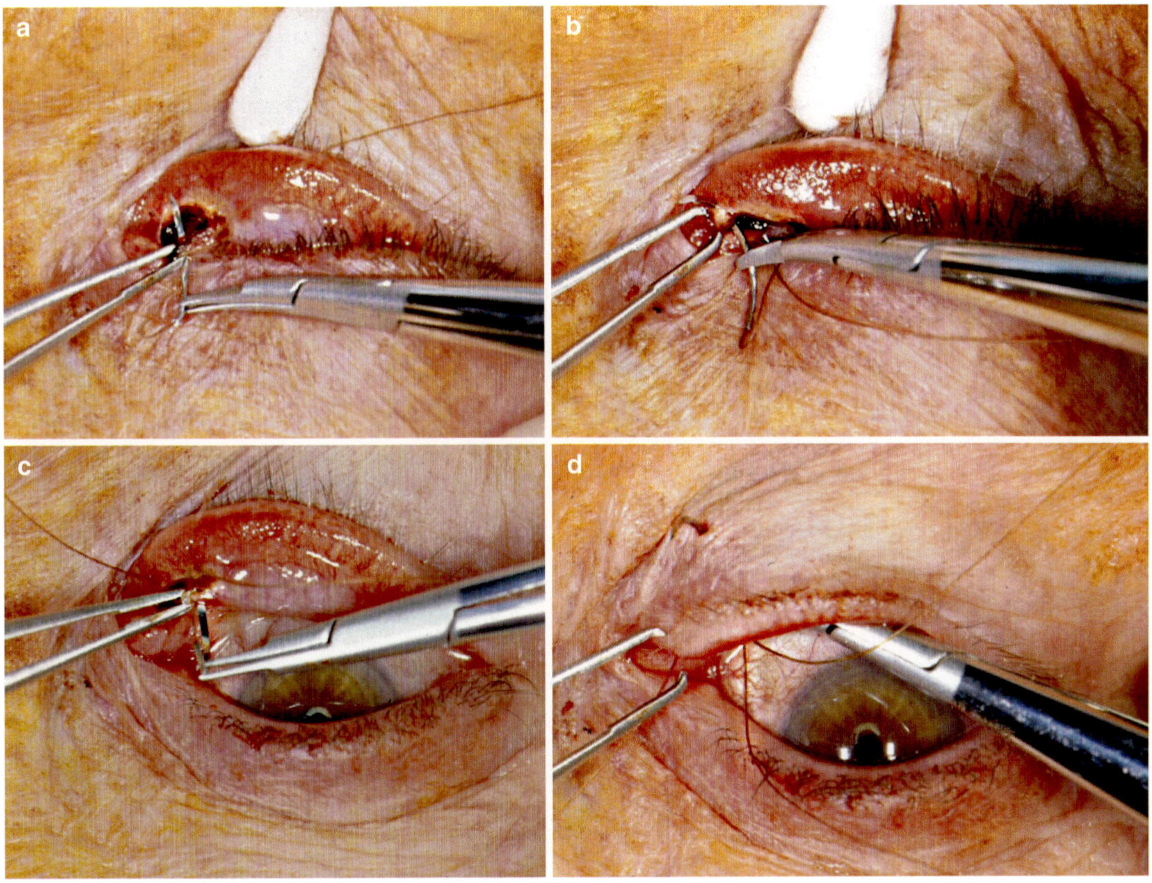

Fig. 39.14 Medial spindle conjunctivoplasty, surgeon view. Each needle is first passed from posterior to anterior through the white inferior retractor layer, with the two passes approximately 3 mm apart (**a**). Each needle is then passed through the inferior tarsal edge (**b**) and looped back through the conjunctival surface of the inferior incision edge (**c**). Both needles exit lower through the eyelid to create a full-thickness scar that inverts the punctum (**d**)

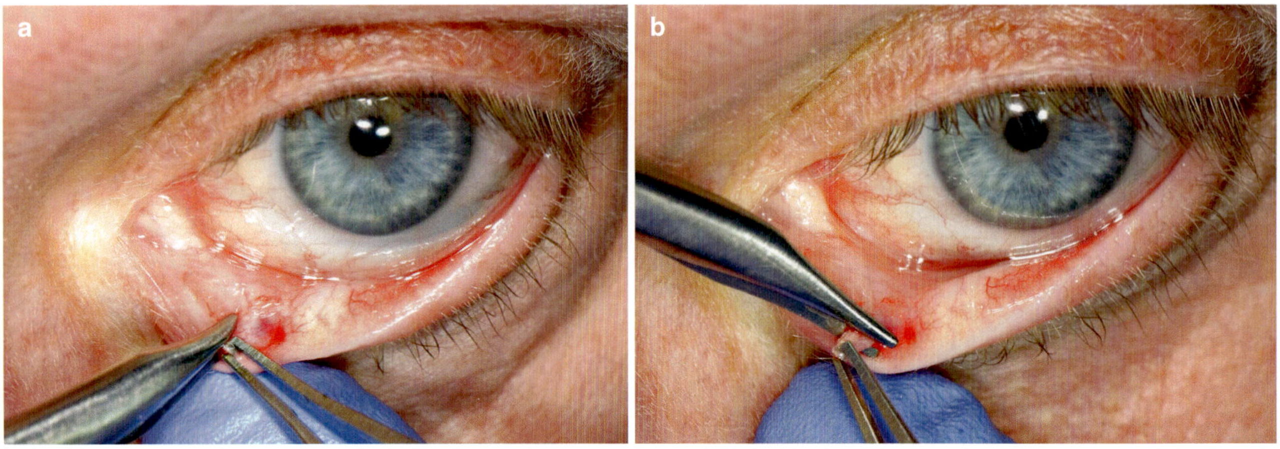

Fig. 39.16 Variation of the three-snip punctoplasty technique used to enlarge the punctum: (**a**) vertical incision starting from the punctum; (**b**) horizontal snip incision connects the two vertical incisions, removing a triangular area of posterior lamellar tissue at the punctum

periosteum. The mucocutaneous margin is then excised along the length of the strip with scissors, taking care to avoid removing the tarsal plate. Some surgeons may also scrape the posterior surface of the strip with a 15 blade to denude the conjunctival epithelium. The tarsal strip is then secured with an absorbable or nonabsorbable 4-0 or 5-0 suture and attached through the periorbita inside the lateral orbital rim at the level of Whitnall's tubercle 2 mm superior to the medial canthus. A double-armed suture may be used or two separate sutures placed through the tarsal strip. Tension is adjusted to optimize the lower eyelid and punctal position with respect to globe, without causing inferior retraction from an overly tight eyelid or excessively shortened tarsal strip [16].

Three-snip punctoplasty can be employed to correct punctal stenosis. The three-snip punctoplasty has been reported to have comparable results when compared to probing and dilation of the punctum with insertion of a silicone stent for 6 weeks [17]. The three-snip punctoplasty allows for creation of wider punctum to facilitate tear excretion. The procedure entails creating a small vertical incision with scissors on the posterior wall of the punctum and the vertical canaliculus. A second incision is made on the posterior lid at the bottom of the vertical cut, extending 2–3 mm medially toward the horizontal canaliculus. A third diagonal or oblique incision is made from the punctum, connecting the previous vertical and horizontal incision (Fig. 39.16a, b). This allows for a small triangular piece of posterior lamellar tissue to be removed, thus successfully widening the punctum. Some surgeons also create a fourth incision from the punctum extending medially along the proximal canaliculus at the eyelid margin, thus excising a rectangular block of tissue. The technique has several variations such as the one-snip and two-snip techniques [18]. The one-snip punctoplasty can be performed at the slit lamp by engaging the posterior wall of the punctum with scissors and creating a small incision. The one-snip punctoplasty has been associated historically with a high failure rate due to reapproximation of the adjacent raw cut edges [19]. A two-snip punctoplasty has been described that utilizes a suture to provide eyelid traction, followed by Vannas scissors inserted into the punctum to create two snips on either side of the suture to excise a small triangular piece of tissue from the posterior aspect of the punctum [20]. Regardless of the precise punctoplasty technique, in some cases the opening may contract and stenose in the early postoperative period and may be treated with redilation with a punctal dilator.

References

1. Hurwitz JJ. Embryology of the lacrimal drainage system. In: Hurwitz JJ, editor. The lacrimal system. Philadelphia: Lippincott-Raven; 1996. p. 9–13.
2. Timlin HM, Keane PA, Day AC, Salam T, Abdullah M, Rose GE, Ezra DG. Characterizing the lacrimal punctal region using anterior segment optical coherence tomography. Acta Ophthalmol. 2016;94(2):154–9. https://doi.org/10.1111/aos.12906. Epub 2015 Dec 9.
3. Chen F, Wang J, Chen W, Shen M, Xu S, Lu F. Upper punctal occlusion versus lower punctal occlusion in dry eye. Invest Ophthalmol Vis Sci. 2010;51:5571–7. https://doi.org/10.1167/iovs.09-5097.
4. Burkat CN, Lucarelli MJ. Tear meniscus level as an indicator of nasolacrimal obstruction. Ophthalmology. 2005;112(2):344–8.
5. Doughty MJ, Laiquzzaman M, Oblak E, Button N. The tear (lacrimal) meniscus height in human eyes: a useful clinical measure or an unusable variable sign? Cont Lens Anterior Eye. 2002;25(2):57–65.
6. Lyons CJ, Rosser PM, Welham RA. The management of punctal agenesis. Ophthalmology. 1993;100(12):1851–5.
7. Soiberman U, Kakizaki H, Selva D, Leibovitch I. Punctal stenosis: definition, diagnosis, and treatment. Clin Ophthalmol (Auckland, NZ). 2012;6:1011–8. https://doi.org/10.2147/OPTH.S31904.
8. Duke-Elder S. The lacrimal apparatus. In: Duke-Elder S, editor. System of ophthalmology. Vol. III Normal and abnormal development. Pt. 2 Congenital deformities. St. Louis: CV Mosby; 1963. p. 911–41.

9. Duke-Elder S, Cook C. The lacrimal passages. In: Duke-Elder S, editor. System of ophthalmology. Vol. III Normal and abnormal development. Pt. 1 Embryology. St. Louis: CV Mosby; 1963. p. 241–6.
10. Cahill KV, Burns JA. Management of epiphora in the presence of congenital punctal and canalicular atresia. Ophthal Plast Reconstr Surg. 1991;7:167–72.
11. Cohen AJ, Mercandetti M. The lacrimal system: diagnosis, management, and surgery. 2nd ed. Cham: Springer; 2014. p. 49–53.
12. Alam MS, Jayshree AMJ. Primary anterior punctal malposition presenting as centurion syndrome. Saudi J Ophthalmol. 2017;31(3):206–7.
13. Francis IC, Wan MK. The punctal apposition syndrome: a new surgical approach. Br J Ophthalmol. 2002;86(11):1256–8.
14. Culbertson WW, Ostler HB. The floppy eyelid syndrome. Am J Ophthalmol. 1981;92(4):568–75.
15. Nowinski TS, Anderson RL. The medial spindle procedure for involutional medial ectropion. Arch Ophthalmol. 1985;103(11):1750–3.
16. Anderson RL, Gordy DD. The tarsal strip procedure. Arch Ophthalmol. 1979;97(11):2192–6.
17. Singh S, Ali MJ, Mohamed A. Comparison of outcomes of 3-snip punctoplasty versus simple punctal dilatation with monocanalicular intubation for acquired punctal stenosis. Ophthal Plast Reconstr Surg. 2017;34(4):375–7.
18. Caesar RH, McNab AA. A brief history of punctoplasty: the 3-snip revisited. Eye (Lond). 2005;19(1):16–8.
19. Bowman W. Methode de traitement applicable a l'epiphora dependent du renversement en dehors ou de l'obliteration des points lacrymaux. Ann Oculist. 1853;29:52–5.
20. Sachdev A, Sagili SR. Suture assisted punctoplasty. Digit J Ophthalmol. 2017;23(3). https://doi.org/10.5693/djo.01.2017.01.001.

Canalicular Obstructions and Management

40

Moisés Enghelberg and Cat Nguyen Burkat

Given the complexity of the lacrimal excretory system of the eyelids, the system can develop abnormalities at any point. Obstruction or stenosis at the level of the canalicular system is common and one of the main causes of epiphora. The canaliculi are divided into two portions: the vertical canaliculus, measuring approximately 2 mm, and the horizontal canaliculus (approximately 8 mm on the upper and 10 mm on the lower eyelid) (Fig. 40.1). The upper and lower horizontal limbs merge into the common canaliculus in over 90% of cases. Normal anatomical variants exist, however, in which the horizontal canaliculi connect directly into the lacrimal sac without a common internal ostium (4–6%). The canaliculi typically angulate posteriorly at the level of the medial canthal tendon. Studies have demonstrated that they then bend at the canaliculi-common canaliculus junction at an angle of 118°, before passing anteriorly and entering the lacrimal sac at a sharp 58° angle [1]. This complex angulation may prevent retrograde flow from the lacrimal sac. The valve of Rosenmüller is located between the common canaliculus and the lacrimal sac, although controversy remains about the presence and physiologic function of this structure [2].

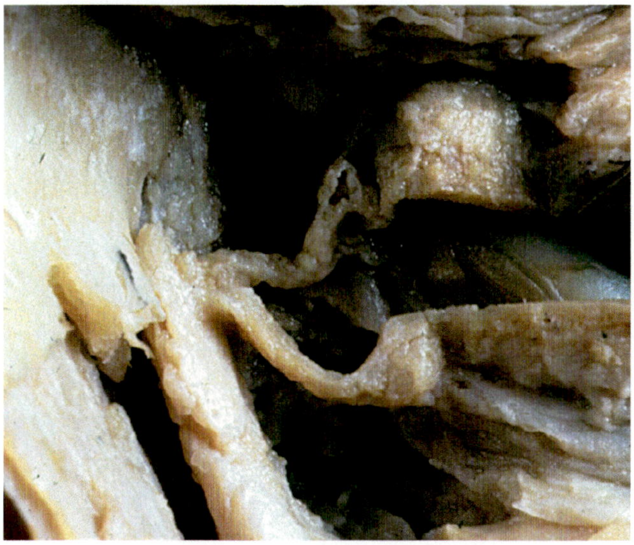

Fig. 40.1 Anatomical dissection of upper and lower eyelid canaliculi merging into a common canaliculus

Other mucosal folds and sinuses reported within the lacrimal drainage system include:

- Valve of Krause—located between the sac and duct
- Valve of Hasner (*plica lacrimalis*)—located at the opening of the duct into the inferior meatus of the nose

Evaluation

The evaluation of epiphora secondary to canalicular obstruction begins with careful observation of the tear meniscus level (Fig. 40.2), as well as the dye disappearance test, also known as the Jones I test. A drop of fluorescein is placed on both ocular surfaces and observed for unequal disappearance from the conjunctival fornix, tear/dye overflow, as well as the duration of time the fluorescein remains on the eye.

The cornerstone of canalicular evaluation in the office is via dilation and irrigation of the lacrimal system. After topical anesthetic, the punctum is dilated, and a Bowman probe (00, 0, or 1 size) is placed through the canaliculus to a hard stop at the nasal bone, which indicates passage through the canaliculus and upper lacrimal sac (Fig. 40.3a, b). Care should be taken to direct the probe in an angled direction, such as slightly superomedially in the lower canaliculus, while also distracting the lower eyelid laterally, in

M. Enghelberg
Department of Ophthalmology, Larkin Community Hospital, South Miami, FL, USA

C. N. Burkat (✉)
Department of Ophthalmology and Visual Sciences, University of Wisconsin-Madison, Madison, WI, USA
e-mail: cburkat@wisc.edu

A. J. Cohen, C. N. Burkat (eds.), *Oculofacial, Orbital, and Lacrimal Surgery*, https://doi.org/10.1007/978-3-030-14092-2_40

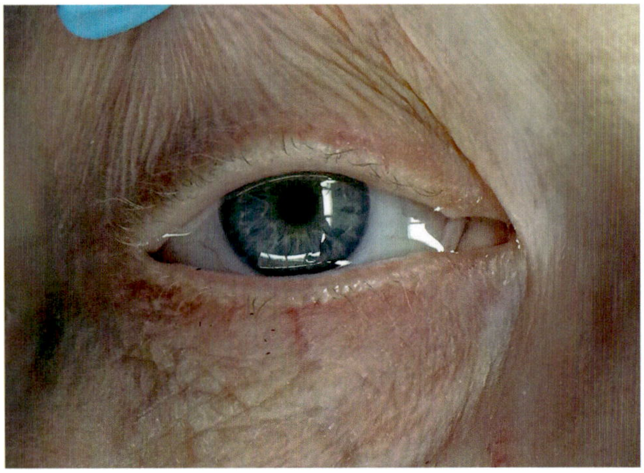

Fig. 40.2 Clinical photo demonstrating an elevated tear meniscus reflected above the lower eyelid margin

order to avoid kinking the canaliculus and creating iatrogenic canalicular injury with a false passage. It is important to gauge any areas of relative stenosis or obstruction along the system during this procedure. Similarly, attention to tactile ease in passing the Bowman probe and soft or hard stops will help assess the overall patency of the canaliculi. Perceptible grittiness to the canaliculus may indicate canalicular concretions or stones. Areas of complete obstruction should also be measured in terms of distance in millimeters from the punctum, by placing a mark or a clamp on the probe at the punctum with the probe up against the focal obstruction, withdrawing the probe, and measuring the length from the clamp to the end of the probe (Fig. 40.4a, b). Focal obstruction or severe stenosis in the proximal canaliculus typically requires conjunctivodacryocystorhinostomy (CDCR) surgery, whereas distal canalicular block-

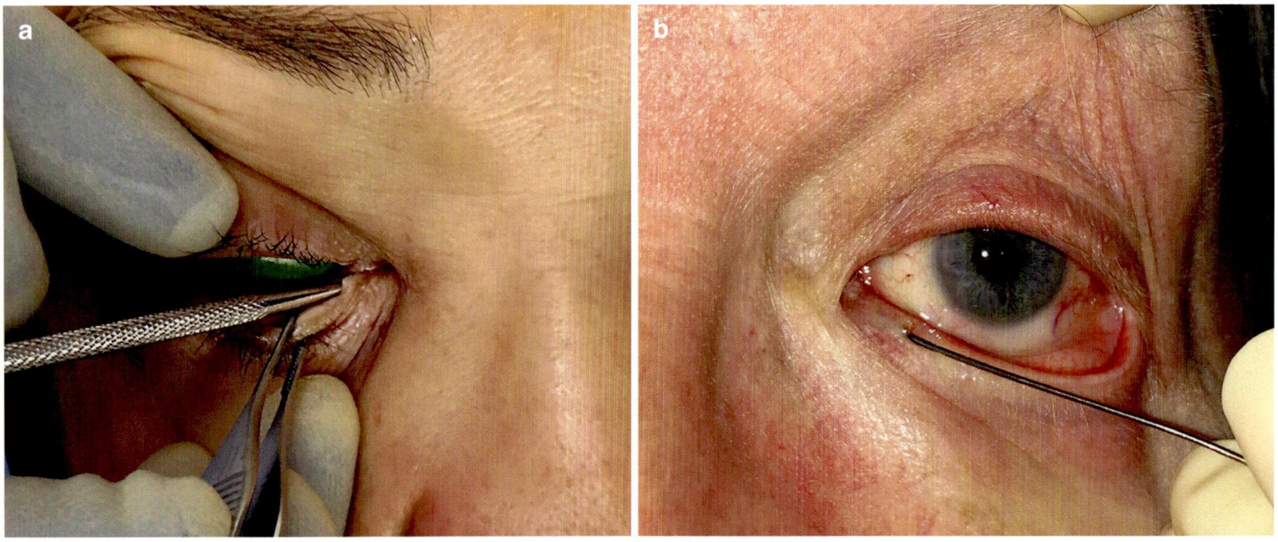

Fig. 40.3 Right inferior punctum is dilated with a punctal dilator (**a**) and a Bowman probe passed through the canaliculus to a hard stop at the bone, indicating passage through the canaliculus to the nasolacrimal sac (**b**)

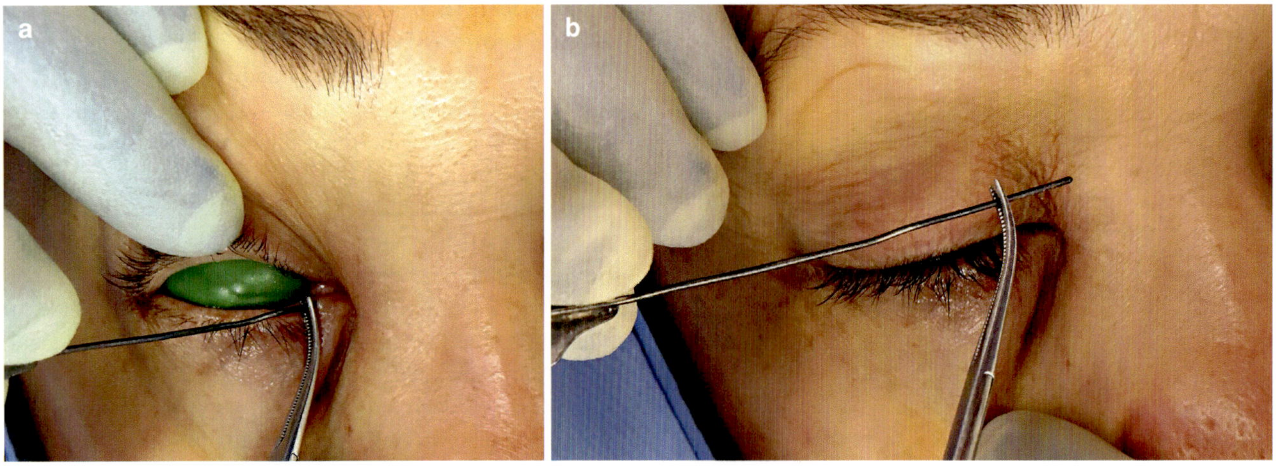

Fig. 40.4 If focal canalicular obstruction is encountered, a clamp is placed on the probe (**a**) and withdrawn to measure the distance from the punctum (**b**)

ages may often be amenable to trephination or excision of scar and placement of silicone intubation past the obstruction.

After thorough assessment of the canaliculi, irrigation of the lacrimal drainage system is performed using a blunt-tipped, straight or angled, lacrimal 23-gauge cannula on a syringe with saline solution (Fig. 40.5). If lower canalicular obstruction is present, solution would reflux back through the same inferior canaliculus (Fig. 40.6a). Likewise, if irrigation is performed through an obstructed upper canaliculus, reflux would occur back through the upper canaliculus. If obstruction is located at the level of the common canaliculus or common internal ostium into the sac, solution would reflux through the path of least resistance, being the opposite canaliculus (Fig. 40.6b). Irrigation that reaches the nasopharynx demonstrates patency, although there may be degrees of concurrent reflux from either the superior or inferior canaliculi, which would suggest partial anatomic obstruction. Reflux through the opposite punctum without any passage into the nose would indicate complete nasolacrimal duct obstruction (Fig. 40.6c). This differs from common canalicular blockage which would also demonstrate a spongy tactile stop with the probe and visible pulling of the medial canthal angle. In contrast, normal passage to a hard bony stop along the medial lacrimal sac with complete reflux would be consistent with nasolacrimal duct obstruction. Lacrimal irrigation also flushes remaining fluorescein dye through the rest of the system, and the dye may be retrieved from the nasal vestibule (Jones II test) [1, 2].

A noninvasive radiologic method of evaluating tear outflow is using lacrimal dacryoscintigraphy. It provides physiologic, rather than anatomic, information using technetium-99 m colloid, or pertechnetate, radionucleotide drops to assess functional tear flow, with multiple images acquired over 15 minutes. Although noninvasive without requiring probing and injection of the canalicular system, this is utilized less frequently due to overall cost and availability of testing. It does not provide precise anatomic location of an obstruction but is most useful in instances of apparently patent systems or dacryocystorhinostomy ostia that appear unobstructed via irrigation, to assess whether a functional abnormality exists [3].

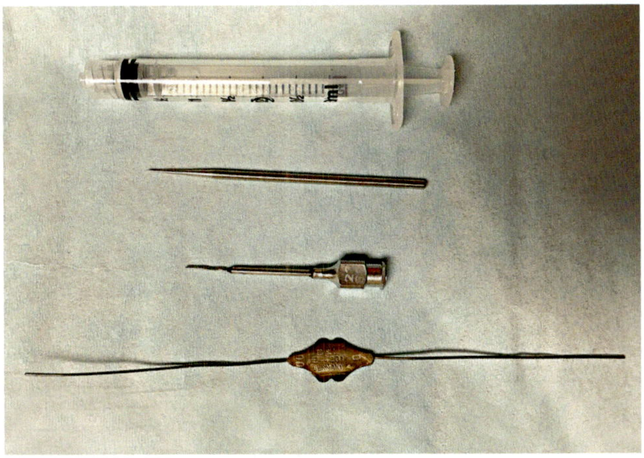

Fig. 40.5 Straight irrigating cannula, syringe, Bowman probe, and punctal dilator used for lacrimal irrigation

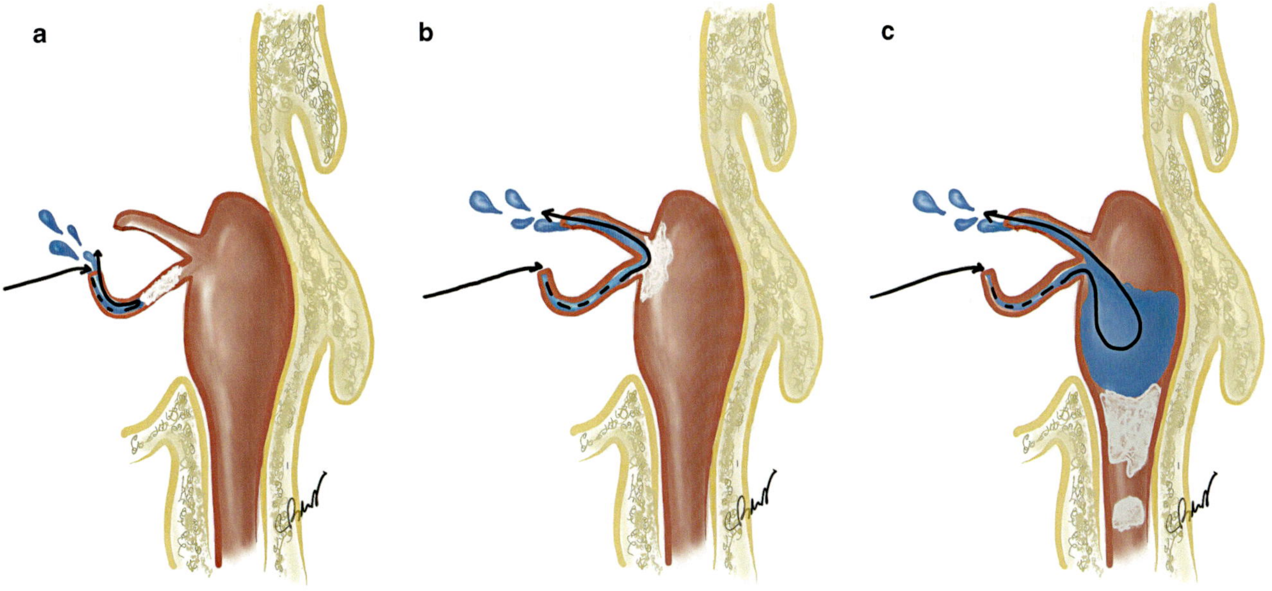

Fig. 40.6 Lacrimal irrigation helps identify the location of stenosis or obstruction. Reflux from the same punctum as being irrigated suggests inferior (or superior) canalicular obstruction (**a**); reflux through the opposite punctum suggests either common canalicular stenosis (**b**) or nasolacrimal duct obstruction (**c**)

Congenital Causes

Congenital nasolacrimal duct obstruction (CNLDO) occurs from incomplete or complete imperforation of the valve of Hasner located at the distal end of the nasolacrimal duct [4]. During embryology, the duct begins to canalize starting from the mid to upper duct and progressing distally toward the nose, although often does not open completely by birth. The valve normally opens spontaneously with conservative treatment (such as warm compresses and manual massage over the lacrimal sac) before 1 year of age in over 90–95% of cases [5]. If obstruction persists beyond 1 year of age, nasolacrimal duct probing is typically recommended to open the membrane. While nasolacrimal duct probing alone is the treatment of choice in children younger than 1 year of age, other studies have demonstrated that adjunctive nasolacrimal silicone intubation or sequential probe dilation increases the success rate in children older than 1 year. Various other modalities used in addition to probing in refractory cases include balloon catheter dilation, monocanalicular intubation, and turbinate infracture [6]. Endoscopic-assisted probing has also been shown to achieve better outcomes for CNLDO, even in older children, with the significantly higher success rates attributed to the ability to visualize and treat associated problems, such as removal of any mucosal flap over the distal duct opening [7].

Monocanalicular intubation has gained popularity as an adjunctive procedure to probing, partly due to ease of procedure and decreased postoperative discomfort [4]. Some studies have found that monocanalicular silicone intubation provides the same success rate as bicanalicular intubation, with less inflammation of the nasolacrimal mucosa [8]. Success rates from 79% to 96% have been reported for intubation as a primary procedure in retrospective case series [9, 10]. More extensive discussion on congenital nasolacrimal duct obstruction is presented in a separate chapter.

Congenital lacrimal fistula or lacrimal anlage is an aberrant developmental connection, which typically forms between the common canaliculus and the medial eyelid skin, occurring in 1 in every 2000 births. The aberrant skin connection may also arise from the lacrimal sac and, less commonly, the nasolacrimal duct. Jones and Wobig termed the cord of cells that normally extended inward from the surface ectoderm during embryonic development the lacrimal anlage, with the nasal end of the anlage forming the sac and the superior aspect creating the canalicular bud that migrates toward the eyelids. Jones and Wobig proposed that this anlage fails to involute in cases of congenital lacrimal fistula and that the cord of cells proliferates and canalizes, forming the fistula. Most fistulae are unilateral, with the ostium located inferonasal to the medial canthus (Fig. 40.7) [11, 12]. Patients can be asymptomatic or present with discharge from the fistula ostium or tearing from the eye. Patients can rarely present with fistulitis, which involves inflammation and tenderness along the fistulous tract.

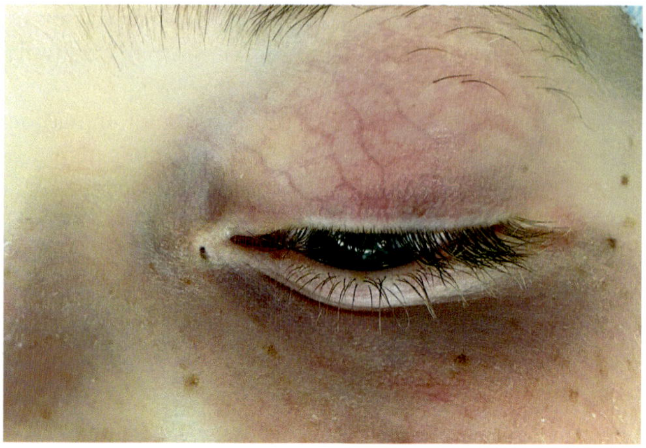

Fig. 40.7 Left-sided congenital lacrimal fistula, with the punctate ostium located inferonasal to the medial canthus

Approximately 29% of patients with a congenital lacrimal fistula will also present with concurrent nasolacrimal duct obstruction. The association between patients with lacrimal fistulae and other congenital developmental abnormalities such as hypospadia, Down syndrome, CHARGE syndrome, and VACTERL association has been reported. Congenital lacrimal fistulae may often be successfully treated with complete excision of the entire fistulous tract, or fistulectomy. An adjunctive dacryocystorhinostomy or silicone intubation may be indicated for those with additional lacrimal outflow tract abnormalities [13].

Congenital rubella syndrome has been documented to be a cause of congenital nasolacrimal duct obstruction. In addition to the classic triad of ocular manifestations (cataracts, glaucoma, and retinopathy), sensorineural deafness, and cardiac abnormalities, the rate of nasolacrimal duct obstruction in those exposed to the rubella virus in utero is higher than in the general population, at close to 14%. Patients often present with a higher rate of nasolacrimal obstruction secondary to imperforation of the valve of Hasner. Complex nasolacrimal duct obstruction secondary to underlying craniofacial malformations has also been described [14]. Patients with congenital rubella syndrome planning to undergo lacrimal probing and dilation should be prophylactically treated with antibiotics, due to the underlying cardiac defects and potential transient bacteremia that may increase the risk of endocarditis [15].

Inflammatory Conditions

*Stevens-Johnson syndrome, graft-*versus-*host disease, ocular cicatricial pemphigoid, or any chronic inflammatory condition* can potentially lead to punctal and canalicular stenosis or obstruction (Fig. 40.8). Systemic inflammatory states may alter

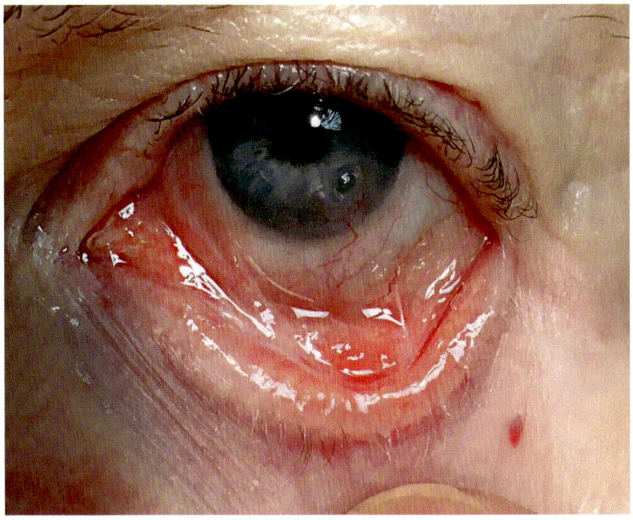

Fig. 40.8 Left inferior punctal and canalicular stenosis associated with ocular cicatricial pemphigoid

the tear composition by diminishing lactoferrin levels. Changes in tear composition subsequently result in inflammation of the canaliculus and scarring of the mucosal tissue. Patients often do not tend to present with epiphora since these conditions tend to decrease tear secretion as well [16–18].

Infectious Causes

Herpes simplex virus (HSV) has been described to cause post-herpetic canalicular obstruction, more commonly in women. Patients typically present in the third decade of life and have a history of vesicular blepharokeratoconjunctivitis. The canalicular pathology tends to be localized to the mid-canaliculus, with the proximal end of the obstruction 2–6 mm from the punctum. Medications used to treat herpetic eye disease, such as 5-iodo-2′-deoxyuridine, trifluorothymidine, and adenine arabinoside, have also been associated with canalicular obstructions. Given the more proximal to midzone site of canalicular involvement, patients with this condition often require canaliculodacryocystorhinostomy or conjunctivodacryocystorhinostomy (CDCR) surgery with placement of a Jones tube [19, 20].

Canaliculitis is an infection of the canaliculus that has been attributed most often to *Actinomyces israelii*, an anaerobic filamentous gram-positive bacteria. *Nocardia asteroides* has also been reported as an offending pathogen in many cases, as well as *Moraxella*, *Staphylococcus aureus*, *Pseudomonas*, and *Streptococcus pneumoniae*. Canaliculitis may also be secondary to a retained foreign body, such as a punctal or canalicular plug. Patients typically present with erythema and tenderness of the punctum and displacement of the swollen punctum away from the globe, described as "pouting" of the punctum (Fig. 40.9). Accompanying erythema and edema over the pericanalicular eyelid margin area is common, in contrast to the focal swelling over the lacrimal sac in acute dacryocystitis. Thick yellow or yellow-green mucous discharge or solid granules can often be expressed from the punctum with manual compression of the canaliculus or lid margin (Fig. 40.10). The sulfur granules once believed to be pathognomonic of *Actinomyces* infection have also been shown to be secondary to *Fusobacterium*, *Staphylococcus aureus*, and other infectious etiologies. The discharge should be sent for culture with gram stain, Grocott-Gomori's methenamine silver stain (GMS), and periodic acid-Schiff (PAS) stains to identify the underlying pathogen in refractory cases. Oral antibiotic therapy is not indicated, and topical antibiotic or antibiotic-steroid treatment is rarely curative over longer follow-up. Similarly, some studies have

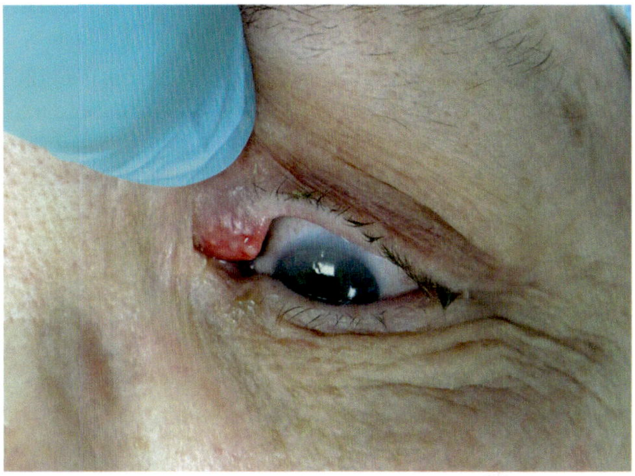

Fig. 40.9 Pouting punctum, canalicular edema, and erythema seen in acute canaliculitis of the upper eyelid

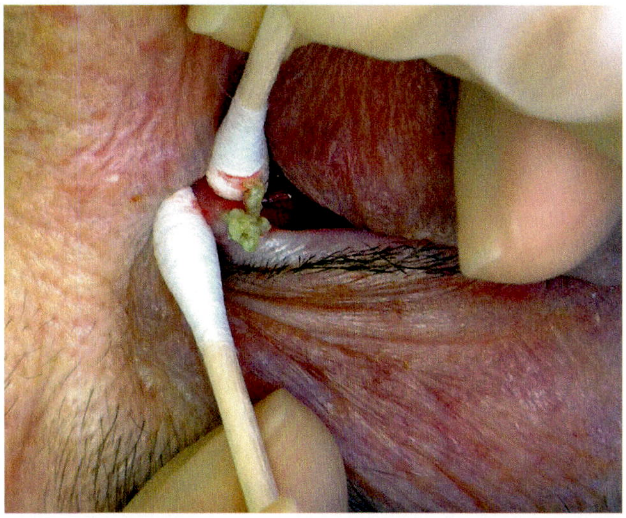

Fig. 40.10 Punctal discharge and granular concretions can be expressed from the canaliculus with digital pressure

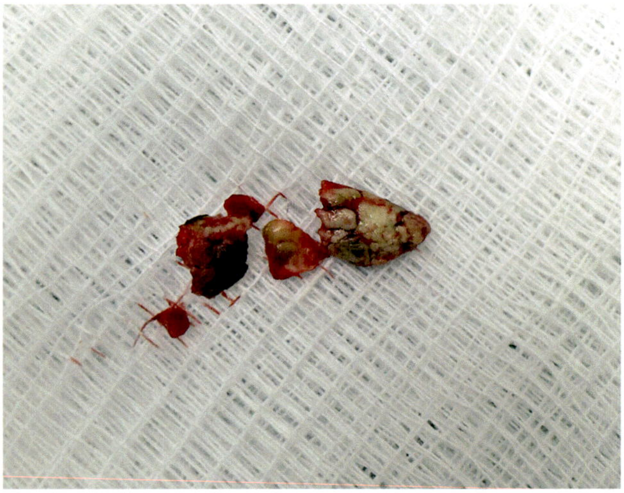

Fig. 40.11 Canalicular stones (concretions, canaliculiths)

suggested benefit with intracanalicular antibiotic irrigation. However, definitive management is most often considered to be canaliculotomy with mechanical debridement and curettage of the canaliculus and extraction of all canalicular stones (also called canaliculiths, concretions, or dacryoliths) (Fig. 40.11). Some surgeons also insert a temporary silicone tube, or short monocanalicular stent, to help maintain patency of the canalicular system during the early healing phase [21].

Canalicular stones can also be indolent for long periods without active signs of inflammation. Studies have demonstrated increased canalicular concretions in older females, with *Actinomyces* being the most commonly isolated pathogen in these stones. In comparison, *dacryoliths,* which are stones found more distally in the lacrimal sac and duct, may be associated more in younger patients with a smoking history. Dacryoliths are often found incidentally during surgery and have equal gender distribution. Although *Actinomyces* has also been cultured from dacryoliths, fungi can also cause dacryoliths but seldomly cause canalicular stones [22].

Medication Induced

Docetaxel (*Taxol*) is a chemotherapeutic agent used most commonly in the treatment of breast malignancies, although also used for ovarian, lung, and prostate cancer. Up to 50% of patients on weekly docetaxel therapy, as compared to an every 3-week regimen, have reported symptoms of epiphora. The onset of epiphora is typically noted starting 12–16 weeks from the initiation of weekly therapy, and usually does not resolve upon cessation of docetaxel therapy. Active secretion of the drug in the tear film has a direct effect on the canalicular mucosa which results in fibrosis of the punctum and canalicular system. Probing, dilation, and irrigation reveal stenosis of the canalicular system, more often than in the nasolacrimal duct. Symptomatic patients on docetaxel therapy should be referred early for placement of bicanalicular silicone stents, to prevent stenosis of the canalicular system. Delayed treatment may lead to more severe canalicular fibrosis that may require CDCR with Jones tube surgery in order to bypass the obstruction. Similar medication-induced canalicular stenosis has been reported in patients undergoing treatment with 5-flurouracil for bowel malignancies and as an adjuvant in breast cancer chemotherapy [23–25].

Surgical Management

Canalicular stenting, or silicone intubation, is performed to treat functional canalicular stenosis, or mild to moderate partial nasolacrimal duct stenosis, as determined by probing and irrigation. Office irrigation that demonstrates more reflux of solution rather than passage into the nasal cavity may indicate that more significant stenosis exists that will require dacryocystorhinostomy (DCR) surgery. Numerous bicanalicular or monocanalicular silicone intubation systems are available that can be placed to maintain patency or dilate the stenotic area. There is a wide discrepancy as to the length of time the stent should be left in place, although a common practice is to leave the tube in place for 2–4 months [26].

Canaliculotomy is typically performed to treat acute or chronic canaliculitis and allows exploration of the canaliculus to remove a suspected foreign body (such as a punctal or canalicular plug), as well as drainage of infection with curettage of granular stones. The procedure is performed by placing a Bowman probe within the canaliculus, which can be seen through the eyelid margin as a light gray line over which the incision is placed to open the canaliculus (Fig. 40.12).

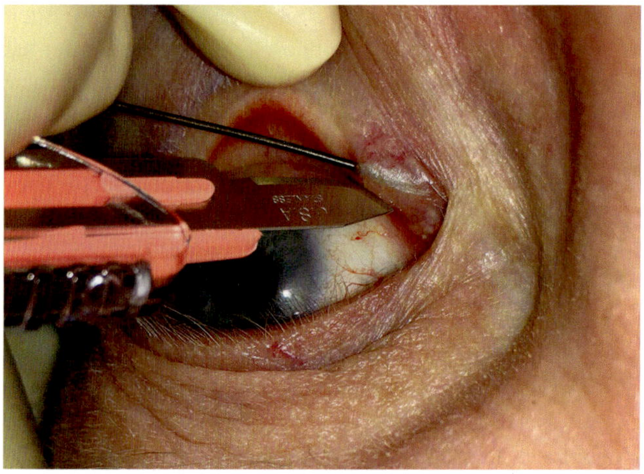

Fig. 40.12 Canaliculotomy: a Bowman probe is placed prior to incising the canaliculus, which can be seen through the eyelid margin as a light gray line over which the incision is placed to open the canaliculus (surgeon's view)

The canaliculus is then incised along the eyelid margin, with or without connecting the punctum (Fig. 40.13a, b). Leaving the punctum intact minimizes the need for lid margin closure and preserves the natural lacrimal pump outflow mechanism as originally described by Rosengren-Döane. A large iatrogenic slit punctum could affect the gradient of negative pressure in the nasolacrimal sac that is required to suction tears from the tear lake into the sac. Cotton tip applicators are used to firmly express the stones or foreign bodies from the canaliculus. A chalazion curette can be used to remove additional concretions that can be sent for pathology. Although some advocate placing a temporary silicone stent, such as a mini-Monoka, for several weeks, other studies have demonstrated good success without placement of tubes or closure of the incision (Fig. 40.14a, b) [27].

Fistulectomy is performed for symptomatic congenital lacrimal fistula. The fistulous tract starting from the skin is carefully dissected from the surrounding tissues. A purse string absorbable suture is placed around the deep origin of the fistula and the remaining tract excised. A silicone stent can sometimes be placed through the canaliculus to maintain patency during healing, if indicated. In cases of concomitant nasolacrimal duct obstruction, a fistulectomy can be performed in conjunction with a dacryocystorhinostomy [11].

Canaliculodacryocystorhinostomy can be attempted if a total obstruction is found distal to the punctum but proximal to the common canaliculus. This technique can be performed prior to placement of a Jones tube. The procedures entails placement of a Bowman probe to the site of obstruction, and a hemostat placed on the probe to mark the area of obstruction.

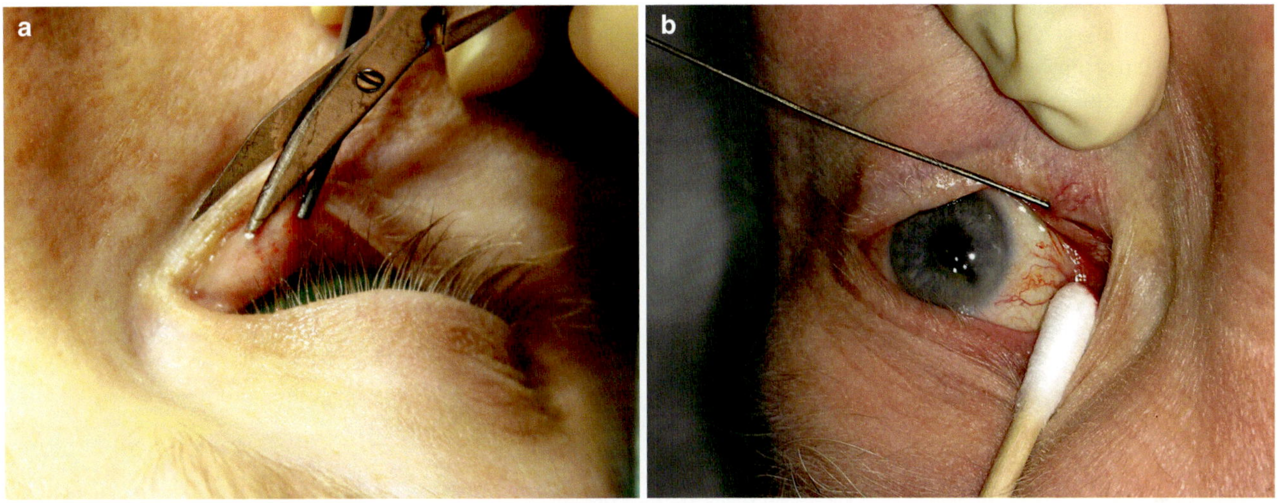

Fig. 40.13 Canaliculotomy: incising the canaliculus along the eyelid margin, with (**a**) or without (**b**) connecting the punctum (note the small area of intact eyelid margin between the punctum and the start of the linear incision) (surgeon's view)

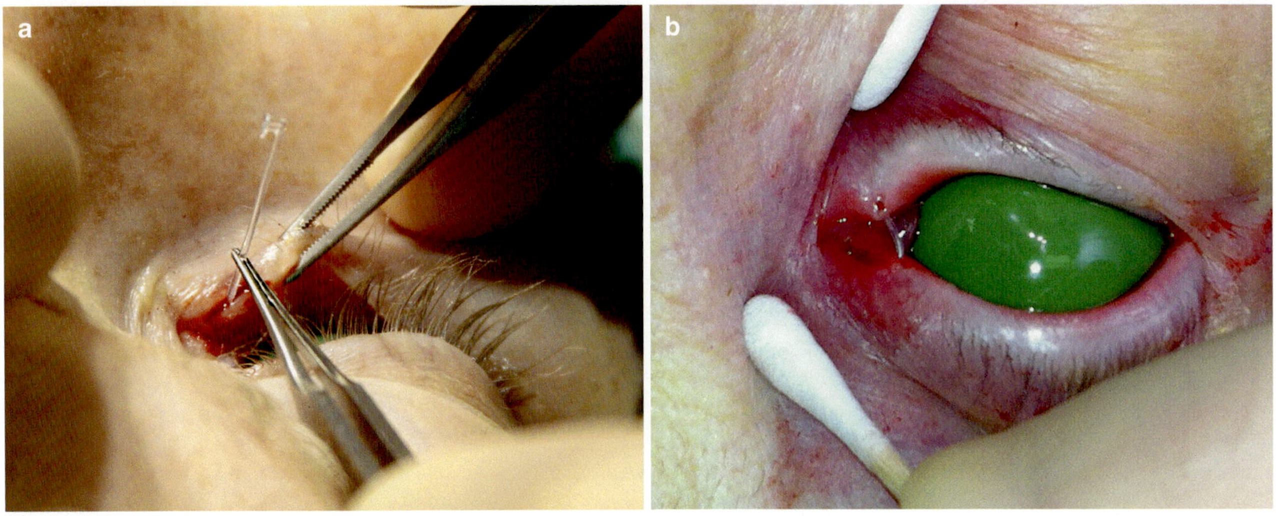

Fig. 40.14 A temporary monocanalicular (**a**) or bicanalicular (**b**) silicone stent may be placed after canalicular curettage, if desired (surgeon's view). Suturing the eyelid margin is not needed

Scissors are used to cut down perpendicular to the eyelid margin and canaliculus to incise and remove the scarred region. The Bowman probe then dilates past the area of obstruction, and a silicone stent is placed past the now patent canaliculus and cut end of the canaliculus. The canalicular ends can be reapproximated and sutured. The stent is subsequently passed down the nasolacrimal duct, or through a DCR ostium, if indicated [28].

Another option of recanalizing a focal canalicular obstruction is to insert a Sisler lacrimal minitrephine (Beaver-Visitec International Ltd., UK) up to the blockage and then remove the protective guard to allow the metal end to core out the obstruction. The Sisler lacrimal trephine has an outer diameter of 0.81 mm and is affixed to a plastic hub for manual grasping and rotating (Fig. 40.15a–d). The intraluminal stylet is round with a domed tip to minimize trauma to the proximal, patent canaliculus while passing to the point of obstruction. The stylet is then removed which allows the stainless steel trephine edge to core out the scar plug. Care is taken to pass the trephine in a twisting forward motion along the proper angle of the normal canaliculus to avoid creating a false passage (Fig. 40.16a, b).

Conjunctivodacryocystorhinostomy (CDCR) is indicated in cases of total canalicular obstruction that are unable to be repaired by canaliculodacryocystorhinostomy, trephination of scar, or dilation with silicone stenting. This surgery is discussed in greater detail in a separate chapter. Briefly, an incision at the level of the caruncle is created to provide space for the Jones tube. A rigid straight instrument, such as an MVR blade, Bowman probe, or specialized introducer, is then directed inferoposteriorly toward the middle turbinate to perforate the area of the proposed tract. The slight posterior angulation also facilitates entry through the posterior portion of the lacrimal sac fossa where the thin lacrimal bone resides behind the maxillary suture line. Various dilators are placed to enlarge the tract, and endoscopic visualization should demonstrate the proper entry into the middle meatus. In early descriptions of this surgery, a Bowman probe would then be placed in the fistulous tract and a hemostat placed on the probe at the caruncle to determine the appropriate length of the Jones tube. Newer systems have specialized sizing devices to assist in selecting the appropriate length and size of the tube. The pyrex tube would then be placed over the guide and advanced into position until the flange rests on the conjunctiva and caruncle (Fig. 40.17). Intranasally, the appropriate position should have the tube end halfway between the lateral nasal wall and nasal septum and rest clear of the middle turbinate (Fig. 40.18). A nonabsorbable or absorbable suture is often placed around the neck of the tube and tied into position at the caruncle to prevent displacement [29].

With proper tube placement, CDCR surgery has relatively high success rates in terms of establishing patency.

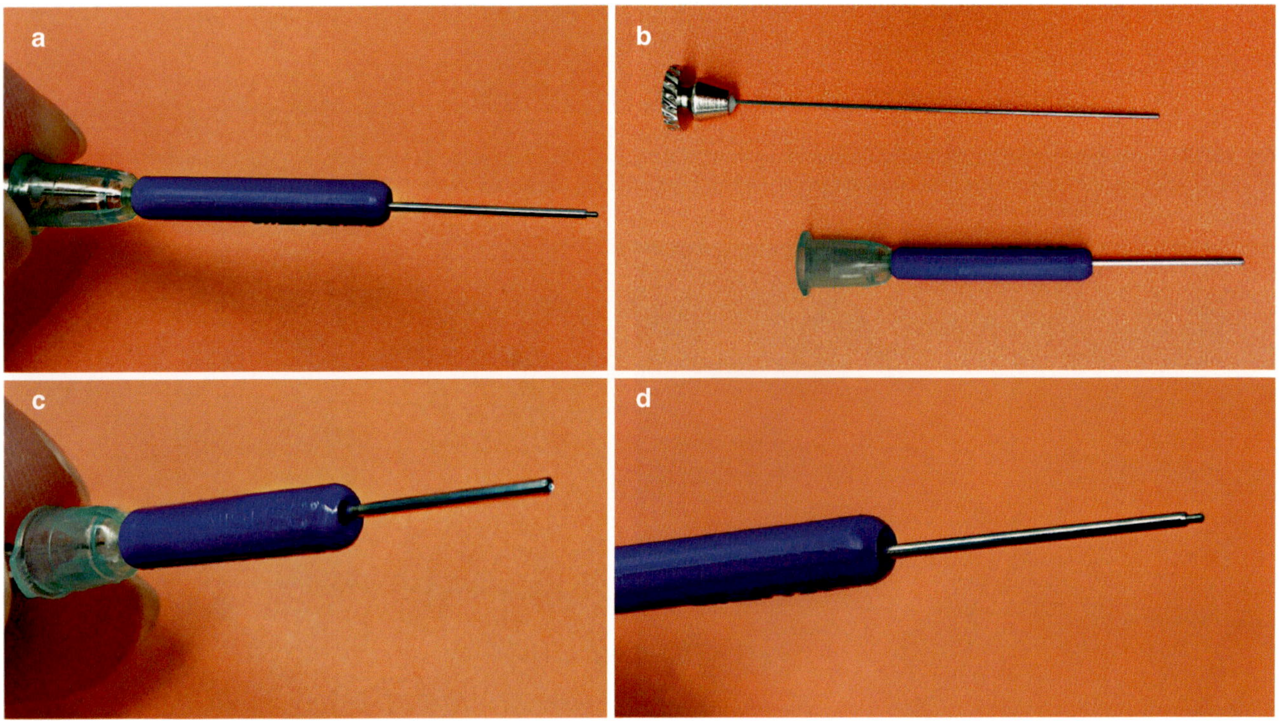

Fig. 40.15 Lacrimal minitrephine with its protective intraluminal stylet prevents false passages until the canalicular blockage is reached (**a**, **b**). When the stylet is removed, the trephine tip is now sharp and able to core out scar (**c**), compared to the rounded blunt stylet that extends past the trephine to avoid false passages (**d**)

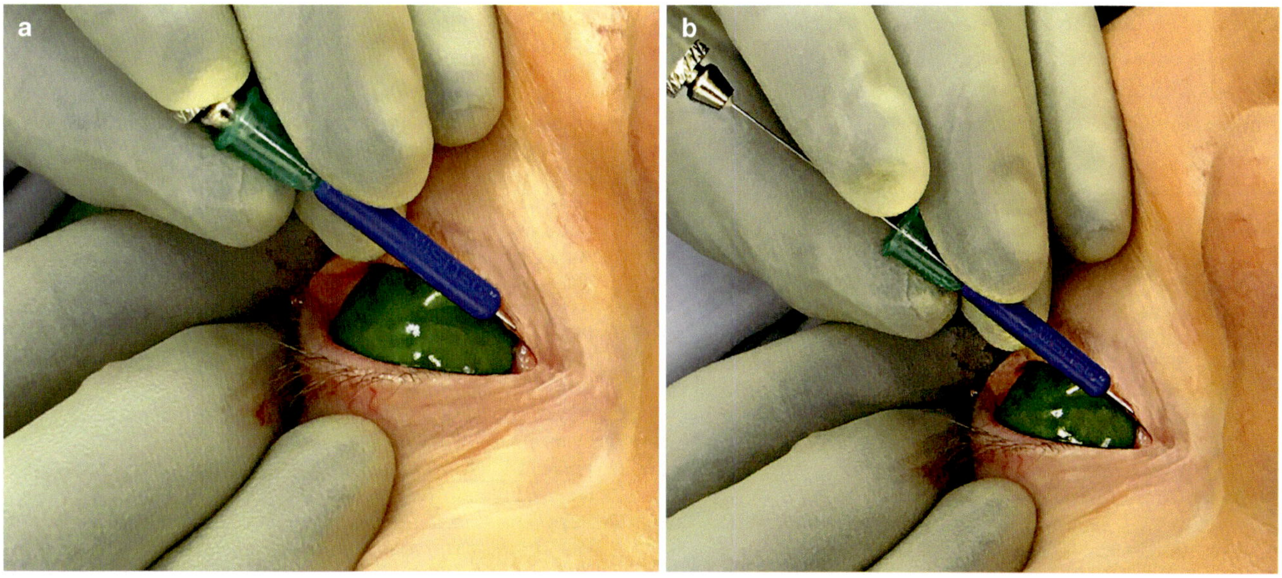

Fig. 40.16 Once the lacrimal trephine is in proper angulation (**a**), the protective stylet is pulled out (**b**), and the trephine is advanced through the scar in a rotating twisting motion

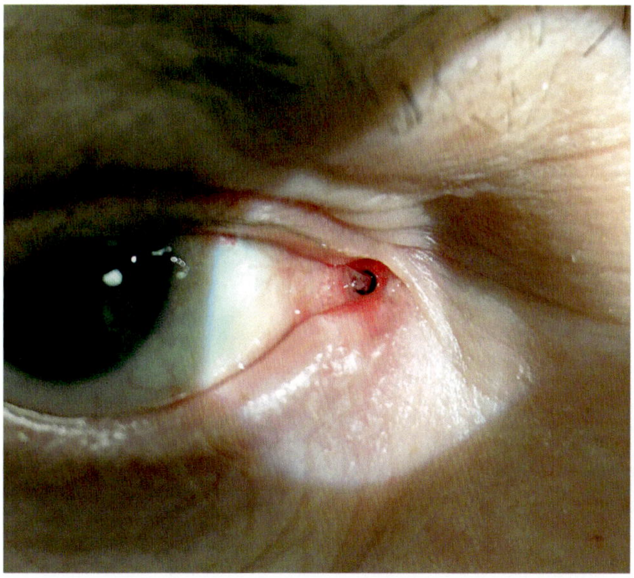

Fig. 40.17 Jones tube rests in position in the inferomedial canthus following conjunctivodacryocystorhinostomy surgery

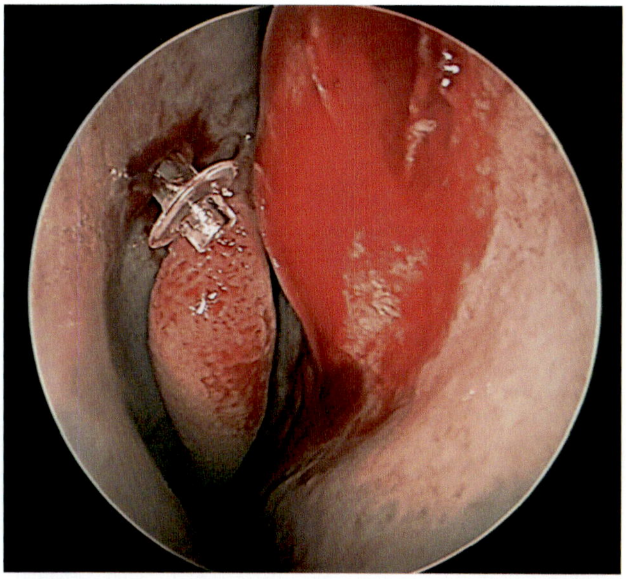

Fig. 40.18 StopLoss Jones tube in position halfway between the lateral nasal wall and septum. Note the internal flange that minimizes tube migration

However, patients should be made aware that lifelong maintenance of the tube is required. Regular clinic visits and cooperation to allow the physician to remove and clean the tube is necessary. Patients may be instructed to clean the tube daily with water flushes, which can become cumbersome or difficult in children [30]. Although symptomatic improvement of epiphora is reported, overall patient satisfaction with this procedure is often decreased due to the need for chronic maintenance and the frequent complications that require additional management. The most common long-term complications following CDCR include ocular surface irritation, tissue overgrowth occluding the flange, pyogenic granuloma, tube breakage, migration, and extrusion and displacement of the tube. Studies have reported that more than 50% require replacement of the tube in the course of 10 years following implantation and even more lifelong [31]. Numerous modifications to the original Lester-Jones tube have been made to minimize the complications of migration and extrusion, including angled tubes, frosted or sleeved tubes, suture fixation techniques, and the addition of a silicone flange on the nasal end (StopLoss

Jones tube). This internal flange opens up similar to an umbrella once inserted to minimize migration of the tube, as demonstrated by significantly lower extrusion rates in some studies (Fig. 40.18) [32].

References

1. Cohen AJ, Mercandetti M. The lacrimal system: diagnosis, management, and surgery. 2nd ed. New York: Springer; 2014. p. 49–53.
2. Kashkouli MB, Pakdel F, Kiavash V. Assessment and management of proximal and incomplete symptomatic obstruction of the lacrimal drainage system. Middle East Afr J Ophthalmol. 2012;19(1):60–9.
3. Guzek JP, Ching AS, Hoang TA, et al. Clinical and radiologic lacrimal testing in patients with epiphora. Ophthalmology. 1997;104(11):1875–81.
4. MacEwen CJ, Young JDH. Epiphora during the first year of life. Eye. 1991;5:596–600.
5. Paul TO. Medical management of congenital nasolacrimal duct obstruction. J Pediatr Ophthalmol Strabismus. 1985;22:68–70.
6. Alañón Fernández MA, Alañón Fernández F, Martínez Fernández A, Cárdenas LM. Treatment of the congenital obstruction of the lachrymal duct, by means of balloon catheter, monocanalicular intubation, and endoscopic control. Acta Otorrinolaringol Esp. 2009;60(6):409–14.
7. Galindo-Ferreiro A, Khandekar R, Akaishi PM, Cruz A, Gálvez-Ruiz A, Dolmetsch A, Schellini S. Success rates of endoscopic-assisted probing compared to conventional probing in children 48 months or older. Semin Ophthalmol. 2017;16:1–8.
8. Andalib D, Gharabaghi D, Nabai R, Abbaszadeh M. Monocanalicular versus bicanalicular silicone intubation for congenital nasolacrimal duct obstruction. J AAPOS. 2010;14(5):421–4. https://doi.org/10.1016/j.jaapos.2010.08.003.
9. Elsawaby EA, El Essawy RA, Abdelbaky SH, Ismail YM. Pushed monocanalicular intubation versus probing as a primary management for congenital nasolacrimal obstruction. Clin Ophthalmol. 2016;10:1487–93.
10. Kaufman LM, Guay-Bhatia LA. Monocanalicular intubation with Monoka tubes for the treatment of congenital nasolacrimal duct obstruction. Ophthalmology. 1998;105(2):336–41.
11. Jones LT, Wobig JL. Surgery of the eyelids and lacrimal system, vol. 67. Birmingham: Aesculapius Publishing Co.; 1976. p. 167–73.
12. Birchansky LD, Nerad JA, Kersten RD, Kulwin DR. Management of congenital lacrimal sac fistula. Arch Oph Thalmol. 1990;108:388–90.
13. Levine J. Congenital fistula of the lacrimal sac. Am J Ophthalmol. 1929;12:745–6.
14. Gupta S, Ali MJ, Naik MN. Lacrimal drainage anomalies in congenital rubella syndrome. Clin Ophthalmol. 2017;11:1975–7.
15. Ganguly A, Ali MJ, Padmaja K, et al. Bacteremia following nasolacrimal duct probing: is there a role of pre-operative antibiotic prophylaxis? Ophthal Plast Reconstr Surg. 2016;32:90–2.
16. Kijlstra A, Jeurissen SH, Koning KM. Lactoferrin levels in normal human tears. Br J Ophthalmol. 1983;67(3):199–202.
17. Tung CI. Graft versus host disease: what should the oculoplastic surgeon know? Curr Opin Ophthalmol. 2017;28(5):499–504.
18. Auran JD, Hornblass A, Gross ND. Stevens-Johnson syndrome with associated nasolacrimal duct obstruction treated with dacryocystorhinostomy and Crawford silicone tube insertion. Ophthal Plast Reconstr Surg. 1990;6(1):60–3.
19. de Koning EW, van Bijsterveld OP. Herpes simplex virus canaliculitis. Acta Ophthalmol. 1983;186(4):173–6.
20. Coster DJ, Welham RN. Herpetic canalicular obstructions. Br J Ophthalmol. 1979;65:259–62.
21. Fulmer NL, Neal JG, Bussard GM, Edlich RF. Lacrimal canaliculitis. Am J Emerg Med. 1999;17:385–6.
22. Repp DJ, Burkat CN, Lucarelli MJ. Lacrimal excretory system concretions: canalicular and lacrimal sac. Ophthalmology. 2009;116(11):2230–5.
23. Esmaeli B, Valero V, Ahmadi MA, Booser D. Canalicular stenosis secondary to docetaxel (taxotere): a newly recognized side effect. Ophthalmology. 2001;108(5):994–5.
24. Mansur C, Pfeiffer ML, Esmaeli B. Evaluation and management of chemotherapy-induced epiphora, punctal and canalicular stenosis, and nasolacrimal duct obstruction. Ophthal Plast Reconstr Surg. 2017;33(1):9–12.
25. Fezza JP, Wesley RE, Klippenstein KA. The treatment of punctal and canalicular stenosis in patients on systemic 5-FU. Ophthalmic Surg Lasers. 1999;30(2):105–8.
26. Park J, Kim H. Sequential probing and dilatation in canalicular stenosis. Graefes Arch Clin Exp Ophthalmol. 2015;253(11):2007–13.
27. Boulze-Pankert M, Roux C, Nkamga VD, Gouriet F, Rojat-Habib MC, Drancourt M, Hoffart L. Aggregatibacter aphrophilus chronic lacrimal canaliculitis: a case report. BMC Ophthalmol. 2016;16:132.
28. Doucet TW, Hurwitz JJ. Canaliculodacryocystorhinostomy in the treatment of canalicular obstruction. Arch Ophthalmol. 1982;100(2):306–9.
29. Steele EA. Conjunctivodacryocystorhinostomy with Jones tube: a history and update. Curr Opin Ophthalmol. 2016;27(5):439–42.
30. Lim C, Martin P, Benger R, Kourt G, Ghabrial R. Lacrimal canalicular bypass surgery with the Lester Jones tube. Am J Ophthalmol. 2004;137(1):101–8.
31. Rose GE, Richard WAN. Jones' lacrimal canalicular bypass tubes: twenty five years' experience. Eye. 1991;5:13–9.
32. Bagdonaite L, Pearson AR. Twelve-year experience of Lester Jones tubes – results and comparison of 3 different tube types. Ophthal Plast Reconstr Surg. 2015;31(5):352–6.

Congenital Lacrimal Gland Disorders and Nasolacrimal Duct Obstruction

41

Michael C. Struck

Introduction

This chapter describes the aspects of the lacrimal apparatus that are important to recognize and evaluate in the treatment of the congenital nasolacrimal disorders. The lacrimal apparatus is composed of the structures responsible for the creation of the tear film and those responsible for adequate drainage and hygiene. A brief discussion of the embryology and anatomy will help guide the surgeon in diagnosis and treatment of these disorders.

Anatomy and Embryology

Lacrimal Gland

The tear-producing structures are the main lacrimal gland and the accessory glands of Krause and Wolfing. Additional essential secretions come from the Meibomian glands, the goblet cells, and the glands of Zeis. These glands originate from the nasal cells of the conjunctiva around 40–45 days of gestation.

The main lacrimal gland consists of two lobes separated by the lateral extension of the lateral horn of the levator. The orbital portion lies over the levator aponeurosis and is often the preferred site of lacrimal gland biopsy. The palpebral portion of the lacrimal gland can often be visualized by everting the lateral upper eyelid, and in this region, there are a multitude of ducts that empty secretions into the superior fossa. Therefore, biopsy of this portion carries the risk of iatrogenic scarring of the excretory ductules.

Lacrimal Drainage System

The lacrimal drainage system consists of a series of effluent structures to provide cleansing functions for the ocular surface. The proximal portion consists of the puncta and canaliculus. These structures are rich in elastic tissue and relatively avascular. Because of this feature, they are normally capable of stretching 2–3 times wider than their normal size. The puncta are normally slightly inverted so that they appose the ocular surface and tear meniscus, but are not occluded by contact with the surface. Each canaliculus first goes perpendicular to the eyelid margin for approximately 2 mm and then turns to run parallel to the eyelid surface of the margin (Fig. 41.1). This superficial pathway makes the canaliculus prone to traumatic rupture from aggressive surgical manipulation or from laterally directed trauma (such as a dog bite injury). The canaliculi enter into the lacrimal sac either separately (4–6%) or through a common canaliculus (94%) [1]. The lacrimal sac rests in the lacrimal fossa, which is just posterior to the infraorbital ridge and lies

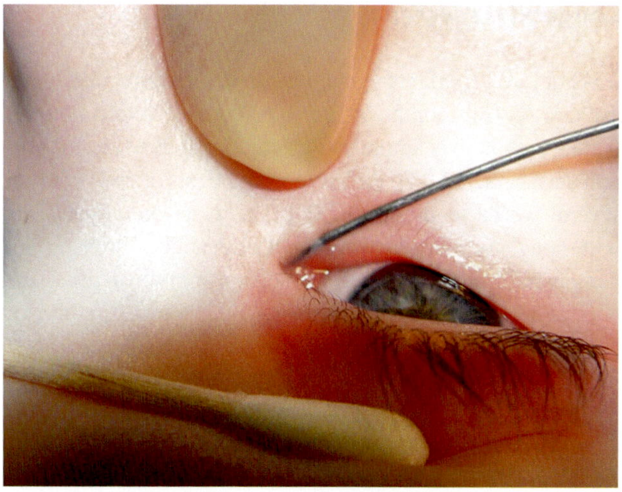

Fig. 41.1 The canaliculus runs parallel to the eyelid margin, with the probe often visible through the thin eyelid margin tissue

M. C. Struck (✉)
University of Wisconsin School of Medicine and Public Health, Madison, WI, USA
e-mail: mcstruck@wisc.edu

A. J. Cohen, C. N. Burkat (eds.), *Oculofacial, Orbital, and Lacrimal Surgery*, https://doi.org/10.1007/978-3-030-14092-2_41

adjacent to the lacrimal bone. Digital manipulation by pressure behind the ridge and against the lacrimal bone (Crigler maneuver) has been associated with consequential opening of an obstructed NLD [2]. The nasolacrimal duct is a continuation of the lacrimal sac, passing vertically and slightly posterolaterally through the maxillary bone to exit into the nasopharynx underneath the inferior turbinate bone. The lining of this structure is pseudostratified columnar epithelium.

The nasolacrimal duct, lacrimal sac, and canaliculi all originate from surface ectoderm at the lateral groove. Surface ectoderm in the nasooptic fissure sends two solid epithelial cords to the rims of the upper and lower eyelids at day 48 of gestation [3]. Canalization of the epithelial cords begins at the lacrimal sac, which is outlined by a connective tissue sheath at 3 months. In the fourth month, the canaliculi and nasolacrimal duct system are formed by branches from the sac that continue to canalize (Hurwitz). Finally, the nasal fossa fuses with the inferior nasolacrimal duct at 6 months. A cellular plug detaches to open the superior and inferior puncta at 7 months.

Abnormalities of the Lacrimal Gland

Congenital Absent Lacrimal Gland

The complete absence of the lacrimal gland is a rare condition, often associated with congenital absence of the trigeminal nerve or facial nerve but also, not surprisingly, in conditions where there is maldevelopment of the conjunctival cells of origin (anophthalmos, cryptopthalmos). Children have features of extreme keratitis sicca and require aggressive treatment.

Congenital Alacrima

It is not rare for infants to manifest deficit in reflex tearing in the first several months of life. Basal tear secretion is unaffected, and there is ample tear production to provide for normal surface health [4]. Reflex tearing begins anywhere from several weeks to months after birth, which is why infants with congenital nasolacrimal duct obstruction often do not demonstrate epiphora until the second month of life. This condition spontaneously resolves, and no investigation or treatment is generally warranted.

Congenital Prolapse

The palpebral lobe of the lacrimal gland, in some instances, may protrude or prolapse under the lateral aspect of the upper eyelid, creating the appearance of a puffy lateral eyelid. The appearance can sometimes appear vascular and mimic a conjunctival hemangioma. Treatment should be conservative observation as the finding is benign. Surgical resection may eliminate the lacrimal ducts that also drain the orbital portion of the lacrimal gland and thus permanently inhibit normal lacrimal gland function. If symptomatic or cosmetically bothersome, the lacrimal gland can be resuspended under the superolateral bony fossa through an upper eyelid anterior orbitotomy approach [5].

Aberrant Lacrimal Tissue

Ectopic lacrimal tissue unassociated with the main lacrimal gland can develop on the surface of the eye. If present at or near the limbus, it can be associated with significant refractive error and secondary amblyopia. Generally this tissue is histopathologically a choristoma of normal lacrimal tissue and can be treated with observation or simple resection.

Abnormalities of Lacrimal Drainage (See Also Chap. 39)

Punctal Atresia and Imperforate Puncta

Absence of the puncta is most often associated with absence of the associated canalicular duct. When this involves the upper eyelid, no treatment is generally required (Fig. 41.2). If, however, the lower eyelid is involved, reestablishing the effluent canal may be necessary (Fig. 41.3) [6]. Occasionally, only a thin membrane of epithelium is present over the puncta which is evident on attempted dilation at the time of surgery. One may attempt

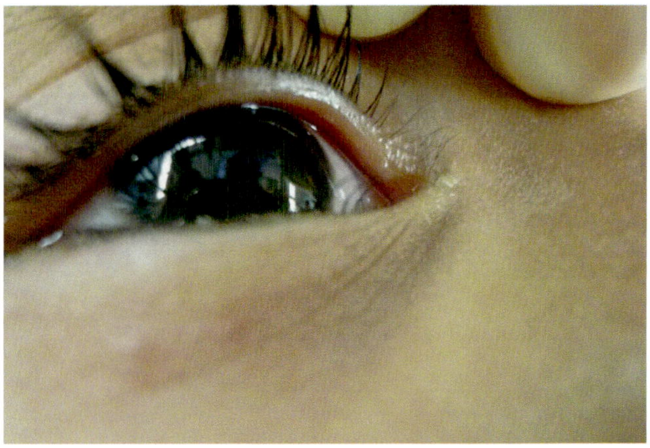

Fig. 41.2 Complete punctal atresia of the right upper eyelid

to carefully pass a pigtail probe from the upper into the lower canalicular system. It may be possible to find the blind canaliculus in this manner and recreate a punctal opening and establish recanalization with silicone tube placement (Fig. 41.4a, b). However, in patients in whom the upper and lower canaliculi do not share a common canaliculus but enter the lacrimal sac separately, the pigtail probe will be less successful and can cause iatrogenic damage to the lacrimal sac and canaliculi. In these instances, a vertical canalicular cutdown performed just medial to the punctal ampulla is often helpful to identify any canalicular mucosa. More often, however, the associated canaliculus is absent in association of true punctal atresia. Retrograde cannulation can be attempted with endoscopy if the remainder of the nasolacrimal duct is present and can be cannulated. Atresia of the canaliculus and associated puncta is most often seen in association with Down syndrome [7, 8].

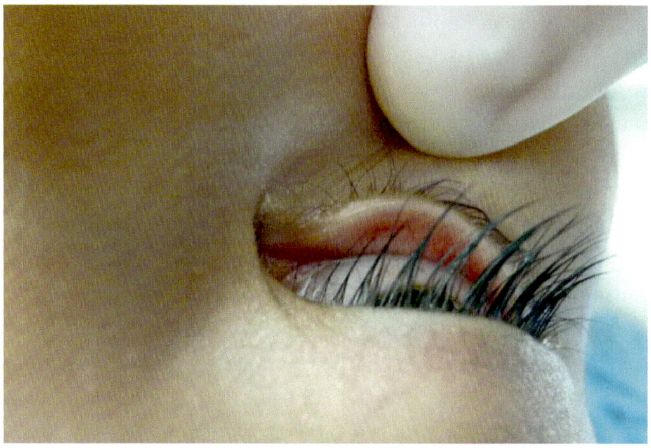

Fig. 41.3 Complete punctal atresia of the right lower eyelid (surgeon's view)

Punctal Stenosis

Stenosis of the puncta can occur congenitally and presents very similar to punctal atresia. This condition can be treated with a simple dilation and/or snip punctoplasty, although recurrence of stenosis may occur. However, as general anesthesia is necessary in young children, monocanalicular or bicanalicular silicone tube placement is often performed and is often sufficient alone to resolve the condition.

Punctal Inversion and Epiblepharon

Inversion of the punctum may create a functional blockage of the tear effluent system because the punctum is incorrectly positioned against the globe. This most often occurs in association with the finding of epiblepharon, in which the eyelid margin is in proper apposition but a fold of hypertrophic orbicularis muscle and skin causes rotation and inversion of the pretarsal tissues and eyelashes. Rotation of the lower eyelid inward, however, can also occur in isolation. An astute clinician will be able to pick up on the symptoms of intermittent blockage with primarily epiphora and view the malposition of the medial aspect of the lower eyelid, simultaneously checking for normal punctal anatomy. Conservative nonsurgical treatment is warranted as this condition generally does not lead to infective dacryocystitis and almost universally resolves with growth of the midface by 3 or 4 years of age.

Dacryocystocele (See Also Chap. 50)

Dacryocystoceles usually present as a firm bluish or bluish-gray mass in the area of the lacrimal sac, below the medial canthal tendon, on the first few days of life. This is a condition whereby mucous, amniotic fluid, and secretions of the

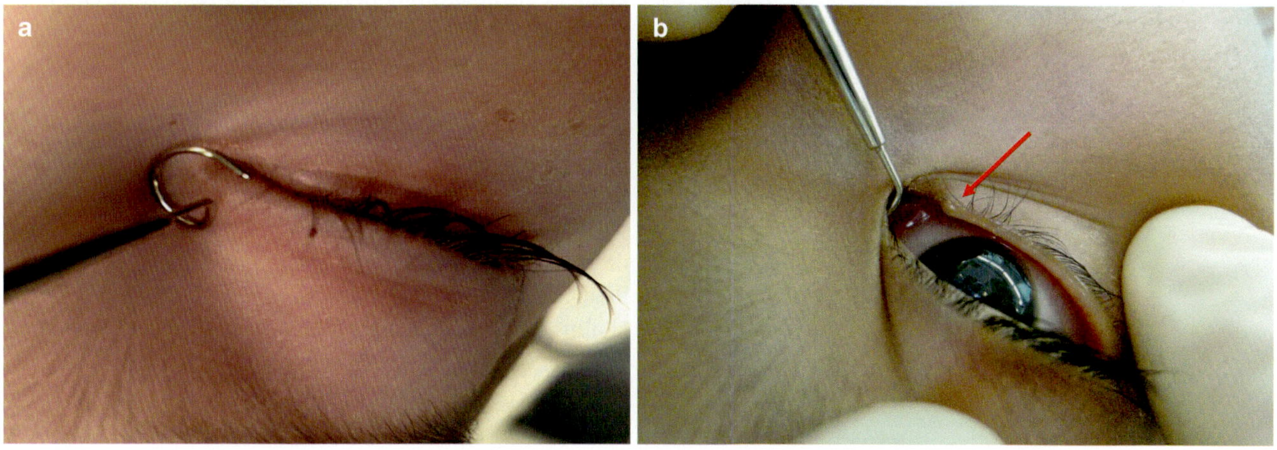

Fig. 41.4 Attempt to pass a pigtail probe from the upper canaliculus into the lower canaliculus to reestablish the inferior punctum

respiratory epithelium fill a blind passage of the lacrimal system. The appearance is generally so classic that no further investigation is necessary. However, a meningocele and meningoencephalocele can present in this location, although typically present as a mass above the level of the medial canthal tendon, and parents may also note slight pulsation of the mass. It is important to always examine the nasal cavity for intranasal extension of the dilated cyst below the turbinate, as large nasal dacryocystoceles can be obstructive. Infants, while feeding, are often considered obligate nasal breathers, and this condition has been reported to cause respiratory compromise, particularly when bilateral [8]. In rare syndromes such as choanal atresia, these infants may be unable to breathe through the nose at all.

Treatment of dacryocystocele varies depending on practice patterns. These are rarely infected at birth; however if they become infected, the potential cellulitis in a newborn can be life threatening (Fig. 41.5). Often conservative management can be achieved with willing and capable parents. Firm pressure on the cyst often will release the contents through a partially patent punctum. Repetitive massage several times a day can convert a dacryocystocele into a more "typical" nasolacrimal duct obstruction. If the contents cannot be expressed, more definitive treatment may be necessary. If conservative treatment fails, opinions vary regarding best course of treatment from a simple probing (which can be performed in the office) to empiric IV antibiotic coverage and nasal endoscopy with complete surgical excision of the nasal cavity cyst structure or dacryocystorhinostomy (see also Chap. 50 on "Congenital Dacryocystocele and Management").

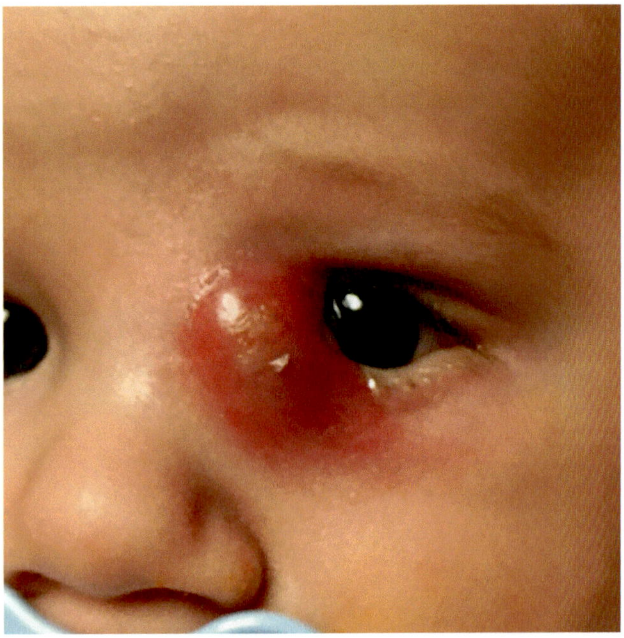

Fig. 41.5 Infected left dacryocystocele in a newborn infant. (Photo courtesy of Cat N Burkat, MD FACS)

Fistula and Diverticulum

Fistulas generally present overlying the lacrimal sac, just inferior to the medial canthal ligament. They can be unilateral or bilateral. Careful history will guide the clinician to the fact that the tear expression is infrequent and minimal and presents on the same portion of the eyelid (over the fistula) every time. The opening of the fistula can be well hidden and initially difficult to find. Treatment involves silicone intubation of the nasolacrimal system followed by excision of the fistula tract with multiple layer closure.

Congenital Nasolacrimal Duct Obstruction

Incidence, History, and Evaluation

Congenital nasolacrimal duct obstruction is a common problem affecting approximately 5–7% of all newborns [9–11]. The prevalence rate increases in children with a history of premature birth and in children delivered by primary cesarean section versus vaginal birth [12, 13]. The spontaneous resolution rate is extremely high and is generally accepted that approximately 90% will resolve without treatment in the first year of life, with the primary care physician caring for a vast majority of these patients (Fig. 41.6).

It is important when the patient presents with signs and symptoms of congenital nasolacrimal obstruction that a through history and physical exam be undertaken to aid in the accurate diagnosis and treatment plan. The typical history of chronic mild discharge, mattering, mild conjunctival injection, dacryocystitis, and chronic dermatitis from skin irritation is supportive of a typical distal obstruction at the entrance to the nasopharynx. The most common obstruction is in the bony, distal portion of the nasolacrimal duct, at the valve of Hasner, distal to the lacrimal sac. This causes stagnation of tear collection and chronic recurrent infection. A history of simple epiphora without recurrent infection should raise a red flag for the clinician. Epiphora alone in a contrary way suggests a more complicated etiology and could suggest a more proximal obstruction, chronic surface eye disease, or congenital glaucoma (particularly in association with photophobia and blepharospasm). Additional history is helpful to predict maldevelopment of the nasolacrimal effluent system which is a feature of several systemic conditions: Down syndrome, ectodermal dysplasia, Hay-Wells syndrome, branchio-oculofacial syndrome, CHARGE, and Treacher Collins syndrome, among others [14]. Additionally, a history of severe mucopurulent discharge, eyelid edema, marked erythema, or obvious acute dacryocystitis should alert the clinician of an unusual etiology such as *Nontypeable Haemophilus influenzae*, *Neisseria gonorrhoeae*, or other virulent organisms [15, 16]. The etiologies of suppurative

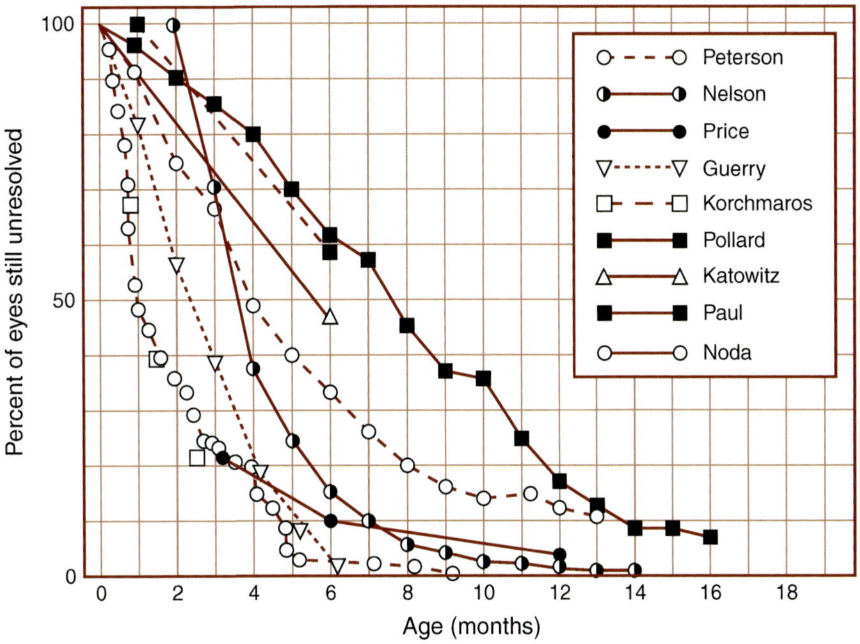

Fig. 41.6 Diagram demonstrating that spontaneous resolution rate without treatment is extremely high within the first year of life. (MacEwen CJ, Young JD Epiphora during the first year of life. Eye 1991;5:596–600)

dacryocystitis are very rare, particularly since the advent of routine *Haemophilus influenzae* type B (Hib) vaccination; however, they still do occur and are reason to culture the discharge in unusual cases [17].

Examination and diagnostic testing should proceed from least to most invasive interventions. Vision and visual development is essential to measure as amblyopia occurs at a significantly higher rate in children with NLDO [18, 19]. Simple observation of the external eyelids and eyelid position can be achieved without intrusiveness. Next eversion of the eyelids can be performed with a simple magnification device (such as a 20D lens) to inspect the puncta and proximal structures. Compression of the lacrimal sac is next at which point cultures can be taken if indicated, and fluorescein dye disappearance test (FDDT) usually follows. This test is performed as follows: (1) instill one drop of 1% fluorescein into the conjunctival sac bilaterally, (2) inspect immediately for fullness of instillation with a cobalt blue light, and (3) inspect again a 5-minute grading for amount of retention (100% = 3) vs complete resolution (none remaining = 0). Advanced radiologic dacryocystography is rarely necessary in the treatment of typical NLDO and in the pediatric population would be performed with sedation at the time of definitive treatment [20]. Ultrasound is a simple noninvasive test for the evaluation of dacryocystocele [21, 22].

Nonsurgical Treatment and Natural History

Early in the course of the obstruction, the management is generally conservative, consisting of empiric antibiotics and massage. Spontaneous resolution is an accepted course in the natural history of congenital nasolacrimal duct obstruction. Paul and Shepherd reviewed the literature and combined the reports of resolution on a graph [23] (Fig. 41.6). This was confirmed in a more contemporary multicenter study by the Pediatric Eye Disease Investigator Group (PEDIG). PEDIG reported that in infants between 6 and 10 months of age, congenital NLDO will resolve within 6 months without surgical management in 66% of eyes [24].

Massage of the lacrimal sac has repeatedly reported to improve spontaneous resolution rates. The correct maneuver for performing the massage is important and often credited to Crigler's report in 1923 and is known colloquially as the "Crigler maneuver" or "Crigler massage" [2]. Kushner preformed a prospective study involving 3 groups with 175 obstructed lacrimal systems. Groups consisted of no massage, simple massage, and hydrostatic massage. The hydrostatic massage group achieved significant resolution of 30%, whereas the simple and no massage groups achieved only 8% resolution [10]. Both the Crigler maneuver and Kushner's hydrostatic massage are designed to increase and transmit fluid pressure down through the bony nasolacrimal canal to the imperforate opening between the canal and the nasopharynx (valve of Hasner).

Timing of Definitive Nasolacrimal Probing on Outcome

Does the timing of probe procedure effect the success rate? From the earliest discussions in the literature, the question of the optimum timing to perform the definitive probing procedure has been proposed and questioned. It was probably

Ffooks in 1962 that suggested from his case series that the cure rate of a simple probing may decrease if initially performed after 9 months of age [9]. Subsequent studies seemed to confirm similar decreased probing success if preformed at ages over 12 or 13 months [25, 26]. However, other early studies seemed to contradict this finding, with El-Mansoury reporting 94% and Robb reporting 92% success with simple probing and irrigation after 13 months of age [27, 28]. It is important to note that all of these studies exclude cases in which there is an associated concurrent acute dacryocystitis, which is known to markedly affect success rate of simple probing. PEDIG attempted to resolve this question in a multicenter study of simple probing procedure performed between 6 months and 4 years of age. Success of initial probing was reported at 78% between 6 and <12 months, 79% between 12 and <24 months, and 79% over 24 months of age [29]. Suggesting that for uncomplicated or "typical" congenital tear duct obstructions without concurrent dacryocystitis, timing of the procedure does not change efficacy of the procedure and success rate of the outcome.

Probing

"Office probing" is the term given to performing a probe of the nasolacrimal system under topical anesthesia in the clinic office without conscious sedation or anesthesia. It is generally a preferred method by parents [30] and has the benefit of avoidance of the potential neurotoxicity risks of general inhalational anesthesia (Fig. 41.7) [31]. Additionally, probing in the office setting has been shown to be a more cost-effective treatment [32, 33]. In an extremely large series involving 2369 eyes, Stager found a success rate of office probing of 94% if performed under 9 months of age [34]. While there is no absolute upper age limit at which an office probing cannot be performed, most clinicians prefer to reserve this technique for children under 12 months old, as children older than this will require more restraint and the globe or fragile lacrimal system can potentially be damaged if the child moves during the procedure. When performing this procedure in the office, it is important that the clinician and staff be experienced that there is sufficient lighting and magnification (surgical loupes) and the staff be aware of the risk for potential aspiration to the lungs from an unprotected infant airway. Because of this risk, irrigation after the office probe procedure is not recommended. Probing in the office should not be done in cases of bilateral dacryocystoceles due to a high risk for a compromised airway secondary to an association with bilateral intranasal cysts [35].

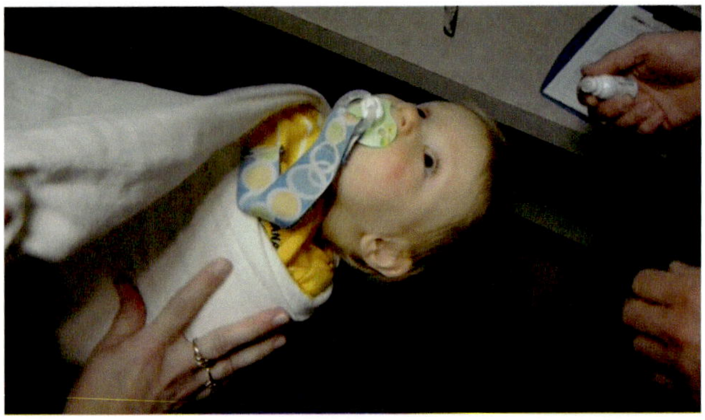

Fig. 41.7 Office probing of the nasolacrimal system requires careful swaddling of the child

Noncomplicated Obstructions

If the child fails conservative management, does not have acute dacryocystitis, and is not candidate for office probing, a procedure under general anesthesia in the operating room should be scheduled.

This procedure, while often labelled "simple," is actually a complex series of important maneuvers that must be completed correctly to provide successful uncomplicated results.

- Step 1 involves dilating the upper and lower puncta with a fine tip dilator that is first passed perpendicular to the eyelid margin (Fig. 41.8) and then rotated to travel parallel to the medial aspect of the eyelid toward the lacrimal bone (Fig. 41.9a, b).
- Step 2, the dilator is replaced with a Bowman probe, and in an identical manner, first perpendicular then parallel to the eyelid, the Bowman probe is advanced while applying mild lateral traction on the associated eyelid.

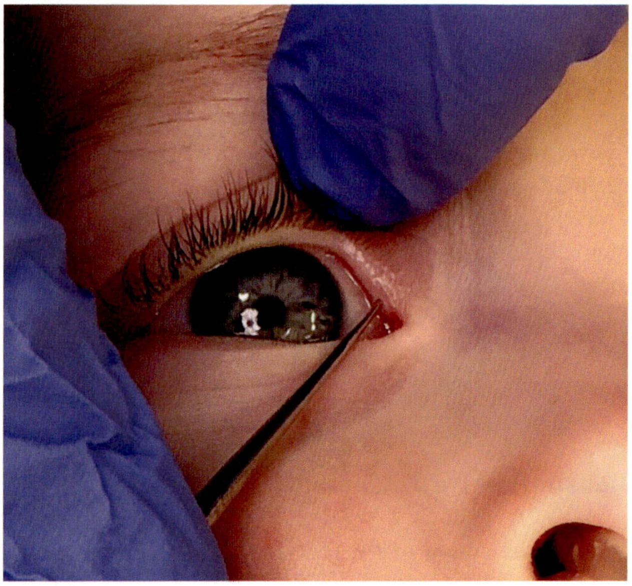

Fig. 41.8 The punctal dilator is first placed perpendicular to the eyelid margin

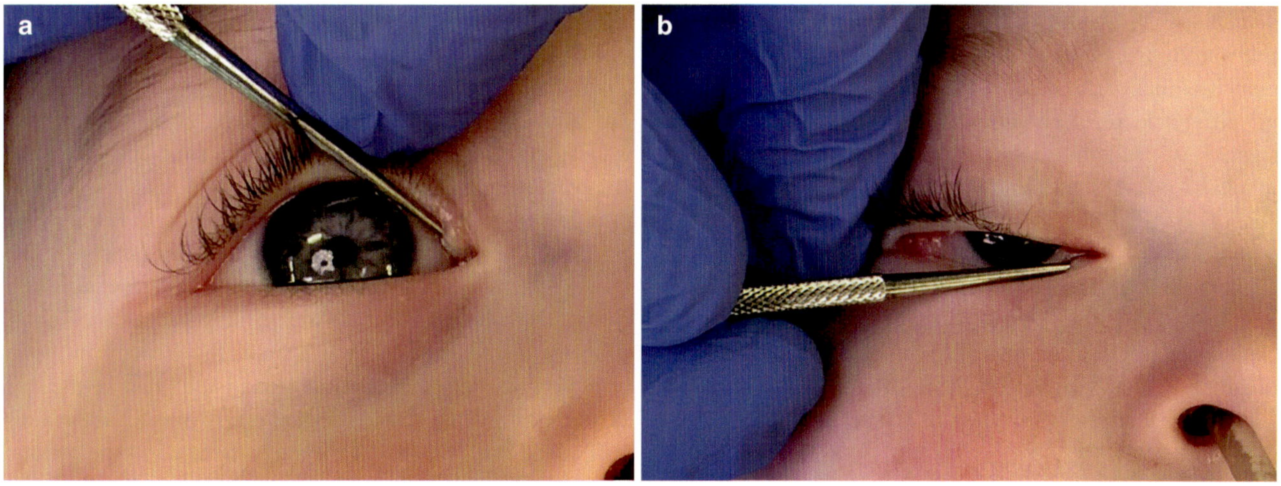

Fig. 41.9 The punctal dilator and probe are then rotated to travel parallel to the medial aspect of the eyelid toward a hard stop along the lacrimal bone. (**a**) Direction in upper eyelid, (**b**) Direction in lower eyelid

- Step 3, when the lacrimal sac is entered, the clinician must recognize the "hard stop" as the Bowman probe encounters the medial wall of the lacrimal sac which is intimate with the lacrimal bone.
- Step 4, eyelid traction is released. Care must be taken to avoid the creation of false passages throughout this procedure.
- Step 5, once the hard stop is confirmed, the probe is rotated 90° inferiorly, taking care to keep contact along the bone, and advanced into the nasolacrimal duct. The probe should rest comfortably on the superior orbital ridge, and two landmarks are important to guide the probe in the correct direction. One landmark is the superior trochlear notch, which if present, lies in a direct line toward the bony nasolacrimal duct. The second landmark is the "eye tooth" (the third tooth from the midline) (Fig. 41.10). The probe should be gently directed inferiorly and slightly posterolaterally along these landmarks, toward the inferior meatus. In a "typical" obstruction of the imperforate valve of Hasner, a second stop can be felt, which can then be punctured with the probe.

Irrigation of the lacrimal system with fluorescein dye is often performed next to ensure patency of the system. An aspiration cannula must be placed before any attempt at irrigation in a sedated patient in order to prevent aspiration. To ensure patency a second probe is advanced from the nasal vestibule posterolaterally to the inferior meatus below the turbinate. Small lateral movements can then be made with the second probe until contact is made with the first probe. Establishment of "metal-to-metal" contact between the two probes is associated with a higher rate of surgical success [36]. If necessary, the inferior turbinate bone may be fractured medially with a blunt end of a Freer periosteal elevator for improved outflow [37]. Prophylactic systemic antibiotics are not indicated in otherwise healthy patients [38–40].

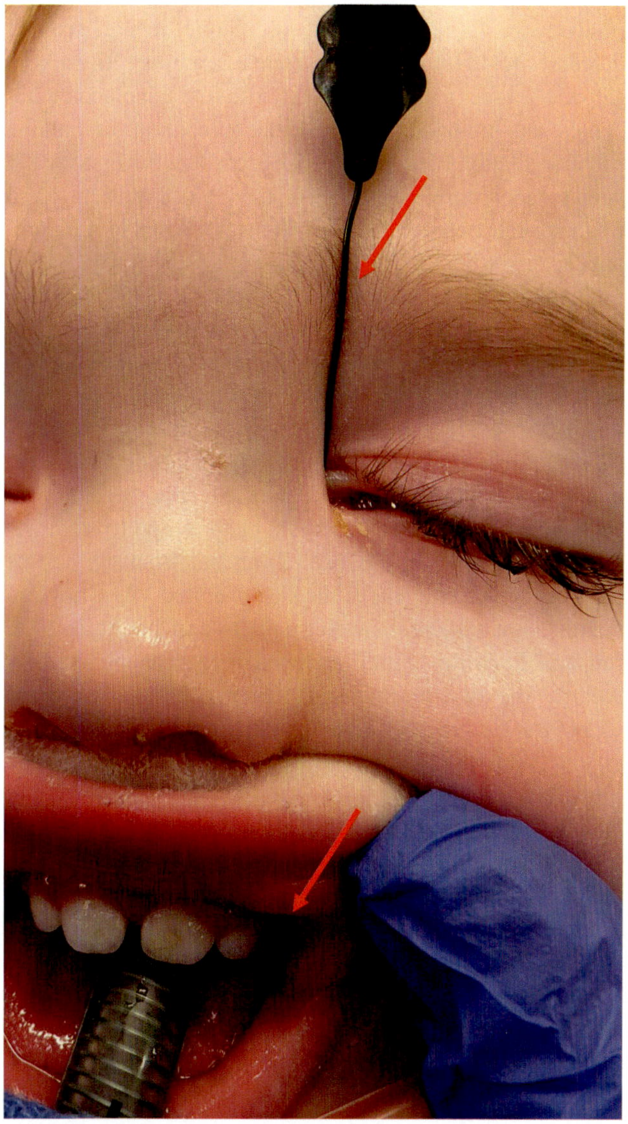

Fig. 41.10 The "eye tooth" position to confirm the correct direction of passage within the nasolacrimal bony duct

Primary NLD intubation or balloon catheter dilation has been promoted by some surgeons. The success rate of primary stenting of the nasolacrimal system is over 90%, with no difference between monocanalicular and bicanalicular stents [29]. Balloon catheter dilation carries a significantly increased cost of materials.

Complex Nasolacrimal Obstructions

In simplest terms, a complex obstruction is either a recurrent obstruction or an obstruction of the system which is not isolated to the location of the valve of Hasner.

Recurrent Obstruction

When a simple probing procedure has failed to resolve the obstruction, the success rate of simple repeat probing decreases to 40–60% with subsequent attempts [26, 34, 41]. Choices for treatment of recurrent obstruction include monocanalicular intubation, bicanalicular intubation, or balloon catheter dilation. The choice of the procedure has historically been surgeon's preference, and all three procedures have had a success rate between 77% and 91% after failed initial probing [33, 42–45].

Bicanalicular nasolacrimal intubation procedure involves (1) packing the nasopharynx with oxymetazoline-soaked pledgets for 5 minutes, (2) performing the standard probing procedure making careful note of the location of the Bowman probe as it exits under the inferior turbinate, (3) replacement of the Bowman probe with the probe of the bicanalicular stent, (4) intubation of the opposite canalicular system using the same retrieval method, and (5) removal of the probe from the silicone tubing and securing the free ends of the silicone tube in the nasopharynx. The Crawford stent system has a probe with a bulbous end that fits into the retrieval hook for "blind" retrieval in the nasopharynx by locking the two mechanisms together. If not using the Crawford system, or if the bulb cannot be locked adequately, the probe can be retrieved using a straight hemostat.

Different methods have been described to secure the free ends. A common method involves pushing the probe through a silicone "bolster" and tying the ends of the tube. The bolster system is designed to "catch" under the inferior turbinate bone for easy retrieval with a muscle hook at the time of removal. Conversely, the free ends can be tied in a square knot and either secured to the lateral aspect of the nasal mucosa with a 6-0 polypropylene suture or attached to a long 4-0 silk suture which is cut long and left freely hanging into the posterior aspect of the nasopharynx. This long thread can be blindly hooked with a muscle hook at the time of removal.

In the monocanalicular intubation procedure, Steps 1 and 2 are identical. In Step 3, a Ritleng probe with central stylet is used to replace the Bowman probe and cannulate the problematic upper or lower system. In Step 4, the stylet is removed, and the hollow probe is used to guide the nylon portion of the Monoka stent into the nasopharynx. The nylon feeder thread is retrieved in the nasopharynx, which pulls the silicone tube into the Ritleng probe. In Step 5, with the nylon portion held secure, the Ritleng probe is removed. In Step 6, the nylon thread is pull taut so the silicone portion of the tube is fed carefully into the nasolacrimal canal until the end of the stent is seated in the puncta. Finally, the nylon thread is cut so that only a portion remains freely hanging in the nasopharynx. The silicone tubing is typically left in place for a period of 3 months (range 6 weeks to 6 months) [42, 46–48].

Balloon catheter dilation (dacryoplasty) is also popular and has the advantage of increased success over probing alone, without the complication of requiring postoperative management and removal of the silicone tube. It also is considered by some to be a simpler and less traumatic procedure; however balloon dacryoplasty does come with additional expense compared with other procedures. Also, when the obstruction lies in the canalicular anatomy, it is unclear if the balloon dilation would be as effective as silicone stent intubation [49]. There is only one commercially available device, the LacriCath system (Atrion, Birmingham, AL). The technique involves using either a 2 mm or 3 mm diameter balloon, which encases a standard flexible probe. The probe with deflated balloon is inserted into the distal nasolacrimal duct and through the valve of Hasner, followed by manual inflation using the included pump to 8 atmospheres for 90 seconds, deflation, and reinflation again to 8 atmospheres for 60 seconds. It is then withdrawn 10 mm proximally and reinflated in a similar fashion, which results in the inflated balloon mechanically dilating the membranous ostium. The probe and balloon come marked with guides which line up at the punctum so the surgeon is aware of the location of the balloon at all times.

The question of whether silicone stent placement or balloon dacryoplasty to treat recurrent obstruction has been studied. The results of both multicenter studies and large clinical practice patterns support an equivalent success rate between stent placement and balloon dacryoplasty [42, 43]. Comparing success of bicanalicular to monocanalicular stent techniques after failed probing is likely technique-dependent, with different surgeons reporting contrary success rates between the two procedures [48, 50].

Acquired Pediatric NLDO and Atypical Obstruction

Acquired non-traumatic pediatric nasolacrimal obstructions can occur for a variety of reasons. The most common etiology, however, is likely an internal stricture formation following an infection with a virus or bacteria that damages the columnar epithelial lining, such as Herpes virus or adenovirus. The location of the obstruction is typically in the proximal canalicular system.

Atypical obstructions are noted at the time of primary probing as frequently as 25–39% [51, 52]. Atypical obstructions include primary stricture of either canalicular system, stricture at the valve of Rosenmüller, narrowing along the length of the bony nasolacrimal canal, or a complex mucosal flap structure covering the opening into the nasopharynx.

Finally, in some instances the lacrimal sac itself is enlarged, dilated, or redundant. This is more typically seen if the child has suffered prolonged recurrent infections. Upon compression of the lacrimal sac, a profound amount of purulent material can be expressed. In this instance, it is often very difficult for the probe to find the inferior/distal entrance to the bony nasolacrimal canal.

There is no consensus on best treatment of atypical or acquired pediatric nasolacrimal obstructions. Conversion from primary probing to silicone stent placement is likely warranted in these cases.

False Passage

Management of false passage: Occasionally the surgeon will encounter a false passage in the nasolacrimal system. These are usually part of the proximal canalicular system and often created surgically at the time of an initial probing procedure. There are two basic methods to approach this condition; both require a stent be placed into the nasolacrimal canal during the healing process. It is rare for this condition to result in the need for DCR. If the false passage is only in one canaliculus, a pigtail probe can be attempted to be passed in a retrograde fashion from the opposite canaliculus. The pigtail probe should have a notched tip which allows a suture to be fastened to it. Once the tip of the pigtail probe is passed, a fine 6-0 prolene suture is secured to the notched end. This suture is then rotated into the canalicular system as the pigtail probe is removed. This prolene suture can then be used as a pilot suture to pass a silicone stent. The second method involves using a fine Bowman probe 000/0000 or a small gauge soft angiocatheter to "fill" the false passage. This fine gauge probe is passed initially and finds its way into the false passage. The subsequent step involves using a Crawford stent with the bulb end removed. The Crawford stent is passed through the same punctum and canaliculus, while the Bowman probe is still present in the false passage. Since the false passage is now occupied, it is often possible for the Crawford stent to find the true canaliculus and lacrimal sac. Once in the lacrimal sac, the initial probe in the false passage can be removed and the system intubated with the silicone stent.

Acute Dacryocystitis

Dacryocystitis is uncommon in infants but is almost exclusively associated with congenital nasolacrimal duct obstruction [16]. Signs of tense edema, erythema, mucopurulent discharge, pain, fever, and leukocytosis are all characteristics of this infection of the lacrimal sac. The prevalence of bacteremia has been reported at approximately 25% [53]. As previously mentioned the success rate of a simple probing procedure with concurrent dacryocystitis is markedly diminished. However, success of probing is increased and need for repeat procedure decreased when initial nasolacrimal duct probing is preceded by IV antibiotic treatment 24 hours in advance [53]. If the initial procedure is unsuccessful, treatment should include preoperative IV antibiotic coverage with potential hospitalization followed by silicone stent placement with or without nasal endoscopic dacryocystorhinostomy.

Dacryocystorhinostomy

Dacryocystorhinostomy (DCR) is generally reserved for patients who have failed multiple other procedures or who have midline facial defects or bony facial anomalies that predispose to failure or traumatic acquired NLDO. Excellent clinical success rates have been documented when performed via external (88–96%) and internal (82–94%) approaches [54–57]. Adjunctive mitomycin C has been shown to be safe in children and is probably most useful in repeat DCR after fibrosis of a previous intranasal osteotomy. It is not typically used for routine cases since the success with this agent (94.4%) in endoscopic DCR does not differ remarkably from the results found in other studies without it [58].

Conclusion

It is important to remember that obstructions can occur at any place along the nasolacrimal system, can be multifactorial, and can be related to other diseases. When symptoms are intolerable and persist, or risk ocular integrity, congenital nasolacrimal duct obstruction can be managed in a stepwise fashion, starting with medical management, progressing to dilation and probing, followed by more invasive surgical procedures. The natural history of congenital NLDO and the appropriate utilization of effective treatment options will typically result in excellent patient outcomes.

References

1. Yazici B, Yazici Z. Frequency of the common canaliculus: a radiological study. Arch Ophthalmol. 2000;118(10):1381–5.
2. Crigler LW. The treatment of congenital dacryocystitis. JAMA. 1923;81:23–4.
3. Hurwitz JJ. In: Hurwitz JJ, editor. The lacrimal system, Embryology of the lacrimal drainage system. Philadelphia: Lippincott-Raven; 1996.
4. Taylor D, editor. Pediatric ophthalmology. 2nd ed. Lacrimal system. Day S, editor. London: Blackwell; 1997.
5. Burkat CN, Lucarelli MJ. Chapter 1 Anatomy of the lacrimal system. In: Cohen AJ, Mercandetti M, Brazzo BG, editors. The lacrimal system. 2nd ed. Cham: Springer; 2015.
6. Soliman M, Lueder GT. Initial management of congenital canalicular atresia. J AAPOS. 2015;19(3):220–2.
7. Shapiro MB, France TD. The ocular features of Down's syndrome. Am J Ophthalmol. 1985;99(6):659–63.
8. Rogister F, Goffart Y, Daele J. Management of congenital dacryocystocele: report of 3 clinical cases. B-ENT. 2016;12(1):83–8.
9. Ffooks OO. Dacryocystitis in infancy. Br J Ophthalmol. 1962;46(7):422–34.
10. Kushner BJ. Congenital nasolacrimal system obstruction. Arch Ophthalmol. 1982;100(4):597–600.
11. Petersen RA, Robb RM. The natural course of congenital obstruction of the nasolacrimal duct. J Pediatr Ophthalmol Strabismus. 1978;15(4):246–50.
12. Lorena SH, Silva JA, Scarpi MJ. Congenital nasolacrimal duct obstruction in premature children. J Pediatr Ophthalmol Strabismus. 2013;50(4):239–44.
13. Spaniol K, et al. Association between congenital nasolacrimal duct obstruction and delivery by cesarean section. Am J Perinatol. 2015;32(3):271–6.
14. Wenger JD. Epidemiology of Haemophilus influenzae type b disease and impact of Haemophilus influenzae type b conjugate vaccines in the United States and Canada. Pediatr Infect Dis J. 1998;17(9 Suppl):S132–6.
15. Murphy TF, et al. Nontypeable Haemophilus influenzae as a pathogen in children. Pediatr Infect Dis J. 2009;28(1):43–8.
16. Ali MJ. Pediatric acute dacryocystitis. Ophthalmic Plast Reconstr Surg. 2015;31(5):341–7.
17. Chhabra MS, Motley WW 3rd, Mortensen JE. *Eikenella corrodens* as a causative agent for neonatal conjunctivitis. J AAPOS. 2008;12(5):524–5.
18. Kipp MA, Kipp MA Jr, Struthers W. Anisometropia and amblyopia in nasolacrimal duct obstruction. J AAPOS. 2013;17(3):235–8.
19. Saleem AA, et al. Anisometropia and refractive status in children with unilateral congenital nasolacrimal duct obstruction. Taiwan J Ophthalmol. 2018;8(1):31–5.
20. Maliborski A, Rozycki R. Diagnostic imaging of the nasolacrimal drainage system. Part I. Radiological anatomy of lacrimal pathways. Physiology of tear secretion and tear outflow. Med Sci Monit. 2014;20:628–38.
21. Kim YH, et al. Dacryocystocele on prenatal ultrasonography: diagnosis and postnatal outcomes. Ultrasonography. 2015;34(1):51–7.
22. Machado MA, et al. Congenital dacryocystocele: diagnosis using ante and post-natal ultrasonography. Arq Bras Oftalmol. 2014;77(4):261–3.
23. Paul TO, Shepherd R. Congenital nasolacrimal duct obstruction: natural history and the timing of optimal intervention. J Pediatr Ophthalmol Strabismus. 1994;31(6):362–7.
24. Pediatric Eye Disease Investigator, G. Resolution of congenital nasolacrimal duct obstruction with nonsurgical management. Arch Ophthalmol. 2012;130(6):730–4.
25. Mittelman D. Probing and irrigation for congenital nasolacrimal duct obstruction. Arch Ophthalmol. 1986;104(8):1125–6.
26. Katowitz JA, Welsh MG. Timing of initial probing and irrigation in congenital nasolacrimal duct obstruction. Ophthalmology. 1987;94(6):698–705.
27. el-Mansoury J, et al. Results of late probing for congenital nasolacrimal duct obstruction. Ophthalmology. 1986;93(8):1052–4.
28. Robb RM. Success rates of nasolacrimal duct probing at time intervals after 1 year of age. Ophthalmology. 1998;105(7):1307–9; discussion 1309–10.
29. Pediatric Eye Disease Investigator, G, et al. Primary treatment of nasolacrimal duct obstruction with probing in children younger than 4 years. Ophthalmology. 2008;115(3):577–584 e3.
30. Goldblum TA, et al. Office probing for congenital nasolacrimal duct obstruction: a study of parental satisfaction. J Pediatr Ophthalmol Strabismus. 1996;33(4):244–7.
31. Good WV. Is anesthesia safe for young children? J AAPOS. 2014;18(6):519–20.
32. Le Garrec J, et al. Nasolacrimal duct office probing in children under the age of 12 months: cure rate and cost evaluation. J Fr Ophtalmol. 2016;39(2):171–7.
33. Eshraghi B, Jamshidian-Tehrani M, Mirmohammadsadeghi A. Comparison of the success rate between monocanalicular and bicanalicular intubations in incomplete complex congenital nasolacrimal duct obstruction. Orbit. 2017;36(4):215–7.
34. Stager D, et al. Office probing of congenital nasolacrimal duct obstruction. Ophthalmic Surg. 1992;23(7):482–4.
35. Levin AV, et al. Nasal endoscopy in the treatment of congenital lacrimal sac mucoceles. Int J Pediatr Otorhinolaryngol. 2003;67(3):255–61.
36. Mocan MC, et al. Prognostic value of metal-metal contact during nasolacrimal duct probing. Can J Ophthalmol. 2015;50(4):314–7.
37. Albert DL, Lucarelli MJ. Clinical atlas of procedures in ophthalmic and oculofacial surgery. 2nd ed. New York: Oxford University Press; 2012.
38. Schaeffer AR, Gordon RA, Sood SK. Bacteremia following nasolacrimal duct probing. Invest Ophthalmol Vis Sci. 1990;31(suppl):610.
39. Venugopalan P, et al. Low frequency of bacteraemia during eye surgery obviates the need for endocarditis prophylaxis. Eye (Lond). 2001;15(Pt 6):753–5.
40. Eippert GA, Burnstine RA, Bates JH. Lacrimal-duct-probing-induced bacteremia: should children with congenital heart defects receive antibiotic prophylaxis? J Pediatr Ophthalmol Strabismus. 1998;35(1):38–40.
41. Pediatric Eye Disease Investigator, G, et al. Repeat probing for treatment of persistent nasolacrimal duct obstruction. J AAPOS. 2009;13(3):306–7.
42. Repka MX, et al. Balloon catheter dilation and nasolacrimal duct intubation for treatment of nasolacrimal duct obstruction after failed probing. Arch Ophthalmol. 2009;127(5):633–9.
43. Goldstein SM, Goldstein JB, Katowitz JA. Comparison of monocanalicular stenting and balloon dacryoplasty in secondary treatment of congenital nasolacrimal duct obstruction after failed primary probing. Ophthal Plast Reconstr Surg. 2004;20(5):352–7.

44. Ali MJ, et al. Simple vs complex congenital nasolacrimal duct obstructions: etiology, management and outcomes. Int Forum Allergy Rhinol. 2015;5(2):174–7.
45. Schnall BM. Pediatric nasolacrimal duct obstruction. Curr Opin Ophthalmol. 2013;24(5):421–4.
46. Migliori ME, Putterman AM. Silicone intubation for the treatment of congenital lacrimal duct obstruction: successful results removing the tubes after six weeks. Ophthalmology. 1988;95(6):792–5.
47. El-Essawy R. Effect of timing of silicone tube removal on the result of duct intubation in children with congenital nasolacrimal duct obstruction. Ophthalmic Plast Reconstr Surg. 2013;29(1):48–50.
48. Eustis HS, Nguyen AH. The treatment of congenital nasolacrimal duct obstruction in children: a retrospective review. J Pediatr Ophthalmol Strabismus. 2018;55(1):65–7.
49. Tao S, et al. Success of balloon catheter dilatation as a primary or secondary procedure for congenital nasolacrimal duct obstruction. Ophthalmology. 2002;109(11):2108–11.
50. Rajabi MT, et al. Bicanalicular versus monocanalicular intubation after failed probing in congenital nasolacrimal duct obstruction. Int J Ophthalmol. 2016;9(10):1466–70.
51. Pediatric Eye Disease Investigator, G, et al. Primary treatment of nasolacrimal duct obstruction with nasolacrimal duct intubation in children younger than 4 years of age. J AAPOS. 2008;12(5):445–50.
52. Pediatric Eye Disease Investigator, G, et al., Primary treatment of nasolacrimal duct obstruction with balloon catheter dilation in children younger than 4 years of age. J AAPOS, 2008. 12(5): p. 451–5.
53. Baskin DE, et al. The timing of antibiotic administration in the management of infant dacryocystitis. J AAPOS. 2008;12(5):456–9.
54. Barnes EA, Abou-Rayyah Y, Rose GE. Pediatric dacryocystorhinostomy for nasolacrimal duct obstruction. Ophthalmology. 2001;108(9):1562–4.
55. Vanderveen DK, et al. Endoscopic dacryocystorhinostomy in children. J AAPOS. 2001;5(3):143–7.
56. Kominek P, Cervenka S. Pediatric endonasal dacryocystorhinostomy: a report of 34 cases. Laryngoscope. 2005;115(10):1800–3.
57. Kominek P, et al. Primary pediatric endonasal dacryocystorhinostomy – a review of 58 procedures. Int J Pediatr Otorhinolaryngol. 2010;74(6):661–4.
58. Dolmetsch AM, Gallon MA, Holds JB. Nonlaser endoscopic endonasal dacryocystorhinostomy with adjunctive mitomycin C in children. Ophthalmic Plast Reconstr Surg. 2008;24(5):390–3.

External Dacryocystorhinostomy

42

Daniele Lorenzano and Geoffrey E. Rose

Introduction

Nasolacrimal duct stenosis or occlusion can give both "flow" symptoms (variable blurring of vision due to excess tear line; tear spillage) and "volume" symptoms due to mucoid debris refluxing from the lacrimal sac debris into the tear lake – causing gross smearing of the vision, recurrent conjunctivitis, dacryocystitis or gummed eyelids on awakening [1].

A *total* cure of volume symptoms and signs is achievable with well-performed external dacryocystorhinostomy (DCR), but flow symptoms and signs will persist (despite a freely patent anastomosis) in a minority of cases – largely dependent on the rate of tear production relative to canalicular conductance and tear evaporation. A "perfect" DCR converts the lacrimal sac into part of the lateral nasal wall, thereby removing any chamber for debris to collect and reflux back into the tear lake – that is, to completely cure any volume symptoms and signs [1] (Fig. 42.1a). Incorporation of the lacrimal sac into the lateral nasal wall is readily achieved with external DCR but requires anterior ethmoidectomy and suturing of both the anterior and posterior mucosal flaps to ensure primary intention healing with minimal scarring. Endonasal DCR emulates the same principles as the external approach, but it cannot achieve the same opening for the lacrimal sac fundus, and it also suffers more secondary-intention healing that leads to ring contracture of the inferiorly biased anastomosis. Continued volume symptoms and signs, due to residual debris within the sac remnant, are fairly common after endonasal procedures or after inadequate external rhinostomy (Fig. 42.1b).

D. Lorenzano
Moorfields Eye Hospital, London, UK

G. E. Rose (✉)
Moorfields Eye Hospital, London, UK

Institute of Ophthalmology, London, UK

City University, London, UK

Anaesthesia for External Dacryocystorhinostomy

External DCR can be performed under general or local anaesthesia, this being decided on the basis of patient preference and systemic medical conditions, but simultaneous bilateral surgery is usually carried out under general anaesthesia.

Local anaesthesia with intravenous sedation provides an excellent operative field, although there may be more post-operative nasal oozing than after general anaesthesia. To ensure maximum vasoconstriction, an epinephrine-containing local anaesthetic should be infiltrated at least 10 minutes before surgery – this being most conveniently prior to surgical gowning.

After optional intravenous sedation, 3–4 puffs of a 4% lidocaine nasal spray are directed into the anterior nasal space – the nostril being pinched closed after each puff to avoid coughing due to inhalation of the spray. The medial lower lid and paranasal area are then subcutaneously injected with 3 ml of 0.5% bupivacaine with epinephrine (1:100,000 to 1:200,000). A 23G needle is then passed backwards from just above the medial canthus, angulated 20° below the axial plane (avoiding damage to the anterior ethmoidal vessels) and 2–3 ml of the same solution placed to achieve an anterior ethmoidal block. The antero-superior nasal cavity is then packed with about 80 cm of 1 cm packing gauze, soaked in 2 ml of a 4% cocaine solution (or, if cocaine not available, use 4% lidocaine with 1:1000 epinephrine), and this packing should be left in place until suturing of the posterior mucosal flaps has been completed. Topical anaesthesia, such as 1% tetracaine, is administered to both eyes before sterile preparation of the face and is supplemented during the surgery.

General anaesthesia with controlled hypotension, suitable for day case surgery, is readily achieved with total intravenous anaesthesia (TIVA) – using, for example, propofol and remifentanil – or with a combination of volatile inhalational agents (such as isoflurane) and titrated small doses of a

A. J. Cohen, C. N. Burkat (eds.), *Oculofacial, Orbital, and Lacrimal Surgery*, https://doi.org/10.1007/978-3-030-14092-2_42

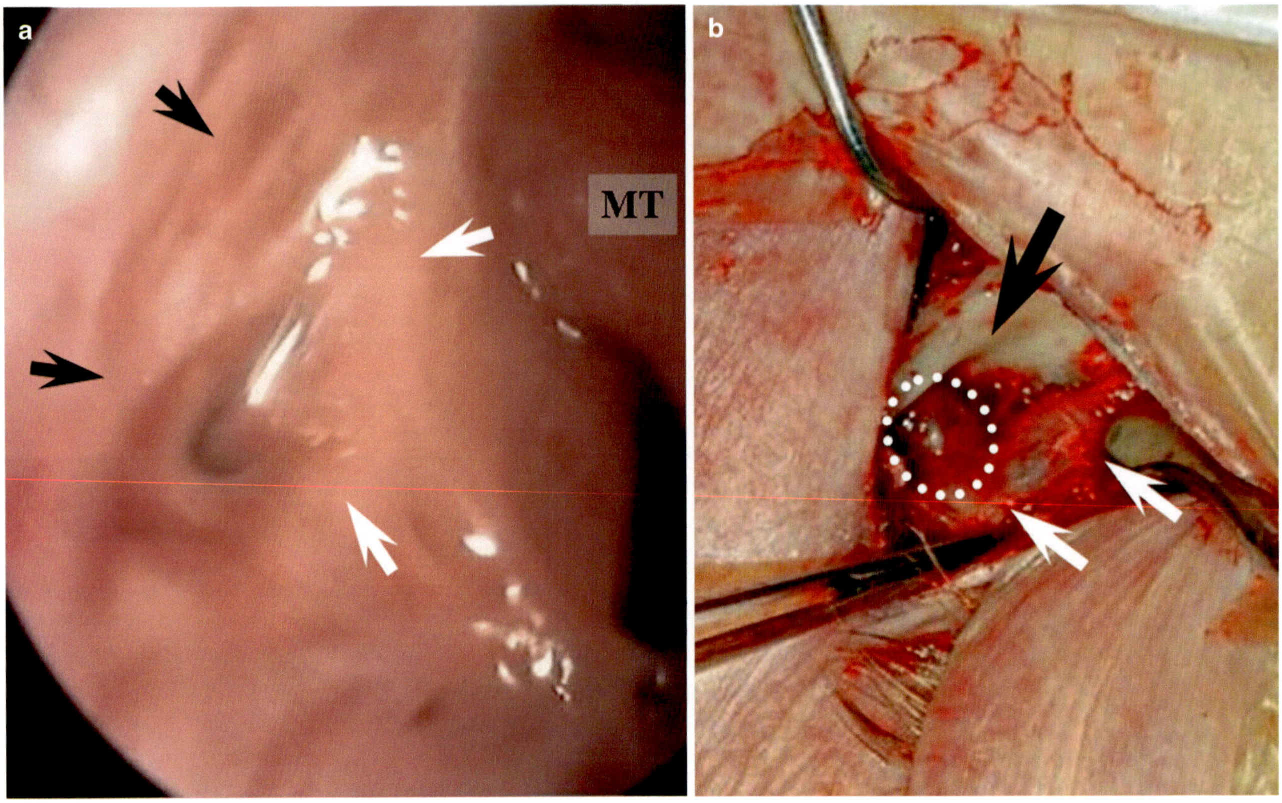

Fig. 42.1 (**a**) Appearance of right lacrimal sac incorporated into lateral nasal wall after successful external dacryocystorhinostomy; the white arrows mark the posterior mucosal anastomosis and the black arrows the anterior mucosal anastomosis ("MT" denotes middle turbinate). (**b**) Failed left endonasal dacryocystorhinostomy with a low, small anastomosis (ring) and significant residual unopened upper sac (white arrows); the black arrow indicates the failure to remove any anterior lacrimal crest

beta-blocker to prevent a compensatory tachycardia [2]. The efficacy of general anaesthesia and the overall drug dosage is markedly reduced if paranasal infiltration of local anaesthetic is performed. Nasal mucosal vasoconstriction is accomplished, after sterile preparation and draping, by placing three cotton tips – moistened in 1:1000 epinephrine – as far superiorly and anteriorly as possible within the nasal space.

To decrease the local venous pressure during either local or general anaesthesia, the headend of the operating table should be raised during surgery.

Surgical Technique for External Dacryocystorhinostomy

A 12–15 mm straight skin incision should be placed on flat paranasal skin about 1 cm in front of the medial canthus, starting just above the canthal tendon (Fig. 42.2a); more posterior incisions should be avoided, as they tend to "bowstring" across the canthal concavity. The skin is separated from the underlying orbicularis oculi (and angular vessels) by spreading with blunt-ended scissors directed backwards towards the anterior limb of the medial canthal tendon. The angular vessels and muscle fibres are then retracted anteromedially using a squint hook, whilst the pretarsal and preseptal portions of orbicularis fibres are separated along the line of the fibres (Fig. 42.2b); separation of the fibres, by spreading them apart with a Rollet's rougine, avoids bleeding and reveals the anterior lacrimal crest. The paranasal periosteum is divided along the anterior lacrimal crest, the periosteal leaf raised to about 12 mm in front of the crest, and the lacrimal sac displaced laterally from its fossa to reveal the posterior lacrimal crest. In some general anaesthetic cases, the surgeon might wish to use two or three fixed traction sutures (2/0 gauge) – these encircling the angular vessels and orbicularis fibres and being clipped to the surgical drapes.

The maxillo-lacrimal suture is exposed by lateral displacement of the lacrimal sac and can usually be entered using an angled periosteal elevator; if this is not possible, the surgeon should perforate the lamina papyracea just behind the posterior lacrimal crest and create the osteotomy by working forwards from this entry site. The periosteal elevator should be moved up and down along the fracture line to facilitate entry of a small up-cutting rongeur into the breach. A large rhinostomy is fashioned by first crossing the thinnest part of the anterior lacrimal crest (close to the skull base;

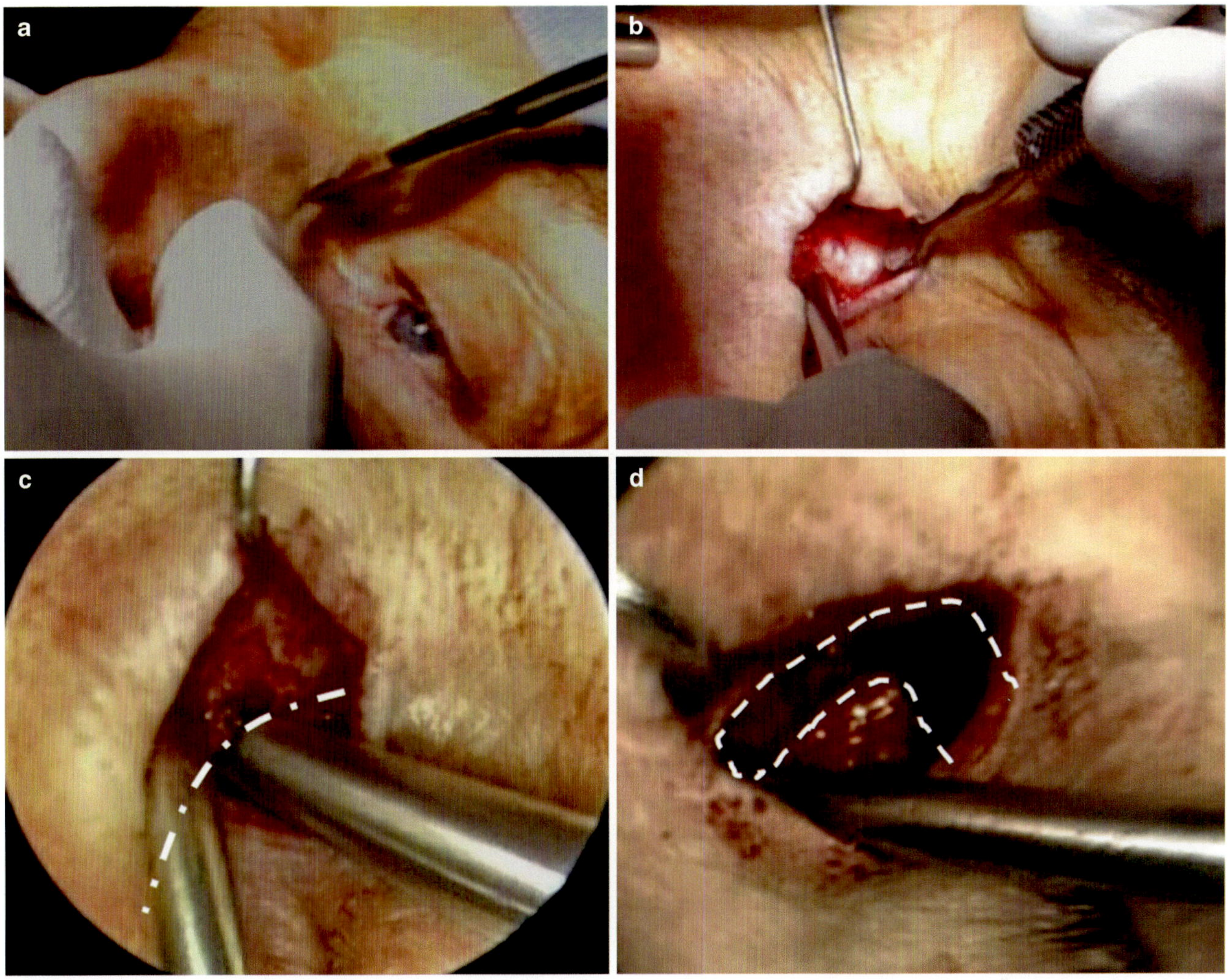

Fig. 42.2 Left external dacryocystorhinostomy: (**a**) Incision placed on the flat area of the nasal bridge; (**b**) spreading between the fibres of orbicularis oculi to minimise haemorrhage; (**c**) initial osteotomy should progress across the anterior lacrimal crest (marked), where it is thinnest in the high fossa; and (**d**) once across the anterior lacrimal crest, bone removal should be directed inferiorly to create an "L-shaped" osteotomy, thereby easing removal of the frontal process of the maxilla

Fig. 42.2c) and then removing bone in an inferior direction in front of the crest (creating an "L-shaped" rhinostomy; Fig. 42.2d). This bone removal isolates the frontal process of the maxilla that should then be removed to create a large osteotomy. The hamular process of the lacrimal bone, between the upper duct and nasal mucosa, is removed using a Jensen bone nibbler, and further bone should be removed from the skull base, to ensure complete clearance to about 6 mm above the common canalicular opening. A partial ethmoidectomy is performed by removing bone fragments and ethmoid sinus mucosa, the residual ethmoid mucosa being cauterised for complete haemostasis.

When removing bone from alongside nasal mucosa, an angled periosteal elevator should be swept around the bone edge every few bites of the rongeur to separate mucosa from the bone, and, where cotton tips have been placed in the nose, these should be temporarily withdrawn to allow the rhinostomy to be fashioned; once the osteotomy is complete, the cotton tips are repositioned in the nasal space. Intranasal gauze packing has sufficient compliance that it can be left undisturbed throughout a local anaesthetic procedure.

A "00" probe is passed to tent the medial wall of the sac, and a No.11 blade is used to enter the system lumen at the antero-medial face of the sac-duct junction (Fig. 42.3a) – thereby avoiding damage to the common canalicular opening. Once the lumen has been identified, curved spring scissors are used to open the medial wall from the skull base to the nasolacrimal canal (Fig. 42.3b), and, once this incision is complete, the sac fundus and the sac-duct junction should be divided to allow the sac to be opened widely (Fig. 42.3c). The surgeon must be aware that, on occasion, only the thick fascia of the lacrimal sac will have been opened and the thin mucosa of the sac remains intact – this leading to DCR failure if not identified.

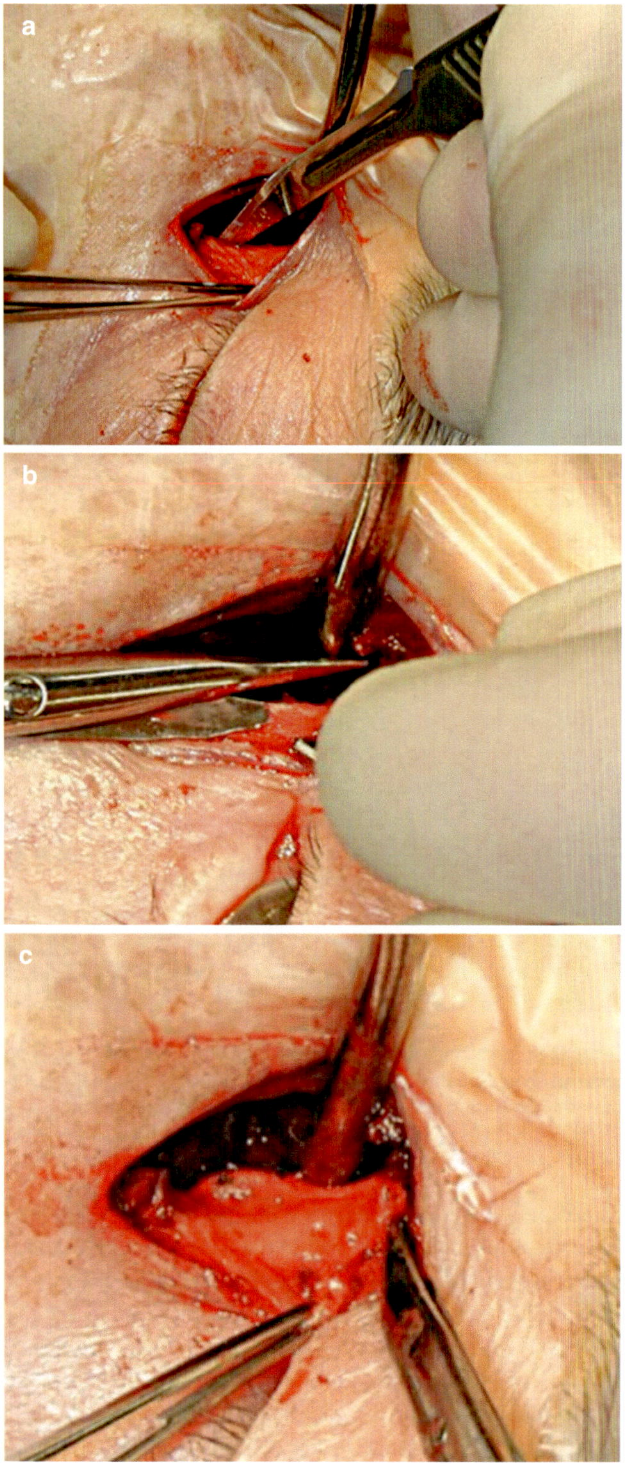

Fig. 42.3 (**a**) Opening the left lacrimal sac should be performed at the sac-duct junction to avoid damage to the common canalicular opening, and (**b**) the sac opened alongside the opening using spring scissors. (**c**) Adequate opening of the sac should be opened "like a book", from the fundus to the upper nasolacrimal duct

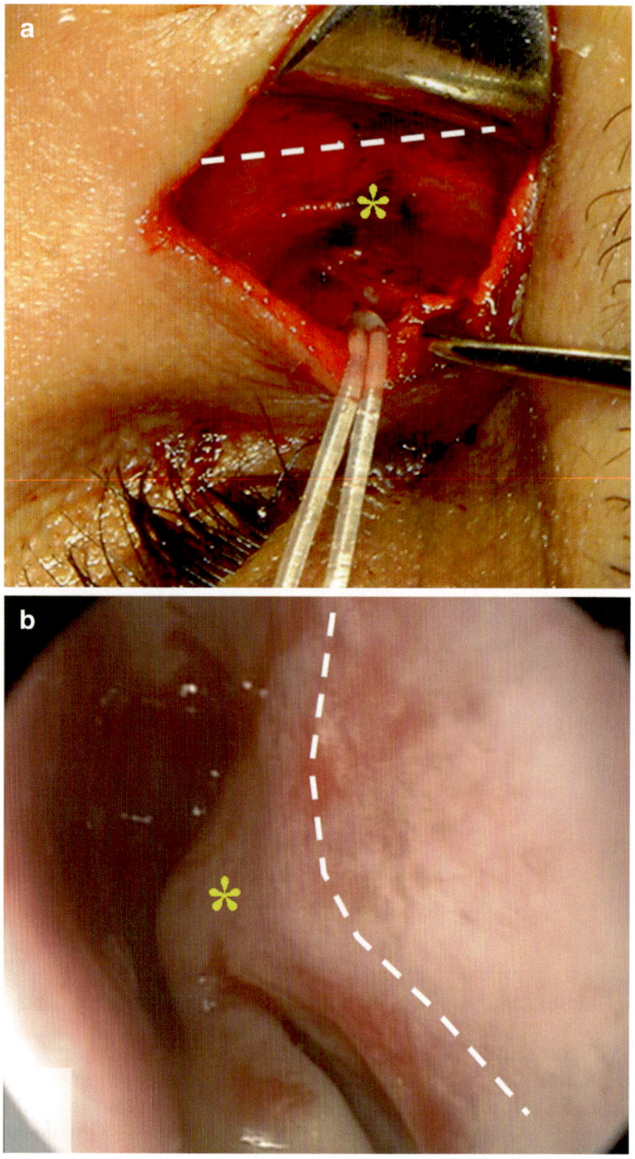

Fig. 42.4 (**a**) Anterior ethmoidectomy reveals the undersurface of nasal mucosa and the very characteristic "arch", with its apex anteriorly (asterisk); this arch is the inside of the middle turbinate, and the apex (asterisk) is the most anterior attachment ("axilla") of the middle turbinate. (**b**) The same area is shown on a left endonasal view, with external pressure applied at the apex of the arch. Knowledge of the "arch" allows best placement of the vertical incision for the posterior flaps, this being about 3–4 mm in front of the arch (dotted lines)

Leaving the nasal packing or cotton tips in place, the nasal mucosa is incised vertically with a No.11 blade, and, for an optimal posterior flap, the incision should be 3–4 mm in front of a mucosal "arch"; this "arch" is revealed only during the anterior ethmoidectomy (Fig. 42.4a) and is formed by the anterior-most attachment of the middle turbinate to the lateral nasal wall (Fig. 42.4b). Anteroposterior relieving horizontal incisions are made at the upper and lower edges of the rhinostomy to create nasal mucosal flaps (Fig. 42.5a).

A 6/0 absorbable suture (8 mm diameter, half-circle needle) is passed through the middle of the previously retracted preseptal orbicularis fibres and through the middle of the

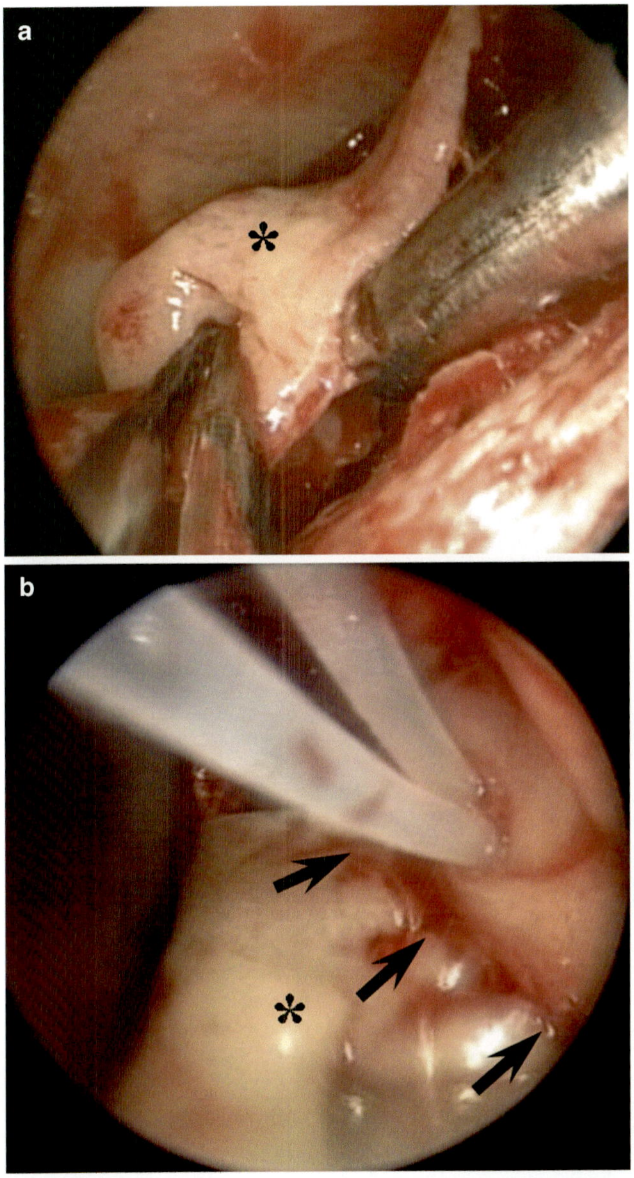

Fig. 42.5 (**a**) View of the posterior nasal mucosal flap after incision 3 mm anterior to the apex of the left "arch"; the asterisk indicates the "axilla" of the middle turbinate. (**b**) The same nasal mucosal flap after continuous suture to the posterior flap of the left lacrimal sac (arrows); the common canalicular opening is clearly seen with emerging silicone intubation

anterior nasal flap, and the two ends hung aside across the nasal bridge to hold the tissues away from the operative site. Likewise, silicone intubation can be placed and gently clipped aside laterally to improve access for suturing of the posterior flaps. The posterior flaps are joined from the fundus to the upper duct using a 6/0 absorbable suture placed as a locked continuous suture, and this is most easy achieved using the whole needle length, with it reverse mounted in a non-locking, angled needle holder; it will be found that these flaps naturally "fall" together with the prior ethmoidectomy and fashioning of mucosa (Fig. 42.5b).

After passing the pre-tied silicone intubation into the nasal space, the preplaced anterior suture is passed through the sac flap directly in front of the internal opening – this effectively "suspending" the anterior mucosal anastomosis from the orbicularis fibres. Another suspended suture is passed through preseptal orbicularis above the first suture, then through the upper anterior nasal flap, through the upper anterior sac mucosa, and finally through the stump of medial canthal tendon; the final suture is passed through orbicularis, through the lower end of the anterior nasal mucosa, through the anterior sac flap near the nasolacrimal duct, and finally through the subdermal tissues lateral to the lower part of the skin incision. Skin closure is achieved with a 6/0 nylon continuous mattress suture, a topical antibiotic instilled, and a firm dressing applied until the following day.

Post-operative Care After External Dacryocystorhinostomy

Nasal packing is not required, but, to reduce nasal venous oozing, the patient should be nursed semierect, hot drinks and hot food avoided for 12 hours after surgery, and nose blowing discouraged for a week. In the rare event of persistent primary or secondary haemorrhage, nasal packing is recommended either with a commercially available nasal tampon or else with about 80 cm of narrow ribbon gauze, moistened with 1:1000 epinephrine. Systemic antibiotics should also be prescribed whilst the pack is left undisturbed for 5–7 days, after which time the pack is very easily removed.

Although there is no evidence for efficacy, a topical antibiotic/anti-inflammatory medication is often prescribed for a few weeks after DCR by any route. Systemic antibiotics are recommended to reduce post-operative soft-tissue infection after external DCR [3], with intraoperative administration providing a more convenient therapy [4]. The dressing is removed on the day after surgery, the skin sutures removed at about 7–10 days, and the intubation at about 4 weeks after surgery.

Additional Procedures During External Dacryocystorhinostomy

With canalicular block, it is possible to perform additional manoeuvres during external DCR – in many cases these not being possible with endonasal DCR.

Medial common canalicular block – due to adherence of the valve of Rosenmuller over the common internal opening (Fig. 42.6a) – is addressed by careful excision of the membrane using a No.11 blade or fine scissors and placement of silicone intubation for a few weeks; simple

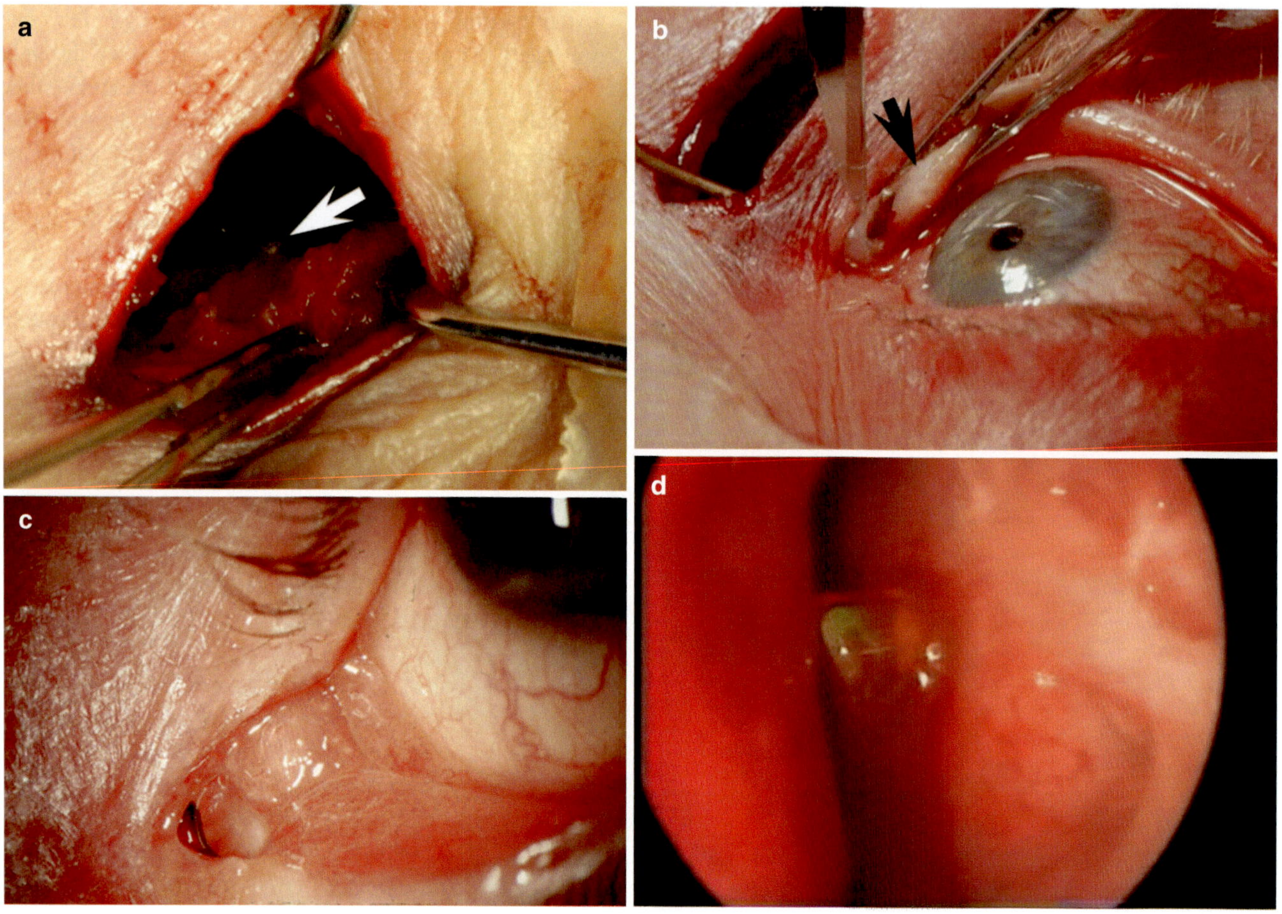

Fig. 42.6 (**a**) Left lacrimal sac with membranous block of the common canalicular opening (arrow). (**b**) Retrograde canaliculostomy on the left upper canaliculus that is obstructed about 5 mm distal to the original punctum (arrow). (**c**) Left glass canalicular bypass tube positioned at site of a partial carunculectomy in a patient with bicanalicular obstruction and (**d**) the internal positioning of a left canalicular bypass tube – being free in the main airspace, but with adequate intranasal length to remain stable during the mucosal swelling of coryza or atopy

perforation of a membranous block will generally fail due to stenosis. Lateral common canalicular block is usually due to a large scar after trauma and may be similarly addressed but in this case by a repeated "cheese-paring" away of scar tissue until the individual (lateral) ends of each canaliculus are revealed.

Where canaliculi are blocked within their first 7 mm or so, a retrograde canaliculostomy should be used to marsupialize any remaining medial canalicular tissue onto the conjunctival surface (Fig. 42.6b) [5]; as the presence of any medial canaliculus can only be established at surgery, the patient should be warned that they might require primary or secondary placement of a glass canalicular bypass tube. If only the common canaliculus is present, it should be opened by retrograde probing into the inner canthus after carunculectomy and the returning intubation passed through one of the punctal annuli and forced medially through the lid tissues; this returns the intubation to the nasal space remote from the canalicular opening. The absence of a punctal annulus with retrograde canaliculostomy renders monocanalicular intubation ineffective. The tubes are removed after 2–3 weeks, or else "cheese wiring" will cause a medial cross-union. Closed placement of a canalicular bypass tube is required if the pseudo-puncta fail to control symptoms.

Primary or secondary placement of a glass Jones' canalicular bypass tube is required where there is no functioning canalicular tissue – the tube being designed for free tear flow, from the medial tear lake into the nose, by way of a false conduit. Primary placement of the tube is undertaken after posterior mucosal suturing during external DCR. The distal end of the tube should be free within the nasal space, anterior to the middle turbinate, and the eye end is positioned at the carunculectomy site, hard behind the lower lid margin (Fig. 42.6c); the tube requires a 30–40° downward tilt for optimum drainage. For secondary placement, a punctal dilator is used to pierce the epithelium at the desired position and a track forced through to the nose using the smallest end of the double-ended ("bullhorn") dilators. An appropriate tube (commonly 11 mm, with a 3.5 mm flange) is placed onto a "1" lacrimal probe. The latter passed along the dilated track, and the tube is forced along the track using the end of the thumbnails. The position of the ocular and nasal ends of the tube should be checked after withdrawing the probe and spontaneous flow of saline verified. Suture of the tube is unnecessary after secondary placement. Endoscopic nasal examination aids secondary placement of bypass tubes (Fig. 42.6d), and the positioning is best performed under a short general anaesthetic, as the vasoconstriction of nasal local anaesthesia creates an artificially capacious nasal space and leads to the incorrect tube positioning.

References

1. Rose GE. The lacrimal paradox: towards a greater understanding of success in lacrimal surgery. Ophthalmic Plast Reconstr Surg. 2004;20:262–5.
2. Hanna IM, Powrie S, Rose GE. Management outcome for day-case open lacrimal surgery, as compared to inpatient management. Br J Ophthalmol. 1998;82:392–6.
3. Walland MJ, Rose GE. Soft tissue infection after open lacrimal surgery. Ophthalmology. 1994;101:608–11.
4. Vardy SJ, Rose GE. Prevention of cellulitis after open lacrimal surgery: a prospective study of three methods. Ophthalmology. 2000;107:315–7.
5. Wearne MJ, Beigi B, Davis G, Rose GE. Retrograde intubation dacryocystorhinostomy for proximal and mid-canalicular obstruction. Ophthalmology. 1999;106:2325–8.

Adult Endoscopic Endonasal Dacryocystorhinostomy

43

Angela Maria Dolmetsch

Abbreviations

CNLDO	Congenital nasolacrimal duct obstruction
CO2	Carbon dioxide
DCR	Dacryocystorhinostomy
EndoDCR	Endonasal dacryocystorhinostomy
ENL-DCR	Endonasal laser dacryocystorhinostomy
Ext-DCR	External dacryocystorhinostomy
KTP	Potassium titanyl phosphate
MMC	Mitomycin C
PANDO	Primary acquired nasolacrimal duct obstruction
RAI	Radioactive iodine therapy
SANDO	Secondary acquired nasolacrimal duct obstruction
YAG	Yttrium aluminum garnet

Introduction

Epiphora or tearing is a common symptom of diverse etiology. One of the causative factors is blockage of the nasolacrimal duct, which provides tear drainage from the lacrimal sac to the nasal cavity. The treatment of choice for nasolacrimal duct obstruction is the dacryocystorhinostomy (DCR) which bypasses the obstruction in the duct by creating a direct aperture from the lacrimal sac to the nose. The traditional approach since its original description by Toti in 1904 has been the transcutaneous or external route, the external dacryocystorhinostomy (Ext-DCR) [1, 2]. Only recently, in the past several decades, has attention been drawn to the endonasal approach.

A. M. Dolmetsch (✉)
Clínica de Oftalmología de Cali, Cali, Valle del Cauca, Colombia

Pontificia Universidad Javeriana, Cali, Valle del Cauca, Colombia

The endonasal dacryocystorhinostomy (EndoDCR) has many advantages over the Ext-DCR including the avoidance of a cutaneous scar, less risk of infection and significant bleeding, minimal disruption of the medial canthal anatomy and lacrimal pump mechanism, less operative time, and faster recovery [3]. Furthermore, the endonasal route can be used safely in the setting of acute dacryocystitis with abscess formation [1, 3–6], and it allows for the simultaneous management of nasal and paranasal sinus abnormalities [3, 7–9]. Nonetheless, EndoDCR has a few potential drawbacks including a relatively steep learning curve and the high cost of endoscopic equipment and instrumentation [3, 8, 10–12].

History

Endonasal dacryocystorhinostomy (or endoscopic intranasal DCR, EndoDCR) is not a recent surgical procedure as is commonly believed. It was first performed by Caldwell, an otolaryngologist, in 1893 [13]. Assisted by a probe placed in one of the canaliculi, he used an electric burr transnasally to create an osteotomy at the level of the lacrimal sac. However, the technique was soon abandoned because of frequent failures, poor results, and recurrences. In 1909, West [14] reattempted the endonasal route but was unable to achieve good success rates mainly because of poor visualization, difficulty achieving effective soft tissue and bone removal, and inadequacy in controlling hemorrhage.

With the advent of rigid endoscopes for nasal and sinus surgery, visualization of the nasal cavity improved considerably, and the EndoDCR acquired renewed popularity. The modern-day EndoDCR was first described with the use of an endoscope by McDonogh and Meiring in 1989 [10, 15, 16]. Their technique involved a 30° rod lens endoscope and a series of forceps and curettes to perform the procedure. In 1990, Massaro et al. [15] introduced a high-powered argon

A. J. Cohen, C. N. Burkat (eds.), *Oculofacial, Orbital, and Lacrimal Surgery*, https://doi.org/10.1007/978-3-030-14092-2_43

blue-green laser coupled to a 300-μm quartz fiber-optic catheter to create an intranasal dacryocystorhinostomy and termed the procedure endonasal laser dacryocystorhinostomy (ENL-DCR). Several groups followed using different types of lasers including carbon dioxide (CO2) and potassium titanyl phosphate (KTP), yttrium aluminum garnet (YAG) [17], and holmium: Yag [18]. The reported success rates were between 59% and 85% with mean follow-up times between 3 and 18 months [7, 11, 19–26]. These results compared unfavorably with the external route or Ext-DCR which at the time was the gold standard for surgical treatment of nasolacrimal duct obstruction obtaining success rates of over 90% [27, 28]. Camara et al. in 2000 obtained a 99.2% success rate in ENL-DCR with the use of mitomycin C (MMC) with no complications and a follow-up period of 30–72 months [29]. However, in further studies, the long-term success rates of ENL-DCR were not sufficiently acceptable (77%) to make the procedure appealing and convincing for oculoplastic surgeons and ophthalmologists to adopt the technique [3, 30–33].

More recently, other endonasal approaches to the lacrimal sac without the use of lasers have been described including radiosurgical incision of the nasal and lacrimal mucosa, mechanically powered, mucosal sparing, and non-mucosal-sparing techniques [8, 34–36]. Most of these techniques have satisfactory success rates, close to 90%, which compare very favorably with the Ext-DCR. In 2003, Tsirbas and Wormald pioneered the mucosal-sparing DCR emphasizing the development of a large powered rhinostomy and preservation of lacrimal sac and nasal mucosa to create mucosal flaps. They reported a success rate of 95% [36].

Current Trends in Endoscopic Endonasal Dacryocystorhinostomy

The ideal surgical technique for EndoDCR is still controversial and under debate. Two types of EndoDCR are favored by most lacrimal surgeons at the present time: EndoDCR with mucosal flaps and EndoDCR without flaps. Both techniques can be performed with or without a drill (powered).

In the EndoDCR with mucosal flaps, a flap of nasal mucosal tissue and the medial wall of the lacrimal sac are preserved and draped together. The principle behind the sparing of nasal and lacrimal mucosa is to form an epithelium-lined fistula that will heal by primary intention without the formation of granulation tissue. Careful handling of the flaps ensures minimal mucosal trauma that helps to attenuate wound contraction and reduce scarring, which is the major factor in DCR failure. Several case series studies have confirmed success rates of over 93% with this technique [33, 37–39]. A recent systematic and critical review of randomized control trials suggests that there may be improved outcomes in EndoDCR when mucosal and lacrimal flaps are preserved [40].

In non-mucosal sparing or EndoDCR without mucosal flap preservation, the nasal mucosa, bone, and medial wall of the lacrimal sac are completely removed with forceps and rongeurs [41]. The mechanical removal of the tissue is technically easier than fashioning mucosal flaps, particularly in tight nasal cavities with septal deviation. The procedure is also faster than the mucosal-sparing technique. Healing occurs by secondary intention with formation of granulation tissue. Minimizing the degree of exposed bone and a careful surgical technique lessen the risk of DCR failure when using this approach. Many investigators have reported good success rates ranging from 92% to 94% [42].

Endoscopic-powered DCR refers to the use of a cutting burr and electric handpiece to remove all the bone on the frontal process of the maxilla that covers the lacrimal sac and the upper part of the nasolacrimal duct. Advocates of this technique maintain that a much larger osteotomy can be performed, which allows for a wider exposure of the lacrimal sac [36].

Another controversial point in EndoDCR is the use of silicone stents. The rationale behind the use of stenting is to maintain the osteotomy patent and impede fibrous closure while healing occurs. Several studies including a recent cumulative meta-analysis revealed that there are no significant differences in success rates between EndoDCR with and without silicone intubation [43–46]. Conversely, another recent study which recruited 300 patients found that there was a statistically significantly higher success rate in EndoDCR with stenting versus no stenting. The non-tube group had a failure rate more than twice as high (12.2%) as the group with tubes (5.3%) [47]. Complications related to silicone intubation include granulomas, punctal and canalicular laceration (cheesewiring), tube displacement or loss, conjunctival irritation, and infection.

The use of MMC and other adjunctives in EndoDCR is routinely used by many lacrimal surgeons to augment the surgical success rate. MMC is an antineoplastic agent that inhibits the synthesis of DNA, cellular RNA, and protein by inhibiting the synthesis of collagen by fibroblasts. MMC is used at the completion of EndoDCR at the osteotomy site in variable concentrations of 0.2–0.5 mg/ml and exposure times from 2 to 15 minutes. Many authors have suggested that the use of intraoperative MMC increases the success rate of primary and revision EndoDCR, particularly if the procedure is technically challenging or if the surgeon is inexperienced [48, 49]. More importantly, no adverse effects or systemic toxicity has been reported with the use of MMC in the range of concentration or time of exposure mentioned previously [50].

Adjunctive mitomycin C:
Concentrations 0.2–0.5 mg/ml
Exposure time range 2–15 minutes

Surgical Anatomy of the Lacrimal Drainage Apparatus and Nasal Cavity

Precise knowledge of the intranasal and lacrimal anatomy is essential for success in EndoDCR. The lacrimal apparatus (Fig. 43.1) is composed of the lacrimal puncta, two openings in the most medial aspect of the lid margins measuring approximately 0.2–0.3 mm in diameter. The puncta sit on a small mound of tissue known as the lacrimal papillae. Once the tears enter the puncta, they travel along the upper and lower canaliculi initially through a 2 mm vertical portion. The canaliculi then change direction horizontally at the level of the ampulla and continue for 8–10 mm more before joining with the canaliculus of the opposite lid to form the common canaliculus. This anatomy is present in 90% of the population. The common canaliculus, measuring 3–5 mm in length, then enters the lacrimal sac at the junction of the upper third with the two lower thirds of the sac. The lacrimal sac lies in the lacrimal fossa, a bony depression limited by the anterior and posterior lacrimal crests. The bony fossa is formed anteriorly by the thick frontal process of the maxilla and posteriorly by the very thin lacrimal bone. The anterior ethmoidal air cells are usually found posterior to the posterior lacrimal crest, but in 10–15% of the population, they may be placed more anteriorly and may sometimes extend all the way past the lacrimal sac to the anterior lacrimal crest. These cells are known as the agger nasi cells and are occasionally encountered in EndoDCR when performing the osteotomy. The sac is 10–15 mm in vertical length and 2–3 mm in width. It narrows down to become the nasolacrimal duct at the level of the entrance of the bony lacrimal canal. The membranous nasolacrimal duct runs vertically 13–15 mm before entering the nasal cavity at the level of the valve of Hasner, which is located in the inferior meatus under the inferior turbinate [51].

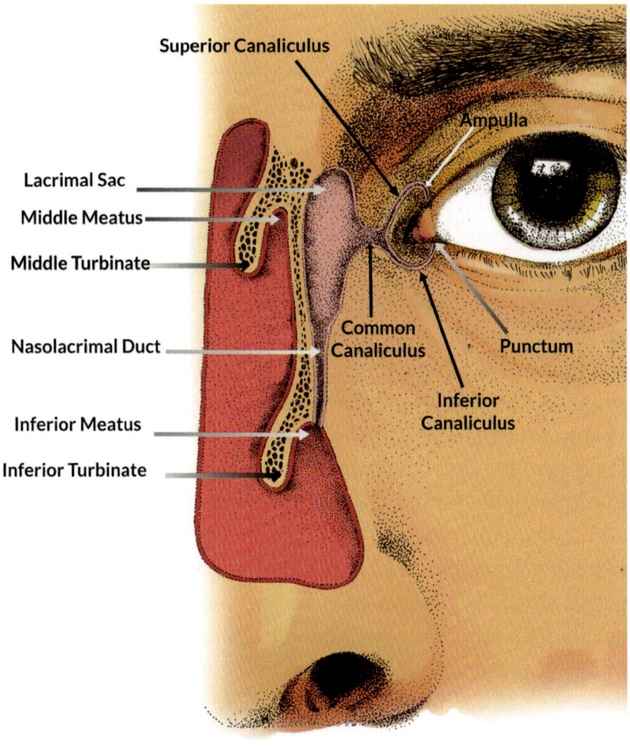

Fig. 43.1 The lacrimal drainage system anatomy

The nasal cavity is divided in two equal spaces by the nasal septum, a bony and cartilaginous structure that extends down the midline from the nasal tip to the choana. The septum is often deviated to one side and can sometimes obstruct adequate view of the internal nasal anatomy. This, however, rarely precludes performing an EndoDCR, unless severe septal deviation is present.

The lateral wall of the nose is a very specialized area (Fig. 43.2). It contains three turbinates (superior, middle, and inferior) which are bony projections covered by nasal mucosa. The turbinates or conchae can cause interference with visualization during endoscopic surgery and always require vasoconstriction [52, 53]. The middle turbinate inserts on the frontal process of the maxilla, and its uppermost anterior portion is called the axilla (Fig. 43.3). Between 2 and 4 mm above the level of the axilla is the cribriform plate. Care must be taken when infracturing or repositioning the middle turbinate to avoid a cerebrospinal fluid (CSF) leak [54].

Anterior to the middle turbinate is the maxillary line which is the anterior projection of the frontal process of the maxilla, an important landmark in EndoDCR surgery. This line runs from the axilla of the middle turbinate to the inferior turbinate. Just posterior to the middle turbinate is the uncinate process, a sickle-shaped flap of mucosa overlying a thin bony layer that extends from the anterior end of the middle meatus and covers the upper aspect of the maxillary sinus. Some surgeons advocate the anterior resection of the uncinate process in order to expose the lacrimal fossa; however this is not always necessary [9]. Behind the uncinate process, the ethmoid bulla, an anterior ethmoidal air cell can often be seen.

The lacrimal sac is positioned in an area 6–10 mm above the axilla of the middle turbinate and 6–8 mm below it (Fig. 43.2). This is the place where the nasal mucosal incision should be performed during EndoDCR.

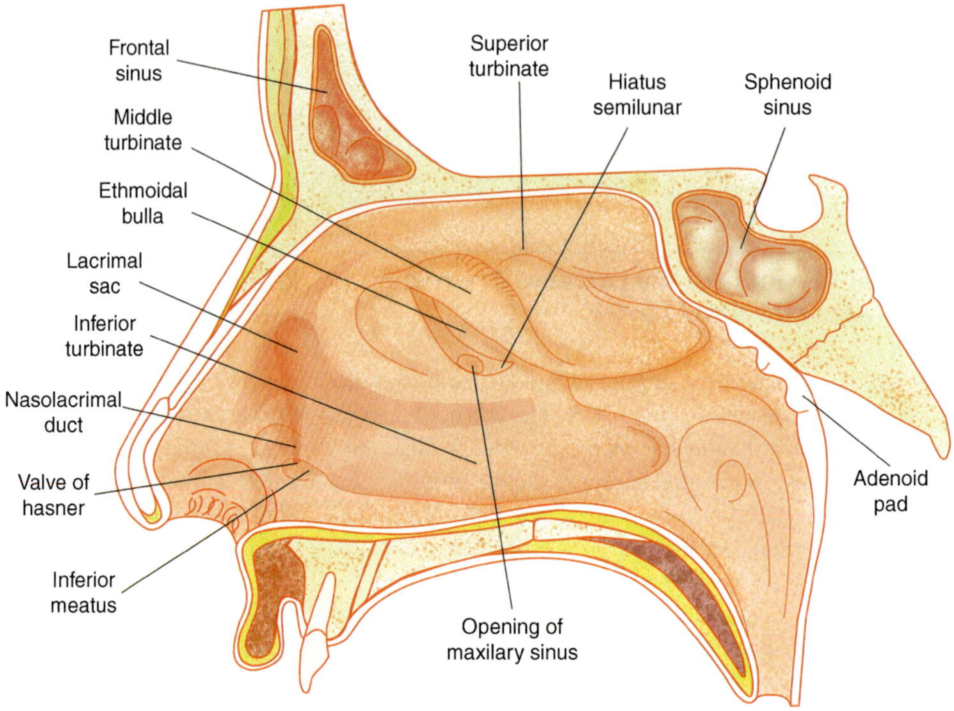

Fig. 43.2 The lateral wall of the nose containing three turbinates

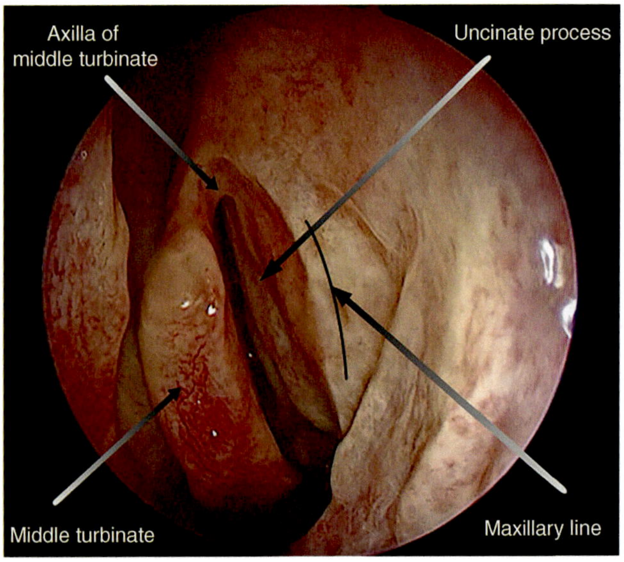

Fig. 43.3 Endoscopic view of normal nasal anatomy (Left nostril)

Indications for EndoDCR

EndoDCR is indicated in nasolacrimal duct obstruction of diverse origin and essentially has the same indications as for Ext-DCR. These include primary acquired nasolacrimal duct obstruction (PANDO), congenital nasolacrimal duct obstruction (CNLDO), and secondary acquired nasolacrimal duct obstruction (SANDO) including midface trauma, granulomatosis with polyangiitis (Wegener's granulomatosis), sarcoidosis, and patients who have received chemotherapy, radioactive iodine therapy (RAI), or high-dose radiation therapy [49, 55]. EndoDCR is particularly useful in revision DCR, acute dacryocystitis with lacrimal abscess, and bilateral simultaneous surgery. In contrast, Ext-DCR has been debatable in the setting of acute infection.

Preoperative Considerations and Contraindications

All patients undergoing EndoDCR require a detailed medical history and complete ophthalmological examination including canalicular evaluation and gentle syringing. A 0 Bowman probe can be carefully inserted in the canaliculi to check for canalicular patency. A "hard stop" should be encountered when the probe reaches the lacrimal sac, which suggests that the nasal bone is being palpated without intervening soft tissue obstruction. Care should be taken to avoid kinking of the canaliculus by pulling the lid temporally when introducing the probe or irrigation cannula.

If canalicular obstruction is present, EndoDCR is not the indicated procedure for the relief of epiphora. Lacrimal irrigation should be performed either through the upper or lower canaliculus to evaluate patency of the nasolacrimal duct. If reflux is present or if there is no passage of fluid into the nose, the nasolacrimal duct is obstructed and an EndoDCR is indicated. Mucus or purulent discharge when palpating an enlarged lacrimal sac also indicates nasolacrimal duct obstruction.

A nasal examination with a speculum and fiber-optic light should be performed in all cases before the surgical procedure. This may reveal the presence of septal deviation, nasal polyps, hypertrophic turbinates, allergic or chronic rhinitis, or intranasal neoplasms. A referral to an otorhinolaryngologist may be warranted in these cases.

In cases with a history of midface trauma, it is imperative to perform imaging studies, preferably CT scans to assess bony abnormalities and presence of fixation hardware. In certain post-traumatic midfacial reconstructions, EndoDCR cannot be performed, and an Ext-DCR is the only option.

EndoDCR should not be performed in patients on anticoagulation medications who are unable to discontinue them perioperatively or when a lacrimal sac neoplasm is suspected.

Operative Techniques

As mentioned earlier, there are several techniques for performing EndoDCR:

- Endoscopic laser-assisted DCR (ENL-DCR)
- Endoscopic radiofrequency endonasal DCR
- Mechanical ("cold steel") endoscopic transnasal DCR with and without mucosal flaps
- Mechanical ("cold steel") transnasal non-endoscopic DCR
- Power-assisted endoscopic transnasal DCR with and without flaps

All techniques follow the same basic principle but vary in the instrumentation utilized, the management of the nasal and lacrimal mucosa, and the way the osteotomy is performed. The basic technique for EndoDCR will be described. The basic instrument set is shown in Table 43.1 and Fig. 43.4. All cases are performed under general endotracheal anesthesia or regional nerve block with sedation.

Table 43.1 Basic instrument set for endonasal DCR

0° and or 30° 4 mm endoscope
Dual-ended punctal dilator
20-gauge disposable vitrectomy light pipe
Nasal speculum
Bayonet forceps
Freer periosteal elevator
Angled 2.0 disposable crescent blade
Yasargil straight scissors
Straight pediatric (true-biting) ethmoid forceps
Frazier suction tube (9 French)
Up-biting (true-biting) pediatric ethmoid forceps
2 mm down-biting Kerrison rongeur
Straight pediatric ethmoid forceps
Up-biting pediatric ethmoid forceps

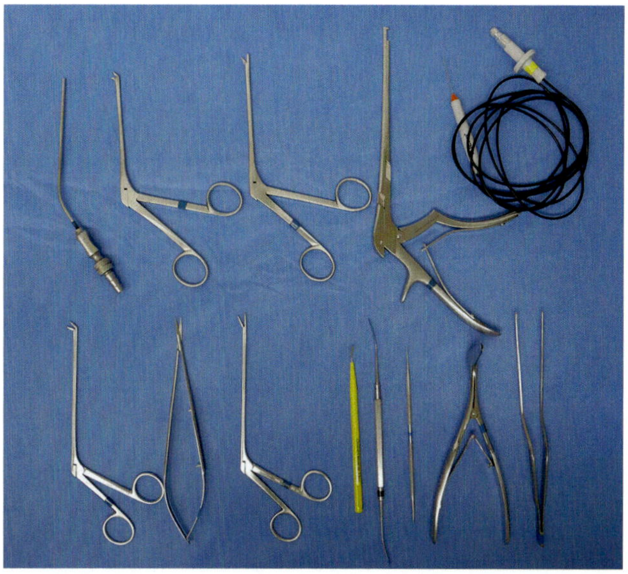

Fig. 43.4 Endonasal dacryocystorhinostomy basic instrument set: (Top row, left to right): Frazier suction tube (9 French), up-biting (true-biting) pediatric ethmoid forceps, straight pediatric (true-biting) ethmoid forceps, 2 mm down-biting Kerrison rongeur, 20-gauge disposable vitrectomy light pipe. (Bottom row, left to right): up-biting ethmoid pediatric forceps, Yasargil straight scissors, straight pediatric ethmoid forceps, angled 2.0 mm disposable crescent blade, Freer straight periosteal elevator, dual-ended punctal dilator, nasal speculum, bayonet forceps

Nasal Preparation

An adequate nose preparation is essential for success and to avoid complications. This can be attained by spraying the nose with oxymetazoline hydrochloride nasal spray twice before starting the procedure (30 and 15 minutes before). Using a nasal speculum, a 1 cm nasal gauze soaked in either 5 cc of 2% cocaine mixed with 5 cc of adrenaline (0.1 mg/cc) or 5 cc of adrenaline (0.1 mg/cc) mixed with 5 cc of oxymetazoline 0.05% is placed between the lateral wall of the nose and the middle turbinate (Fig. 43.5). If the procedure is bilateral, both nostrils are packed at this time. This is left for 10 minutes.

Surgical Technique

The superior punctum is then dilated, and a 20-gauge disposable vitrectomy light pipe is passed through the superior canaliculus into the lacrimal sac. The light pipe is taped to the forehead with sterile tape. The nasal packing is then removed, and a 4 mm, 0° rigid nasal endoscope attached to an endoscopic video camera is introduced into the nostril. The position of the light pipe is viewed endonasally by transillumination of the nasal mucosa at the intended osteotomy site. This corresponds to the location of the lacrimal sac.

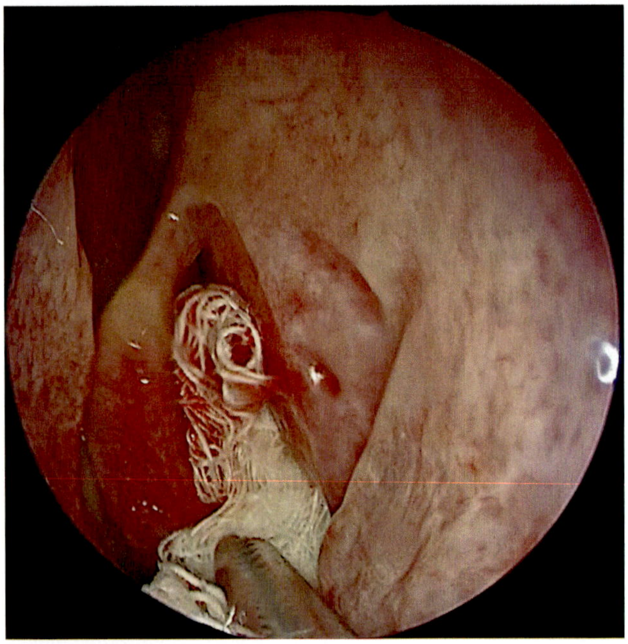

Fig. 43.5 Nasal packing is placed between the lateral wall of the nose and the middle turbinate

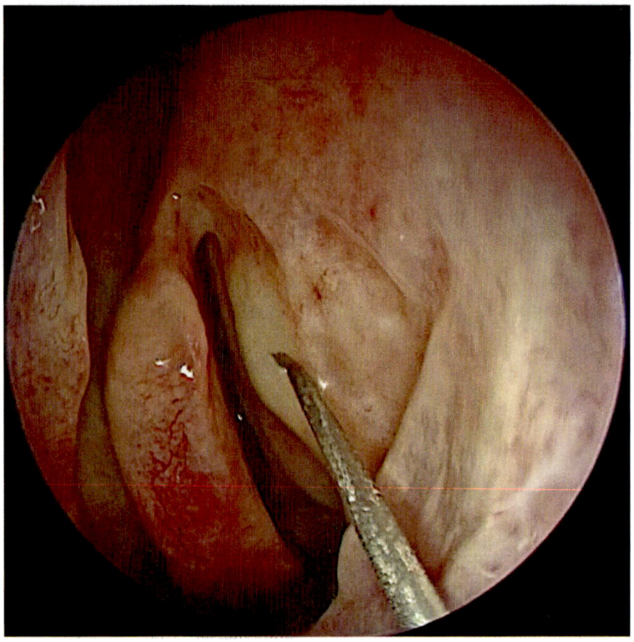

Fig. 43.6 Infiltration of nasal mucosa with 1–2 ml of 2% lidocaine with 1:100,000 epinephrine

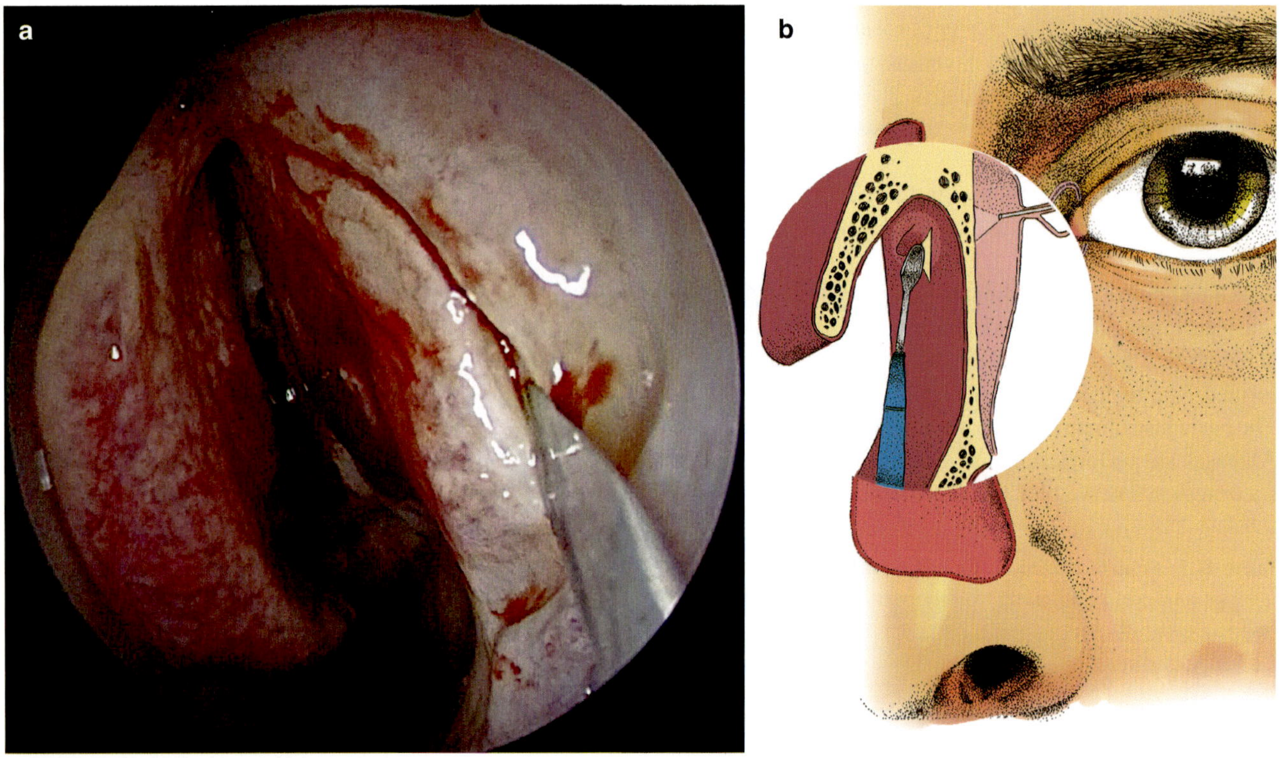

Fig. 43.7 (a) and (b). Anterior incision created on the nasal mucosa with a crescent blade

This area is infiltrated with 1–2 ml of 2% lidocaine with 1:100,000 epinephrine (Fig. 43.6). The nostril is repacked with nasal gauze soaked in the same solution of either 2% cocaine and 0.1 mg/cc adrenaline or 5 cc of adrenaline (0.1 mg/cc) mixed with 5 cc of oxymetazoline 0.05% for 5 minutes.

Using a two-handed technique, with the endoscope attached to a video camera display, two incisions are made on the nasal mucosa with a crescent blade, one anterior to the area of maximal illumination (Fig. 43.7) and the other just posterior to the same zone forming an ellipse. If the middle

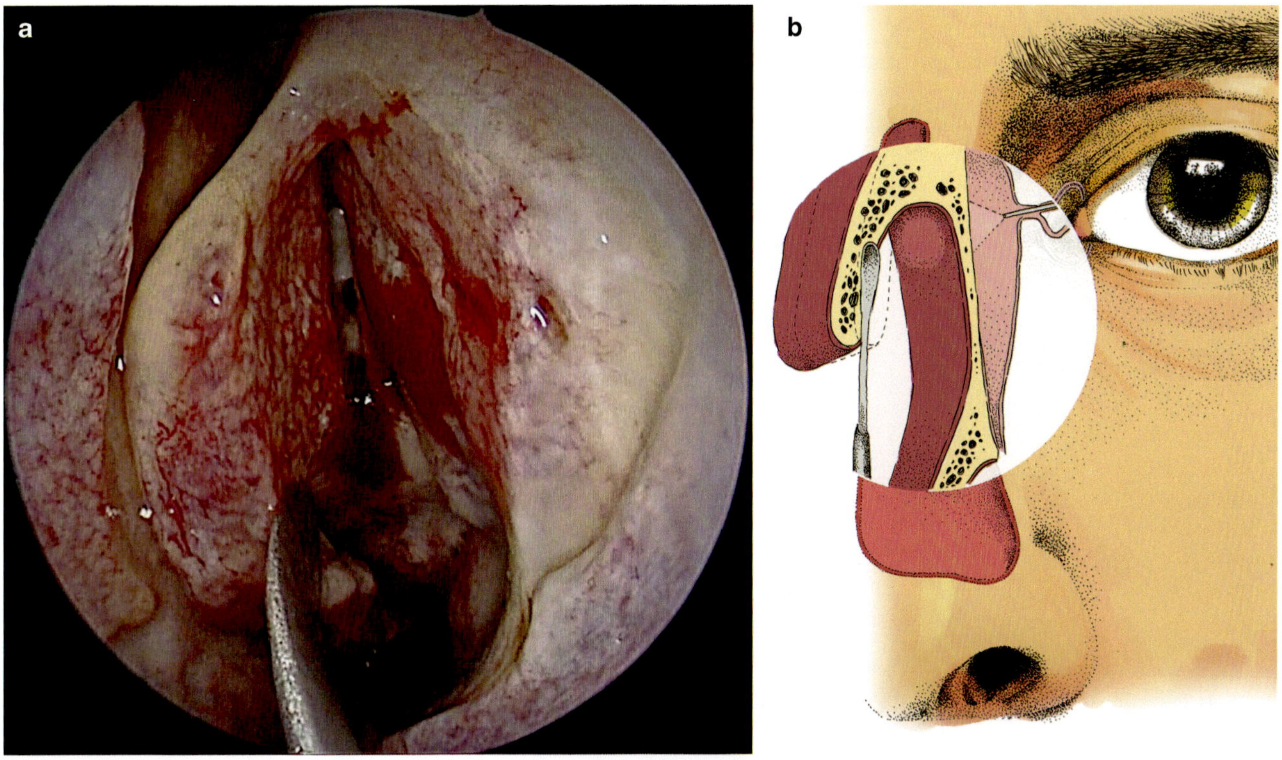

Fig. 43.8 (**a**) and (**b**). The middle turbinate is gently infractured with a periosteal or Freer elevator

turbinate is obstructing the view, it is gently infractured with a periosteal or Freer elevator (Fig. 43.8). If additional intranasal procedures such as septoplasty or turbinectomy are needed, they are performed at this point.

The ellipse of nasal mucosa and periosteum are then lifted from the underlying bone with the periosteal elevator (Fig. 43.9) and completely resected with an up-biting true-biting pediatric ethmoid forceps (Fig. 43.10). The frontal process of the maxilla is well exposed at this point. If performing an EndoDCR with mucosal preservation, the incision is made just anterior to the insertion of the middle turbinate and extended about 1 cm along the frontal process of the maxilla to an area superior to the insertion of the inferior turbinate. Two perpendicular incisions are created at the upper and lower edges of the initial incision. The mucosa is elevated with the periosteal elevator and the flap hinged posteriorly [38]. The uncinate process is generally left untouched in either technique.

Using the periosteal elevator, the thin lacrimal bone overlying the lacrimal sac is infractured by placing the elevator just beneath the frontal process of the maxilla and displacing it medially (Fig. 43.11). This sheet of bone is then removed with a straight pediatric nonbiting ethmoid forceps (Fig. 43.12).

The osteotomy is then performed using a variety of techniques depending on surgeon preference. In the mechanical EndoDCR (author's preferred method), a 2 mm Kerrison upbiting rongeur is placed behind the frontal process of the maxilla and used to remove bone superiorly and anteriorly (Fig. 43.13). Some bone covering the upper part of the nasolacrimal duct is also removed. Approximately 4–5 bites of bone are removed which is equivalent to an 8–10 mm osteotomy. The light pipe can then be easily visualized behind the lacrimal sac (Fig. 43.14). When performing a powered-assisted EndoDCR, a straight or curved high-speed burr is

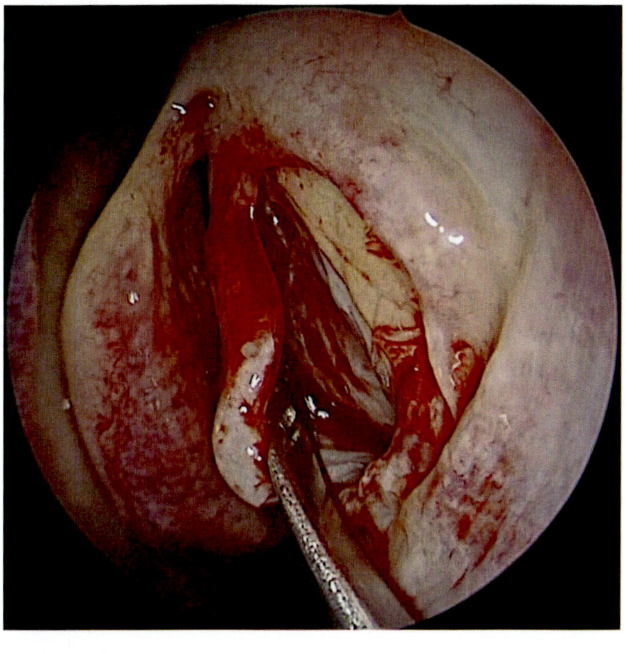

Fig. 43.9 The nasal mucosa and periosteum are gently lifted from the underlying bone with the periosteal elevator

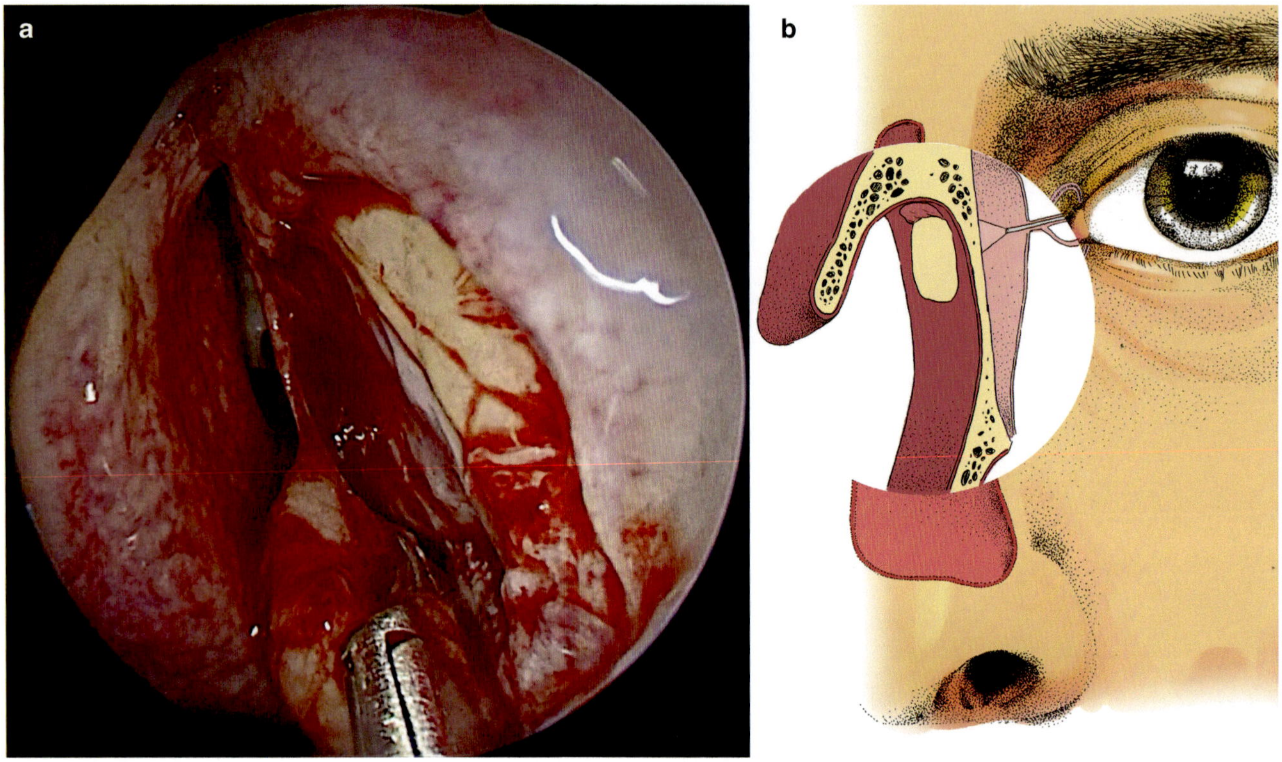

Fig. 43.10 (**a**) and (**b**) Resection of nasal mucosal flap with an up-biting true-biting pediatric ethmoid forceps

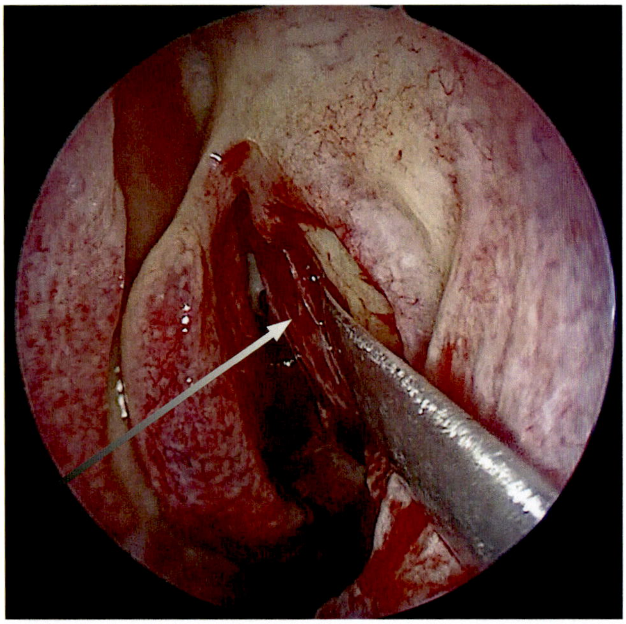

Fig. 43.11 The lacrimal bone overlying the lacrimal sac is infractured by placing the elevator just beneath the frontal process of the maxilla and displacing it medially. The arrow points to the thin lacrimal bone

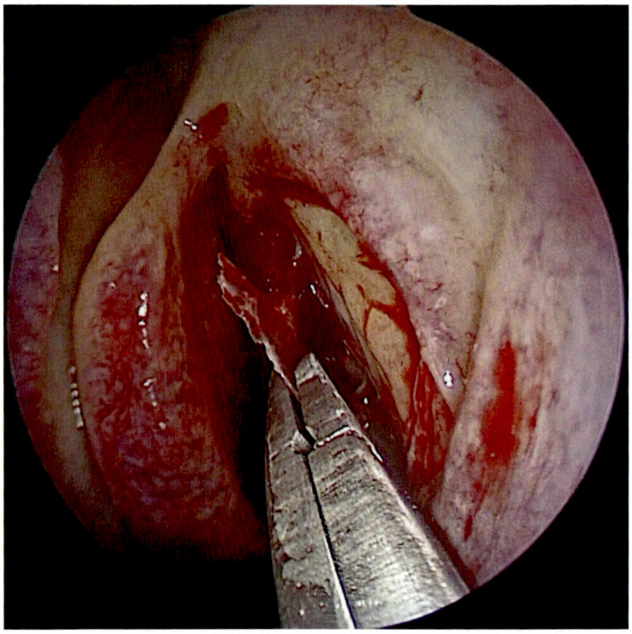

Fig. 43.12 Removal of thin sheet of lacrimal bone with straight pediatric nonbiting ethmoid forceps

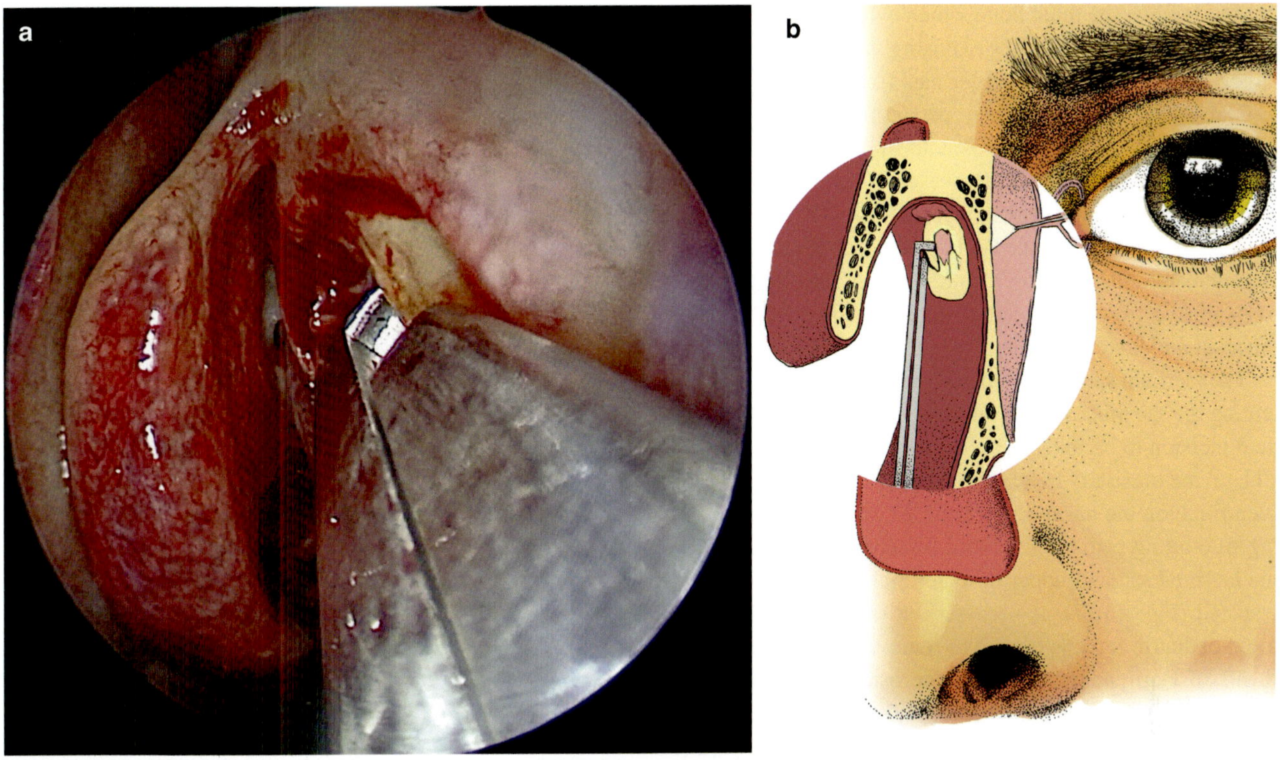

Fig. 43.13 (**a**) and (**b**). Osteotomy with a 2 mm Kerrison up-biting rongeur, placed behind the frontal process of the maxilla to remove bone superiorly and anteriorly

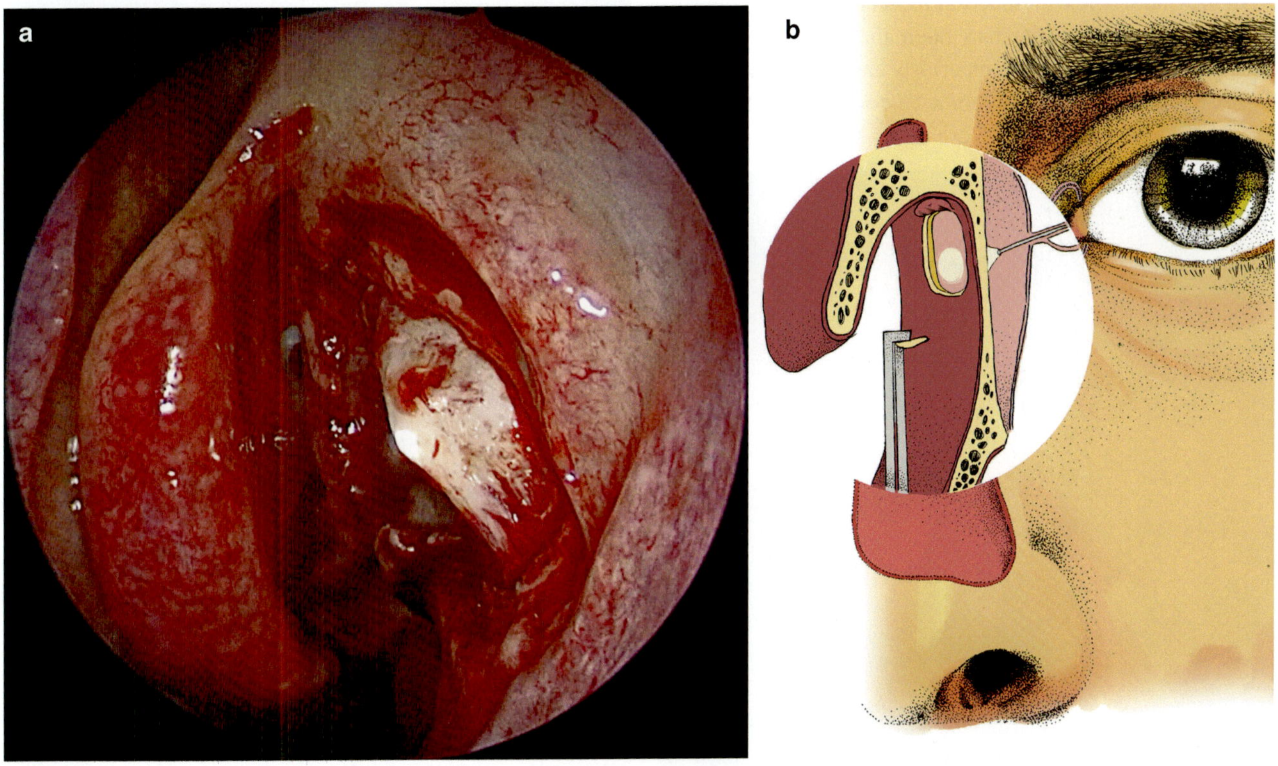

Fig. 43.14 (**a**) and (**b**) Lacrimal sac completely exposed with the light pipe visualized within the sac

used to remove the thick bone which extends up to the axilla of the middle turbinate, thus exposing the lacrimal sac completely and very often the agger nasi (the most anterior ethmoidal air cells) [56]. When performing a laser-assisted EndoDCR (ENL-DCR), the osteotomy is completed with a YAG/KTP or similar device. However, in several comparative studies, as mentioned previously, the ENL-DCR was found to be less effective than the "cold steel" techniques with success rates ranging from 64% to 85%. This may be the result of extensive fibrosis secondary to heat generated from the mucosal and bone ablation [57].

The lacrimal sac is now opened with the crescent blade by tenting the sac mucosa with the light pipe which allows a vertical incision to be made. This must be done as close as possible to the maxillary bone (Fig. 43.15). The light pipe is then seen freely in the nasal cavity (Fig. 43.16). Using the up-biting true-biting pediatric ethmoid forceps, the medial wall of the lacrimal sac and upper nasolacrimal duct are completely resected (Fig. 43.17). If necessary, a smaller up-biting ethmoid pediatric forceps is used to remove the remaining fragments of lacrimal sac visible at the osteotomy sight. When using MMC, a neurosurgical cottonoid is cut into a small triangular shape with all sides measuring approximately 0.8 cm and soaked in MMC at a concentration of 0.5 mg/ml. The cottonoid is placed at the osteotomy site for 5–10 minutes. No flushing or irrigation is needed after the cottonoid is removed.

In the EndoDCR with mucosal preservation, once the vertical incision is performed to open the lacrimal sac, two relaxing incisions are made superiorly and inferiorly, and the flap is hinged posteriorly to come in contact with the nasal

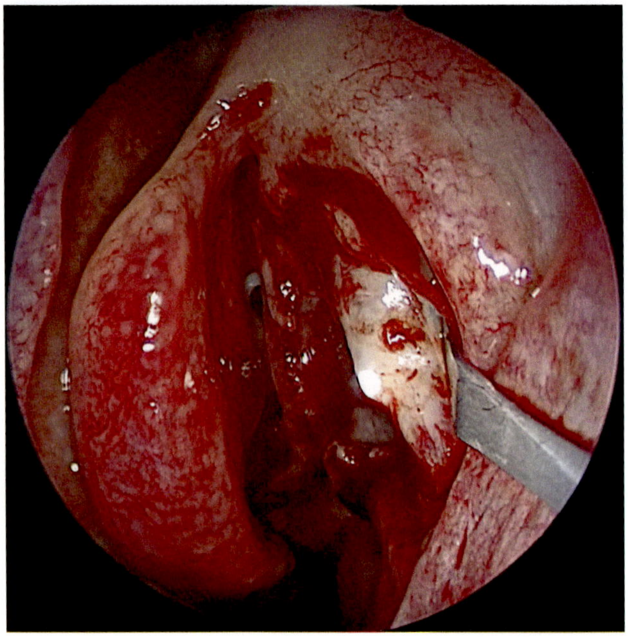

Fig. 43.15 The lacrimal sac is incised vertically with the crescent blade as close as possible to the maxillary bone

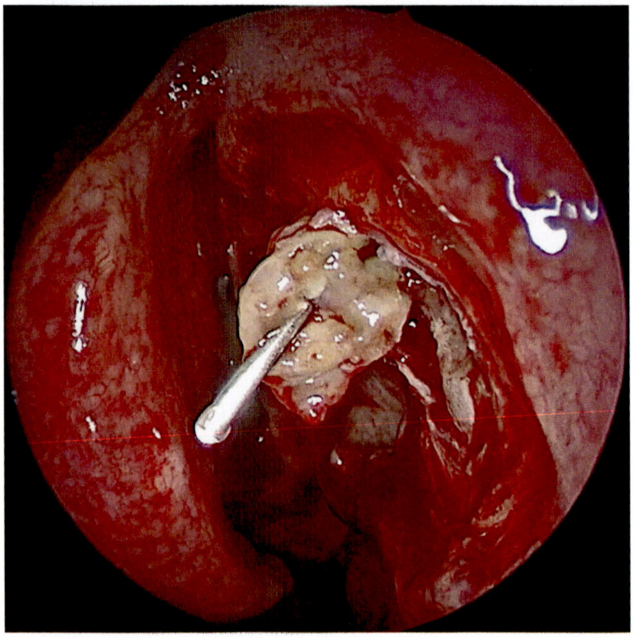

Fig. 43.16 The lacrimal sac is open and the light pipe seen freely in the nasal cavity

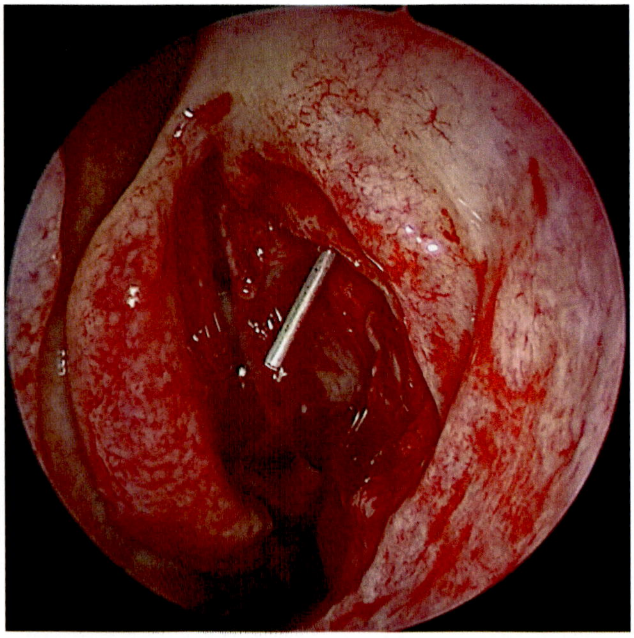

Fig. 43.17 The medial wall of the lacrimal sac and upper nasolacrimal duct are completely resected

mucosal flap. If silicone stents are used, bicanalicular intubation is performed at this point (Fig. 43.18). If this is impossible because of absence or obstruction of one of the canaliculi, monocanalicular intubation (Monoka®, FCI Ophthalmics) can also be performed.

Postoperatively, all patients are prescribed a steroid nasal spray twice a day and a combination of tobramycin-

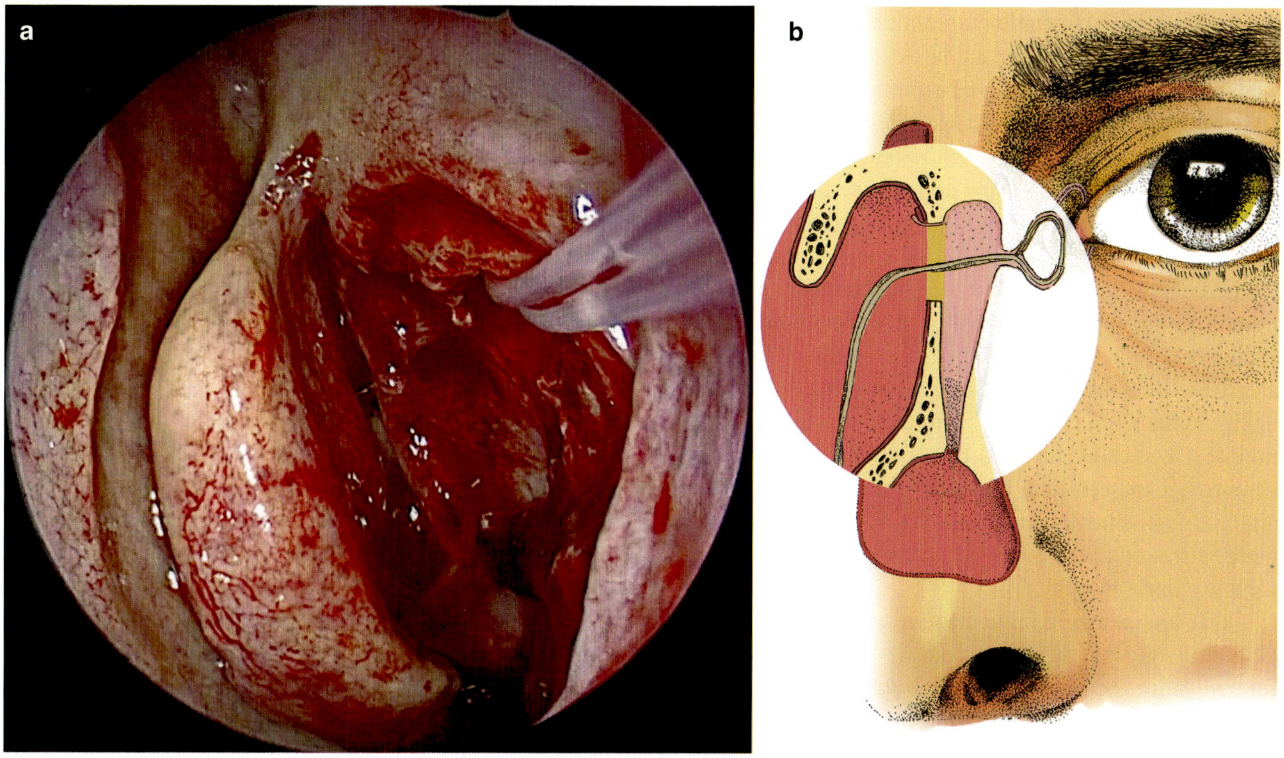

Fig. 43.18 (**a**) and (**b**) Bicanalicular intubation placed through the new ostium

dexamethasone eye drops four times a day. The nasal spray is discontinued after 2 weeks and the eye drops tapered over 3 weeks. Patients should be seen 2 days after surgery, after 1 week, after 1 month, and at 3 and 6 months. At each follow-up visit, lacrimal irrigation should be performed. At 6 weeks, the silicone intubation stent is removed under topical anesthesia through the upper or lower lacrimal punctum and irrigation done to confirm patency of the ostium. If the silicone tube prolapses before 6 weeks, an attempt to reposition it can be performed in the office. If unsuccessful, the tube is removed under local anesthesia with two drops of topical anesthetic.

If tearing or gross lacrimal discharge associated with lacrimal obstruction on irrigation develops at any point during follow-up, an endoscopic revision can be performed using the same technique described. EndoDCR revisions most often reveal osteotomy closure and fibrosis, synechiae between the middle turbinate and the lateral wall of the nasal cavity or between the nasal septum and middle turbinate, and pyogenic granulomas.

Complications

Although EndoDCR is considered a safe procedure, complications can occur. Precise knowledge of the lacrimal and nasal anatomy and technical considerations of the surgical procedure are crucial in preventing complications. It is generally accepted that the complication rate is usually less than 5% and major complications less than 2% [57].

Intraoperative complications are generally associated with excessive bleeding (which obstructs adequate visualization of the intranasal anatomy) and lack of expertise. If dissection is carried to posteriorly or when the uncinate process is aggressively removed, there is a high risk of orbital penetration with fat prolapse, hematoma, and injury of the medial rectus muscle with subsequent diplopia [36]. Fat prolapse can be managed with minimal bipolar cautery which produces retraction into the orbit and avoids further complications. In no circumstances should fat be pulled and resected, since this may lead to more fat prolapse and intraorbital hematoma. Fat extrusion has also been associated with a 5.3-fold higher risk of EndoDCR failure [58].

Medial orbital wall injury can also lead to ecchymosis, eyelid edema, and emphysema. Although these complications are mild and self-limited, they are uncomfortable to the patient and if possible should be avoided. Periocular and palpebral emphysema occurs because of an increase in positive air pressure in the nasal cavity which forces air into the orbit, through the breach in the medial wall [57]. It can be prevented by asking the patient not to blow his nose or avoid blocking the nostrils when sneezing. Cold compresses and rest for a few days can alleviate these problems.

Intraoperative bleeding can be minimized by adequate nose preparation before the surgical procedure as was mentioned previously and by discontinuing anticoagulant medications [54]. Warfarin, clopidogrel, and NSAIDS should be stopped 7 days before the procedure, and aspirin and similar products 10 days. The primary care physician should take the decision of withdrawing medications for the perioperative period, if he considers that it is safe and appropriate to do so. Herbal remedies such as garlic, green tea, ginseng, gingko biloba, vitamin E, and others should also be stopped 10 days before the procedure. If active, mild to moderate bleeding occurs intraoperatively, it can generally be controlled with the placement of pledgets or neurosurgical cottonoids soaked in a mixture of diluted 1:5000 adrenaline and oxymetazoline 0.05% in the nasal cavity for 5 minutes. If available, a solution of 4% cocaine can also be used. Very rarely, copious hemorrhage may ensue if a branch of the anterior ethmoidal artery is inadvertently sectioned. Bipolar cautery and nasal packing soaked in the previously mentioned solution can be used to control bleeding.

Other less common intraoperative complications include CSF leak (0.04%) which occurs when dissection is performed above the insertion of the middle turbinate [59] and punctal and/or canalicular injury during insertion of a Bowman probe or the vitrectomy light pipe [60]. When using a drill in powered EndoDCR, there is also a risk of eyelid/cheek bruise and nostril burn [61].

Early postoperative complications include infection and epistaxis. Infection is extremely rare in EndoDCR and is probably related to chronic, unsuspected rhinosinusitis. It can be adequately treated with systemic antibiotics [57]. Epistaxis is usually transient and self-limited and can be treated with cold compresses, local pressure, and oxymetazoline 0.05% spray. However, if bleeding is persistent, it may be necessary to check hemostasis and use bipolar cautery with endoscopic visualization under local or general anesthesia. Nasal packing is not recommended, since it can cause damage to the mucosal flaps if used and/or scarring of the osteotomy.

Late complications of EndoDCR include persistent epiphora, lacrimal sump syndrome, canalicular obstruction, nasal synechiae, osteotomy scarring, and obstruction (DCR failure).

Persistent epiphora can present with a fully patent ostium and normal lacrimal irrigation. This occurs in approximately 5–10% of patients and is termed *functional failure* [62]. In these patients, there are no underlying etiological factors such as ocular surface disorders or eyelid malposition. In a recent study, the authors found that management of this complication with silicone stenting and eyelid tightening offers relatively good success rates (72%) [62].

Lacrimal sump syndrome occurs because of inadequate marsupialization of the inferior lacrimal sac leaving a pouch where tears and discharge accumulate. Inadequate opening of the bone of the inferior lacrimal sac fossa can also contribute to a sump syndrome. Typically, lacrimal irrigation is fully patent. Treatment of this complication is revision EndoDCR removing the remnants of the inferior lacrimal sac and/or bone adjacent to the sac [62–64].

Canalicular obstruction after EndoDCR is rare but can occur at the level of the common canaliculus, upper or lower canaliculi. When the common canaliculus is obstructed, a silicone stent or revision EndoDCR can be attempted. Occasionally, a conjunctivorhinostomy with a Jones tube is necessary [57].

Nasal synechiae usually occur between the middle turbinate and the osteotomy site or between the middle turbinate and the septum. Synechiae per se are not problematic unless they produce obstruction of the ostium or reduction of airflow. In these cases as in DCR failure, a revision EndoDCR must be performed. The incidence of ostium scarring and obstruction varies widely according to surgical technique, surgeon expertise, etiology of nasolacrimal duct obstruction, chronic sinonasal inflammation/disease, use of silicone intubation, and use of adjunctive agents. However, success rates for EndoDCR parallel, in some studies, surpass Ext-DCR success rates averaging between 79% and 97% in the past decade [5, 31–33, 37–42, 44, 45, 47–50, 55, 57, 65].

Summary

Endonasal DCR is a successful and safe procedure for the treatment of nasolacrimal duct obstruction in adults. Precise knowledge of the lacrimal and intranasal anatomy is critical for success and to avoid complications.

References

1. Wu W, Yan W, MacCallum JK, Tu Y, Jiang AC, Yang Y, Xiao T, Li J, Wang Q, Qu J. Primary treatment of acute dacryocystitis by endoscopic dacryocystorhinostomy with silicone intubation guided by a soft probe. Ophthalmology. 2009;116(1):116–22.
2. Toti A. Nuovo metodo conservatore di cura radicale delle suppurazioni croniche del sacco lacrimale (dacriocistorinostomia). Clin Mod. 1904;10:385–7.
3. Woog JJ, Kennedy RH, Custer PL, Kaltreider SA, Meyer DR, Camara JG. Endonasal dacryocystorhinostomy. A report by the American Academy of Ophthalmology. Ophthalmology. 2001;108:2369–77.
4. Madge SN, Chan W, Malhotra R, Ghabrial R, Floreani S, Wormald PJ, Tsirbas A, Selva D. Endoscopic dacryocystorhinostomy in acute dacryocystitis: a multicenter case series. Orbit. 2011;30(1):1–6.
5. Jain S, Ganguly A, Singh S, Mohapatra S, Tripathy D, Rath S. Primary nonendoscopic endonasal versus delayed external dacryocystorhinostomy in acute dacryocystitis. Ophthalmic Plast Reconstr Surg. 2017;33(4):285–8.
6. Lee TS, Woog JJ. Endonasal dacryocystorhinostomy in the primary treatment of acute dacryocystitis with abscess formation. Ophthalmic Plast Reconstr Surg. 2001;17(3):180–3.
7. Szubin L, Papageorge A, Sacks E. Endonasal laser-assisted dacryocystorhinostomy. Am J Rhinol. 1999;13:371–4.

8. Dolman PJ. Comparison of external dacryocystorhinostomy with nonlaser endonasal dacryocystorhinostomy. Ophthalmology. 2003;110:78–8.
9. Fayet B, Racy E, Assouline M. Systematic unciformectomy for a standardized endonasal dacryocystorhinostomy. Ophthalmology. 2002;109(3):530–6.
10. McDonogh M, Meiring JH. Endoscopic transnasal dacryocystorhinostomy. J Laryngol Otol. 1989;103:585–7.
11. Kong YT, Kim TI, Kong BW. A report of 131 cases of endoscopic laser lacrimal surgery. Ophthalmology. 1994;101:1793–800.
12. Lee JJ, Lee HM, Lim HB, Seo SW, Ahn HB, Lee SB. Learning curve for endoscopic endonasal dacryocystorhinostomy. Korean J Ophthalmol. 2017;31(4):299–305.
13. Caldwell GW. Two new operations for obstruction of the nasal duct, with preservation of the canaliculi, and with an incidental description of a new lachrymal probe. Am J Ophthalmol. 1893;10: 189–93.
14. West JM. A window resection of the nasal duct in cases of stenosis. Trans AM Opthalmol Soc. 1909–1911;12:654–8.
15. Massaro BM, Gonnering S, Harris GJ. Endonasal laser dacryocystorhinostomy. A new approach to nasolacrimal duct obstruction. Arch Ophthalmol. 1990;108:1172–6.
16. Harish V, Benger RS. Origins of lacrimal surgery, and evolution of dacryocystorhinostomy to the present. Clin Exp Ophthalmol. 2014;42(3):284–7.
17. Gonnering RS, Lyon DB, Fisher JC. Endoscopic laser-assisted lacrimal surgery. Am J Ophthalmol. 1991;111:152–7.
18. Woog JJ, Metson R, Puliafito CA. Holmium:YAG endonasal laser dacryocystorhinostomy. Am J Ophthalmol. 1993;116:1–10.
19. Reifler DM. Results of endoscopic KTP laser-assisted dacryocystorhinostomy. Ophthal Plast Reconstr Surg. 1993;9:231–6.
20. Metson R. The endoscopic approach for revision dacryocystorhinostomy. Laryngoscope. 1990;100:1344–7.
21. Seppa H, Grenman R, Hartikainen J. Endonasal CO2-Nd:YAG laser dacryocystorhinostomy. Acta Ophthalmol. 1994;72:703–6.
22. Tutton MK, O'Donnell NP. Endonasal laser dacryocystorhinostomy under direct vision. Eye. 1995;9:485–7.
23. Sadiq SA, Hugkulstone CE, Jones NS, Downes RN. Endoscopic holmium:YAG laser dacryocystorhinostomy. Eye. 1996;10: 43–6.
24. Mickelson SA, Kim DK, Stein IM. Endoscopic laser assisted dacryocystorhinostomy. Am J Otolaryngol. 1997;18:107–11.
25. Hartikainen J, Grenman R, Puukka P, Seppa H. Prospective randomized comparison of external dacryocystorhinostomy and endonasal laser dacryocystorhinostomy. Ophthalmology. 1998;105: 1106–13.
26. Hehar SS, Jones NS, Sadiq SA, Downes RN. Endoscopic holmium:YAG laser dacryocystorhinostomy – safe and effective as a day-case procedure. J Laryngol Otol. 1997;111:1056–9.
27. Tarbet KJ, Custer PL. External dacryocystorhinostomy: surgical success, patiente satisfaction, and economic cost. Ophthalmology. 1995;102:1065–70.
28. Walland MJ, Rose GE. Factors affecting the success rate of open lacrimal surgery. Br J Ophthalmol. 1994;78:888–91.
29. Camara JG, Bengzon AU, Henson RD. The safety and efficacy of mitomycin C in endonasal endoscopic laser-assisted dacryocystorhinostomy. Ophthal Plast Reconstr Surg. 2000;16:114–8.
30. Knisely A, Harvey R, Sacks R. Long-term outcomes in endoscopic dacryocystorhinostomy. Curr Opin Otolaryngol Head Neck Surg. 2015;23(1):53–8.
31. Zengin MO, Eren E. The return of the jedi: comparison of the outcomes of endolaser dacryocystorhinostomy and endonasal dacryocystorhinostomy. Int Forum Allergy Rhinol. 2014;4:480–3.
32. Huang J, Malek J, Chin D, et al. Systematic review and meta-analysis on outcomes for endoscopic versus external dacryocystorhinostomy. Orbit. 2014;33:81–90.
33. Marcet MM, Kuk AK, Phelps PO. Evidence based review of surgical practices in endoscopic endonasal dacryocystorhinostomy for primary acquired nasolacrimal duct obstruction and other new indications. Curr Opin Ophthalmol. 2014;25:443–8.
34. Javate RM, Campomanes BS Jr, Co ND, et al. The endoscope and the radiofrequency unit in DCR surgery. Ophthal Plast Reconstr Surg. 1995;11:54–8.
35. Moore WM, Bentley CR, Olver JM. Functional and anatomic results after two types of endoscopic endonasal dacryocystorhinostomy: surgical and holmium laser. Ophthalmology. 2002;109: 1575–82.
36. Tsirbas A, Wormald PJ. Endonasal dacryocystorhinostomy with mucosal flaps. Am J Ophthalmol. 2003;135:76–83.
37. Trimarchi M, Resti AG, Bellini C, et al. Anastomosis of nasal mucosal and lacrimal sac flaps in endoscopic dacryocystorhinostomy. Eur Arch Otorhinolaryngol. 2009;266:1747–52.
38. Codere F, Denton P, Corona J. Endonasal dacryocystorhinostomy: a modified technique with preservation of the nasal and lacrimal mucosa. Ophthalmic Plast Reconstr Surg. 2010;26:161–4.
39. Sonkhya N, Mishra P. Endoscopic transnasal dacryocystorhinostomy with nasal mucosal and posterior lacrimal sac flap. J Laryngol Otol. 2009;123:320–6.
40. Green R, Gohil R, Ross P. Mucosal and lacrimal flaps for endonasal dacryocystorhinostomy: a systematic review. Clin Otolaryngol. 2017;42:514–20.
41. Ramakrishnan VR, Hink EM, Durairaj VD, Kingdom TT. Outcomes after endoscopic dacryocystorhinostomy without mucosal flap preservation. Am J Rhinol. 2007;21(6):753–7.
42. Hodgson N, Bratton E, Whipple K, Priel A, Oh SR, Fante RG, Kikkawa DO, Korn BS. Outcomes of endonasal dacryocystorhinostomy without mucosal flap preservation. Ophthalmic Plast Reconstr Surg. 2014;30(1):24–7.
43. Xie C, Zhang L, Liu Y, Ma H, Li S. Comparing the success rate of dacryocystorhinostomy with and without silicone intubation: a trial sequential analysis of randomized control trials. Sci Rep. 2017;7(1):1936.
44. Chong KK, et al. Randomized trial on silicone intubation in endoscopic mechanical dacryocystorhinostomy (SEND) for primary nasolacrimal duct obstruction. Ophthalmology. 2013;120:2139–45.
45. Smirnov G, Tuomilehto H, Terasvirta M, et al. Silicone tubing is not necessary after primary endoscopic dacryocystorhinostomy: a prospective randomized study. Am J Rhinol. 2008;22:214–7.
46. Feng YF, Cai JQ, Zhang JY, Han XH. A meta-analysis of primary dacryocystorhinostomy with and without silicone intubation. Can J Ophthalmol. 2011;46(6):521–7.
47. Fayers T, Dolman PJ. Bicanalicular silicone stents in endonasal dacryocystorhinostomy: results of a randomized clinical trial. Ophthalmology. 2016;123(10):2255–9.
48. Dolmetsch AM. Nonlaser endoscopic endonasal dacryocystorhinostomy with adjunctive mitomycin C in nasolacrimal duct obstruction in adults. Ophthalmology. 2010;117:1037–40.
49. Cheng SM, Feng YF, Xu L, Li Y, Huang JH. Efficacy of mitomycin C in endoscopic dacryocystorhinostomy: a systematic review and meta-analysis. PLoS One. 2013;13:8(5).
50. Li EY, Cheng AC, Wong AC, Sze AM, Yuen HK. Safety and efficacy of adjunctive intranasal mitomycin C and triamcinolone in endonasal endoscopic dacryocystorhinostomy. Int Ophthalmol. 2016;36(1):105–10.
51. Dutton JJ. Atlas of oculoplastic and orbital surgery. 1st ed. Philadelphia: Lippincott Williams & Wilkins; 2013. p. 216–9.
52. Neskey D, Eloy JA, Casiano RR. Nasal, septal and turbinate anatomy and embryology. Otolaryngol Clin N Am. 2009;42(2):193–205.
53. Oneal RM, Beil RJ. Surgical anatomy of the nose. Clin Plast Surg. 2010;37(2):191–211.
54. Nerad JA. Clinical anatomy. In: Techniques in ophthalmic plastic surgery. 1st ed. Philadelphia: Saunders; 2010. p. 27–80.

55. Sweeney AR, Davis GE, Chang SH, Amadi AJ. Outcomes of endoscopic dacryocystorhinostomy in secondary acquired nasolacrimal duct obstruction: a case-control study. Ophthalmic Plast Reconstr Surg. 2018;34(1):20–5.
56. Ali MJ, Psaltis AJ, Murphy J, Wormald PJ. Powered endoscopic dacryocystorhinostomy. Ophthalmic Plast Reconstr Surg. 2015;31(3):219–21.
57. Mattavelli D, Lombardi D, Ferrari M, Nicolai P. Complications of endoscopic DCR. In: Presutti L, Mattioli F, editors. Endoscopic surgery of the lacrimal drainage system. Cham: Springer; 2016.
58. Hammoudi DS, Tucker NA. Factors associated with outcome of endonasal dacryocystorhinostomy. Ophthal Plast Reconstr Surg. 2011;27:266–9.
59. Friedel ME, Earley MA, Eloy JA. Skull base defect in a patient with ozena undergoing dacryocystorhinostomy. Allergy Rhinol (Providence). 2011;2:36–9.
60. Zuercher B, Tritten JJ, Friedrich JP, Monnier P. Analysis of functional and anatomic success following endonasal dacryocystorhinostomy. Ann Otol Rhinol Laryngol. 2011;120:231–8.
61. Herzallah I, Alzuraiqi B, Bawazeer N, Marglani O, Alherabi A, Mohamed SK, Al-Qahtani K, Al-Khatib T, Alghamdi AJ. Endoscopic dacryocystorhinostomy (DCR): a comparative study between powered and non-powered technique. Otolaryngol Head Neck Surg. 2015;44:56.
62. Shams PN, Chen PG, Wormald PJ, Sloan B, Wilcsek G, McNab A, Selva D. Management of functional epiphora in patients with an anatomically patent dacryocystorhinostomy. JAMA Ophthalmol. 2014;132(9):1127–32.
63. Jordan DR, McDonald H. Failed dacryocystorhinostomy: the sump syndrome. Ophthalmic Surg. 1993;24:692–3.
64. Migliori ME. Endoscopic evaluation and management of the lacrimal sump syndrome. Ophthal Plast Reconstr Surg. 1997;13:281–4.
65. Coumou AD, Genders SW, Smid TM, Saeed P. Endoscopic dacryocystorhinostomy: long-term experience and outcomes. Acta Ophthalmol. 2017;95:74–8.

Pediatric Endonasal Dacryocystorhinostomy

44

Krista Stewart and Andrew R. Harrison

Indications

Symptomatic nasolacrimal duct obstruction (NLDO) in children is most commonly due to a congenital obstruction at the level of the valve of Hasner. Symptoms resolve spontaneously by 12 months of age in 85–95% of patients [1]. Of those patients, whose symptoms do not resolve spontaneously, the vast majority respond to a single probing. A small percentage of children with NLDO require a second probing with or without silicone intubation or balloon dacryoplasty [2]. If these measures fail to resolve the symptoms, dacryocystorhinostomy (DCR) is indicated. Earlier surgical intervention may be considered in cases of post-traumatic scarring or cases of chronic or recurrent dacryocystitis as the rate of failure of probing and stenting is lower in these patients [3]. Historically, external DCR has been performed in children with a success rate between 83% and 96% [3–5]. The advent of smaller endoscopic instrumentation and techniques along with the reported equal efficacy of endonasal compared to external DCR in adults has led many surgeons to consider endonasal DCR in children. Several case series have demonstrated an overall success rate of 87–92% for pediatric endonasal DCR [6–10]. Advantages of endonasal DCR over standard external DCR in children include shorter recovery time, minimizing facial scarring from a skin incision, and preservation of the orbicularis oculi muscle portion of the lacrimal pump mechanism [10].

Anatomic Considerations

Generally, the anatomic landmarks of pediatric endonasal DCR are similar to those in an adult but with a narrower nasal space and smaller overall dimensions. There are a few important anatomic differences to be aware of between adults and children when performing endonasal DCR. Most notably, the cribriform plate inserts slightly lower in children than in adults. The lacrimal sac is typically just anterior to the insertion of the middle turbinate because in children the agger nasi air cells are not well pneumatized [11]. Occasionally, middle turbinate infracture is necessary to create an adequate ostium [9]. The frontal process is softer and thinner in children making bone removal easier but increasing the risk of overlying skin or nasal vestibule injury during bone removal [6]. In cases of craniofacial anomaly or significant facial trauma, maxillofacial and orbital imaging is often useful preoperatively. In these patients, a joint approach with otolaryngology and ophthalmology may be beneficial.

Surgical Technique

General anesthesia is typically required for endonasal DCR in children. The patient should be positioned and draped so both the nose and surgical eye are fully exposed. The surgical side of the nose should be packed with cottonoids soaked with a topical vasoconstrictive agent such as 0.05% oxymetazoline hydrochloride solution. After 5–10 minutes of topical vasoconstriction, the middle turbinate and lateral nasal wall should be infiltrated with 1% lidocaine with 1:100,000 epinephrine to provide pain control and more robust hemostasis. Cottonoids soaked in oxymetazoline hydrochloride solution should be available on the surgical field for additional intraoperative hemostasis. Other instrumentations that should be available on the surgical field include both a 4.0 mm and a 2.7 mm endoscope with either a 0° or 30° view, an angled keratome, crescent knife or sickle blade, Freer elevator, punctal dilator, Bowman probes, suction, and either a Sonopet ultrasonic aspirator (Stryker, Kalamazoo, MI), bone drill, or angled neurosurgical microrongeurs for bone removal (Fig. 44.1).

K. Stewart · A. R. Harrison (✉)
Department of Ophthalmology, University of Minnesota, Minneapolis, MN, USA
e-mail: stewartk@umn.edu; harri060@umn.edu

A. J. Cohen, C. N. Burkat (eds.), *Oculofacial, Orbital, and Lacrimal Surgery*, https://doi.org/10.1007/978-3-030-14092-2_44

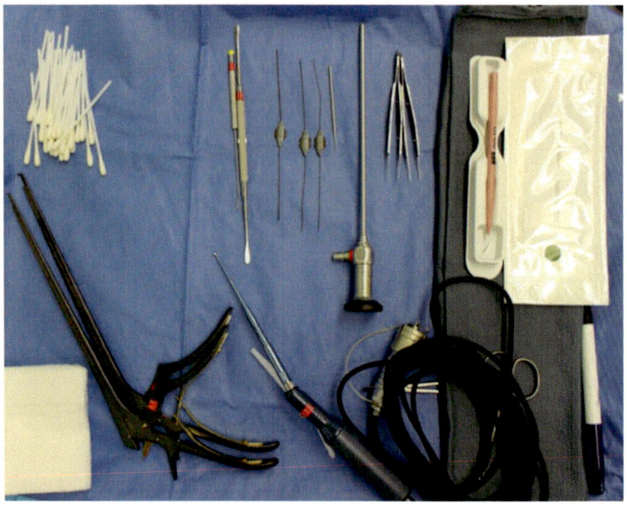

Fig. 44.1 Instrumentation required for pediatric endonasal dacryocystorhinostomy

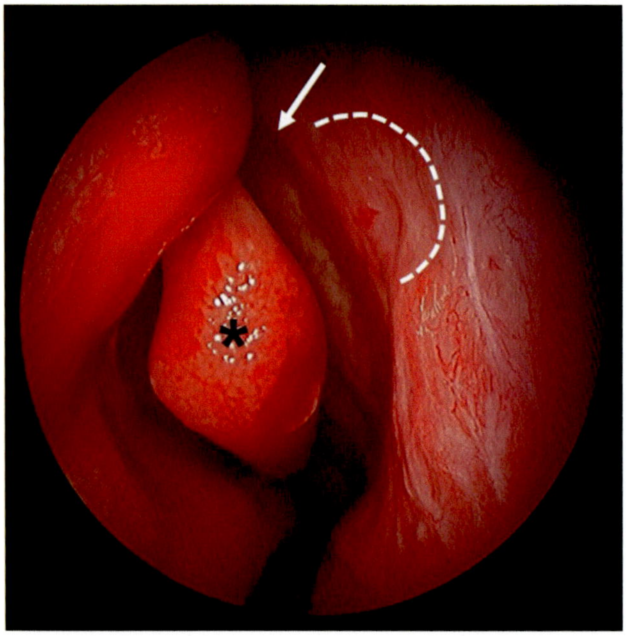

Fig. 44.2 Endonasal anatomy relevant to pediatric endonasal dacryocystorhinostomy. The asterisk overlies the middle turbinate, and the solid arrow points anterior to the root of the middle turbinate

The first step of endonasal DCR is identification of the anatomic landmarks and the lacrimal sac (Fig. 44.2). This can be aided by passage of either a Bowman probe or a vitrectomy light pipe (20 gauge disposable) through the puncta into the lacrimal sac. With a light pipe, the transilluminated lacrimal sac can easily be viewed through the lateral nasal wall. If the sac position is posterior to the anterior-most portion of the middle turbinate, infracture or a small partial turbinectomy may be required. Once the location of the lacrimal sac is identified, an angled blade can be used to make a curvilinear incision into the nasal mucosa. A Freer or otologic canal wall elevator is then used to lift the mucosal flap anteriorly to posteriorly to expose the underlying bone. The nasal mucosal flap should be removed using a cut-through or Blakesley forceps to prevent occlusion of the ostium. There are reports of the mucosal flap being creased with laser ablation or radiofrequency desiccation [12, 13]. Removal of bone can be initiated once the mucosa is adequately cleared. A high-speed drill using a hooded tip burr may be used to create the ostium. Alternatively, a Sonopet (Stryker, Kalamazoo, MI) ultrasonic aspirator can be used for bone removal, which may provide improved control and minimize surrounding soft tissue damage. The ostium should measure approximately 1.0–1.5 cm in diameter once completed.

Once the ostium is formed, a dacryocystorhinostomy is performed. A Bowman probe can be inserted through the superior punctum into the lacrimal sac and then used to tent the medial wall of the lacrimal sac through the ostium. An angled blade is then used to vertically open the medial lacrimal sac. If adequate edges of the nasal mucosa and medial lacrimal sac are preserved, the mucosal flap can be tucked into the lacrimal sac flaps. Alternatively, the flaps can be excised and the ostium allowed to heal primarily, or the nasal mucosa and lacrimal sac flaps may be sutured together, although this is difficult from the endonasal approach [14, 15].

At this point, the Bowman probe should be freely mobile within the DCR opening. Patency can be confirmed with lacrimal system irrigation. At this point, some authors recommend the use of 0.5 mg/mL mitomycin-C (MMC) soaked in a cottonoid to be applied to the ostium for 5 minutes [16]. This may limit scar formation to improve long-term patency; however evidence is limited. Bicanalicular silicone intubation through the newly formed nasolacrimal fistula is performed, and the ends of the silicone tube are tied in a square knot and may or may not be secured to the lateral nasal wall with a single suture (Fig. 44.3). Removal of the silicone stent may be performed in the clinic setting if the patient is cooperative or in the operating room with general anesthesia if uncooperative. Timing of stent removal is controversial but typically ranges from 2 to 6 months postoperatively.

Following surgery, the patient should be placed on steroid-antibiotic combination drops and saline nasal spray as tolerated. Steroid nasal spray may also be considered especially in patients prone to scar formation. Nasal packing is usually not necessary unless there are concerns for postoperative bleeding or excessive intraoperative bleeding.

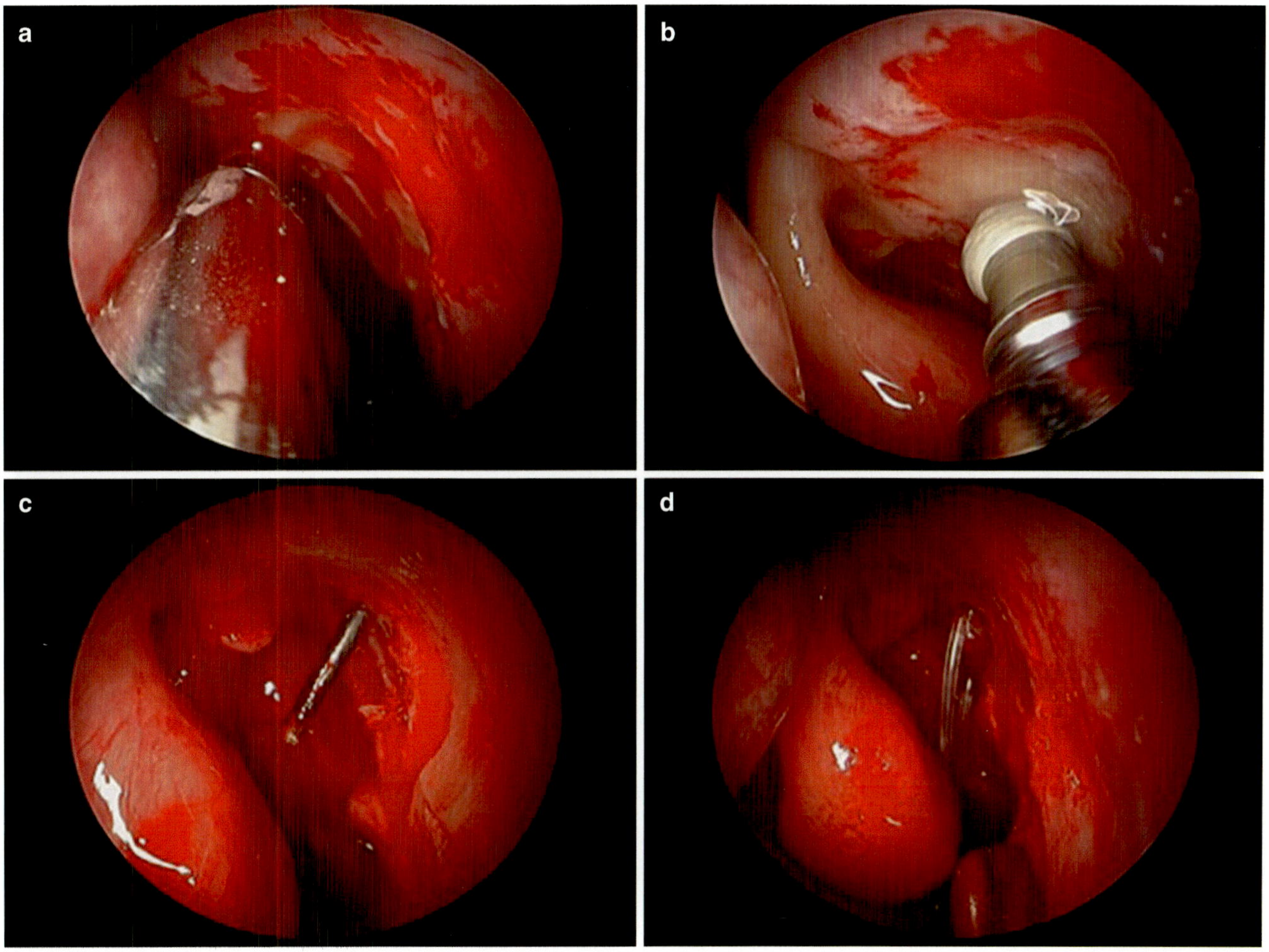

Fig. 44.3 Steps of endonasal dacryocystorhinostomy. First a nasal mucosal flap is created anterior to the middle turbinate (**a**), and then the exposed bone is drilled to form an ostium (**b**). A Bowman probe is inserted into the nasal cavity after the lacrimal sac is exposed (**c**), and silicone tubes are placed through the superior and inferior canaliculi and tied in the nose (**d**)

Outcomes

Clinical success of endonasal DCR is determined by the resolution of symptoms. This may be confirmed anatomically with irrigation and nasal endoscopy, although it is often difficult to perform in young children without general anesthesia. In those children who cannot tolerate nasal endoscopy or irrigation, the dye disappearance test may be used to assess anatomic patency. The overall success rate of endonasal DCR in children is reported to be between 87% and 94% [6–10, 17]. Patients with craniofacial abnormalities have a success rate reported around 78% [6]. Other risk factors for endonasal DCR failure that have been identified include early removal of silicone tube, craniofacial anomalies, septal deviation, inadequate ostium size, prior canaliculitis or dacryocystitis, and African descent [16, 18].

Complications

The overall complication rate for pediatric endonasal DCR is approximately 5–10% [6, 11]. Serious complications such as CSF leak or vision loss have not been reported in any case series of pediatric endonasal DCR but are possible and have been reported in adult endonasal DCR. Extreme care should be taken when creating the bony ostium as the cribriform plate inserts more inferiorly in children, as previously mentioned. The most common complication of pediatric endonasal DCR is early extrusion of the silicone tube. This does not often lead to any further complications, but premature loss of the silicone tube may be associated with a higher rate of failure long-term. Other common complications include synechiae or granuloma formation which can lead to failure and may require a repeat surgery. Infection and abscess formation are less common but possible. Slitting of the puncta may occur if the stent is tied too tightly. One complication unique to endonasal DCR in comparison to external DCR is nasal vestibule or skin abrasion secondary to drill shaft rotation [6].

References

1. Petersen RA, Robb RM. The natural course of congenital obstruction of the nasolacrimal duct. J Pediatr Ophthalmol Strabismus. 1978;15(4):246–50.
2. Paul TO, Shepherd R. Congenital nasolacrimal duct obstruction: natural history and the timing of optimal intervention. J Pediatr Ophthalmol Strabismus. 1994;31(6):362–7.
3. Hakin KN, Sullivan TJ, Sharma A, Welham RA. Paediatric dacryocystorhinostomy. Aust N Z J Ophthalmol. 1994;22(4):231–5.
4. Welham RA, Hughes SM. Lacrimal surgery in children. Am J Ophthalmol. 1985;99(1):27–34.
5. Nowinski TS, Flanagan JC, Mauriello J. Pediatric dacryocystorhinostomy. Arch Ophthalmol (Chicago, Ill 1960). 1985;103(8):1226–8.
6. Chan W, Wilcsek G, Ghabrial R, Goldberg RA, Dolman P, Selva D, et al. Pediatric endonasal dacryocystorhinostomy: a multicenter series of 116 cases. Orbit. 2017;36(5):311–6.
7. de Souza CE, Nisar J, de Souza RA. Pediatric endoscopic dacryocystorhinostomy. Otolaryngol Neck Surg. 2012;147(2):335–7.
8. Komínek P, Červenka S, Matoušek P, Pniak T, Zeleník K. Primary pediatric endonasal dacryocystorhinostomy – a review of 58 procedures. Int J Pediatr Otorhinolaryngol. 2010;74(6):661–4.
9. Leibovitch I, Selva D, Tsirbas A, Greenrod E, Pater J, Wormald PJ. Paediatric endoscopic endonasal dacryocystorhinostomy in congenital nasolacrimal duct obstruction. Graefes Arch Clin Exp Ophthalmol. 2006;244(10):1250–4.
10. Gupta AK, Bansal S. Primary endoscopic dacryocystorhinostomy in children – analysis of 18 patients. Int J Pediatr Otorhinolaryngol. 2006;70(7):1213–7.
11. Celenk F, Mumbuc S, Durucu C, Karatas ZA, Aytaç I, Baysal E, et al. Pediatric endonasal endoscopic dacryocystorhinostomy. Int J Pediatr Otorhinolaryngol. 2013;77(8):1259–62.
12. Javate RM, Campomanes BS, Co ND, Dinglasan JL, Go CG, Tan EN, et al. The endoscope and the radiofrequency unit in DCR surgery. Ophthal Plast Reconstr Surg. 1995;11(1):54–8.
13. Kong YT, Kim TI, Kong BW. A report of 131 cases of endoscopic laser lacrimal surgery. Ophthalmology. 1994;101(11):1793–800.
14. Tsirbas A, Wormald PJ. Endonasal dacryocystorhinostomy with mucosal flaps. Am J Ophthalmol. 2003;135(1):76–83.
15. Codère F, Denton P, Corona J. Endonasal dacryocystorhinostomy: a modified technique with preservation of the nasal and lacrimal mucosa. Ophthalmic Plast Reconstr Surg. 2010;26(3):161–4.
16. Dolmetsch AM, Gallon MA, Holds JB. Nonlaser endoscopic endonasal dacryocystorhinostomy with adjunctive mitomycin C in children. Ophthalmic Plast Reconstr Surg. 2008;24(5):390–3.
17. Gioacchini FM, Alicandri-Ciufelli M, Kaleci S, Re M. The outcomes of endoscopic dacryocystorhinostomy in children: a systematic review. Int J Pediatr Otorhinolaryngol. 2015;79(7):947–52.
18. Jones DT, Fajardo NF, Petersen RA, VanderVeen DK. Pediatric endoscopic dacryocystorhinostomy failures: who and why? Laryngoscope. 2007;117(2):323–7.

Adjunctive Endonasal Procedures During Dacryocystorhinostomy

45

Alkis J. Psaltis

Endoscopic dacryocystorhinostomy (DCR) has become a common procedure for the management of certain lacrimal conditions. Its high success rate and negligible cosmetic morbidity have made it an attractive alternative to traditional external approaches. To perform this procedure well, the surgeon must have a sound understanding of endoscopic endonasal anatomy and its normal anatomic variants and be well trained in the use of the nasal endoscope for adjunctive turbinectomy or septoplasty procedures, if indicated. Figure 45.1 highlights important normal endoscopic anatomy that will be referenced in the chapter.

Preoperative Assessment

Prior to endoscopic surgery, all patients should undergo a complete endoscopic assessment of their nasal cavity. This examination will allow the preoperative identification of normal anatomical variants such as a deviated nasal septum or pneumatized middle turbinate that may hinder visualization and access to the lacrimal sac during endoscopic surgery. The decision on whether adjunctive endonasal procedures will be required at the time of lacrimal surgery should therefore occur in the preoperative setting to facilitate the informed consent process and optimize surgical planning. Figure 45.2 represents the basic office setup required to perform the preoperative examination.

A. J. Psaltis (✉)
Department of Otolaryngology Head and Neck Surgery, The Queen Elizabeth Hospital, Adelaide, South Australia

Department of Surgery, The University of Adelaide, Adelaide, South Australia

Topical Anesthesia

The preoperative examination occurs in the ambulatory clinic setting under topical anesthesia. Topical agents are most commonly administered in an aerosolized form or on presoaked packing materials and usually contain a rapid-onset anesthetic agent, such as lidocaine (xylocaine or lignocaine), and a vasoconstrictor agent, such as phenylephrine or oxymetazoline. Commercially available combination sprays are available and provide an easy and effective way of preparing the nose for the examination. One such example of this is the product Cophenylcaine Forte (ENT Technologies, Melbourne Victoria, Australia) which contains 50 mg/ml of lidocaine hydrochloride and 5 mg/ml of phenylephrine. Figure 45.3 shows this product with the patented single-use disposable nozzle that allows delivery deep with the nasal cavity. The use of these agents will not only increase the comfort of the endoscopy but also improve the overall visibility and access by reducing mucosal edema.

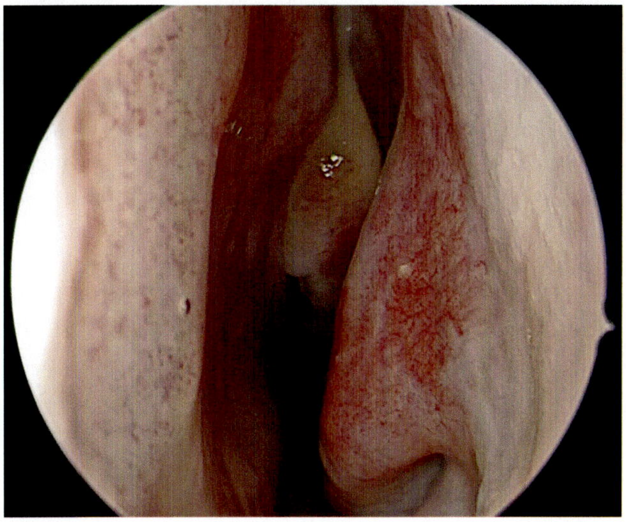

Fig. 45.1 Endoscopic view of the normal nasal anatomy

A. J. Cohen, C. N. Burkat (eds.), *Oculofacial, Orbital, and Lacrimal Surgery*, https://doi.org/10.1007/978-3-030-14092-2_45

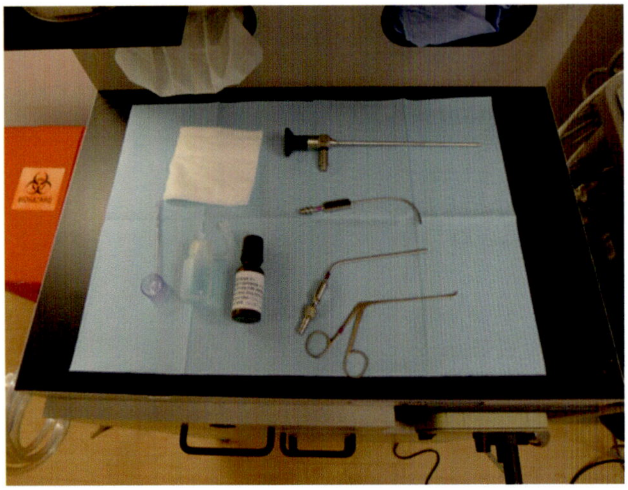

Fig. 45.2 Basic instrumentation includes topical anesthetic, rigid endoscope, angle and straight suctions, and endoscopic forceps

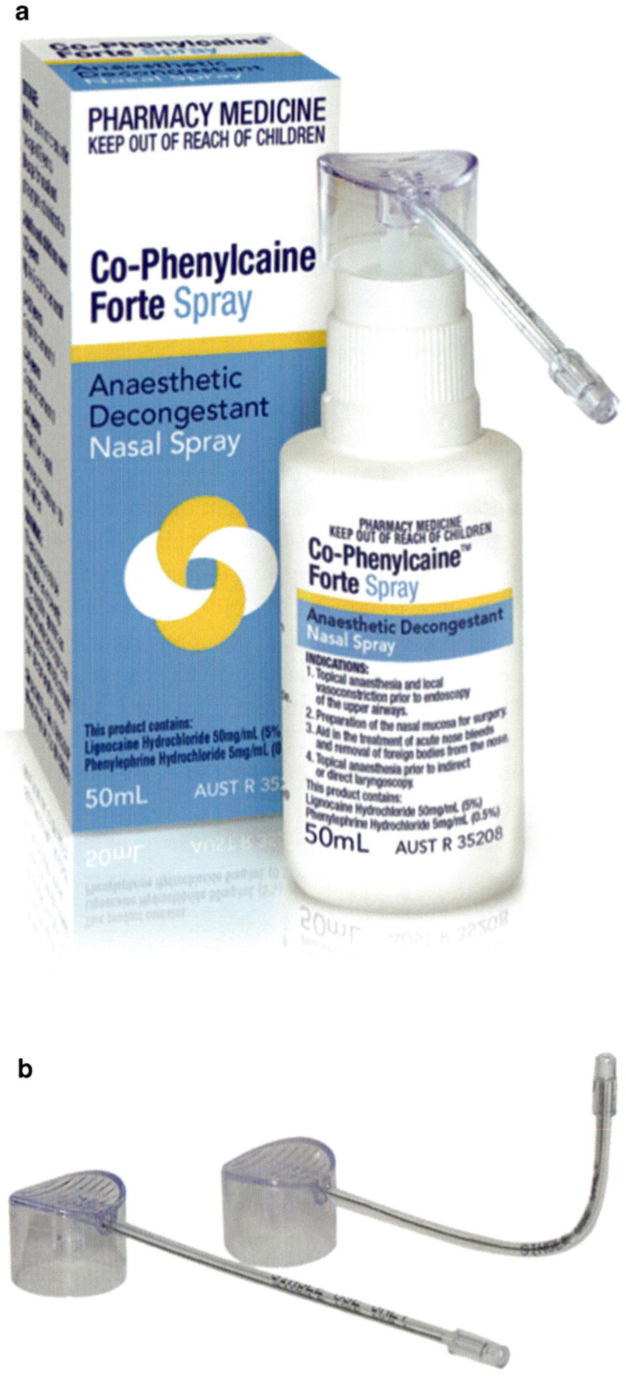

Fig. 45.3 (a) Commercially available Cophenylcaine Forte ™ (ENT Technologies, Melbourne, Australia) is a combination spray containing a vasoconstrictor agent (phenylephrine hydrochloride) and an anesthetic agent (lignocaine hydrochloride). (b) Using a flexible extended nozzle, this agent can adequately decongest and anesthetize the nose

Basic Nasal Endoscopy

The patient should be positioned comfortably in an upright position with the head supported by a firm headrest. Ideally, the neck should be in the neutral position with minimal flexion or extension. Figure 45.3 demonstrates the typical office setup and equipment needed to perform rigid nasal endoscopy. For adults a 3-mm or 4-mm 0° or 30° rigid endoscope is typically well tolerated, while in younger children, a 2.7-mm endoscope may be preferred to navigate the smaller nasal cavity. The scope lens is first prepared with a thin layer of antifog solution to prevent the warm expired nasal air clouding the field of vision. Although commercially available preparations are available, cetrimide solution typically works just as well. Endoscopy should then be performed in a structured systematic fashion. The endoscope is introduced into the nasal cavity and anchored at the apex of the nostril superiorly to add stability to the procedure. Contact with the nasal mucosa should be avoided at all times. Employing a three-pass technique, the first pass is made along the nasal floor to visualize the inferior meatus as well as the postnasal space. The second pass is then made between the inferior and middle turbinates to visualize the middle meatus. Edema, purulence, and polypoid disease should be looked for as possible markers of concomitant sinus disease. If present, then further imaging should be organized typically comprising of a fine-cut computerized tomography of the paranasal sinuses. Close inspection of the shape and size of the middle turbinate will also be performed during this pass to exclude a concha bullosa or paradoxically curved middle turbinate that may need to also be dealt with at the time of DCR surgery to improve access. The third pass should then be performed to visualize the olfactory cleft and swept superiorly to visualize the axilla of the middle turbinate. This will not only allow visualization of any polyps within the sphenoethmoidal recess but will also allow the surgeon to assess whether the patient has a septal deviation that may preclude access to the lateral nasal wall during surgery. If the axilla cannot be visualized completely or the access is deemed too narrow for an obstructed endoscopic DCR, then the patient should be counseled preoperatively of the highly likelihood of also requiring a septoplasty as part of their lacrimal procedure. Having identified all of the anatomical variations on preoperative endoscopy, a clear surgical plan can be conveyed to the patient and an appropriate informed consent obtained.

Surgery

Patient Positioning

Proper patient positioning is critical to the safety of the patient, the surgical field attainable, and the ergonomics of surgery. The surgery is often performed with the surgeon seated on the right of the patient. The operating bed is typically reversed to allow the surgeon to have their legs under the bed while in this sitting position. The surgeon's left elbow can be supported on an arm board anchored to the operative bed to increase the stability of the scope held in the non-dominant hand. The patient is positioned supine, with the head in a neutral position and the bed placed in a reverse Trendelenburg position. Head elevation has been shown to reduce the mean arterial pressure in the elevated region by 2 mmHg for every 2.5 mm above cardiac level [1]. Cerebral perfusion studies have also demonstrated that the ideal angle of tilt is between 20° and 30° above the horizontal as this decreases venous congestion without affecting cerebral perfusion [2]. The endoscopic tower is positioned in the surgeon's straight line of sight to increase surgeon comfort and avoid needless rotation of the surgeon's neck. The monitor should be positioned at eye level to minimize extension of the surgeon's neck. Figure 45.4 demonstrates the ideal bed positioning and the operating room setup.

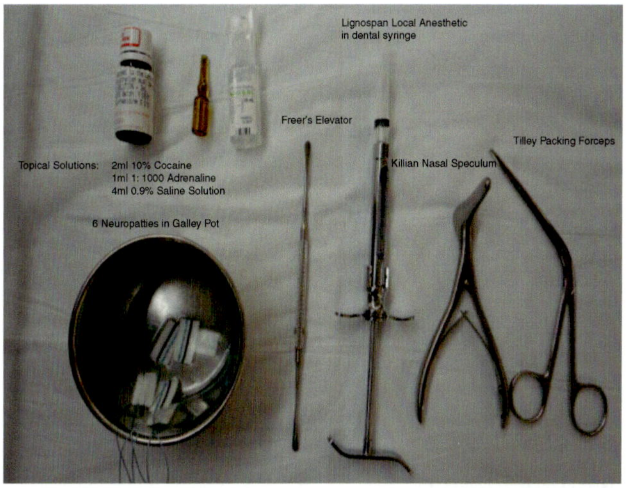

Fig. 45.5 Instruments and solutions required for topicalization of the nasal mucosa prior to performing endoscopic nasal surgery

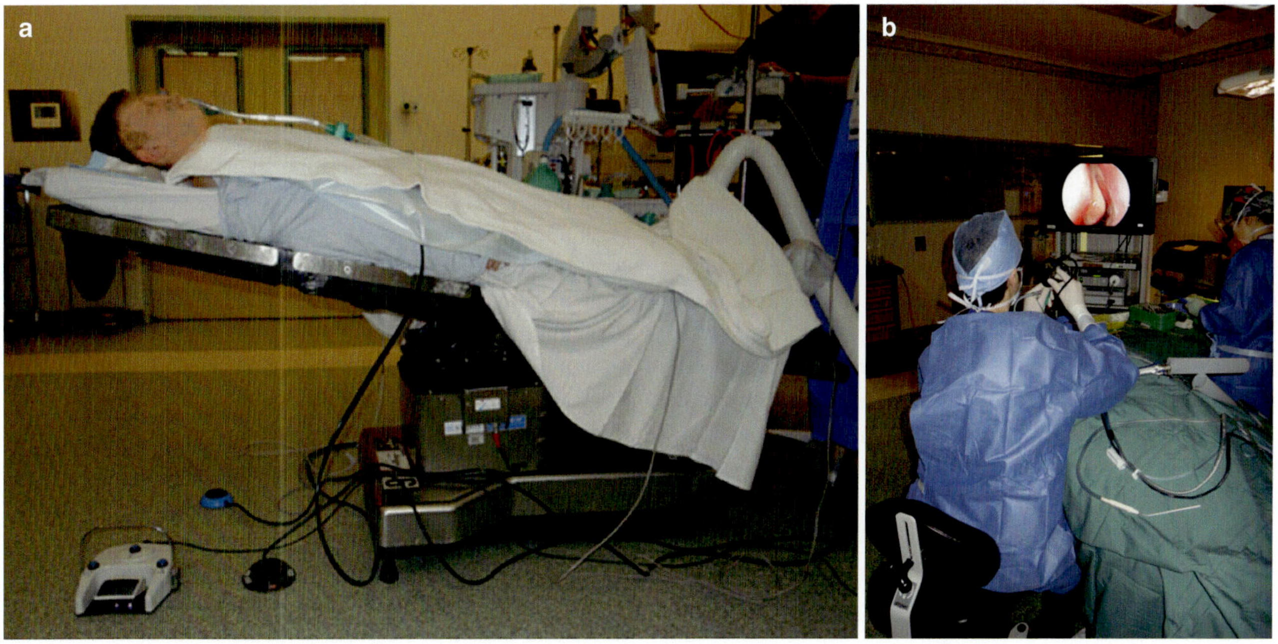

Fig. 45.4 (**a**) Positioning of the patient. The operating bed is reversed to allow the surgeons to sit and placed in a reverse Trendelenburg position to increase venous drainage away from the surgical field. (**b**) The surgeon is seated with his left elbow supported on an arm board. The monitor is placed directly across at eye level for comfort

Table 45.1 Endoscopic DCR instrumentation

Basic endoscopic equipment
0° and 30° 4-mm rigid endoscope
Endo-Scrub 2 lens cleaning sheaths (Medtronic ENT, Jacksonville, Fl, USA)
#15 blade scalpel or monopolar needle-tip Bovie for mucosal incisions
Malleable suction Freer elevator (Medtronic ENT)
Malleable suction curette (Medtronic ENT)
Hajek-Koffler forward-biting punch
Freer dissector
Tilley-Henkel forceps
Variable-sized osteotomes
Endoscopic sinoscopy scissors
DCR instrumentation
Microdebrider instrumentation (Medtronic ENT)
Medtronic Integrated Power Console
M4 or M5 handpiece
25° curved 2.5 mm rough diamond DCR burr
Wormald Dacryocystorhinostomy Set (Medtronic ENT)
Spear knife
Microsickle knife
Lusk MicroBite Forceps
Lacrimal punctal dilator
Bowman lacrimal probes
O'Donoghue lacrimal intubation tubes (Beaver-Visitec International Waltham, MA, USA)

Instrumentation

Table 45.1 summarizes a list of the endoscopic surgical instruments required for endoscopic DCR surgery and adjunctive nasal procedures. Items produced only by a single company also include the manufacturer details. Using a bimanual technique, the surgeon holds the rigid endoscope in his/her left hand, with their elbow firmly positioned on the arm rest. The endoscope is inserted into the nostril retracting the apex of the nasal vestibular skin. Tenting the nostril in this way not only adds further stability to the endoscope but increases the working space for the second surgical instrument held in the dominant hand. The surgeon should consciously avoid any instrument cross by always maintaining the endoscope in a superior position to the operating instrument. Nasal procedures including septoplasty, middle turbinate surgery, and anterior ethmoid surgery will typically require the use of a 0° endoscope, while the majority of the DCR procedure itself is performed with the 30° endoscope given the lateral location of the lacrimal sac on the nasal wall.

Surgical Field

Nasal Preparation

Optimizing the surgical field is critical to the performance of safe and efficient endoscopic endonasal surgery. This commences with the preparation of the nasal mucosa. After induction of general anesthetic, the surgeon injects 1–2 ml of 2% lidocaine with 1:100,000 epinephrine into the region of the axilla of the middle turbinate and the adjoining lateral nasal wall. Injection continues until blanching of the mucosa is seen. The use of prefilled anesthetic syringes can eliminate the inadvertent injection of higher concentrations of epinephrine. This injection can be performed with the use of a headlight or under direct endoscopic visualization if access is difficult. If a septoplasty or middle turbinate surgery is to be performed for surgical access, the surgeon should also inject the caudal septal mucosa and head of the middle turbinate, respectively, at the site of the likely incisions. For DCR surgery the lateral nasal wall is injected around the insertion of the middle turbinate. To ensure adequate topicalization of the entire nasal mucosa, the surgeon then places three ½ inch × 1 inch cottonoid pledgets soaked in a mixture of 2 ml of 10% cocaine solution, 1 ml of 1:100,000 epinephrine, and 4 ml normal saline into each nasal cavity. If there is a contraindication to cocaine or difficulty in obtaining cocaine solution, 1:100,000 units of epinephrine can be used alone. For endoscopic lacrimal surgery, we typically recommend placing one pledget along the septal mucosa, one into the middle meatus between the middle turbinate and lateral nasal wall, and one along the lateral nasal wall overlying the axilla. Any solution leftover from the initial mixture is handed over to the scrub nurse for later use if required.

Anesthetic

The manner in which general anesthesia is induced and maintained is critical in the surgical field. Ideally for nasal surgery, a laryngeal mask airway (LMA) is preferred over endotracheal intubation. It is associated with less respiratory and cardiovascular reflex responses due to reduced stimulation of the larynx as compared to endotracheal intubation. Moreover, LMA facilitates controlled hypotension, allows for a lighter depth of anesthesia, and is associated with less coughing and strain upon emergence. The use of a small throat pack above the mask can minimize the risk of any contamination of the upper airway by blood during the case [3]. Total intravenous anesthesia (TIVA) utilizing propofol and an opioid such as remifentanil has been shown to be an effective way of delivering controlled hypotensive general anesthetic. TIVA avoids the use of inhalational agents that typically cause end arteriolar vasodilation and may increase surgical bleeding.

Ideally, if not medically contraindicated, pulse rate should be maintained between 60 and 70 beats per minute to increase venous return by increasing end-diastolic filling time, and mean arterial blood pressure should be maintained around 65–70 mmHg to avoid organ and cerebral hypoperfusion [4].

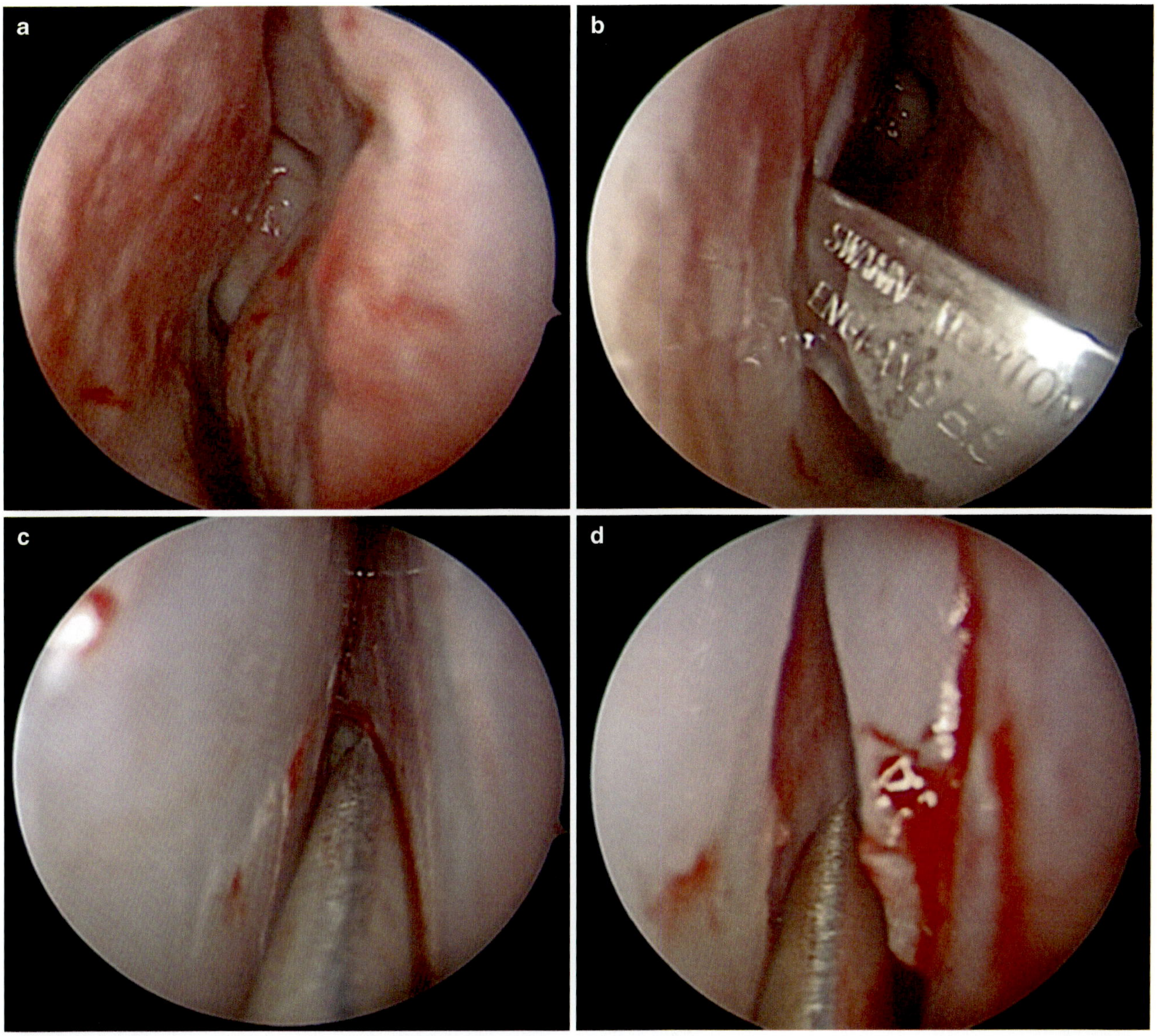

Fig. 45.6 The steps of an endoscopic septoplasty performed through the left nostril. (**a**) Demonstrates how the high deviation of the septum prevents visualization and access to the axilla of the middle turbinate. (**b**) Killian incision with a #15 blade scalpel at the mucocutaneous junction. (**c**) Identification of the submucoperichondrial plane using the sharp end of a malleable suction curette. (**d**) Raising of the submucoperichondrial mucosa flap with the suction freer instrument. Note the pearly white appearance of the underlying cartilage. The cartilage is transected just anterior to the deviation. (**e**) Raising of a contralateral submucoperichondrial mucosal flap with isolation of the cartilage and bone centrally. (**f**) Superior "safety" cut with the turbinectomy scissors to prevent injury of the skull base on removal of the ethmoid bone. (**g**) Removal of the cartilage using a grasping instrument. (**h**) Suction freer demonstrating the residual soft tissue of the septal mucosa that can now be easily retracted to allow visualization of the axilla of the middle turbinate and direct access to the frontal process of the maxilla for DCR surgery

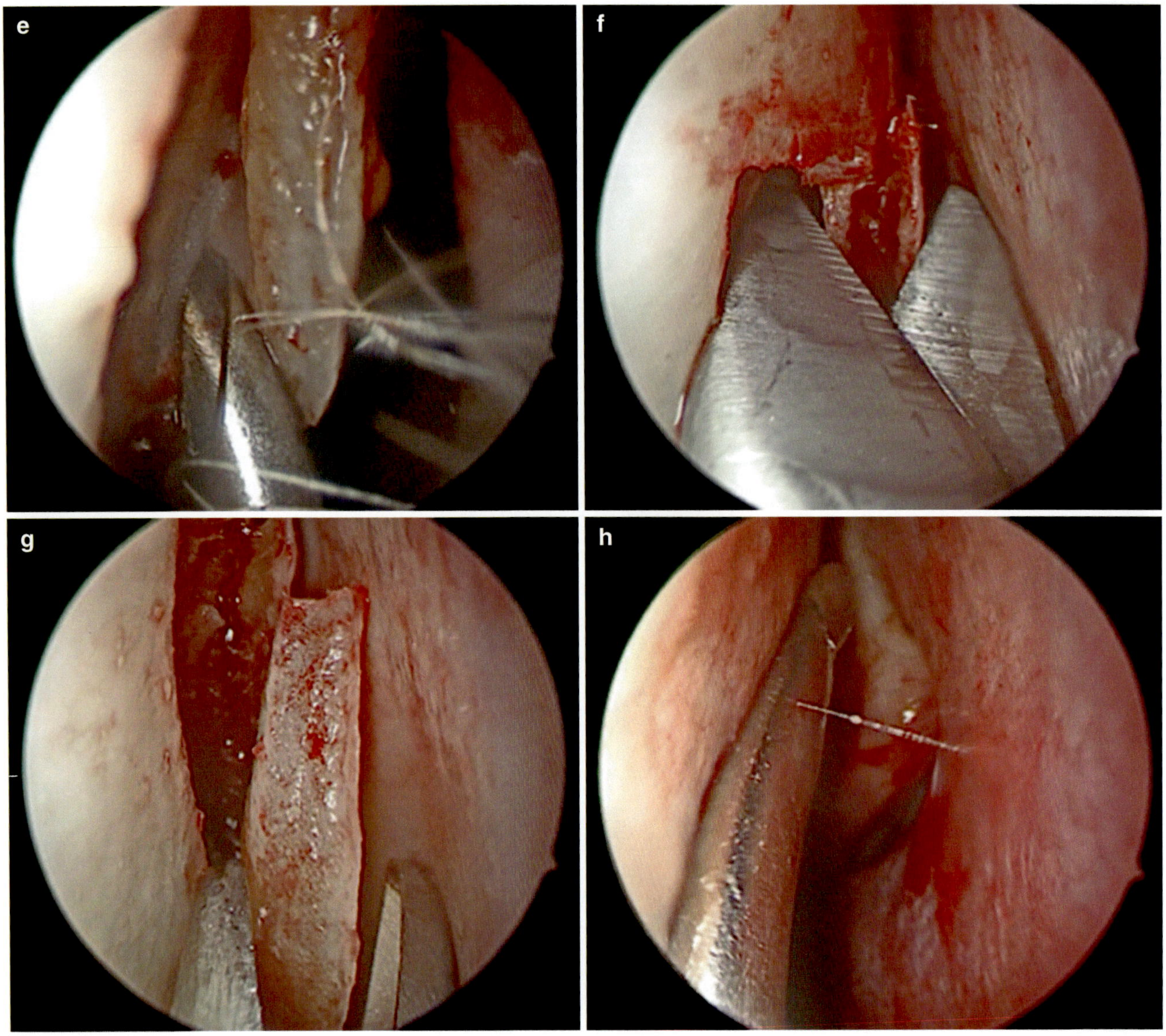

Fig. 45.6 (continued)

Surgical Technique: Adjunctive Nasal Procedures

A recent review by our department revealed that additional adjunctive procedures are required in approximately half of the patients undergoing endoscopic DCR [5]. These procedures range from those aimed at improving access to the lateral nasal wall such as septoplasty and middle turbinoplasty (or turbinectomy), as well as for performing functional endoscopic sinus surgery (FESS) for concomitant sinus disease. The next section describes in detail the surgical steps involved in performing an endoscopic septoplasty and concha bullosa reduction. Oculoplastic surgeons wishing to perform endoscopic lacrimal surgery should be skilled in these two procedures.

Endoscopic Septoplasty

Exposure and access are the two primary indications for performing a septoplasty during endonasal lacrimal surgery. Deviations precluding complete visualization of the axilla of middle turbinate should be addressed. By performing a septoplasty, early, inadvertent trauma to the septal mucosa can be avoided. This further reduces the risk of synechiae formation that may compromise success rates. Before performing this procedure, the operating surgeon should be familiar with the anatomy of the septum and important regions that must be respected to avoid compromising structural support.

The septum is composed of cartilage anteriorly and bone posteriorly. The cartilaginous component is formed by the quadrilateral cartilage that articulates posteriorly with the perpendicular plate of the ethmoid, inferiorly with the maxillary crest, posterosuperiorly with the nasal bones, and posteroinferiorly with the vomer. It is lined by the mucosa that firmly attaches to the cartilage by a mucoperichondrial layer and the bone by a mucoperiosteal layer. These layers are not continuous but rather fuse inferiorly to insert into the septum as decussating fibers. When performing a septoplasty, at least 1.5 cm of dorsal and caudal cartilage must be preserved in order to preserve its support and structure. Violation of this can compromise function as well as lead to cosmetic abnormalities such as saddling of the nasal dorsum or ptosis of the nasal tip.

Septoplasty was traditionally performed using a headlight and nasal speculum. The performance of this procedure with an endoscope confers many advantages including improved magnification and illumination. Irrespective of the technique employed, the principles of surgery remain the same. The procedure commences with the mucosal incision. Broad anterior deviations are best addressed through a hemitransfixion incision, while more posterior deflections can be addressed through a Killian incision, placed just beyond where the septum starts. The advantage of the Killian incision is that it can be performed with the endoscope, while the hemitransfixion incision still requires the use of a headlight and nasal speculum at the beginning of the procedure. The Killian incision is placed at the mucocutaneous junction and is typically performed with a #15 blade scalpel. It should be broad based extending from the dorsum of the nose, inferiorly onto the maxillary crest. Curving the incision posteriorly at its most inferior extent may prevent the septal mucosal flap from tearing during the procedure. The depth of the incision should traverse all the soft tissue layers of the mucosa down to the cartilage to facilitate early identification of the submucoperichondrial plane. Identification of this plane is critical to the entire procedure, as dissecting beneath it yields an avascular surgical plane and maximizes flap vascularity and strength [6]. Given its adherence to the cartilage, this plane can be difficult to identify and raise. The use of a sharp instrument such as the sharp end of a freer dissector, a suction curette, sharp-tapered iris scissors, or the back of the #15 blade can help identify the cartilaginous surface. This surface typically is pearly white with a blue tinge when viewed under the endoscope and feels slightly less smooth than the mucoperichondrium. Once identified, the flap is further raised to allow the endoscope to be inserted. The surgeon can then proceed to raise the entire submucoperichondrial plane in a sweeping motion from superior to inferior using a suction freer instrument. The tip of the freer should always be angled toward the septum and kept in close contact with the septum to avoid causing inadvertent perforation of the mucosal flap. The flap should be raised beyond the deviation and beyond the osseocartilaginous fusion of the quadrilateral cartilage with the ethmoid plate.

Once ipsilateral dissection has been performed, the cartilage is then transected carefully using a freer to allow a contralateral mucosal flap to be elevated. This cartilaginous incision is placed anterior the deviation and should not extend higher than 1.5 cm beneath the dorsal edge of the septum. In this way the dorsal support of the septum will be maintained, and the risk of "saddling" will be minimized. Once the transection incision has been carried through the cartilage, the freer will enter the submucoperichondrial plane on the contralateral side, and the contralateral mucosa can then be elevated off the cartilage and ethmoid bone in the same fashion. This will isolate the cartilage/bone from the mucosa bilaterally and allow it to be resected without injuring the mucosa.

Prior to removing the cartilage/bone, a superior cut should be performed parallel, but inferior to, the dorsum using an endoscopic scissor. This will safeguard against inadvertently fracturing the skull base at the insertion of the ethmoid plate when the ethmoid bone is removed. The deviated cartilage/bone can then be removed using a grasping instrument such as Irwin-Moore or Tilley-Henkel forceps. Following removal of the deviation, the bilateral mucosal flaps can then be reposited back down. If completely intact, a unilateral drainage hole placed as posteriorly as possible in a dependent position should be created to allow drainage of blood from the surgical site and prevent a septal hematoma. The two flaps can then be approximated using a quilting stitch with a dissolvable suture such as a 4-0 polyglactin (Vicryl). The anterior incision site can be incorporated into this closure or closed separately. The purpose of the quilting stitch is to remove as much "dead space" as possible and allow the two mucosal flaps to closely adhere to each other.

Complications

All patients undergoing septoplasty should be consented prior to surgery regarding the possible complications. Complications include bleeding, infection, septal hematoma or abscess formation, septal perforation, cosmetic complications, loss of structural support, tip ptosis, paresthesia of the upper teeth, and cerebrospinal fluid leak. The rate of perforation varies considerably between studies. Older studies employing more extensive submucosal resection of the septal cartilage quote up to 25%, whereas modern septoplasty techniques aimed at conserving as much cartilage as possible report lower rates, closer to 5%. The risk of perforation can be minimized by meticulous surgical technique, dissecting beneath the submucoperichondrial/submucoperiosteal plane and ensuring that at least one mucosal flap remains completely intact during the procedure.

Concha Bullosa Reduction

Pneumatization of the middle turbinate is not an uncommon occurrence. The reported incidence of concha bullosa ranges anywhere between 14% and 53% with the variation in incidence reflective of differing anatomical definitions [7]. Although most commonly occurring unilaterally, bilateral pneumatization can be present in up to 20% of patients [8]. Although considered a normal anatomical variant, concha bullosa appears significantly associated with a contralateral septal deviation and may require reduction if particularly large or if it interferes with endoscopic access during a DCR (Fig. 45.7). A recent study by Ali et al. reported the necessity for a concurrent middle turbinoplasty in up to 6% of endoscopic DCR cases [5].

Numerous techniques for reducing a middle turbinate concha bullosa have been described. All share a common principle of resection of the lateral aspect or lamella, with preservation of as much of the medial lamella as possible. Excessive manipulation of this medial portion should be avoided at all times given its insertion into the skull base. Our preferred technique is described as follows. Using a #15 blade scalpel, a vertical stab incision is made into the head of the middle turbinate. Using a sawing motion, this incision is extended superiorly and inferiorly. Endoscopic scissors can then be inserted and rotated 90° to further distract the lateral and medial lamellae. The surgeon can then use the scissors or knife to continue the incision posteriorly along the inferior and superior margins of the middle turbinate to their lateral insertion. Once removed, the straight microdebrider can be used in forward high-speed motion to tidy up the mucosa edges, ensuring preservation of the anteromedial mucosa (Fig. 45.8).

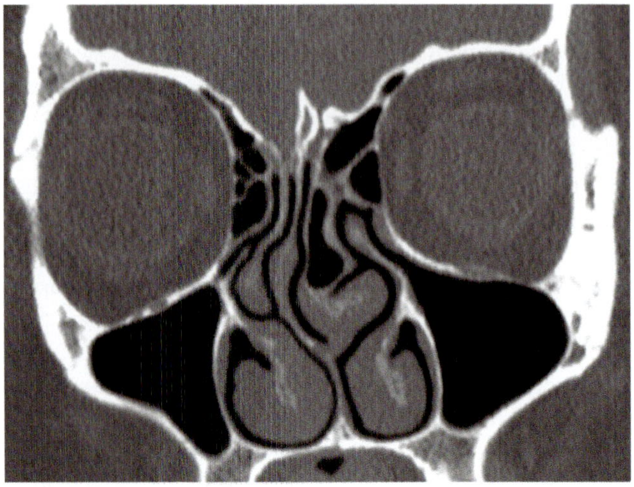

Fig. 45.7 Coronal CT of the sinuses showing pneumatization of the left middle turbinate (concha bullosa) with a corresponding deviation of the nasal septum to the right

After reducing a concha bullosa, destabilization of the middle turbinate may occur. If this occurs and there is any risk of lateralization, the remaining middle turbinate should be sutured with a 4-0 polyglactin (Vicryl) suture to the septum. This will minimize the risk of a postoperative adhesion to the lateral nasal wall that may interfere with the drainage of the ostiomeatal unit.

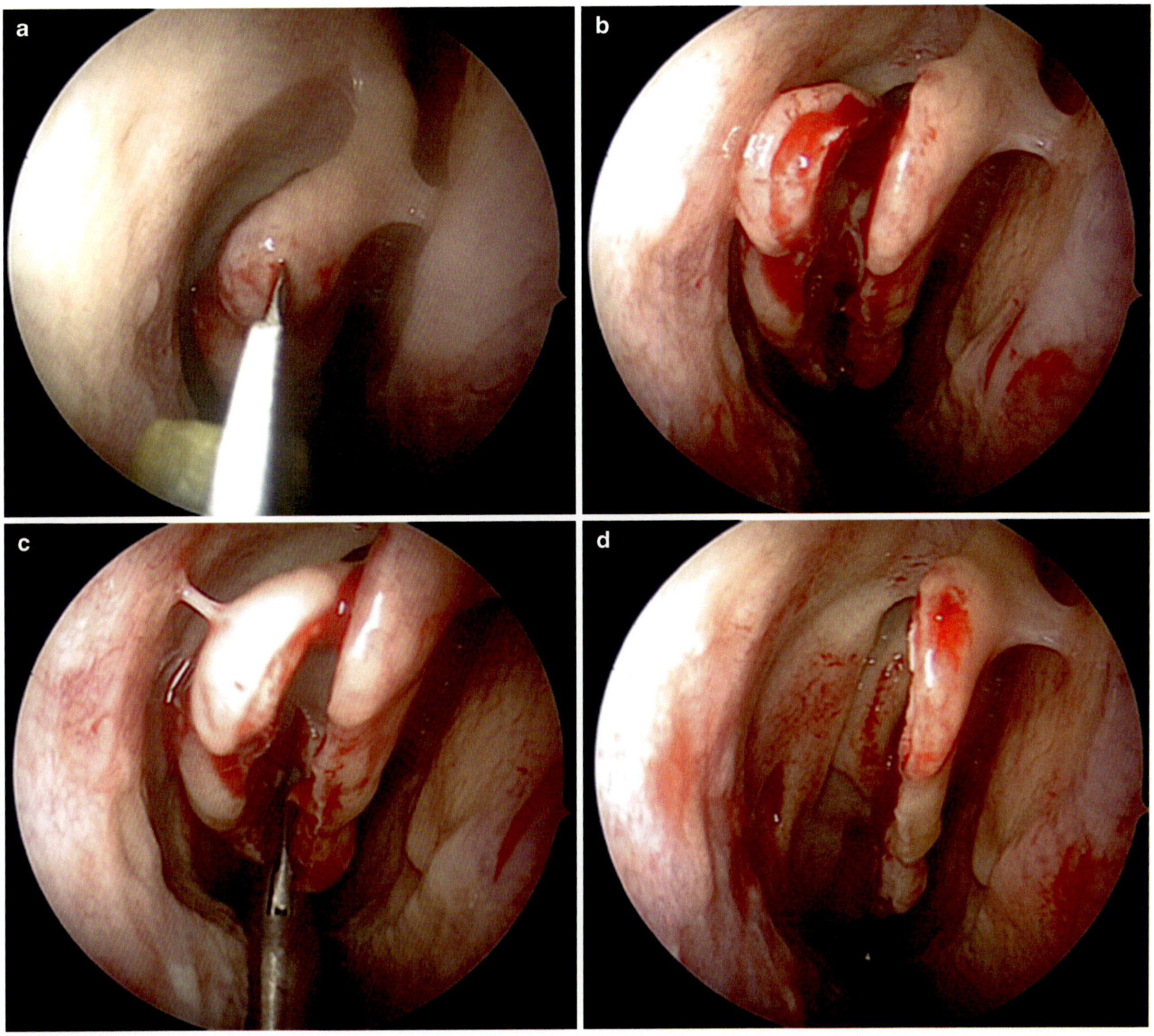

Fig. 45.8 Resection of concha bullosa. (**a**) Stab incision is made in the head of the middle turbinate with a #15 blade scalpel. (**b**) Incision is extended superior and inferiorly to distract the two leaflets of the middle turbinate. (**c**) Endoscopic scissors are used to complete the cut posteriorly. (**d**) Completion of the concha bullosa resection. The medial leaflet is preserved and access to the lateral nasal wall increased

References

1. Simpson P. Perioperative blood loss and its reduction: the role of the anesthetist. Br J Anesth. 1992;69:498–507.
2. Palazon JH, Asensi PD, Lopez SB, Bautista FP, Candel AG. Effect of head elevation on intracranial pressure, cerebral perfusion pressure, and regional cerebral oxygen saturation in patients with cerebral hemorrhage. Revista espanola de anestesiologia y reanimacion. 2008;55:289–93.
3. Atef A, Fawaz A. Comparison of laryngeal mask with endotracheal tube for anesthesia in endoscopic sinus surgery. Am J Rhinol. 2008;22:653–7.
4. Ha TN, van Renen RG, Ludbrook GL, Valentine R, Ou J, Wormald PJ. The relationship between hypotension, cerebral flow, and the surgical field during endoscopic sinus surgery. Laryngoscope. 2014;124:2224–30.
5. Ali MJ, Psaltis AJ, Wormald PJ. The frequency of concomitant adjunctive nasal procedures in powered endoscopic dacryocystorhinostomy. Orbit. 2015;34:142–5.
6. Kim DW, Egan KK, O'Grady K, Toriumi DM. Biomechanical strength of human nasal septal lining: comparison of the constituent layers. Laryngoscope. 2005;115:1451–3.
7. Lloyd GA. CT of the paranasal sinuses: study of a control series in relation to endoscopic sinus surgery. J Laryngol Otol. 1990;104:477–81.
8. Stallman JS, Lobo JN, Som PM. The incidence of concha bullosa and its relationship to nasal septal deviation and paranasal sinus disease. AJNR Am J Neuroradiol. 2004;25:1613–8.

Transcanalicular Laser-Assisted Dacryocystorhinostomy

46

Pelin Kaynak

Introduction

Epiphora, due to primary and secondary nasolacrimal duct obstructions (NLDO), is generally managed by dacryocystorhinostomy (DCR) techniques aiming to reconstruct the lacrimal drainage system. The obstructed outflow pathway is redirected by connecting the lacrimal sac to the middle nasal cavity to relieve symptoms. External dacryocystorhinostomy (EX-DCR) is the standard surgical technique for the treatment of NLDO, described first by Toti in 1904 [1]. Dupuy-Dutemps and Bourguet modified it in 1921 with the introduction of the anastomosis of the lacrimal sac and nasal mucosal linings [2]. Despite the published high success rates of EX-DCR exceeding 90% [3–5], the search for a scarless DCR technique that can be performed quickly and with high success rates has continued [6–12].

Development of high-resolution fiber-optic endoscopes and fine endonasal surgical tools in the late 1980s intensified the interest in endoscopic management of lacrimal obstructions, where laser energy could be used to rapidly create a precise and bloodless rhinostomy opening during a scarless technique [13, 14]. Laser energy can be delivered either nasally, as in endonasal laser-assisted DCR (ENL-DCR), or via a probe passed through the canaliculus, referred to as transcanalicular laser-assisted DCR (TCL-DCR). Both techniques allow the surgeon to create the alternative route for lacrimal drainage; however, TCL-DCR is likely safer than ENL-DCR, as the laser beam is directed toward the nose and away from the orbit. In Fig. 46.1a, TCL-DCR is schematically presented.

Endoscopic DCR procedures avoid the external scar as well but necessitate additional surgical equipment and visualization systems. Laser delivery systems facilitate the precise removal of bone and soft tissues and minimize bleeding while creating the rhinostomy during endoscopic lacrimal techniques. However, the cost and maintenance of these devices are high. Laser safety measures also deserve maximum attention in surgical rooms.

Historical Perspective

Jack published the first transcanalicular DCR in 1963 [15]. In 1992, Levin and Silkiss studied laser endocanalicular DCRs on cadavers [16, 17], while Christenbury performed the first TCL-DCR with argon laser assistance on patients with NLDO [18]. Various laser wavelengths have been utilized to create the rhinostomy in lacrimal surgery, such as neodymium:YAG (Nd:YAG) laser [19–24], holmium:yttrium-aluminum-garnet (Ho:YAG) laser [25–27], potassium-tytanyl-phosphate (KTP) laser [28, 29], and erbium:YAG (Er:YAG) laser [30].

The use of solid-state diode laser for lacrimal surgery was first reported in 1994 by Mchugh, and an interventional case series of TCL-DCR with high success was reported by Eloy in 2000 [31, 32]. The diode laser subsequently gained popularity among other laser delivery devices, possibly due to relatively lower costs of buying and maintenance. TCL-DCR continues to remain the subject of many ongoing studies [26, 32–39].

Management of Epiphora via TCL-DCR

Transcanalicular laser-assisted DCR is performed with the assistance of nasal endoscopy to visualize the aiming beam and laser probe in the middle meatus during lacrimal surgery. The laser delivers focal energy to open the rhinostomy site, for the management of NLDO as explained below. The major advantages of TCL-DCR are briefly listed in Table 46.1.

P. Kaynak (✉)
Rufus Eye Microsurgical Center, Ophthalmic Plastic and Reconstructive Surgery Division, Istanbul, Turkey

A. J. Cohen, C. N. Burkat (eds.), *Oculofacial, Orbital, and Lacrimal Surgery*, https://doi.org/10.1007/978-3-030-14092-2_46

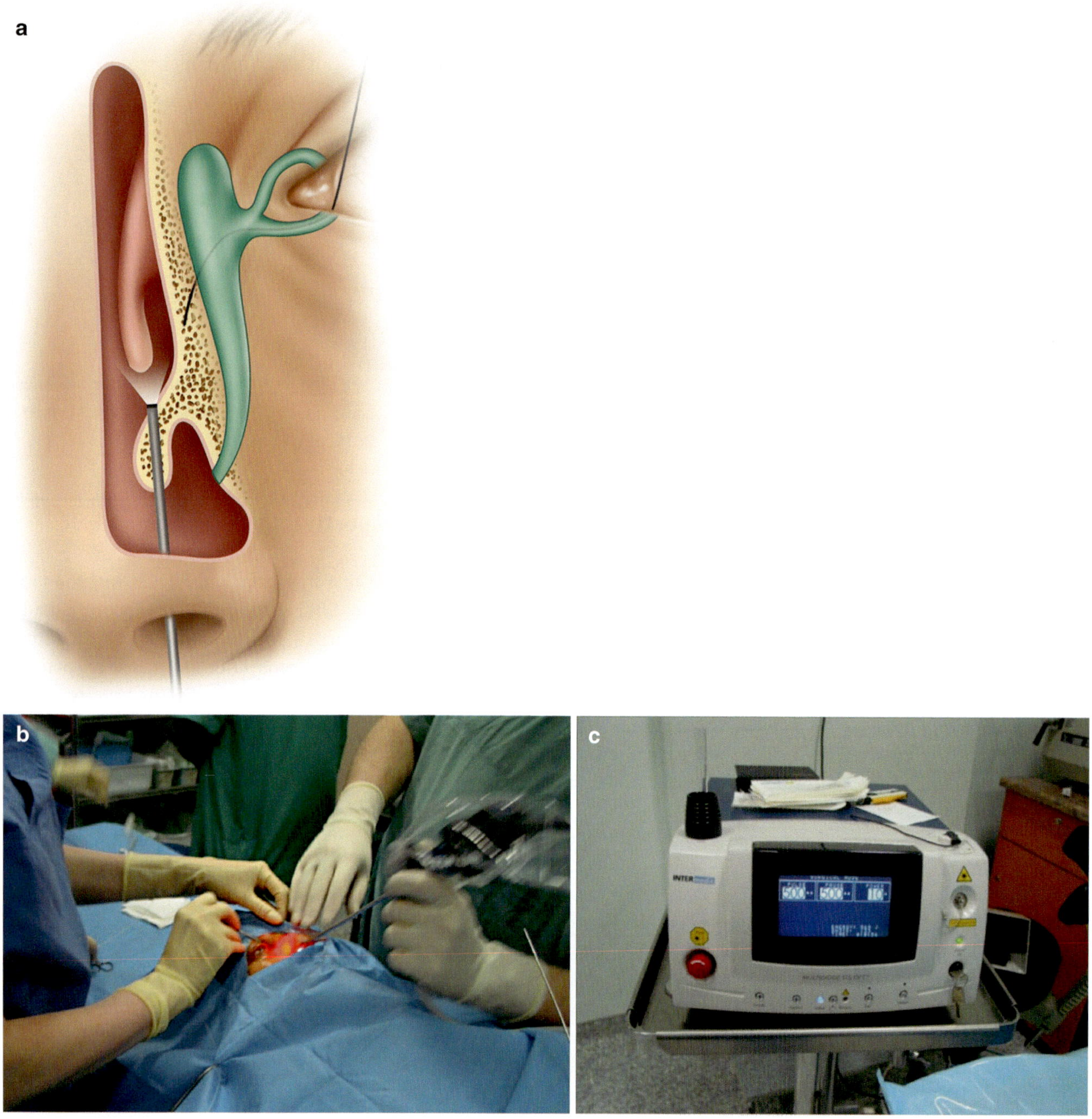

Fig. 46.1 (**a**) Schematic illustration of the transcanalicular laser DCR. The laser fiber-optic probe is introduced through the inferior punctum and canaliculus until a hard bony stop is felt. The aiming beam is turned on and visualized transmucosally in the nasal cavity with the endoscope, typically at the level anterior to the middle turbinate. (**b**) Performing TCL-DCR surgery with the Multidiode S30 OFT (INTERMEDIC Inc., Spain). (**c**) Multidiode S30 OFT (INTERMEDIC Inc., Spain)

Table 46.1 Advantages of transcanalicular laser-assisted dacryocystorhinostomy (TCL-DCR)

Avoids a facial scar
Minimal trauma to medial canthal structures
Less bleeding, particularly useful in patients on anticoagulation
Faster intraoperative time
Shorter recovery time

Diagnostic Evaluation and Patient Selection for TCL-DCR

Patients with nasolacrimal drainage system obstructions typically present to clinic with epiphora and/or dacryocystitis. A large tear lake with mucoid or purulent discharge is a common sign of nasolacrimal duct obstruction. All patients with a history of tearing and/or dacryocystitis must be evaluated via a clinical work-up and ophthalmic examination to rule out other causes of epiphora, such as blepharitis, conjunctivitis, keratitis, eyelid malpositions or laxity, and orbicularis oculi muscle weakness. The lacrimal sac area should be palpated for a mass and/or copious mucopurulent reflux, indicating a dacryocele (dacryocystocele). If a dacryocele is evident, it would be anticipated that the enlarged lacrimal sac flaps would need to be trimmed down for a successful DCR. Therefore, such patients may not be appropriate candidates for minimally invasive techniques, or the sac flaps would require adequate shortening transnasally during the endoscopic surgery.

The puncta and lacrimal canaliculi must be evaluated if canaliculitis is suspected. Definitive treatment of this condition typically requires canaliculotomy for drainage and curettage.

When considering the transcanalicular approach, office lacrimal irrigation to evaluate its patency and to determine the level of any obstruction in the proximal drainage system is mandatory.

Nasal cavity examination by the surgeon may identify intranasal pathologies such as hypertrophic or bullous middle turbinate, nasal polyps, and septal deviation. In patients with narrow nasal cavities, endoscopic surgery may be more challenging to perform.

A ^{99m}Tc-DTPA (diethylenetriaminepentaacetic acid) dacryoscintigraphy scan can be considered for patients with a history of tearing despite patent lacrimal irrigation, as this may detect functional epiphora in addition to a prolonged dye disappearance test. In contrast, dacryocystography (DCG) can be helpful to diagnose an anatomic etiology for outflow obstruction, such as a filling defect from a lacrimal sac mass, foreign bodies, or dacryolith. Dilated or undersized fibrotic sacs can be detected by DCG and be helpful in the differential diagnosis.

Punctal and/or canalicular stenosis, history of nasal and/or lacrimal surgery, naso-orbital trauma, congenital nasolacrimal duct occlusion, and previous transconjunctival blepharoplasty are important risk factors to elicit before TCL-DCR.

In some instances, TCL-DCR may not be easily performed in patients with prominent frontal processes and wide dorsum nasi, as the manipulation of the laser probe is limited. The use of pediatric TCL-DCR surgery is controversial due to the risk of significant fibrosis caused by heat convection. Table 46.2 summarizes the contraindications for TCL-DCR.

Table 46.2 Contraindications for transcanalicular laser-assisted dacryocystorhinostomy (TCL-DCR)

Suspected lacrimal system and midfacial neoplasms
Proximal lacrimal drainage apparatus pathology
Nasal pathologies that limit visualization
Suspected dacryolithiasis or intrasaccal foreign body
Granulomatous diseases
Collagen tissue disorders
Acute dacryocystitis[a] and lacrimal sac abscess[a]
Large dacryoceles[a]
Lacrimal fistulae[a]
Children[a]
Previous lacrimal surgery of unknown indication[a]
Accidental and/or surgical trauma to midface and orbital bony structures[a]
Allergic and/or atrophic rhinitis[a]

[a]Denotes relative contraindications for TCL-DCR

Surgery

TCL-DCR surgery with diode laser assistance has become increasingly popular worldwide (Fig. 46.1a–c). This technique can be performed under local anesthesia, with or without sedation, or under general anesthesia.

Preoperative Preparation Premedication to aid in hemostasis and analgesia is performed with 0.05% xylometazoline +1% lidocaine nasal spray and nasal cavity packing using absorbent sponges soaked in xylometazoline 0.05% with 1:200,000 epinephrine. The uncinate process mucosa and medial canthal area are infiltrated with approximately 1–4 ml of 1:1 volume 1% lidocaine HCl with 0.0125 mg/ml adrenaline and 0.05% bupivacaine HCl. An acrylic corneal protector is placed to protect cornea. Laser safety rules must be strictly applied to prevent operating room hazards and patient or staff injuries.

Surgical Steps

Surgery is performed with a clean setup and sterile draping. The 980 nanometer (nm) wavelength diode laser is delivered via a silica-silica polyamide laser fiber optic. The Multidiode S30 OFT laser delivery device (INTERMEDIC Inc., Spain), equipped with a 600 μm silica-silica polyamide laser fiber optic is displayed in Fig. 46.1c.

The preferred total caliper of the probe with the sleeve is between 300 and 600 microns. Laser settings are adjusted for each patient, ranging between 8 and 12 W power range, 350–500 milliseconds pulse time, and 350–500 milliseconds pause duration between pulses to use the lowest amount of energy sufficient to create an osteotomy.

The diode laser fiber optic is passed through the canaliculus into the lacrimal sac, until the bright transillumination of the aiming beam can be seen via a nasal endoscope with a 0° or 30° angle (Fig. 46.2a). An anteriorly located ethmoidal cell may prevent direct access to the nasal cavity, or ethmoidal

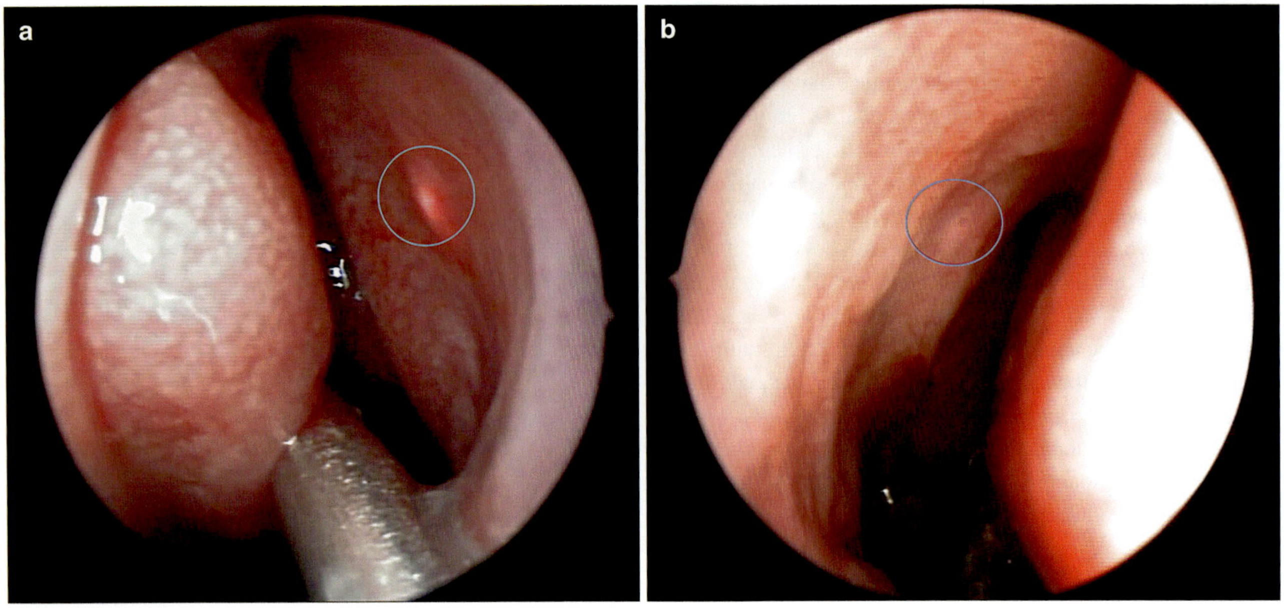

Fig. 46.2 (**a**) Bright transillumination of the aiming beam (in blue circle) is seen when the tip is in the lacrimal sac posterior to the uncinate process. (**b**) The aiming beam (in blue circle) is dull when not in the sac, or there is an intervening ethmoidal air cell between the sac and nasal cavity

cells may be entered instead. The aiming beam is dull in these cases (Fig. 46.2b).

The surgical steps of TCL-DCR are demonstrated in Fig. 46.3a–d. The upper canaliculus is typically the preferred entrance as long as the aiming beam is clearly visible across the middle turbinate. Infracture or medialization of the middle turbinate may be necessary in some cases for better view of the lateral nasal wall (Fig. 46.4). A bullous or large middle concha may be partially resected to debulk its volume to prevent functional blockage of the ostium (Fig. 46.5).

Laser energy is the delivered until the large bony opening is created, at least 5 mm in diameter. The ostium can then be further enlarged with rongeurs through the nasal cavity to decrease the amount of laser energy delivered. A can opener type of laser application (Fig. 46.6) may also decrease the total laser energy. The rhinostomy is opened by the removal of the sac mucosa-lacrimal bone-nasal mucosa button created.

In a patient with a wide dorsum nasi, the frontal process of the maxillary bone is generally thick. In these patients, it should be kept in mind that the total laser energy delivered to open a large enough rhinostomy would be quite high and could cause extensive thermal damage to the neighboring tissues.

It is also recommended to minimize the in-out maneuvers with the laser probe through the canaliculi in order to avoid trauma to the delicate endothelial lining of the proximal drainage system. The debris around the osteotomy is preferably removed transnasally with a Takahashi endo-forceps and backbiting rongeur. Once the carbonized debris (Fig. 46.7) is cleared around the ostium, bicanalicular silicone intubation is performed to facilitate healthy endocanalicular epithelialization.

Adjunctive antifibrotic agents applied during TCL-DCR should be applied precisely to the ostium via an irrigation cannula, followed by copious irrigation of the ocular surface. A dry surgical sponge is placed in the nasal ostium during this procedure to minimize contact of the healthy nasal mucosa from the antifibrotic agent. The lacrimal tract can then be irrigated with 0.2% dexamethasone and 2% gentamycin mixture or 0.9% NaCl solution.

Occasionally, the surgeon may choose to convert to a conventional external DCR with skin approach if an adequately sized bony ostium could not be created via TCL-DCR. The common technical and intraoperative difficulties in performing TCL-DCR are listed in Table 46.3.

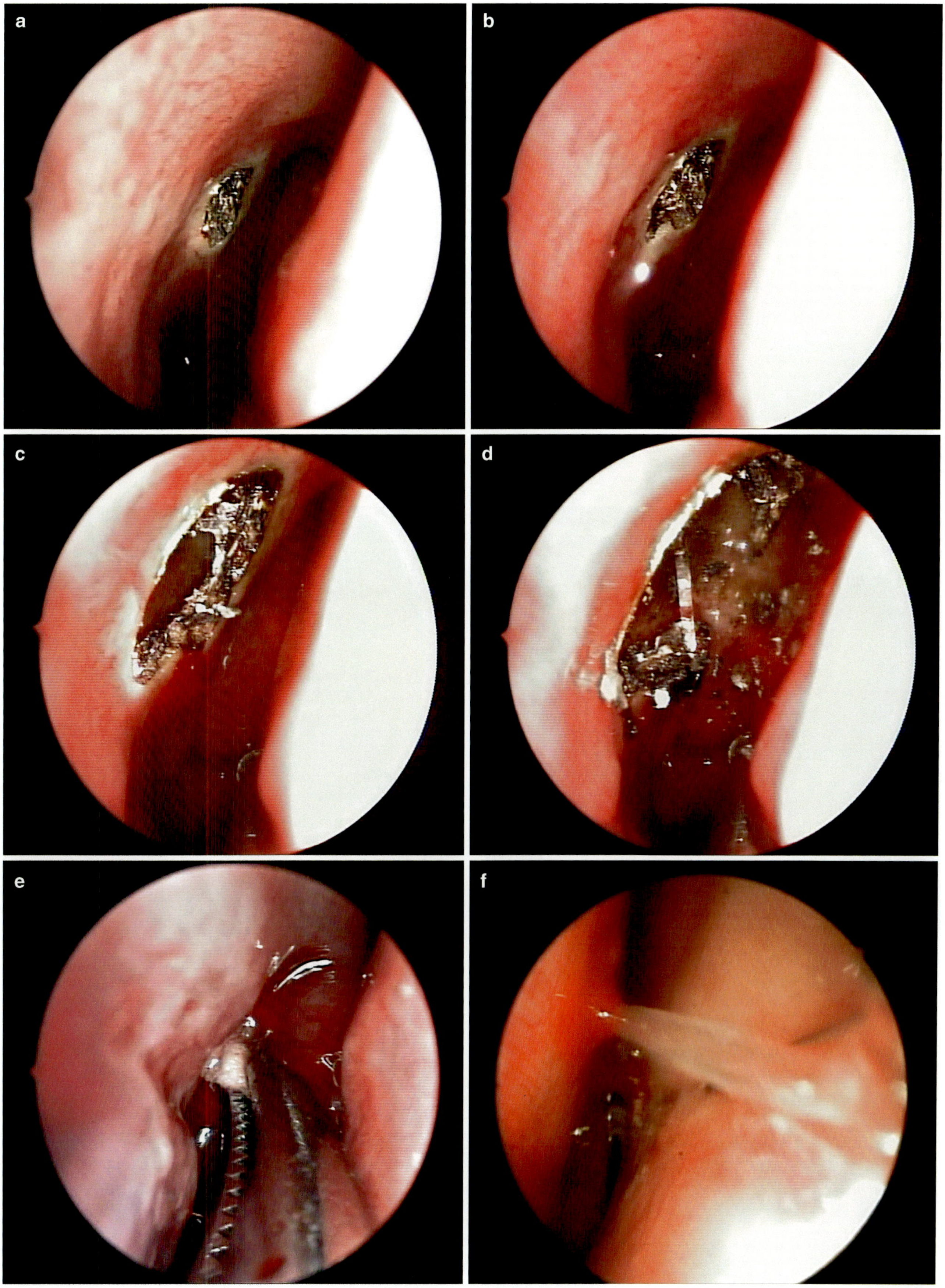

Fig. 46.3 Surgical steps of TCL-DCR: (**a**) rhinostomy, initial opening; (**b**) aiming beam in the lacrimal sac; (**c**) rhinostomy, mid-surgery; (**d**) probe tip in the lacrimal sac entering the nasal cavity next to the middle turbinate; (**e**) antifibrotic agent application to the rhinostomy site; (**f**) rhinostomy site and silicone tube

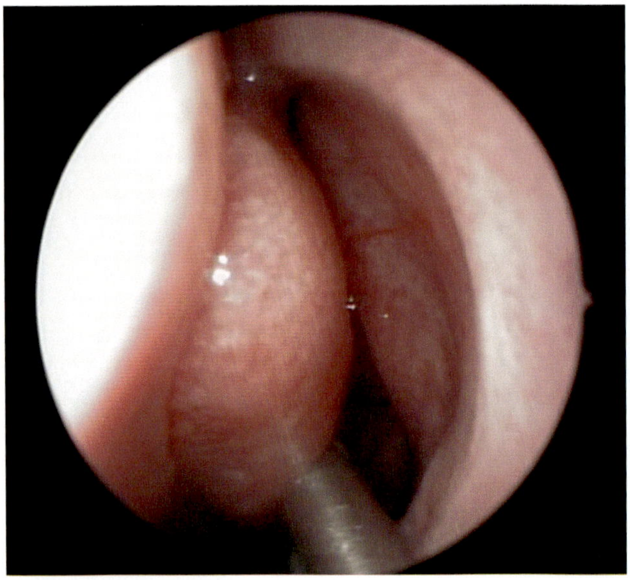

Fig. 46.4 Middle turbinate is medialized

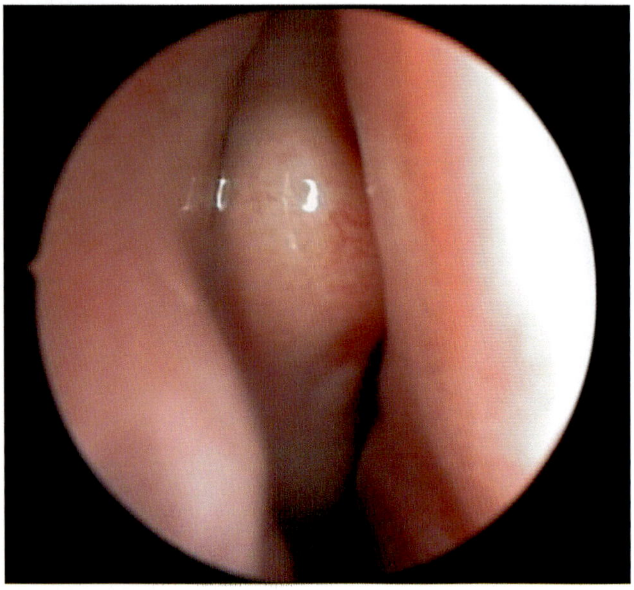

Fig. 46.5 A large bullous concha is seen

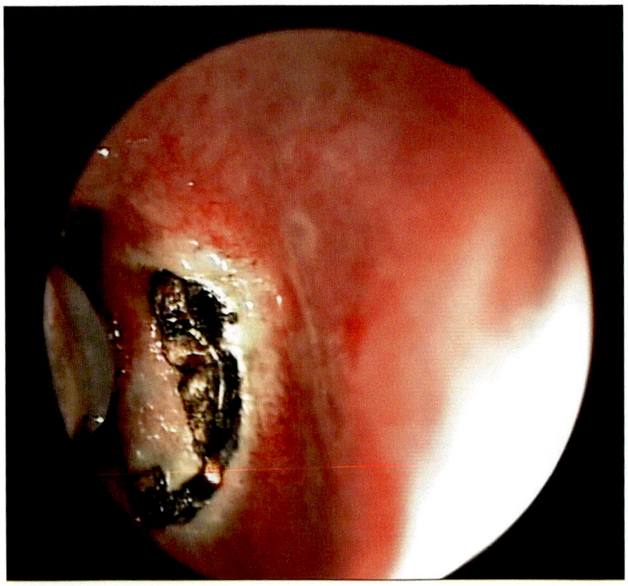

Fig. 46.6 A can opener-type laser application is shown

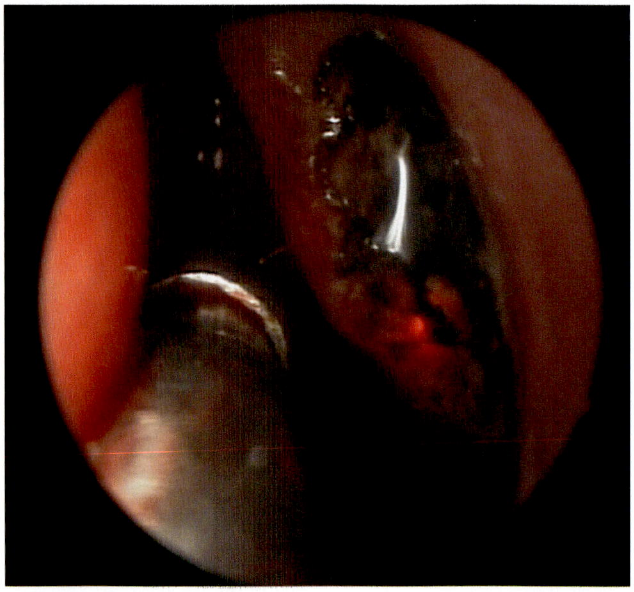

Fig. 46.7 Enlarging the rhinostomy following laser ablation. The carbonized debris is cleared around the ostium

Table 46.3 Difficulties in performing TCL-DCR

Requires additional equipment and tools
Indirect visualization of surgical site
Limited surgical space
Nasal and canalicular pathologies may affect the surgical outcome
Prominent frontal process of maxilla and/or saddle nose may limit probe manipulation

Postoperative Care

After surgery, eye patching for 4 hours with sterile antibiotic and corticosteroid drops is often advised. Although rarely necessary, nasal packing can be removed later that day or the following day if used. Cold compresses used frequently in the first 24 hours after surgery help decrease pain and edema. Topical, and occasionally systemic, antibiotics are prescribed for 1 week. Nasal and ocular steroids and nasal saline spray are continued for 3 weeks postoperatively. Follow-up visits are recommended at postoperative day 1, day 3, week 1, month 1, and every 3 months until the end of the first postoperative year to check for recurrence of symptoms or infection. The ostium is examined, and any debris clogging the ostium removed if still present after the first postoperative week. The patency of the new rhinostomy is assessed by dye disappearance test (DDT), or lacrimal irrigation if the DDT is fluorescein-negative intranasally. Bicanalicular stents are typically removed between 1 and 3 months postoperatively.

Tissue Response to Laser in TCL-DCR

Laser wavelength, laser power and energy, method of application (contact or noncontact), application mode (continuous, burst, or pulsed), and tissue properties play important roles in the tissue response to laser [39]. Several studies have assessed the histological effects of different wavelength lasers on various tissues [40–44]. Scanning electron microscopy studies revealed large coagulation zones underneath the ablated hypertrophic inferior nasal turbinates following Nd:YAG and diode lasers. The coagulation effect was noted to be minimal with CO_2 lasers, whereas the ablative effect of CO_2 was the most precise [45].

In vitro thermal tissue effects induced by contact application of fiber-guided lasers, such as Ho:YAG, Nd:YAG, and diode lasers (830, 940 nm), which are similar to those used for endocanalicular DCR approaches, revealed that the 830 nm diode laser created the widest ablation zones.

Although the 810–980 nm diode laser, operating in wavelengths near the infrared part of the light spectrum, is highly absorbed by melanin and hemoglobin to provide good hemostasis, the coagulative effect of the contact mode was less than the noncontact mode of the 830 nm diode laser and contact mode of the Ho:YAG laser [41, 44].

Histopathologically, inflammation and reepithelialization are delayed when lasers are used, as compared to the steel scalpel, as shown on guinea pig oral mucosa. Complete reepithelialization occurred by the end of the first week with the scalpel, compared to the fourth week with CO_2 laser. Resolution of inflammation was also delayed up to 4 weeks with lasers and bipolar cautery, compared to resolution of inflammation by the second week when using the scalpel [42, 43, 46]. The most extensive coagulation damage with delayed reepithelialization was noted with Nd:YAG applications, and more prominent inflammatory infiltration was seen in Nd:YAG and combined CO2-Nd:YAG wounds compared to CO_2 and non-laser wounds [43, 47].

Briefly, the 2940 nm Er:YAG and 2140 nm Ho:YAG lasers have good bone ablation properties with limited coagulative effects [48]. The 532 nm KTP laser has both good cutting and coagulating properties. The 1064 nm Nd:YAG laser can lead to significant collateral damage in spite of its good ablative effect. Diode lasers in the 830–980 nm wavelength segment have demonstrated both good cutting and coagulating effects with less collateral damage and are more effective in the noncontact mode. Due to these characteristics, combined with its applicability via fiber probes ranging between 0.4 and 1.0 mm and fiber-optic tips that confine the laser energy to the tip, the diode laser has gained popularity in endocanalicular nasolacrimal surgery [49]. Newer compact and more easily operated diode laser delivery systems are also available, which enable the surgeon to mobilize the device if needed (Fig. 46.1c).

However, based on the current data available in peer-reviewed literature, it is unclear whether a particular laser source provides a significant advantage over the others with respect to clinical outcomes [24, 39, 49]. Practically speaking, laser assistance in lacrimal surgery enables precise, bloodless, easy, and fast ablation of the mucosa-bone-mucosa tissues at the rhinostomy site with minimal trauma to adjacent tissues. Adequate coagulation is achieved in the well-vascularized nasal mucosa; however, some degree of heat is conveyed to the vicinity of the surgical site.

The advantages of diode lasers are therefore reported as its ability to deliver a sufficiently powerful laser beam via a relatively narrow optical fiber with less collateral heat spread and less residual thermal damage to tissue.

Surgical Outcome of TCL-DCR

Functional success after lacrimal drainage surgery is assessed by the recovery of patency by lacrimal irrigation and the resolution of epiphora and dacryocystitis. Anatomical success describes an unobstructed ostium and lacrimal pathway but may be paradoxically accompanied by ongoing symptoms of obstruction.

Success rates reported for TCL-DCR with erbium:YAG [30], neodymium:YAG, and holmium:YAG lasers are 75%, between 64% and 85%, and between 47% and 82.5%, respectively [19–26]. However, these studies are not comparable due to the variable demographics of the study groups, number of patients, and follow-up periods.

Despite the limited number of published articles involving laser-assisted lacrimal surgery, the increasing number of solid-state diode laser delivery devices in ophthalmology and otolaryngology worldwide has led to more studies of diode laser-assisted TCL-DCR since first published by Eloy in 2000 [33–37]. The success rates of diode laser-assisted TCL-DCR for treating primary NLDO in adults range from

34% [50] to 95.2% [51]. The majority of these interventional case series report the success rates of TCL-DCR higher than 80%, close to the success rates of EX-DCR of 90–98% [3, 52] and endonasal DCR, which are between 61% and 100% [53–60]. Several studies comparing the outcome of EX-DCR and TCL-DCR with diode laser assistance revealed functional success of 89–95.4% for EX- DCR versus 73.7–84% for TCL-DCR [61–63]. A similar study by Ajalloueyan reported 92.6% success for EX-DCR and 93.4% for TCL-DCR, with less hemorrhage and shorter surgical times (19 versus 67 minutes) noted in the diode laser TCL-DCR group [64]. The shorter operative time of diode laser-assisted TCL-DCR (approximately 20 minutes) versus EX- DCR (60–90 minutes) has also been confirmed by others [61, 62, 65]. Piedrola compared diode laser-assisted techniques for transcanalicular and transnasal DCRs with similar outcomes [66].

Piaton then introduced the use of mitomycin-C (MMC) as an adjunct in Ho:YAG and Nd:YAG laser-assisted TCL-DCR [19, 23]. Henson used 0.4 mg/ml MMC for 5 minutes during 40 diode laser TCL-DCR procedures and reported a success rate of 87.5% after 12 months [67]. Henson then stated that "the cicatricial closure of the ostium can still occur even with a single intraoperative application of MMC." By applying multiple applications of MMC (0.4 mg/ml for 5 minutes) postoperatively after TCL-DCR, he then found higher success rates of 92.8% after 12 months in 125 diode laser-assisted TCL-DCR surgeries [68]. In general, although antifibrotic agents such as MMC and 5-FU have demonstrated potential benefits, the published data in laser-assisted DCR are not consistent, and high doses of adjunctive MMC applications during and/or after TCL-DCR may damage ocular and nasal surfaces [69–72].

Kaynak et al. reported a 60.3% functional success with diode laser-assisted TCL-DCR with intraoperative 0.2 mg/ml MMC applied at the rhinostomy site in a large series of patients with PANDO with 2-year follow-up. The relatively high failure rate was attributed to the overall greater total energy delivered, when compared to similar studies [38].

Low-level diode laser irradiation of cultured human oral mucosa fibroblasts in vitro has been found to lead to an increase in DNA synthesis [73]. In a similar study, laser-patterned microcoagulation using the 980 nm diode laser on the oral mucosa of healthy rabbits demonstrated stimulation of gingival and oral mucosal tissue regeneration. The study concluded that "laser-patterned microcoagulation treatment with the 980nm diode laser is a promising method for treating degenerative diseases of the oral soft tissues," such as gingivitis and gingival recession [74]. With these studies in mind, it can be postulated that the high amount of laser energy used to create a large bony ostium in TCL-DCR may cause increased fibroblastic activity and wound healing, thus contributing to ostium fibrosis and surgical failure. Theoretically, laser delivery systems with irrigating ports may decrease the thermal effect of ablative lasers on the surgical site and surrounding tissues; however, published data is lacking in the ophthalmic literature. One study using a diode laser with an irrigation port for TCL-DCR yielded 83.3% functional success with an average of 245 joules of total energy delivered [37]. The higher success rates may be attributed to the lower heat delivered due to the irrigation system attached to the laser probe, which decreases thermal injury to the rhinostomy site and neighboring tissues.

In TCL-DCR, an inferiorly located rhinostomy of at least 7 mm diameter may sometimes be difficult to achieve by laser ablation only. Aggressive attempts may lead to higher energy delivery and subsequent thermal damage to both mucosal surfaces that may lead to fibrosis and failed TCL-DCR. To decrease the energy delivered and to place the rhinostomy more inferiorly, endonasal mechanical enlargement of the ostium have shown increased success rates. The mechanical removal of the composite mucosal tissue and bone along the rhinostomy circumference also removes the charred tissues as well, leaving raw rhinostomy edges for healing by secondary intention [75, 76].

Middle turbinectomy during TCL-DCR, if necessary, may also increase the success from 71% to 88% [77]. TCL-DCR can also be performed with anastomosed flaps with good success rates, although technically this is much more challenging [78].

The functional success rate of secondary diode laser TCL-DCR has been reported as 80% for treating failed external DCR (27.3-month follow-up). Similarly, patients who had failed TCL-DCR may be treated via subsequent external DCR with 80% success [79].

Uysal reported 100% anatomical success and 85% functional success at the end of 20-month follow-up in a study group of 18 children with NLDO between the ages of 4 and 10 years treated with TCL-DCR [80]. Çakmak reported an 87.5% success rate in eight children with a shorter follow-up of 9 months [81]. It may be that iatrogenic canalicular injury by the laser probe to the delicate proximal drainage system in children may lead to robust fibrosis and proximal lacrimal system obstruction. Generally, the success rate of TCL-DCR for the younger population is lower when compared with an elderly population [82]. TCL-DCR may therefore be considered as a relative contraindication in the pediatric population.

Table 46.4 summarizes the data from studies where various lasers are used in TCL-DCR.

Table 46.4 Outcome of TCL-DCR with various lasers

Author(s)	Year	Laser assisted	No. of eyes	Follow-up (months)	Success rate (%)
Christenbury	1992	Argon	12	–	50
Piaton	1994	Nd:YAG	41	6	75
Dalez et al.	1996	Ho:YAG	26	7	47
Rosen et al.	1997	Nd:YAG	14	20	64
Pearlman et al.	1997	Nd:YAG	49	24	85
Eloy et al.	2000	Diode	26	–	65
Muellner et al.	2001	KTP	48	6	83
Caversaccio et al.	2001	Er:YAG	12	19	75
Piaton et al.	2001	Nd:YAG[a]/Ho:YAG[b]	317	6	63.2
Hofmann et al.	2003	KTP	78	12	83
Alanon et al.	2004	Diode	34	11	94.1
Hong et al.	2005	Nd:YAG	102	9.5	73.6
Alanon et al.	2006	Diode[a]/diode	150[a]/50	15	92[a]/78.2
Henson et al.	2007	Diode[a]	40	12	87.5[a]
Plaza et al.	2007	Diode	25	36	88
Ajalloueyan et al.	2007	Diode	122	18	93.4
Maeso and Sellarès	2007	Diode/diode[a]	75/75[a]	16	92/97[a]
Narioka and Ohashi	2008	Diode	15	27.3	80[c]
Cintra and *A. Lima*	2008	Diode	32	6	88
Cakmak and Yildirim	2010	Diode	8	9	87.5[d] (mean age: 11.25 years)
Uysal et al.	2011	Diode	20	20.5	85[d] (mean age: 6.11 years)
Basmak et al.	2011	Diode/diode[e]	44/47[e]	11/9.2[e]	71/88[e]
Henson et al.	2012	Diode[a]	125[a]	12	92.8[a]
Drnovsek-Olup et al.	2010	Diode	126	6	83.3
Nuhoglu et al.	2012	Diode	42	42	95.2
Derya et al.	2013	Diode	25	7	68
Dogan et al.	2013	Diode/diode[a]	27/30[a]	24	80/84.3[a]
Robert et al.	2013	Diode[f]	7[f]	10	89[f]
Kaynak et al.	2014	Diode[a]	125[a]	24.3	68.2[a](60.3[a])[g]
Taşkıran-Çomez et al.	2014	Diode[a]	34/28[a]	6	79.4[a]
Uludağ et al.	2015	Diode	19	12	73.7
Goel et al.	2016	Diode	30	12	90
Mourya and Rijal	2017	Diode	79[81]	–	90.1

DCR dacryocystorhinostomy, *KTP* potassium titanyl phosphate, *Nd:YAG* neodymium:yttrium-aluminum-garnet, *Er:YAG* erbium:yttrium-aluminum-garnet
[a]Intraoperative adjunctive MMC is applied
[b]Intraoperative adjunctive 5FU is applied
[c]Revision TDL-DCR for failed EX-DCR
[d]Pediatric age group
[e]TCL-DCR with partial anterior middle turbinectomy
[f]Mucosal flaps are done after laser ablation
[g]Functional success rate in the same group

Complications and Failure of TCL-DCR

Canalicular lacerations, punctal slitting, and punctal adhesions are not rare in TCL-DCR (Fig. 46.8a, b).

Due to the oval shape of the lacrimal sac, which is narrower inferiorly, the ability of the surgeon to move the laser probe anteriorly and posteriorly during TCL-DCR becomes more restricted as the probe is advanced more inferiorly, and punctal and canalicular lacerations can occur due to the forced manipulation. Therefore, the final ostium is usually wider superiorly and narrower inferiorly (Fig. 46.9a–f). The narrow inferior part can be easily occluded with mucosal proliferation forming a residual lacrimal sac leading to a sump syndrome. The patient may exhibit a patent ostium by irrigation (due to flow through the opening superiorly) but have functional epiphora. Closure of the ostium due to fibrosis and/or adhesions between the middle turbinate and the ostium are other causes of failure. Excessive thermal injury is a well-known risk factor for nasal mucosal and ostium adhesions.

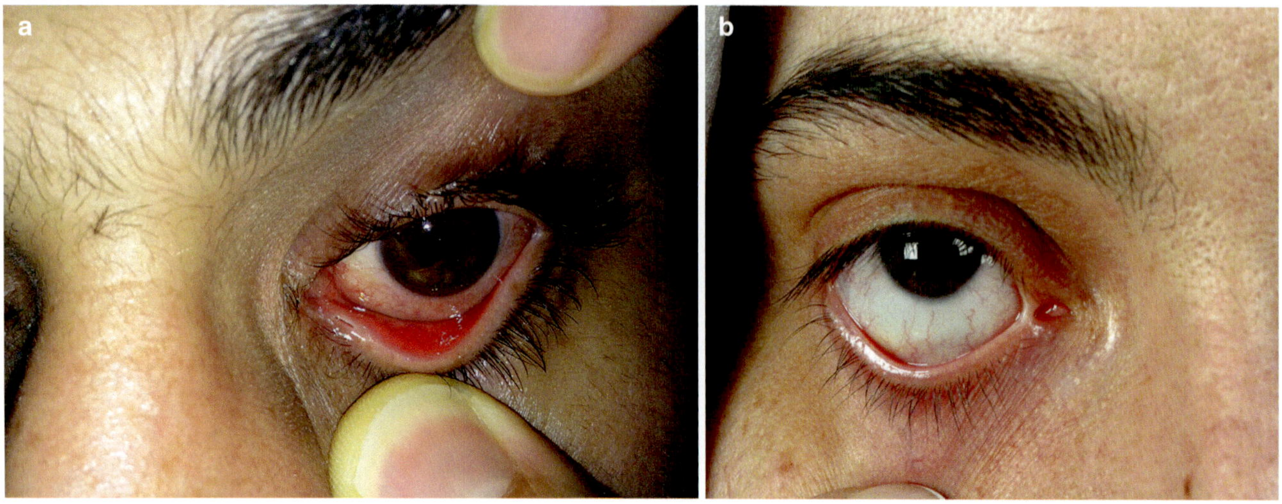

Fig. 46.8 (**a**) Eyelid complications: inferior punctal slitting due to TCL-DCR. (**b**) Eyelid complications: punctal adhesions following TCL-DCR with tight silicone intubation

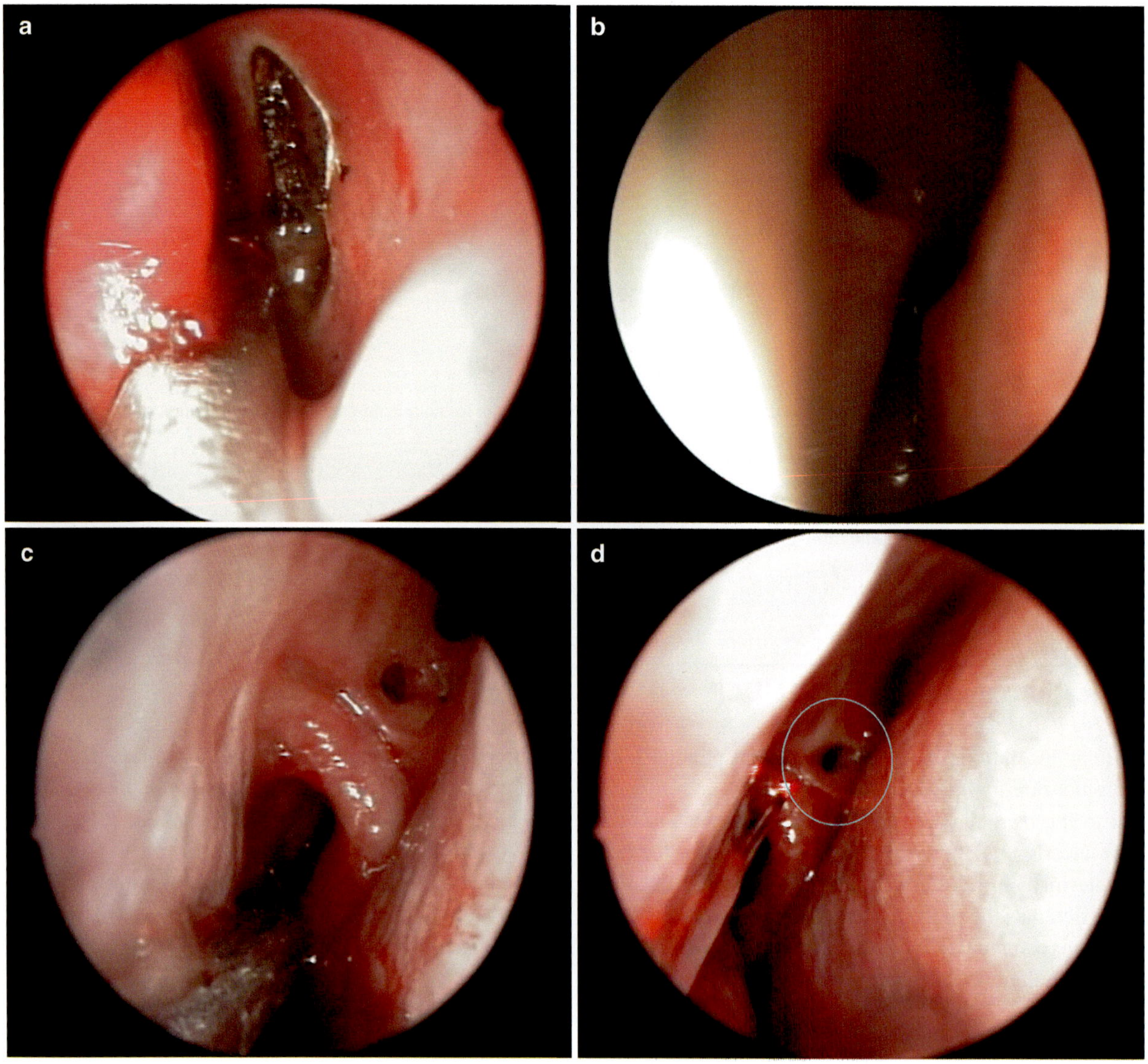

Fig. 46.9 Failure after TCL-DCR: (**a**) the typical upside-down pear-shaped ostium of laser-assisted TCL-DCR; (**b**) sump syndrome in TCL-DCR; (**c**) middle turbinate adhesion to the rhinostomy; (**d**) small pinhole ostium at the 3rd postoperative month; (**e**) false ostium in the anterior ethmoidal cell; (**f**) total closure of the ostium (in blue circle)

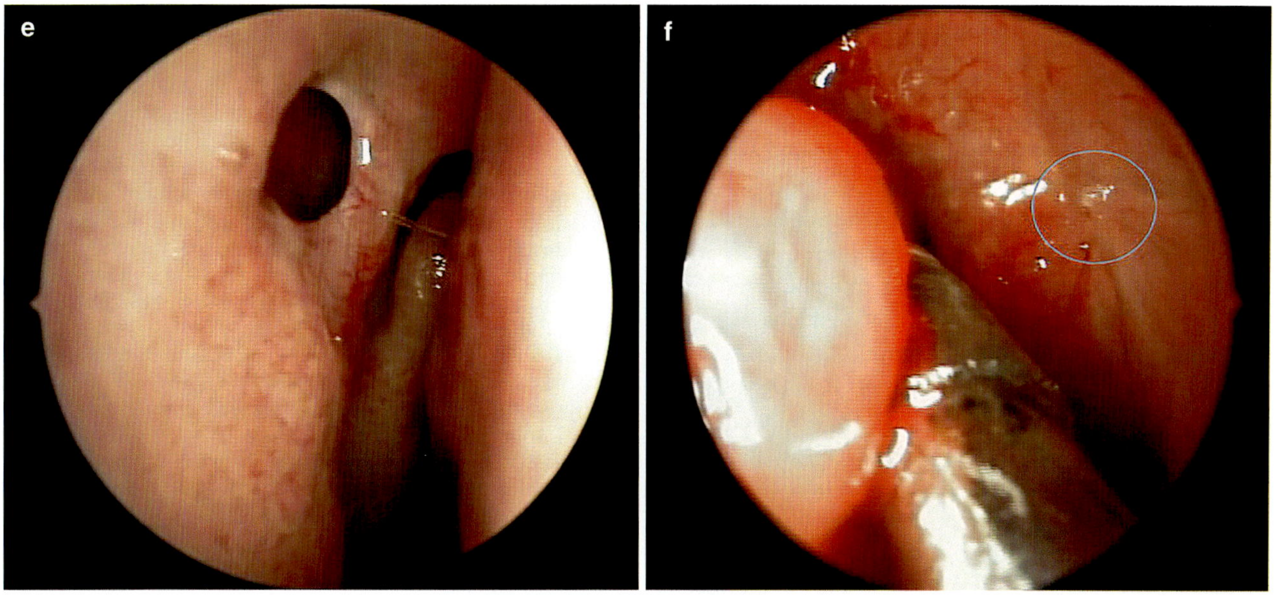

Fig. 46.9 (continued)

Lacrimal system tumors and dacryoliths may be missed using the TCL-DCR approach. Thus, a patient with a missed dacryolith during the TCL-DCR may postoperatively report persistent infection, regional pain, and functional epiphora, and therefore additional exploration is warranted. TCL-DCR would be contraindicated if these etiologies are suspected prior to surgery.

Although the transcanalicular route is a safer method of laser delivery in lacrimal surgery due to its direction away from the eye, there are risks of iatrogenic mechanical injury to the puncta, canaliculi, and/or the common canaliculus by the laser probe and sleeve. Dilating the puncta to enable the passage of the laser probe and/or maneuvering the probe to reach the maximum limits of the sac may cause small tears that subsequently enlarge to canalicular lacerations by the presence of the silicone tubes.

The lasers may also cause thermal canalicular burns and fibrosis that result in narrowing or occlusion of the upper lacrimal drainage system. Such complications may necessitate recanalization surgery with a conjunctivodacryocystorhinostomy with Jones tube.

Kaynak reported tube prolapse or stent loss in 17.7% of patients, which was speculated to be due to the absence of a visible wound that keeps the patient away from the medial canthal area (Fig. 46.10) [38].

Less commonly, tissue necrosis, nasocutaneous fistula at the nasojugal sulcus, and orbital infarction syndrome following diode laser-assisted TCL-DCR have been reported [83, 84].

The possible complications of TCL-DCR are listed in Table 46.5.

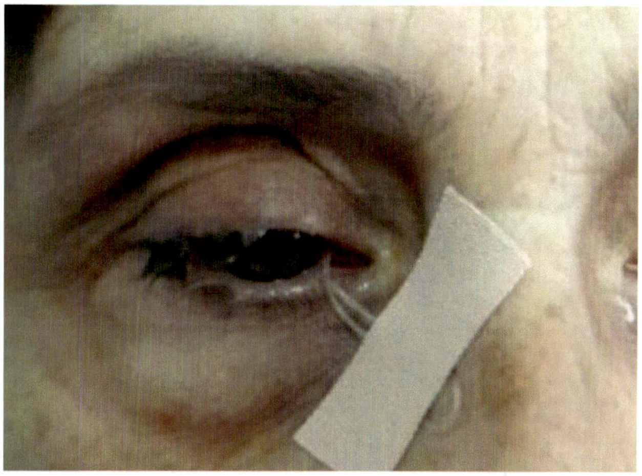

Fig. 46.10 Postoperative patient with tube prolapse after TCL-DCR

Table 46.5 Complications of transcanalicular laser-assisted dacryocystorhinostomy (TCL-DCR)

Thermal and/or mechanical injury to periocular area
Thermal and/or mechanical injury to proximal lacrimal drainage system
Creating false rhinostomy
Thermal injury and subsequent obstruction of maxillary sinus ostium
Intranasal laser injury and consequent adhesions that cause respiratory problems
Undiagnosed or misdiagnosed lacrimal sac pathologies and foreign materials
Trauma to olfactory receptors on nasal mucosae
Permanent desensitization of intranasal mucosa
Orbital infarction syndrome

Conclusion

The relative technical ease, shorter surgery, and rapid recovery time associated with TCL-DCR compared to external DCR have attracted the attention of many surgeons in recent years. The published success rate of TCL-DCR varies widely from 34% to 95.2%. The differences in the number of cases, follow-up time, definition of success, and surgeon variations in the TDL-DCR technique make it difficult to compare these results. The use of silicone stents, endonasal instrumentation, newer lasers, and antifibrotic agents have been reported to increase the success rate of TCL-DCR for the management of NLDO. Failure of TCL-DCR is often due to adhesions between middle turbinate and the ostium, closure of the rhinostomy site due to significant heat spread with resultant fibrosis, or sump syndrome from occlusion of the inferior ostium in the majority of patients. Among the complications of this surgery, patients should also be informed of the possibility of thermal or mechanical injury to the proximal lacrimal drainage apparatus.

Financial Disclosures The author has *no financial interest* in any of the materials or equipment used in the chapter.

References

1. Toti A. Nuovo metodo conservatore di cura radicale delle suporazioni chroniche del sacco lacrimale. Clin Mod Firenze. 1904;10:385–9.
2. Dupuy-Dutemps L, Bourguet J. Procédé plastique de dacryocystorhinostomie et ses resultats. Ann Ocul J. 1921;158:241–61.
3. Tarbet KJ, Custer PL. External dacryocystorhinostomy. Surgical success, patient satisfaction, and economic cost. Ophthalmology. 1995;102:1065–70.
4. Warren JF, Seiff SR, Kavanagh MC. Long term results of external dacryocystorhinostomy. Ophthalmic Surg Lasers Imaging. 2005;36:446–50.
5. Fayers T, Laverde T, Tay E, Olver JM. Lacrimal surgery success after external dacryocystorhinostomy: functional and anatomical results using strict outcome criteria. Ophthal Plast Reconstr Surg. 2009;25:472–5.
6. Caldwell GW. Two new operations for obstruction of the nasal duct with preservation of the canaliculi, and an incidental description of a new lachrymal probe. NY Med J. 1893;57:581.
7. Krasnov MM. Ultrasonic dacryocystorhinostomy. Am J Ophthalmol. 1971;72:200–1.
8. Javate RM, Campomanes BS, Co ND, et al. The endoscope and the radiofrequency unit in DCR surgery. Ophthal Plast Reconstr Surg. 1995;11:54–8.
9. Ibrahim HA, Noble JL, Batterbury M, Johnson CP, Williams R. Endoscopic-guided trephination dacryocystorhinostomy (Hesham DCR): technique and pilot trial. Ophthalmology. 2001;108:2337–45.
10. Wormald PJ. Powered endonasal DCR. Laryngoscope. 2002;112:69–71.
11. Adenis JP, Robert PY. Retrocaruncular approach to the medial orbit for dacryocystorhinostomy. Graefes Arch Clin Exp Ophthalmol. 2003;241:725–9.
12. Kaynak-Hekimhan P, Yilmaz OF. Transconjunctival dacryocystorhinostomy: scarless surgery without endoscope and laser assistance. Ophthal Plast Reconstr Surg. 2011;27:206–10.
13. Massaro BM, Gonnering RS, Harris GJ. Endonasal laser dacryocystorhinostomy. A new approach to nasolacrimal duct obstruction. Arch Ophthalmol. 1990;108:1172–6.
14. Gonnering RS, Lyon DB, Fisher JC. Endoscopic laser-assisted lacrimal surgery. Am J Ophthalmol. 1991;111:152–7.
15. Jack MK. Dacryocystorhinostomy: description of a transcanalicular method. Am J Ophthalmol. 1963;56:974–7.
16. Levin PS, Stormogipson DJ. Endocanalicular laser- assisted dacryocystorhinostomy. An anatomic study. Arch Ophthalmol. 1992;110(10):1488–90.
17. Silkiss RZ, Axelrod RN, Iwach AG, et al. Transcanalicular THC: YAG dacyrocystorhinostomy. Ophthalmic Surg. 1992;23:351–3.
18. Christenbury JD. Translacrimal laser dacrycystorhinostomy [letter]. Arch Opthalmol. 1992;110:170–1.
19. Piaton JM, Limon S, Ounnas N, et al. Transcanalicular endodacryocystorhinostomy using Neodynium:YAG laser. J Fr Ophthalmol. 1994;17(10):555–67.
20. Pearlman SJ, Michalos P, Leib ML, et al. Translacrimal transnasal laser-assisted dacryocystorhinostomy. Laryngoscope. 1997;107:1362–5.
21. Rosen N, Barak A, Rosner M. Transcanalicular laser-assisted dacryocystorhinostomy. Ophthalmic SurgLasers. 1997;28:723–6.
22. Fay AM, Michalos P, Rubin PA. Endocanalicular Nd: YAG laser dacryocystorhinostomy [review]. Int Ophthalmol Clin. 1999;39:177.
23. Piaton JM, Keller P, Limon S, et al. Holmium:YAG and neodymium:YAG laser assisted trans-canalicular Dacryocystorhinostomy. Results of 317 first procedures. J Fr Ophthalmol. 2001;24:253–64.
24. Hong JE, Hatton MP, Leib ML, et al. Endocanalicular laser dacryocystorhinostomy: an analysis of 118 consecutive surgeries. Ophthalmology. 2005;112(9):1629–33.
25. Dalez D, Lemagne JM. Transcanalicular dacryocystorhinostomy by pulse Holmium-YAG laser. Bull SocBelge Ophthalmol. 1996;263:139–40.
26. Kaynak P, Çelikoyar M, Göker S, Küçüksümer Y, Yılmaz ÖF. Endoskopik Ho:YAG laser dakriyosistorinostomi. Türk Oftalmoloji Gazetesi. 2002;32:332–6. (Article in Turkish).
27. Kaynak Hekimhan P, Yılmaz ÖF. Holmium:YAG LASER lacrimal by-pass surgery. Techin Ophthalmol. 2006;4:39–44.
28. Muellner K, Wolf G, Luxenberger W, et al. Laser-assisted transcanalicular dacryocystorhinostomy. Initial results Ophthalmologe. 2001;98:174–7.
29. Hofmann T, Lackner A, Muellner K, et al. Endolacrimal KTP laser-assisted dacryocystorhinostomy. Arch Otolaryngol Head Neck Surg. 2003;129(3):329–32.
30. Caversaccio M, Frenz M, Schar P, et al. Endonasal and transcanalicular Er:YAG laser dacryocystorhinostomy. Rhinology. 2001;39:28–32.
31. Mchugh JDA, Rose GE, Marshall J. The application of high-power diode lasers in ophthalmology. Laser Light Ophthalmol. 1994;6:229–38.
32. Eloy P, Trussart C, Jouzdani E, et al. Transcanalicular didoe laser assisted Dacryocystorhinostomy. Acta Otohinolaryngol Belg. 2000;54:157–63.
33. Alanon FFJ, Alanon FMA, Martinez FA, et al. Transcanalicular dacryocystorhinostomy technique using diode laser. Arch Soc Esp Oftalmol. 2004;79(7):325–30.
34. Plaza G, Betere F, Noquiera A. Transcanalicular dacryocystorhinostomy with diode laser: long-term results. Ophthal Plast Reconstr Surg. 2007;23(3):179–82.
35. Maeso RJ, Sellarès FMT. Trans-canalicular diode laser dacryocystorhinostomy: technical variations and results. Acta Otorrinolaringol Esp. 2007;58(1):10–5.

36. Cintra PPVC, Anselmo-Lima WT. Endocanalicular diode laser-assisted dacryocystorhinostomy. Otolaryngol Head Neck Surg. 2008;139:159–61.
37. Drnovšek-Olup B, Beltram M. Transcanalicular diode laser-assisted dacryocystorhinostomy. Indian J Ophthalmol. 2010;58:213–7.
38. Kaynak P, Ozturker C, Yazgan S, Ozturk Karabulut G, Akar S, Demirok A, Yilmaz OF. Transcanalicular diode laser assisted dacryocystorhinostomy ın primary acquired nasolacrimal duct obstruction: 2-year-follow up. Ophthal Plast Reconstr Surg. 2014;30:28–33.
39. Dowd T, Jones N, Eloy P, Oswal V. Laser assisted dacryocystorhinostomy. In: Oswal V, Remacle M, editors. Principles and practice of lasers in otorhinolaryngology and head and neck surgery. The Hague: Kugler Publishers; 2002. p. 187–219.
40. Janda P, Sroka R, Tauber S, et al. Diode laser treatment of hyperplastic inferior nasal turbinates. Lasers Surg Med. 2000;27:129–39.
41. Sroka R, Janda P, Killian T, et al. Comparison of long term results after Ho:YAG and diode laser treatment of hyperplastic inferior nasal turbinates. Lasers Surg Med. 2007;39:324–31.
42. Goharkhay K, Mortiz A, Wilder-Smith P, et al. Effects on oral soft tissue produced by diode laser in vitro. Lasers Surg Med. 1999;25:401–6.
43. Zborayova K, Ryska A, Lansky M, et al. Histomorphologic study of nasal turbinates after surgical treatment: a comparison of laser surgery and radiofrequency-induced thermotherapy effects in animals. Acta Otolaryngol. 2009;129:550–5.
44. Janda P, Sroka R, Mundweil B, et al. Comparison of thermal tissue effects induced by contact application of fiber guided laser systems. Lasers Surg Med. 2003;33:93–101.
45. Janda P, Sroka R, Betz CS, et al. Comparison of laser induced effects on hyperplastic inferior nasal turbinates by means of scanning electron microscopy. Lasers Surg Med. 2002;30:31–9.
46. Sinha UK, Gallagher LA. Effects of steel scalpel, ultrasonic scalpel, bipolar electrosurgery on wound healing in guinea pig oral mucosa. Laryngoscope. 2003;113:228–36.
47. Luomanen M, Rauhamaa-Mäkinen R, Meurman JH, et al. Healing of rat mucosa after irradiation with CO2, Nd:YAG, Co2-Nd:YAG combination lasers. Scand J Dent Res. 1994;102:223–8.
48. Kuchaer A, Novak P, et al. Endoscopic laser recanalisation of presaccal canalicular obstruction. Br J Ophthalmol. 1999;83(4):443–7.
49. Ali MJ. Primary endocanalicular laser dacryocystorhinostomy. In: Ali MJ, editor. Principles and practice of lacrimal surgery. New Delhi: Springer; 2015. p. 219–28.
50. Joshi RS. Conventional dacryocystorhinostomy in a failed transcanalicular laser-assisted dacryocystorhinostomy. Indian J Ophthalmol. 2011;59:383–5.
51. Nuhoglu F, Gurbuz B, Eltutar K. Long-term outcomes after transcanalicular laser dacryocystorhinostomy. Acta Otorhinolaryngol Ital. 2012;32:258–62.
52. Welham RA, Henderson PH. Results of dacryocystorhinostomy analysis of causes for failure. Trans Ophthalmol Soc U K. 1973;93:601–9.
53. Ben Simon GJ, Joseph J, Lee S, et al. External versus endoscopic dacryocystorhinostomy for acquired nasolacrimal duct obstruction in a tertiary referral center. Ophthalmology. 2005;112:1463–8.
54. Woog JJ, Kennedy RH, Custer PL, et al. Endonasal dacryocystorhinostomy: a report by the American Academy of Ophthalmology. Ophthalmology. 2001;108:2369–77.
55. Hartikainen J, Grenman R, Puukka P, Seppa H. Prospective randomized comparison of external dacryocystorhinostomy and endonasal laser dacryocystorhinostomy. Ophthalmology. 1998;105:1106–13.
56. Moore WM, Bentley CR, Olver JM. Functional and anatomic results after two types of endoscopic endonasal dacryocystorhinostomy: surgical and holmium laser. Ophthalmology. 2002;109:1575–82.
57. Maini S, Raghava N, Youngs R, et al. Endoscopic endonasal laser versus endonasalsurgical dacryocystorhinostomy for epiphora due to nasolacrimal duct obstruction: prospective, randomized, controlled trial. J Laryngol Otol. 2007;121:1170–6.
58. Lester SE, Robson AK, Bearn M. Endoscopic 'cold steel' versus laser dacryocystorhinostomy: completing the audit cycle. J Laryngol Otol. 2008;122:924–7.
59. Mirza S, Al-Barmani A, Douglas SA, et al. A retrospective comparison of endonasal KTP laser dacryocystorhinostomy versus external dacryocystorhinostomy. Clin Otolaryngol Allied Sci. 2002;27:347–51.
60. Lee S, Yen MT. Laser-assisted dacryocystorhinostomy: a viable treatment option? Curr Opin Ophthalmol. 2011;22:413–8.
61. Taşkıran Çömez A, Karadağ O, Arıkan S, Gencer B, Kara S. Comparison of transcanalicular diode laser dacryocystorhinostomy and external dacryocystorhinostomy in patients with primary acquired nasolacrimal duct obstruction. Lasers Surg Med. 2014;4:275–80.
62. Mourya D, Rijal RK. Transcanalicular laser-assisted dacryocystorhinostomy with diode laser. Orbit. 2017;36:370–4.
63. Uludag G, Yeniad B, Ceylan E, Yildiz-Tas A, Kozer-Bilgin L. Outcome comparison between transcanalicular and external dacryocystorhinostomy. Int J Ophthalmol. 2015;18:353–7. https://doi.org/10.3980/j.issn.2222-3959.2015.02.25.
64. Ajalloueyan M, Fartookzadeh M, Parhizgar H. Use of laser for dacryocystorhinostomy. Arch Otolaryngol Head Neck Surg. 2007;133:340–3.
65. Derya K, Demirel S, Doganay S, Orman G, Cumurcu T, Gunduz A. Endoscopic transcanalicular diode laser dacryocystorhinostomy: Is it an alternative method to conventional external dacryocystorhinostomy? Ophthal Plast Reconstr Surg. 2013;29:15–7.
66. Piédrola Maroto D, Franco SJ. Endonasal versus transcanalicular endoscopic dacriocystorhinostomy using diode laser. Surgical techniques and outcomes. Acta Otorrinolaringolo Esp. 2008;59(6):283–7.
67. Henson RD, Henson RG Jr, Cruz HL Jr, et al. Use of the diode laser with intraoperative Mitomycin C in endocanalicular laser dacryocystorhinosotmy. Ophthal Plast Reconstr Surg. 2007;23:134–7.
68. Henson RD, Cruz HL, Henson RG Jr, et al. Postoperative application of mitomycin-C in endocanalicular laser dacryocystorhinostomy. Ophthal Plast Reconstr Surg. 2012;28:192–5.
69. Camara JG, Bengzon AU, Henson RD. The safety and efficacy of mitomycin C in endonasal endoscopic laser-assisted dacryocystorhinostomy. Ophthal Plast Reconstr Surg. 2000;16:114–8.
70. Alanon FMA, Alanon FFJ, Martinez FA, et al. Results of the application of Mitomycin-c during endonasal and endocanalicular dacryocystorhinostomy by diode laser. Acta Otorhinolaryngol Esp. 2006;57:355–8.
71. Ali MJ, Mariappan I, Maddileti S, et al. Mitomycin C in dacryocystorhinostomy: the search for the right concentration and duration – a fundamental study on human nasal mucosa fibroblasts. Ophthal Plast Reconstr Surg. 2013;29:469–74.
72. Kamal S, Ali MJ, Naik MN. Circumostial injection of Mitomycin C (COS-MMC) in external and endoscopic dacryocystorhinostomy: efficacy, safety profile and outcomes. Ophthal Plast Reconstr Surg. 2014;30:187–90.
73. Loevschall H, Arenholt-Bindslev D. Effect of low level diode laser irradiation of human oral mucosa fibroblasts in vitro. Lasers Surg Med. 1994;14:347–54.
74. Romanos GE, Gladkova ND, Feldchtein FI, et al. Oral mucosa response to laser patterned microcoagulation (LPM) treatment. An animal study. Lasers Med Sci. 2013;28:25–31.
75. Basmak H, Caklı H, Sahin A, Gursoy H, Ozer A, Altun E, Yildirim N. Comparison of endocanalicular laser dacryocystorhinostomy

with and without endonasal procedures. Graefes Arch Clin Exp Ophthalmol. 2011;249(5):737–43.
76. Goel R, Nagpal S, Kumar S, Meher R, Kamal S, Garg S. Transcanalicular laser-assisted dacryocystorhinostomy with endonasal augmentation in primary nasolacrimal duct obstruction: Our experience. Ophthalmic Plast Reconstr Surg. 2017;33:408–12.
77. Basmak H, Cakli H, Sahin A, et al. What is the role of partial middle turbinectomy in endocanalicular laser- assisted endonasal dacryocystorhinostomy? Am J Rhinol Allergy. 2011;25:160–5.
78. Robert MC, Maleki B, Boulos P. Endocanalicular laser dacryocystorhinostomy with mucosal flaps. Ophthal Plast Reconstr Surg. 2013;29:294–7.
79. Narioka J, Ohashi Y. Transcanalicular-endonasal semiconductor diode laser-assisted revision surgery for failed external dacryocystorhinostomy. Am J Ophthalmol. 2008;146(1):60–8.
80. Cakmak SS, Yildirim M. Use of endocanalicular dacryocystorhinostomy with multidiode laser in children. Int J Pediatr Otorhinolaryngol. 2010;74:1320–2.
81. Uysal IO, Ozçimen M, Yener HI, Kal A. Pediatric endocanalicular diode laser dacryocystorhinostomy: results of a minimally invasive surgical technique. Eur Arch Otorhinolaryngol. 2011;268:1283–8. https://doi.org/10.1007/s00405-011-1585-z.
82. Ayintap E, Buttanri IB, Sadıgov F, Serin D, Ozsutcu M, Umurhan Akkan JC, Tuncer K. Analysis of age as a possible prognostic factor for transcanalicular multidiode laser dacryocystorhinostomy. J Ophthalmol. 2014;2014:913047. https://doi.org/10.1155/2014/913047.
83. Yeniad B, Bilgin LK, Cagatay A, et al. A rare complication after transcanalicular dacryocystorhinostomy: tissue necrosis and nasal-cutaneous fistula. Ophthal Plast Reconstr Surg. 2011;27(5):112–3.
84. Yeniad B, Tuncer S, Kir N, et al. Orbital infarction syndrome after transcanalicular dacryocystorhinostomy with diode laser. Ophthalmic Surg Lasers Imaging. 2012;25:43.

Revision Dacryocystorhinostomy

47

Emmy Y. Li

Introduction

Dacryocystorhinostomy (DCR), with the aim to establish a patent fistula between the lacrimal sac and the nasal cavity by removal of intervening bone, is the procedure of choice for management of primary nasolacrimal duct obstruction (NLDO). Over the years, the indications have expanded to include NLDO in patients with history of trauma, tumor, chemotherapy or radiotherapy, acute dacryocystitis with lacrimal sac abscesses, and common canalicular obstructions. Dacryocystorhinostomy via the external approach (EXT-DCR), first described by Toti in 1904 [1], has been the gold standard for many years. The endonasal approach (EN-DCR) described over 120 years ago, initially limited by quality of instruments, was reintroduced in 1989 and gained popularity [2]. With the introduction of sophisticated instruments, newer techniques, and adjuvant measures, surgical outcomes were enhanced while maintaining patient safety.

The success of DCR can be gauged by functional success and anatomical success. Functional success refers to a lack of tearing 3 months after surgery, a good indicator of successful surgery as suggested by the Royal College of Ophthalmologists. Anatomical success can be confirmed by patency on lacrimal irrigation, visualization of the ostium on nasal endoscopy, positive functional endoscopic dye test, scintigraphy, or contrast dacryocystography. The success rate of DCR varies with the surgical approach adopted. In the meta-analysis by Huang et al., there is an overall result favoring EXT-DCR, with a success rate of 84% for EN-DCR and 87% for EXT-DCR. In fact, the success rate of mechanical DCR with powered drills was 87%, comparable to that of EXT-DCR, yet the success for the laser-assisted EN-DCR was only 77%, thus inferior to EXT-DCR. When it comes to revision DCR, outcomes seem to be more favorable for EN-DCR, with 7% endoscopic cases versus 8% external cases requiring a further revision [3]. However, direct comparison of success rates is difficult given the significant variation in techniques, definition of success, and follow-up duration across studies.

In managing a failed DCR, the options are mainly surgical, though some patients may opt for observation. A failed primary EXT-DCR can be revised externally or endoscopically; likewise, a failed primary EN-DCR can be amended endoscopically or externally. Various adjunctive measures including intraoperative application of mitomycin-C (MMC) and intubation with silicone tubing have been proposed to enhance the success rate of revision surgery. Less traumatic procedures like probing and intubation and balloon dacryoplasty have also been suggested as an alternative in selected cases to salvage a failed primary surgery.

Causes of Failure in Dacryocystorhinostomy

Before deciding the best approach for revision DCR, it is important to understand the causes of failure in DCR. The common causes of failure are inadequately sized osteotomy, inadequate sac opening, common canalicular obstruction, intervening ethmoid air cell, inappropriately placed osteotomy with respect to the lacrimal sac leading to sump syndrome [4], scarred internal ostium (Fig. 47.1), ostium stenosis (Fig. 47.2), granulation tissue (Fig. 47.3), or synechiae formation at the ostium (Fig. 47.4) [5]. Not uncommonly, multiple causes for failure were noted [4, 5]. Other less common causes of failure include a deviated nasal septum and inadequately excised middle turbinate. Rare causes may be occult carcinoma, bony obstruction caused by Paget

E. Y. Li (✉)
Department of Ophthalmology, Hong Kong Eye Hospital, Kowloon City, Hong Kong

A. J. Cohen, C. N. Burkat (eds.), *Oculofacial, Orbital, and Lacrimal Surgery*, https://doi.org/10.1007/978-3-030-14092-2_47

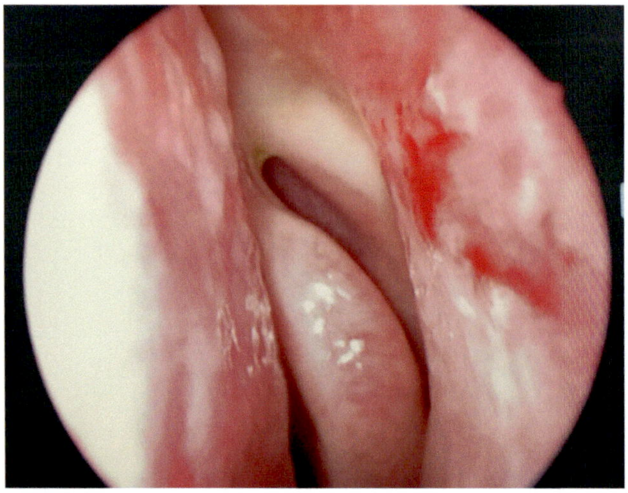

Fig. 47.1 Scarred and closed internal ostium

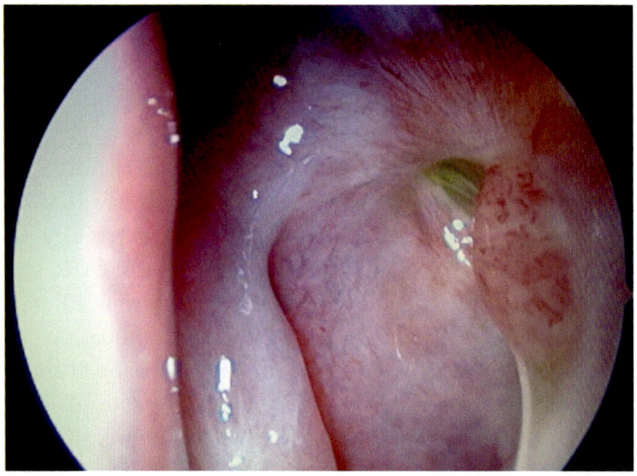

Fig. 47.2 Internal ostium stenosis

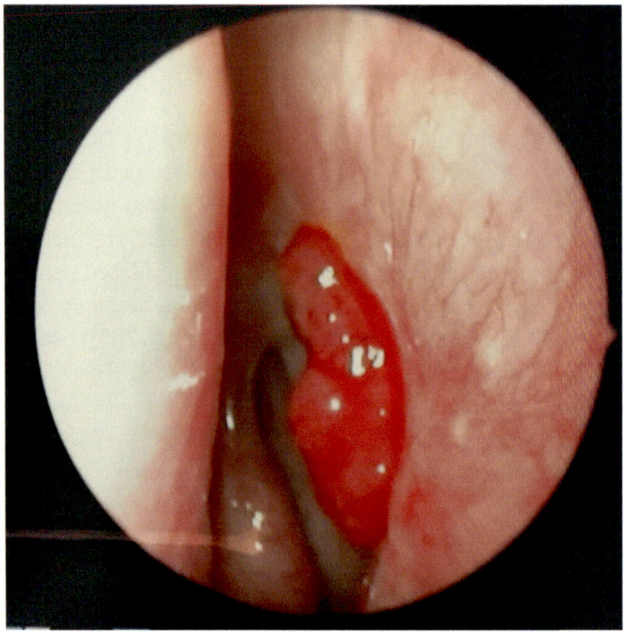

Fig. 47.3 Granulation tissue at the internal ostium

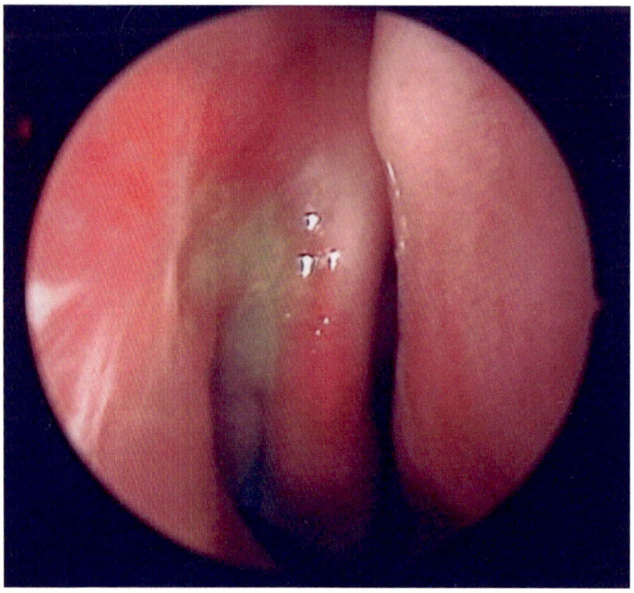

Fig. 47.4 Synechiae formation at the internal ostium

disease, ethmoidal sinus osteoma, and soft tissue obstruction caused by inflammatory diseases like sarcoidosis and Wegener granulomatosis [6–8].

Surgical factors that have been reported to be associated with a higher risk of failure include a small lacrimal sac opening intraoperatively and prolapse of orbital fat [9]. It was also proposed that excessive thermal damage to the sac or nasal mucosa/septum may increase the risk of fibrosis and failure [10]. In a study exploring prognostic factors for outcome, it was suggested that younger patient age at the time of surgery was associated with a higher failure rate, likely related to the high regenerative power leading to increased fibrosis and scarring in the younger group [11]. Surgeon experience is also a factor. Fayers et al. reported an overall lower rate of surgical success for trainees, both in terms of functional and anatomic improvement, as compared to that for attending/consultant surgeons [12]. Dacryocystorhinostomy in the pediatric group is less commonly performed. In the small case series published [13, 14], the most important cause of failure is complex congenital NLDO with associated craniofacial abnormalities, which are known to carry a poor prognosis.

DCR failures usually occur in early postoperative period. The average time to failure reported is 4.9 months after surgery, although failure can occur as early as 1 week postoperatively. It has been reported that the first 4 weeks after surgery was the period when the ostium size reduction was the greatest (79% of total shrinkage). However, the same group noted that the final ostium size did not predict the ultimate success rate [15]. Early obstruction was frequently found proximal to the common internal ostium [16]. Late failure, defined as recurrence of symptoms at least 12 months after surgery, is uncommon (<1%), and most of the obstruction occurred at the common canaliculus [17].

Preoperative Evaluation

Before considering revision surgery, the patient with a failed primary DCR must be reexamined to determine the etiology of symptoms and to rule out other causes of tearing, such as blepharitis, trichiasis, eyelid malposition such as lower eyelid laxity, entropion, ectropion, punctal abnormalities, and canalicular obstruction. Systemic inflammatory disease should also be excluded. Standard preoperative evaluation includes dye disappearance testing, lacrimal irrigation, and probing, and endoscopic evaluation of the internal ostium and nasal cavity are essential. If the ostium is found to be patent on irrigation or nasal endoscopy, the diagnosis of functional NLDO should be considered. Acquired NLDO can be divided into anatomic NLDO and functional NLDO. Functional NLDO is defined as delayed tear clearance on scintigraphy or dacryocystography in the absence of anatomic obstruction. It is thought to be caused by a narrowing of the nasolacrimal duct or failure of the lacrimal pump mechanism [18, 19]. Functional NLDO has a greater incidence of surgical failure, and patients may experience persistent symptoms despite adequate surgery. Unfortunately, revision surgery in this subset of patients has been shown to be of little value [20].

In most cases, the causes of failed DCR can be determined by lacrimal probing and nasal endoscopy. Syringing will be non-patent in cases of failed DCR, and probing should be repeated to identify the site of obstruction. For a scarred internal ostium, a negative endoscopic dye test will be observed. The use of imaging studies like scintigraphy or dacryocystography (DCG) with plain films may provide further information in delineation of the lacrimal drainage tract and determination of the exact site and nature of obstruction, thus helping to formulate a surgical revision strategy. DCG can also be performed with computed tomography (CT) or magnetic resonance imaging (MRI).

Typically, a patent fistulous tract confirmed by lacrimal probing and irrigation gives a characteristic "Y-on-its-side" configuration of the soft tissue on CT. Occlusion of the osteotomy by soft tissue corresponds to a mucocele-like soft tissue density with a central lucency and soft tissue obstruction. Occlusion of the osteotomy by inadequately excised bone is evident by the bone in the region of the osteotomy and would therefore warrant additional bone removal [6]. Using the spiral technology, high-resolution CT-dacryocystography (CT-DCG) allows measurement of the diameter of the osteotomy window, evaluation of osteotomy position relative to the lacrimal sac. Imaging should also assess carefully for any abnormal findings around the ostium, such as extension of ethmoidal air cells medial to the lacrimal sac, concha bullosa, nasal polyp, or a medial canthal mass that may contribute to the DCR failure [21].

Alternatively, dacryoendoscopy can provide direct visualization of the obstruction and the appearance of the obstructed space in failed DCR. It is particularly useful to identify a common canalicular obstruction, as conventional dacryocystography may not adequately outline the lacrimal canaliculi. If the DCR failure is due to an adhesive obstruction, endoscopic revision would be difficult without causing orbital fat prolapse as the dissection is performed toward the orbit; thus revision via the external approach may be preferred. However, if no such adhesive occlusion is observed, an endoscopic revision is a safe alternative [22].

Management

A failed primary EXT-DCR can be revised externally or endoscopically; likewise, a failed primary EN-DCR can be amended endoscopically or externally. Adjunctive measures, such as intraoperative application of MMC and silicone intubation may also be used to enhance surgical success rates.

Surgical Technique for Revision Endoscopic DCR

In the setting of revision EN-DCR, the keys to success include a thorough understanding of intranasal endoscopic anatomy, especially the location and extent of the lacrimal sac, efficient bone removal to achieve complete exposure of the lacrimal sac, and a complete incision and marsupialization of the lacrimal sac mucosa. At the beginning of the procedure, the nasal mucosal flap is incised slightly more anteriorly over the frontal process of maxilla than typically placed for primary cases. This allows the mucosal incision to be made onto the bone, and when this flap is elevated off the bone, it allows the correct surgical plane to be established for dissection of the mucosal flap off the underlying scar tissue. The bony osteotomy is then expanded, if indicated, with a rongeur until the lacrimal sac is completely exposed. Care is taken to be sure the inferior sac is exposed and opened, in order to avoid a lacrimal sump that continues to cause outflow obstruction. If the sac is relatively normal in size, standard mucosal flaps are fashioned. In cases when the sac is scarred and contracted and it is difficult to fashion mucosal flaps, the mucosal apposition between the nasal and lacrimal mucosa can be obtained by trimming correspondingly less of the nasal mucosal flap. One may also consider to use the agger nasi mucosa as a free graft to create functional mucosa surrounding the common canaliculus–sac junction [23]. Concomitant procedures, such as uncinectomy, septoplasty, polypectomy, anterior middle turbinectomy, or anterior ethmoidectomy, can be performed to allow adequate surgical exposure and to optimize canalicular clearance [5]. Anatomic and radiographic studies have demonstrated that the anterior ethmoid air cells not uncommonly extend forward to lie medial to the posterior, and even anterior, lacrimal sac fossa. Lastly, MMC can be applied to the ostium to inhibit fibrosis, and silicone intubation may be placed for several months.

Surgical Technique for Revision External DCR

A skin incision is made through the original scar. Orbicularis muscle is separated at the junction of the orbital and palpebral portions. Bowman lacrimal probes are placed to check the patency of both the inferior and superior canaliculi. The medial palpebral tendon, if present, is divided. A combination of sharp and blunt dissection is used to separate the scar above and below the probes. Great care is taken not to enter the lumen of the common canaliculi. The anterior edge of the original dacryocystorhinostomy is identified, and the periosteum is freed from the bone for approximately 4 mm anterior to the bony edge of the original ostium. The bony opening is enlarged to allow adequate exposure of the sac and to expose virgin nasal mucosa. A trapdoor incision based on the newly exposed original nasal mucosa is cut so that the lateral free edge is close to the previously identified common canaliculus and the upper and lower edges are next to the edges of the newly enlarged rhinostomy. The nasal mucosal flap is reflected anteriorly with traction sutures. The interior of the dacryocystorhinostomy is then examined, to remove any intervening bone, ethmoid air cell, turbinate, stones, or scar. Anterior and posterior mucosal flaps are sutured with fine absorbable suture, such as Dexon or polyglactin (Vicryl).

If common canalicular obstruction is present, an incision is made lateral to the obstruction to expose healthy canalicular mucosa, the abnormal segment removed, and the end anastomosed to the remaining sac or nasal mucosa. Canalicular flaps should be sutured under slight tension so that they do not adhere internally and form an obstruction. Silicone tubes should be placed if there is canalicular pathology or if the sac is small, scarred, or inflamed. Lastly, the orbicularis muscle and canthal tendon are repositioned with absorbable sutures, and the skin closed [4].

Endoscopic Revision Versus External Revision

Apart from the established advantages for endoscopic primary DCR, namely, the avoidance of cutaneous scar and preservation of the pump action of the orbicularis muscle, some authors have suggested that the endonasal approach is preferred for revision surgery. Reasons typically cited were its ability to better identify the etiology of failure, improved visualization of the ostium position relative to the lacrimal sac, direct access to the residual lacrimal sac hence allowing more complete sac marsupialization, easier hemostasis, and the capacity to address concurrent intranasal pathologies [24]. However, similar to the primary procedure, the potential drawbacks are a steep learning curve and high equipment costs.

The success rates for revision endoscopic DCR are in the range of 76–100% [23, 25–27], comparable to that reported for external revision DCR, which varied from 80% to 90% [4, 28]. Direct comparisons of the endoscopic and external techniques have also been reported [23]. Revision endoscopic DCR surgery was successful in 77% of cases, and external revision was successful in 85%, yet this difference was not statistically significant. In a meta-analysis comparing EN-DCR and EXT-DCR, 7% endoscopic revision cases versus 8% external revision cases required a further revision, although again the difference was not statistically significant [3]. In a study by Paik [29], which included 82 endoscopic revision DCR, a success rate of 84% was achieved for those with failed primary EXT-DCR and 81% for those who failed a primary EN-DCR. In the preoperative nasal endoscopy, it was observed that more of those who underwent primary EXT-DCR exhibited a hypertrophic middle turbinate or severe septal deviation, whereas more of those who underwent primary endoscopic DCR exhibited a small ostium.

The success rates of revision surgery are also lower if there is scarring and cicatrization of the lacrimal sac. This is because even with adequate bony ostium and full sac exposure, only a small amount of lacrimal mucosa can be marsupialized. This leads to a higher risk of repeated scarring and stenosis. This may also partly explain why patients who fail the first revision surgery are likely to fail additional revision [30]. In the presence of proximal canalicular obstruction, conjunctivodacryocystorhinostomy with the insertion of a Lester Jones tube, or similar variant, would be required to achieve surgical success.

Transcanalicular laser-assisted revision DCR has been advocated less as a simple office-based procedure to re-establish a patent drainage tract when soft scar tissue was the cause of failed DCR. In this procedure, the laser probe was carefully inserted through the upper canaliculus into the nasal cavity. The laser energy was applied until the tip of the laser probe was recognized by nasal endoscopy. Theoretically, the targeted application of laser energy allows effective tissue dissection with minimal collateral damage and retrograde damage of the lacrimal drainage system. Other advantages include short operative time, avoidance of skin incision, minimal risk of hemorrhage, less surgical trauma, and a rapid postoperative recovery. Both the use of diode laser and continuous wave neodymium-doped yttrium-aluminum-garnet (Nd:YAG) laser have been studied, with some studies demonstrating that the diode laser was able to achieve a higher success rate [31, 32]. Careful patient selection would also help to optimize the success rate. Lee reported that success rates were 100% in cases with membranous or synechial obstruction at the internal ostium, but only 50% in cases with granulomatous obstruction. A 100% failure rate was observed in cases with sump syndrome [31].

Therefore, preoperative assessment to identify the cause of DCR failure is most essential to determine the preferred surgical approach for revision.

Adjunctive Use of Mitomycin-C

The adjunctive use of intraoperative mitomycin-C (MMC) is a popular choice to enhance the success rate, particularly in revision surgery. Being an antibiotic isolated from *Streptomyces caespitosus*, MMC impedes the synthesis of DNA, cellular RNA, and protein by inhibiting collagen synthesis by fibroblasts. A histological study showed that MMC could enhance the success rate of DCR by decreasing the density and cellularity of nasal mucosa, thus reducing scar formation at the internal ostium, which is recognized as a major cause of DCR failure [33].

Many studies have attempted to define the role of MMC in DCR. It was, in general, recognized to be a safe adjunct, but may not necessarily increase the success rate in primary DCR [34]. However, the role of MMC is more definite in revision surgery. Success rates ranging from 89% to 93% were noted for revision endoscopic DCR with intraoperative application of MMC, much higher compared to success rates of 56–60% when MMC was not used, with the difference statistically significant [35, 36]. In a meta-analysis by Xue, the overall failure rate of revision EN-DCR with MMC was 13.2%, which was significantly lower compared to 30.4% in the control group [34]. The reported concentration of intraoperative MMC ranged from 0.02 to 0.75 mg/ml, and the duration of application ranged widely from 2 to 30 minutes. However, there is no consensus on the optimal concentration and duration of MMC established in the literature yet. In our center, MMC at a concentration 0.4 mg/ml, applied to the edges of the ostium for 5 minutes, has the standard practice for more than a decade, and no related complications have been observed.

Silicone Lacrimal Intubation

The role of lacrimal intubation (typically silicone stents) in enhancing the surgical success of primary or revision DCR is still controversial. Theoretically, the intubation prevents obliteration of the fistulous tract during the early postoperative period, yet some have reported that it may cause granulation tissue formation, infection, biofilms, canalicular laceration, and patient discomfort [37, 38]. In a randomized controlled trial by Chong, the success rate of primary EN-DCR was almost the same (96% vs 95%) with and without intubation [39].

There is no study in the existing literature to specifically define the efficacy of silicone intubation in revision DCR. In the subgroup analysis of Smirnov's study, revision surgery was successful in 100% with silicone tubing and 85% without silicone tubing. However, the sample size was small, and the difference was not statistically significant [40]. Silicone tube placement seems to be more important in setting of common canalicular obstruction. Some surgeons may also utilize larger caliber tubes or double intubation to further minimize closure of the ostium. The duration of silicone tube placement is also highly controversial. Some surgeons may keep the tube in place for up to 6 months or longer. In general, many surgeons opt to keep the silicone tubes in place for 2–4 months postoperatively in revision cases.

Probing and Silicone Intubation

Late failure after primary DCR is rare. It can be considered as a distinct clinical entity, and for the majority of patients, the level of obstruction has been shown to be at the common canaliculus. McMurray reported that all patients with secondary common canalicular obstruction underwent probing with either common canalicular membranotomy or membranectomy followed by silicone intubation for an average of 8 weeks. The outcomes were favorable and can be considered as a less invasive surgical alternative to a repeated DCR [17].

Balloon Dacryoplasty

Balloon dacryoplasty has been introduced for over two decades. Using specially designed balloon catheters of various diameters and lengths (LacriCATH, Quest Medical Products, Inc., Allen, TX, USA), targeted dilatation at different sites of the lacrimal outflow tract can be performed. The use of endoscopically assisted balloon dacryoplasty was initially proposed for congenital NLDO in children [41] and incomplete NLDO in adults [42]. In a highly selected group of patients with internal ostium stenosis, (Fig. 47.3) defined as minimal dye passage through a tiny internal ostium on irrigation as visualized on nasal endoscopy, and resistance on syringing, together with partially relieved tearing symptoms, balloon dacryoplasty could achieve an anatomical success of 84% and functional success of 74% [43]. This provides another less trauma alternative to revision DCR with advantages of shorter operative time, quick recovery, and performed under local anesthesia.

Conclusion

The most common causes of failed DCR include inadequately sized bony ostium or lacrimal sac opening, inappropriately placed osteotomy, scarring causing contracture, granulation tissue or synechiae formation at the ostium, and common canalicular obstruction. Meticulous primary surgery and intraoperative adjunctive techniques may prevent the occurrence of some of these factors. Most failed primary procedures can be readily managed with revision endoscopic or external DCR with relatively high success rates. Laser-assisted revision EN-DCR is particularly useful for cases in which the cause of failure is membranous obstruction at the internal ostium. Mitomycin-C, an antifibrotic agent, can help enhance the success of revision cases. Silicone tube placement can be considered especially in the presence of common canalicular obstruction. Balloon dacryoplasty, in carefully selected patients, can achieve reasonably good results. It should be noted, however, that patients with functional NLDO may not improve with revision surgery.

It is also important to discuss with the patient that those who have undergone multiple surgeries will likely have a decreased chance of success with additional revision procedures. Appropriate clinical and intraoperative assessment to identify the cause of DCR failure is critical to determine the preferred surgical approach for revision and to optimize the clinical outcome.

References

1. Toti A. Nuovo metodo conservatore di cura radicale delle suppurazioni croniche del sacco lacrimale (Dacriocistorinostomia). Clin Mod Firenze. 1904;10:385–7.
2. Woog JJ, Kennedy RH, Custer PL, Kaltreider SA, Meyer DR, Camara JG. Endonasal dacryocystorhinostomy: a report by the American Academy of Ophthalmology. Ophthalmology. 2001;108:2369–77.
3. Huang J, Malek J, Chin D, Snidvongs K, Wilcsek G, Tumuluri K, Sacks R, Harvey RJ. Systematic review and meta-analysis on outcomes for endoscopic versus external dacryocystorhinostomy. Orbit. 2014;33(2):81–90.
4. Welham RA, Wulc AE. Management of unsuccessful lacrimal surgery. Br J Ophthalmol. 1987;71(2):152–7.
5. Hull S, Lalchan SA, Olver JM. Success Rates in powered endonasal revision surgery for failed dacryocystorhinostomy in a tertiary referral center. Ophthal Plast Reconstr Surg. 2013;29:267–71.
6. Mauriello JA Jr, Vahedra V, Fleckner M, Shah C. Correlation of orbital computed tomographic findings with office probing and irrigation in 17 patients after successful and failed dacryocystorhinostomy. Ophthal Plast Reconstr Surg. 1999;15(2):116–20.
7. Konuk O, Kurtulmusoglu M, Knatova Z, Unal M. Unsuccessful lacrimal surgery: causative factors and results of surgical management in a tertiary referral center. Ophthalmologica. 2010;224(6):361–6.
8. Gupta N. Improving results in endoscopic DCR. Indian J Otolaryngol Head Neck Surg. 2011;63(1):40–4.
9. Hammoudi DS, Tucker NA. Factors associated with outcome of endonasal dacryocystorhinostomy. Ophthal Plast Reconstr Surg. 2011;27(4):266–9.
10. Garcia Vilaro M, Vásquez L, Marin A, Burés A, Medel R. Thermal damage influences endonasal dacryocystorhinostomy success. Ophthalmic Res. 2013;49(4):209–14.
11. Mak ST, Io IY, Wong AC. Prognostic factors for outcome of endoscopic dacryocystorhinostomy in patients with primary acquired nasolacrimal duct obstruction. Graefes Arch Clin Exp Ophthalmol. 2013;251:1361–7.
12. Fayers T, Laverde T, Tay E, Olver JM. Lacrimal surgery success after external dacryocystorhinostomy: functional and anatomical results using strict outcome criteria. Ophthal Plast Reconstr Surg. 2009;25(6):472–5.
13. Dietrich C, Mewes T, Kühnemund M, et al. Long-term follow-up of patients with microscopic endonasal dacryocystorhinostomy. Am J Rhinol. 2003;17:57–61.
14. Zenk J, Karatzanis AD, Psychogios G, et al. Long-term results of endonasal dacryocystorhinostomy. Eur Arch Otorhinolaryngol. 2009;266:1733–8.
15. Chan W, Selva D. Ostium shrinkage after endoscopic dacryocystorhinostomy. Ophthalmology. 2013;120:1693–6.
16. McLachlan DL, Shannon GM, Flanagan JC. Results of dacryocystorhinostomy: analysis of the reoperations. Ophthalmic Surg. 1980;11(7):427–30.
17. McMurray CJ, McNab AA, Selva D. Late failure of dacryocystorhinostomy. Ophthal Plast Reconstr Surg. 2011;27(2):99–101.
18. Wormald PJ, Tsirbas A. Investigation and endoscopic treatment for functional and anatomical obstruction of the nasolacrimal duct system. Clin Otolaryngol Allied Sci. 2004;29:352–6.
19. Mansour K, Blanksma LJ, Vrakking H, et al. Scintigraphic evaluation for tear drainage, after dacryocystorhinostomy, in relation to patient satisfaction. Eye. 2008;22:414–9.
20. Brewis C, Yung M, Merkonidis C, et al. Endoscopic dacryocystorhinostomy in functional lacrimal obstruction. J Laryngol Otol. 2007;27:1–3.
21. Gökçek A, Argin MA, Altintas AK. Comparison of failed and successful dacryocystorhinostomy by using computed tomographic dacryocystography findings. Eur J Ophthalmol. 2005;15(5):523–9.
22. Takahashi Y, Nakamura Y, Kakizaki H. Dacryoendoscopic findings in the lacrimal passage in failed dacryocystorhinostomy. Ophthal Plast Reconstr Surg. 2013;29(5):373–5.
23. Tsirbas A, Davis G, Wormald PJ. Revision dacryocystorhinostomy: a comparison of endoscopic and external techniques. Am J Rhinol. 2005;19(3):322–5.
24. Orcutt JC, Hillel A, Weymuller EA. Endoscopic repair of failed dacryocystorhinostomy. Ophthal Plast Reconstr Surg. 1990;6:197–202.
25. El-Guindy A, Dorgham A, Ghoraba M. Endoscopic revision surgery for recurrent epiphora occurring after external dacryocystorhinostomy. Ann Otol Rhinol Laryngol. 2000;109(4):425–30.
26. Demarco R, Strose A, Araújo M, et al. Endoscopic revision of external dacryocystorhinostomy. Otolaryngol Head Neck Surg. 2007;137:497–9.
27. Ramakrishnan VR, Durairaj VD, Kingdom TT. Revision endoscopic dacryocystorhinostomy. Oper Tech Otolaryngol. 2008;19(3):177–81.
28. Rose GE, Walland MJ. Factors affecting the success rate of open lacrimal surgery. Br J Ophthalmol. 1994;78:888–91.
29. Paik JS, Cho WK, Yang SW. Comparison of endoscopic revision for failed primary external versus endoscopic dacryocystorhinostomy. Clin Exp Ophthalmol. 2013;41(2):116–21.
30. Ben Simon GJ, Joseph J, Lee S, Schwarcz RM, McCann JD, Goldberg RA. External versus endoscopic dacryocystorhinostomy for acquired nasolacrimal duct obstruction in a tertiary referral center. Ophthalmology. 2005;112(8):1463–8.
31. Lee J, Choi SY, Lee H, Chang M, Park M, Baek S. The clinical effectiveness of transcanalicular diode laser-assisted revision surgery for failed endoscopic endonasal dacryocystorhinostomy. Br J Ophthalmol. 2015;99(8):1130–3.
32. Patel BCK, Phillips B, McLeish WM, et al. Transcanalicular neodynium: YAG laser for revision of dacryocystorhinostomy. Ophthalmology. 1997;104:1191–7.
33. Ugurbas SH, Zilelioglu G, Sargon MF, Anadolu Y, Akiner M, Aktürk T. Histopathologic effects of mitomycin-C on endoscopic transnasal dacryocystorhinostomy. Ophthalmic Surg Lasers. 1997;28(4):300–4.

34. Xue K, Mellington FE, Norris JH. Meta-analysis of the adjunctive use of mitomycin C in primary and revision, external and endonasal dacryocystorhinostomy. Orbit. 2014;33(4):239–44.
35. Ozkiriş M, Ozkiriş A, Göktaş S. Effect of mitomycin C on revision endoscopic dacryocystorhinostomy. J Craniofac Surg. 2012;23(6):e608–10.
36. Penttilä E, Smirnov G, Seppä J, Kaarniranta K, Tuomilehto H. Mitomycin C in revision endoscopic dacryocystorhinostomy: a prospective randomized study. Am J Rhinol Allergy. 2011;25(6):425–8.
37. Unlu HH, Toprak B, Aslan A, et al. Comparison of surgical outcomes in primary endoscopic dacryocystorhinostomy with and without silicone intubation. Ann Otol Rhinol Laryngol. 2002;111:704–9.
38. Woog JJ, Kennedy RH, Custer PL, et al. Endonasal dacryocystorhinostomy: a report by the American Academy of Ophthalmology. Ophthalmology. 2001;108:2369–77.
39. Chong KK, Lai FH, Ho M, Luk A, Wong BW, Young A. Randomized trial on silicone intubation in endoscopic mechanical dacryocystorhinostomy (SEND) for primary nasolacrimal duct obstruction. Ophthalmology. 2013;120(10):2139–45.
40. Smirnov G, Tuomilehto H, Teräsvirta M, Nuutinen J, Seppä J. Silicone tubing after endoscopic dacryocystorhinostomy: is it necessary? Am J Rhinol. 2006;20(6):600–2.
41. Maheshwari R. Balloon catheter dilation for complex congenital nasolacrimal duct obstruction in older children. J Pediatr Ophthalmol Strabismus. 2009;46(4):215–7.
42. Couch SM, White WL. Endoscopically assisted balloon dacryoplasty treatment of incomplete nasolacrimal duct obstruction. Ophthalmology. 2004;111(3):585–9.
43. Lee A, Ali MJ, Li EY, Wong AC, Yuen HK. Balloon dacryoplasty in internal ostium stenosis after endoscopic dacryocystorhinostomy. Ophthal Plast Reconstr Surg. 2014;30(1):7–10.

48 Conjunctivodacryocystorhinostomy: Indications, Tubes, and Techniques

C. Blake Perry and Eric A. Steele

Conjunctivodacryocystorhinostomy (CDCR) with placement of a Jones tube remains the gold standard treatment for upper lacrimal outflow obstruction. Since the original description by Dr. Lester Jones in the 1960s, there have been numerous variations in the surgical technique proposed and an ever-increasing number of tubes available for use [1–9]. Yet the fundamental principle remains constant: a surgical ostium connecting the caruncle to the nose, with a glass tube to provide capillary flow of tears.

Indications

CDCR is the treatment of choice in cases where both canaliculi are absent or obliterated. It is also useful in cases of flaccid canaliculi with poor tear drainage and in those with dysfunction of the normal tear pump mechanism [10].

Tubes

The original tube developed by Dr. Lester Jones and Mr. Gunther Weiss in Portland, Oregon, in the 1960s was a pyrex tube with an internal diameter of 0.8 mm and an angled 30° tip. The tubes had collars of varying sizes, ranging from 3.0 to 4.0 mm. The 0.8 mm internal diameter and 30° angled tip was chosen based on optimizing the capillary flow characteristics. Typically, a 4.0 mm collar is placed at the time of surgery to prevent inward migration of the tube during the immediate postoperative period. This could be exchanged for a smaller diameter collar after the surgical tract is healed if the appearance or comfort of the larger collar were objectionable to the patient.

Because the tube was designed to be removed and cleaned on a regular basis to avoid the accumulation of mucus crusting and tear salts, migration and extrusion are potential complications of the procedure. Reported extrusion rates range from 5% to 50% in the literature [11]. Subsequently, this has led to the development of several tube design variations. These have included the Putterman-Gladstone tube that has an additional intranasal dilation of the glass tube [5], frosted tubes that have a textured outer surface aimed to increase friction with surrounding tissue [3, 8], extended angled tubes that conform differently to the nasal anatomy [7], porous polyethylene-coated (Medpor) tubes designed to promote fibrovascular ingrowth [4], and the StopLoss Jones tube that has an intranasal silicone flange to minimize migration and extrusion [2]. It remains controversial, however, whether these modifications to the original tube have demonstrated statistically significant improvements [12, 13]. Additional studies with long-term follow-up would be helpful in determining usefulness.

Surgical Technique

The conjunctivodacryocystorhinostomy (CDCR) procedure can be performed from an external or endoscopic approach. The first portion of the procedure is identical to standard dacryocystorhinostomy, with a slight modification at the end to create a tract from the caruncle to the nasal passageway to allow for placement of a Jones tube.

Procedure: External CDCR

This surgery is typically performed using infiltration of local anesthetic with monitored anesthesia care (MAC) or general anesthesia. The local anesthetic often used is a 1:1 mixture of

C. B. Perry
Aesthetic Surgery Centre, Tacoma, WA, USA

E. A. Steele (✉)
Casey Eye Institute, Oregon Health & Science University, Portland, OR, USA
e-mail: steeleer@ohsu.edu

A. J. Cohen, C. N. Burkat (eds.), *Oculofacial, Orbital, and Lacrimal Surgery*, https://doi.org/10.1007/978-3-030-14092-2_48

1% lidocaine with 1:100,000 epinephrine and 0.5% bupivacaine. Epinephrine aids in hemostasis due to its vasoconstrictive properties. Neurosurgical cottonoids are saturated in either cocaine hydrochloride 4% solution or adrenaline 1:1000 solution in preparation to pack the nose to vasoconstrict the nasal mucosa. This solution is often mixed with fluorescein dye to properly identify the clear liquid.

After parenteral sedation is successfully administered, topical proparacaine is instilled on the ocular surface. The local anesthetic is then infiltrated subcutaneously in the medial canthal area, taking care to avoid intravascular injection into the angular vessels. The cottonoids are placed in the nose with a bayonet forceps to the area just anterior to the attachment of the middle turbinate. The same infiltration of local anesthesia and nasal packing are performed if the patient is placed under general anesthesia.

Similar to a dacryocystorhinostomy (DCR) surgery, the skin incision is made 11 mm medial to the medial commissure, with the superior border in level with the medial canthal tendon and extending approximately 18 mm inferiorly and slightly lateral toward the ala of the nose. The incision placed within the thin lower eyelid skin and nasojugal groove is often better camouflaged with less scarring than an incision within the thicker upper cheek skin (Fig. 48.1). A sharp Stevens scissors is used to divide the remaining subcutaneous tissue, and an Agricola self-retaining retractor can be placed for exposure of the operative field. Alternatively, an assistant can use a rake or Desmarres retractor to retract the soft tissues. A Freer or Cottle elevator is used to dissect through the periosteum down to the maxillary bone anterior to the anterior lacrimal crest. The angular vessels are typically encountered during this process and can be avoided or cauterized at the surgeon's discretion. Hemostasis is achieved using a handheld battery cautery unit or monopolar/bipolar cautery.

The Freer elevator is used to lift the periosteum posteriorly to expose the anterior lacrimal crest. There is often a small vessel in a bony groove (sutura notha) just anterior to the crest that can be cauterized. The periosteum is lifted off the lacrimal sac fossa to the posterior lacrimal crest and inferiorly as far as possible to the nasolacrimal canal (Fig. 48.2). The medial canthal tendon can also be elevated superiorly if greater exposure is needed.

At this point, local anesthetic is infiltrated in the lacrimal sac. A small cottonoid or pledget with adrenaline or cocaine is placed in the space between the lacrimal sac and the fossa to protect the lacrimal sac. The intranasal cottonoids are also removed to avoid damage to nasal mucosal tissues during the next step of bone removal.

The Agricola retractor is replaced with a Goldstein retractor, which has longer teeth to provide better exposure. A 4 mm burr on a high-speed drill is used to remove an oval window of bone anterior to the lacrimal crest, taking care not to damage the nasal mucosa. The nasal mucosa is infiltrated with local anesthetic, and a dental burnisher is passed through the bony window to separate the nasal mucoperiosteum from the underside of the bone (Fig. 48.3). If a high-speed drill is not available, a freer elevator or blunt hemostat can be used to gently break through the thinner lacrimal bone just posterior to the maxillary-lacrimal suture line of the fossa.

A 90° Kerrison rongeur is used to enlarge the bony opening. The osteotomy should include removal of the anterior lacrimal crest and the entire lacrimal sac fossa from the level of the medial canthal tendon superiorly to the superior aspect

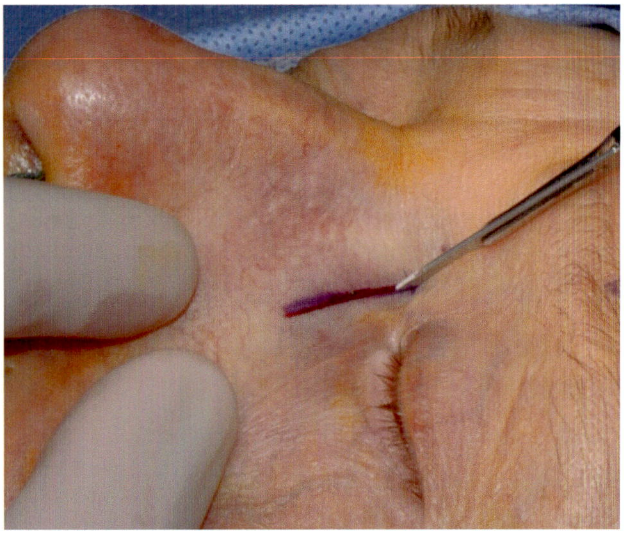

Fig. 48.1 The skin incision of an external DCR is made 11 mm medial to the medial commissure, with the superior border in the plane of the medial canthal tendon and extending approximately 18 mm inferiorly and slightly lateral toward the ala of the nose

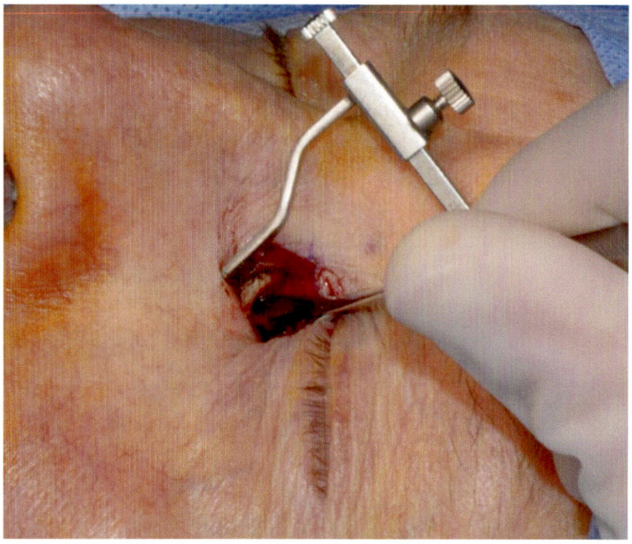

Fig. 48.2 A Freer elevator is used to lift the periosteum off the lacrimal sac fossa

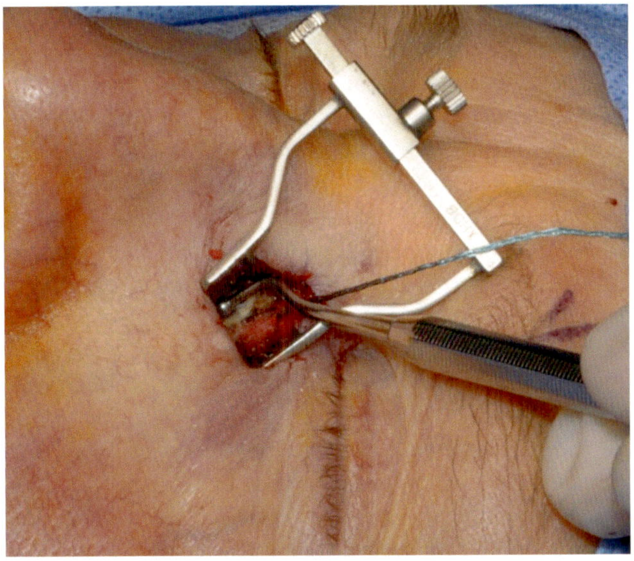

Fig. 48.3 A dental burnisher is passed through the created bony window to separate the nasal mucoperiosteum from the underside of the bone

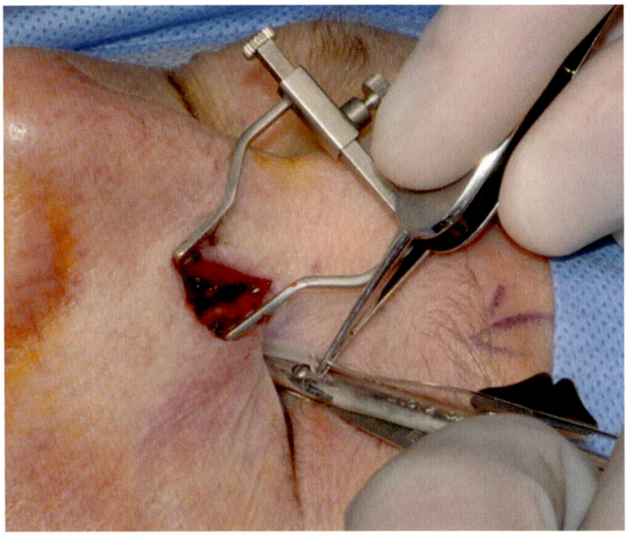

Fig. 48.4 A Bowman probe loaded with the appropriate length Jones tube in place is passed immediately anterior to the scissors. The Jones tube is pressed forward using forceps as the scissors are slowly removed

of the nasolacrimal canal/duct inferiorly. Care is taken to remove enough bone in this area to provide at least a 5 mm distance from the level of the common canaliculus. Occasionally during this process, there may be an anteriorly placed ethmoid air cell that needs to be removed to provide entry into the nasal cavity.

A Bowman probe can be placed through the superior canaliculus to gently tent the medial sac wall away from the common internal ostium. The lacrimal sac is then vertically incised along its entire length with a #11 blade (or Westcott scissors), and anterior and posterior flaps are created with backcuts. A corresponding vertical incision is made through the nasal mucosa, with creation of anterior and posterior flaps via an "H-shaped" incision (the initial vertical incision in the nasal mucosa corresponds to the central bridge of the "H"). Both posterior flaps are then excised or sutured together using 5-0 polyglactin suture on a small curved P-2 needle.

Attention is then directed to the caruncle. If it is prominent, it is conservatively debulked with a scissors taking care not to excise the surrounding conjunctiva. A sharp Stevens scissors is inserted in the area of the caruncle and gently advanced in a slightly downward trajectory into the previously created opening into the nose, taking care to angle anterior to the middle turbinate. If the middle turbinate interferes, the anterior tip can be judiciously resected. The scissors are slightly opened by an assistant, and a Bowman probe with the appropriate length Jones tube (Gunther Weiss Scientific Glass Blowing Company, Portland, Oregon) in place is passed immediately anterior to the scissors. The scissors are slowly removed, with the blades still slightly open, as the Jones tube is pressed forward using forceps (Fig. 48.4). The tip of the tube should rest approximately halfway between the lateral wall of the nose and the septum or should be replaced with a tube of a different length. Typically, a 4 × 16 mm tube is initially placed. Alternatively, the length of the scissors from its tips to the medial canthal angle can be measured to help calculate the appropriate tube length. The anterior mucosal flaps are then sutured together anterior to the Jones tube using 5-0 polyglactin suture on a small curved needle. The orbicularis muscle is closed with an interrupted or running 6-0 polyglactin suture, followed by closure of the skin with a running 6-0 fast-absorbing plain gut suture. A 6-0 polyglactin suture is wrapped around the collar of the tube and secured to the medial canthal tissue to prevent migration of the tube in the early postoperative period.

Procedure: Endoscopic CDCR

This surgery can also be performed with monitored sedation. But unlike the external approach, the surgery starts with manipulation of the nasal mucosa, which can produce intraoperative bleeding from the very beginning of the procedure that can interfere with surgical progress. This procedure is therefore typically performed with general anesthesia, which allows for protection of the airway during the procedure.

Local anesthesia is used consisting of a 1:1 mixture of 1% lidocaine with 1:100,000 epinephrine and 0.5% bupivacaine. This is infiltrated into the medial canthal and lacrimal sac areas externally. A control syringe on a 25 gauge, 3.5 inch, spinal needle with the guide wire removed is used to infiltrate the maxillary line, the uncinate process, and the axilla and anterior portions of the middle turbinate. Neurosurgical cottonoids, saturated in either cocaine hydrochloride 4% solution or adrenaline 1:1000 solution, are placed in the nose with bayonet forceps in the area just anterior to the middle turbinate, adjacent to the previously anesthetized nasal mucosa. The nasal packing is placed before the endoscopic setup to allow time for adequate vasoconstriction of the nasal mucosa. Once the operative field is completely set up, the cottonoids are removed.

A zero-degree endoscope, attached to a fiber-optic light source and external video monitor, is used for visualization. It is advanced through the nares using the nasal tip as a fulcrum. A curvilinear incision is made with a crescent knife or sharp edge of a Freer elevator that outlines the lacrimal sac and mirrors the middle turbinate. A Freer or Cottle elevator is then used to elevate the mucosa off the nasal wall and removed using grasping forceps. Alternatively, the nasal mucosa can be removed using a microdebrider if available. A 90° Kerrison rongeur is used to create the bony osteotomy by first removing the frontal process of the maxilla. Care is taken to insert the rongeurs between the bone and lacrimal sac to avoid distorting the anatomy. Enough bone is removed to completely uncover the lacrimal sac. Toward the axilla the maxillary bone can become difficult to remove with a Kerrison rongeur. If this is the case, a Ferris-Smith rongeur or diamond burr can be helpful. A keratome blade is then used to incise the vertical length of the lacrimal sac. If possible, a Bowman probe can be advanced down the canalicular system and used to tent out the lacrimal sac. Once incised, a dental burnisher is inserted inside the sac and used to enlarge the opening to allow visualization of the interior portions of the sac. The anterior and posterior leaflets of the lacrimal sac are then excised using a grasping forceps (such as a Takahashi forceps) or microdebrider. Care is taken to avoid damage to the common canaliculus ostium (Fig. 48.5).

Attention is then directed toward the insertion of the Jones tube. The caruncle is conservatively debulked, if needed. A sharp Stevens scissors is inserted in the area of the caruncle and gently advanced in a slightly downward trajectory through the previously made ostium. Endoscopic visualization of the scissors tips through the ostium is confirmed. The scissors are slightly opened, and a Bowman probe with the appropriate length Jones tube in place is passed immediately anterior to the scissors. The scissors are slowly removed, with the blades still slightly open, as the Jones tube is pressed forward using blunt forceps. The tip of the tube should rest halfway between the lateral wall of the nose and the septum or should be replaced with a tube of a different length. If the middle turbinate interferes, it can be judiciously resected.

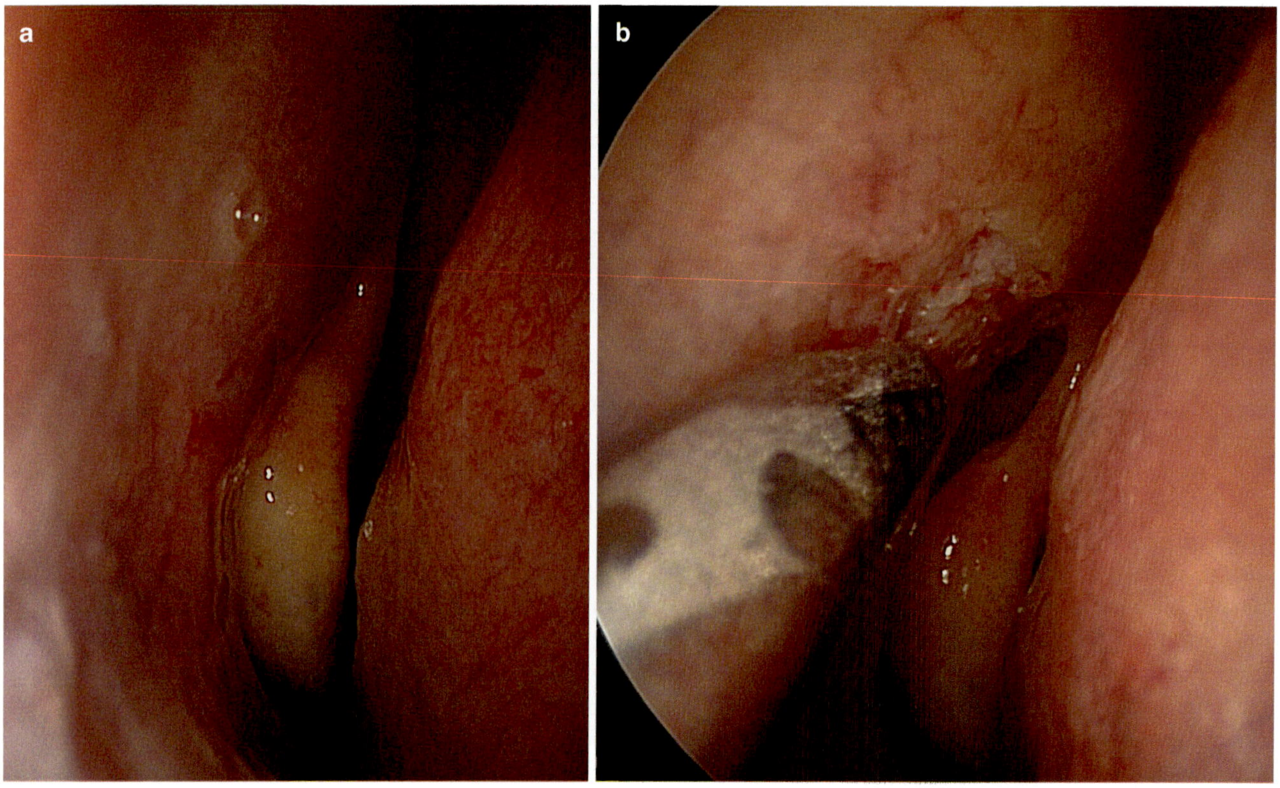

Fig. 48.5 (**a**) Endoscopic view of the right middle turbinate. (**b–d**) The nasal mucosa mirroring the middle turbinate is removed using a microdebrider. (**e**) An osteotomy is created using a 90-degree rongeur. (**f**) Enough bone is removed to completely uncover the lacrimal sac. (**g**, **h**) A keratome blade is used to incise the vertical length of the lacrimal sac. (**i**) The anterior and posterior leaflets of the lacrimal sac are removed, followed by insertion of a Bowman probe

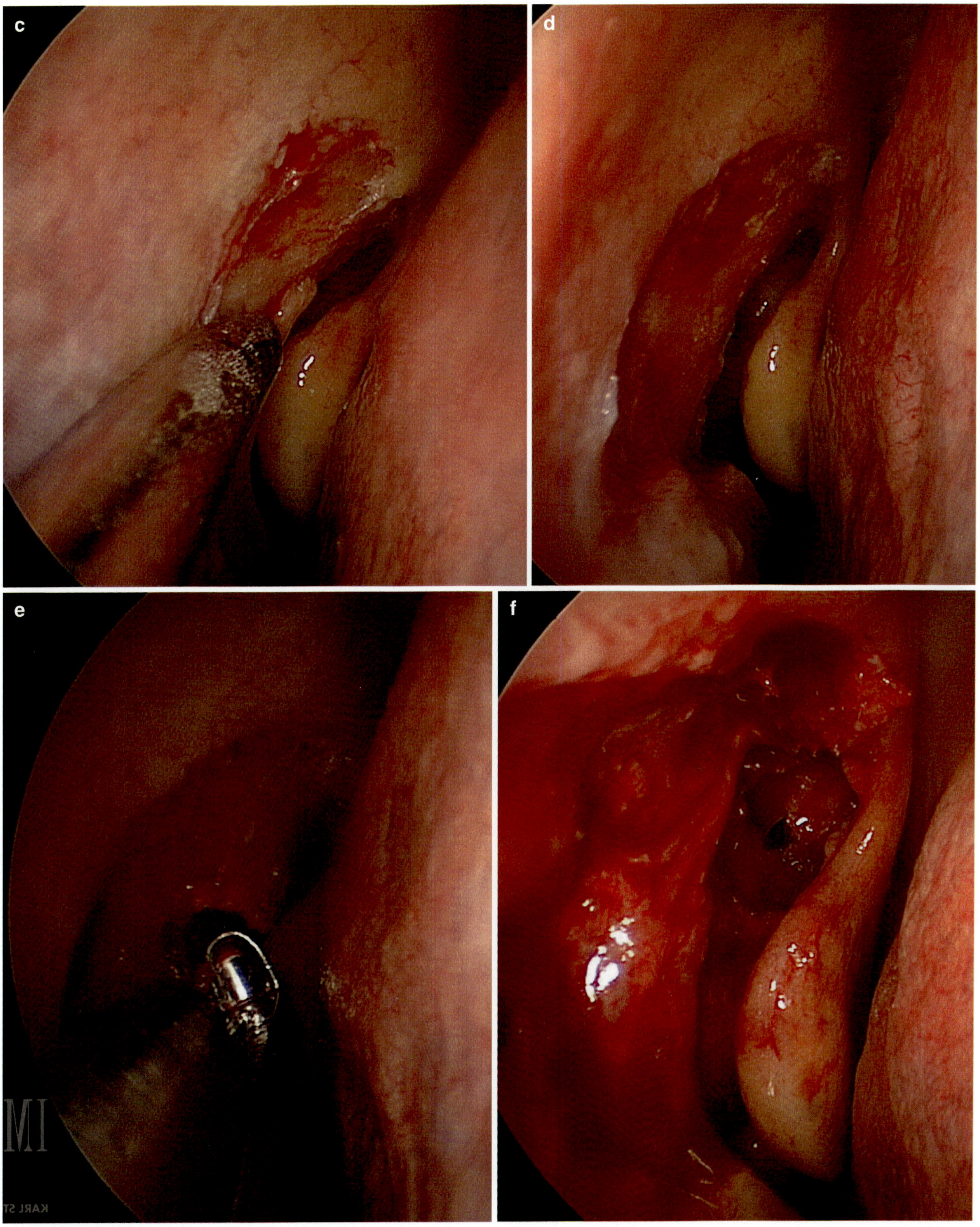

Fig. 48.5 (continued)

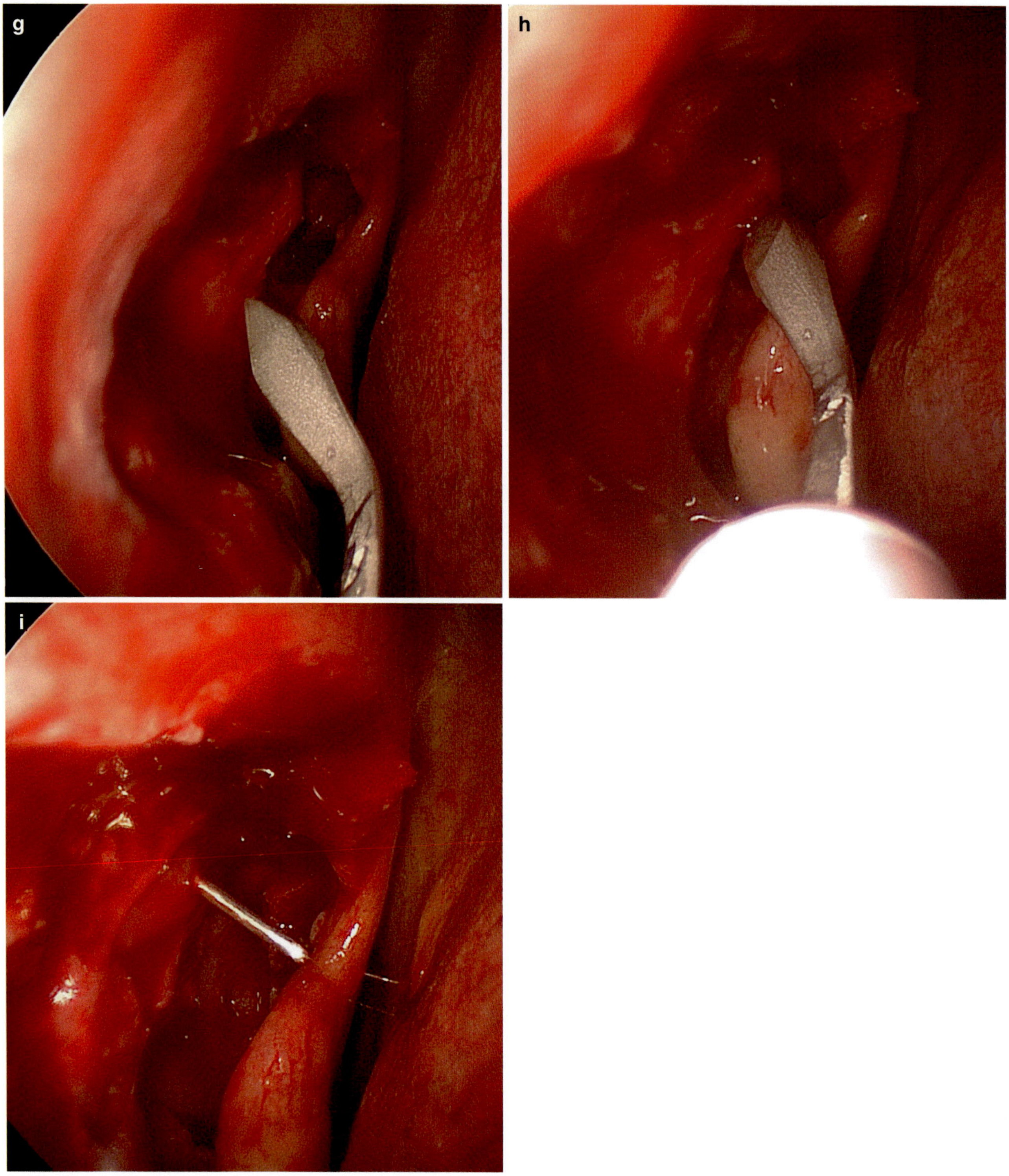

Fig. 48.5 (continued)

A 6-0 polyglactin suture is wrapped around the collar of the tube and secured to the medial canthal tissue.

Endoscopic visualization of the tube length is again checked. A piece of notched Hemcon (HemCon Medical Technologies, Portland OR) or trimmed PosiSep (Hemostasis, Saint Paul, MN) can be placed at the conclusion of the procedure for additional hemostasis (Fig. 48.6).

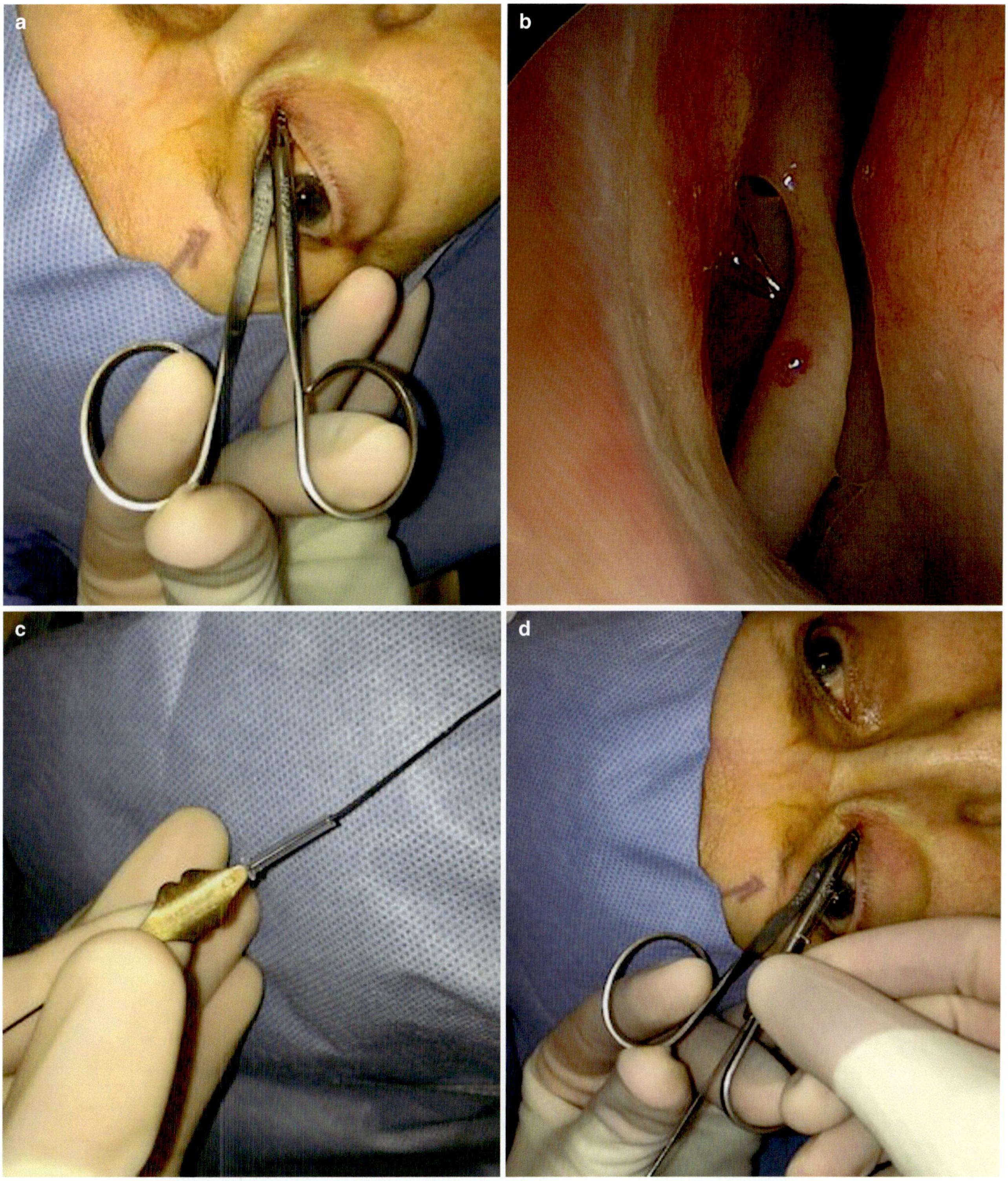

Fig. 48.6 (**a**) A Stevens scissors is inserted in the area of the caruncle in a slightly downward trajectory aiming for the previously created opening into the nose. (**b**) Endoscopic view of the position of scissors through the osteotomy. (**c**) Bowman probe loaded with the appropriate-sized Jones tube. (**d**) The scissors are slightly opened, and the loaded Bowman probe is passed immediately anterior to the scissors. (**e**) Endoscopic view demonstrating proper location of scissors and Bowman probe. (**f**) The Jones tube is then advanced over the Bowman probe as the scissors are removed. (**g**) The Bowman probe is removed once the Jones tube is advanced into the proper position. (**h**) Endoscopic view of the distal end of Jones tube halfway between the lateral nasal wall and septum. (**i**) 6-0 polyglactin suture is wrapped around the collar of the tube and secured to the medial canthal tissue.

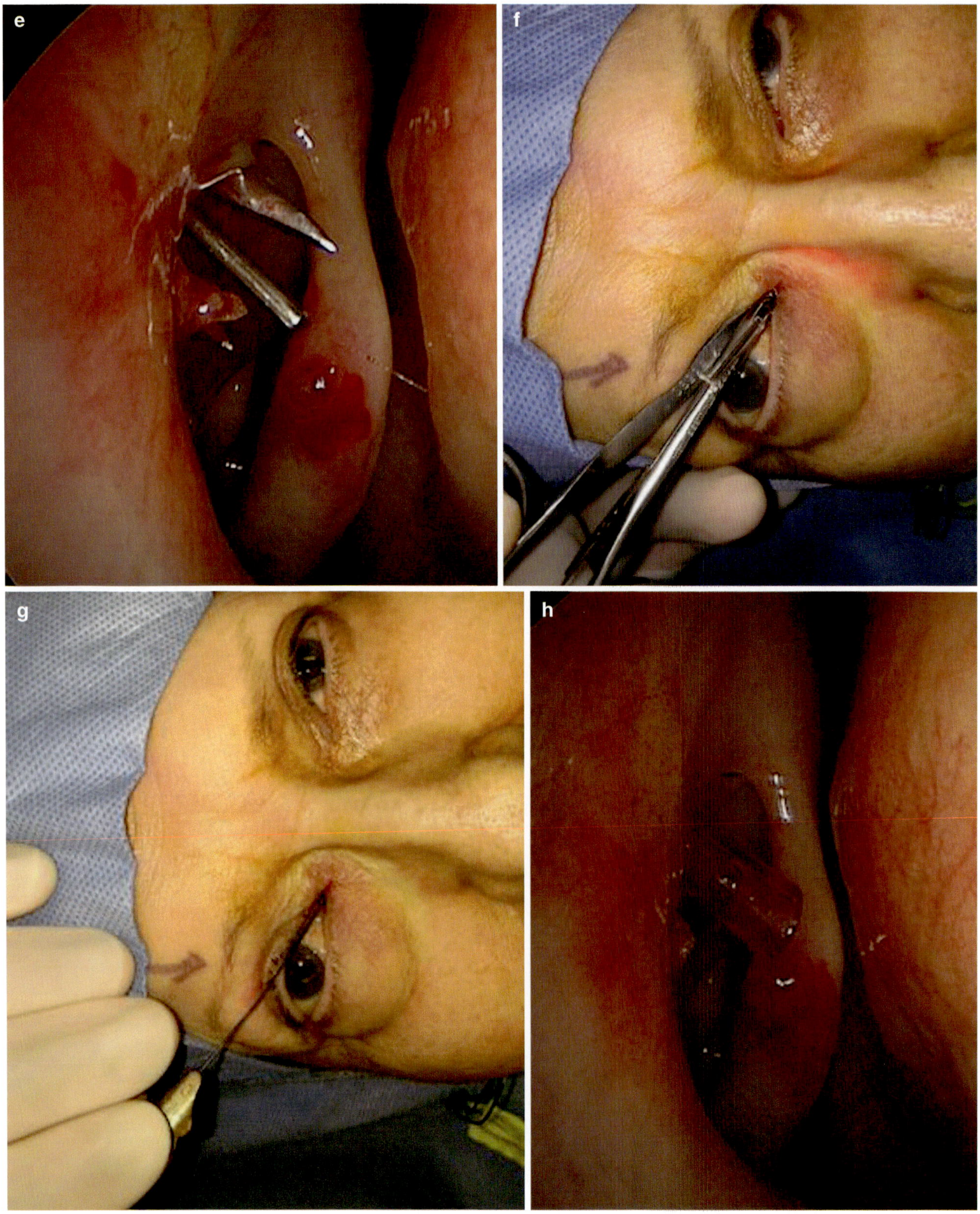

Fig. 48.6 (continued)

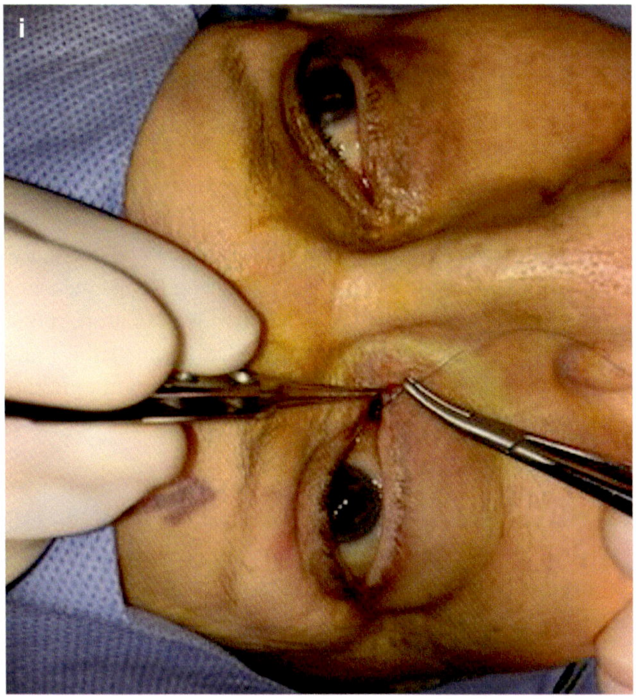

Fig. 48.6 (continued)

Post DCR Patient

In patients who have previously undergone a dacryocystorhinostomy, it is important to ensure adequate bone removal has been performed. This can be done through an external incision or endoscopically. Once adequate bone removal is ensured, the Jones tube is placed as previously described.

Postoperative Care

For the most optimum function, the Jones tube requires maintenance from the surgeon and patient after CDCR:

A. Home Care
   The Jones tube is prone to develop obstruction over time due to deposition of mucous and tear salts. In an effort to prevent this, patients are instructed to place an artificial tear in the eye on a daily basis and "snuff" it through the tube by pinching their nose and inspiring. This irrigates the internal aspect of the tube and helps prevent buildup of debris. Similarly, the patient can use saline nasal irrigation or corticosteroid spray if they have issues with nasal crusting or congestion. At the same time of the artificial tear placement, the patient should make sure the tube collar is visible with no significant change in position.
B. Office Cleaning
   Jones tubes are routinely scheduled for in-office cleaning on a semiannual or annual basis. However, the frequency of follow-up is often dictated by the patient, with earlier visits for those experiencing sluggish outflow. If properly performed, the tube cleaning is generally well tolerated. Atomized anesthetic is sprayed in the appropriate naris followed by instillation of topical anesthetic to the eye. The Jones tube collar is then grasped with forceps and removed. A Weiss (gold) dilator (Gunther Weiss Scientific Glass Blowing Company, Portland, Oregon) (Fig. 48.7) is immediately placed in the tract to avoid contracture while the tube is being cleaned.

   The tube is cleaned by rubbing the tube under running water or with an alcohol wipe taking care to remove any external debris. A piece of alcohol-soaked cotton is then pushed through the tube using a Bowman probe to clean the internal lumen. Alternatively, ultrasonic cleaning may be used.

   The tube is then "loaded" on a Bowman probe. The Weiss dilator is removed, and the Bowman probe is

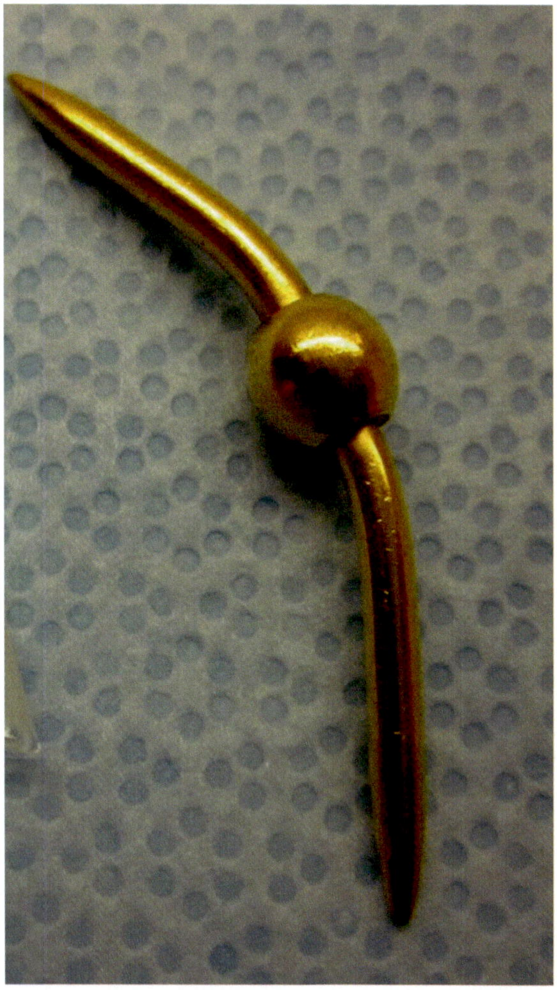

Fig. 48.7 A Weiss (gold) dilator (Gunther Weiss Scientific Glass Blowing Company, Portland, Oregon)

passed into the nose, followed by gentle pressure with forceps to advance the Jones tube into proper position. If the patient is squeezing their eyelids tightly, having an assistant pull the medial canthus toward the nose with the lids held open can improve exposure. Injection of local anesthetic is rarely needed. Proper placement in the nose is confirmed by examination with a headlight and a nasal speculum. The patient is asked to "snuff" in to check tube function. An audible suction noise confirms patency. Patency can also be demonstrated to the patient by irrigation through the Jones tube with a lacrimal cannula, but is not necessary.

At each visit, the proximal and distal position of the tube should be evaluated. The collar size and length can be adjusted according to any patient issues that may arise.

Patients are educated to call with any blockage in the tube or any change in position. If blockage of the tube occurs, the patient should be examined to check tube function, inspect medial canthal and intranasal position, and ensure no proximal or distal obstruction. If the tube is no longer visible, the patient is instructed to call to be seen as soon as possible to try to replace the tube. Within the first 24 hours, it is usually possible to dilate the tract with the Weiss (gold) dilator and replace the tube. If the dilator cannot be passed, an attempt can be made to re-establish the tract using local anesthetic in the office, or a new tract can be created in the operating room with intravenous sedation for patient comfort.

Given the chronic maintenance required and the potential lifelong complications that may arise, appropriate patient selection is necessary to avoid CDCR surgery in those with poor follow-up or limited cooperation.

Complications of Jones Tubes

A. Air Flow
Jones tubes are not tolerated by all patients and occasionally require removal. One of the most common complaints is related to the bi-directional nature of the tube [14–19]. Patients are often bothered by air puffing onto their eye when they blow their nose or describe a splattering of tears on their glasses. Patients with obstructive sleep apnea who use a CPAP machine can be especially bothered in this regard. Attempts can be made to adjust the type of mask or settings on the CPAP machine, but this may still not provide a satisfactory solution. A mask that fits over both the nose and the tube can sometimes be beneficial as this produces equivalent air pressure on either side of the tube. If the patient continues to have problems, bone wax can be placed to provide temporary closure or the tube can be removed.

B. Chronic Conjunctival Inflammation
Occasionally, the patient will develop a chronic conjunctivitis in the medial canthal area. This usually occurs from debris deposition on the outside of the tube that can be scraped off of the tube during the routine cleaning process to improve the patient's symptoms. The conjunctivitis will typically respond nicely to a 2-week course of an antibiotic/steroid drop administered twice daily. Chronic inflammation may also be secondary to mechanical pressure and irritation from the tube collar. Rarely a pyogenic granuloma can develop adjacent to the tube. This can be treated conservatively with an antibiotic/steroid drop or excised in the office.

C. Infection
Over time, the tube may serve as a nidus for infection as it accumulates bacterial debris and biofilms [20, 21]. This can usually be treated sufficiently with tube cleaning and a short course of a topical antibiotic/steroid drop.

D. Tube Obstruction
Proximal mechanical blockage of the upper tube by a flap of conjunctiva or caruncle can occur. This is generally resolved with tissue excision or a larger collar size. In rare instances, the tube may need to be repositioned if the angle of the bypass tract does not allow the proximal tube to have sufficient clearance.

E. Tube Extrusion/Migration
Extrusion or migration of the tube is not uncommon, due to its design that allows for periodic removal. Extrusion rates vary greatly depending on surgical technique and type of tube and can occur anytime throughout the life of the patient [2, 3, 9, 11, 22]. If the tube demonstrates inward migration, the collar size can be increased by 0.5 mm increments with the tube length left the same or slightly longer. If extrusion is an issue, the tube can be lengthened by 1–2 mm or a smaller diameter collar can be used. The StopLoss Jones tube design now incorporates a soft umbrella at the distal tube inside the nose that may minimize the upward extrusion of the tube while still permitting removal for cleaning if necessary.

F. Breakage
Although uncommon, the tube may fracture in the setting of blunt facial trauma.

Conclusion

Conjunctivodacryocystorhinostomy (CDCR) with insertion of a Jones tube remains the gold standard for treatment of upper lacrimal system disorders. By creating a new outflow pathway for tears, symptomatic epiphora can be greatly improved. Appropriate postoperative care including tube maintenance, patient education, and regular follow-up remains essential for optimal outcomes and patient satisfaction.

References

1. Jones LT, Wobig JL. Surgery of the eyelids and lacrimal system. Birmingham: Aesculapius Pub. Co; 1976. p. 241.
2. Bagdonaite L, Pearson AR. Early experience with the StopLoss Jones tube. Orbit. 2015;34(3):132–6.
3. Dailey RA, Tower RN. Frosted jones pyrex tubes. Ophthal Plast Reconstr Surg. 2005;21(3):185–7.
4. Fan X, Bi X, Fu Y, Zhou H. The use of Medpor coated tear drainage tube in conjunctivodacryocystorhinostomy. Eye (Lond). 2008;22(9):1148–53.
5. Gladstone GJ, Putterman AM. A modified glass tube for conjunctivodacryocystorhinostomy. Arch Ophthalmol. 1985;103(8):1229–30.
6. Massry GG, Larian B. A novel technique of Jones tube fixation for refractory tube extrusion. Ophthal Plast Reconstr Surg. 2012;28(6):e150–1.
7. Mombaerts I, Colla B. Modified Jones' lacrimal bypass surgery with an angled extended Jones' tube. Ophthalmology. 2007;114(7):1403–8.
8. Steele EA, Dailey RA. Conjunctivodacryocystorhinostomy with the frosted jones pyrex tube. Ophthal Plast Reconstr Surg. 2009;25(1):42–3.
9. Witters E, Mombaerts I. The survival of an angled extended Jones' tube. Br J Ophthalmol. 2015;99(11):1523–6.
10. Wobig JL, Dailey RA. Oculofacial plastic surgery: face, lacrimal system, and orbit. New York: Thieme; 2004. xi, 290
11. Lim C, Martin P, Benger R, Kourt G, Ghabrial R. Lacrimal canalicular bypass surgery with the Lester Jones tube. Am J Ophthalmol. 2004;137(1):101–8.
12. Shin DH, Kim YD, Lee CH, Johnson ON 3rd, Woo KI. Restrictive strabismus and diplopia 2 years after Conjunctivodacryocystorhinostomy with Medpor-coated tear drain. Ophthal Plast Reconstr Surg. 2015;31(6):e159–62.
13. Tawfik HA, Abdulhafez MH. Re: "twelve-year experience of Lester Jones tubes-results and comparison of three different tube types". Ophthal Plast Reconstr Surg. 2016;32(2):156.
14. Ginat DT, Freitag SK. Orbital emphysema complicating jones tube placement in a patient treated with continuous positive airway pressure. Ophthal Plast Reconstr Surg. 2015;31(1):e25.
15. Goldberg DS. Management of air regurgitation through a jones tube in a patient using continuous positive airway pressure. Ophthal Plast Reconstr Surg. 2011;27(3):e76–7.
16. Kreis AJ, Mehat MS, Madge SN. Periorbital emphysema: an unusual complication of lacrimal canalicular bypass surgery with the Lester-Jones tube. Clin Exp Ophthalmol. 2014;42(2):201–2.
17. Longmire MR, Carter KD, Allen RC. Intolerance of jones tube placement in a patient using continuous positive airway pressure. Ophthal Plast Reconstr Surg. 2010;26(1):68–9.
18. Servat JJ, Black EH, Gladstone GJ. A solution to the Jones tube continuous positive airway pressure (CPAP) dilemma? Ophthal Plast Reconstr Surg. 2012;28(6):e151–2.
19. Vicinanzo MG, Allamneni C, Compton CJ, Long JA, Nabavi CB. The prevalence of air regurgitation and its consequences after conjunctivodacryocystorhinostomy and dacryocystorhinostomy in continuous positive airway pressure patients. Ophthal Plast Reconstr Surg. 2015;31(4):269–71.
20. Costerton JW, Stewart PS, Greenberg EP. Bacterial biofilms: a common cause of persistent infections. Science. 1999;284(5418):1318–22.
21. Parsa K, Schaudinn C, Gorur A, Sedghizadeh PP, Johnson T, Tse DT, et al. Demonstration of bacterial biofilms in culture-negative silicone stent and jones tube. Ophthal Plast Reconstr Surg. 2010;26(6):426–30.
22. Bagdonaite L, Pearson AR. Twelve-year experience of Lester Jones tubes-results and comparison of 3 different tube types. Ophthal Plast Reconstr Surg. 2015;31(5):352–6.

Dacryocystectomy

49

Jane Olver

Definitions

Dacryocystectomy (DCT) is defined as the excision of the lacrimal sac wall.

Rethinking DCT in the Twenty-First Century

Dacryocystectomy (DCT) had been regarded in the past as a mutilating type of surgery and reserved mainly for the excision of lacrimal sac tumors or severe chronic dacryocystitis in elderly frail persons. However, DCT can have other indications [1–3].

Removal of the lacrimal sac, or DCT, is performed much more often then we realize. We often erroneously assume that DCT means the total excision of the lacrimal sac by an external approach. However, it can also apply to the surgical removal of only part of lacrimal sac in which case it is called a partial dacryocystectomy as opposes to a total DCT. In addition, DCT can be performed either via an external skin incision or endonasally, depending on the indications.

We now have a new approach to the term and use of DCT (dacryocystectomy), including an encompassing classification and spectrum of indications.

Indications for and Types of Dacryocystectomy (DCT)

A. External approach DCT
   I. Partial dacryocystectomy (PExt-DCT)
      (a) Lacrimal sac outpouching
      (b) Segmented sac with partial dacryocystitis
   II. Total dacryocystectomy (TExt-DCT)
      (a) Chronic dacryocystitis
      (b) Lacrimal sac tumor
   III. Extended dacryocystectomy (EExt-DCT) with nasolacrimal duct, surrounding soft tissue and bone
      (a) Lacrimal sac tumors
      (b) Extrinsic tumors involving the lacrimal fossa and nasolacrimal duct
B. Endoscopic endonasal DCT
   I. Partial dacryocystectomy (PEnd-DCT)
      (a) Biopsy of lacrimal sac
   II. Subtotal dacryocystectomy (STEnd-DCT)
      (a) Large lacrimal sac with diverticuli
   III. Total dacryocystectomy (TEnd -DCT)
      (a) Planned removal of the entire lacrimal sac, often with the common canaliculus and partial excision of the canaliculi
      (b) Performed inadvertently during dacryocystorhinostomy
      (c) Planned for removal of secondary scarred/fibrotic or inflamed lacrimal sac
   IV. Extended dacryocystectomy (EEnd-DCT)
      (a) Removal of all the lacrimal sac, nasolacrimal duct (NLD), and lateral nasal wall structures for lacrimal sac tumor extending into the NLD

J. Olver (✉)
Oculoplastic and Lacrimal, Clinica London, London, UK
e-mail: Jane.Olver@clinicalondon.co.uk

Dacryocystorhinostomy (DCR)

DCR was originally performed through an external skin incision and can be dated to the early part of the eighteenth century, described by Woolhouse in 1724 [4].

The term dacryocystorhinostomy (DCR) indicates making an opening between the tear lake (dacryo), the lacrimal scar (cysto), and the nose via a hole in the nose (rhinostomy). DCR makes no mention of whether the lacrimal sac wall is left completely intact, partially excised, or totally removed.

A. J. Cohen, C. N. Burkat (eds.), *Oculofacial, Orbital, and Lacrimal Surgery*, https://doi.org/10.1007/978-3-030-14092-2_49

DCR (dacryocystorhinostomy) can include DCT (dacryocystectomy) whenever the lacrimal sac or part of it is excised.

Canaliculo-rhinostomy-DCT is the term used for a DCT in which the sac and lacrimal fossa bone is removed along with the common canaliculus and even part of the canaliculi.

History of Dacryocystectomy (DCT)

DCT was one of the earliest and easiest operations to do for chronic dacryocystitis with lacrimal fistulas and also for certain indications such as malignant lacrimal sac tumors. Historically, DCT was regarded as a gold standard for chronic dacryocystitis in the eighteenth, nineteenth, and early twentieth centuries, particularly where there were lacrimal fistulas.

Once DCR was introduced, external approach DCT remained but with a limited role for elderly frail patients with dacryocystitis, for patients with lacrimal sac tumors, and where the systemic disease was affecting the lacrimal sac such as granulomatosis with polyangiitis (Wegener's granulomatosis) or mucocutaneous leishmaniasis. Although these remain indications, our understanding of DCT is changing, and it is again becoming a more mainstream option.

Many ophthalmologists regard DCT for chronic dacryocystitis as a potential primary procedure in individuals over 70 years old because the surgery done via an external approach has a very low risk particularly when there are other associated comorbidities related to their age [5].

DCT has an important role in Wegener's granulomatosis and chronic dacryocystitis because it gets rid of the troublesome discharge and has a good functional result with relief of the dacryocystitis. In patients with Wegener's granulomatous and chronic dacryocystitis, the patients' symptoms of discharge and suppuration from the skin are often more greatly distressing than the epiphora; therefore, an operation that removes the dacryocystitis is likely to provide relief even if a watery eye remains in approximately 25% of those who undergo DCT [6].

Historical Shift in Our Perspective

Lacrimal surgery existed in the middle ages for the treatment of dacryocystitis from a blocked nasolacrimal duct. It was then restricted to a crude external drainage of abscess and extirpation of lacrimal sac. This was the original dacryocystectomy (DCT) and represented a very much pre-antibiotic era where the blockage of a nasolacrimal duct could result in chronic recurrent dacryocystitis and fistula. However, the sophistication of lacrimal surgery with the advent of endoscopic endonasal DCR using precise and delicate surgical techniques with miniature powered intranasal tools and FESS (functional endoscopic sinus surgery) instruments has shifted us away from external DCR to an endoscopic, endonasal dacryocystorhinostomy.

With many centers performing lacrimal surgery endonasally and endoscopically, and using power tools, microscopes, or functional endoscopic sinus surgery (FESS) instruments in adults and children, these techniques are being applied to DCT (dacryocystectomy) as well [7].

Dacryocystectomy (DCT) is shifting from an external approach with total removal of sac to endonasal DCT with partial or total removal of the lacrimal sac [7].

This shift in perspective is very similar to the shift in cataract surgery techniques, which was seen toward the end of the twentieth century in the 1980s with intracapsular to extracapsular cataract extraction where the spectrum of disease changed from dense white cataracts or dark nuclear sclerosis to lighter, subtler lenticular opacities. The approach then further changed to phacoemulsification extraction in the 1990s and more recently laser treatment and other options for mild lenticular opacity.

Patient expectations of surgery have also changed and indeed increased. A real quality of life benefit for patients with watery sticky eyes can be attained by not only DCR but also DCT by an external or endonasal approach.

Current Concepts and Techniques of Dacryocystectomy

DCT can be done either via an external excision under local anesthetic or can be done via an endonasal approach either under local anesthetic with sedation or with general anesthetic.

Similar to our philosophy about DCR versus nasolacrimal duct (NLD) intubation, we are changing our way of thinking about the spectrum of lacrimal disease from a true "black and white" picture of total nasolacrimal duct obstruction to partial nasolacrimal duct obstruction and milder forms of epiphora. The indications for external DCR versus indication for endonasal graded DCR and NLD surgery are based on each individual assessment and the differing spectrum of disease. These small variations include doing degrees of DCT as well, as indicated by suspected tumor or abnormal mucosa requiring DCT biopsy.

Types of DCT (Dacryocystectomy)

The prevailing perception of DCT is external approach removal for chronic dacryocystitis and for lacrimal sac tumor, particularly if it affects the elderly. However, we need to examine the more extensive use of DCT or partial DCT. Surgeons are often performing a partial DCT, either externally or endonasally, without really appreciating this.

Case Example 1: External DCT

For instance, when a medial canthal basal cell carcinoma is invading the caruncle and medial canthal tendon, there is often excision of the medial canthus with removal of the lacrimal sac and possibly bone in the lacrimal fossa. This is a DCT (dacryocystectomy). Following initial oculoplastic reconstruction, a secondary surgery of formal DCR and placement of a Jones bypass tube may be required to relieve persistent epiphora.

Case Example 2: Endoscopic Endonasal Partial DCT

A patient with suspected lacrimal pathology has a DCR via an endonasal approach, and a specimen of the lacrimal sac is taken for histopathological analysis. This is a partial DCT biopsy.

As in DCR surgery, there has been a change in concept from external approach DCT to an endoscopic endonasal approach DCT. Although an endoscopic endonasal DCT involves a DCR in so much that the bone between the nose and the lacrimal sac has to be removed, it indeed can be a DCT. It is a DCT if the lacrimal sac is either partially or totally removed, or extirpated, leaving either a remnant of lacrimal sac and common canaliculus or merely the common canalicular opening into the nasal space.

Expanding on the second case above, if all of the sac is removed for whatever purpose, be it biopsy or because small and scarred, and a canalicular DCR is done endonasally, this constitutes a total endoscopic endonasal DCT.

Case Example 3: Extended Endonasal Endoscopic DCT

A patient with an intrinsic lacrimal sac tumor extending into the lacrimal sac requires an extended DCT, in which the NLD and structures of the lateral nasal wall are also excised.

Aims of All Dacryocystectomy (DCT) Approaches

The surgical goals of DCT are to remove the entire lacrimal sac or part of the lacrimal sac if it is partial DCT while preserving the periorbita. If necessary, the bone may need to be traversed if through an endonasal approach DCT.

A complete or total DCT involves complete excision of the sac leaving the canaliculi, the nasolacrimal duct, and the surrounding tissues such as the medial canthal tendon intact. However, variations exist as there may be situations where it is necessary to remove the canaliculi or they are removed via Mohs micrographic surgery or en bloc removal of a medial canthal tumor.

An extended DCT may be indicated if there is involvement of the sac by an intrinsic or extrinsic tumor, and the nasolacrimal duct is also involved. In such a case, an extended DCT with extirpation of the nasolacrimal duct and any involved surrounding tissue is required.

Categories and Subcategories of DCT

First Category

A. External approach DCT
   I. Partial external dacryocystectomy (less common) (PExt-DCT) for lacrimal sac outpouching and segmented sac with partial dacryocystitis
   II. Total external dacryocystectomy (TExt-DCT) for chronic dacryocystitis and lacrimal sac tumor
   III. Extended external dacryocystectomy (EExt-DCT) with the nasolacrimal duct, surrounding soft tissue, and bone as indicated particularly for lacrimal sac tumors and extrinsic tumors involving the lacrimal fossa and nasolacrimal duct, such as malignant melanoma of the nasolacrimal duct

Second Category

B. Endoscopic endonasal DCT
   IV. Partial endonasal dacryocystectomy (PEnd-DCT) for biopsy of lacrimal sac and for diagnostic purposes, particularly when a possible lacrimal sac tumor is suspected but not yet diagnosed.
   V. Subtotal endonasal dacryocystectomy (STEnd-DCT) when there is an enlarged lacrimal sac with diverticuli where the lacrimal sac has to be removed as much as possible, but leaving a small sac remnant will not be detrimental to success as long as the lacrimal sac mucosa is draining intranasally.
   VI. Total endonasal dacryocystectomy (TEnd-DCT) when there is planned removal of the entire lacrimal

sac, often with the common canaliculus and partial excision of the canaliculi. This is typically performed for removal of extremely scarred/fibrotic or inflamed lacrimal sacs, for complete excision of tumors isolated within the sac, or inadvertently during dacryocystorhinostomy.

VII. Extended endonasal dacryocystectomy (EEnd-DCT) where not only all the lacrimal sac but also the nasolacrimal duct and lateral nasal wall structures are removed due to lacrimal sac or sinonasal tumors extending into the NLD.

External DCT Surgical Technique

External approach DCT is typically reserved for adults, although there have been reports of it being performed in children such as in a case report of posttraumatic nasolacrimal drainage obstruction following nasoorbitoethmoid (NOE) fracture [8].

The main benefit of an external approach DCT is that it is a relatively avascular and quick technique that can be performed under local anesthetic. It is relatively noninvasive, does not enter the nose or risk bleeding within the nasopharynx, and has rapid recovery in most cases.

(a) Type of anesthesia

External approach DCT can be done under local anesthetic, intravenous sedation, or general anesthetic. Careful injection of local anesthetic (lidocaine with epinephrine) with infiltration around the sac and medial canthus assists in hemostasis. If required, an infratrochlear nerve block, as well as a medial anterior orbital and/or infraorbital nerve block, can be utilized.

(b) Incision for Ext-DCT

The tear trough incision or lateral nasal wall incision is used, with the length of incision dependent on the pathology. In the setting of chronic dacryocystitis, surgery may be preferred from a more remote site such as the lateral nasal wall rather than directly over the dacryocystitis, particularly if it is quite ulcerated or fistulous. If imaging demonstrates a malignant lacrimal sac tumor, the incision may be made longer in order to facilitate complete removal of the sac and any further excision of the nasolacrimal duct and surrounding tissue, such as a lateral rhinostomy.

(c) Isolation of the lacrimal sac in Ext-DCT

The main aim of the external approach dacryocystectomy is to isolate part of the sac, or the whole lacrimal sac, within the lacrimal sac fossa.

The anterior lacrimal crest of the maxillary bone and the posterior lacrimal crest on the lacrimal bone must be identified and the sac gently teased with Freer elevators from the bone. Then its superior attachments to the medial canthal tendon are divided, and the inferior connection to the nasolacrimal duct must be divided and cauterized. Once released, the entire sac and periorbita can be reflected laterally, and the sac is dissected out and divided from the common canaliculus.

(d) Use of viscoelastic to inflate and identify the lacrimal sac

A useful tip for DCT is to use a viscoelastic to inflate the lacrimal sac [9]. Viscoelastic injected through the punctum into the lacrimal sac helps the surgeon see the dilated lacrimal sac during dissection for DCT. One article described performing DCT with bone preservation for a patient with Wegener's granulomatosis, using canalicular clamps during DCT to keep the viscoelastic substance confined within the lacrimal sac.

(e) Canalicular cauterization

The common canaliculus, or canalicular ends, must be cauterized well in order to prevent tears draining into the soft tissues of the surgical area.

(f) Wound closure

Once the sac has been removed, the wound is closed in the usual fashion.

Endoscopic Endonasal DCT Surgical Technique

This is similar to external approach DCT but is performed endonasally with endoscopic visualization. The advantages are the lack of skin incision and greater endonasal visibility; however, the operative field is narrower and requires a greater learning curve to perform with expertise. Surgical anastomoses of the mucosal flaps are also more difficult.

(a) Removal of lacrimal fossa bone is an essential and unavoidable step in this surgical approach

The bone and lacrimal sac are removed from the endonasal approach. Although this involves a bony rhinostomy similar to a DCR, it is classified as a DCT if the lacrimal sac is removed fully or a partial DCT if the sac is partially removed. We are, therefore, often performing an endoscopic endonasal DCT without realizing it during a DCR.

(b) Consideration of the canaliculi at endonasal DCT

Whether dacryocystectomy is performed via the external or endonasal approach, management of the distal canaliculi is necessary to consider. Preservation of the canaliculi for drainage of tears (DCR element) may be considered, particularly if the patient is elderly and/or has significant dry eye syndrome.

Similar to external approach DCT, it is customary to cauterize the common canalicular opening if a total endoscopic endonasal DCT for tumor has been performed. In contrast, this is not necessary if a partial DCT was performed for simple lacrimal sac biopsy with normal canaliculi, and drainage of tears is desired.

Canalicular Variations of DCT

If the common canaliculus or part of the canaliculi are removed during DCT, it is referred to as a canalicular DCT or a canaliculorhinostomy DCT if there is also bone removal with a DCR. This is irrespective of whether the DCT is approached via an external, endonasal, or combined approach.

The common canaliculus and any amount of canaliculi can be removed at the same time as DCT or subsequently, or the common canaliculus opened directly into the lateral nasal wall [10]. Olga et al. described a case of a lacrimal sac that was initially biopsied and found to have a benign fibrous histiocytoma. Subsequently, a dacryocystectomy was performed as a DCR had already been performed with a bone opening. They identified the common canaliculus and attached it to a nasal mucosal flap via an external approach, along with silicone intubation with good results. This is a good example of a planned secondary external DCT status post dacryocystorhinostomy, where drainage was also possible with the canaliculi opened into the nose. It especially shows us the range of DCT possible.

Hemostasis in Dacryocystectomy

Hemostasis is not generally a problem with a standard external or endonasal endoscopic DCT but may be encountered with more extended DCT surgery.

Postoperative Care

Postoperative follow-up of DCT is similar to that of the standard external approach DCR or endoscopic endonasal DCR if the indication for removal of part of or all of the lacrimal sac is benign. However, if the indication for DCT is lacrimal sac tumor, either from within the lacrimal sac or from without, then follow-up is dictated by the nature and spread of the tumor. A multidisciplinary team approach is recommended in order to plan further therapy and monitoring.

Effectiveness of DCT

Since there are many various indications for DCT, there are limited studies demonstrating overall results. In addition, if the surgical indication was for a lacrimal sac tumor, the outcome is dependent on the nature of the tumor and its stage at removal [11]. Lee et al. described a case of local DCT excision that resulted in an aesthetically satisfying result and a long cancer-free period, which exemplifies the diverse use of dacryocystectomy. Alkatan et al. performed a retrospective review of all lacrimal sac specimens received over a 12-year period, which included 498 specimens from 459 patients. Although the incidence of pathology was low, biopsy (partial DCT) is considered useful at DCR in order to avoid missing incidental malignancy [12].

Risks of DCT and Surgical Consent

There has been a single recorded episode of visual loss during DCT in 2006 [13].

This was a case report of a 65-year-old patient who underwent bilateral DCT, complicated by pain and loss of vision to light perception from a retrobulbar hemorrhage. Although rare, all patients undergoing DCT should thus be aware of the real, but extremely low, risks of losing eyesight with any surgery around the eye.

Summary

Dacryocystectomy is a much more commonly used lacrimal procedure than we realize. Whereas it was historically performed for mainly lacrimal sac tumors or chronic dacryocystitis in elderly patients unable to undergo general anesthesia, it has become more common as we perform more graded surgery specifically tailored to each patient.

References

1. Matayoshi S, Van Baak A, Cozak A, Sardinha M, Fernandes JB, da Mota Moura E. Dacryocystectomy indications and results. Orbit. 2004;23(3):169–73.
2. Cook HL, Olver JM. Dacryocystectomy as a treatment of chronic dacryocystitis in a frail elderly patient. Eye. 2004;18(3):334–6.

3. Boynton JR, Anawis MA. Role of dacryocystectomy in the management of failed dacryocystorhinostomy associated with chronic dacryocystitis. Ophthalmic Surg Lasers. 1996;27(2):133–6.
4. Ali MJ. Dacryocystectomy: goals, indications, techniques and complications. Ophthalmic Plast Reconstr Surg. 2014;30(6):512–6.
5. Meireles MN, Viveiros MMH, Meneghin RLFS, Galindo-Ferreiro A, Markques MEA, Schellini SA. Dacryocystectomy as a treatment of chronic dacryocystitis in the elderly. Orbit. 2017;36:419–21.
6. Wegener's Granulomatosis Dacryocystectomy Case Report, Holds JB, Anderson RL, Wolin MJ. Dacryocystectomy for the treatment of dacryocystitis patients with Wegener's granulomatosis. Ophthalmic Surg. 1989;20(6):443–4.
7. Shams PN, Selva D. An endoscopic endonasal approach to dacryocystectomy. Orbit. 2013;32(2):134–6.
8. Varghese SM, Varghese AM, Syed KA, Paul RR. Dacryocystectomy an uncommon Indication, a case report. Int J Pediatr Otorhinolaryngol. 2014;78(1):139–41.
9. Baddeley PA, Lewis GD, Lane CM. A novel technique to facilitate dacryocystectomy using viscoelastic substances. Orbit. 2011;30(3):158–9.
10. Olga JJ, Sims LM. Canaliculorhinostomy following dacryocystectomy for removal of a benign fibrous histiocytoma of the lacrimal SAC. Ophthalmic Surg. 1993;24(11):753–4.
11. Lee SB, Kim KN, Lee SR, Bernardino CR. Mucoepidermoid carcinoma of the lacrimal sac after dacryocystectomy for squamous papilloma. Ophthalmic Plast Reconstr Surg. 2011;27:E44–6.
12. Discussion on Histopathological Examination of Lacrimal Sac Specimens, Alkatan H, Al-Qurashi M. Is routine histopathological examination of dacryocystorhinostomy/dacryocystectomy specimens necessary? A tertiary eye hospital experience. Can J Ophthalmol. 2017;52(1):34–41.
13. Pai VH, Rao DK. Bhandary synergy report. Visual loss following dacryocystectomy. Ophthalmic Surg Lasers Imaging. 2006;37(6):494–6.

Congenital Dacryocystocele: Diagnosis and Management

50

Pelin Kaynak

Introduction

Congenital dacryocystocele (also known as dacryocele, amniocele, amniotocele) is a diffuse, nonneoplastic, cystic dilation of the lacrimal sac, which generally appears as a bluish-gray swelling below the medial canthal tendon seen at the time of birth or within the early perinatal period [1–5] (Fig. 50.1). It occurs in newborns with congenital nasolacrimal duct obstruction (CNLDO) as a result of consequent obstruction of proximal opening of the enlarged lacrimal sac, where the Rosenmuller valve acts as a one-way valve, in addition to the incomplete canalization of the distal aperture of the lacrimal drainage apparatus at the level of Hasner's valve [2, 5–7]. The functional obstruction at the proximal opening may also be caused by compression of the dilated lacrimal sac onto the internal common canaliculus and the canaliculi so that these short and fine structures plicate or collapse at the junction site with the sac (Fig. 50.2) [2, 6, 8]. This causes the lacrimal sac compartment to become isolated, with the outflow of fluid blocked. Accumulation of fluid in the drainage system eventually dilates the lacrimal sac into a dacryocystocele. The distal obstruction is anatomical, where the proximal obstruction is functional [2, 9–11]. Occasionally, punctal agenesis or atresia, an anatomical maldevelopment or obstruction, can be the cause of congenital dacryocystocele [12, 13]. Two patients with congenital punctal agenesis and CNLDO with dacryocystoceles that slowly enlarged

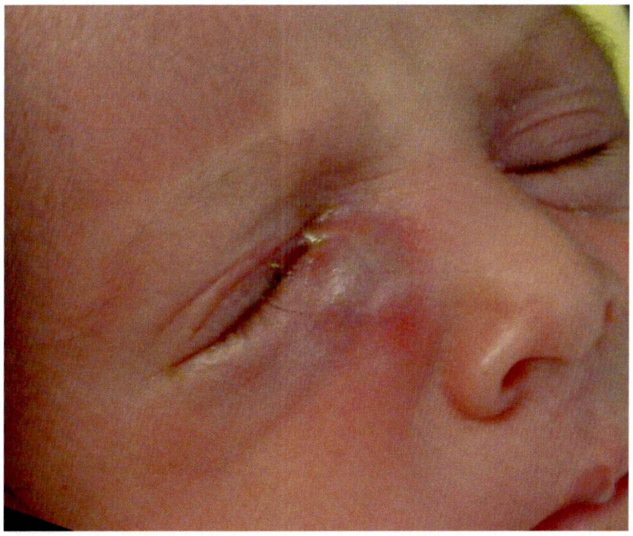

Fig. 50.1 Congenital dacryocystocele in a newborn

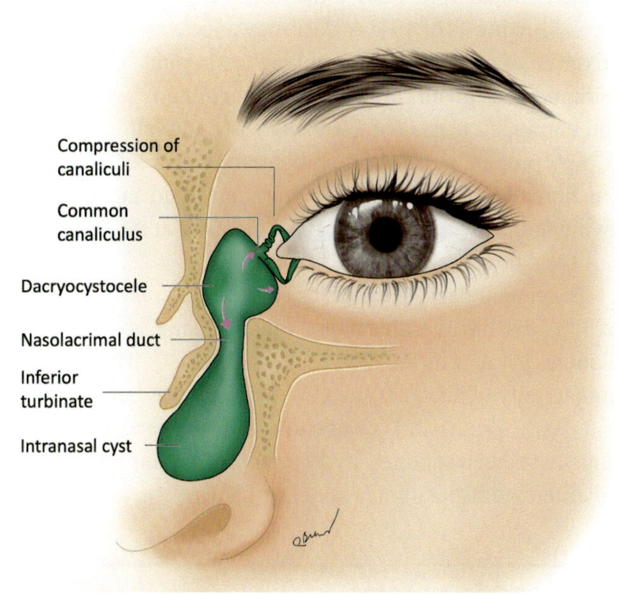

Fig. 50.2 Schematic representation of dacryocystocele formation in CNLDO. Kinking of the canaliculi at the canaliculo-saccal junction (pink arrow) and cystic protrusion of membranous lacrimal mucosa at the level of the uncanalized valve of Hasner (purple arrow). (Illustration courtesy of Cat N. Burkat, MD)

P. Kaynak (✉)
Rufus Eye Microsurgical Center, Ophthalmic Plastic and Reconstructive Surgery Division, Istanbul, Turkey

A. J. Cohen, C. N. Burkat (eds.), *Oculofacial, Orbital, and Lacrimal Surgery*, https://doi.org/10.1007/978-3-030-14092-2_50

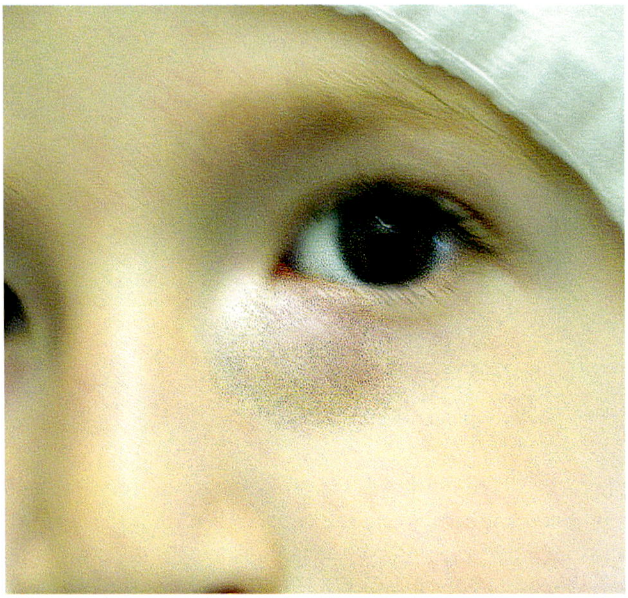

Fig. 50.3 Late-onset enlargement of an uninfected dacryocystocele in a 6-year-old boy with lower punctal atresia

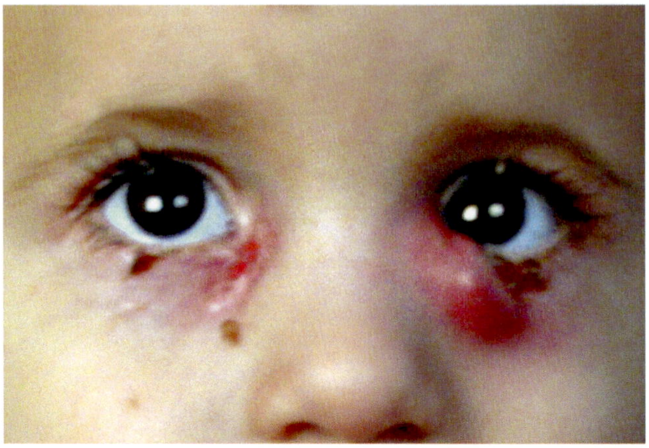

Fig. 50.4 Dacryocystitis (right side) and dacryocystocele (left side) in a 2-year-old child

over years during childhood (Fig. 50.3) have been reported in two publications [14, 15]. One of these patients had alacrima related to lacrimo-auriculo-dento-digital (LADD) syndrome [15].

The terms amniotocele, or amniocele, were also used for dacryocystoceles present at birth referring to the probable presence of amniotic fluid in the lacrimal sac as a result of in utero blinking [16, 17]. A dacryocystocele is filled with a mixture of secretions of goblet cells and submucosal seromucinous glands of the inner epithelium of lacrimal tract and entrapped tears. The clear fluid is light yellow in color. A high protein and potassium content differs it from amniotic fluid. It reflects the transmembranous fluid and ion fluxes owing to the presence of apical cellular villi at the lumen and cell breakdown products [18, 19].

Congenital dacryocystoceles are seen in approximately 1 of 3900 live births with a higher incidence in Caucasian populations [4] and in females up to 73% [2, 4]. The reported unilaterality of dacryocystoceles in neonates is between 86% and 100% [4, 20–22]. Congenital dacryocystoceles in siblings have been reported by Wang and Cunningham, but an inherited predisposition is not clear [23].

Signs and Symptoms

The most common symptoms of dacryocystocele in the newborn are epiphora and difficulty breathing. Respiratory distress may worsen during breastfeeding, particularly in bilateral cases if an intranasal extension of the dacryocystocele obstructs the nasal cavity. An elevated tear meniscus height and/or overflow of tears in the affected eye in the presence of a bluish-gray, firm, nontender mass located at or below the medial canthus denotes a sterile distension of the lacrimal sac [2, 5, 7, 11, 24].

Secondary infection may begin within days or weeks if the condition is left untreated. Acute dacryocystitis occurs as the retained stagnant fluid becomes infected by microorganisms, generally of bacterial origin. The previously clear secretions then become an opaque yellow-green color consistent with purulence. Crusting of the eyelid margin and eyelashes is common. With dacryocystitis, the lacrimal sac area becomes tender and demonstrates erythema, edema, and calor. Neighboring structures and soft tissues may become inflamed, resulting in secondary preseptal or orbital cellulitis (Fig. 50.4). The dye disappearance test is positive with increased accumulation of fluorescein (limited drainage) in the affected eye. Occasionally, transillumination of the fluid-filled cystic sac can be helpful in determining the diagnosis.

Complications of Congenital Dacryocystoceles

Dacryocystitis is the most common complication, seen in 14–75% of infants with congenital dacryocystoceles, and generally necessitates surgical intervention [4, 20–22]. According to Becker's study of 29 lacrimal sides of 27 patients, 34.5% of lacrimal systems developed dacryocystitis alone, and an additional 37.9% developed dacryocystitis and cellulitis requiring intravenous antibiotic therapy (Fig. 50.5a, b) [10]. Other studies have reported similar high rates of infection [4, 20, 25, 26], although others have shown lower rates of infection [2, 22, 27, 28].

Other common complications of dacryocystoceles are the formation of nasal cysts that may cause respiratory dis-

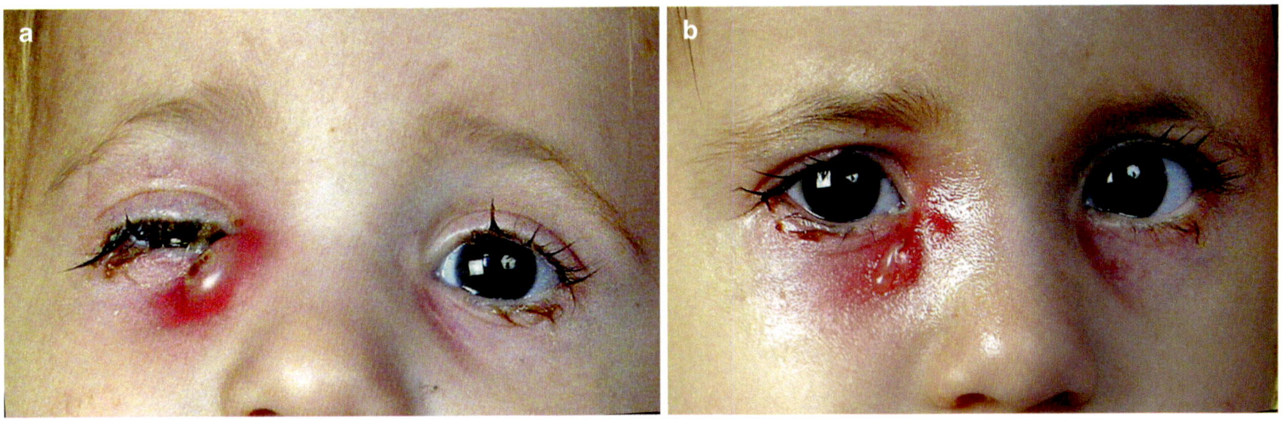

Fig. 50.5 Lacrimal sac abscess in a 2-year-old girl with untreated CNLDO, before (**a**) and after (**b**) antibiotic therapy and probing without marsupialization, with ongoing abscess and cutaneous fistulization

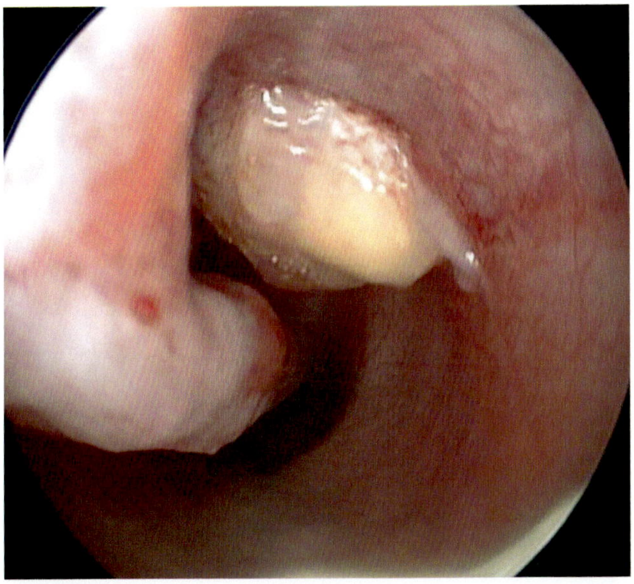

Fig. 50.6 Endoscopic view of an intranasal cyst extension of a dacryocystocele (Courtesy of Y. Özkan Arat)

tress (Fig. 50.6), cutaneous fistulae (Fig. 50.7a–c), and eyelid and orbital abscesses [5, 7, 10, 29, 30]. Rarely, intraorbital enlargement of the dacryocystocele may result in acute proptosis and distortion of the globe. In a case series of four children with dacryoceles that extended to the orbit, the authors discussed the mechanism of congenital dacryocystocele expansion. With an abnormal increase in hydraulic pressure within the sac, the sac most commonly expands in a newborn anteriorly toward the eyelid where it is covered only by the skin and orbicularis muscle. This manifests as the typical bluish-gray mass appearance of an external dacryocystocele. The second potential direction of sac distension is inferiorly through the nasolacrimal duct, resulting in an intranasal cystic expansion. A third direction of expansion has been postulated that may occur due to anatomical variations of the lacrimal sac fossa with less posterior resistance, resulting in cystic expansion of the sac posteriorly into the orbit. In the setting of an infected sac, the already thin walls become even more fragile due to the inflammatory response and may be more prone to unpredictable routes of expansion. Maturing bones forming the nasolacrimal sac fossa and duct may prevent the sac from evaginating inside the nose, initially forcing an anterior, cutaneous route, with recurring episodes of spontaneous external drainage through a fistulous tract (Fig. 50.7a–c). Additionally, if the eyelid skin becomes more scarred, increased resistance to anterior distension may cause the sac to expand posteriorly into the orbit as seen in Fig. 50.8a, b [31]. Severe orbital infections may progress to orbital cellulitis, meningitis, and rarely sepsis. Eyelid disorders such as ectropion, cicatrix formation, lagophthalmos, trichiasis, and corneal erosions and keratitis may ensue. Theoretically, the mass effect of the dilated sac on the globe may induce astigmatism and diplopia and may cause amblyopia if prolonged and untreated.

Diagnostic Imaging

The typical clinical presentation of congenital dacryocystoceles and the relatively short course prior to management minimize the need for imaging studies in the majority of infants [32]. However, ultrasound (US), computerized tomography (CT) scanning, and magnetic resonance imaging (MRI) can be informative if orbital invasion, with or without infection is suspected, and/or neoplasms or meningoencephaloceles are in the differential diagnosis.

Ultrasound (US) is a noninvasive method that can be used in infants, mostly without sedation to distinguish dacryocystoceles from other pathologies [11, 33, 34].

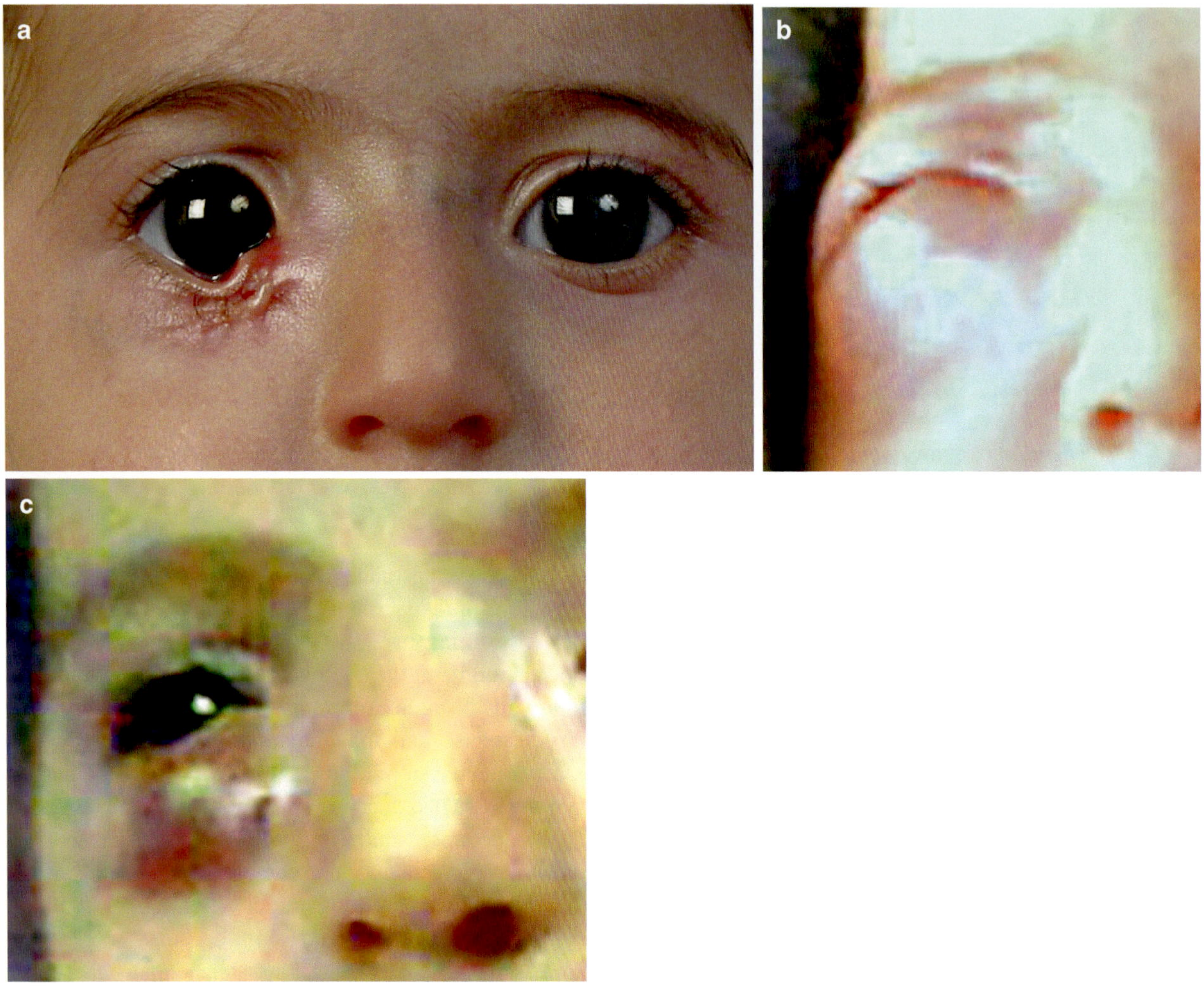

Fig. 50.7 (**a**) Right dacryocystocele swelling below the medial canthal tendon and cicatricial ectropion due to intermittent repeating fistulization of an untreated dacryocystocele in a 7–month-old child. (**b**) Swelling involving the right lower eyelid and cheek of the patient in Fig. 50.7a, several weeks after birth. (**c**) Large dacryocystocele with intraorbital extension and cellulitis after 1 week of massaging

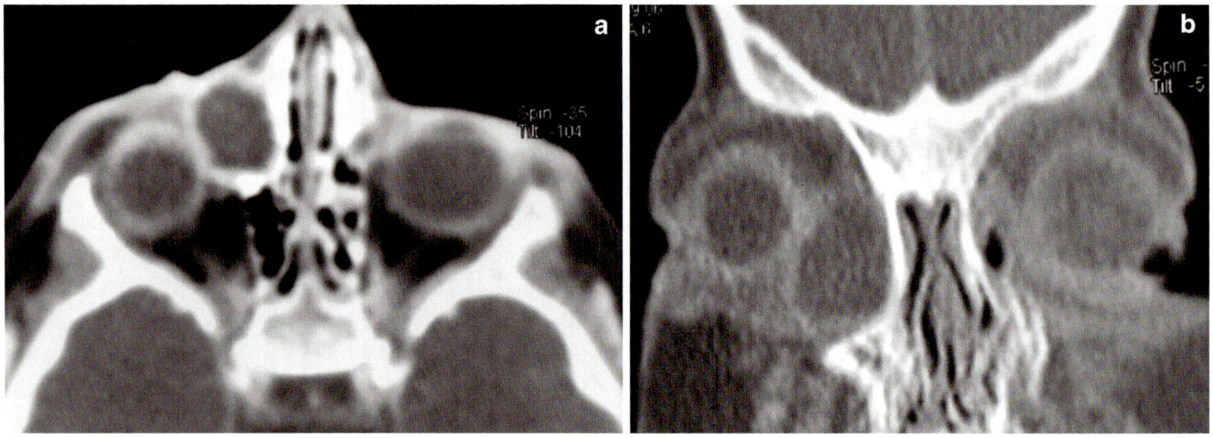

Fig. 50.8 Axial (**a**) and coronal (**b**) CT images of the infant in Fig. 50.7, demonstrating intraorbital extension of the dacryocystocele

Since any fluid-filled structure and any accessible adnexal structure that is close to the surface can be examined by ultrasonic biomicroscopy (UBM), this tool is also used for lacrimal drainage system evaluation. It has also been reported to be able to noninvasively visualize the canaliculosaccal junction and distal lacrimal duct opening, but the need to use a liquid media limits its frequent use in infants [35, 36].

CT imaging has the advantage of detecting bone changes with precision, whereas MRI is more precise in visualizing the soft tissue and the cyst contents without ionic radiation exposure [11, 33, 34, 37, 38]. Contrast material in the lacrimal drainage system as in CT-DCG (DCG = dacryocystography) and MR-DCG also provides more definitive results [11, 34]. Gadolinium chelate drops instilled in the cul-de-sac in MR-DCG avoid catheterization of the lacrimal system with improved detail [39]. The sonographic appearance of a dacryocystocele is a medial cystic mass with a fluid content communicating with the dilated nasolacrimal duct [33–35, 40, 41]. In utero ultrasonography and MRI can diagnose dacryocystoceles [42, 43], with in utero MRI demonstrating superior results when compared with prenatal ultrasound [43]. Preterm diagnosis of a bilateral dacryocele may alert the physician and family to respiratory difficulties after birth.

The appearance of a prenatal dacryocystocele on MR imaging without contrast enhancement on T2-weighted images is a homogenous, hyperintense cystic mass within the medial canthal region [44]. In the postnatal period, CT can reveal the dilated duct, cystic changes in the inferior meatus and nasal submucosa, and the bony contour changes [33, 37, 45]. MR imaging of simple dacryocystoceles and dacryocystomucopyoceles reveals fluid-filled cysts without solid components or a sac lumen accompanied by a thin rim of wall enhancement with contrast injection. The cystic fluid content is of low signal intensity on T1-weighted MRI images but displays high signal intensity in T2-weighted images, similar to the appearance of the vitreous body as reported by Farrer et al. The dilated sac was centered in the region of the medial canthus and extended inferiorly into the nasal cavity and elevated the inferior turbinate [38]. Dacryoendoscopy has been described by Kakizaki et al. to view the internal wall of a dacryocystocele in an infant who did not respond to initial probing, as well as to aid in the biopsy and marsupialization of the cyst. Using dacryoendoscopy, injection and hemorrhages on the inner cyst wall with inflammatory debris were noted. Histopathologically, the submucosal tissue demonstrated fibrous thickening with an infiltration of mononuclear leukocytes [46].

Differential Diagnosis

The differential diagnosis of medial canthal swellings includes diverticula of the lacrimal drainage apparatus, supernumerary sacs, epidermoid and dermoid cysts, mucoceles of paranasal sinuses, anterior encephaloceles or meningoencephaloceles, vascular aneurysms, and tumors impinging on the sac [47, 48]. Diverticulae of the lacrimal drainage apparatus, or supernumerary sacs, are often diagnosed at the time of intervention or by imaging studies [49]. Dermoid cysts may seldom be present at birth. They generally become apparent during the first decade of life, and a deeper orbital dermoid cyst may occasionally remain asymptomatic until later in life. Eighty five percent of dermoid cysts are located in the frontozygomatic area, with rare sites in the frontoethmoidal and lacrimal area. CT scans demonstrate the chronic bony erosion and well-circumscribed walls of dermoid cysts, as well as any potential orbital component such as through a bony opening. There is no communication with the intranasal cavity or lacrimal system [47, 50, 51].

Orbital cephaloceles (meningocele, encephalocele according to contents) are relatively rare in the orbit, occurring in only 2 out of 764 consecutive orbital masses of all types in a series published in 1994 by the Mayo Clinic [57]. The Wills Eye Hospital in 1997 published only one cephalocele among a series of 250 orbital biopsies in children [51, 52]. The two general types that involve the orbit are the anterior (ethmoidal) cephalocele and the posterior (sphenoidal) cephalocele. The incidence of orbital cephaloceles may be slightly higher as the majority of these cystic masses are managed by neurosurgeons or otolaryngologists. Encephaloceles or menigoceles can present as subtle pulsating proptosis and a mass typically above the medial canthal level. On CT, the orbital cyst with or without solid tissue contents and the osseous defect can usually be demonstrated. If there is no osseous defect, the lesion is considered ectopic brain tissue within the orbit [47].

Mucoceles of the paranasal sinuses can occur from chronic inflammation, trauma, or surgery of these structures. They are extremely rare in childhood and commonly associated with cystic fibrosis [53, 54]. A nontender fluctuant mass may displace the globe in an inferior and/or lateral direction. Diagnostic changes on CT scans are opacification of the affected sinuses, erosion of adjacent orbital bones, and herniation of the cyst through the defect into the orbit [55]. These lesions are typically managed by complete excision with repair of the bone defect and often obliteration of the sinus cavity with fat.

A sudoriferous cyst, the apocrine gland cyst of Moll, is a choristomatous congenital lesion, which becomes clinically apparent in early life. It appears as a fluctuant swelling beneath the lower eyelid similar to dacryocystitis without inflammation. CT and MRI sections show only a small cystic lesion without bone involvement, making it difficult to differentiate it from other orbital cysts [56, 57]. Aneurysms and neoplasms are mostly solid firm masses best diagnosed using MRI with contrast enhancement.

Management of Congenital Dacryocystoceles

Congenital dacryocystoceles are conservatively addressed with warm compresses, massaging, and topical antibiotics during the postnatal several weeks. Resolution rate with conservative therapy is reported from 17% to 80% according to multiple studies [4, 10, 20–22, 27, 58, 59]. The Crigler method of finger pressure applied on the sac and massaging inferiorly down the side of the nose over the nasolacrimal sac several times daily is described. However, some controversy exists in regard to massaging, as there is felt to be a possibility of spreading the contents of the dacryocystocele into the orbit. The frequency and method of massaging overall still remain vague. Typically, firm pressure on the dacryocystocele by an experienced ophthalmologist at the first visit is advocated, in order to direct the fluid content inferiorly, aiming to break the membranous tissue open at the valve of Hasner by hydraulic pressure [31, 60, 61]. If the pressure overcomes the resistance at the inferior meatal soft tissues, the cyst immediately decompresses, and the lacrimal sac becomes nonpalpable beneath the medial canthal tendon with resolution of symptoms. If conservative measures are unsuccessful, lacrimal probing, preferably with a 00 to 0 Bowman probe, is the first step surgical intervention and can be performed as early as possible [10, 30, 41]. Probing should be performed with care to the kinked canaliculi so that a false passage and canalicular trauma are avoided. In some cases, if the canalicular kink is straightened adequately, the contents of the sac may regurgitate from the puncti. Then, probing should proceed through the sac and nasolacrimal duct to open the membranous mucosa at the valve of Hasner and marsupialize the nasal cystic protrusion if present. Successful probing through the obstructing membrane can prevent the incidence of secondary dacryocystitis and cellulitis, which typically presents in the second week after birth (between 3rd and 43rd days) if treatment is delayed [10]. Urgent probing is recommended if dacryocystitis occurs. Mansour et al. reported a 78% success rate with probing in 36 of 54 infants with dacryocystoceles complicated with dacryocystitis [4]. Balloon catheter dilatation of the nasolacrimal duct can also aid in marsupialization of the nasal cyst [10]. Endoscopic visualization of the inferior turbinate and nasal antrum during probing is most optimal to detect intranasal cysts and to prevent a false opening. Often, a membranous flap can also be visualized and directly removed that would otherwise remain hinged in place if probing alone was performed. Direct visualization can give valuable intranasal information as well, when an endoscope is not available. Inspection of the inferior turbinate and intranasal structures should be performed prior to the application of topical decongestants that could distort the anatomy. In children, 0.05% oxymetazoline hydrochloride solution is generally used.

The debate of probing under general anesthesia is still ongoing, with many surgeons performing initial probing in the office in young children. Ideally, it is preferable to perform lacrimal probing for this condition under general anesthesia with endoscopic visualization, as this allows the advantages of detailed visualization of the anatomy and cyst, precise manipulation of delicate lacrimal tissues, and the ability to change the surgical plan if additional pathologies are detected. The success rate can be as high as 98% after the first probing and/or silicone intubation with nasal endoscopy under general anesthesia. [Unpublished data by Kaynak et al.] Silicone stenting of the lacrimal drainage system is performed if a significant stenosis within the duct or canaliculi is encountered, with self-stabilizing monocanalicular or bicanalicular stents simplifying the stent removal in infants. Intranasal cysts caused by extension of dacryocystoceles into the inferior nasal cavity require marsupialization of the cysts under direct or endoscopic visualization. Recurrence with mucocele may occur if marsupialization of the cyst wall is not done at the time of probing [65]. Interestingly, a unilateral dacryocystocele does not exclude the possibility of bilateral intranasal cysts, and therefore both nasal cavities should always be evaluated [26, 62–64].

In a large series of 27 infants with congenital dacryoceles, Becker reported a 100% success rate after early probing (mean, 5.9 days of age; range, 1–12 days) in all surgical patients who did not develop infection. The only patient who did not have probing and did not develop infection was treated with intravenous gentamicin and ampicillin, with the lacrimal sac manually decompressed into the nose at the first examination at day 2 of age. Fifty-three percent patients developed infection in this study group and were generally older at the time of initial probing [10]. A smaller series of five patients by Cavazza described one patient responding to massage and topical antibiotics, with the remaining four patients requiring probing under endoscopy with 100% success. One child required marsupialization of the intranasal cyst. One patient developed postoperative dacryocystitis that improved with systemic antibiotics. No recurrences were seen in the follow-up period (mean: 18 months) [41].

Intraorbital extension of congenital dacryocystoceles must be handled with care and promptly managed. Massaging is not recommended in long-standing cases with concurrent dacryocystitis. Extreme bony thinning from chronic inflammation may potentially predispose to intraorbital extension

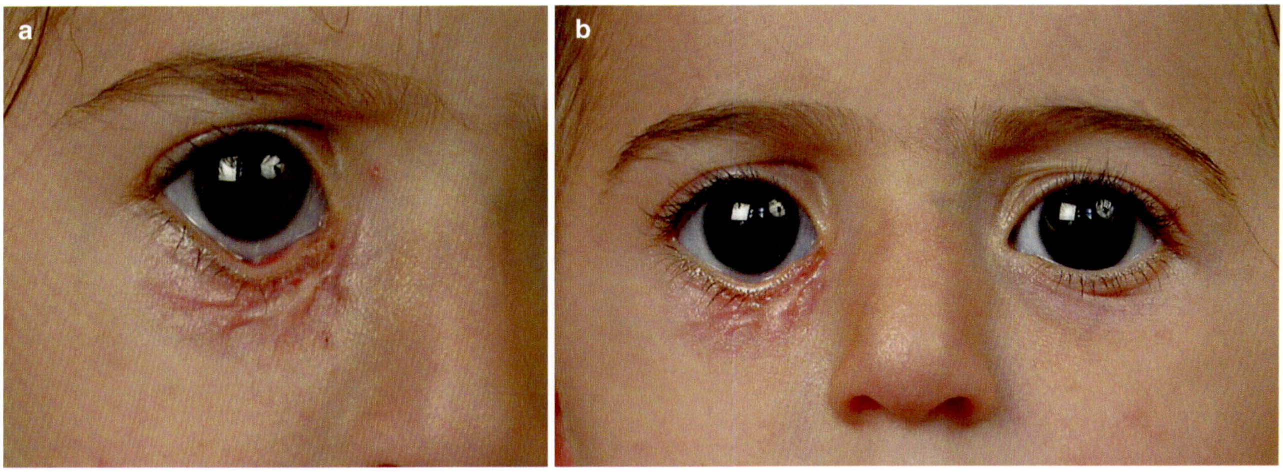

Fig. 50.9 Patient in Fig. 50.7 after external DCR at postoperative weeks 1 and 4. Scatricial ectropion is a complication of repeated numerous fistulization of the dacryocele. DCR incision is 5mm along the superomedial tear trough

of the sac contents with manual pressure on the sac. Two iatrogenic cases of intraorbital dacryocystocele extension and abscess formation have been reported following digital massage [31, 60]. CT or MRI imaging should be considered when intraorbital extension is suspected. In addition, probing must be performed with care to prevent a false entry to the orbit and secondary introduction of infectious agents into the orbit [31]. In cases of orbital extension, a transconjunctival approach with marsupialization of the dacryocystocele, followed by probing, can be utilized.

In severe refractory, or untreated, cases of recurrent dacryocystitis within a dacryocystocele, a lacrimal-cutaneous fistula can develop, which may lead to cicatricial changes or ectropion of the lower eyelid (Fig. 50.7a–c). Intraorbital extension of a dacryocystocele in communication with the nasolacrimal duct can also occur (Fig. 50.8a, b), requiring marsupialization of the dacryocystocele, lacrimal probing, and intranasal cyst marsupialization. Accumulation of fluid in the enlarged sac compartment may sometimes persist, however, and cause dacryocystitis despite the drainage of some tears. Both endonasal and external DCR approaches can be used for recurrent dacryocystitis or when the sac volume does not return to normal after establishing patency of the lacrimal drainage apparatus [65–67]. During dacryocystorhinostomy, a partial dacryocystectomy to reduce the dilated sac walls should be performed to allow anastomosis of more properly sized sac flaps to the nasal flaps (Fig. 50.9a, b).

In rare cases, dacryocystoceles in the setting of significant congenital punctal agenesis may require conjunctivodacryocystorhinostomy (CDCR) [14, 68]. In another patient with lacrimo-auriculo-dento-digital syndrome with alacrima and agenesis of the lacrimal punctae, a transconjunctival orbitotomy was performed to excise the dacryocystocele, in conjunction with endonasal antrostomy [15].

Summary

The management of congenital dacryocystoceles differs according to the presence of infection, extent of the cyst, and other anatomic findings or complications. The main purpose of management is to establish the drainage of tears through a patent and functional lacrimal system and to resolve infection, via interventions ranging from conservative therapy to CDCR. Fortunately, the majority of infants with congenital dacryocystoceles respond to conservative therapy and probing with or without marsupialization of the sac.

Financial Disclosures The author has *no financial interest* in any of the materials or equipment mentioned in the chapter.

References

1. Scott WE, Fabre JA, Ossoinig KC. Congenital mucocele of the lacrimal sac. Arch Ophtalmol. 1979;97:1656–8.
2. Harris GJ, DiClementi D. Congenital dacryocystocele. Arch Ophthalmol. 1982;100:1763–5.
3. Weinstein GS, Biglan AW, Patterson JH. Congenital lacrimal sac mucoceles. Am J Ophthalmol. 1982;94:106–10.
4. Mansour AM, Cheng KP, Mumma JV, Stager DR, Harris GJ, Patrinely JR, Lavery MA, Wang FM, Steinkuller PG. Congenital dacryocele. A collaborative review. Ophthalmology. 1991;98: 1744–51.
5. Perry LJ, Jakobiec FA, Zakka FR, Rubin PA. Giant dacryocystomucopyocele in an adult: a review of lacrimal sac enlargements with clinical and histopathologic differential diagnoses. Surv Ophthalmol. 2012;57(5):474–85.
6. Zoumalan CI, Joseph JM, Lelli GJ Jr, et al. Evaluation of the canalicular entrance into the lacrimal sac: an anatomical study. Ophthal Plast Reconstr Surg. 2011;27:298–303.
7. Kapadia MK, Freitag SK, Woog JJ. Evaluation and management of congenital nasolacrimal duct obstruction. Otolaryngol Clin North Am. 2006;39(5):959–77, v. ii.

8. Yazici B, Yazici Z. Anatomic position of the common canaliculus in patients with a large lacrimal sac. Ophthal Plast Reconstr Surg. 2008;24:90–3.
9. Jones LT, Wobig JL. Surgery of the eyelids and lacrimal system. Birmingham: Aesculapius; 1976. p. 162–4.
10. Becker BB. The treatment of congenital dacryocystocele. Am J Ophthalmol. 2006;142:835–8.
11. Kamal S, Ali MJ, Gauba V, et al. Congenital nasolacrimal duct obstruction. In: Ali MJ, editor. Principles and practice of lacrimal surgery. New Delhi: Springer; 2015. p. 148–59.
12. Lyons CJ, Rosser PM, Welham RA. The management of punctal agenesis. Ophthalmology. 1993;100:1851–5.
13. Woo KI, Kim YD. Four cases of dacryocystocele. Korean J Ophthalmol. 1997;11:65–9.
14. Ong CA, Prepageran N, Sharad G, et al. Bilateral lacrimal sac mucocele with punctal and canalicular agenesis. Med J Malaysia. 2005;60:660–2.
15. Santo RO, Golbert MB, Akaishi PM, Cruz AA, Cintra MB. Giant dacryocystocele and congenital alacrimia in lacrimo-auriculo-dento-digital syndrome. Ophthal Plast Reconstr Surg. 2013;29(3):e67–8.
16. Levy NS. Conservative management of congenital amniotocele of the nasolacrimal sac. J AAPOS. 1979;16:254–6.
17. George JL, Badonnel Y, Kissel C. Congenital lacrimal mucocele or amniotocele? Bull Soc Ophtalmol Fr. 1984;84:263–6.
18. Paulsen FP, Corfield AP, Hinz M, et al. Characterization of mucins in human lacrimal sac and nasolacrimal duct. Invest Ophthalmol Vis Sci. 2003;44:1807–13.
19. Paulsen F. Cell and molecular biology of human lacrimal gland and nasolacrimal duct mucins. Int Rev Cytol. 2006;249:229–79.
20. Boynton JR, Drucker DN. Distention of the lacrimal sac in neonates. Ophthalmic Surg. 1989;20(2):103–7.
21. Petersen RA, Robb RM. The natural course of congenital obstruction of the nasolacrimal duct. J Pediatr Ophthalmol Strabismus. 1978;15(4):246–50.
22. Sullivan TJ, Clarke MP, Morin JD, et al. Management of congenital dacryocystocele. Aust N Z J Ophthalmol. 1992;20(2):105–8.
23. Wang JC, Cunningham MJ. Congenital dacryocystocele: is there a familial predisposition? Int J Pediatr Otorhinolaryngol. 2011;75:430–2.
24. Buerger DG, Schaefer AJ, Campbell CB, et al. Congenital lacrimal disorders. In: Nesi F, Levine MR, editors. Smith's ophthalmic plastics and reconstructive surgery. St. Louis: Mosby; 1998. p. 649–60.
25. Paysse EA, Coats DK, Bernstein JM, et al. Management and complications of congenital dacryocele with concurrent intranasal mucocele. J AAPOS. 2000;4:46–53.
26. Grin TR, Mertz JS, Stass-Isern M. Congenital nasolacrimal duct cysts in dacryocystocele. Ophthalmology. 1991;98:1238–42.
27. Schnall BM, Christian CJ. Conservative treatment of congenital dacryocele. J Pediatr Ophthalmol Strabismus. 1996;33:219–22.
28. Shashy RG, Durairaj V, Holmes JM, et al. Congenital dacryocystocele associated with intranasal cysts: diagnosis and management. Laryngoscope. 2003;113:37–40.
29. Edmond JC, Keech RV. Congenital nasolacrimal sac mucocele associated with respiratory distress. J Pediatr Ophthalmol Strabismus. 1991;28:287–9.
30. Lueder GT. Neonatal dacryocystitis associated with nasolacrimal duct cysts. J Pediatr Ophthalmol Strabismus. 1995;32:102–6.
31. Bernardini FP, Cetinkaya A, Capris P, Rossi A, Kaynak P, Katowitz JA. Orbital and periorbital extension of congenital dacryocystoceles: suggested mechanism and management. Ophthal Plast Reconstr Surg. 2016;32(5):e101–4.
32. Nagi KS, Meyer DR. Utilization patterns for diagnostic imaging in the evaluation of epiphora due to lacrimal obstruction: a national survey. Ophthal Plast Reconstr Surg. 2010;26(3):168–71.
33. Hurwitz JJ, Edward Kassel EE, Jaffer N. Computed tomography and combined CT-dacryocystography (CT-DCG). In: Hurwitz JJ, editor. The lacrimal system. New York: Raven Press; 1996. p. 83–5.
34. Lefebvre DR, Freitag SK. Update on imaging of the lacrimal drainage system. Semin Ophthalmol. 2012;27(5–6):175–86.
35. Schlenck B, Unsinn K, Geley T, Schon A, Gassner I. Sonographic diagnosis of congenital dacryocystocele. Ultraschall Med. 2002;23:181–4.
36. Al-Faky YH. Anatomical utility of ultrasound biomicroscopy in the lacrimal drainage system. Br J Ophthalmol. 2011;95:1446–50.
37. Rand PK, Ball WS, Kulwin DR. Congenital nasolacrimal mucoceles: CT evaluation. Radiology. 1989;173:691–4.
38. Farrer RS, Mohammed TL, Hahn FJ. MRI of childhood dacryocystocele. Neuroradiology. 2003;45:259–61.
39. Goldberg RA, Heinz GW, Chiu L. Gadolinium magnetic resonance imaging dacryocystography. Am J Ophthalmol. 1993;115(6):738–41.
40. Oksala A. Diagnosis by ultrasound in acute dacryocystitis. Acta Ophthalmol. 1959;37:176–9.
41. Cavazza S, Laffi GL, Lodi I, Tassinari G, Dall'olio D. Congenital dacryocystocele: diagnosis and treatment. Acta Otorhinolaryngol Ital. 2008;28:298–301.
42. Sepulveda W, Wojakowski AB, Elias D, et al. Congenital dacryocystocele: prenatal 2- and 3- dimensional sonographic findings. J Ultrasound Med. 2005;24:225–30.
43. Yazici Z, Kline-Fath BM, Yazici B, et al. Congenital dacryocystocele: prenatal MRI findings. Pediatr Radiol. 2010;40:1868–73.
44. Bianchini E, Zirpoli S, Righini A, et al. Magnetic resonance imaging in prenatal diagnosis of dacryocystocele: report of 3 cases. J Comput Assist Tomogr. 2004;28:422–7.
45. Menestrina LE, Osborn RE. Congenital dacryocystocele with intranasal extension: correlation of computed tomography and magnetic resonance imaging. J Am Osteopath Assoc. 1990;90:264–8.
46. Kakizaki H, Takahashi Y, Sa H-S, Ichinose A, Iwaki M. Congenital dacryocystocele: comparative findings of dacryoendoscopy and histopathology in a patient. Ophthal Plast Reconstr Surg. 2012;28(4):e85–6.
47. Shields JA, Shields CL. Orbital cysts of childhood – classification clinical features, and management. Surv Ophthalmol. 2004;49:281–99.
48. Gunalp I, Gunduz K. Cystic lesions of the orbit. Int Ophthalmol. 1996;20:273–7.
49. Kim JH, Chang HR, Woo KI. Multilobular lacrimal sac diverticulum presenting as a lower eyelid mass. Korean J Ophthalmol. 2012;26:297–300.
50. Nugent RA, Lapointe JS, Rootman J, et al. Orbital dermoids: features on CT. Radiology. 1987;165:475–8.
51. Shields JA, Kaden IH, Eagle RC Jr, Shields CL. Orbital dermoid cysts. Clinicopathologic correlations, classification, and management. Josephine E. Schueler Lecture. Ophthal Plast Reconstr Surg. 1997;13:265–76.
52. Henderson JW, Campbell RJ, Farrow GM, Garrity JA. Cysts. In: Henderson JW, Campbell RJ, Farrow GM, Garrity JA, editors. Orbital tumors. 3rd ed. New York: Raven Press; 1994. p. 53–88.
53. Levine MR, Kim Y, Witt W. Frontal sinus mucopyocele in cystic fibrosis. Ophthal Plast Reconstr Surg. 1988;4:221–5.
54. Sharma GD, Doershuk CF, Stern RC. Erosion of the wall of the frontal sinus caused by mucopyocele in cystic fibrosis. J Pediatr. 1994;124:745–7.

55. Perugini S, Pasquini U, Menichelli F, et al. Mucoceles in the paranasal sinuses involving the orbit: CT signs in 43 cases. Neuroradiology. 1982;23:133–9.
56. Mims J, Rodrigues M, Calhoun J. Sudoriferous cyst of the orbit. Can J Ophthalmol. 1977;12:155–6.
57. Rosen WJ, Li Y. Sudoriferous cyst of the orbit. Ophthal Plast Reconstr Surg. 2001;17:73–5.
58. Lueder GT. Pediatric lacrimal disorders. In: M. Edward Wilson • Richard A. Saunders Rupal H. Trivedi (Eds.) Pediatric ophthalmology: current thought and a practical guide. Berlin/Heidelberg Springer; 2009.
59. Dagi LR, Bhargava A, Melvin P. Associated signs, demographic characteristics, and management of dacryocystocele in 64 infants. J AAPOS. 2012;16:255–60.
60. Baker MS, Allen RC. Re: "orbital and periorbital extension of congenital dacryocystoceles: suggested mechanism and management". Ophthal Plast Reconstr Surg. 2015;31:248–9.
61. Bernardini FP, Katowitz JA, Capris P. Reply re: "orbital and periorbital extension of congenital dacryocystoceles: suggested mechanism and management". Ophthal Plast Reconstr Surg. 2015;31(3):249–50.
62. Teixeira CC, Dias RJ, Falcao-Reis FM, Santos M. Congenital dacryocystocele with intranasal extension. Eur J Ophthalmol. 2005;145:126–8.
63. Roy D, Guevara J, Castillo L. Endoscopic marsupialization of congenital duct cyst withdacryocoele. Clin Otolaryngol. 2002;27:167–70.
64. Ali MJ, Psaltis AJ, Brunworth J, et al. Congenital dacryocele with large intranasal cysts. Efficacy of cruciate marsupialization, adjunctive procedures and outcomes. Ophthal Plast Reconstr Surg. 2014;30:346–51.
65. Leibovitch I, Selva D, Tsirbas A, et al. Paediatric endoscopic endonasal dacryocystorhinostomy in congenital nasolacrimal duct obstruction. Graefes Arch Clin Exp Ophthalmol. 2006;244:1250–4.
66. Raflo GT, Horton JA, Sprinkle PM. An unusual intranasal anomaly of the lacrimal drainage system. Ophthalmic Surg. 1982;13:741–4.
67. Plaza G, Nogueira A, González R, et al. Surgical treatment of familial dacryocystocele and lacrimal puncta agenesis. Ophthal Plast Reconstr Surg. 2009;25:52–3.
68. Allen RC, Nerad JA. Re: "surgical treatment of familial dacryocystocele and lacrimal puncta agenesis". Ophthal Plast Reconstr Surg. 2010;26:67; author reply 67.

Part IV
Orbit

Orbital Anatomy

51

Humbert Massegur, Juan-Ramon Gras-Cabrerizo, and Jacinto García-Lorenzo

Anatomy of the Orbit

Understanding orbital pathology and its consequences requires precise knowledge of the anatomy of the orbit. Careful study of the relationship of the orbit with nearby structures will help us manage orbital complications and is essential for surgical planning [1–4].

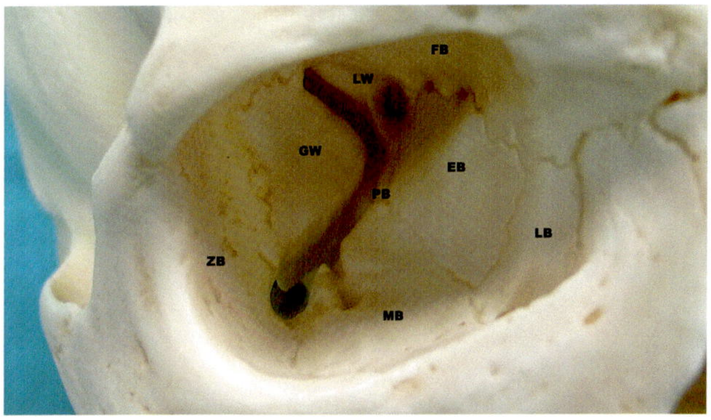

Fig. 51.1 Right orbital cavity. The seven bones: *FB* frontal bone, *LW* lesser wing of sphenoid bone, *GW* greater wing of sphenoid bone, *PB* palatine bone (orbital process), *EB* ethmoid bone (lamina papyracea), *MB* maxillary bone, *ZM* zygomatic bone

Osteology

The orbital cavity has the shape of a quadrangular pyramid pointing posteriorly. The base of this pyramid is anterior measuring 3.5 cm wide and 4 cm high. The depth of the orbit is 4 cm in an adult, what makes a total volume of 30 cc. It is made by seven bones: the frontal bone, the ethmoid bone, the lacrimal bone, the sphenoid bone, the zygomatic bone, the palatine bone, and the maxillary bone [5] (Fig. 51.1).

Orbital Opening (Fig. 51.2)
The orbital opening is limited by three bones joined by three sutures. This square has four margins: superior, lateral, inferior, and medial.

The superior or supraorbital margin is made by the frontal bone. The passage of neurovascular elements originates two distinctive notches in this margin. The lateral branch of the supraorbital nerve and the supraorbital artery carve a supraorbital notch, while the medial branch of the supraorbital nerve and the supratrochlear artery (or medial frontal artery) carve the frontal notch (Fig. 51.3).

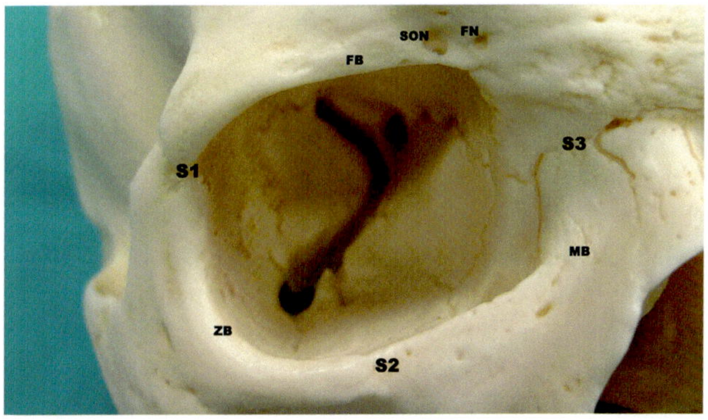

Fig. 51.2 Right orbital cavity. Orbital opening: *S1* fronto-zygomatic suture, *S2* maxillo-zygomatic suture, *S3* fronto-maxillary suture, *FB* frontal bone, *ZB* zygomatic bone, *MB* maxillary bone, *SON* superior orbital notch, *FN* frontal notch

H. Massegur (✉)
Otorhinolaryngology Department, Hospital de Sant Pau, Barcelona, Spain

Medical School of Girona University, Girona, Spain
e-mail: info@humbertmassegur.com

J.-R. Gras-Cabrerizo · J. García-Lorenzo
Otorhinolaryngology Department, Hospital de Sant Pau, Barcelona, Spain

A. J. Cohen, C. N. Burkat (eds.), *Oculofacial, Orbital, and Lacrimal Surgery*, https://doi.org/10.1007/978-3-030-14092-2_51

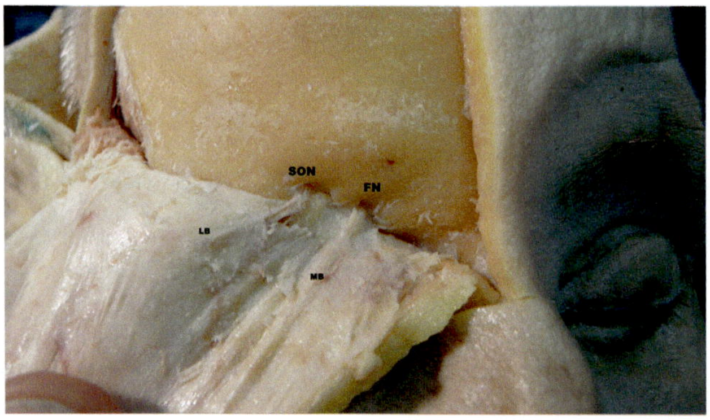

Fig. 51.3 Right orbit. Superior orbital margin with superior orbital notch and frontal notch with supraorbital nerve branches: *SON* supraorbital notch, *FN* frontal notch, *LB* lateral branch of supraorbital nerve, *MB* medial branch of supraorbital nerve

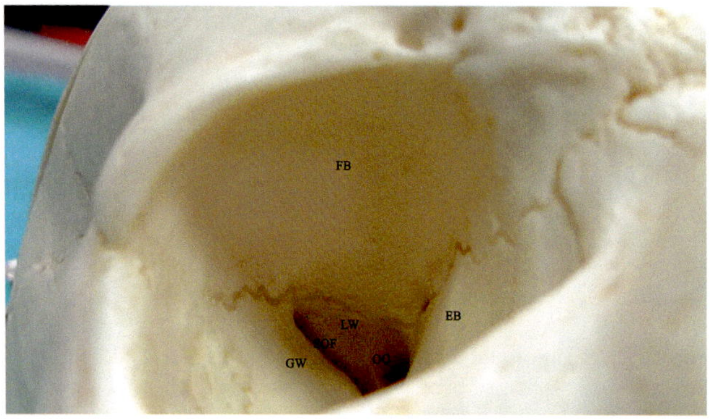

Fig. 51.4 Right orbital cavity. Superior wall: *FB* frontal bone, *LW* lesser wing of the sphenoid bone, *GW* greater wing of the sphenoid bone, *EB* ethmoid bone (lamina papyracea), *SOF* superior orbital fissure, *OC* optic canal

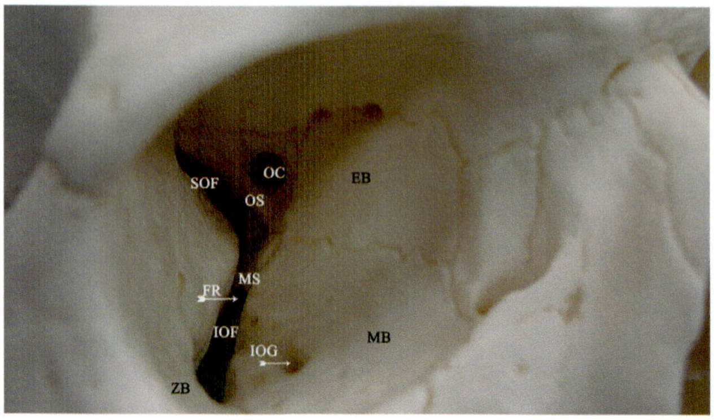

Fig. 51.5 Right orbital cavity. Inferior wall: *MB* maxillary bone, *ZB* zygomatic bone, *IOG* infraorbital groove, *IOF* inferior orbital fissure, *FR* foramen rotundum, *MS* maxillary strut, *SOF* superior orbital fissure, *OS* optic strut, *OC* optic canal, *EB* ethmoid bone (lamina papyracea)

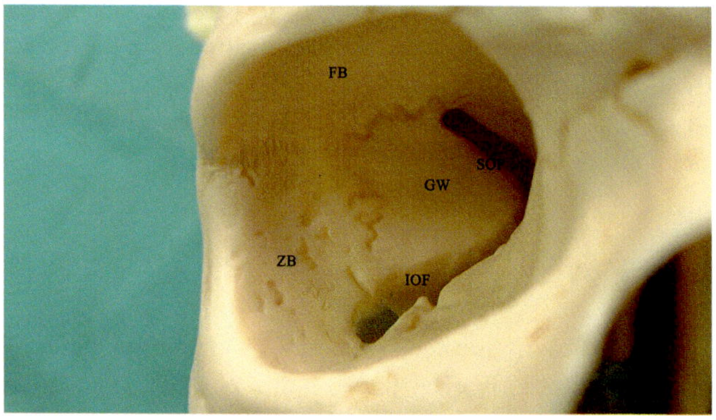

Fig. 51.6 Right orbital cavity. Lateral wall: *FB* frontal bone, *ZM* zygomatic bone, *GW* greater wing of the sphenoid bone, *SOF* superior orbital fissure, *IOF* inferior orbital fissure

The lateral margin is made by the zygomatic process of the frontal bone and the frontal process of the zygomatic bone. A small orbital tubercle in the zygomatic bone marks the attachment of the lateral palpebral ligament.

The inferior or infraorbital margin is formed by the zygomatic bone laterally and the maxilla medially.

The medial margin is formed by the frontal bone superiorly and the frontal process of the maxilla inferiorly.

The infraorbital margin curves upward to become the anterior lacrimal crest of the frontal process of the maxillary bone, while the supraorbital margin bends down toward the lacrimal crest, posterior to the lacrimal bone.

Orbital Walls

Roof of the Orbit (Fig. 51.4)

The roof of the orbit is, at the same time, the floor of the anterior cranial fossa. It is formed by the orbital plate of the frontal bone anteriorly and by the lesser wing of the sphenoid bone posteriorly. The orbital plate of the frontal bone shows two depressions: the lacrimal fossa in the anterolateral aspect and the trochlear fossa in the anteromedial aspect. The latter serves as insertion for the superior oblique muscle.

Floor of the Orbit (Fig. 51.5)

The floor of the orbit is composed of three bony structures: the orbital plate of the maxillary bone, the orbital surface of the zygomatic bone, and the orbital process of the palatine bone.

There are three openings in the floor of the orbit that allow the passage of neurovascular and glandular structures. The nasolacrimal canal is placed anteromedially in the orbital plate of the maxilla. The inferior orbital fissure separates the floor from the lateral wall of the orbit. The infraorbital groove allows the passage of the infraorbital nerve and the infraorbital artery.

Lateral Wall (Fig. 51.6)

It is the thickest wall of all. It forms a 45° angle with the medial wall and a 90° angle with the contralateral lateral wall.

It is formed by two main structures: the greater wing of the sphenoid bone and the frontal process of the zygomatic bone.

The greater wing of the sphenoid bone separates the middle cranial fossa from the orbit. The lacrimal foramen opens in the posterior end of the greater wing of the sphenoid bone to allow the passage of the anastomosis to the orbital branch of the middle meningeal artery.

The zygomatic-orbital foramen opens in the anterior end of the frontal process of the zygomatic bone. It serves as entrance of the zygomatic nerve into the orbit.

The superior orbital fissure separates the lateral wall from the roof of the orbit.

The lateral tubercle is 3–4 mm posterior to the orbital rim. It serves as insertion for the elevator muscle, the lateral canthal tendon, and the ligament to the rectus lateralis muscle.

Medial Wall (Fig. 51.7)

The medial wall is formed by four bony structures: from anterior to posterior, the frontal process of the maxilla, the lacrimal bone, the lamina papyracea of the ethmoid bone, and the body of the sphenoid bone.

The lacrimal groove sits between the frontal process of the maxilla and the lacrimal bone. It is limited by the anterior and posterior lacrimal crests.

The lamina papyracea of the ethmoid bone inserts in the lateral part of the body of the sphenoid bone, immediately anterior to the optic canal.

The medial wall is articulated with the roof of the orbit by the frontoethmoidal suture and with the floor of the orbit by the maxilloethmoidal suture.

The frontoethmoidal suture has two foramina for the anterior and posterior ethmoidal arteries and for the ethmoidal branches of the nasociliary nerve. These foramina mark the division of the orbit in three anatomical regions: bulbar, retrobulbar, and apical. The bulbar region is anterior to the anterior ethmoidal artery, the retrobulbar region is limited by the two ethmoidal foramina, and the apical region is posterior to the posterior ethmoidal artery.

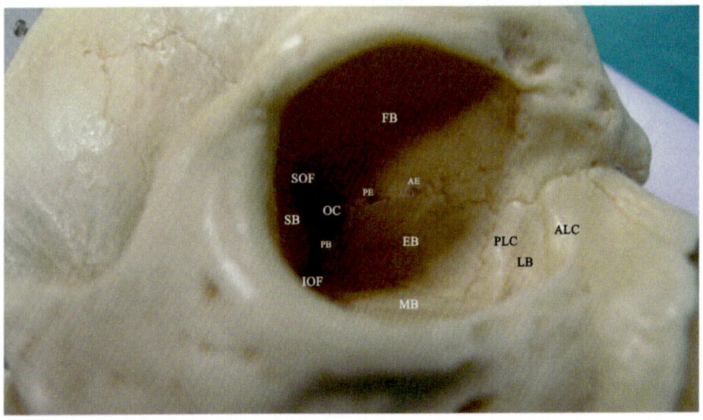

Fig. 51.7 Right orbital cavity. Medial wall: *FB* frontal bone, *EB* ethmoidal bone (lamina papyracea), *PE* posterior ethmoid artery canal, *AE* anterior ethmoid artery canal, *PLC* posterior lacrimal crest, *LB* lacrimal bone, *ALC* anterior lacrimal crest, *MB* maxillary bone, *PB* palatine bone (orbital process), *OC* optic canal, *SOF* superior orbital fissure, *IOF* inferior orbital fissure, *SB* sphenoid bone

Orbital Apex (Fig. 51.8)

The orbital apex is situated 4.5 cm deep from the orbital margin. Through the apex, the orbit communicates with the cranial cavity through the superior orbital fissure and the optic foramen and with the pterygopalatine fossa through the inferior orbital fissure.

The main structures in the apex are the optic canal, the optic strut, the superior orbital fissure, and the common annular tendon (annulus of Zinn.) (Fig. 51.9).

The optic canal is crossed by the optic nerve and the ophthalmic artery. It is carved between the body and the roots of the lesser wing of the sphenoid bone, in the most superior and medial region of the orbit. The posterior

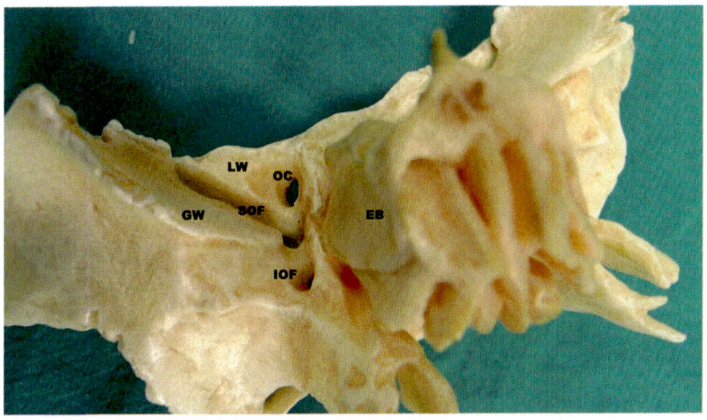

Fig. 51.8 Right orbital apex: *EB* ethmoid bone, *OC* optic canal, *LW* lesser wing of the sphenoid bone, *GW* greater wing of the sphenoid bone, *SOF* superior orbital fissure, *IOF* inferior orbital fissure

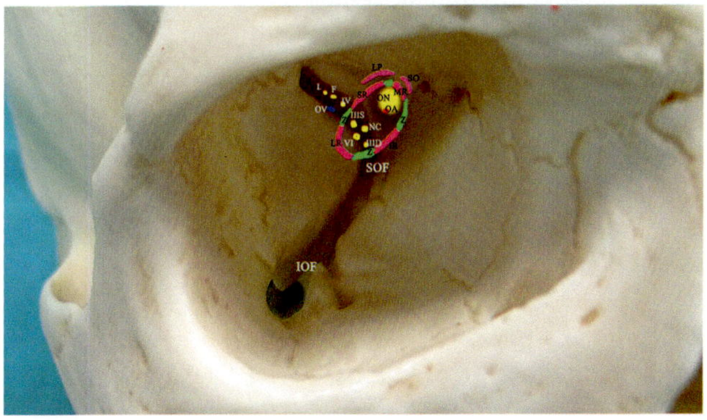

Fig. 51.9 Right orbital apex. Common annular tendon: *LP* levator palpebrae muscle, *SO* superior orbital muscle, *MR* medial rectus muscle, *IR* inferior rectus muscle, *LR* lateral rectus muscle, *SR* superior rectus muscle, *Z* annulus of Zinn, *ON* optic nerve, *OA* ophthalmic artery, *OV* ophthalmic vein, *L* lacrimal nerve, *F* frontal nerve, *IV* trochlear nerve, *IIIS* oculomotor nerve (superior branch), *IIID* oculomotor nerve (inferior branch), *NC* nasociliary nerve, *VI* abducens nerve, *SOF* superior orbital fissure, *IOF* inferior orbital fissure

ethmoidal cells form the medial wall of the optic canal in many cases.

The optic strut is the posterior root of the lesser wing of the sphenoid bone. It forms the inferolateral border of the optic canal and separates the optic canal from the superior orbital fissure.

The superior orbital fissure opens between the body of the sphenoid bone (medial), the greater wing of the sphenoid bone (inferior), and the lesser wing of the sphenoid bone (superior). It is usually narrower in the laterosuperior end and widens inferomedially under the optic foramen.

The common annular tendon inserts around the optic foramen and across the superior orbital fissure. It can serve to divide the superior orbital fissure in two compartments, namely, intraconal and extraconal.

The intraconal compartment is crossed by [6]:

- The optic nerve
- The ophthalmic artery
- The superior and inferior divisions of the oculomotor nerve (III)
- The nasociliary branch of the abducens nerve (VI)
- The trunk of the abducens nerve (VI)

The extraconal compartment is crossed by:

- The trochlear nerve (IV)
- The frontal nerve
- The lacrimal nerve
- The superior ophthalmic veins

Branches of the carotid sympathetic plexus enter the orbit inferior to the common annular tendon.

The maxillary strut separates the inferior end of the superior orbital fissure from the foramen rotundum.

The inferior orbital fissure sits between the greater wing of the sphenoid bone (posterior), the orbital processes of the palatine bone and the maxilla (anterior), the zygomatic bone (lateral), and the body of the sphenoid bone (medial). The zygomatic and infraorbital branches of the maxillary artery and the inferior ophthalmic vein access the orbit through the inferior orbital fissure.

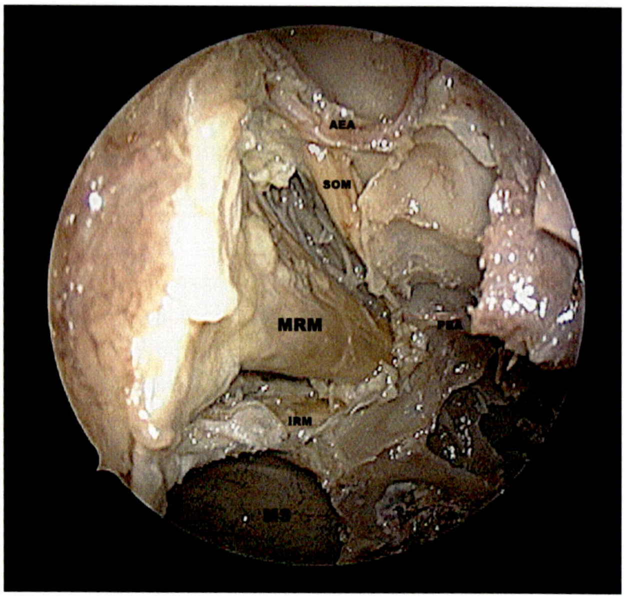

Fig. 51.10 Right orbit seen from nasal fossa. *MS* maxillary sinus, *IRM* inferior rectus muscle, *MRM* medial rectus muscle, *SOM* superior oblique muscle, *AEA* anterior ethmoidal artery, *PEA* posterior ethmoidal artery

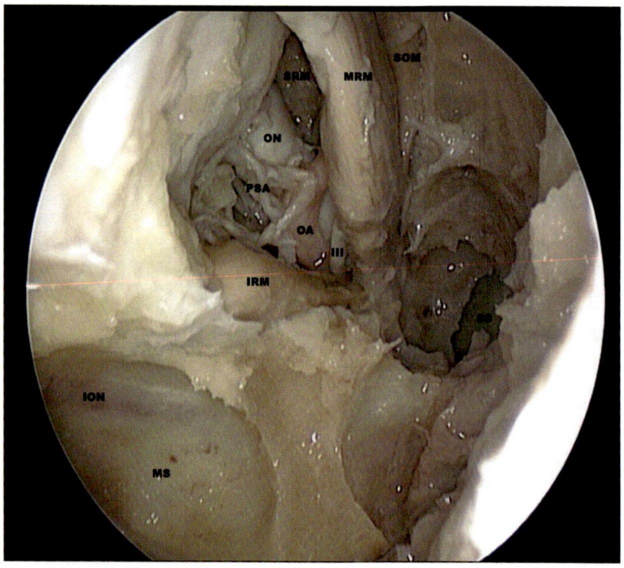

Fig. 51.11 Right orbit seen from nasal fossa after removal of orbital fat: *SRM* superior rectus muscle, *SOM* superior oblique muscle, *MRM* medial rectus muscle, *IRM* inferior rectus muscle, *ON* optic nerve, *III* oculomotor nerve (inferior branch), *ION* infraorbital nerve, *OA* ophthalmic artery, *MS* maxillary sinus, *SS* sphenoid sinus

Muscles and Tendons (Figs. 51.10, 51.11, 51.12, and 51.13)

Orbicular Muscle (Orbicularis Oculi)

The orbicular muscle inserts around the orbital rim. It can be divided into three portions: orbital, palpebral, and lacrimal.

The orbital part inserts medially in the nasal process of the frontal bone, in the frontal process of the maxilla, in the palpebral ligament, and laterally in the occipitofrontalis muscle and in the corrugator muscle.

The palpebral part inserts in the medial palpebral ligament and in the surrounding bone. The tarsi are located in the deep portion of the palpebral part. They insert in the palpebral ligament in the anterior lacrimal crest, in the frontal process of the maxilla, in the lateral palpebral ligament, and in a small tubercle of the zygomatic process. The superior tarsus receives fibers from the levator palpebrae superioris muscle.

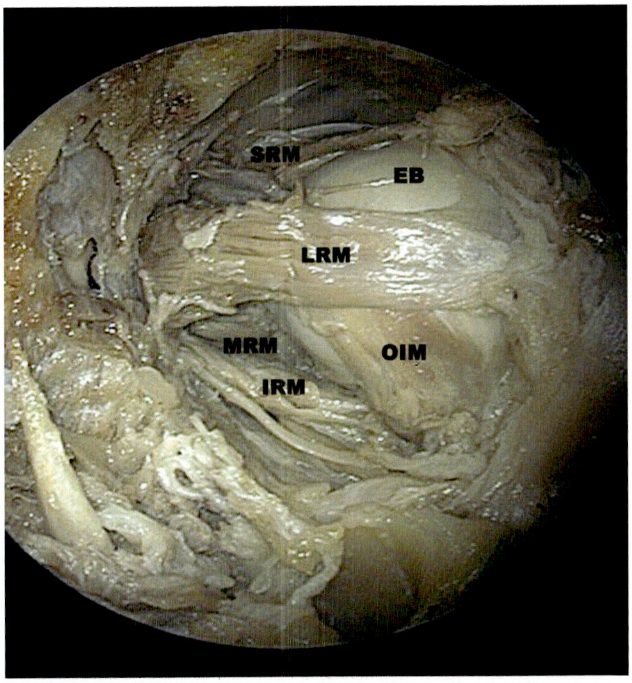

Fig. 51.12 Right orbit, lateral view: *SRM* superior rectus muscle, *LRM* lateral rectus muscle, *IRM* inferior rectus muscle, *MRM* medial rectus muscle, *IOM* oblique inferior muscle, *EB* eye ball

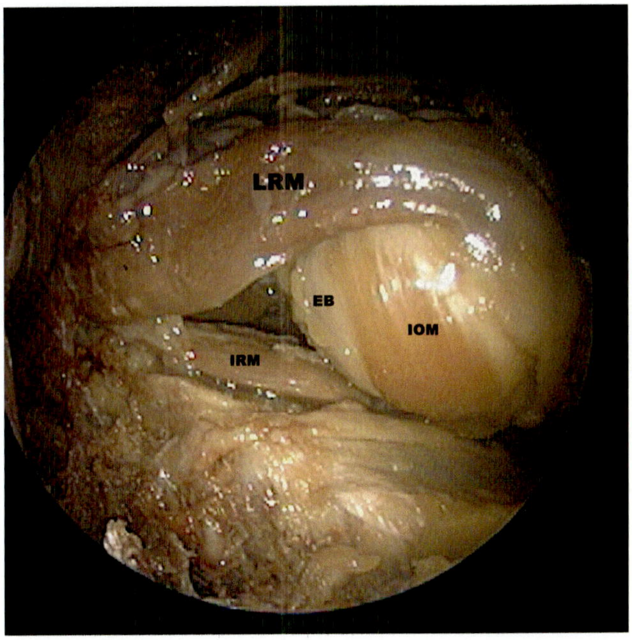

Fig. 51.13 Right orbit, lateral view: *LRM* lateral rectus muscle, *IOM* inferior oblique muscle, *IRM* inferior rectus muscle, *EB* eye ball

The lacrimal part inserts in the posterior lacrimal crest of the lacrimal bone, immediately posterior to the lacrimal sac.

Recti Muscles

The four recti muscles of the orbit share a common characteristic. They are wide in the middle portion, becoming progressively narrow at the posterior insertion in the common annular tendon. The four recti muscles and the intermuscular septa limit the intraconal space.

Anteriorly, the recti muscles insert in the sclera. The sclera is a dense membrane that maintains the spherical shape of the eyeball.

The external and medial recti are in a horizontal plane, while the superior and inferior recti are in a vertical plane.

Superior Rectus

The superior rectus is slightly wider than the rest of the straight muscles. It expands from the common annular tendon to the posterior sclera, at the level of the spiral of Tillaux, which represents the meridian of the eyeball. The contraction of the superior rectus produces elevation, adduction, and external rotation of the eye. It is innervated by the superior branch of the oculomotor nerve (III).

Medial Rectus

The medial rectus is the shortest and the strongest of the straight muscles. It runs very close to the lamina papyracea, extending from the common annular tendon to the sclera. It produces adduction of the eye. It is innervated by the inferior branch of the oculomotor nerve (III).

Lateral Rectus

The lateral rectus inserts in the common annular tendon, in the greater wing of the sphenoid bone along the border of the superior orbital fissure, and in a tendinous portion of the common annular tendon that expands from the lesser wing to the greater wing of the sphenoid bone. It is cushioned from the lateral wall by some adipose tissue. Its scleral insertion is close to the corneal border.

The ciliary ganglion, the lacrimal nerve, and the lacrimal artery are situated superior to the lateral rectus.

The contraction of the lateral rectus produces abduction of the eye. It is innervated by the abducens nerve (VI).

Inferior Rectus

The inferior rectus runs very close to the orbital floor in the posterior portion. The anterior portion is cushioned by adipose tissue. It produces depression, adduction, and external rotation of the eyeball, together with the superior oblique muscle. The contraction of the inferior rectus achieves a certain depression of the inferior eyelid.

It is innervated by the inferior branch of the oculomotor nerve (III).

Oblique Muscles

Superior Oblique Muscle

The superior oblique muscle originates in the common annular tendon and extends superomedially to the trochlea. The trochlea is a fibrous cartilage that forms a pulley-like structure that reflects the body of the superior oblique. From the trochlea, it angles posteriorly and inferolaterally to reach the sclera between the insertions of the superior and lateral recti. It becomes narrower and more tendinous as it approaches the margins of the orbit.

The superior oblique muscle produces abduction and elevation of the posterior pole of the eyeball. The cornea is then depressed and rotated internally.

It is innervated by the trochlear nerve (IV).

Inferior Oblique Muscle (Figs. 51.12 and 51.13)

It inserts on the floor of the orbit, lateral to the lacrimal duct. From this insertion, it runs laterally and posteriorly between the inferior rectus and the floor of the orbit to the sclera between the insertions of the lateral rectus and the superior rectus. It is covered by fibers of the capsulopalpebral fascia and by the inferior suspensory ligament of the orbit (Lockwood's ligament).

It produces depression of the posterior pole of the eyeball, elevating the cornea. Synergistically with the superior oblique and the lateral rectus, it produces abduction and lateral rotation.

It is innervated by the inferior branch of the oculomotor nerve (III).

Levator Palpebrae Superioris

The levator palpebrae superioris originates in the lesser wing of the sphenoid bone, superior and medial to the superior rectus. From here it runs above the superior rectus to insert in the superior tarsal plate and in the skin of the upper eyelid. The levator palpebrae opens the eye, elevating the superior eyelid exposing the cornea. It antagonizes the action of the orbicularis muscle.

It is innervated by the superior branch of the oculomotor nerve (III).

Superior Tarsal Muscle

The superior tarsal muscle is composed of smooth muscle fibers located between the tendon of the levator palpebrae superioris muscle and the superior tarsus. It helps in the elevation of the eyelid. It is innervated by sympathetic fibers.

Orbital Muscle

The orbital muscle is a thin layer of muscle that runs from the superior margin of the infraorbital groove and sphenomaxillary fissure to the periosteum of the maxilla and the perineurium of the infraorbital nerve.

Ciliary Muscle

The ciliary muscle is a ring of smooth muscle located in the ciliary body. It controls accommodation for close vision. It is innervated by the short ciliary fibers.

The term Müller's muscle is indistinctly used in the literature to refer to these three muscles (superior tarsal, orbital, or ciliary). Therefore, the use of this term should be discouraged to avoid the frequent confusion.

Nerves

Optic Nerve (CN II) (Fig. 51.17)

The optic nerve has three layers that are continuations of the meninges:

- The external layer is a continuation of the dura mater. It is imbricated with the sclera of the eyeball.
- The middle layer is a continuation of the arachnoid mater.
- The inner layer is a continuation of the pia mater.

The course of the optic nerve can be divided into four segments: intracranial, intracanalicular, intraorbital, and intraocular. It measures around 4 cm in length. The intraorbital segment is the longest, measuring 3 cm. The intraorbital segment is slightly longer than the distance between the eyeball and the orbital apex due to the sinuous course of the optic nerve that allows the movements of the eyeball.

The optic nerve enters the orbit through the optic canal, medial to the common annular tendon and beneath the superior rectus muscle and the levator palpebrae muscle, and then runs between the medial rectus and the inferior rectus, surrounded by the orbital fat.

Motor Nerves

The motor nerves for the eyeball are the oculomotor nerve (CN III), the abducens nerve (CN IV), and the trochlear nerve (CN VI). All three of them cross the cavernous sinus in their way to the orbit. The oculomotor nerve (CN III) innervates most of the extraocular muscles except for the lateral rectus muscle, innervated by CN VI, and the superior oblique muscle, innervated by CN IV [7].

Oculomotor Nerve (CN III)

The oculomotor nerve emerges from the isthmus of the encephalus medial to the cerebral peduncle. It courses between the posterior cerebral artery and the superior cerebellar artery, crossing the interpeduncular cistern. The oculomotor nerve pierces the dura mater external to the posterior clinoid process and crosses the cavernous sinus [8]. The oculomotor nerve enters the orbit through the common annular ring in the central part of the superior orbital fissure, close to the lateral aspect of the optic strut. It then divides in two branches, superior and inferior.

The superior branch curves upward under the insertion of the superior rectus. Then it progresses anteriorly under the belly of the superior rectus and the lesser wing of the sphenoid bone. It remains superior and lateral to the optic nerve and divides into terminal branches for the superior rectus and the levator palpebrae muscle.

The inferior branch enters the orbit through the superior orbital fissure. It is located medial to the nasociliary nerve and the abducens nerve (CN VI), and inferior to the optic nerve. It divides into three terminal branches: one for the medial rectus, one for the inferior rectus and one for the inferior oblique. The branch of the inferior oblique carries parasympathetic fibers that connect with the ciliary nerves and innervate the ciliary body and the iris.

Trochlear Nerve (CN IV)

The trochlear nerve originates on the dorsum of the encephalic isthmus. It is the only motor nerve, spinal or cranial, that arises from the dorsal aspect of the nervous system.

The trochlear nerve contours the cerebral peduncle between the posterior cerebral artery and the superior cerebellar artery. It runs caudal to the tentorium cerebelli and pierces the dura mater. Then, it progresses lateral to the cavernous sinus, running below the oculomotor nerve and over the ophthalmic nerve. It enters the orbit through the superior orbital fissure, being the nerve situated in the most cranial position. It continues over the common annular tendon and the levator palpebrae superioris muscle becoming medial to the frontal nerve and to the lacrimal nerve. After a short intraorbital trajectory, the trochlear nerve reaches its only muscle, the superior oblique muscle.

The trochlear nerve divides in two branches in 72% of the cases. In 15%, it has a single trunk, and in the remaining 13%, it has three or four branches.

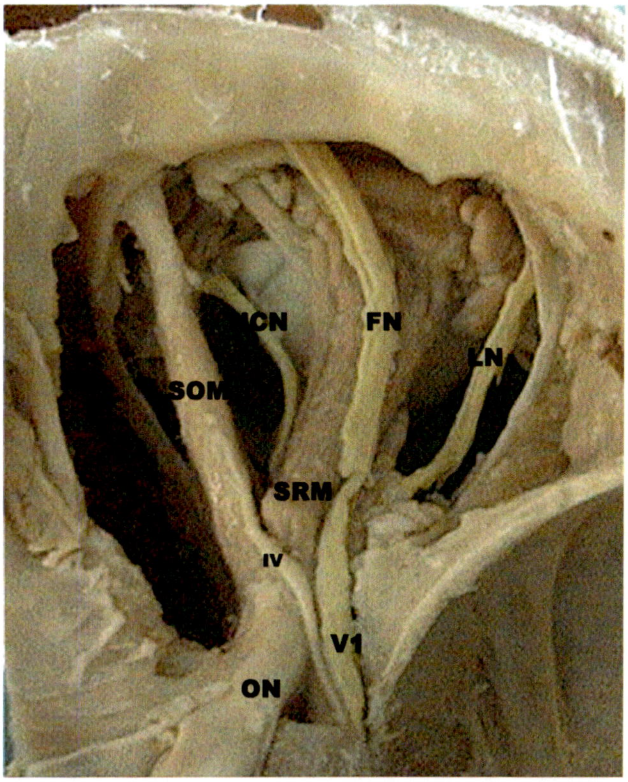

Fig. 51.14 Right orbit, superior view: *ON* optic nerve, *V1* ophthalmic nerve, *FN* frontal nerve, *LN* lacrimal nerve, *NCN* nasociliary nerve, *IV* trochlear nerve, *SOM* superior oblique muscle, *SRM* superior rectus muscle

Abducens Nerve (CN VI)

The abducens emerges from the isthmus between the protuberance and the bulb. It crosses the subarachnoid cistern in an anterior, superior, and lateral direction. The abducens pierces the dura mater below the posterior clinoid process and crosses the inferior petrous sinus. Then, it crosses between the apical portion of the temporal and the dorsum of the sella turcica. At this point, it enters the cavernous sinus medial to the ophthalmic nerve and below the nasociliary nerve. It enters the orbit through the superior orbital fissure, medial to the common annular tendon, together with fibers of the sympathetic plexus, to reach the medial surface of the lateral rectus muscle.

Sensitive Nerves

Trigeminal Nerve (CN V) (Fig. 51.14) [9]

Ophthalmic Nerve (V1)

The ophthalmic nerve runs lateral the cavernous sinus and enters the orbit through the superior orbital fissure. It divides in three branches: lacrimal, frontal, and nasociliary.

Both the lacrimal and the frontal branches enter the orbit through the superior part of the superior orbital fissure, outside the common annular tendon and below the superior ophthalmic vein.

The lacrimal nerve runs superior to the lateral rectus, carrying secretory fibers from the pterygopalatine ganglion to the lacrimal gland. It also innervates the skin and the conjunctiva.

The frontal nerve is situated medial to the lacrimal nerve and to the superior ophthalmic vein and inferior to the trochlear nerve. It crosses between the levator palpebrae superioris muscle and the periorbit. It divides in two branches inside the orbit: supraorbital and supratrochlear. The supraorbital branch splits in two branches, medial and lateral, that innervate the eyebrow, the lateral part of the forehead, and the scalp back to the vertex. The supratrochlear branch innervates the conjunctiva, the skin of the superior eyelid, and the rest of the forehead.

The nasociliary nerve enters the intraconal superior orbital fissure medial to the ophthalmic nerve and superior to the optic nerve. It reaches the medial part of the orbit, where it divides in anterior and posterior ethmoidal branches and in an infratrochlear branch. This infratrochlear branch innervates the medial canthus and the tip of the nose. It also carries sensory branches for the ciliary gland and sympathetic fibers.

Maxillary Nerve (V2)

The maxillary nerve enters the orbit through the inferior orbital fissure and penetrates the pterygopalatine fossa through the foramen rotundum. There it divides into four branches: sphenopalatine, posterosuperior alveolar, zygomatic, and infraorbital. It also gives connections to the sphenopalatine ganglion.

The infraorbital branch runs through the floor of the orbit, lodged in the infraorbital groove, to reach the infraorbital foramen. It innervates the skin of the inferior eyelid, the cheek, and the superior incisor teeth.

The zygomatic branch runs on the lateral wall of the orbit. It gives two branches, zygomaticofacial and zygomaticotemporal. These branches exit the orbit through independent foramina. The zygomatic branch innervates the skin over the lateral orbit and the zygoma. It also carries secretory-motor fibers for the lacrimal gland that connect to the branches of the lacrimal nerve.

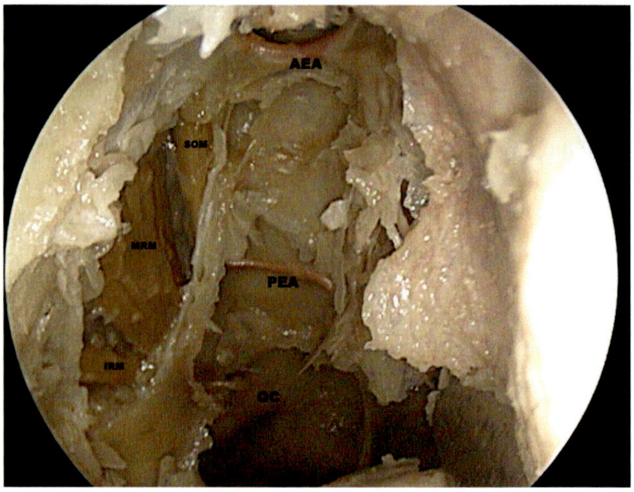

Fig. 51.15 Right orbit seen from the nasal fossa. The ethmoid cells, the lamina papyracea, the periorbita, and the orbital fat have been removed. *SOM* superior oblique muscle, *MRM* medial rectus muscle, *IRM* inferior rectus muscle, *AEA* anterior ethmoidal artery, *PEA* posterior ethmoidal artery, *ON* optic nerve

Ciliary Ganglion

The ciliary ganglion is located in the dorsal region of the orbit, close to the orbital apex.

It is situated anterior and lateral to the ophthalmic artery, inferior and lateral to the optic nerve, and medial to the lateral rectus muscle.

The ciliary ganglion receives three inputs: parasympathetic fibers from the oculomotor nerve for the iris sphincter muscle, sensory fibers from the nasociliary nerve, and sympathetic fibers from the carotid plexus for the iris dilator muscle.

Sympathetic Fibers

The sympathetic fibers for the eyeball originate in the superficial plexus of the internal carotid artery. They enter the orbit through the medial end of the superior orbital fissure and through the oculomotor foramen, following the course of the abducens nerve, the ophthalmic nerve, and the ophthalmic artery.

There is an independent branch that follows the abducens nerve to reach the inferior division of the oculomotor nerve. Some fibers reach the nasociliary nerve and distribute in the pupil.

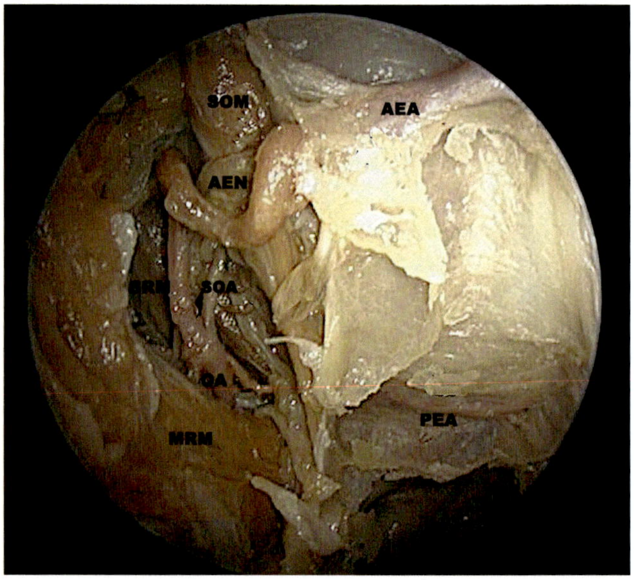

Fig. 51.16 Right orbit seen from the nasal fossa. The ethmoid cells, the lamina papyracea, the periorbita and the orbital fat have been removed. *SOM* superior oblique muscle, *SRM* superior rectus muscle, *MRM* medial rectus muscle, *AEA* anterior ethmoidal artery, *AEN* anterior ethmoid nerve, *PEA* posterior ethmoidal artery, *OA* ophthalmic artery

Arteries (Figs. 51.15, 51.16, and 51.17) [10]

The arterial network of the orbit is extremely complex and has a myriad of interindividual variations. Therefore, any attempt of classification turns into a mere schematic approximation to reality.

Ophthalmic Artery [11]

The ophthalmic artery and its branches are the main arterial supply of the orbit together with the infraorbital artery and the orbital branch of the middle meningeal artery. The latter are branches of the maxillary artery.

The ophthalmic artery is a branch of the internal carotid artery (ICA). It arises from the ophthalmic segment of the ICA in the subarachnoid space, above the cavernous sinus. In rare cases it can arise from the middle meningeal artery and, exceptionally, it can be a branch of the middle cerebral artery, of the anterior cerebral artery, of the anterior communicating artery, or of the basilar artery.

It runs medial to the anterior clinoid process, below the optic nerve. Then, it enters the orbit lateral to the optic

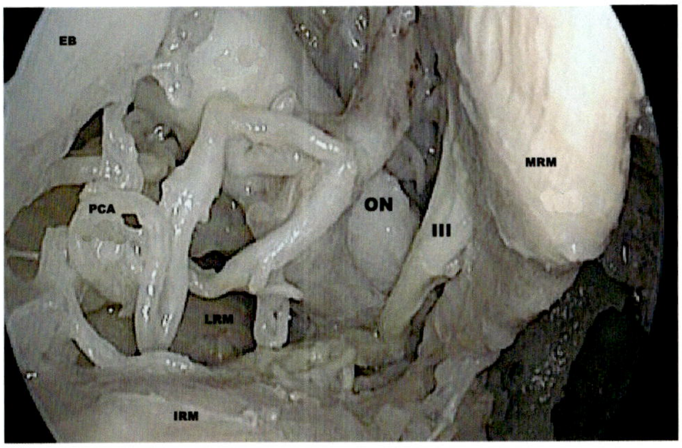

Fig. 51.17 Endoscopic view of the contents of the right orbit after removal of the orbital fat: *ON* optic nerve, *III* inferior branch of oculomotor nerve, *PCA* posterior ciliary artery, *EB* eye ball, *MRM* medial rectus muscle, *LRM* lateral rectus muscle, *IRM* inferior rectus muscle

nerve at the level of the optic canal. It becomes inferior to the optic nerve at the level of the orbital apex, crossing through the common annular tendon. In 8% of the cases, it can emerge from the superior orbital fissure. Occasionally, the ophthalmic artery divides in two branches that enter the orbit separately, one through the superior orbital fissure, and the other through the optic canal. Exceptionally, the artery can enter the orbit through an accessory ophthalmic foramen.

The intraorbital path of the ophthalmic artery contours the external and superior sides of the optic nerve to reach the inferior border of the superior oblique muscle in 66–88% of the cases. In the remaining cases, the artery runs below the optic nerve. The ophthalmic artery gives off a significant number of branches:

- Central retinal artery. It arises near the orbital apex and enters the optic nerve in its ventral aspect. It is a terminal branch of the ophthalmic artery and the most important branch in clinical terms.
- Long posterior ciliary arteries. They irrigate the optic nerve, the choroid, the ciliary body, and the iris.
- Short posterior ciliary arteries that pierce the sclera to reach the choroid.
- Anterior and posterior ethmoidal arteries. They are located along the medial wall of the orbit. The anterior ethmoidal artery runs below the superior oblique muscle, while the posterior ethmoidal artery runs over it.
- Lacrimal artery. It gives off zygomatic branches, lateral palpebral branches, and the recurrent meningeal artery. The latter anastomoses with the middle meningeal artery.
- Muscular branches for the extraocular muscles. They arise from the inferior part of the ophthalmic artery and divide into superior and inferior branches. The medial rectus and the inferior rectus are usually supplied by the inferomedial branch. The muscular branches end in the anterior ciliary arteries, which pierce the sclera to form the anterior conjunctival arteries.
- Supraorbital artery. It runs over the levator palpebrae muscle to reach the supraorbital notch. In some cases, it forms a common trunk with the posterior ethmoidal artery.
- Medial palpebral arteries. They anastomose with the lateral palpebral arteries and give off the posterior conjunctival arteries.
- Supratrochlear artery. It supplies the forehead and the scalp.
- Dorsal nasal artery. It supplies the nasal root and the lacrimal sac. It anastomoses with the facial artery.
- Meningeal branches.

Infraorbital Artery

The infraorbital artery is a terminal branch of the maxillary artery. It enters the orbit through the inferior orbital fissure. It gives off branches for the inferior oblique muscle, for the orbicular muscle, and for the lacrimal sac and the lacrimal duct and an anterior superior alveolar branch that supplies the anterior incisor teeth and the anterior region of the maxillary sinus.

The infraorbital artery also supplies the inferior eyelid, the cheek, the superior lip, and the nasal pyramid.

Middle Meningeal Artery

The middle meningeal artery is a branch of the maxillary artery. It gives off an orbital branch that anastomoses with the lacrimal artery to supply the lacrimal gland.

Veins

As opposed to other territories, the veins of the orbit are not parallel to the arteries. They usually present in inconstant patterns with high variability. Only the superior ophthalmic vein has certain correspondence to the ophthalmic artery. The venous systems of the orbit anastomose with the facial vein, with the pterygoid plexus and with the cavernous sinus.

Superior Ophthalmic Vein

The superior ophthalmic vein is the largest vein of the orbit. It originates behind the trochlea by the confluence of supratrochlear, supraorbital and angular veins. It then enters the orbit lateral to the superior oblique muscle, crossing over the optic nerve to reach the lateral orbit.

It has three parts: one that travels along the medial border of the superior rectus; a second one that travels under the superior rectus; and a third one that travels along the lateral border of the superior rectus exiting the orbit outside the common annular tendon. It usually reaches the inferior ophthalmic vein before entering the cavernous sinus.

Inferior Ophthalmic Vein

It arises from a venous plexus that drains the inferior rectus, the inferior oblique muscle, the lacrimal sac, and the eyelids in the inferior medial orbital fat. Then, it runs between the inferior rectus and the lateral rectus, where it communicates with the pterygoid plexus. It exits the orbit under the common annular tendon to enter the cavernous sinus next to the superior ethmoidal artery. In the anterior orbit, it anastomoses with branches from the angular and facial veins, connecting them with the venous plexus of the infratemporal fossa.

Central Retinal Vein

The central retinal vein enters directly in the cavernous sinus. Occasionally, it can drain in either of the ophthalmic veins.

There are some inconstant veins, such as the middle ophthalmic vein, the collateral veins, and the medial ophthalmic veins.

Periorbital Fat and Periorbita

The function of the orbital is to protect the eyeball and, at the same time, to allow the movement of the orbital structures.

It is more compact in the anterior part as it is reinforced by connective tissue septa. The posterior part is less dense to better allow displacement of the nerves and muscles.

The orbital fat is contained in a fibrous membrane called the periorbita. Anteriorly, the periorbita condenses in the orbital rim to form the orbital septum.

Orbital Septum (Fascia Palpebralis)

The orbital septum is a membranous sheath that separates the orbital structures from the facial structures. It inserts in the orbital rim and extends to the eyelids.

Acknowledgments Prof Rosa Mirapeix PhD. Unit of anatomy and Human Embriology. Universidad Autónoma de Barcelona. Spain.

References

1. Lund VJ, Stammberger H, Fokkens WJ, Beale T, Bernal-Sprekelsen M, Eloy P. European position paper on the anatomical terminology of the internal nose and paranasal sinuses. Rhinol Suppl. 2014;24:1–34.
2. Dauber W. Feneis: Nomenclaturaanatómicailutrada/Wolfgang Dauber. 5th ed. Barcelona: Elsevier Masson; 2007.
3. Drake L, Gray H. Gray's atlas of anatomy. 1st ed. Philadelphia: Churchill Livingstone; 2008.
4. René C. Update on orbital anatomy. Eye (Lond). 2006;20(10):1119–29.
5. Martins C, Costa e Silva IE, Campero A, Yasuda A, Aguiar LR, Tatagiba M, Rhoton A Jr. Microsurgical anatomy of the orbit: the rule of seven. Anat Res Int. 2011;468727:1–14.
6. Bleier BS, Healy DY Jr, Chhabra N, Freitag S. Compartmental endoscopic surgical anatomy of the medial intraconal orbital space. Int Forum Allergy Rhinol. 2014;4(7):587–91.
7. Zhang Y, Liu H, Liu EZ, Lin YZ, Zhao SG, Jing GH. Microsurgical anatomy of the ocular motor nerves. SurgRadiol Anat. 2010 Aug;32(7):623–8.
8. Iaconetta G, de Notaris M, Cavallo LM, Benet A, Enseñat J, Samii M, Ferrer E, Prats-Galino A, Cappabianca P. The oculomotor nerve: microanatomical and endoscopic study. Neurosurgery. 2010;66(3):593–601.
9. Joo W, Yoshioka F, Funaki T, Mizokami K, Rhoton AL Jr. Microsurgical anatomy of the trigeminal nerve. Clin Anat. 2014;27(1):61–88.
10. Hayreh SS. Orbital vascular anatomy. Eye. 2006;20:1130–44.
11. Erdogmus s GF. Accurate course and relationship of the intraorbital part of the ophthalmic artery in sagital plane. Minim Invasive Neurosurg. 2007;50(4):2002–8.

Imaging for Orbital Diseases: Traditional Modalities and Newer Concepts

52

Miral Jhaveri and Murali Nagarajan

Radiological imaging in ophthalmology plays an important role to complement a thorough clinical examination. Imaging of the orbit involves two distinct areas, i.e., the globe and the bony orbit and orbital and periorbital soft tissues. Ultrasound, computed tomography (CT), and magnetic resonance imaging (MRI) are mainstays in orbital imaging, supplemented in certain situations with more advanced or specific imaging. Radiography, for the most part, has been superseded by advances in CT imaging techniques.

Ultrasound [1]

By virtue of having very high resolution for superficial structures, ultrasound (US) provides detailed evaluation of intraocular lesions. It is often the first-line modality following a funduscopic examination. It is particularly helpful in conditions which limit direct visualization such as dense cataract or vitreous hemorrhage. Usefulness of US ranges from providing measurements of the globe for intraocular lens implantation and measurement of the angle to assess posterior segment pathology such as retinal detachment, intraocular neoplasms, and foreign body. It is inexpensive and readily available and does not involve ionizing radiation. However, it has very limited usefulness when it comes to extraocular orbital pathology. It is also contraindicated when open globe injury is suspected.

Computed Tomography

Natural contrast provided by bone, fat, air, and soft tissues of the orbit in conjunction with high spatial resolution makes CT an ideal modality for imaging the orbit. By providing excellent bony details, CT is superior to MRI for orbital trauma and for orbital lesions that arise from or directly affect the bones, such as osteocartilaginous tumors, osteodystrophic processes, benign masses that cause bony scalloping, and aggressive tumors that cause bony destruction. Rapid acquisition helps in evaluating uncooperative patients and children. It is also the ideal modality to evaluate foreign bodies.

Multidetector CT (MDCT) is commonplace and provides isotropic imaging with excellent multiplanar reformatting and 3D volume rendering capabilities. CT protocol consists of axial 1–2 mm sections with sagittal and coronal 1–2 mm reformats in soft tissue and bone algorithms. Intravenous contrast may be administered to evaluate infectious or vascular lesions when MR is not contemplated. The major disadvantage of CT is ionizing radiation.

MRI

MRI has superior soft tissue contrast resolution compared to CT. This is reinforced with fat suppression technique and contrast administration. These features make MR the ideal modality for evaluating complex soft tissue lesions such as malignant tumors and complex inflammatory processes. Important features visible on MR include perineural tumor spread, optic nerve pathology, hematogenous or cerebrospinal fluid (CSF) disseminated metastases, and intracranial extension. MR provides exquisite characterization of the globe itself, which is particularly useful in circumstances where funduscopic evaluation is obscured.

Typical imaging protocol includes thin sections (2–3 mm) and small field of view (12–16 cm) scans. Stronger gradients, faster sequences, and surface coils are used. Precontrast T1, fat-suppressed T2, and post-contrast T1 with fat suppression images are obtained in axial and coronal planes from above the orbital roof to the orbital floor and from the back of the pons through the globe. Axial FLAIR and post-contrast images through the brain may be acquired as needed.

M. Jhaveri (✉) · M. Nagarajan
Rush University Medical Center, Chicago, IL, USA
e-mail: Miral_D_Jhaveri@rush.edu

A. J. Cohen, C. N. Burkat (eds.), *Oculofacial, Orbital, and Lacrimal Surgery*, https://doi.org/10.1007/978-3-030-14092-2_52

The major disadvantage is the longer scan time, thus limiting its usefulness in pediatric and uncooperative patients and also in the setting of trauma. MRI is not safe when metallic foreign bodies are suspected.

Advanced Imaging

Optical coherence tomography (OCT) provides much higher resolution compared to ultrasound. Similar to US, it uses backscatter to generate images, but in OCT, high-frequency pulsed laser is used instead of ultrasonic waves. It is most commonly used to image the macula and optic nerve [2].

Magnetic resonance imaging of the retina, using high-resolution sequences such as balanced steady-state free precession, small field of view, and small eye-shaped surface coils on a 3 T scanner, brings out detailed anatomy of the retina. Incorporation of arterial spin labeling technique also provides dynamic flow information of the retinal vessels [3]. It can potentially help in diagnosing and monitoring diabetic retinopathy, glaucoma, and retinal degeneration [4]. However, OCT is superior in terms of providing better anatomic detail with resolution as high as 4 microns vs 100 × 200 microns of high-resolution MRI [5].

Diffusion-weighted imaging uses a fast echoplanar sequence (EPI) to identify areas of ischemia. It can help in the early diagnosis of posterior ischemic optic neuropathy in which the funduscopic exam is usually normal [6]. Because of the susceptibility artifacts which occur in this region due to bone and air interfaces, specialized techniques such as thinner slices, parallel imaging, and non-echoplanar sequences may be necessary.

Magnetization transfer contrast is a technique which creates contrast between structures depending upon their myelin content. This technique can help in diagnosing conditions which result in the loss of myelination, such as optic neuritis [7].

Diffusion tensor imaging (DTI) works on the principle that myelinated axons restrict diffusion of water along certain directions. Neuronal tracts oriented in a particular direction, for example, optic radiation, can be mapped out separately. On diffusion tensor tractography (DTT), this information is visually represented in a three-dimensional space [8]. Even more specialized techniques such as diffusion spectrum imaging and high angular resolution diffusion imaging (HARDI) help to get better resolution of regions with crossing fibers, with sharp angles, and within intratumor segments. DTI can be used for presurgical planning in order to navigate through the surgical field without injuring vital structures [9].

Functional MRI is a special technique which is employed to image brain activity. It works on the principle of blood oxygen level dependence (BOLD). Brain activity results in local changes in blood flow, blood volume, and oxygen saturation which help to map out the metabolically active regions. An ultrafast echoplanar (EPI) sequence is used for high temporal resolution [10]. Cortical mapping of the visual field is obtained which helps in preoperative planning as well as evaluation of neurodegenerative diseases such as glaucoma and macular degeneration [11].

Time-resolved MR imaging with contrast kinetics (TRICKS) is an excellent modality useful for dynamic vascular studies with high resolution and temporal correlation. As it allows the evaluation of the rapidity and degree of vascular circulation into and drainage from a particular lesion, it can differentiate lesions such as cavernous malformations, hemangiopericytomas, and arteriovenous malformations (AVM).

Anatomy [12]

Major portions of the bony orbital walls are contributed by the frontal bone superiorly, zygomatic bone laterally, maxillary bone inferiorly, and ethmoid bone medially. Smaller contributions medially include the lacrimal bone, nasal bone, and a tiny portion of the palatine bone. The sphenoid bone makes up a large portion of the orbit posteriorly and laterally, forming the complex foramina at the orbital apex.

The globe is divided into anterior aqueous and posterior vitreous segments by the lens and ciliary body. The anterior segment is divided into anterior and posterior chambers by the iris. The cornea constitutes the transparent outer layer of the anterior segment and, with the sclera, comprises the outer layer of the globe. The uveal tract, which includes the choroid, iris, and ciliary body, comprises the middle layer. The deepest layer is the retinal layer. These individual layers are usually not differentiated on CT or MR imaging in the normal globe.

The orbital septum is a fascial layer arising from the orbital periosteum which inserts onto the aponeurosis of the tarsal plates of the lids, providing a barrier between the anterior periorbita and the intraorbital contents. The septum is readily evident when a disease process is contained on one side of the barrier.

The four rectus muscles originate from the annulus of Zinn at the apex and insert on the corneoscleral surface. This muscle cone divides the postseptal space into intraconal and extraconal compartments. The superior oblique has a similar origin and insertion but courses through the trochlea at the superomedial orbital rim toward the trochlea. The inferior oblique has a short, more direct course originating from the anteroinferior orbital rim. The levator palpebrae superioris originates at the annulus, coursing just above the superior rectus to insert on the upper eyelid tarsus.

The optic nerve traverses the optic canal to insert at the optic nerve head. The surrounding dural sheath is contiguous with the intracranial dura and the sclera. A thin layer of CSF surrounding the nerve is typically visible on MR and is contiguous with CSF in the suprasellar cistern.

The 3rd, 4th, 5th, and 6th cranial nerves are not consistently identifiable within the orbit. However, knowledge of their course allows localization of pathology that involves these nerves. The 3rd, 4th, and 6th nerves and ophthalmic division of trigeminal nerve pass through the superior orbital fissure. The maxillary division of trigeminal nerve passes through the foramen rotundum and inferior orbital fissure and exits through the infraorbital foramen.

The ophthalmic artery enters the orbit within the optic nerve. It is frequently visible in the orbit as it exits the nerve near the apex. The superior ophthalmic vein is found between the superior rectus muscle and the optic nerve. Enlargement of this vein can be highly suggestive for carotid-cavernous fistula, most commonly, as well as ophthalmic vein varix, Graves' orbitopathy, retrocavernous meningioma, and increased intracranial pressure.

The lacrimal gland lies in a bony fossa superolaterally in the anterior orbit. Lacrimal drainage is via canaliculi and lacrimal sac at the inferomedial orbit, and from there through the nasolacrimal duct, which drains via the inferior meatus.

The orbital fat acts as a filler for the orbital cavity and provides intrinsic imaging contrast, making other structures and disease processes more conspicuous.

Orbital Pathology

Orbital Trauma

Certain characteristic traumatic fracture patterns involve the orbits. CT with multiplanar reformats help in accurate assessment of these fractures.

Blow-Out Fracture

A blow-out fracture refers to a displaced fracture of an orbital wall directed away from the orbit with or without involvement of the orbital rim, typically involving the floor. It often results from increased intraorbital pressure (hydraulic mechanism) or less commonly from transmission of force through orbital rim (bone conduction mechanism) [13]. The inferior orbital wall is the weakest and involved more commonly. Although the medial wall is the thinnest, it is supported by the bones of the ethmoid sinuses and is affected less often. Herniation of orbital fat, extraocular muscles, degree of enophthalmos, and involvement of the infraorbital canal need to be assessed on CT.

A special type of the orbital blow-out fracture is the trapdoor fracture in which the inferior rectus muscle or infraorbital fat herniates through the fracture defect into the underlying maxillary sinus with return of the fracture fragment back to its original position. CT will show a non-displaced fracture with a possibly entrapped inferior rectus. This is more common in younger patients in whom the bones are more pliable.

Blow-In Fracture

Direct blow to the forehead results in downward displacement of the superior orbital wall which is termed as blow-in fracture. It is often associated with a fracture of the frontal sinus. It may result in proptosis, diplopia, orbital emphysema, cerebrospinal fluid (CSF) leak, or brain herniation [14]. Often a fragment of the superior orbital bone will be seen resting on the superior muscle complex, which contributes to diplopia.

LeFort Fractures

These are complex fractures that result in varying degrees of craniofacial dislocation. There are three types and all of these, by definition, involve the pterygomaxillary junction. Type I fracture does not involve the orbits. Type II is a pyramid-shaped fracture with its apex at the nasofrontal suture and laterally extending into the medial and inferior orbital walls. Type III is complete craniofacial dissociation in which the fracture runs from the nasofrontal suture into the medial and lateral orbital walls and into the zygomatic arches—the bony face is attached by soft tissue only. Multiplanar reformats from CT accurately classify these fractures [15].

Zygomatico-maxillary Complex (ZMC) Fracture

A ZMC fracture is a diastatic fracture involving the four sutures that connect the zygomatic bone to the surrounding cranial and facial bones, including the zygomatic arch [16]. The zygoma forms portions of the inferior and lateral orbital walls. Displaced ZMC fractures or concomitant orbital floor blow-out fractures can result in enophthalmos, lateral canthal angle dystopia, trismus, and malar flattening.

Naso-orbito-ethmoid (NOE) Complex Fracture

High-impact force over the nasal region results in comminuted fracture of the nasal bones, nasal septum, ethmoid sinuses, cribriform plate, and medial orbital walls [16]. Complications include proptosis, exophthalmos, hemorrhage (due to laceration of the ethmoidal arteries), and CSF rhinorrhea. Comminuted fracture through the medial wall and medial canthal tendon injury can result in telecanthus. If the lacrimal sac or nasolacrimal duct is injured, future dacryocystorhinostomy surgery may be indicated.

Orbital Apex Fracture

Fractures of the orbital apex [17] can extend through the optic canal or superior orbital fissure, resulting in damage to the cranial nerves that traverse these structures. When the superior orbital fissure alone is involved, it results in injury to III, IV, and VI nerves and the ophthalmic division of V nerve which manifest as ophthalmoplegia, diplopia, and ptosis, termed superior orbital fissure syndrome. When the optic nerve is also involved, it may be referred to as an orbital apex syndrome [18], which can also be seen with infectious etiologies. CT or MRI can show obliteration of fat in the optic canal. Optic nerve edema is better demonstrated on MRI. Prognosis for vision is very guarded in orbital apex fractures.

Traumatic Soft Tissue Injury

Traumatic hemorrhage can occur in various compartments. Hyphema, hemorrhage within the anterior chamber, appears as dense blood-fluid level on CT. Diffuse heterogeneous hyperdensity is seen in the posterior segment in vitreous hemorrhage [19]. Subhyaloid hemorrhage, that is the hemorrhage between hyaloid membrane covering the vitreous and retina, appears as pooling hyperdensity anterior to the optic disc with a sharp margin against the vitreous. Retinal detachment due to hemorrhage between the choroid and retina appears as lentiform-shaped collections which extend to, but do not cross, the optic disc, with a V-shaped appearance on CT or MRI [20]. Choroidal detachment occurs when there is hemorrhage between the choroid and sclera. On imaging, this appears as lentiform collections as well but does not extend to the posterior third of the globe and can reach more anteriorly beyond the ora serrata, unlike retinal detachment [21]. Subtenon hemorrhage is situated between the sclera and Tenon capsule. On CT, subtenon hemorrhage appears as a lentiform-shaped hyperdensity along the outer surface of the globe and may be difficult to distinguish from retrobulbar hematoma. Subperiosteal hematoma is seen as a hyperdense collection along the orbital wall projecting into the orbit.

Traumatic lens subluxation, dislocation, and extrusion are readily evident on imaging. With subluxation, the lens is in normal location but shows abnormal angulation. Dislocated lens more commonly settles down in the vitreous, but anterior dislocations can also occur. Traumatic cataract results from edema and is seen as a decrease in density of the lens on CT [22].

Open globe injury, which is a full-thickness tear of sclera, cornea, or both, results in loss of volume of the globe and loss of its normal spherical shape. Lens injury, foreign body, vitreous hemorrhage, and intraocular air may be associated [23].

Orbital emphysema usually results from an orbital fracture communicating with the paranasal sinuses. It is generally benign; however, air extending into the optic nerve sheath may result in optic nerve ischemia. Edema or hemorrhage of the extraocular muscles can occur with trauma which is seen as swelling or increased density on CT. Inferior rectus or orbital fat herniation can be seen prolapsing through a blow-out fracture.

Optic nerve injury can occur due to compression from a hematoma or optic canal fracture. The affected segment may show restricted diffusion on MRI [24]. Severe trauma can result in rare transection of the nerve, which is seen as a discontinuity along the nerve with an intact nerve sheath.

Foreign Bodies

Foreign bodies can be metallic such as iron or copper, nonmetallic such as glass or plastic, or organic such as wood. Characterization of foreign bodies is important for preoperative planning. For example, organic foreign bodies often contain microorganisms and need to be removed. CT is the best modality to identify, localize, and characterize the foreign bodies. MRI is reserved for suspected nonmetallic foreign body, if CT is negative. Plain radiographs are only used to rule out metallic foreign bodies prior to MR imaging. Metallic foreign bodies have high density, appearing brighter than bones. Nonmetallic foreign bodies are denser than soft tissues but less dense than metal. Organic foreign bodies can have variable densities. For example, wood can have air density. Air density conforming to a particular geometric shape or air density in dependent position is suggestive of wood [25, 26]. Wood can be demonstrated on both CT and MRI, with proper notification of the radiologist if wood is suspected so that the parameters of CT imaging can be adjusted.

Abnormal densities such as calcifications secondary to optic nerve drusen, phthisis bulbi, and postoperative conditions such as silicone gel implantation and scleral bands should not be confused with foreign bodies [27, 28].

Congenital Lesions

Coloboma [29–31]

Coloboma is a developmental abnormality that occurs as a result of failure of closure of the embryonic choroidal fissure and presents as a cleft in the inferonasal quadrant. Typically, these are optic disc or choroidoretinal types and may also involve any or all structures of the embryonic fissure including the iris, ciliary body, lens, or eyelid.

On imaging, these are seen as a focal defect with outpouching at the posterior pole of the globe with the vitreous contiguous with the defect. These are usually small, ranging from a few to several millimeters. Associated findings may include microcornea, microphthalmia, optic tract and chiasm atrophy, retrobulbar colobomatous cyst, retinal detachment, and cataract. Morning glory disc anomaly is a related but distinct entity where the disc is posteriorly displaced in a deep funnel-shaped excavation at the optic nerve head.

Colobomas are unilateral when sporadic but often bilateral when associated with syndromes such as trisomy 13 and 18, CHARGE, Aicardi, COACH, Meckel, Warburg, and Lenz, among others.

Persistent Hyperplastic Primary Vitreous (PHPV) [29, 32, 33]

PHPV is a congenital lesion that results when the portion of the hyaloid artery, which traverses the vitreous region from the optic nerve head to the lens, and the fibrovascular tissue of the primary vitreous fail to degenerate and resorb.

Presence of an enhancing triangular retrolental soft tissue and a central tissue stalk of hyaloid remnant is characteristic, seen as a "martini glass" appearance. Isolated anterior and posterior forms can also occur but are less common. PHPV is generally unilateral and rarely shows calcification. Bilateral lesions are associated with syndromes such as Warburg and Norrie. The vitreous is hyperdense on CT, is T1 and T2 hyperintense on MRI, and shows contrast enhancement depending on the degree of persistent vascularity. Hemorrhage and layering of debris can be seen in the vitreous. PHPV is usually associated with a small globe. Retinal detachment is common.

Presence of a small globe and the absence of calcification help differentiate PHPV from retinoblastoma, a commonly misdiagnosed entity.

Coats Disease [32]

This is an idiopathic primary retinal vascular disease, characterized by telangiectasias, neovascularization, beading, and tortuosity of retinal vessels, with progressive accumulation of lipoproteinaceous exudate leading to retinal detachment. It is generally unilateral but bilateral when syndromic. The affected globe is slightly small.

Typical V-shaped contour of retinal detachment is seen. Subretinal exudate is hyperdense on CT and T1 hyperintense on MRI due to blood products and proteinaceous material. Calcification is very uncommon. Lack of calcification and contrast enhancement and the small size of the globe help to differentiate it from retinoblastoma, an important differential consideration.

Vascular Lesions [34]

These can be true neoplasms such a capillary hemangioma or vascular malformations which are present at birth or shortly after birth. Vascular malformations grow commensurately with age, show normal mitotic activity, and do not involute. Vascular malformations are classified based on flow. Lymphatic malformations show no flow. Venous flow is seen in venous/venolymphatic malformations. Arterial flow malformations can be of slow-flow, such as typical in cavernous hemangioma, or high-flow, such as an arteriovenous malformation.

Capillary Hemangioma

Also called infantile hemangiomas, these are the most common orbital vascular tumor, appearing just before, or shortly after, birth. The lesion grows rapidly in infancy during the phase of endothelial proliferation and has an involutional phase with spontaneous regression of most lesions in childhood during the next 5–7 years.

Most hemangiomas are entirely or largely extraconal in location. In the proliferative phase, the tumor shows strong contrast enhancement. Fatty replacement occurs in the involutional phase. Calcification is not seen. CT may show orbital enlargement or bony scalloping. On MRI, the lesion is isointense to mildly hyperintense on T1 and hyperintense on T2 with flow voids of enlarged arterial feeders and draining veins in or around the lobulated lesion.

Venolymphatic Malformations

Venolymphatic malformations are poorly demarcated, multilocular, cystic, and trans-spatial masses with variable amount of venous and lymphatic elements. They are often confined to the conjunctiva, and when postseptal extension is present, it is more often in the extraconal space. Fluid-fluid levels when present are characteristic. Blood products and proteinaceous contents appear hyperdense on CT and hyperintense on T1 on MRI. CT may show remodeling of bony orbit with large lesions. Phleboliths are uncommon. Contrast enhancement is seen along the margins of the cystic areas. Diffuse enhancement can be seen if prominent venous components are present.

Venous Varix

Venous varix is a low-flow venous malformation with dynamically distensible wall. It appears as an intensely enhancing mass that distends with increased venous pressure and can occur anywhere in the orbit. It may be small and undetectable on quiet breathing. Phleboliths may be present. On MRI, it shows complex signal with blood products and fluid-fluid levels. The best imaging modality is dynamic contrast-enhanced CT scan with Valsalva maneuver.

Orbital Cavernous Venous Malformation (Hemangioma)

Orbital cavernous venous malformation is a low-flow vascular malformation characterized by endothelial-lined cavernous spaces. It is the most common orbital mass in adults often detected incidentally on brain imaging. It appears as a circumscribed ovoid, avidly enhancing mass. Most lesions are intraconal although they can occur anywhere in the orbit. On CT, it is homogeneously isodense, and bone remodeling can be seen with larger lesions. On MRI, it is hyperintense on T2 with a pseudocapsule. Internal septations can be seen in larger lesions. On dynamic contrast-enhanced MRI (TRICKS), it shows a characteristic enhancement pattern with early patchy central enhancement and homogeneous filling on delayed images. CT is diagnostic in appropriate clinical setting. Dynamic contrast-enhanced MRI can be obtained for doubtful cases.

Dermoid and Epidermoid [31, 35, 36]

These are the most common space-occupying lesions of the orbit in the pediatric age group. These are inclusion cysts which arise from rests of sequestered embryonic ectoderm entrapped in the orbital bony sutures. Both epidermoid and dermoid lesions are lined by keratinizing stratified squamous epithelium, with dermoids also containing the skin adnexa including hair and sebaceous glands.

These appear as cystic, well-circumscribed lesions adjacent to orbital periosteum near suture lines with the majority located at the frontozygomatic suture. They can be superficial or deep and even extend through the lateral orbital wall to have both an orbital and external component. Superficial lesions are small with subtle bony changes, while deep lesions are larger and complicated and show extensive bony changes. Epidermoids are homogeneous and show fluid density and signal, whereas dermoids are more heterogeneous and typically contain fat. Fat-fluid/fluid-fluid levels can be seen in some cases. The cyst walls demonstrate thin rim enhancement, but thick irregular enhancement is seen when there is rupture and inflammation. Epidermoids show restricted diffusion on diffusion-weighted MRI. CT is generally adequate for diagnosis, while MRI may be useful for deep complicated lesions.

Neurofibromatosis Type 1 [37, 38]

Neurofibromatosis is a phakomatoses that can affect the orbit in multiple ways. The constellation of features includes plexiform neurofibroma, optic nerve glioma, sphenoid dysplasia, buphthalmos, and optic nerve sheath ectasia. Plexiform neurofibroma is typically a serpentine, non-encapsulated, infiltrative mass. It may involve cranial nerves, muscles, optic nerve sheath, and sclera. On CT, it appears hypodense. Bone remodeling and widening of the skull base foramina can be seen. On MRI, it is T2 hyperintense with central hypointensity- "target" sign. Variable contrast enhancement is present. Optic nerve glioma can affect any segment of the optic nerve and may involve the chiasm and brainstem. On MRI, it appears as a T2 hyperintense fusiform mass with variable enhancement. Sphenoid wing dysplasia presents as bony defects, decalcification, remodeling of greater wing of sphenoid, and enlargement of middle cranial fossa with herniation of intracranial contents into the orbit. Optic nerve sheath ectasia is enlargement of the dural sheath with increased CSF space around the optic nerve.

Infectious and Inflammatory Lesions

Orbital Infection [39]

Imaging (contrast-enhanced CT or MRI) is usually performed to differentiate preseptal cellulitis from the more vision-threatening orbital cellulitis. Preseptal cellulitis is characterized by soft tissue swelling, stranding, and patchy enhancement of the soft tissues superficial to the orbital septum. Orbital cellulitis will demonstrate inflammatory stranding and enhancement posterior to the orbital septum. A subperiosteal abscess is a rim-enhancing fluid collection along the orbital wall with adjacent paranasal sinus infection, which is most commonly seen along the medial orbital wall with associated acute ethmoid sinusitis. On MR imaging, subperiosteal or intraorbital abscesses will demonstrate rim enhancement with internal T2 hyperintensity and restricted diffusion. Invasive fungal sinusitis can involve the orbits and may be associated with osseous destruction. Intracranial complications of orbital cellulitis include cavernous sinus thrombosis, intracranial abscess, subdural empyema, and meningitis.

Scleritis or uveitis when it affects the posterior segment is difficult to diagnose clinically. The inflamed layers will show thickening and contrast enhancement which can be focal, nodular, or diffuse. Endophthalmitis or panophthalmitis can result in increased density of the vitreous. MRI may show increased signal in vitreous on FLAIR images, restricted diffusion within the globe, ocular wall thickening and enhancement, and periorbital inflammatory changes.

Ocular Toxocariasis [40]

Infection with toxocara species results in granulomatous sclerosing endophthalmitis. Imaging may reveal a moderately enhancing retinal nodule which typically lacks calcification. Intravitreal membranes and retinal detachment may be present.

Idiopathic Orbital Inflammation [41, 42]

This is a nonspecific inflammation without any known etiology and is a diagnosis of exclusion. It can involve any part of the orbit, and depending on the part affected, it can be classified into myositic, lacrimal, anterior (involving globe or retrobulbar region), apical (orbital apex), or diffuse. MRI is the modality of choice, although CT can be used. The disease is typically unilateral but can be bilateral in 25% cases. Occasionally, a poorly marginated, enhancing soft tissue mass may be seen. In the myositic form, the extraocular muscles are enlarged with a tubular configuration typically involving the tendon as well. In contrast, muscle enlargement secondary to thyroid eye disease tends to spare the muscle tendinous insertion onto the globe. The lesions are iso-intense to slightly T2 hyperintense. The T2 signal decreases with increase in fibrotic component. Tolosa-Hunt syndrome is a variant when the disease extends through the superior orbital fissure into the cavernous sinus.

Orbital Sarcoidosis [43]

Sarcoidosis is a noncaseating granulomatous inflammation which can involve multiple sites in the orbit including the lacrimal gland, optic nerve sheath, extraocular muscles, orbital fat, uvea, and preseptal soft tissues. It can be seen as an orbital mass or diffuse enlargement of the involved structure. On CT, the lesions appear isodense. On MRI, they are variably T2 hyperintense and demonstrate diffuse homogeneous contrast enhancement. Ga-67 scintigraphy shows increased uptake.

Thyroid Orbitopathy [44]

Thyroid orbitopathy, or thyroid eye disease, is an autoimmune inflammatory condition where antibodies target thyrotropin receptors which are seen in the thyroid gland and orbit. It results in diffuse enlargement of the muscle bellies with typical sparing of the tendons. Involvement of the muscles is nonuniform with inferior, medial, superior, and lateral recti and superior oblique muscles being affected in the order of decreasing severity. Bilateral and symmetric involvement is seen in most cases, although asymmetric muscle involvement is also frequently seen. The muscles are isodense on CT. During acute phase, they show T2 hyperintensity on MRI and hypointensity during the chronic phase due to fibrosis. An increase in orbital fat, exophthalmos, stretching/straightening of the optic nerve, and lacrimal gland enlargement may be seen. Some studies have shown that volumetric analysis of muscles can be used to monitor treatment response.

Optic Neuritis [45]

Optic neuritis is an autoimmune inflammatory condition which can be focal or segmental and is more often unilateral. Any segment of the nerve can be affected. Enhancement and focal enlargement of the optic nerve are seen, which are best assessed on MRI. Enhancement may be central or diffuse. Nerve sheath enhancement may be present. Presence of white matter lesions in the brain or spinal cord is a strong predictor for multiple sclerosis. Optic neuritis is also a characteristic feature and one of the diagnostic criteria for neuromyelitis optica (NMO), which is an inflammatory CNS disorder distinct from multiple sclerosis [46].

Orbital Tumors

Optic Pathway Glioma [47]

There are three subtypes: childhood lesions with NF1 (syndromic type), sporadic childhood lesions, and adult type. Child tumors are far more common and are typically low-grade gliomas. Adult lesions are either anaplastic astrocytoma or glioblastoma. It is typically unilateral, but bilateral lesions can be seen in syndromic type. MRI is the preferred modality. Any part of the optic pathway, from optic nerve to optic radiation, can be affected. Fusiform enlargement and kinking of the involved segment are seen. They are iso- to mildly hypointense on T1 and variably hyperintense on T2. Focal cystic spaces can be seen. Contrast enhancement is variable. Syndromic type shows no or minimal enhancement. Moderate to intense enhancement is seen in sporadic type and moderate heterogeneous enhancement in adult type. In syndromic type, other orbital manifestations of NF1 can be present. Spontaneous regression can occur with syndromic lesions.

Optic Nerve Sheath Meningioma [48]

Optic nerve sheath meningioma is a benign tumor arising from arachnoid cap cells in the optic nerve sheath. It is relatively small at presentation due to early visual symptoms. On imaging, it appears as a solid, well-defined tubular mass encasing the optic nerve. Eccentric or pedunculated type of growth can occur but less commonly. Linear or punctate calcification is characteristic and is seen in almost half the cases. On MRI, it is T1 isointense and variably hyperintense to hypointense on T2. Perioptic cysts can be seen between the distal optic nerve and the globe. It shows moderate to intense homogeneous contrast enhancement. Circumferential contrast enhancement gives the characteristic "tram track" appearance on cross section. Optic nerve sheath meningioma should not be confused with the spheno-orbital meningioma, which is a larger intracranial tumor with orbital extension.

Lacrimal Gland Tumors [49]

Benign mixed tumor, also known as pleomorphic adenoma, is the most common benign tumor of the lacrimal gland. It appears as a solid, well-circumscribed mass in the anterior superotemporal extraconal space. It is hypo- to isointense on T1 and iso- to hyperintense on T2 and shows moderate to intense enhancement. Chronic bony remodeling of the lacrimal fossa can occasionally be seen.

In contrast, lacrimal gland carcinoma appears as an irregular lacrimal fossa mass with bone erosion. Adenoid cystic carcinoma is the most common type, which often shows perineural spread.

Retinoblastoma [62]

Retinoblastoma is the most common intraocular tumor of childhood. It is a malignant, primitive neuroectodermal tumor arising from the retina. It is unilateral in 60% and bilateral in 40% cases. Trilateral tumors, i.e., bilateral retinoblastoma with pineal neuroblastoma, or quadrilateral tumors with pineal and suprasellar tumors, are rare. Retinoblastoma may show endophytic growth (growth into the vitreous) or exophytic growth (outward growth into the subretinal space) or a mixed pattern. On imaging, it appears as an irregular mass. Punctate calcification is seen in most cases (90–95%). It is mildly T1 hyperintense and moderate to markedly hypointense on T2. Moderate to intense heterogeneous contrast enhancement is seen. Enhancement of the anterior chamber indicates neoangiogenesis which is seen in aggressive tumors. The involved globe is generally larger. Subretinal fluid or vitreous hemorrhage may be present.

MRI is optimal to assess for tumor invasion, which can be intraocular with involvement of the choroid or sclera or extraocular into the optic nerve, orbit, or intracranial cavity.

Ocular Melanoma [50]

Ocular melanoma is the most common intraocular tumor in adults. It is a malignant tumor arising from the melanocytes within the uveal layer. Most tumors originate from the choroid, although the ciliary body and iris can also be affected. The temporal region posterior to the equator is the most common site of involvement. On imaging, these appear as dome-shaped lesions with a broad base along the choroid. It becomes a mushroom shape when it penetrates the Bruch membrane. These are typically solid in appearance and show moderate homogeneous enhancement. Calcification is rare. MRI typically shows mild to strong T1 hyperintensity and strong T2 hypointensity when compared to vitreous. Tumors with a higher content of melanin pigment are more hyperintense on T1. Associated retinal detachment is common. The subretinal fluid shows T1 hyperintensity and iso- or hypointensity on T2 secondary to blood products or proteinaceous content. Extraocular tumor extension is best assessed with MRI.

Orbital Lymphoma [51]

Orbital lymphoma is commonly a low-grade small B-cell lymphoma although more aggressive lesions can occur. It can occur anywhere in the orbit, with the anterior extraconal compartment and lacrimal gland most commonly involved. Lymphoma can also be seen in the eyelid and conjunctiva. When present in the orbit, tumor plasticity allows the lesion to characteristically conform to the shape of other structures, which results in minimal symptoms initially as the mass molds to, rather than compresses, the optic nerve or muscles. Due to high cellularity, it appears iso- to mildly hyperdense on CT and only mildly hyperintense to muscle on T2-weighted MR images. Homogeneous moderate to strong contrast enhancement is seen. Bone remodeling or destruction can occur depending on the aggressiveness of the lesion.

Postoperative Orbital Imaging

Recognizing the normal postoperative appearance of commonly encountered orbital procedures is important to eliminate false-positive reads and also help in early detection of postoperative complications.

1. Intraocular lens implants are visible as thin, disc-shaped hyperdense structures on CT and T2 hypointense on MRI [52].
2. Glaucoma shunting implants are generally placed in the upper quadrants of the globe and less often in the lower quadrants. These consist of a plate placed within a scleral pocket, which connects to a tube that extends into the anterior chamber. The shunted aqueous collects around the plate, forms an encapsulated bleb, and gets absorbed by the surrounding tissues. The implants may be made of silicone which appear hyperdense on CT or polypropylene or polyethylene which are hypodense. These implants are hypointense on MRI [52, 53].
3. Retinal detachment can be treated with retinopexy, scleral buckling, or vitrectomy. In pneumatic retinopexy, sterile room air, sulfur hexafluoride, or perfluoropropane is used to create a tamponade effect to keep the retina against the walls of the globe. It gets gradually resorbed over a few days to few weeks depending on the type of gas used. Air attenuation is seen on CT and should not be mistaken for infection. A scleral buckle is a smooth synthetic band sutured to the sclera that exerts pressure to appose the detached layers of the retina together [54]. Scleral buckles are oriented either parallel or perpendicular to the rectus muscles and are focal, segmental, or circumferential. Porous silicone sponges appear as bands with air attenuation on CT, whereas the solid silicone rubber bands show hyperattenuation. Both are hypointense on MRI [20].

Following vitrectomy, silicone oil can be used as a tamponade agent. Silicone oil appears homogeneously hyperdense on CT and should not be mistaken for vitreous hemorrhage. It is hyperintense to normal vitreous on T1 and variably hyperintense to hypointense on T2-weighted images. The presence of chemical shift artifact can be used to differentiate silicone oil from vitreous hemorrhage. Occasionally, silicone may migrate outside the globe [20, 55].

4. An orbital implant is placed following evisceration or enucleation. Appearance of the implant on CT depends upon the material used. The majority of implants used are spheres, although other shapes are available. Polyethylene implants are hypodense. Acrylic and silicone implants are homogeneously hyperdense. Hydroxyapatite is very hyperdense with a characteristic lattice pattern [52, 56]. The extraocular muscles can be seen to be reattached to the anterior face of the implant.
5. Eyelid weights are used to enable eyelid closure in patients with lagophthalmos. These rectangular weights are implanted subcutaneously and typically secured to the anterior tarsus. Gold is the commonly used material and is MR compatible, although platinum weights are preferred in some cases. Metallic density is seen on CT [57].
6. In cases of nasolacrimal duct surgery, a silicone stent can be placed down the nasolacrimal duct to exit into the inferior meatus of the nose. In dacryocystorhinostomy, the stent travels through the lacrimal sac and into the nose through the new ostium anterior to the middle turbinate. These plastic stents appear as hyperdense tubular structures on CT [58].
7. Decompression for thyroid eye disease may be seen as bony fenestrations of the medial, lateral, or inferior orbital wall, with or without removal of the intraorbital fat [59].
8. Orbital wall reconstruction is commonly necessary after facial trauma or removal of extensive tumors. Surgical exploration and reconstruction allow for release of entrapped tissues, restoration of orbital volume and contour, avoidance of late enophthalmos, and improvement of cosmetic deformity. 3D-volume-rendered CT reconstruction provides the best evaluation of orbital volume, contour, and bony anatomy prior to surgery and following reconstruction [60]. Orbital implants used to bridge the fractures can be seen lying along the surface of the orbital walls. Implants and screws used to repair the orbital rim or facial bones are often metallic, such as titanium.
9. In cases of certain malignant tumors of the orbit or eyelid, surgery with an orbital exenteration with or without free-flap reconstruction may be necessary. Imaging is crucial to evaluate the extent of tumor resection, monitor the response to chemoradiation, and assess for tumor recurrence after reconstruction. The muscle flap can show T2 hyperintensity and contrast enhancement due to vascular disruption, revascularization, or muscular denervation. A vascularized scar shows contrast enhancement. In the case of radiation treatment, contrast enhancement in the surgical bed may persist for years. Stability or a gradual loss of volume of the enhancing flap/scar over time distinguishes them from a recurrent or growing tumor [61].

Summary

This chapter discusses a wide spectrum of orbital diseases commonly encountered in clinical practice. CT and MRI are highly valuable in lesion characterization and in providing a differential diagnosis.

References

1. Kendall CJ, Prager TC, Cheng H, Gombos D, Tang RA, Schiffman JS. Diagnostic ophthalmic ultrasound for radiologists. Neuroimaging Clin N Am. 2015;25(3):327–65.
2. Schiffman JS, Patel NB, Cruz RA, Tang RA. Optical coherence tomography for the radiologist. Neuroimaging Clin N Am. 2015;25(3):367–82.

3. Peng Q, Zhang Y, Nateras OS, et al. MRI of blood flow of the human retina. Magn Reson Med. 2011;65(6):1768–75.
4. Zhang Y, Harrison JM, Nateras OS, et al. Decreased retinal-choroidal blood flow in retinitis pigmentosa as measured by MRI. Doc Ophthalmol. 2013;126(3):187–97.
5. Zhang Y, Nateras OSE, Peng Q, et al. Lamina-specific anatomic magnetic resonance imaging of the human retina. Invest Ophthalmol Vis Sci. 2011;52:7232–7.
6. Bender B, Heine C, Danz S, et al. Diffusion restriction of the optic nerve in patients with acute visual deficit. J Magn Reson Imaging. 2014;40(2):334–40.
7. Wang Y, van der Walt A, Paine M, et al. Optic nerve magnetisation transfer ratio after acute optic neuritis predicts axonal and visual outcomes. PLoS One. 2012;7(12):e52291.
8. Zhang Y, Wan SH, Wu GJ, et al. Magnetic resonance diffusion tensor imaging and diffusion tensor tractography of human visual pathway. Int J Ophthalmol. 2012;5(4):452–8.
9. Winston GP, Yogarajah M, Symms MR. Diffusion tensor imaging tractography to visualize the relationship of the optic radiation to epileptogenic lesions prior to neurosurgery. Epilepsia. 2011;52(8):1430–8.
10. Warnking J, Dojat M, Guerin-Duque A, et al. fMRI retinotopic mapping – step by step. NeuroImage. 2002;17(4):1665–83.
11. Reitsma DC, Mathis J, Ulmer JL, et al. Atypical retinotopic organization of visual cortex in patients with central brain damage: congenital and adult onset. J Neurosci. 2013;33(32):13010–24.
12. Go JL, Vu VN, Lee KJ, Becker TS. Orbital trauma. Neuroimaging Clin N Am. 2002;12(2):311–24.
13. Waterhouse N, Lyne J, Urdang M, et al. An investigation into the mechanism of orbital blowout fractures. Br J Plast Surg. 1999;52:607–12.
14. Antonyshyn O, Gruss M, Kassel E. Blow-in fractures of the orbit. Plast Reconstr Surg. 1989;84:10–20.
15. Rhea J, Novelline R. How to simplify the CT diagnosis of Le fort fractures. AJR Am J Roentgenol. 2005;184:1700–5.
16. Hopper R, Salemy S, Sze R. Diagnosis of midface fractures with CT: what the surgeon needs to know. Radiographics. 2006;26:783–93.
17. Unger J. Orbital apex fractures: the contribution of computed tomography. Radiology. 1984;150:713–7.
18. Yeh S, Foroozan R. Orbital apex syndrome. Curr Opin Ophthalmol. 2004;15:490–8.
19. Kubal W. Imaging of orbital trauma. Radiographics. 2008;28:1729–39.
20. Lane JI, Watson RE Jr, Witte RJ, et al. Retinal detachment: imaging of surgical treatments and complications. Radiographics. 2003;23(4):983–94.
21. Mafee M, Peyman G. Choroidal detachment and ocular hypotonia: CT evaluation. Radiology. 1984;153:697–703.
22. Segev Y, Goldstein M, Lazar M, et al. CT appearance of a traumatic cataract. AJNR Am J Neuroradiol. 1995;16:1174–5.
23. Yuan W, Hsu H, Cheng H, et al. CT of globe rupture: analysis and frequency of findings. AJR Am J Roentgenol. 2014;202:1100–7.
24. Bodanapally U, Kathirkamanathan S, Geraymovych E, et al. Diagnosis of traumatic optic neuropathy: application of diffusion tensor magnetic resonance imaging. J Neuroophthalmol. 2013;33:128–33.
25. Ho V, McGuckin J, Smergel E. Intraorbital wooden foreign body: CT and MR appearance. AJNR Am J Neuroradiol. 1996;17:134–6.
26. Lin T, Liao T, Yuan W, et al. Management and clinical outcomes of intraocular foreign bodies with the aid of orbital computed tomography. J Chin Med Assoc. 2014;77:433–6.
27. Shriver E, McKeown C, Johnson T. Trochlear calcification mimicking an orbital foreign body. Ophthal Plast Reconstr Surg. 2011;27:e143–4.
28. Ramirez H, Blatt E, Hibri N. Computed tomographic identification of calcified optic nerve drusen. Radiology. 1983;148:137–9.
29. Gujar SK, Gandhi D. Congenital malformations of the orbit. Neuroimaging Clin N Am. 2011;21(3):585–602.
30. Hopper KD, Sherman JL, Boal DK, et al. CT and MR imaging of the pediatric orbit. Radiographics. 1992;12:485–503.
31. Bilaniuk LT, Farber M. Imaging of developmental anomalies of the eye and orbit. AJNR Am J Neuroradiol. 1992;13:793–803.
32. Edward DP, Mafee MF, Garcia-Valenzuela E, et al. Coats' disease and persistent hyperplastic primary vitreous. Role of MR imaging and CT. Radiol Clin N Am. 1998;36(6):1119–31.
33. Smirniotopoulos JG, Bargalio N, Mafee MF. Differential diagnosis of leukokoria: radiologic-pathologic correlation. Radiographics. 1994;14:1059–79.
34. Smoker WR, Gentry LR, Yee NK, et al. Vascular lesions of the orbit: more than meets the eye. Radiographics. 2008;28:185–204.
35. Kaufman LM, Villablanca JP, Mafee MF. Diagnostic imaging of cystic lesions in the child's orbit. Radiol Clin N Am. 1998;36(6):1149–63.
36. Gorospe L, Royo A, Berrocal T, et al. Imaging of orbital disorders in pediatric patients. Eur Radiol. 2003;13:2012–26.
37. Jacquemina C, Bosleyb TM, Svedbergc H. Orbit deformities in craniofacial Neurofibromatosis type 1. AJNR Am J Neuroradiol. 2003;24(8):1678–82.
38. Barkovich AJ. The phakomatoses. In: Barkovich AJ, editor. Pediatric neuroimaging. 5th ed. Philadelphia: Lippincott Williams & Wilkins; 2011. p. 569–636.
39. Winegar BA, Gutierrez JE. Imaging of orbital trauma and emergent non-traumatic conditions. Neuroimaging Clin N Am. 2015;25(3):439–56.
40. Kadom N, et al. Radiological reasoning: leucocoria in a child. AJR Am J Roentgenol. 2008;191(3 Suppl):S40–4.
41. Mendenhall WM, et al. Orbital pseudotumor. Am J Clin Oncol. 2010;33(3):304–6.
42. Schuknecht B, et al. Tolosa-hunt syndrome: MR imaging features in 15 patients with 20 episodes of opthalmoplegia. Eur J Radiol. 2009;69(3):445–53.
43. Simon EM, et al. Systemic sarcoidosis with bilateral orbital involvement: MR findings. AJNR Am J Neuroradiol. 1998;19(2):336–7.
44. Kirsch E, et al. Imaging in Graves' orbitopathy. Orbit. 2009;28(4):219–25.
45. Swanton JK, et al. Early MRI in optic neuritis: the risk for clinically definite multiple sclerosis. Mult Scler. 2010;16(2):156–65.
46. Wingerchuk DM, Banwell B, et al. International consensus diagnostic criteria for neuromyelitis optica spectrum disorders. Neurology. 2015;85(2):177–89.
47. Chateil JF, et al. MRI and clinical differences between optic pathway tumours in children with and without neurofibromatosis. Br J Radiol. 2001;74(877):24–31.
48. Mafee MF, Goodwin J, Dorodi S. Optic nerve sheath meningiomas. Role of MR imaging. Radiol Clin N Am. 1999;37(1):37–58, ix.
49. Vaidhyanath R, et al. Lacrimal fossa lesions: pictorial review of CT and MRI features. Orbit. 2008;27(6):410–8.
50. Mafee MF. Uveal melanoma, choroidal hemangioma and simulating lesions. Role of MR imaging. Radiol Clin N Am. 1998;36(6):1083–99.
51. Weber AL, et al. Lymphoproliferative disease of the orbit. Neuroimaging Clin N Am. 1996;6(1):93–111.
52. Adams A, Mankad K, Poitelea C, et al. Post-operative orbital imaging: a focus on implants and prosthetic devices. Neuroradiology. 2014;56(11):925–35.
53. Patel S, Pasquale LR. Glaucoma drainage devices: a review of the past, present, and future. Semin Ophthalmol. 2010;25(5–6): 265–70.

54. Chan CK, Lin SG, Nuthi AS, et al. Pneumatic retinopexy for the repair of retinal detachments: a comprehensive review (1986–2007). Surv Ophthalmol. 2008;53(5):443–78.
55. Mathews VP, Elster AD, Barker PB, et al. Intraocular silicone oil: in vitro and in vivo MR and CT characteristics. AJNR Am J Neuroradiol. 1994;15(2):343–7.
56. Su GW, Yen MT. Current trends in managing the anophthalmic socket after primary enucleation and evisceration. Ophthal Plast Reconstr Surg. 2004;20(4):274–80.
57. Kartush JM, Linstrom CJ, McCann PM, et al. Early gold weight eyelid implantation for facial paralysis. Otolaryngol Head Neck Surg. 1990;103(6):1016–23.
58. Learned KO, Nasseri F, Mohan S. Imaging of the postoperative orbit. Neuroimaging Clin N Am. 2015;25(3):457–76.
59. Leong SC, Karkos PD, Macewen CJ, et al. A systematic review of outcomes following surgical decompression for dysthyroid orbitopathy. Laryngoscope. 2009;119(6):1106–15.
60. Kolk A, Pautke C, Schott V, et al. Secondary posttraumatic enophthalmos: high-resolution magnetic resonance imaging compared with multislice computed tomography in postoperative orbital volume measurement. J Oral Maxillofac Surg. 2007;65(10):1926–34.
61. Lee PS, Sedrak P, Guha-Thakurta N, et al. Imaging findings of recurrent tumors after orbital exenteration and free flap reconstruction. Ophthal Plast Reconstr Surg. 2014;30(4):315–21.
62. de Graaf P, et al. Retinoblastoma: MR imaging parameters in detection of tumor extent. Radiology. 2007;244(1):273–80.

Transcutaneous and Transconjunctival Surgical Approaches to the Orbit

53

Raymond I. Cho

Introduction

The orbit is the bony compartment which houses the globe and its supporting structures, including the optic nerve, extraocular muscles, lacrimal gland, sensory and motor nerves, vascular structures, and orbital fat. The anatomy of the orbit is complex, and surgery within its confines must be undertaken with an intimate knowledge of and consideration for this anatomy. Additionally, orbital surgeons must be very familiar with the anatomy of the craniofacial structures surrounding the orbit, such as the paranasal sinuses, temporalis fossa, and anterior and middle cranial fossae.

There are numerous indications for performing surgery in the orbit. These include, but are not limited to, repair of orbital fractures, biopsy or excision of orbital tumors, drainage or debridement of orbital abscesses or fungal infections, removal of orbital foreign bodies, correction of congenital or acquired orbital deformities, and orbital decompression for thyroid orbitopathy or other congestive disorders. Regardless of the indications, all orbital surgery should be performed in such a manner as to preserve as much as possible the normal function of the globe and its supporting structures. This is easier said than done, as the challenge of operating within a deep, tightly enclosed space containing numerous vital structures enveloped by fat can be daunting.

The choice of surgical approach must take into account several factors. Foremost among these factors is the anatomic location of the process to be addressed. Anterior orbitotomies can be conceptually divided into inferior, medial, lateral, superior, and intraconal approaches (Table 53.1). Both transconjunctival and transcutaneous incisions can be considered, depending on location (Figs. 53.1 and 53.2). Other considerations include the goals of surgery, the degree

Table 53.1 Summary of common anterior orbital approaches

Location	Transconjunctival	Transcutaneous
Inferior	Inferior fornix	Subciliary
Medial	Transcaruncular	Lynch Medial canthal tendon
Lateral	N/A	Lateral upper eyelid crease Lateral canthotomy
Superior	N/A	Upper eyelid crease Lid split
Intraconal	Medial rectus disinsertion Inferior fornix	Medial upper eyelid crease

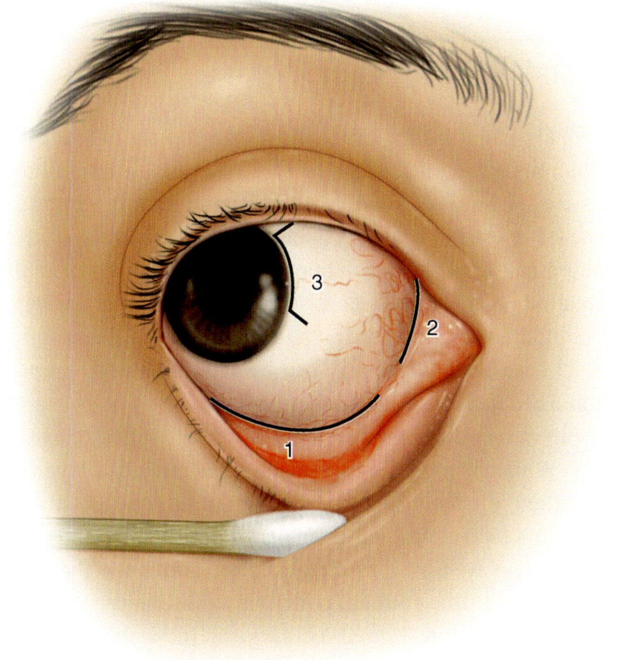

Fig. 53.1 Transconjunctival incisions used for anterior orbitotomy, right eye. 1, inferior fornix incision; 2, transcaruncular incision; 3, nasal peritomy for disinsertion of medial rectus muscle

R. I. Cho (✉)
Department of Ophthalmology and Visual Science, The Ohio State University Wexner Medical Center, Columbus, OH, USA
e-mail: raymond.cho@osumc.edu

A. J. Cohen, C. N. Burkat (eds.), *Oculofacial, Orbital, and Lacrimal Surgery*, https://doi.org/10.1007/978-3-030-14092-2_53

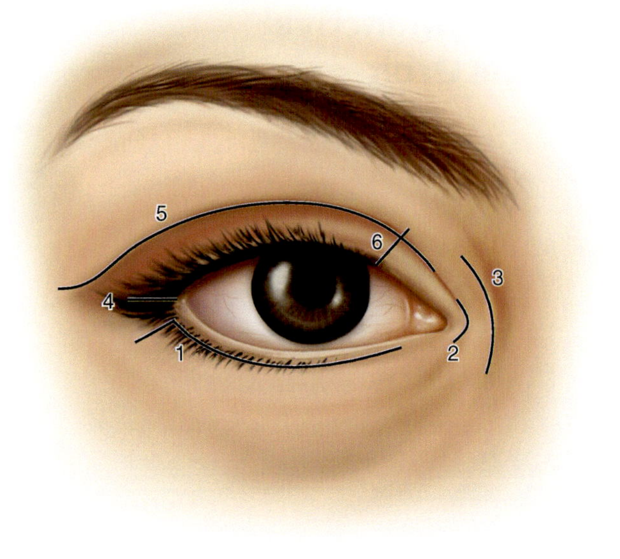

Fig. 53.2 Transcutaneous incisions used for anterior orbitotomy, right eye. 1, subciliary lower eyelid incision, 2, medial canthal tendon (Nunery) incision; 3, Lynch incision; 4, lateral canthotomy; 5, upper eyelid crease incision; 6, upper eyelid splitting

of exposure or access required, relative risks of each approach, patient-specific factors, and aesthetic preferences.

Operative Planning

Preoperative planning for orbital surgery should address numerous issues, including informed consent with a full discussion of the risks, benefits, and alternatives to surgery; the type of anesthesia; anticoagulation status; optimization of the patient's medical condition prior to surgery; and the potential need for postoperative admission. The majority of orbitotomies are done under general anesthesia, although in select cases, orbital surgery can be safely performed under monitored anesthesia care with sedation.

Preoperative orbital imaging is essential, with rare exception. While in most cases, imaging has already played an important role in the decision to undergo surgery, it is always advisable to review such imaging while devising an operative plan, as well as immediately before going into the orbit.

Although the routine administration of prophylactic antibiotics within 1 hour of surgical incision is recommended by the Surgical Care Improvement Project [1], practice patterns still vary widely among orbital surgeons. Antibiotics tend to be more commonly administered in cases of trauma, if there is a communication with the paranasal sinuses, or if an alloplastic implant is being placed in the orbit. The use of postoperative systemic antibiotics is also controversial, but topical antibiotics are routinely prescribed by most surgeons [2].

Intraoperative Strategies

As previously mentioned, orbital surgery can be fraught with challenges. In the operating room, certain steps can be taken to minimize those challenges. Of paramount importance is adequate illumination of the surgical field, which in the case of orbital surgery requires a headlamp. Numerous types and designs of headlamps utilizing halogen, xenon, or LED light sources are available. Headband-mounted lamps are commonplace, but are difficult to wear for surgeons who also use loupe magnification. For said surgeons, loupe-mounted headlights are an excellent choice due to their ease of use and comfort.

For fracture repair and other bone work, such as orbital decompression, the goal should be to create a subperiosteal dissection plane and maintain the integrity of the periorbita for the duration of the case. An intact periosteum virtually guarantees the safety of the orbital contents, at least from direct trauma. When it is necessary to enter the orbit proper (e.g., to remove a tumor), staying in the subperiosteal space initially and then opening the periosteum directly over the tumor can sometimes decrease the amount of obfuscating fat encountered during the approach, as well as decrease the risk of damage to other orbital structures.

As with all other surgery, adequate hemostasis in the orbit is critical. When possible, the use of insulated bipolar cautery is preferred to monopolar cautery when in the orbital space to minimize thermal spread and inadvertent cauterization of vital structures. Careful attention should be paid to the cautery settings, utilizing the minimum energy level necessary to achieve hemostasis. Local anesthetics with epinephrine can also help with hemostasis, as well as improve postoperative pain control. However, the use of epinephrine-containing solutions within the intraconal space should be avoided, as they can cause vision-threatening vasospasm of the ophthalmic or central retinal arteries. Intraoperative blood pressure control can also help to decrease the risk of hemorrhage.

While not used routinely, consideration can be given to perioperative corticosteroid administration, which often ameliorates orbital edema and congestion. The potential benefits of steroids must be weighed against the risks, which include increased susceptibility to infection, derangements in blood glucose, and numerous other side effects.

Many recent technological advances offer the potential to increase the margin of safety and the chances of success in the orbit. Intraoperative imaging (including fluoroscopy and computed tomography), surgical navigation, ultrasonic bone removal, endoscopy, and other technologies can provide a tactical advantage to the orbital surgeon [3–6]. Also, use of the very low-tech corneal shield can prevent corneal exposure and damage to the globe during orbital surgery.

It is worth noting that orbital surgery is in large part a solitary endeavor. Even with a room full of assistants, scrub techs, and circulators, the primary surgeon is usually the only person who can see exactly what is happening deep in the orbit during surgery. Even the most skilled and attentive assistant may have difficulty providing retraction, suction, and other maneuvers that are often taken for granted in other surgical settings. Therefore, effective and efficient communication becomes that much more critical to achieving successful outcomes.

Postoperative Considerations

Patient monitoring in the immediate postoperative period is advisable to rule out the presence of hemorrhage, optic nerve damage, or other vision-threatening complications. Overnight admission is advocated by some surgeons for all orbital cases, while others consider admission on a case by case basis.

Patient instructions in the early postoperative period are tailored for each case, but typically include activity restrictions, cold compresses, elevating the head of the bed, topical antibiotics, medications for pain control, and instructions to call for decreased vision, worsening pain, or signs of infection. Nonabsorbable sutures are usually removed 5–7 days postoperatively, and subsequent follow-up visits are scheduled at the surgeon's discretion.

Complications of Orbital Surgery

The risk of complications is inherent in all surgery, and the orbit is no exception. In addition to the ubiquitous risks of bleeding, infection, pain, and scarring, orbital surgery can also lead to numerous other complications including vision loss, diplopia, globe malposition, facial deformity, eyelid malposition, cerebrospinal fluid (CSF) leaks, mucocele or meningoencephalocele, dry eyes, epiphora, and numbness.

Causes of vision loss include direct damage to the globe or optic nerve; ischemia due to compression of or damage to the vascular supply to the globe or optic nerve; orbital compartment syndrome from hemorrhage, emphysema, or third spacing; and posterior ischemic optic neuropathy.

Diplopia can result from damage to the extraocular muscles or cranial nerves III, VI, and VI; extraocular muscle impingement by incompletely reduced fractures or malpositioned implants; postoperative scarring or adhesions to the extraocular muscles; trochlear damage (traumatic Brown's syndrome); or herniation of orbital contents into paranasal sinuses.

Globe malpositions include enophthalmos, exophthalmos, or displacement of the globe in any vertical or horizontal direction. These typically are the result of incompletely reduced fractures or improperly positioned implants that restrict or entrap the soft tissues. Progressive atrophy of orbital fat from trauma, ischemia, or radiation can also produce enophthalmos.

Eyelid malpositions include blepharoptosis, lagophthalmos, eyelid retraction, ectropion, and entropion. These are usually related to the surgical approach used and typically are a result of damage to the anterior lamellar, posterior lamella, orbital septum, or levator muscle. Cicatricial damage to the posterior lamella can be particularly difficult to treat, and strategies to mitigate such damage are addressed below.

CSF leaks during orbital surgery result from violation of the dura beneath the greater sphenoid wing, orbital roof, fovea ethmoidalis, or cribriform plate. The literature suggests that risk of CSF leak is highest with orbital exenteration (0.6–16.7%) and relatively low (1–3%) with orbital decompression through standard anterior approaches [7].

Sensory loss from damage to branches of the ophthalmic or maxillary divisions of the trigeminal nerve (V-1 and V-2, respectively) can affect the globe, lacrimal gland, periocular regions, midface, and scalp. Nasociliary nerve damage can lead to corneal anesthesia with resultant neurotrophic keratopathy and possible corneal melting. Loss of parasympathetic innervation of the lacrimal gland, which runs through the zygomaticotemporal and lacrimal nerves, can lead to aqueous tear insufficiency and keratoconjunctivitis sicca.

Anterior Surgical Approaches
- Inferior orbitotomy
- Medial orbitotomy
- Lateral orbitotomy
- Superior orbitotomy
- Intraconal approaches

Inferior Orbitotomy

Common indications for inferior orbitotomy include orbital floor fracture repair, biopsy or excision of tumors in the inferior orbit, lower eyelid blepharoplasty, orbital fat decompression, and orbital volume augmentation [8, 9]. The inferior orbit can be approached through either transconjunctival or transcutaneous incisions.

The *inferior transconjunctival incision* is undoubtedly one of the most commonly used approaches to the orbit. It can be performed quickly, does not create any visible external scarring, and provides excellent access to the inferior orbit. In select cases, a lateral canthotomy and inferior cantholysis (discussed in the lateral orbitotomy section) can be combined with this incision to improve surgical exposure – also known as the "swinging eyelid" approach. If a canthotomy/cantholysis is planned, it is typically performed before creating the conjunctival incision. Another strategy is to proceed initially with the conjunctival incision alone, and only perform a canthotomy/cantholysis if exposure is found to be inadequate during the course of the orbitotomy. This is entirely a matter of surgeon preference.

The conjunctival incision can be made anywhere between the inferior border of the tarsus and the inferior fornix. A more superior incision facilitates a preseptal approach to the inferior orbital rim, which many surgeons prefer to minimize orbital fat prolapse, particularly in the setting of fracture repair. On the other hand, a postseptal approach through a more inferior incision can be performed more quickly and potentially minimizes damage to the anterior lamella and orbital septum, decreasing the risk of cicatricial eyelid retraction and ectropion. However, unless there is a specific reason to expose the tarsus (e.g., retractor reinsertion or spacer graft placement), it is advisable to keep the incision well clear of the tarsus, at least 3 mm below its inferior border. Regardless of its placement, the incision should be created in a manner that limits postoperative scarring of the posterior lamella (tarsus, conjunctiva, and lower eyelid retractors). Using a scalpel blade or scissors eliminates the risk of thermal injury, but cautery provides better hemostasis. If monopolar cautery is used, it should be placed on a needle tip on pure cut mode with the energy set to the minimum level necessary to create an incision. Once the conjunctiva and retractors are divided and the orbital septum is cleared, the settings can be increased as desired.

When utilizing the preseptal approach, following incision of the conjunctiva and retractors, blunt dissection is carried between orbicularis and septum to the inferior orbital rim with cotton-tipped applicators or other blunt instruments. Some surgeons place a traction suture through the inferior edge of the incision to provide countertraction and improve visualization. Excessive manipulation or cauterization of the septum should be avoided during the dissection. For bony work, the periosteum over the rim is incised and subperiosteal dissection is carried over the orbital floor. While incising the periosteum medially, it is critical to stay anterior to the inferior oblique muscle, whose origin is immediately posterior to the inferomedial orbital rim.

If a postseptal approach is preferred, an efficient method of creating an inferior fornix incision [10] is to retract the lower eyelid anteriorly with a Desmarres retractor while compressing the forniceal tissues over the floor just behind orbital rim with a malleable ribbon retractor (Fig. 53.3). This essentially places all the eyelid structures and the orbital septum in front of the rim, while pushing the orbital contents, including the inferior orbital fat, behind the rim. When done correctly, a thin layer of tissue comprised of only conjunctiva and capsulopalpebral fascia is seen over the bone between the two retractors. The incision is made with the surgeon's instrument of choice directly down to the rim. Again, care should be taken medially to avoid damaging the inferior oblique muscle.

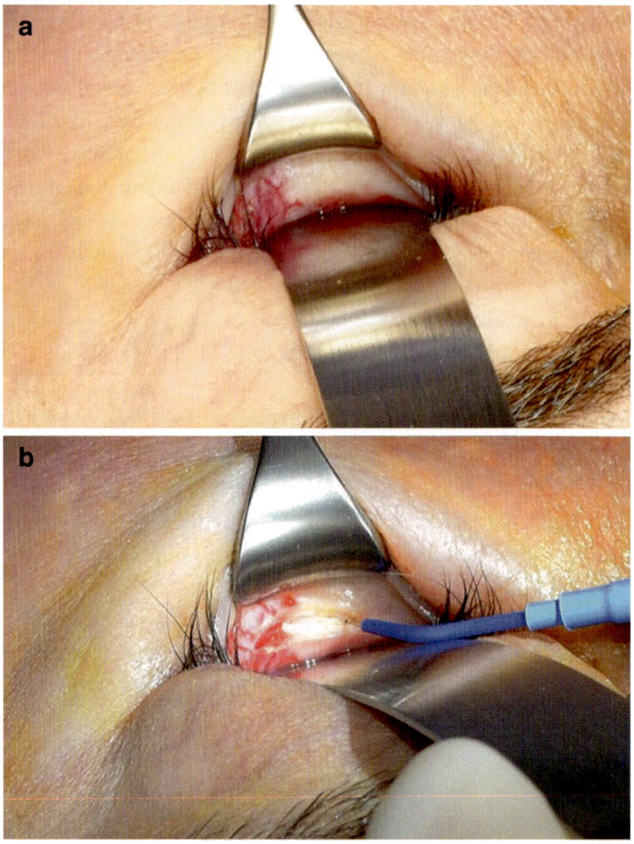

Fig. 53.3 Intraoperative photograph, left inferior orbitotomy for floor fracture repair through conjunctival fornix incision, surgeon's view. The lower eyelid is retracted while the forniceal tissues and orbital fat are compressed with a ribbon retractor behind the orbital rim (**a**). A horizontal incision is made with low-energy needle-tipped cautery through conjunctiva, lower eyelid retractors, and periosteum (**b**). The incision is made at least 4 mm below the inferior border of tarsus

Incision closure following the transconjunctival approach must be performed judiciously. Layered closure is usually unnecessary and may actually increase the risk of complications such as eyelid retraction and entropion [11]. The pitfall with layered closure is that, following the tissue manipulation that occurs throughout the case, it may be difficult to make a clear distinction between eyelid retractors, orbital septum, periosteum, and other tissues. If tissues are mismatched (e.g., the retractors are sutured to the orbital septum, or the periosteum to the conjunctiva), complications are likely to result (Fig. 53.4). The safest option for closure is to simply approximate the conjunctival edges with a few buried interrupted absorbable sutures. The tissues are not under significant tension, and proper mucosal alignment is all that is typically needed.

The preferred transcutaneous approach to the inferior orbit is the *subciliary incision*. The most common application for this approach is for lower eyelid blepharoplasty with orbital fat sculpting/repositioning and skin removal. A horizontal skin incision is made across the lower eyelid immediately

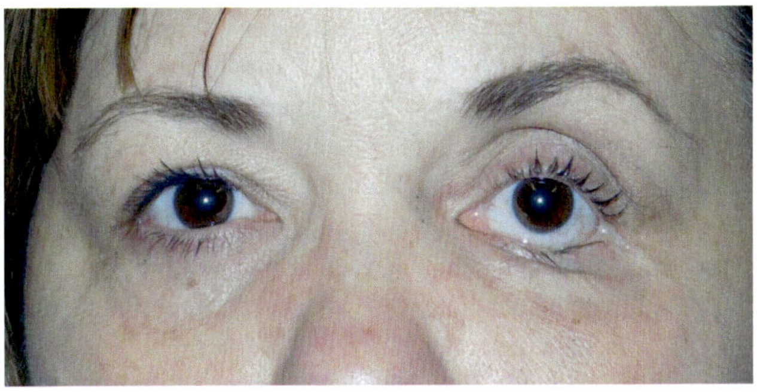

Fig. 53.4 Left lower eyelid retraction with tethering to the inferior orbital rim following "layered closure" of inferior transconjunctival incision which presumably incorporated orbital septum

below the lashes, and is often continued inferotemporally in a hockey stick pattern through the lateral canthus along natural skin tension lines. The orbicularis muscle is opened at or below the level of the skin incision, and blunt preseptal dissection is carried inferiorly to the orbital rim. The orbital septum or the periosteum is then opened to provide access to the orbit, depending on the procedure being performed.

The primary advantage of the subciliary incision is that it facilitates surgery on the anterior lamella while creating the least objectionable postoperative scar compared to other transcutaneous approaches. Infratarsal and orbital rim incisions are highly discouraged due to inferior aesthetic outcomes and the risk of anterior lamellar tethering to the orbital rim.

For the majority of oculofacial surgeons, the transconjunctival approach to the inferior orbit is preferred over transcutaneous incisions, with the exceptions noted above. The potential for surgical exposure is better, especially with the availability of lateral canthotomy/inferior cantholysis, there is no visible scar, and there is less trauma to the anterior lamella. An additional advantage of the transconjunctival incision is that in cases of lower eyelid retraction or cicatricial entropion, it can also serve as the incision through which a posterior lamellar spacer graft can be placed. The primary downside to transconjunctival surgery is the risk of damage to the posterior lamella, which can lead to cicatricial entropion and/or retraction (Fig. 53.5). However, this risk can be minimized by a thorough knowledge of anatomy and adherence to the tenets described above.

Medial Orbitotomy

Common indications for medial orbitotomy include medial orbital decompression, medial orbital wall fracture repair, drainage of subperiosteal abscess, biopsy or excision of tumors in the medial orbit, and retrieval of a "lost" medial rectus muscle [12–14]. Like the inferior orbit, the medial orbit can also be approached through transconjunctival or transcutaneous approaches.

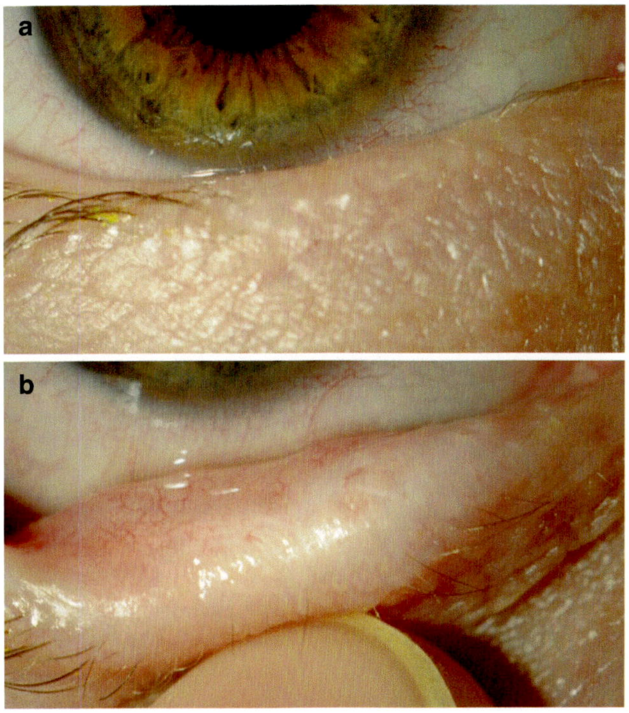

Fig. 53.5 Right lower eyelid cicatricial entropion following inferior transconjunctival orbitotomy (**a**). Eversion of the eyelid (**b**) reveals scarring over the palpebral surface of the tarsus caused by monopolar cautery

The *transcaruncular incision* is essentially a transconjunctival approach to the medial orbit. Since publication of the technique in 2000 [14], it has become the preferred medial approach for many orbital surgeons. A vertical 10–12 mm incision is made with scissors through the lateral one-third of the caruncle (as originally described) or between the caruncle and the plica semilunaris. Ring scissors are placed through the incision in a posteromedial direction to the posterior lacrimal crest and spread to bluntly dissect a path to the medial orbital wall (Fig. 53.6). Narrow ribbon retractors and/or muscle hooks are then placed through the dissection plane to improve exposure. As the surgical opening stretches during the case, ribbon retractors of increasing width can be placed to improve exposure. In cases of fracture repair, orbital decompression, or subperiosteal abscess drainage, the periosteum behind the posterior lacrimal crest is opened vertically with a blade or needle-tipped cautery, and subperiosteal dissection is performed to create the surgical plane. Through this relatively small incision, access can be obtained to the entire medial orbital wall, the inferomedial strut, the medial orbital floor, the anterior and posterior ethmoidal neurovascular bundles, and even the superomedial orbital wall.

At the conclusion of the case, the incision is typically closed with buried absorbable sutures, although some surgeons forego suture closure completely. In the vast majority

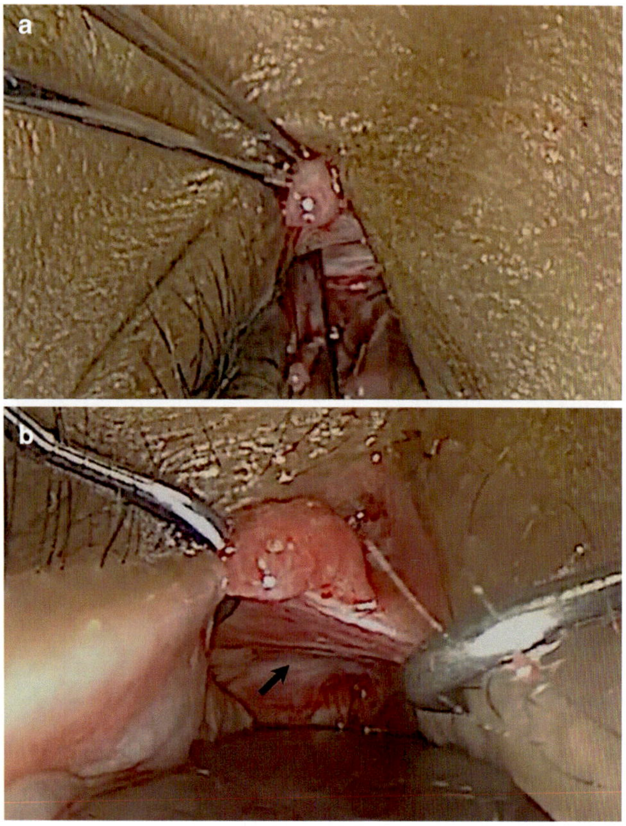

Fig. 53.6 Intraoperative photograph, right transcaruncular orbitotomy for medial orbital decompression. An incision is made with Westcott scissors between the caruncle (grasped with the forceps) and the plica semilunaris, and blunt dissection is performed with tenotomy scissors in a posteromedial direction to the medial orbital wall (**a**). Muscle hooks and a malleable ribbon retractor provide exposure to the site (**b**) where the periosteum will be opened behind the posterior lacrimal crest (arrow). The pictures were obtained with an endoscope for photographic documentation only

of cases, the patient will be left with an imperceptible scar which is only visible under slit lamp magnification, if in fact it is visible at all.

Prior to the introduction of the transcaruncular approach, the *Lynch incision* was the most commonly used approach to the medial orbit [15]. This incision is made transcutaneously in a curvilinear fashion over the medial orbital rim. Once the rim is exposed, dissection is carried either subperiosteally or through the orbital septum into the medial orbit, depending on the purpose of the surgery. If additional exposure is needed inferiorly, the anterior crus of the medial canthal tendon can be disinserted from the anterior lacrimal crest and the lacrimal sac dissected from the lacrimal sac fossa to the level of the nasolacrimal duct. The main anatomic structures limiting exposure through this incision are the nasolacrimal duct inferiorly and the trochlea superiorly. Another disadvantage of this approach is the resultant scar, which is not well-camouflaged and can sometimes lead to medial canthal webbing. A Z-plasty modification has been described to mitigate the unsightliness and webbing that can result from the traditional curvilinear scar [16]. Most orbital surgeons favor the transcaruncular over the Lynch incision for access to the orbit, but it can still be a useful approach for repair of naso-orbital-ethmoid fractures and transnasal wiring.

The *medial canthal tendon incision* (also known as the Nunery incision) is an alternative transcutaneous approach to the medial orbit [17]. A 15–20 mm skin incision is created over the insertion of the anterior crus of the medial canthal tendon (Fig. 53.2), which is disinserted from the anterior lacrimal crest. The lacrimal sac is then dissected from the lacrimal sac fossa, and dissection is continued past the posterior lacrimal crest into the medial orbit. The external scar is reported to be favorable to that created by the Lynch incision.

Lateral Orbitotomy

Indications for lateral orbitotomy include lateral orbital decompression, repair of zygomaticomaxillary fractures, and biopsy or excision of orbital tumors, especially lacrimal gland tumors. The lateral orbit is typically approached transcutaneously or through a lateral canthotomy and inferior cantholysis. The lateral orbitotomy is considered by most to have been first reported by Krönlein in 1888 [18, 19], but the incision placement as first described has undergone significant modifications since then [20, 30].

The *lateral lid crease incision* is essentially the lateral half of an upper eyelid blepharoplasty incision. Depending on the degree of exposure desired, it can start anywhere from the central to lateral upper eyelid and extend in a curvilinear fashion across the lateral orbital rim through the lateral canthus (Fig. 53.7). The lateral limit of the incision should be no more than 25 mm from the lateral commissure, as extending beyond this point places the temporal branch of the facial nerve at risk. Dissection is carried superior to the incision in the preseptal plane to the superolateral orbital rim. Inferior to the incision, preperiosteal dissection is performed over the inferolateral orbital rim.

If the orbital space is to be entered, such as for lacrimal gland tumor excision, the orbital septum can be opened to gain access to the orbit. Alternatively, as mentioned in the introduction, subperiosteal dissection can be performed as far posteriorly as is deemed necessary to reach the orbital process in question.

For bony work, the periosteum over the lateral orbital rim is incised and subperiosteal dissection is carried over the lateral orbital wall with elevators. If a bone flap is being created or wide exposure of the greater sphenoid wing is required, such as with lateral orbital decompression, the periosteum is dissected from the lateral rim to the temporalis fossa, and the superficial and deep layers of the temporalis fascia are

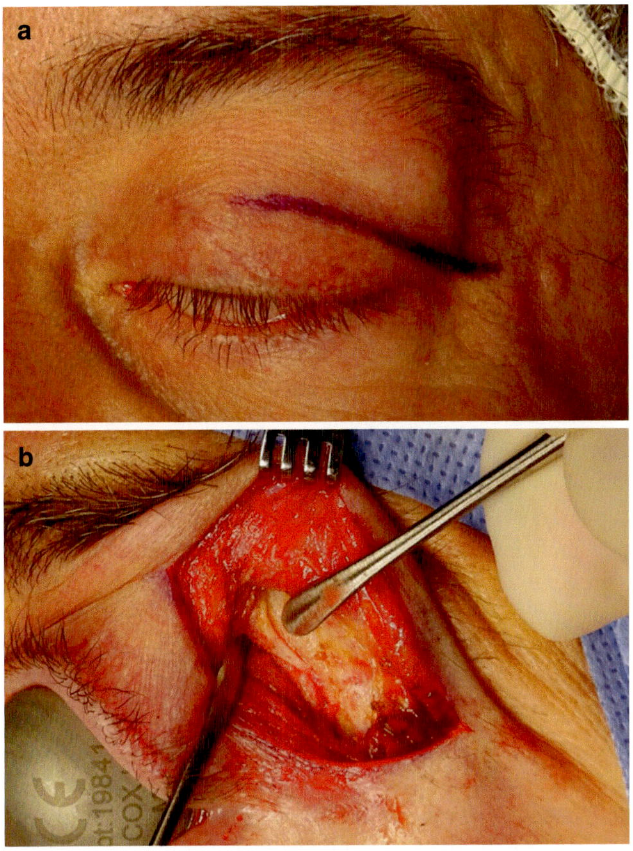

Fig. 53.7 Left lateral upper eyelid crease incision marked for lateral orbital decompression (**a**). Intraoperative photograph (**b**). Following preseptal dissection and exposure of the lateral orbital rim, subperiosteal dissection is carried into the orbit

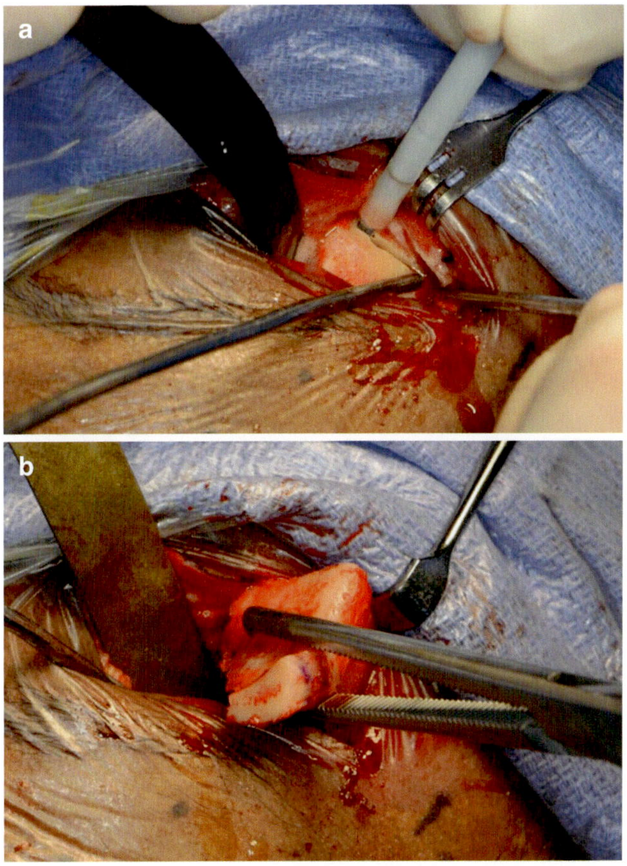

Fig. 53.8 Intraoperative photographs, right lateral orbitotomy with bone flap for tumor resection, superior view. A cut is made through the inferolateral orbital rim with an ultrasonic bone curette (**a**). Following a second cut through the superolateral orbital rim, the lateral rim segment is grasped with a bone clamp, fractured from the lateral wall, and removed (**b**)

separated from the bone with a sharp periosteal elevator. A horizontal incision can be made through the temporalis fascia if desired to improve exposure, but should not extend more than 25 mm posterior to the rim. If needed, the temporalis muscle can be dissected from the underlying bone with sharp periosteal elevators.

Bone flaps can dramatically improve exposure in select cases, such as removal of large tumors or extensive drilling over the greater sphenoid wing. The decision to use them is highly surgeon dependent, and the benefits of improved exposure should be weighed against the risks of using powered instruments in the orbit, the potentially increased operative time, and the need for refixation of the bone flap. The bone cuts are usually made with a reciprocating or sagittal saw through the superior and inferior portions of the lateral orbital rim – at or just above the frontozygomatic suture and just above the level of the zygomatic arch. Cutting drill bits or an ultrasonic bone remover with a serrated knife tip can also be used (Fig. 53.8). After the bone cuts are made, the rim segment is grasped with a bone clamp, fractured from the sphenoid bone, and kept in a safe location wrapped in saline-soaked gauze until the conclusion of the case. The bone is refixated with plates and screws, or alternatively with sutures passed through predrilled holes.

Closure of the periosteum over the lateral rim is usually performed with buried absorbable monofilament or braided sutures. Deep closure of the soft tissues can be performed if desired, and the skin is closed with running monofilament sutures. Long-term healing and aesthetic outcomes of the lateral eyelid crease incision are generally excellent, similar to what is seen after upper eyelid blepharoplasty (Fig. 53.9).

Lateral canthotomy and cantholysis has already been mentioned as an adjunct to inferior orbitotomy, but it can also be used to access the lateral orbital rim and to some extent the lateral orbit. The canthotomy is performed by making a horizontal cut from the lateral commissure to the lateral orbital rim, separating the lateral canthal tendon into superior and inferior limbs (Fig. 53.10). Either limb can then be detached from the lateral orbital tubercle by distracting the eyelid anteriorly, strumming the tendon, and cutting the tendon vertically as close to the lateral rim as possible. While it is more common to perform an inferior cantholysis,

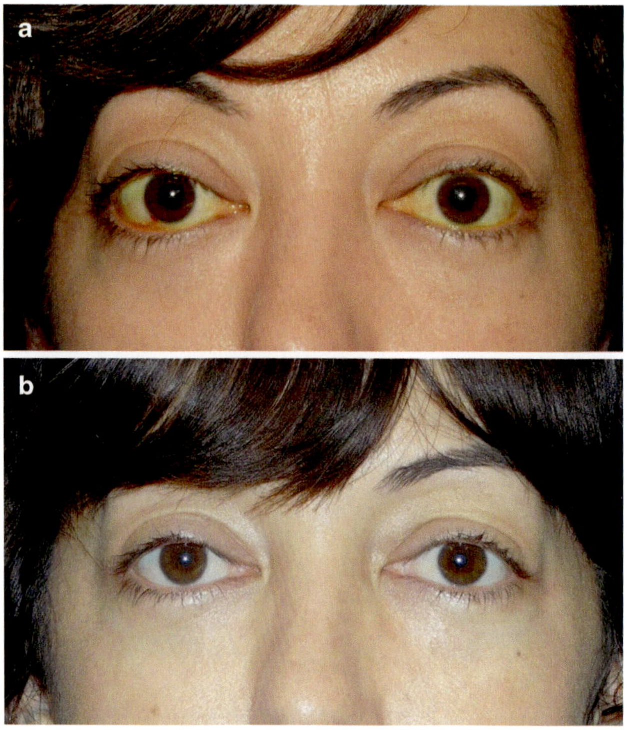

Fig. 53.9 Bilateral lateral orbital decompression. Preoperative (**a**) and postoperative (**b**) photographs show significant proptosis reduction and excellent aesthetic appearance of the lateral upper eyelid crease incisions

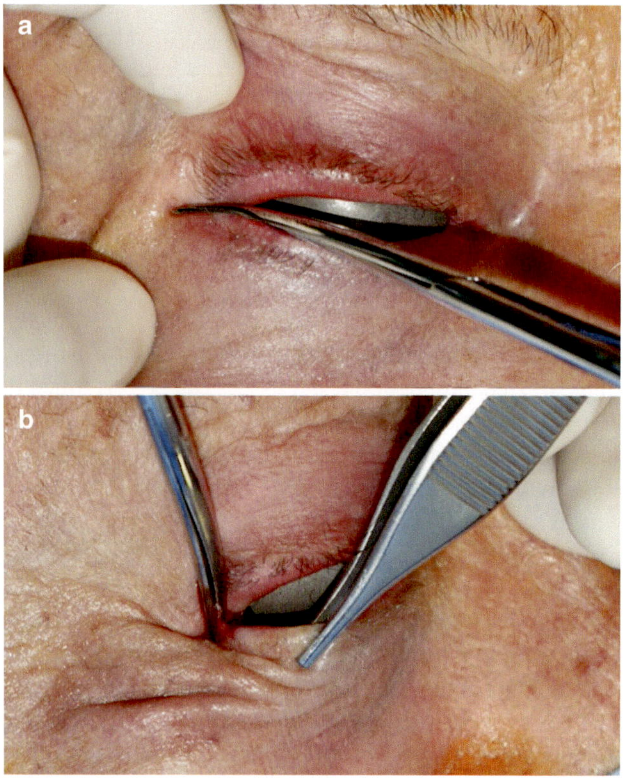

Fig. 53.10 Intraoperative photographs, right lateral canthotomy and inferior cantholysis. Tenotomy scissors are used to create a horizontal incision from the lateral commissure to the lateral orbital rim (**a**). As the lower eyelid is retracted away from the rim, tenotomy scissors are used to separate the inferior limb of the lateral canthal tendon from the lateral orbital wall (**b**)

a superior cantholysis can also be performed instead of or in addition to the lower.

Upon conclusion of the orbitotomy, the lateral canthal tendon is resuspended from the bone in an anatomic position. Sturdy monofilament or braided absorbable sutures on a short half-circle needle are typically used for this purpose. Care should be taken to ensure that the tendon is securely anchored to periosteum over or slightly above the lateral orbital tubercle, which is a few millimeters posterior to the lateral orbital rim. The lateral canthal angle is reformed with a braided absorbable suture in a buried fashion, and the skin is closed with the surgeon's choice of suture.

The degree of exposure achievable with a canthotomy/cantholysis is generally not as great as that provided by the lateral eyelid crease incision, unless inferior and superior cantholysis are both performed. However, if the operative plan includes horizontal eyelid tightening or repositioning of the lateral canthal tendon, then the use of this approach may make more sense.

More recently, a *lateral canthotomy orbitotomy* without cantholysis has been reported as a simple and efficient approach to the lateral orbit and intraconal space [21]. Following the horizontal canthotomy as described above, traction sutures are placed through both limbs and retracted craniocaudally to increase exposure, and blunt dissection is carried directly into the lateral extraconal or intraconal space. Closure is accomplished by simple approximation of the upper and lower limbs of the lateral canthal tendon and the skin incision. While surgical exposure may be relatively limited with this approach, it can be an effective option for select cases.

Superior Orbitotomy

Indications for superior orbitotomy include biopsy or excision of tumors in the superior orbit, repair of orbital roof fractures or meningoencephaloceles, and drainage of subperiosteal hemorrhage or abscess. The majority of superior orbitotomies are performed through a transcutaneous approach, utilizing the versatile upper eyelid crease incision [22]. A superior transconjunctival approach is not practical, due to the risk of damage to the levator palpebrae superioris and the lacrimal gland ductules.

The *upper lid crease incision* is identical to a blepharoplasty incision. In most cases, the eyelid crease is clearly visible and can be marked with a marking pen prior to local anesthetic infiltration. If the eyelid crease is absent or in an abnormal position, the incision can be marked to match the contralateral side or placed at 8–10 mm above the eyelid margin centrally (typically lower for men and higher for women). The incision is made through skin and orbicularis, and preseptal dissection is carried to the superior orbital rim. Care is taken to identify the supraorbital neurovascular

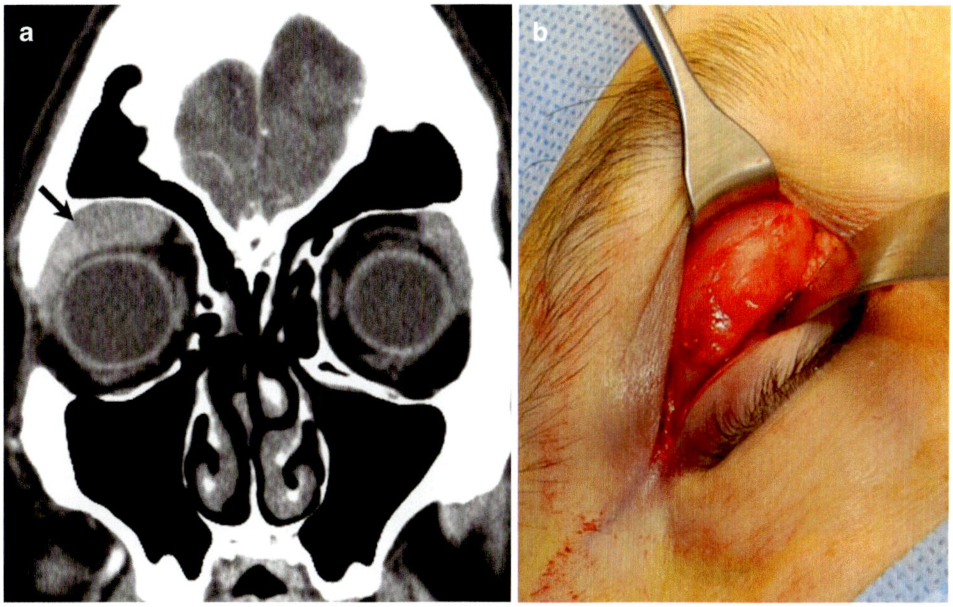

Fig. 53.11 Right orbital lymphoma (arrow), coronal CT scan image (**a**). Intraoperative photograph (**b**) showing tumor being exposed through an upper lid crease incision

bundle (Fig. 53.11). The orbit proper can be entered by opening the orbital septum, preferably just inferior to the arcus marginalis. Subperiosteal dissection can begin by incising the periosteum over the superior orbital rim, beginning just lateral to the supraorbital notch/foramen and extending as far laterally as necessary.

An alternative approach to the superior orbit is the *lid-splitting incision*, whereby a full-thickness incision is made vertically through the upper eyelid [23]. By dividing all layers of the anterior, middle, and posterior lamella, access is gained to the postseptal space above the levator aponeurosis, whose long-term function is ostensibly not affected due to the longitudinal direction of the cut. This maneuver may provide a large amount of surgical freedom, but it requires meticulous repair of the full-thickness incision at the conclusion of the case, and carries the attendant risks of postoperative eyelid deformity and trichiasis.

Intraconal Approaches

Surgery for intraconal or optic nerve processes can be particularly challenging for the orbital surgeon. The potential for damage to vital structures such as the optic nerve, rectus muscles, ciliary ganglion, and ophthalmic artery is high. Due to its central position in the orbit, any of the above approaches could be considered when addressing the intraconal space.

An additional option not yet addressed is a transconjunctival incision with *disinsertion of the medial rectus muscle*. Commonly applied for optic nerve sheath fenestration [24], this is the same approach utilized by strabismus surgeons for medial rectus muscle recession/resection. A peritomy incision is created through conjunctiva and Tenon's capsule near the nasal corneoscleral limbus, and sub-Tenon's dissection is carried to the medial rectus insertion. The medial rectus muscle is isolated with muscle hooks and the Tenon's and tendon sheath cleanly dissected from the tendon with cotton-tipped applicators. The tendon is then tagged with a double-armed 6–0 braided absorbable suture on spatulated needles and disinserted from the globe. Blunt dissection can then be carried beneath the muscle into the intraconal space. At the conclusion of the case, the tendon is reattached to the globe using the preplaced muscle suture, and the conjunctiva is closed with buried 7–0 braided absorbable sutures.

Another approach commonly used for optic nerve sheath fenestration (Fig. 53.12) and intraconal tumors is the *medial upper eyelid crease incision* [25]. A 10 mm incision is created over the medial upper eyelid within the natural eyelid crease. After incision of the skin and orbicularis, the orbital septum is opened and blunt dissection is carried into the orbit in an inferolateral direction, between the superior oblique tendon and the medial horn of the levator aponeurosis, until the superomedial intraconal space is encountered. Care should be taken during the dissection to avoid damage to the superior ophthalmic vein. Approaching the optic nerve from the medial direction avoids damage to the ciliary ganglion, which is situated on the lateral aspect of the optic nerve.

For well-encapsulated intraconal tumors, such as cavernous hemangiomas or schwannomas, it is common to utilize the inferior transconjunctival approach due to its ease of use and the relative absence of vital structures in the inferolateral orbit. A lateral canthotomy and inferior cantholysis can improve exposure, and a cryoprobe can also be helpful in the removal of such lesions [26]. Blunt dissection is carried through the inferolateral fat and intermuscular septum to expose the tumor, and the tip of the cryoprobe is applied to the tumor surface. Once the ice ball has formed an adequate seal between the tumor and the cryoprobe, gentle anterior

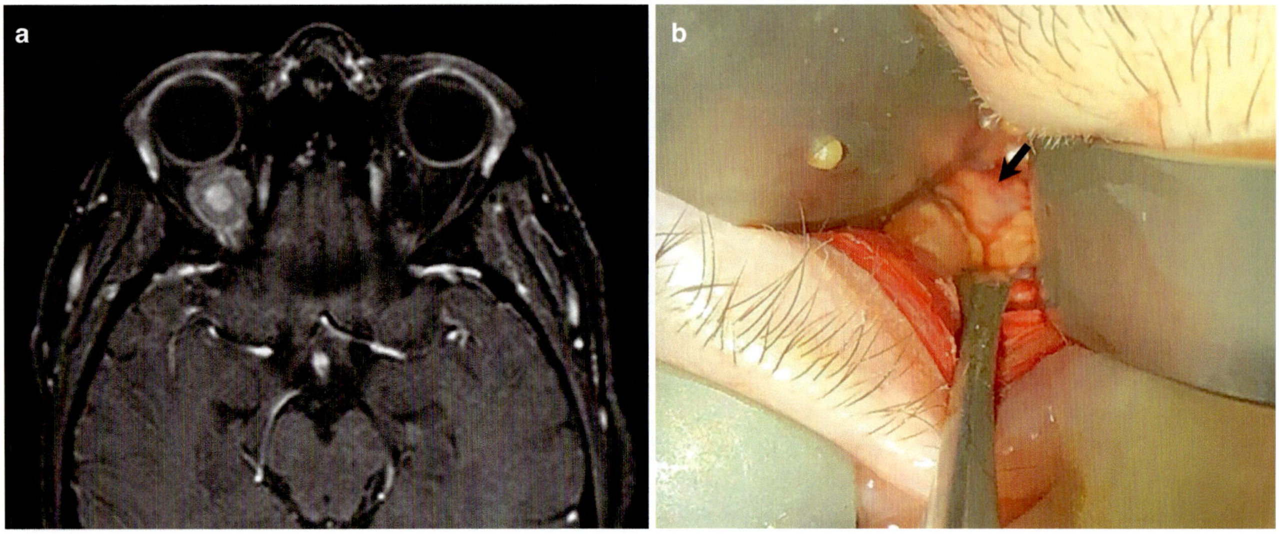

Fig. 53.12 Right intraconal diffuse large B-cell lymphoma, T-1 fat-suppressed gadolinium-enhanced axial MRI image (**a**). Intraoperative photograph (**b**) of medial upper lid crease approach for incisional biopsy of tumor (arrow)

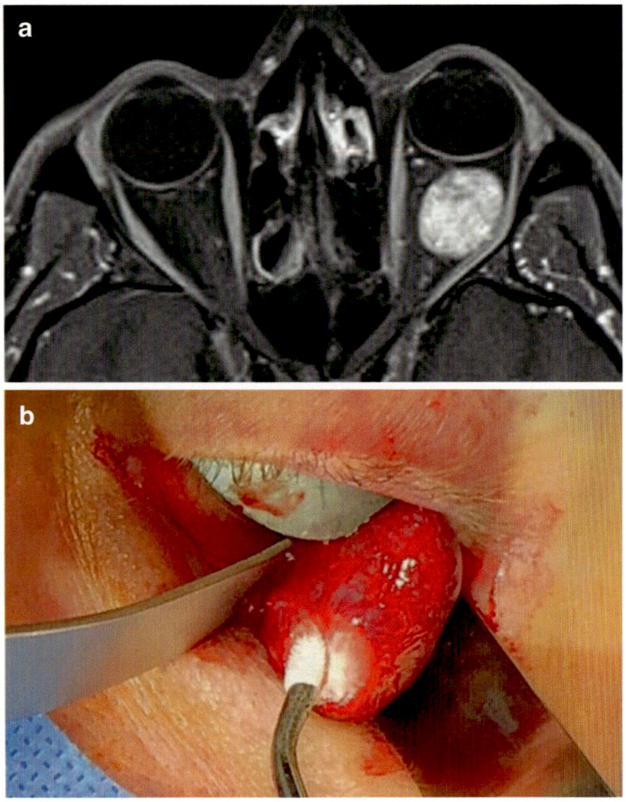

Fig. 53.13 Left intraconal cavernous hemangioma, T1 fat-suppressed gadolinium-enhanced axial MRI image (**a**). Intraoperative photograph (**b**), tumor removal through "swinging eyelid" approach (inferior fornix incision with lateral canthotomy/inferior cantholysis). The tumor is engaged with a cryoprobe and placed on gentle traction while blunt dissection is performed with malleable ribbon retractors

traction is applied while dissection is carried out around the tumor capsule with cotton-tipped applicators or other blunt instruments until the tumor is completely free (Fig. 53.13). This method of delivery minimizes tissue manipulation within the muscle cone, decreasing the risk of vision loss, diplopia, and other complications.

Combination Approaches

In some orbital cases, the use of multiple approaches may be advantageous. For example, a combined fracture of the orbital floor and medial wall can be approached through transconjunctival and transcaruncular incisions. The incisions are made contiguously through the conjunctiva, preseptal or postseptal tissues, and periosteum. The subperiosteal dissection planes over the floor and medial wall can then be combined into a single surgical plane to greatly improve visualization and exposure. If additional exposure or wider access is needed, such as in the case of a very large implant covering the floor and medial wall, the origin of the inferior oblique muscle can be disinserted from its bony attachment [14, 27]. Another example of a commonly combined approach is an inferior transconjunctival incision and lateral orbitotomy for reduction and two-point fixation of a zygomaticomaxillary complex fracture.

Transantral Approach

Although rarely utilized today, the *transantral approach* deserves brief mention due to its common use in the recent past for orbital decompression [28]. This approach, which is the same one used for the *Caldwell-Luc procedure*, utilizes an upper gingivobuccal sulcus incision to expose the anterior wall of the maxillary sinus, which is removed with a bone rongeur or a high-speed drill. The orbital floor and/or medial orbital wall is then removed from below through the maxillary sinus, and the periorbita is incised to decompress the orbit. Enlargement of the maxillary outflow tract is typically performed prior to closure of the gingivobuccal sulcus incision with absorbable sutures. The anterior wall of the maxillary sinus is left unreconstructed. Several decades ago, this was the most common decompression performed by orbital surgeons [29]. However, due to the relatively high rate of postoperative diplopia and globe dystopia, the procedure has been largely abandoned in favor of other decompression techniques.

Existing Lacerations

In occasional cases of trauma, an existing laceration may be large enough and in an appropriate position to provide access to the orbit. When utilizing such lacerations, however, care must be taken to avoid exacerbating the soft tissue damage that has already occurred. If excessive manipulation or enlargement of the laceration is necessary for adequate access or exposure, a more standard approach should be considered.

References

1. Rosenberger LH, Politano AD, Sawyer RG. The surgical care improvement project and prevention of post-operative infection, including surgical site infection. Surg Infect. 2011;12:163–8.
2. Fay A, Nallasamy N, Bernardini F, et al. Multinational comparison of prophylactic antibiotic use for eyelid surgery. JAMA Ophthalmol. 2015;133:778–84.
3. Bevans SE, Moe KS. Advances in the reconstruction of orbital fractures. Facial Plast Surg Clin North Am. 2017;25:513–35.
4. Cho RI, Kahana A, Patel B, et al. Intraoperative fluoroscopy-guided removal of orbital foreign bodies. Ophthalmic Plast Reconstr Surg. 2009;25:215–8.
5. Sivak-Callcott JA, Linberg JV, Patel S. Ultrasonic bone removal with the Sonopet Omni: a new instrument for orbital and lacrimal surgery. Arch Ophthalmol. 2005;123:1595–7.
6. Wilde F, Schramm A. Intraoperative imaging in orbital and midface reconstruction. Facial Plast Surg. 2014;30:545–53.
7. Limawararut V, Valenzuela AA, Sullivan TJ, et al. Cerebrospinal fluid leaks in orbital and lacrimal surgery. Surv Ophthalmol. 2008;53:274–84.
8. Davies BW, Hink EM, Durairaj VD. Transconjunctival inferior orbitotomy: indications, surgical technique, and complications. Craniomaxillofac Trauma Reconstr. 2014;7:169–74.
9. McCord CD, Moses JL. Exposure of the inferior orbit with fornix incision and lateral canthotomy. Ophthalmic Surg. 1979;10:53–63.
10. Bernardini FP, Nerad J, Fay A, et al. The revised direct transconjunctival approach to the orbital floor. Ophthalmic Plast Reconstr Surg. 2017;33:93–100.
11. Westfall CT, Shore JW, Nunery WR, et al. Operative complications of the transconjunctival inferior fornix approach. Ophthalmology. 1991;98:1525–8.
12. Goldberg RA. Is there a "lost" rectus muscle in strabismus surgery? Am J Ophthalmol. 2001;132:101–3.
13. Leone CR, Lloyd WC, Rylander G. Surgical repair of medial wall fractures. Am J Ophthalmol. 1984;97:349–56.
14. Shorr N, Baylis HI, Goldberg RA, Perry JD. Transcaruncular approach to the medial orbit and orbital apex. Ophthalmology. 2000;107:1459–63.
15. Lynch RC. The technique of a radical frontal sinus operation which has given me the best results. Laryngoscope. 1921;31:1–5.
16. Esclamado RM, Cummings CW. Z-plasty modification of the Lynch incision. Laryngoscope. 1989;99:986–7.
17. Timoney PJ, Sokol JA, Hauck MJ, Lee HB, Nunery WR. Transcutaneous medial canthal tendon incision to the medial orbit. Ophthalmic Plast Reconstr Surg. 2012;28:140–4.
18. Krönlein RU. Zur pathologie und operative behandlung der dermoidcysten der orbita. Bruns Beitr Klin Chir. 1888;4:149–63.
19. Stallard HB. Lateral orbitotomy (Krönlein's operation). Br J Ophthalmol. 1946;30:250.
20. Harris GJ, Logani SC. Eyelid crease incision for lateral orbitotomy. Ophthalmic Plast Reconstr Surg. 1999;15:9–18.
21. Hamed-Azzam S, Verity DH, Rose GE. Lateral canthotomy orbitotomy: a rapid approach to the orbit. Eye. 2017; https://doi.org/10.1038/eye.2017.173.
22. Pelton RW. The anterior eyelid crease approach to the orbit. Curr Opin Ophthalmol. 2009;20:401–5.
23. Kersten RC, Kulwin DR. Vertical lid split orbitotomy revisited. Ophthalmic Plast Reconstr Surg. 1999;15:425–8.
24. Galbraith JEK, Sullivan JH. Decompression of the perioptic meninges for relief of papilledema. Am J Ophthalmol. 1973;76:6887–92.
25. Pelton RW, Patel BCK. Superomedial lid crease approach to the medial intraconal space: a new technique for access to the optic nerve and central space. Ophthalmic Plast Reconstr Surg. 2001;17:241–53.
26. Rosen N, Priel A, Simon GJ, Rosner M. Cryo-assisted anterior approach for surgery of retroocular tumors avoids the need for lateral or transcranial orbitotomy in most cases. Acta Ophthalmol. 2010;88:675–80.
27. Cho RI, Davies BW. Combined orbital floor and medial wall fractures involving the inferomedial strut: repair technique and case series using preshaped porous polyethylene/titanium implants. Craniomaxillofac Trauma Reconstr. 2013;6:161–70.
28. Walsh TE, Ogura JH. Transantral orbital decompression for malignant exophthalmos. Laryngoscope. 1957;67:544–68.
29. McCord CD. Current trends in orbital decompression. Ophthalmology. 1985;92:21–33.
30. Maroon JC, Kennerdell JS. Surgical approaches to the orbit: indications and techniques. J Neurosurg. 1984;60:1226–35.

Endonasal and Transcranial Surgical Approaches to the Orbit

54

Kyle VanKoevering, Alexandre Bossi Todeschini, Daniel L. Prevedello, Ricardo L. Carrau, and Raymond I. Cho

Introduction

Most orbital processes can be surgically addressed using one of the standard anterior orbitotomy approaches detailed in the preceding chapter. However, for complex pathology located in the posterior orbit or involving the extraorbital compartments, a transnasal or transcranial approach may be indicated to provide adequate exposure and access. In this chapter, we highlight a variety of extended orbital exposures and discuss key technical concepts and potential pitfalls.

Fundamental concepts of orbital surgery such as preoperative surgical planning, intraoperative strategies, and postoperative care mirror those described in the anterior orbitotomy chapter. However, the use of an extraorbital approach introduces numerous additional considerations. For endonasal surgery, for example, specialized equipment is required, different bacterial flora affect the choice of prophylactic antibiotics, and postoperative sinonasal hygiene is generally required. Transcranial approaches are also associated with additional challenges and the potential complications associated with craniotomy procedures. A detailed discussion of these considerations falls outside the scope of this text, but they are foundational to the practice of skull base surgeons, be they otolaryngologists or neurosurgeons. This highlights the importance of a comprehensive, multidisciplinary skull base team in dealing with such cases. Working collaboratively, the skull base team can provide complete surgical and non-surgical treatment options for many orbital pathologies.

K. VanKoevering · R. L. Carrau
Department of Otolaryngology – Head and Neck Surgery, The Ohio State University Wexner Medical Center, Columbus, OH, USA

A. B. Todeschini · D. L. Prevedello
Department of Neurological Surgery, The Ohio State University Wexner Medical Center, Columbus, OH, USA

R. I. Cho (✉)
Department of Ophthalmology and Visual Science, The Ohio State University Wexner Medical Center, Columbus, OH, USA
e-mail: raymond.cho@osumc.edu

Endonasal Approaches to the Orbit

- Endoscopic orbital decompression
- Optic canal decompression
- Endonasal orbitotomy
- Combined anterior/endoscopic approach

The orbital floor and medial orbital wall are thin bony partitions separating the sinonasal cavity from the orbital contents. The development of modern endoscopic sinus surgery introduced new corridors to access the orbital contents and the opportunity to improve visualization and address lesions that might be considered high-risk if approached by a conventional orbitotomy. Applications for transnasal approaches include medial orbital decompression, optic canal decompression, tumors in the medial orbit or orbital apex, primary sinonasal pathologies with intraorbital extension, invasive fungal sinusitis, and subperiosteal abscesses arising from acute sinusitis.

There are numerous factors to consider when deciding between external and endoscopic orbital surgery. Anterior orbitotomy requires less specialized equipment, can often be performed more quickly, and allows for direct visualization of orbital structures and direct access to the ethmoidal arteries. Conversely, endonasal surgery provides excellent magnification and visualization of the sinuses, requires no external incisions, obviates the need for globe retraction, limits fat herniation into the field of visualization, and can minimize direct trauma to orbital structures. Both approaches, however, require extensive training to perform safely and effectively.

A. J. Cohen, C. N. Burkat (eds.), *Oculofacial, Orbital, and Lacrimal Surgery*, https://doi.org/10.1007/978-3-030-14092-2_54

Endoscopic Orbital Decompression

Orbital decompression is most commonly performed in the setting of thyroid-related orbitopathy [20, 32], but it can also be used in the treatment of any congestive orbital process causing proptosis and/or vision compromise. While any wall or compartment of the orbit can be accessed through standard anterior approaches, the medial wall and orbital floor are particularly amenable to the endonasal approach. The current techniques of endoscopic orbital approaches stem from orbital decompression techniques described in the early 1990s by Kennedy et al. [10] and Metson et al. [19]. Standard equipment and instrumentation used for endoscopic sinus surgery are required. Image guidance is a useful tool, but it does not replace a comprehensive knowledge of the anatomy and surgical landmarks and can be utilized at the surgeon's discretion.

The nasal cavity is prepared by inserting cottonoids soaked in a vasoconstricting agent such as epinephrine 1:10,000 solution or oxymetazoline 0.05%. The ipsilateral middle turbinate is medialized or removed under endoscopic guidance, as needed to obtain adequate access. This is followed by a comprehensive ethmoidectomy, exposing the skull base and lamina papyracea from the frontal sinus outflow anteriorly to the orbital apex posteriorly.

Once the lamina papyracea is exposed, a periosteal elevator can usually be used to out-fracture and remove it with forceps, ideally without disrupting the periorbita. If the lamina is too thick to be easily fractured, a 3- or 4-mm endonasal drill can be used to thin the lamina to eggshell thickness, allowing it to be removed while preserving the periorbita. The dissection can be carried from the lacrimal sac back to the orbital apex. If the orbital floor is to be removed, it is usually necessary to first remove the inferonasal strut (the ethmoid-maxillary suture, also known as the orbital strut) with a drill and forceps. A wide maxillary antrostomy may also be performed to allow a more extensive removal of the floor (Fig. 54.1). The remainder of the floor can then be removed from the strut to the infraorbital canal. The anterior third of the orbital floor is typically spared to reduce the risk of postoperative diplopia and globe dystopia.

At this point, it is important to note that the anatomic definition of an orbital decompression may differ between surgeons. Technically, a medial decompression entails removal of the medial orbital wall (lamina papyracea) alone. If the orbital floor (or a portion thereof) is removed, this entails a combined medial/floor decompression. However, some surgeons remove the orbital floor and medial wall routinely. It is therefore critical for surgical team members to clearly communicate the intended decompression target(s) preoperatively.

If the periorbita is violated during bone removal, orbital fat can herniate into the surgical field and obstruct the view. In this event, the orbital fat can be gently cauterized with bipolar cautery, but exquisite care must be taken to avoid injury to the medial rectus muscle. Once all intended bone is removed and the periorbita is exposed, a sickle or 90 ° knife can be used to open the periorbita in a posterior to anterior fashion for a better visualization of the cuts, avoiding the medial rectus muscle, which lies just deep to the periorbita. Following this, the contents of the orbit should prolapse into the nasal cavity and/or maxillary sinus, maximizing the decompressive effect.

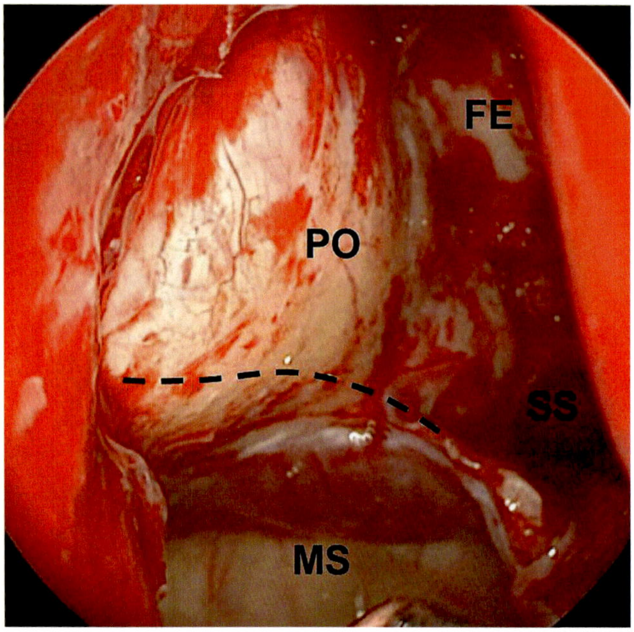

Fig. 54.1 Intraoperative photograph, right endoscopic orbital decompression following ethmoidectomy and removal of the lamina papyracea and prior to incision of the medial periorbita (PO). The inferomedial orbital strut (dashed line) and medial floor have also been removed, exposing the maxillary sinus (MS). (*FE* fovea ethmoidalis, *SS* sphenoid sinus; Courtesy of Alexander Farag, MD, FARS)

Optic Canal Decompression

Decompression of the intracanalicular portion of the optic nerve can be performed endoscopically through a transsphenoidal approach or via frontotemporal craniotomy (see below) [18]. Indications for this procedure include tumors of the lesser sphenoid wing or sinonasal cavity causing optic nerve compression, tumors of the intracanalicular optic nerve, and traumatic optic neuropathy (TON), although the efficacy of optic canal decompression for the treatment of TON is controversial [3, 5, 11, 13, 23]. Decompression of the optic canal is not generally helpful in the setting of thyroid-related compressive optic neuropathy.

To perform an optic nerve decompression, an endoscopic ethmoidectomy is performed as described above, widely exposing the lamina papyracea back to the sphenoid sinus. The anterior wall of the sphenoid sinus is then removed,

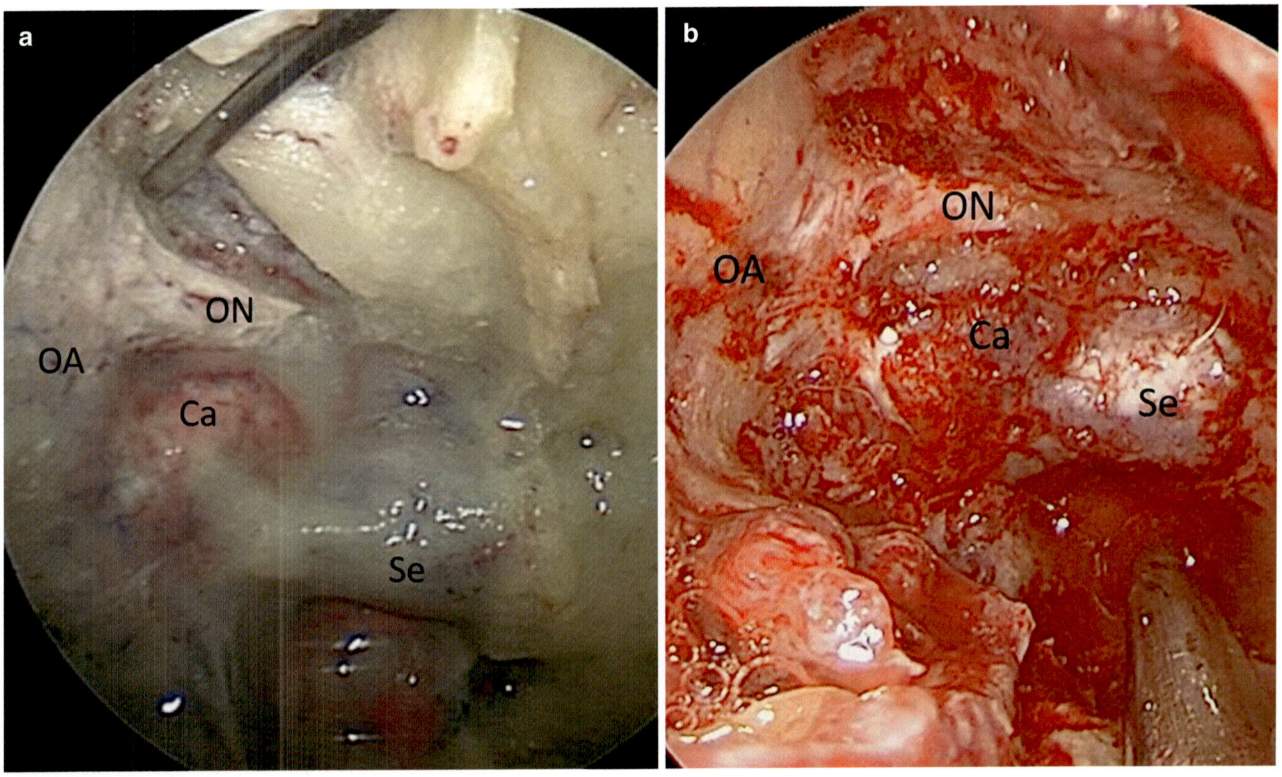

Fig. 54.2 Endoscopic right optic nerve decompression demonstrated in cadaveric dissection (**a**) and comparable intraoperative photograph (**b**) of a patient with a large cavernous sinus meningioma requiring orbital apex (OA) and optic nerve (ON) decompression. Note the proximity of the carotid artery (Ca) as the optic nerve passes superior to the carotid protuberance, and the relationship of both structures to the sella (Se)

creating a wide sphenoidotomy. The sphenoid rostrum is drilled flush to the orbit, and the optic canal, superior orbital fissure, carotid artery, sella turcica, and lateral opticocarotid recess are then identified within the sphenoid sinus. Using the techniques described above, the medial wall of the posterior orbit and orbital apex are then decompressed to define the periosteal layer of the orbit. This is traced back to the optic canal. Using a 3- or 4-mm drill, the medial wall of the optic canal is then gently drilled to eggshell thickness overlying the optic nerve. The drill should be moved parallel to the direction of the optic nerve as the bone is thinned, and exquisite care is taken as the nerve courses just superior to the carotid protuberance (Fig. 54.2). Using a cottle elevator, the bone is atraumatically elevated off the medial canal. This can allow for 180° decompression of the medial optic canal.

Endonasal Orbitotomy

Removal of lesions in the orbital apex through standard anterior orbital approaches can be challenging and high-risk. A transnasal endoscopic approach can potentially provide safer access with improved visualization of such lesions, largely bypassing many of the critical structures and most of the obstructing fat that orbital surgeons must contend with [17, 33]. The approach described above is first used to expose the medial orbital wall, remove as much of the lamina papyracea as is required to access the lesion, and open the periorbita. For extraconal lesions in the medial orbit, minimal dissection should be required. Intraconal lesions can be accessed by bluntly dissecting between the medial rectus muscle and the inferior or superior rectus muscle. The lesion is gently grasped, delicately dissected from the orbital contents, and removed. Adherence to the tenets of microsurgery is critical to avoid complications. A bimanual endonasal approach to the posterior orbit has also been described, whereby a posterior nasal septectomy is performed to allow access for a second instrument through the contralateral nares during the procedure [8]. Reconstruction of the medial wall is not typically required unless the defect is particularly large and there is significant orbital prolapse into the ethmoid sinus. In such cases, repair can be accomplished with a nasal mucosal flap or with an alloplastic implant placed through a separate anterior orbitotomy incision.

Combined Anterior/Endoscopic Approach

In some cases, a simultaneous anterior orbitotomy and endonasal approach can be helpful. For example, if an aggressive sinonasal tumor involving the ethmoid sinus is invading the medial orbit, a transcaruncular medial orbitotomy can facilitate resection of the orbital portion of the tumor by direct visualization while protecting the globe and medial rectus, after which a malleable ribbon or cottonoids can be placed along the medial aspect of the orbit to protect the orbital tissues. This provides a definitive barrier between the orbit and ethmoid sinus, allowing for endonasal resection of the sinonasal portion of the tumor to be safely performed without inadvertent damage to orbital structures. For complex pathology involving the orbit and paranasal sinuses, a thorough knowledge of anatomy and the limitations of each surgical approach, coupled with a high degree of creativity and flexibility, can have a tremendously positive impact on patient outcomes.

Transcranial Orbitotomy

- Minimally invasive unilateral subfrontal approach
- Frontotemporal approach
- Orbitozygomatic approach
- Bilateral subfrontal (transbasal) approach

A transcranial approach can be considered for large or high-risk lesions of the medial, superior, or lateral orbit, and for conditions that affect both the orbit and anterior or middle cranial fossae. Examples of such pathologies include but are not limited to high-flow vascular lesions or infiltrating tumors of the orbit, meningoencephaloceles, frontal sinus mucoceles, spheno-orbital meningiomas, lesions that involve both the intraorbital and intracanalicular or intracranial portions of the optic nerve, orbital roof fractures, and orbital roof decompression [9, 12, 16, 21, 29]. Different incisions and craniotomies can be used to reach the orbit and may or may not include osteotomies of the orbital rim, depending on the need for access to the anterior orbit [26]. The following discussion will start with the least invasive and proceed to progressively more invasive approaches.

Minimally Invasive Unilateral Subfrontal Approach

For processes involving the anterior cranial fossa and superior orbit, such as orbital roof fractures or meningoencephaloceles, and meningiomas invading the orbital roof or superior periorbita, a minimally invasive subfrontal approach may be useful [25]. An eyebrow incision is created, running laterally from the supraorbital notch and following within the brow. It can be extended a few millimeters over the lateral projection of the brow into the frontozygomatic area. The frontal skin flap is dissected upward following a subcutaneous plane exposing the orbicularis oculi, frontalis and temporalis muscles. The frontalis muscle is incised, and the temporalis muscle is elevated from its bony insertion (Fig. 54.3a). A frontobasal burr hole posterior to the temporal line is initially performed and a straight osteotomy across the frontal bone just superior to the orbital rim is then performed. The craniotomy is then completed by performing a C-shaped superior osteotomy back to the initial burr hole, creating a small supraorbital craniotomy (Fig. 54.3b). The dura is elevated from the floor of the anterior cranial fossa and the bone is drilled to expose the periorbita beneath the orbital roof. It is important to avoid entry into the frontal sinus with the medial extension of the craniotomy, for which surgical navigation can be used to plan the osteotomies. If a small sinusotomy is created, this can often be plugged with a small patch of muscle or temporalis fascia. However, if a large sinusotomy is inadvertently created, the sinus may need to be obliterated. Patients with significant lateral extension of the frontal sinus may be poor

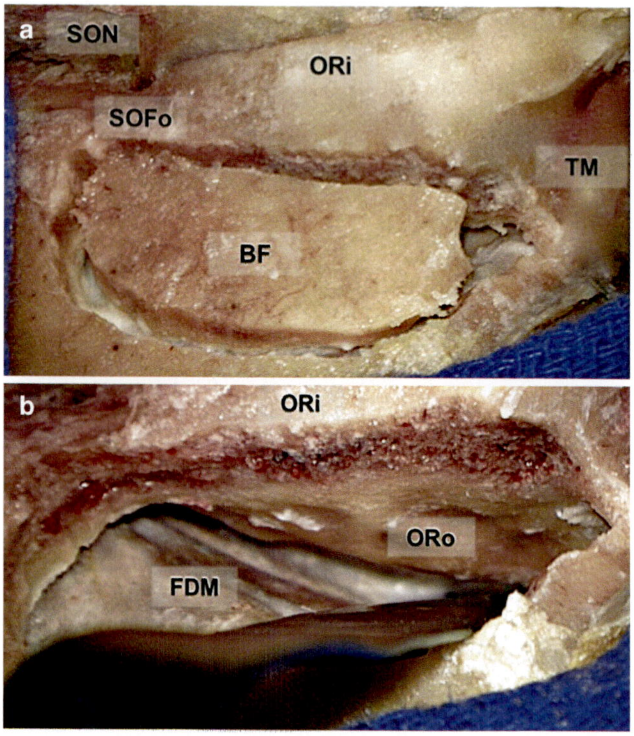

Fig. 54.3 Cadaver dissection demonstrating the exposure provided by a frontal craniotomy through an eyebrow incision (right orbit, surgeon's view). The brow is reflected over the orbital rim (ORi) and a frontal bone flap (BF) is created superior to the rim (**a**). The supraorbital nerve (SON) is seen exiting the supraorbital foramen (SOFo). (*TM* temporalis muscle). The bone flap has been removed and the frontal dura mater (FDM) has been elevated from the orbital roof (ORo) (**b**)

candidates for this approach. However, for properly selected patients, this approach provides wide access to the superolateral orbit and, with minimal frontal lobe retraction, it also provides exposure of the orbital apex and optic nerve including its foramen and canal.

A limited subfrontal craniotomy can also be performed through an upper eyelid crease incision [22], as described in the anterior orbitotomy chapter. However, the inferior placement of this incision limits the superior extent of the craniotomy, and it may be a more useful approach if the superior orbital rim is to be removed. The orbital rim osteotomy must be created lateral to the supraorbital fissure in order to spare the supraorbital nerve.

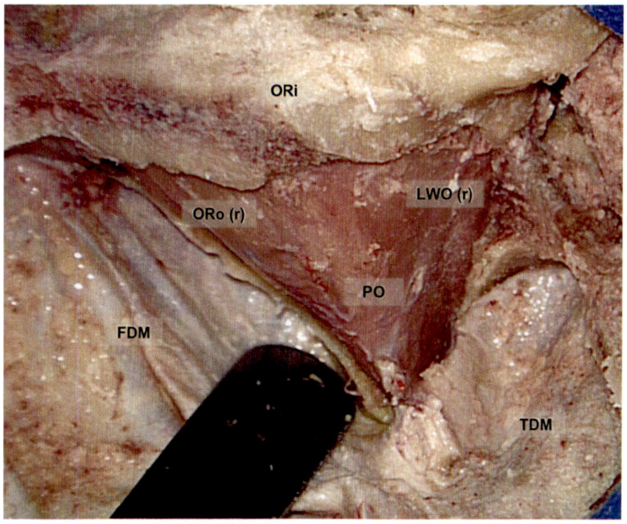

Fig. 54.4 Cadaver dissection demonstrating the exposure provided by a frontotemporal approach (right orbit, surgeon's view). Following dissection of the scalp and temporalis muscle, the frontotemporal bone flap is removed, leaving the superior orbital rim (ORi) in place. The frontal dura (FDM) and temporal dura (TDM) have been dissected, and the orbital roof (ORo) and lateral wall of the orbit (LWO) have been removed, exposing the periorbital (PO) over the superior and lateral orbit

Frontotemporal Approach

A frontotemporal craniotomy is a useful approach to the superior and lateral orbit. It is particularly well-suited for lesions of the greater wing of the sphenoid and/or frontal bone, such as sphenoid wing meningiomas [27]. A curvilinear scalp incision is created behind the hairline, extending from the helical root superiorly through the temple and curving anteriorly across the forehead. After elevating the scalp flap, the temporalis muscle is dissected from the temporalis fossa, and a key burr hole is performed at the junction of the frontal, temporal and sphenoid bones. A second burr hole is typically placed at the junction of the superior temporal line and coronal suture. A wide craniotomy is then performed to expose the frontal and temporal lobes. The dura is elevated from the orbital roof, following an anterolateral to posterior direction. Next, protecting the temporal lobe as needed, the sphenoid wing and crest are drilled away, exposing the lateral orbit (Fig. 54.4). Drilling can be extended to expose the superior orbital fissure and anterior clinoid process as needed on a case by case basis. The roof and lateral wall can be removed through this approach. While this approach provides excellent extraorbital exposure of the entire superior and lateral orbit, it is limited in its anterior exposure by the orbital rim. If the anterior orbit needs exposure, an orbitozygomatic approach is indicated.

Orbitozygomatic Approach

The orbitozygomatic approach provides wide exposure of the entire superior, lateral, and potentially inferior orbit [28, 30]. This approach is facilitated by an extended frontotemporal incision, or alternatively a coronal incision for maximal exposure. The scalp flap is elevated subperiosteally and the dissection continues lateral to the supraorbital notch. The periosteum is dissected from the orbital rim, identifying and preserving the supraorbital neurovascular bundle. This dissection is carried down to fully expose the lateral orbital rim and zygomatic arch. The deep temporalis fascia is incised following an imaginary line connecting the root of the zygoma and the superior orbital rim, usually exposing the interfascial fat pad. A dissection plane deep to the superficial layer of the deep temporalis fascia protects the facial nerve, while exposing the zygomatic arch.

Once the orbitozygomatic complex is fully exposed (Fig. 54.5a), a frontotemporal craniotomy is performed as described above. Three key osteotomies are performed: (1) the malar eminence (at the level of the zygomaticofacial foramen), (2) the superolateral orbital rim (frontozygomatic suture), and (3) the zygomatic arch (temporozygomatic suture). This is followed by an osteotomy at the posterior aspect of the lateral orbital wall toward the inferior orbital fissure, which is difficult to see directly, but can be palpated using a small dissector (Fig. 54.5b). Completing these osteotomies allows the en bloc translocation of the orbitozygomatic complex, including the orbital rim, body of the zygoma, and zygomatic arch (Fig. 54.5b inset). The superior osteotomy may be modified to include the orbital roof (usually the portion lateral to the supraorbital notch) extending posteriorly toward the superior orbital fissure.

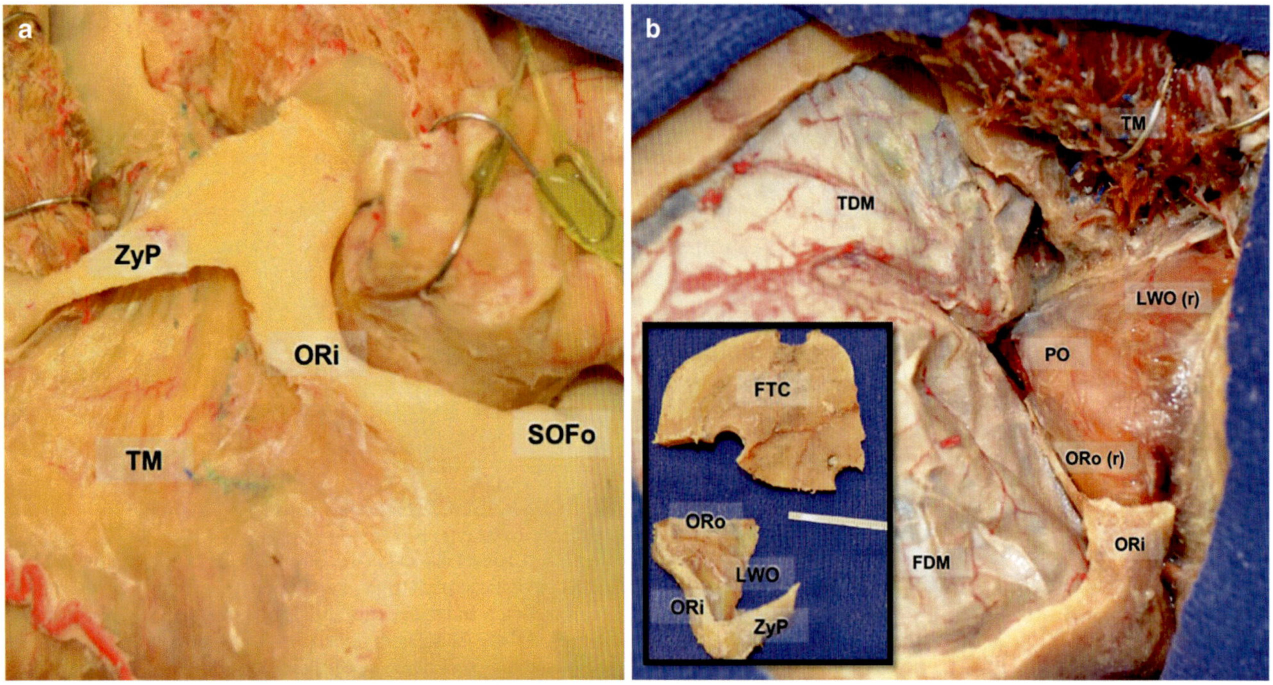

Fig. 54.5 Cadaver dissection demonstrating the exposure provided by an orbitozygomatic approach (left orbit, surgeon's view). The scalp flap is dissected as in the frontolateral approach (**a**) exposing the orbital rim (ORi), supraorbital foramen (SOFo), zygomatic arch (ZyP), and temporalis muscle (TM). Following dissection of the temporalis muscle, the frontotemporal bone flap (FTC) is removed (**b**), and the orbital roof (ORo), lateral orbital rim (ORi), lateral wall of the orbit (LWO), and zygomatic process of the zygomatic arch (ZyP) are removed en bloc (**b**, inset). The periorbita (PO) over the superior and lateral orbit is exposed to a greater extent than with the frontolateral approach

Bilateral Subfrontal (Transbasal) Approach

If exposure of the anterior cranial fossa, superior/medial orbits, and/or sinonasal cavity is required, a bilateral subfrontal approach, also known as the transbasal approach, can be utilized [7]. First, a bicoronal incision is carried extending from the level of the ipsilateral zygomatic arch to the level of the contralateral helical root according to the exposure needed. The scalp flap is elevated from the frontal bone, down to the nasal bones medially and the orbital rims laterally (Fig. 54.6a). The supraorbital notches or foramina are identified, and their corresponding supraorbital neurovascular bundles are carefully dissected and released. A complete foramen requires an inverted V osteotomy to allow the inferior mobilization of the bundle with the periorbita [31]. A large bifrontal craniotomy is then performed just above the orbital rim (Fig. 54.6b), transecting the frontal sinus (which is subsequently cranialized). This provides extradural exposure of the orbital roof back to the intracranial portion of the optic nerves. The frontal bar (both superior orbital rims and the nasion) is then removed while protecting the supraorbital neurovascular bundles. Removal of the frontal bar requires a series of osteotomies to mobilize the bony complex en bloc. The anterior two-thirds of the orbital roof can be removed with the frontal bar or removed separately with a drill. Once the superior periorbita has been exposed, the frontal nerve and the levator palpebrae superioris muscle can be visualized through it, and an incision is created through the periorbita parallel to the levator muscle. This provides clear and wide access to the entire superior orbit, as well as the lateral and medial orbital compartments (Fig. 54.6c). As mentioned before, this approach also provides access to the sinonasal cavity in the midline. If access to only one orbit is required without the need for sinus exposure, the ipsilateral half of the frontal bar can be removed (Fig. 54.7a, b).

Reconstruction

With each of these transcranial approaches, a craniotomy bone flap is temporarily removed to provide exposure and access to the brain and orbit. Adequate bony reconstruction of the orbital walls and cranial vault is essential. If the periorbita has been resected, the missing portions can be replaced with free fascia

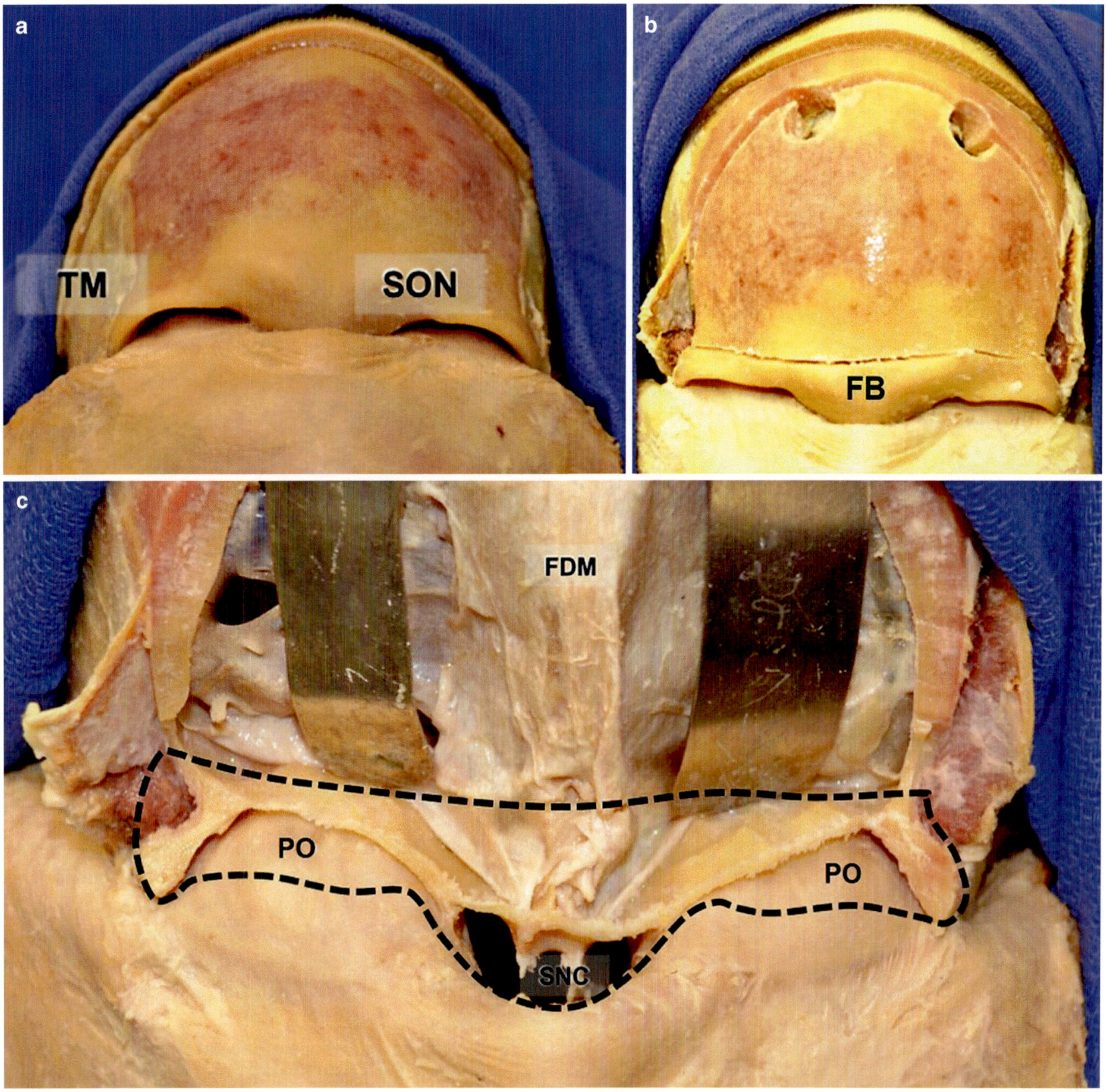

Fig. 54.6 Cadaver dissection demonstrating the exposure provided by a bicoronal subfrontal approach (frontal view). A bicoronal scalp flap is reflected inferiorly to expose the superior orbital rims and nasion (**a**). Burr holes are drilled through the frontal and temporal bones and the frontal bone flap is cut with a saw (**b**). The frontal bone flap is removed (**c**), exposing the anterior cranial fossa bilaterally and the frontal sinus (FS). The frontal bar (dashed line) has been removed en bloc (**c**), exposing the periosteum over the superior orbits bilaterally, as well as the sinonasal cavity (SNC) in the midline. (*FDM* frontal dura mater)

or acellular dermis grafts to prevent tethering of the extraocular muscles. Large bony defects of the orbit can lead to orbital pulsations or meningoencephaloceles, especially if the periorbital has been violated, and should be reconstructed with bone grafts or alloplastic implants (Fig. 54.8). Any skull base defect must be repaired with multilayered closure to prevent a cerebrospinal fluid leak, which often entails a pedicled pericranial flap. The craniotomy bone flap is then plated back into position to restore the cranial contour, and the scalp incision is closed using a multilayered technique.

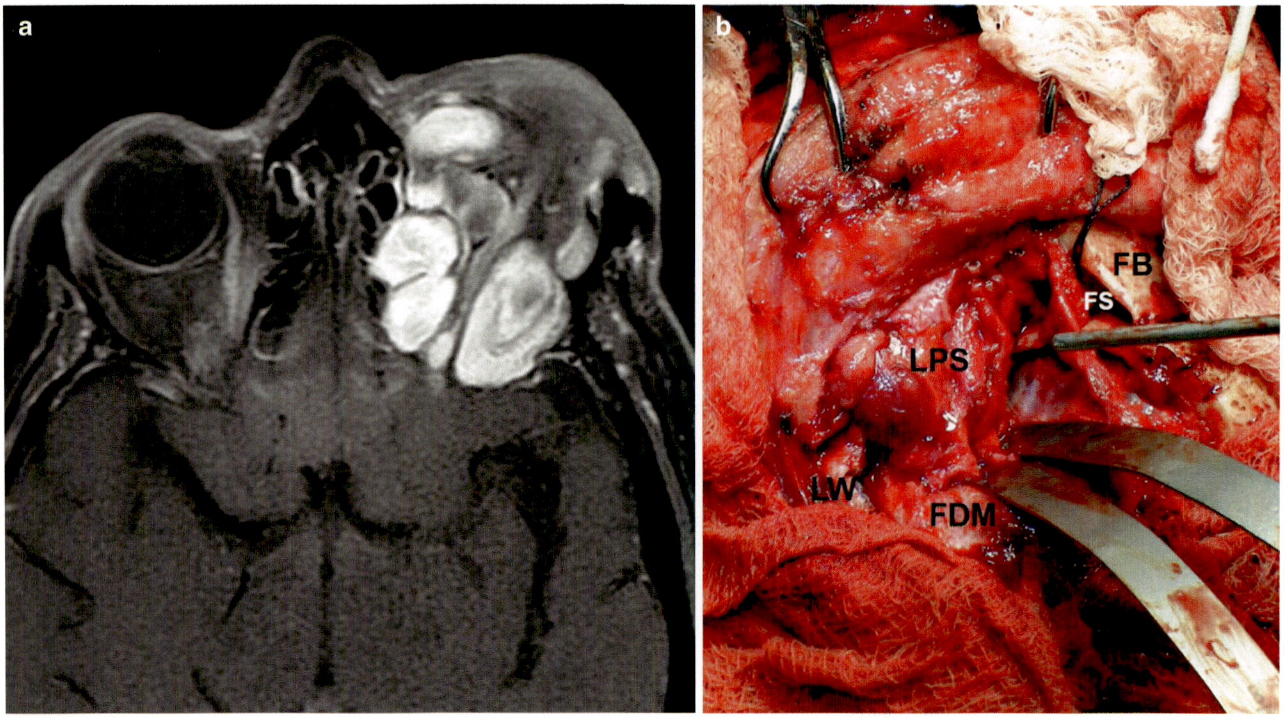

Fig. 54.7 Large recurrent solitary neurofibroma of the left superior orbit, T1 fat-suppressed axial MRI (**a**). Intraoperative photograph (**b**) (superior surgeon's view) following tumor resection through a trans-basal craniotomy with removal of the left half of the frontal bone flap and frontal bar (FB). (*FDM* frontal dura mater, *LW* lateral wall of the orbit, *LPS* levator palpebrae superioris muscle)

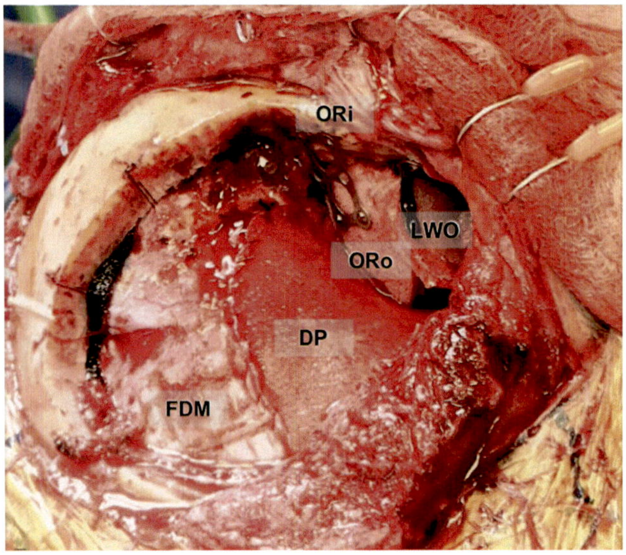

Fig. 54.8 Intraoperative photograph, right frontotemporal craniotomy for resection of a spheno-orbital meningioma. The orbital rim (ORi) was left intact, and the orbital roof (ORo) and lateral wall of the orbit (LWO) have been reconstructed with a pre-shaped porous polyethylene implant fixated with titanium plates and screws. The frontal dura mater (FDM) has been repaired with an acellular dermis patch graft (DP)

Transorbital Skull Base Surgery

While the orbit can be approached through transcranial approaches, the converse is also true, in that the anterior cranial fossa, middle cranial fossa, cavernous sinus, and suprasellar region can be accessed through transorbital approaches [1, 2, 14]. These cases can be performed open or endoscopically, depending on the approach and pathology to be addressed.

In selected cases, lesions of the cavernous sinus or anterior portion of the middle cranial fossa can be approached through a lateral orbitotomy [4]. The greater wing of the sphenoid is removed in a similar manner as a lateral orbital decompression with deep bone removal, with or without and lateral orbital rim bone flap. Complete removal of the greater sphenoid wing all the way back to the superior orbital fissure can provide exposure to the anterior tip of the temporal lobe and access to the cavernous sinus.

Similarly, the anterior cranial fossa can be approached through a superior orbitotomy, typically utilizing an upper lid crease incision. A large lid crease incision facilitates an open approach with wide removal of the orbital roof using a drill or ultrasonic bone removal. Additionally, several groups have recently reported the successful use of endoscopic techniques through a limited upper lid crease incision and subperiosteal plane dissection to fully access the optic nerve and anterior and middle cranial fossae [6, 15, 24]. These techniques potentially allow for a minimally invasive approach to areas of the skull base previously accessible only by a craniotomy incision. While promising, these techniques remain in their early stages of development, and further studies are needed to prove safety and standardization of the approaches.

Conclusion

Extraorbital approaches can be utilized for orbital pathology that is extensive, high risk, or extending into the paranasal sinuses, cranial fossa, or inferotemporal fossa. Endonasal techniques provide excellent access to and visualization of the medial and posterior orbit. Transcranial approaches provide wide access to the orbit and cranial contents as dictated by the extent of the pathology. All of these approaches require a comprehensive multidisciplinary skull base team combining neurosurgery, otorhinolaryngology, and oculoplastic surgery to optimize outcomes.

References

1. Allen RC. The evolving role of the oculoplastic surgeon in skull base surgery. Curr Opin Ophthalmol. 2016;27:420–7.
2. Balakrishnan K, Moe KS. Applications and outcomes of orbital and transorbital endoscopic surgery. Otolaryngol Head Neck Surg. 2011;144(5):815–20.
3. Berhouma M, Jacquession T, Abouaf L, et al. Endoscopic endonasal optic nerve and orbital apex decompression for nontraumatic optic neuropathy: surgical nuances and review of the literature. Neurosurg Focus. 2014;37:E19.
4. Chabot JD, Gardner PA, Stefko ST, et al. Lateral orbitotomy approach for lesions of the middle fossa: a retrospective review of thirteen patients. Neurosurgery. 2017;80:309–22.
5. Chaon BC, Lee MS. Is there treatment for traumatic optic neuropathy? Curr Opin Ophthalmol. 2015;26:445–9.
6. Dallan I, Sellari-Franceschini S, Turri-Zanoni M, et al. Endoscopic transorbital superior eyelid approach for the management of selected spheno-orbital meningiomas: preliminary experience. Oper Neurosurg (Hagerstown). 2018;14(3):243–51.
7. Feiz-Erfan I, Spetzler RF, Horn EM, Porter RW, Beals SP, Lettieri SC, Joganic EF, DeMonte F. Proposed classification for the transbasal approach and its modifications. Skull Base. 2008;18(1):29.
8. Healy DY, Lee NG, Freitag SK, Bleier BS. Endoscopic bimanual approach to an intraconal cavernous hemangioma of the orbital apex with vascularized flap reconstruction. Ophthalmic Plast Reconstr Surg. 2014;30:e104–6.
9. Jian T, Sun F, Tang D, Wang S, Wu T, Zhao L. Clinical analysis of transcranial orbitotomy approach on cranio-orbital tumors. J Craniofac Surg. 2015;26(2):441–6.
10. Kennedy DW, Goodstein ML, Miller NR, Zinreich SJ. Endoscopic transnasal orbital decompression. Arch Otolaryngol Head Neck Surg. 1990;116:275–82.
11. Kumuran AM, Sundar G, Lim TC. Traumatic optic neuropathy: a review. Craniomaxillofac Trauma Reconstr. 2015;8:31–41.
12. Leone CR, Wissinger JP. Surgical approaches to diseases of the orbital apex. Ophthalmology. 1988;95:391–7.
13. Levin LA, Beck RW, Joseph MP, et al. The treatment of traumatic optic neuropathy: the international optic nerve trauma study. Ophthalmology. 1999;106:1268–77.
14. Lim JH, Sardesai MG, Ferreira M Jr, Moe KS. Transorbital neuroendoscopic management of sinogenic complications involving the frontal sinus, orbit, and anterior cranial fossa. J Neurol Surg B Skull Base. 2012;73(6):394–400.
15. Locatelli D, Pozzi F, Turri-Zanoni M, et al. Transorbital endoscopic approaches to the skull base: current concepts and future perspectives. J Neurosurg Sci. 2016;60:514–25.
16. Maroon JC, Kennerdell JS. Surgical approaches to the orbit: indications and techniques. J Neurosurg. 1984;60:1226–35.
17. McKinney KA, Snyderman CH, Carrau RL, et al. Seeing the light: endoscopic endonasal intraconal orbital tumor surgery. Otolaryngol Head Neck Surg. 2010;143:699–701.
18. Mesquita Filho PM, Prevedello DM, Prevedello LM, Carrau RL, et al. Optic canal decompression: comparison of 2 surgical techniques. World Neurosurg. 2017;104:745–51.
19. Metson R, Dallow RL, Shore JW. Endoscopic orbital decompression. Laryngoscope. 1994;104(8):950–7.
20. Michel O, Bresgen K, Rüssmann W, Thumfart WF, Stennert E. Endoskopisch kontrollierte endonasale Orbitadekompression beim malignen Ophthalmus. Laryngo-Rhino-Otologie. 1991;70(12):656–62.
21. Naffziger HC. Progressive exophthalmos following thyroidectomy: its pathology and treatment. Ann Surg. 1931;94:582–6.
22. Owusu Boahene KD, Lim M, Chu E, Quinones-Hinojosa A. Transpalpebral orbitofrontal craniotomy: a minimally invasive approach to anterior cranial vault lesions. Skull Base. 2010;20:237–44.
23. Pletcher SD, Sindani R, Metson R. Endoscopic orbital and optic nerve decompression. Otolaryngol Clin N Am. 2006;39(3):551–61, ix.
24. Ramakrishna R, Kim LJ, Bly RA, Moe K, Ferreira M Jr. Transorbital neuroendoscopic surgery for the treatment of skull base lesions. J Clin Neurosci. 2016;24:99–104.
25. Reisch R, Perneczky A. Ten-year experience with the supraorbital subfrontal approach through an eyebrow skin incision. Oper Neurosurg. 2005;57(suppl_4):ONS-242.
26. Rhoton AL, Natori Y. The orbit and sellar region: microsurgical anatomy and operative approaches. New York: Thieme; 1996.
27. Ringel F, Cedzich C, Schramm J. Microsurgical technique and results of a series of 63 spheno-orbital meningiomas. Neurosurgery. 2007;60:214–21.

28. Seçkin H, Avci E, Uluc K, et al. The work horse of skull base surgery: orbitozygomatic approach. Technique, modifications, and applications. Neurosurg Focus. 2008;25:E4.
29. Shriver EM, Ragheb J, Tse DT. Combined transcranial-orbital approach for resection of optic nerve gliomas: a clinical and anatomical study. Ophthalmic Plast Reconstr Surg. 2012;28:184–91.
30. van Furth WR, Agur AM, Woolridge N, Cusimano MD. The orbitozygomatic approach. Neurosurgery. 2006;58(1 Suppl):ONS103-107; discussion ONS103-107.
31. Webster RC, Gaunt JM, Hamdan US, et al. Supraorbital and supratrochlear notches and foramina: anatomical variations and surgical relevance. Laryngoscope. 1986;96:311–5.
32. Wehrmann D, Antisdel JL. An update on endoscopic orbital decompression. Curr Opin Otolaryngol Head Neck Surg. 2017;25:73–8.
33. Yao WC, Bleier BS. Endoscopic management of orbital tumors. Curr Opin Otolaryngol Head Neck Surg. 2016;24:57–62.

Eyelid Trauma: Principles of Management and Repair

55

Suzanne W. van Landingham and Cat Nguyen Burkat

Introduction

Eyelid trauma spans a spectrum from easily managed abrasions to complex injuries that involve the deeper orbital tissue and globe. Eyelid trauma often is not isolated, and care of these patients may require coordination with neurosurgery and otolaryngology services, depending on the degree involvement of other organ systems. This chapter reviews the epidemiology, evaluation, and management of eyelid trauma, focusing on eyelid lacerations. This chapter also addresses key components of the acute management of eyelid burns. Of note, canalicular trauma and injuries involving the lateral canthal tendon are beyond the scope of this chapter and are more thoroughly addressed in the other chapters of this text.

Epidemiology of Eyelid Trauma

Eyelid injuries are commonly encountered by oculoplastic surgeons and other ophthalmologists. A study using the National Trauma Data Base National Sample Program, which contains data from sequential traumatic encounters voluntarily submitted from American emergency departments, reported that 0.39–1.36% of all trauma admissions between 2003 and 2007 suffered from eyelid lacerations, and 0.95–2.48% had contusions and other superficial periocular injuries [1]. Mechanisms of injury are diverse and vary quite a bit by geographic location, so it is difficult to quantify the prevalence of different causes. Assault, dog bites, automobile accidents, and workplace-related injuries are common etiologies. Eyelid lacerations in the pediatric population are most often secondary to dog bites, and commonly include periocular lacerations, punctures, and canalicular injury.

S. W. van Landingham · C. N. Burkat (✉)
Department of Ophthalmology and Visual Sciences, University of Wisconsin-Madison, Madison, WI, USA
e-mail: svanlandingh@wisc.edu; cburkat@wisc.edu

Evaluation of Eyelid Trauma

Eyelid injuries often occur as part of polytrauma. In these cases, the first steps in the care of the patient must be to evaluate the patient systemically and ensure that the patient is hemodynamically and neurologically stable. Once this initial phase has occurred, a careful history and physical examination should be performed.

History

The clinical history for a patient with an eyelid wound is geared toward identifying factors that may affect management of the patient, such as infection risk, likelihood of ocular injury, presence of foreign body, and contamination with chemicals. The patient should be asked about symptoms of eye injury, such as eye pain, blurred vision, diplopia, and flashes of light, which will help guide the comprehensive ocular examination. As with any trauma case, the clinician should inquire about the mechanism and timing of the injury. If the injury involved any chemicals, irrigation of the ocular surface should be initiated promptly, and the type and concentration of chemical should be determined. If the mechanism of injury was an animal bite, the risk of rabies transmission must be considered, and local animal control authorities should be contacted. Typically, if the animal has documentation of a recent rabies vaccine and can be observed following the injury for abnormal behavior, rabies vaccination is not needed. However, if the animal cannot be identified, prophylactic vaccination against rabies should be given.

From a logistical standpoint, the patient should be asked if the injury occurred at his or her workplace, and if they were using safety goggles at the time, as proper documentation of these items may be important for obtaining workers' compensation. Additionally, the tetanus vaccination status should be determined, and a booster given if the date of the most recent tetanus vaccine is unknown or many years ago.

A. J. Cohen, C. N. Burkat (eds.), *Oculofacial, Orbital, and Lacrimal Surgery*, https://doi.org/10.1007/978-3-030-14092-2_55

Patients can be considered up to date on their tetanus vaccination if they have had three or more tetanus vaccinations total and the most recent has been within 10 years (for a clean wound) or 5 years (for a dirty wound) [2]. Of note, three tetanus vaccinations are given within the first year of life on the standard vaccination schedule, so if the patient was "fully vaccinated" as a child, they likely have had three in their lifetime.

Physical Examination

Evaluation of eyelid trauma starts with a thorough ophthalmic examination, including dilation, to rule out injury to the globe. Any open globe injury must be repaired prior to addressing eyelid wounds as the pressure placed on the globe during repair could cause further damage via expulsion of the intraocular contents. The wound should be irrigated and examined closely.

Lacerations should be assessed for involvement of the eyelid margin (Fig. 55.1), lacrimal canaliculus (Fig. 55.2), lateral canthal tendon, or tissue loss, as each of these findings may make repair more challenging and, depending on the patient, may necessitate taking the patient to the operating room rather than treating them at the bedside. For lacerations that extend medial to the punctum, the examiner should have a very low threshold for probing the canaliculi with a 0-0 Bowman probe to assess involvement of the lacrimal canaliculus (Fig. 55.2). In cases where tissue loss is suspected,

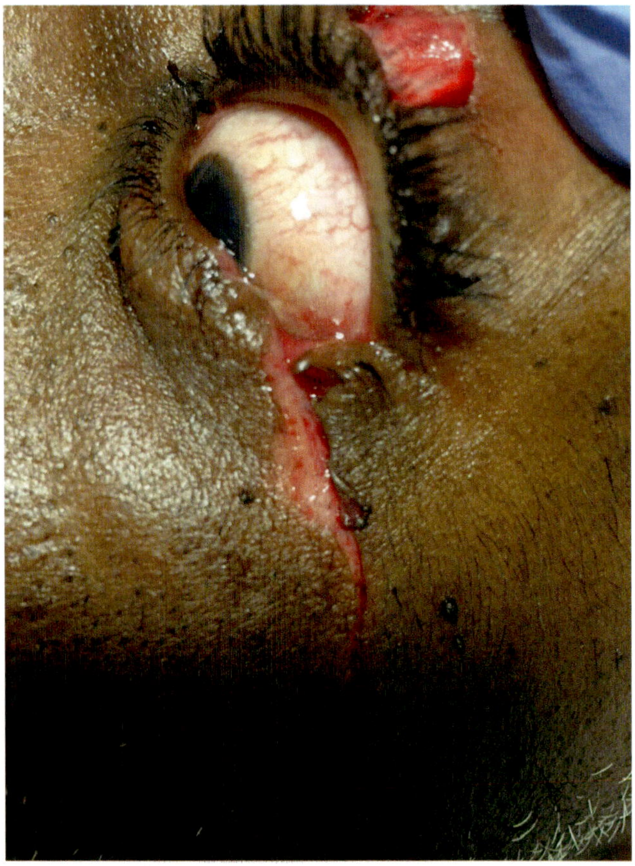

Fig. 55.1 Eyelid laceration involving the lower eyelid margin. This patient was the victim of an attack with a box cutter. Note that the examiner is elevating the upper eyelid

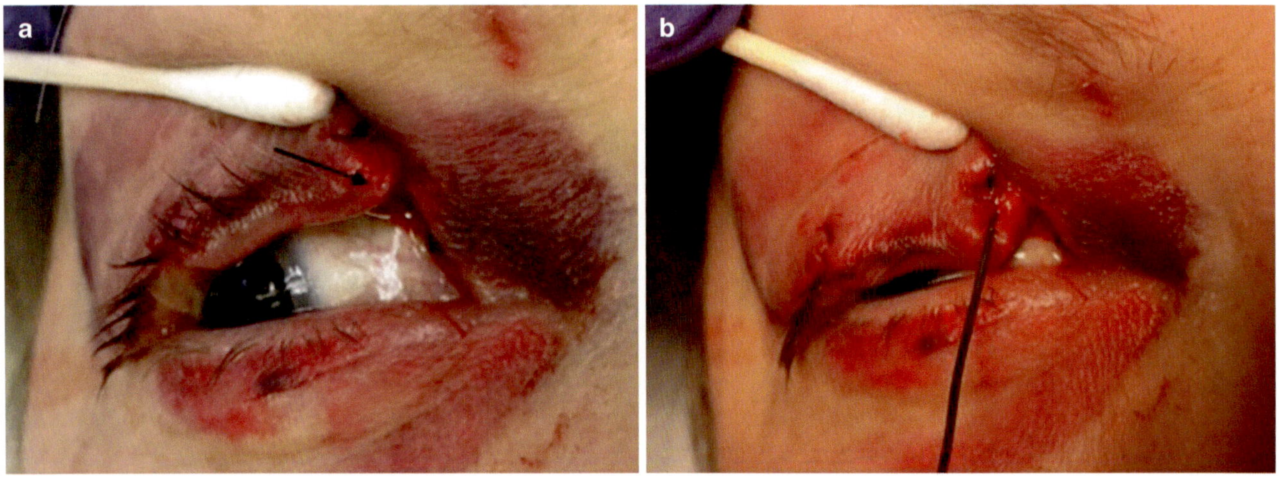

Fig. 55.2 Eyelid laceration involving the lacrimal canaliculus. This patient sustained a complex upper eyelid laceration when she was scratched by her dog. (**a**) The location of the laceration medial to the punctum suggests that it may involve the canaliculus. The arrow indicates the punctum. (**b**) Probing with a 0-0 Bowman probe confirms canalicular injury. Of note, the punctum and ampulla were transected in this injury. (Image courtesy of Alana D. Trotter, MD)

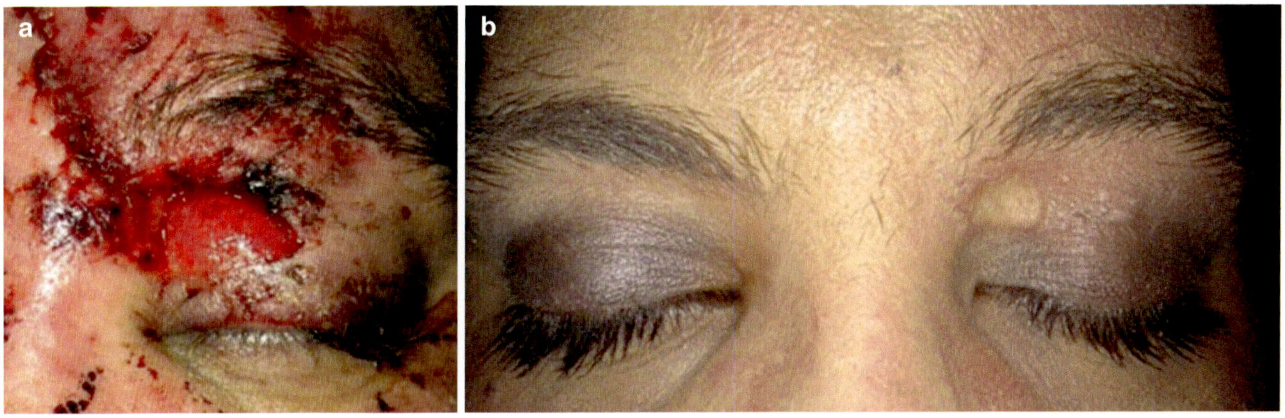

Fig. 55.3 Eyelid laceration with missing skin. This patient sustained a laceration involving the forehead and left upper eyelid during a motor vehicle collision. (**a**) After closure of the forehead laceration and as much of the eyelid laceration as possible, she was found to have a 12 mm × 10 mm area of missing tissue, which was repaired using a full-thickness preauricular skin graft. (**b**) 4 months postoperatively, she was doing well without eyelid malposition

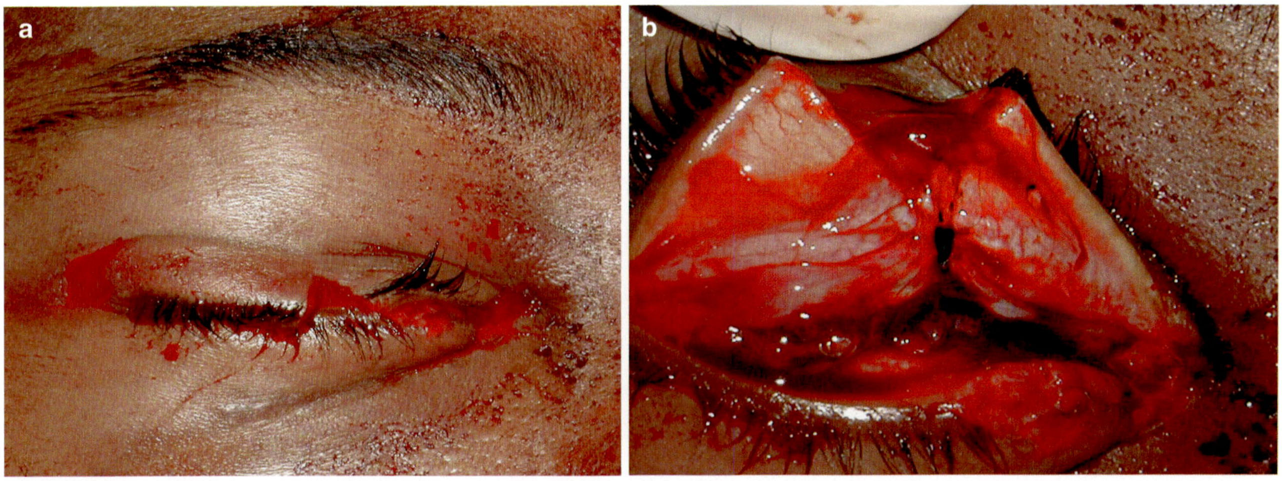

Fig. 55.4 Occult tarsal plate laceration. The eyelid should be everted carefully if indicated, as a small superficial wound may occasionally mask a larger laceration to the deeper structures, such as the tarsal plate

the examiner can assess for missing tissue by gently repositioning the skin at the edges of the wound. Consider whether or not the mechanism is consistent with tissue loss, as often edema, hematoma, or furled skin edges can exaggerate the extent of a skin defect. In most cases, the tissues can be brought together in normal anatomical position; rarely, there may be tissue loss that may require a skin graft (Fig. 55.3).

Additionally, the wound should be gently probed to determine the depth. The eyelid should be everted carefully if indicated, as a small superficial laceration may occasionally mask a larger laceration to the deeper structures, such as the tarsal plate (Fig. 55.4) or orbital septum. A deep wound may also conceal a foreign body, or may indicate damage to important orbital (or even intracranial) structures. Visible fat in the wound suggests violation of the orbital septum and typically represents protrusion of the preaponeurotic fat pad in the upper eyelid (Fig. 55.5). This warrants further exploration for any injury to the levator complex, as well as may increase the risk of orbital cellulitis. If the upper eyelid orbital septum has been violated and levator function is noted to be decreased compared to the contralateral eyelid, surgical exploration should be performed to evaluate for damage to the *levator palpebrae superioris* muscle (Fig. 55.6). However, soft tissue edema and/or hematoma may also lead to decreased levator function measurements as well as temporary ptosis. If frank laceration or transection of the levator complex is noted, the edges should be carefully reapproximated to avoid persistent ptosis.

Finally, if there is a mechanism of injury or exam findings consistent with occult foreign body, the physician should have a low threshold to obtain imaging. Particular caution should be observed with blast injuries, such as those caused by fireworks, firearms, and other explosives, as shrapnel may have tiny entry wounds and can travel a good distance within

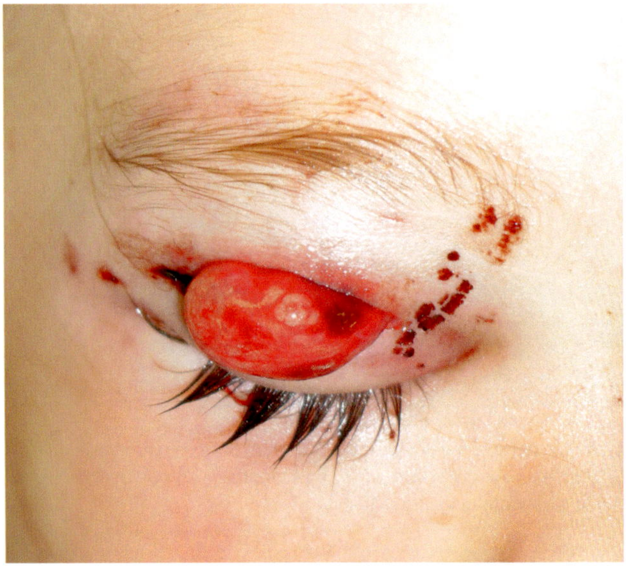

Fig. 55.5 Eyelid laceration with violation of the orbital septum. The presence of fat in this upper eyelid laceration indicates violation of the orbital septum. The wound should be explored for injury to deeper orbital structures and foreign bodies

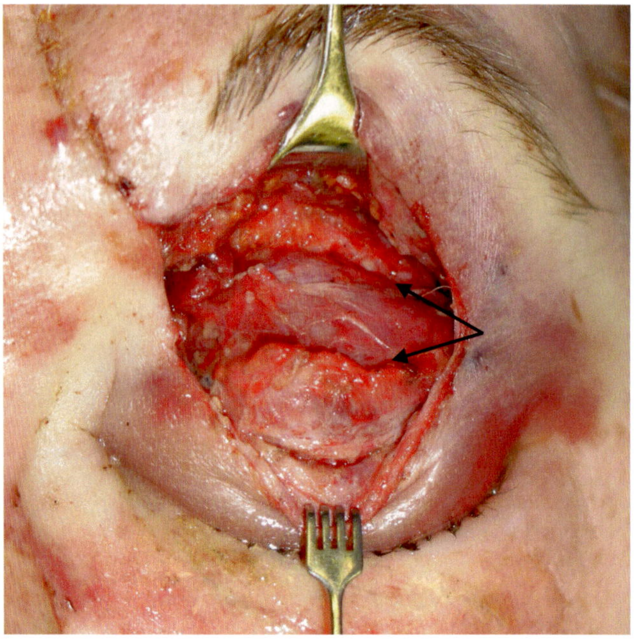

Fig. 55.6 Eyelid laceration with complete levator muscle transection. The arrows indicate the cut ends of the levator muscle complex

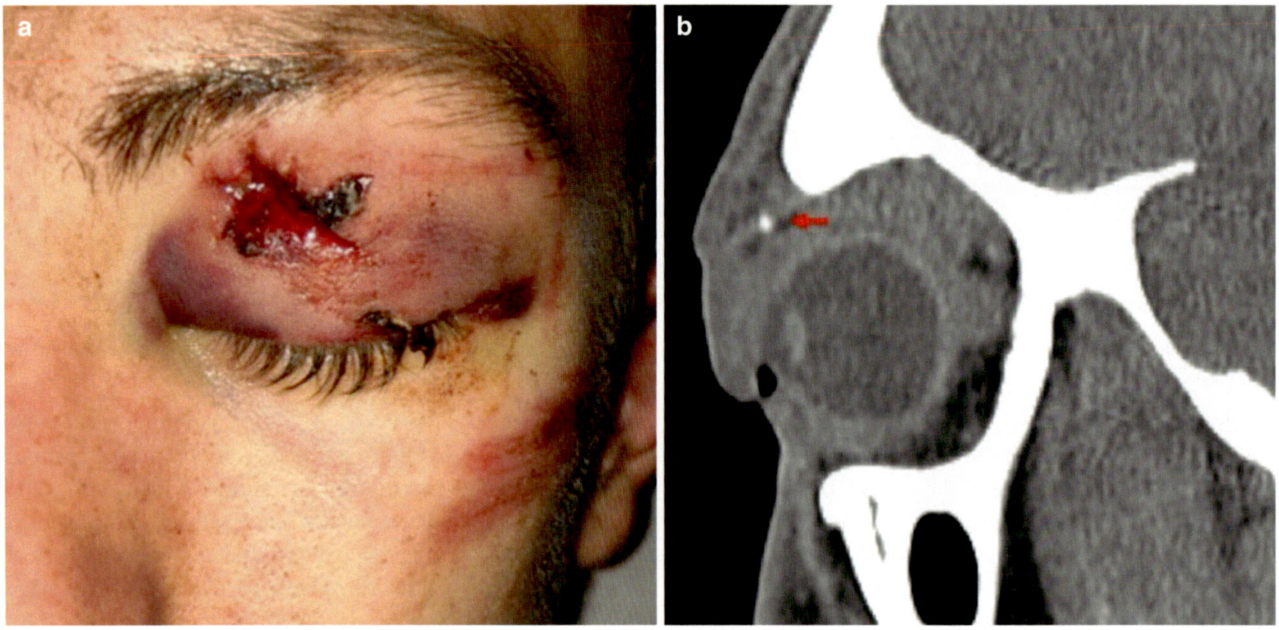

Fig. 55.7 Eyelid laceration containing an occult foreign body. This injury was sustained in a motor vehicle collision. (**a**) The wound did not violate the orbital septum, but had an exaggerated depth due to the surrounding hematoma. (**b**) A CT scan of the head performed to rule out intracranial injury revealed a hyperintense foreign body in the wound. Careful deep exploration revealed a 2.5 mm piece of windshield glass. (Image courtesy of Alana D. Trotter, MD)

tissue. Computed tomography (CT) scan with fine cuts through the orbits is the typical starting place, and is ideal for identifying metallic foreign bodies and most glass (commonly found in automobile injuries) (Fig. 55.7) [3]. It can be difficult to identify some materials, including wood and plastic, that have a similar radiodensity to orbital soft tissues. A CT finding of intraorbital air may be a clue to the presence of an occult foreign body. Close consultation with the reading radiologist or neuroradiologist may also be helpful, particularly if wood is suspected, as manipulation of the window settings can result in reliable identification of wooden foreign bodies even with CT. If CT imaging has ruled out a metallic object but the suspicion for an occult foreign body remains high, magnetic resonance imaging (MRI) may be obtained. Orbital ultrasound can also be very useful for identifying foreign bodies in experienced hands.

Treatment of Non-burn Eyelid Trauma

Superficial eyelid abrasions may be cleansed and covered with antibiotic ointment, and hematomas may be treated with ice. The remainder of this section will focus on the management of lacerations, which are more complex and depend on the extent of the injury.

Closure of Eyelid Lacerations

Anesthesia

Most eyelid lacerations in cooperative adults can be repaired at the bedside using local anesthesia and, if needed, an oral sedative (e.g., diazepam). Studies have not demonstrated any statistically significant improvement in outcome for repairs performed at the bedside in the emergency room versus in the operating room. Small children typically require general anesthesia for repair of a complex laceration, although if the laceration is simple and repair will be quick, monitored sedation may be an alternative option.

Anterior Lamellar Repair

The goal of laceration repair is always meticulous layered closure with physiologic reapproximation of tissues. Simple eyelid lacerations involving only the anterior lamella can be repaired using the following steps:

1. Inject local anesthetic, preferably with epinephrine for vasoconstriction.
2. Irrigate wound thoroughly with saline solution or if the laceration is deep or contaminated, with 5% betadine or antibiotic solution.
3. Meticulously remove all foreign bodies and debris.
4. Debride as little tissue as possible. Given the excellent vascularity of eyelid tissue, even dusky skin is likely to survive.
5. Place 6-0 or 7-0 polyglactin (Vicryl, Ethicon) sutures subcutaneously in a buried interrupted fashion, starting centrally and then bisecting the wound on either side, until the skin edges are well approximated. In jagged wounds, it is helpful to start by reapproximating the points first to avoid creating standing cutaneous defects (Fig. 55.8). These sutures can be replaced later in the repair if the wound does not seem to be coming together well [4].
6. Reapproximate the skin edges with 6-0 fast absorbing plain gut suture placed in a running or interrupted fashion.

The authors favor absorbable sutures for laceration repair because many patients find suture removal unpleasant, and if the patient fails to follow-up, there is little consequence. Others favor permanent suture, such as nylon or polypropylene, citing more durable materials and less tissue reactivity. Studies addressing the question of whether to use absorbable or permanent suture for blepharoplasty incision closure do not conclusively indicate a difference in outcomes between the two [5, 6].

In simple, linear wounds that are not under tension, tissue adhesive such as 2-octyl cyanoacrylate, known as

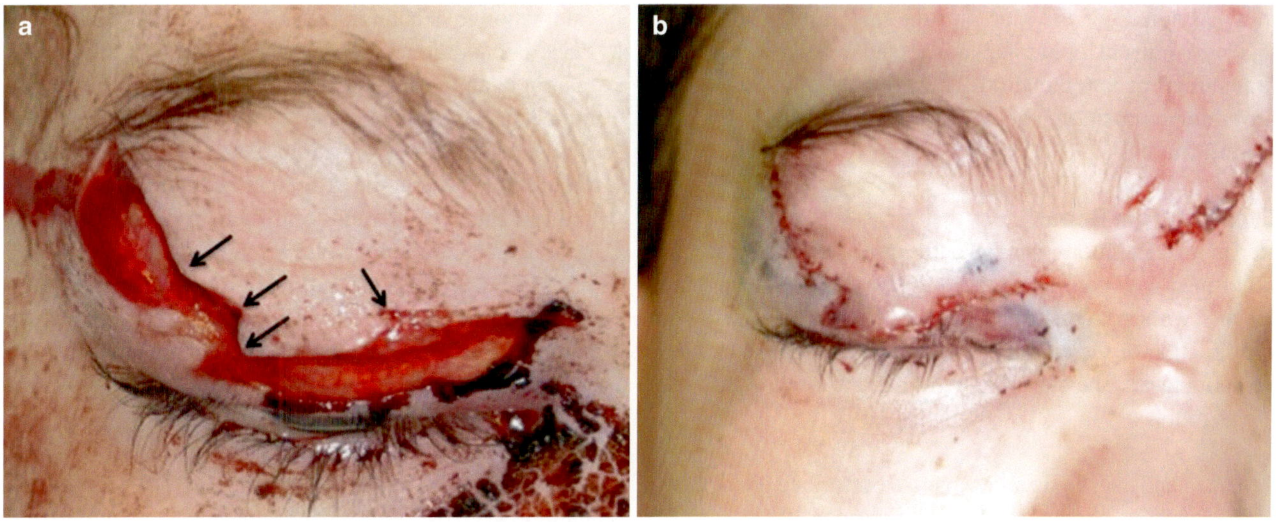

Fig. 55.8 Eyelid laceration with jagged edges. (**a**) The jagged points of this wound, indicated by arrows superiorly, were identified and reapproximated first before repairing the rest of the wound with running sutures (**b**)

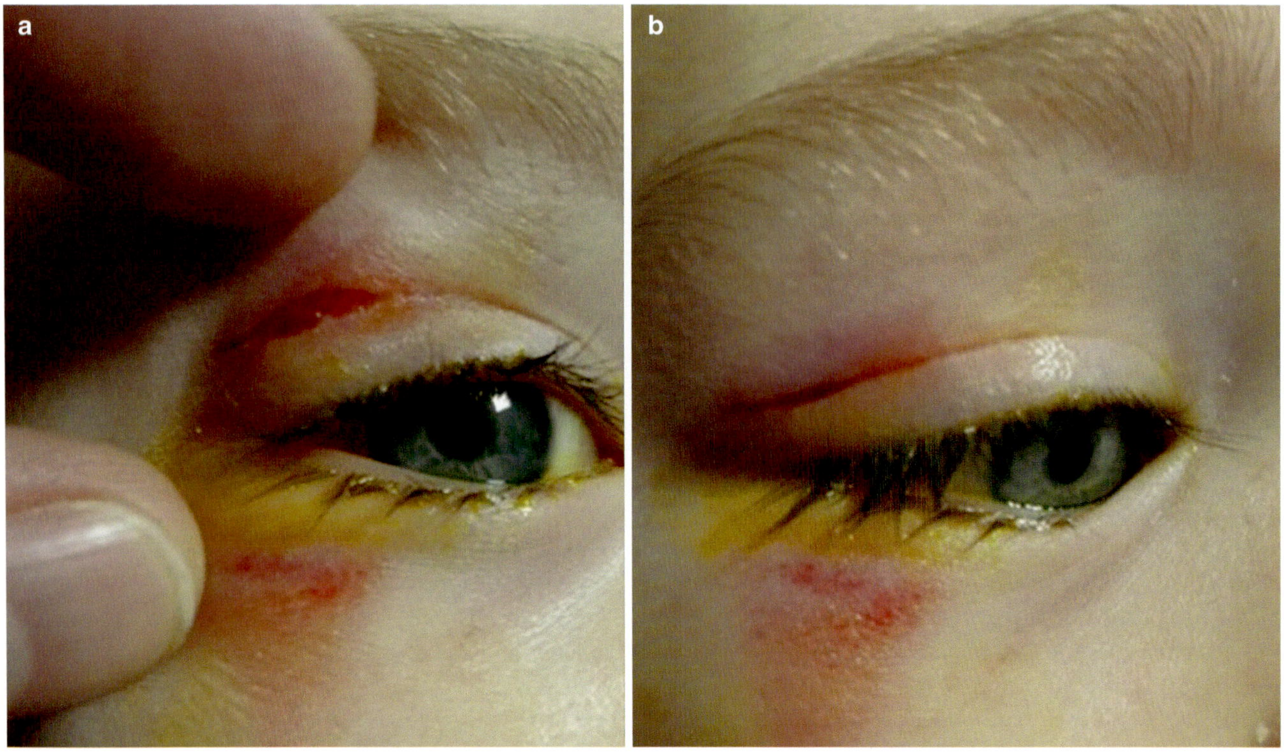

Fig. 55.9 Eyelid laceration amenable to closure with tissue adhesive. (a) This small, linear, laceration located in the lateral right upper eyelid crease lies in physiologic position without tension and thus was a good candidate for closure with tissue adhesive (b). This can be easily accomplished without sedation for small children

Dermabond (Ethicon), may be used in lieu of sutures (Fig. 55.9). The major advantage of tissue adhesive is that it does not require local anesthetic or the use of any sharp instruments, so it may be used at the bedside on children who would otherwise have to be repaired in the operating room under general anesthesia. The wound edges must be reapproximated using cotton tipped applicators while adhesive is placed in a thin layer over the skin edges. Take care to avoid spread of the glue into the underlying tissues, as this will prevent epidermal union and risk postoperative granulomas or inflammation. The wound should be held in physiologic position for the duration specified by the manufacturer.

Eyelid Margin Repair

Repair of lacerations involving the eyelid margin must be performed with care to avoid notching of the eyelid margin (occurs with inadequate eversion of the margin tissues) or misdirection of the cilia (occurs with poor alignment of the wound edges). The steps of eyelid margin laceration repair are as follows:

1. Clean and anesthetize the wound as described previously. A protective corneal shield is also placed.
2. Minimally freshen the edges, if needed, so that the laceration edges are smooth and viable for optimal closure.
3. Reapproximate the eyelid margin by placing a 6-0 polyglactin (Vicryl) suture through the gray line or meibomian gland orifices in a buried vertical mattress fashion. Use of a vertical mattress suture helps to optimally evert the tissue edges to avoid postoperative margin notching (Fig. 55.10a, b). After tightening the suture to ensure proper alignment of the margin, leave it untied to facilitate the next step. The suture can then be placed on vertical traction to help align the rest of the eyelid tissues.
4. Place 1-2 additional 6-0 polyglactin sutures at the eyelid margin in an interrupted vertical mattress or buried interrupted fashion, taking care to cut the suture ends very short to avoid corneal abrasion. Ideally, the margin sutures should be placed at the gray line, meibomian gland line, and lash line. Two margin sutures are also an option if the lacerated edges preclude placement of the third one.
5. Place a 6-0 polyglactin suture in the tarsus in an interrupted, horizontal lamellar fashion as close to the eyelid margin as possible. This suture adjacent to the eyelid margin provides much of the closure strength and is also key for margin alignment.
6. The remainder of the tarsus is reapproximated with several additional interrupted lamellar 6-0 polyglactin sutures. Keep the sutures partial thickness and not extending to the posterior conjunctiva in order to avoid corneal abrasion.

7. If the laceration extends vertically past the tarsus, additional sutures may be needed to close the inferior retractor layer or levator complex.
8. The overlying orbicularis muscle and skin are closed as described previously.

It should be noted that traditionally the eyelid margin repair is described using fine gauge silk sutures with the tails left long and sutured to the anterior lamella. The authors have found that the tails often dislodge and irritate the ocular surface, and the removal of tight silk sutures from the eyelid margin is unpleasant for even the most cooperative patient. Additionally, trauma patients may fail to follow up for many reasons, and therefore the use of absorbable sutures makes follow-up less essential. Avoiding the need for suture removal is also beneficial for the pediatric population.

Repair of Lacerations Deep to the Orbital Septum

In cases where the orbital septum has been violated, the wound should be repaired as follows:

1. Inject local anesthetic and place a corneal shield.
2. Irrigate and explore the wound carefully, as these deeper wounds are especially capable of hiding foreign bodies (Fig. 55.4).
3. If injury to the levator complex was suggested by the preoperative examination, the wound should be explored to identify the lacerated ends of the levator (Fig. 55.6). If the case is being performed under local anesthetic, the surgeon should limit the amount of local anesthesia given to avoid paralyzing the muscle. The patient can be asked to look up, which will contract and elevate the levator and aid in identification.

a

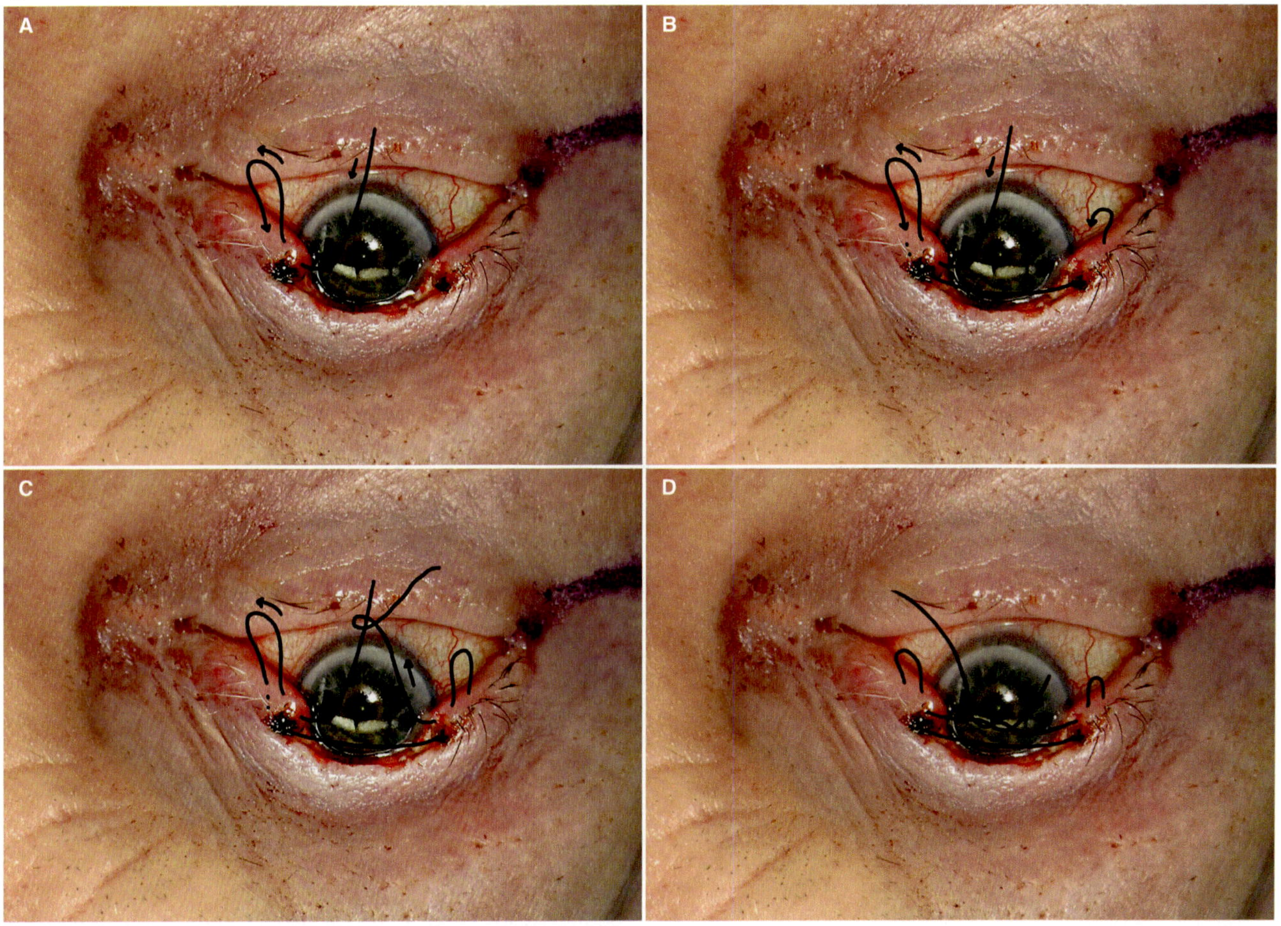

Fig. 55.10 Placement of a buried vertical mattress suture for eyelid margin closure (surgeon view of right upper eyelid): (**a**, **b**) illustrate the intraoperative and schematic steps, respectively. (A) The 6-0 polyglactin suture first enters from within the incision and is placed approximately 2–3 mm deep, to exit 2–3 mm along the gray line in the middle of the eyelid margin. (B) The suture is passed on the same defect side but farther from the previous suture and exiting deeper to avoid cutting the suture. (C) The suture is passed through the opposite wound edge to match the deeper pass and exits at the margin away from the wound edge to match the farther suture on the first side. (D) On the same eyelid side, the suture is directed a few millimeters nearer to the wound edge and shallower, taking care to match the depth of passes in both the "near" and "far" passes so the margin is aligned properly. The suture is finally tied and cut, resulting in a buried knot within the defect that avoids corneal irritation. Ideally, these sutures should be placed in the gray line, posterior line, and anterior eyelash line, with good wound edge eversion

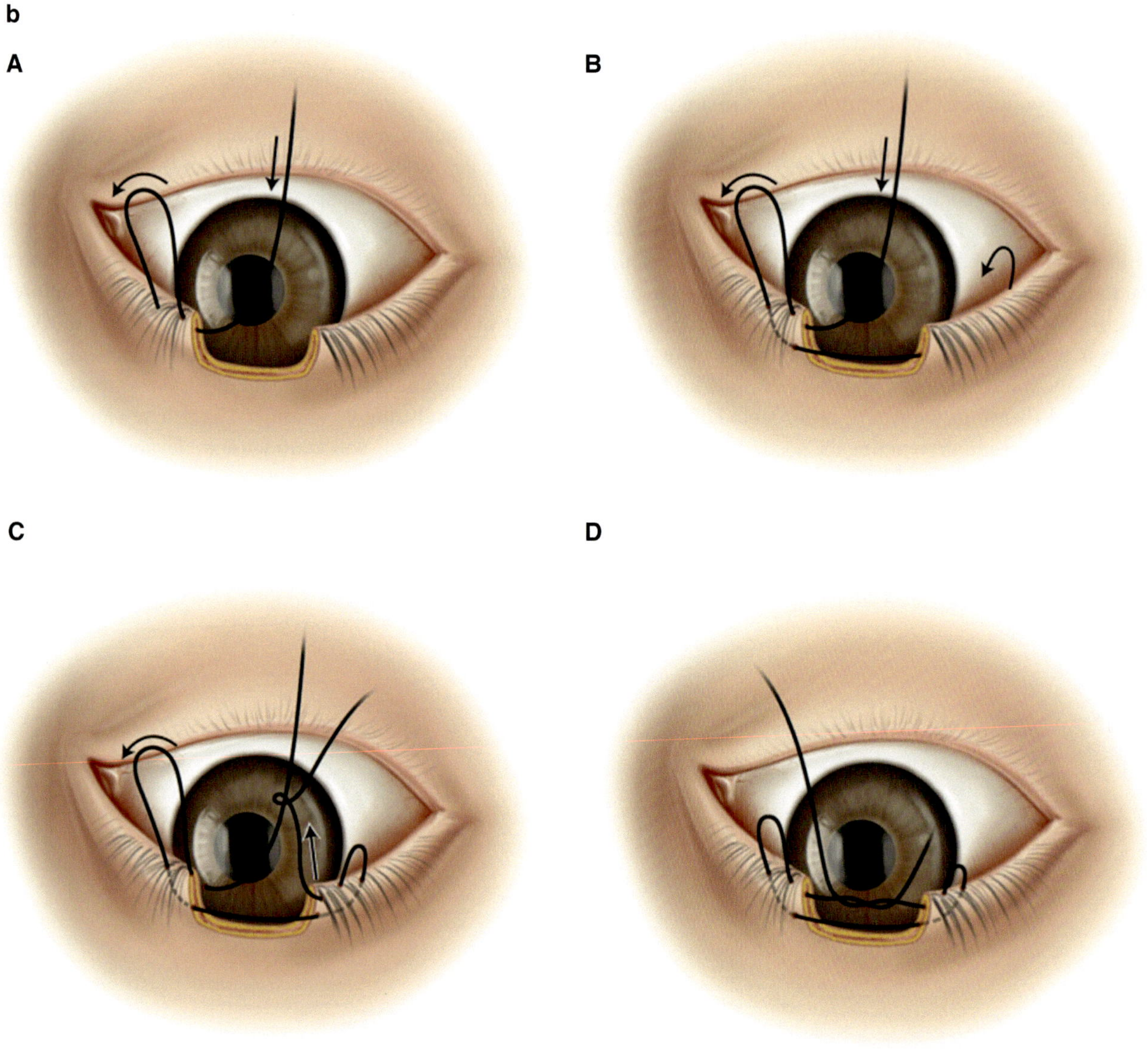

Fig. 55.10 (continued)

4. If the cut edges of the levator muscle can be identified, they can be reapproximated using 6-0 polypropylene or polyglactin sutures placed in an interrupted fashion, taking care to avoid shortening the levator that could result in upper eyelid retraction.
5. Prolapsed fat may be reposited into normal position and the wound closed as described previously. The orbital septum itself should not be repaired, as this may result in eyelid retraction, lagophthalmos, and/or infection [7, 8].

If blepharoptosis is identified in follow-up, the eyelid is typically allowed to heal for at least 3–6 months to allow for maximum return of eyelid function following the injury before attempting surgical repair [4].

Lacerations with Missing Tissue

Lacerations that are missing tissue are unusual, and may require some creativity to repair. Surgeons who are familiar with the repair of post-Mohs surgery defects can approach these wounds similarly. Large skin defects may require full-thickness skin grafting using grafts from the contralateral eyelid, preauricular or postauricular region, or the supraclavicular region, depending on patient and recipient site factors (Fig. 55.3). Recall that skin edges are often curled under, retracted, or stretched due to underlying hematoma, so a wound that initially appears to have missing skin may actually reapproximate well without grafting – careful bedside manipulation with cotton tip applicators or forceps before creating a surgical plan is helpful.

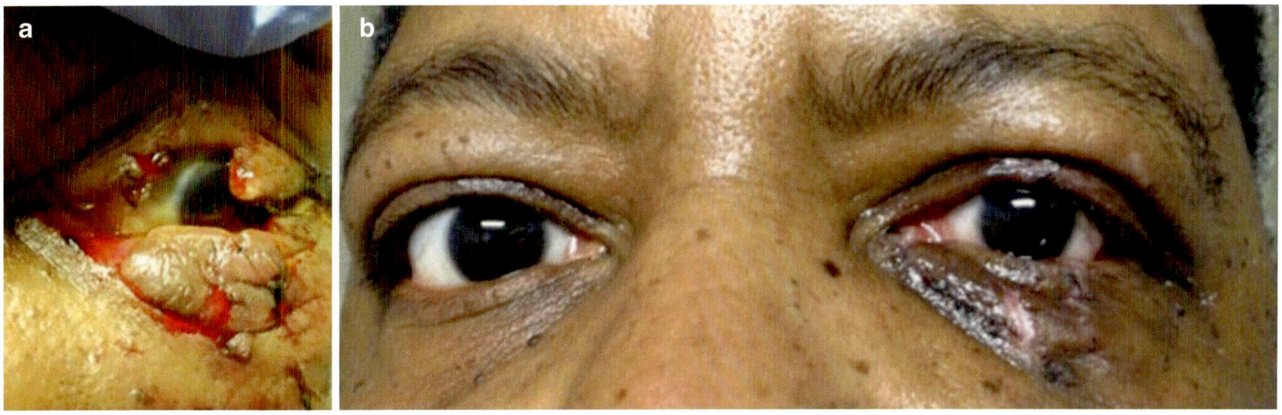

Fig. 55.11 Eyelid laceration with full-thickness tissue defect. This patient suffered an eyelid laceration by an unknown mechanism while intoxicated. (**a**) Note the full-thickness tissue defect in the central upper eyelid. He also has lacerations involving the canaliculus and margin of the lower eyelid. (**b**) 1 week after the wound was repaired

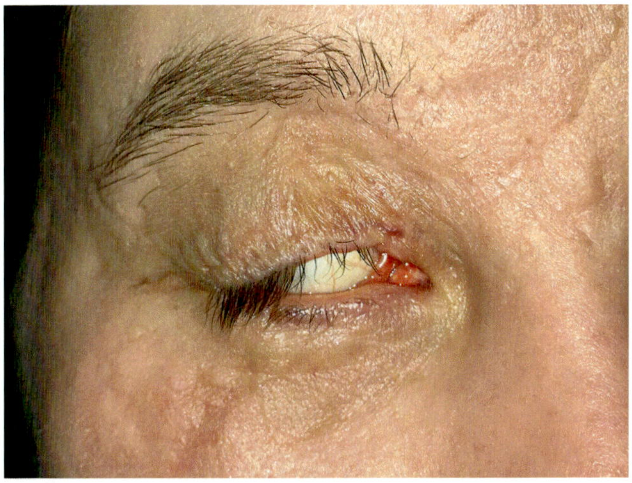

Fig. 55.12 Cicatricial retraction and lagophthalmos. Patient is shown at 5 months after repair of significant upper eyelid tissue loss from a motor vehicle accident. There are right cicatricial upper eyelid retraction, lagophthalmos, and exposure keratopathy

An uncommon, but complex injury is a full-thickness defect of the eyelid margin (missing tarsus and orbicularis in addition to skin.) The laceration depicted in Fig. 55.11 was repaired using a wedge resection technique – the wound was trimmed into a pentagonal shape and then closed using the technique described in the section on eyelid margin repair. In cases of severe tissue loss, significant cicatricial changes can result in eyelid retraction, lagophthalmos, and exposure keratopathy (Fig. 55.12). Aggressive lubrication is needed to protect the ocular surface, as it is preferable to wait at least 6 months to allow fibrosis to mature and soften. If at any point the corneal integrity is compromised, earlier intervention with release of scar, tissue grafting or flaps, or tarsorrhaphy may be performed until more definitive repair can be undertaken.

Postoperative Care

Standard eyelid postoperative instructions can be given following eyelid laceration repair. The patient should rest and elevate the head for a week, and apply cold compresses to the region as much as possible during the first 2 days. Topical antibiotic or combination antibiotic-steroid ointment may be applied over the wound. Oral antibiotics may be prescribed if the wound is contaminated, such as a bite wound, or if the patient is at high risk for infection, or is immunocompromised. The patient is typically seen in 5–14 days, where any nonabsorbable sutures are removed. Subsequently, the patient may return on an as-needed basis.

Periorbital Burns

Ocular and periorbital burns can cause substantial morbidity. Sequelae may range from dry eye and corneal abrasion (Fig. 55.13) to severe exposure keratopathy resulting in loss of the globe. Of note, while some patients may have burns isolated to the periorbital region or face, many have burns involving a large portion of the body's surface area. Management of ocular and periorbital injuries in these severely injured patients must be coordinated with management of the potentially life-threatening complications of their wounds, such as hemodynamic instability via volume loss, airway compromise, or sepsis. This section will review the basics of acute periorbital burn care. More thorough discussions of periorbital burns, including the subacute and chronic phases of burn care, can be found in other references [9, 10].

Severe burn wounds are best managed at burn centers, where program oversight by national and international organizations supports appropriate and timely interventions [11,

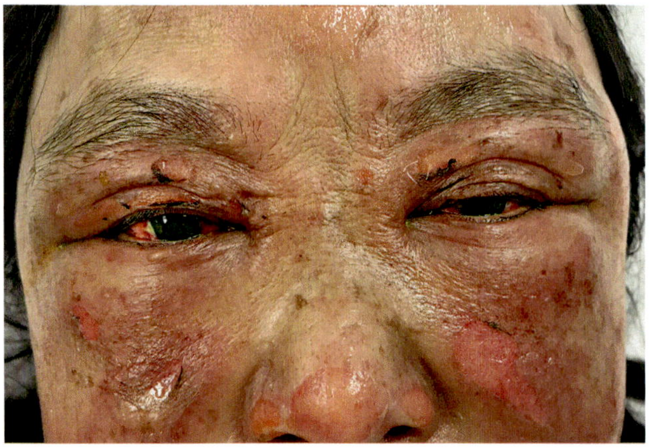

Fig. 55.13 Periocular superficial burns and corneal burn. Careful ophthalmic examination demonstrates fluorescein uptake on both eyes, consistent with corneal abrasions from thermal burns. (Image courtesy of Braden A. Burckhard, MD)

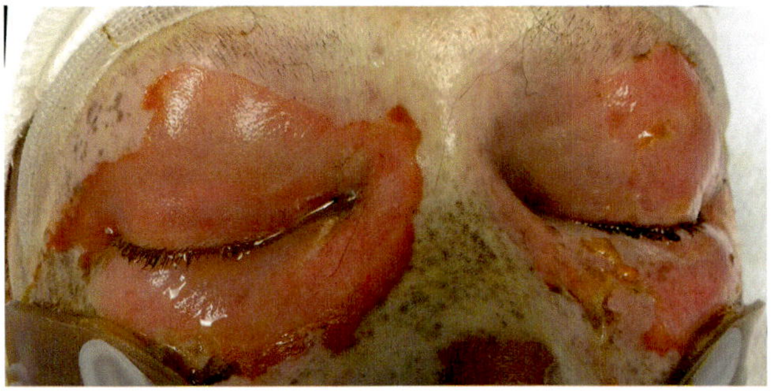

Fig. 55.14 Eyelid edema in the setting of acute facial/eyelid burn injury. This patient suffered a thermal burn within 24 h of taking this photograph. Note effacement of the eyelid crease due to edema and the singed eyelashes and eyebrows

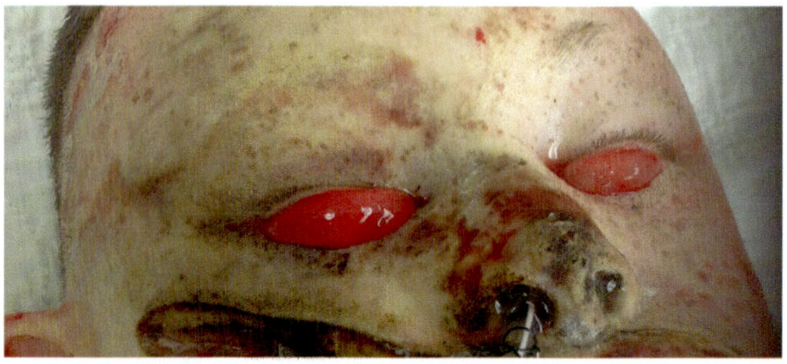

Fig. 55.15 Orbital compartment syndrome. This patient suffered a severe electrical burn during a motor vehicle collision resulting in a deep full-face burn. Note the impressive bilateral chemosis and tense-appearing eyelids. He was treated with bilateral lateral canthotomy/cantholysis soon after this photograph was taken. (Image courtesy of Mark J. Lucarelli, MD)

12]. Burn centers verified by the American Burn Association have been found to have comparable mortality to nonverified centers despite caring for patients with more severe injuries [13]. The degree of involvement of the ophthalmology service in facial burn management varies by institution – some burn surgeons are skilled at examining the eye and operating on the eyelids whereas others rely heavily on consulting ophthalmologists. One study showed that early referral for ophthalmic assessment actually decreased the subsequent need for ophthalmic surgery [14].

Initial burn management is aimed at fluid resuscitation, airway protection, and infection prevention. The globe should be examined early in the patient's hospital course to rule out injury. Globe injuries may be vision-threatening if not treated promptly, and marked periorbital edema often develops in burn patients that may make evaluation of the globe challenging (Fig. 55.14). Elevation of the head may help to limit this edema. A rare but potentially devastating consequence of massive early fluid resuscitation is orbital compartment syndrome, which has been reported in some patients with burns involving over 25% of their total body surface area, with periorbital burns being an independent risk factor (Fig. 55.15) [10, 15]. Malhotra et al. advocate for daily intraocular pressure checks for the first 72 h of these patients' care and performance of urgent canthotomy/cantholysis if needed.

The natural history of eyelid burns involves severe eyelid edema in the acute phase (onset within 24 h of injury), followed by scarring and wound contracture in the subacute and chronic phases (onset within 2 weeks of injury) [10]. The end stage of this healing process depends, of course, on the extent of the wound and may include cicatricial ectropion, entropion, eyelid retraction, and/or lagophthalmos with exposure keratopathy (Fig. 55.16).

Treatment of eyelid burns is aimed at preventing these consequences and protecting the globe. Facial burns may be managed conservatively initially, in part because the face only comprises 4% of the body surface area and even a total facial burn, in isolation, is unlikely to cause severe systemic consequences such as sepsis [12]. Initial management is focused on prevention of desiccation and infection via regular cleansing of the wound with gentle soap and water and application of ophthalmic antibiotic ointment such as bacitracin. Superficial first-degree or partial-thickness second-degree eyelid burns (Fig. 55.17) often heal well without permanent sequelae with these conservative, but essential, measures.

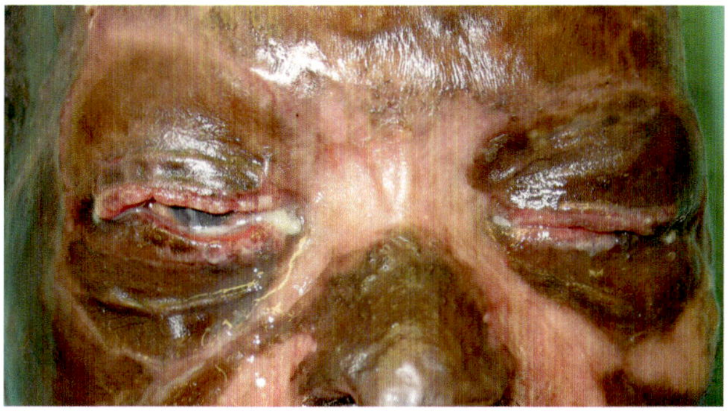

Fig. 55.16 Sequelae of severe facial burn injury. This patient had severe facial and body burns and had undergone multiple periorbital reconstructive surgeries by this stage. Note the remaining right, worse than left, cicatricial eyelid ectropion, retraction, and lagophthalmos, among other sequelae of the facial burn

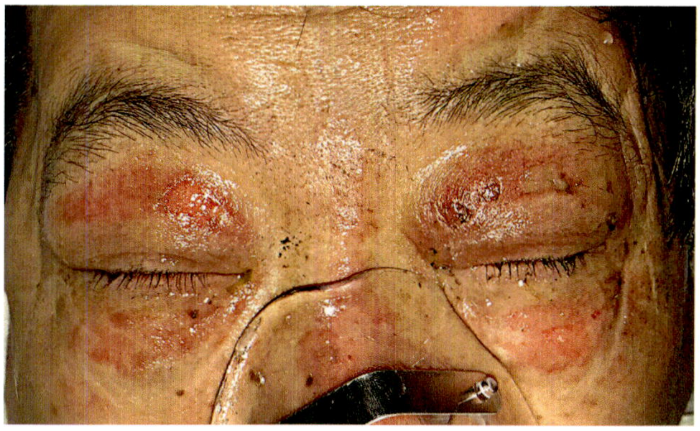

Fig. 55.17 Superficial or partial-thickness eyelid burns. Thermal injuries involving the epidermis or superficial dermis may blister but can heal without permanent sequelae if adequately lubricated

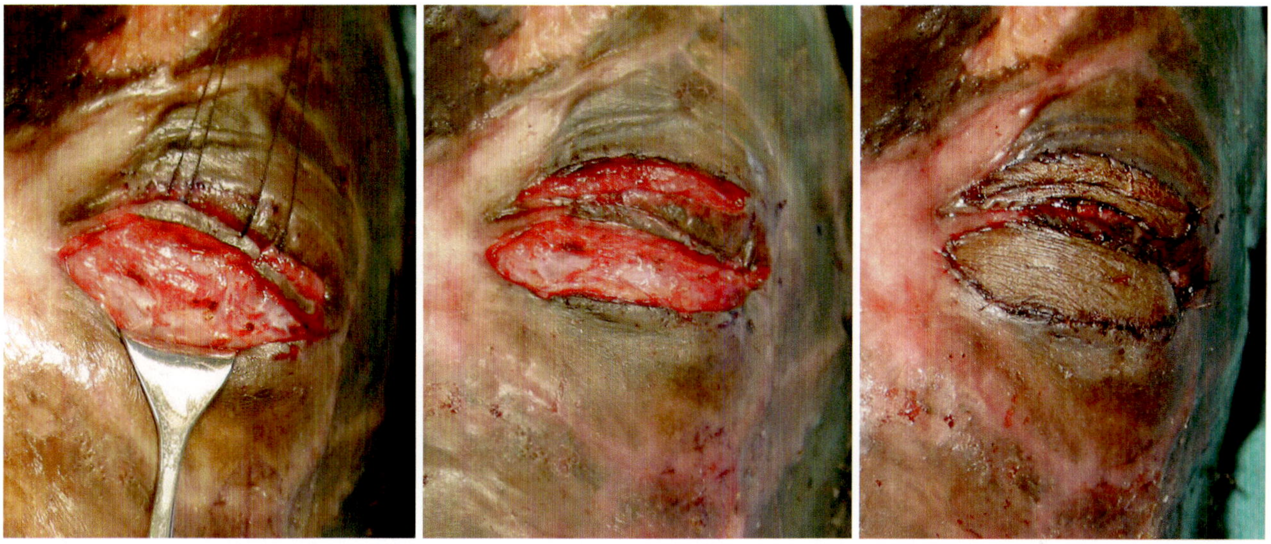

Fig. 55.18 Repair of cicatricial retraction. In more severe cases of eyelid retraction with corneal compromise, early upper and lower eyelid surgery with cicatrix release and skin graft placement may be considered (surgeon view)

As eyelid edema recedes, mild exposure keratopathy may be treated with lubricating ointment. A temporary tarsorrhaphy may be placed if the exposure keratopathy is resistant to this conservative management, particularly if the patient has other risk factors for exposure such as a poor Bell's phenomenon. However, tarsorrhaphy provides temporary protection of the cornea only and does not halt progression of the cicatrization and lid retraction; therefore, these patients must be followed closely. If the tarsorrhaphy is under great tension as cicatrization worsens, the sutures should be removed to avoid cheese-wiring through the eyelid margin. In these more severe cases of eyelid retraction, early eyelid surgery with cicatrix release and skin graft placement may be considered, although graft failures and persistent retraction are not uncommon (Fig. 55.18). Some argue that split-thickness skin grafts should be used for the upper lid and full-thickness grafts should be used in the lower lid in these cases – this is an ongoing controversy [9]. Tarsorrhaphy or bolster dressing may be used to ensure postoperative lid closure.

Discussion of the management of chronic burn-related malpositions such as cicatricial ectropion and eyelid retraction is beyond the scope of this chapter.

Conclusions

Eyelid trauma has many causes and phenotypes. Management with thorough examination of the globe, exploration of the wound to rule out deep injury and foreign bodies, proper sanitation, and meticulous layered closure (in the case of eyelid lacerations) typically yields good results. Eyelid burns are treated with attentive cleansing and lubrication in the short term and early surgical intervention only in certain cases of exposure keratopathy. Reoperations are unfortunately common in significant burn injuries. Additional discussion of eyelid trauma can be found in the other chapters regarding canalicular, lateral canthal tendon, and orbital trauma.

References

1. Scruggs D, Scruggs R, Stukenborg G, Netland PA, Calland JF. Ocular injuries in trauma patients: an analysis of 28,340 trauma admissions in the 2003–2007 National Trauma Data Bank National Sample Program. J Trauma Acute Care Surg. 2012;73(5):1308–12.
2. Kim DK, Riley LE, Harriman KH, Hunter P, Bridges CB. Advisory committee on immunization practices. Recommended immunization schedule for adults aged 19 years or older, United States, 2017. Ann Intern Med. 2017;166(3):209–19.
3. de Santana Santos T, Avelar RL, Melo AR, de Moraes HHA, Dourado E. Current approach in the management of patients with foreign bodies in the maxillofacial region. J Oral Maxillofac Surg. 2011;69(9):2376–82.
4. Nelson CC. Management of eyelid trauma. Aust N Z J Ophthalmol. 1991;19(4):357–63.
5. Jaggi R, Hart R, Taylor SM. Absorbable suture compared with nonabsorbable suture in upper eyelid blepharoplasty closure. Arch Facial Plast Surg. 2009;11(5):349–52.
6. Joshi AS, Janjanin S, Tanna N, Geist C, Lindsey C. Does suture material and technique really matter? Lessons learned from 800 consecutive blepharoplasties. Laryngoscope. 2007;117(6):981–4.
7. Burkat CN, Punja KG, Kim N. Eyelid and canalicular trauma. In: Clinical atlas of procedures in ophthalmic and oculofacial surgery. 2nd ed. New York: Oxford University Press; 2012. p. 1002–14.
8. Beadles KA, Lessner AM. Management of traumatic eyelid lacerations. Semin Ophthalmol. 1994;9(3):145–51.
9. Sheridan R, Perry J, Burns CR. Diseases and disorders of the orbit and ocular adnexa. 1st ed. Edinburgh: Elsevier; 2016. p. 677–91.
10. Malhotra R, Sheikh I, Dheansa B. The management of eyelid burns. Surv Ophthalmol. 2009;54(3):356–71.
11. Sheridan RL. Burn care: results of technical and organizational progress. JAMA. 2003;290(6):719–22.
12. Sheridan R, Weber J, Prelack K, Petras L, Lydon M, Tompkins R. Early burn center transfer shortens the length of hospitalization and reduces complications in children with serious burn injuries. J Burn Care Rehabil. 1999;20(5):347–50.
13. Palmieri TL, London JA, O'Mara MS, Greenhalgh DG. Analysis of admissions and outcomes in verified and nonverified burn centers. J Burn Care Res. 2008;29(1):208–12.
14. Spencer T, Hall AJH, Stawell RJ. Ophthalmologic sequelae of thermal burns over ten years at the Alfred Hospital. Ophthal Plast Reconstr Surg. 2002;18(3):196–201.
15. Singh CN, Klein MB, Sullivan SR, Sires BS, Hutter CM, Rice K, et al. Orbital compartment syndrome in burn patients. Ophthal Plast Reconstr Surg. 2008;24(2):102–6.

Lacrimal Trauma: Principles of Management and Repair

56

Chirag M. Shah, Seanna R. Grob, Christina Kong, and Jeremiah Tao

Introduction

The lacrimal system is commonly injured in the context of facial injuries. Adult canalicular injuries are most commonly due to traction from assault or similar altercation (31%), while childhood injuries are usually secondary to eyelid avulsion from a dog bite (39.5% of all causes). Conservative estimates are that 35.6% of eyelid lacerations secondary to a dog bite may result in damage to the lacrimal apparatus [1, 2]. More than 70% of adult and pediatric lacrimal system trauma occurs in males [1]. Lacrimal sac and nasolacrimal duct injuries are more frequently seen with nasoethmoid fractures and midfacial soft tissue trauma.

While it is debated whether both the upper and lower canaliculi are required for adequate drainage, patients with monocanalicular damage do frequently complain of epiphora. Studies have shown that tear elimination through the upper and lower canalicular systems is nearly equivalent [3]. Thus, the upper and lower canaliculus should be given equal consideration for repair. Delayed diagnosis and loss to follow-up may lead to permanent loss of adequate natural drainage and may require repair with a Pyrex (Jones) tube if the canaliculus cannot be repaired. Hence, a prompt and careful examination of the lacrimal system is warranted when the mechanism of injury or constellation of symptoms imply involvement.

C. M. Shah · S. R. Grob · J. Tao (✉)
Division of Oculofacial Plastic and Orbital Surgery, Gavin Herbert Eye Institute, Irvine, CA, USA

Department of Ophthalmology, University of California, Irvine, School of Medicine, Irvine, CA, USA
e-mail: chirags@uci.edu; jeremiat@uci.edu

C. Kong
University of California, Irvine School of Medicine, Irvine, CA, USA

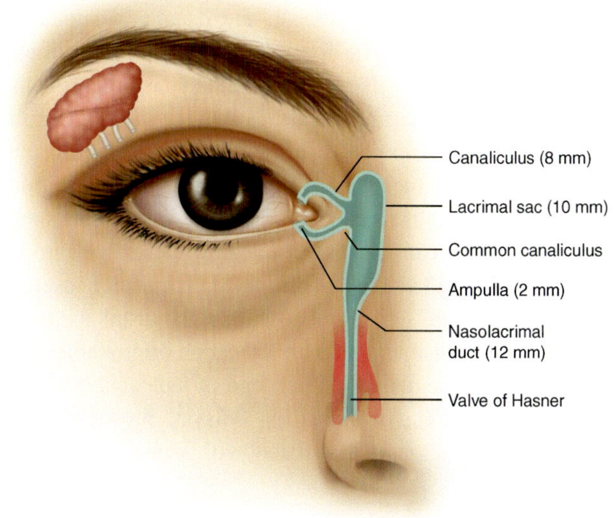

Fig. 56.1 Lacrimal drainage schematic. Approximate anatomy and dimensions of the lacrimal excretory system

Anatomy

The lacrimal system begins at the upper and lower puncta and terminates at the inferior meatus. From the puncta, canaliculi enveloped in a thin layer of orbicularis underlie the surface of the medial eyelid and unite to form a common canaliculus in 90% of patients (Fig. 56.1) [4, 5].

The common canaliculus drains into the lacrimal sac supero-posterior to the anterior limb of the medial canthal tendon (MCT). The anterior and posterior limbs of the MCT surround the lacrimal sac via attachments on the anterior and posterior lacrimal crest, respectively. The lacrimal sac itself is 12–15 mm long, 4–8 mm deep, and 3 mm wide and drains into the nasolacrimal duct (NLD). The NLD has both a proximal fibrous intraosseous and a distal membranous portion, which are 12 mm and 2–5 mm long, respectively. The NLD empties into the inferior meatus.

A. J. Cohen, C. N. Burkat (eds.), *Oculofacial, Orbital, and Lacrimal Surgery*, https://doi.org/10.1007/978-3-030-14092-2_56

Preoperative Evaluation and Management

An ophthalmic examination is of utmost importance in periocular trauma to evaluate for any ocular injury. Depending on the nature of the injury, a full trauma workup might be necessary as well. Globe trauma should be addressed prior to eyelid or periocular injury.

A high index of suspicion ought to be maintained with even superficial abrasions near or involving the medial eyelids, as these may belie deeper injuries demanding intervention by a specialist comfortable with canalicular reconstruction, such as an oculoplastic surgeon. A close inspection of the medial soft tissues and eyelids is necessary. A laceration medial to the upper or lower eyelid punctum should raise suspicion for canalicular or lacrimal system injury. In order to confirm canalicular involvement, the canaliculi should be probed (Fig. 56.2a, b). The upper and lower puncta are dilated with a punctal dilator. Then, the canaliculus is probed with a Bowman wire or lacrimal probe. Following the structure of the canaliculus, the probe is initially inserted vertically into the punctum and then turned approximately 90 ° to point nasally toward the medial canthus. Gentle lateral traction on the lower eyelid can help insert the Bowman probe into the canaliculus. Should there be difficulty completely inserting the probe to a hard stop at the nose, or if the distal end of the probe becomes visible, this is an indication of probable canalicular injury. The distal (medial) end of the canalicular laceration is important to identify. Delayed presentation or delayed examination is associated with wound contraction that can make finding the distal cut end more difficult. A headlight or magnification can help.

The canaliculus can be injured either from direct laceration or trauma to the canaliculus or as a result of avulsion from lateral tension of the eyelid. Direct laceration can often be easier to repair compared to an avulsion injury, as the distal end of the canaliculus is often easier to find and re-anchoring of the medial eyelid to follow the contour of the globe is not required.

Burns may also cause punctal or canalicular stenosis, and careful dilation followed by probing ought to be performed in these scenarios as well. A stent may need to be placed in these situations in order to prevent scarring, canalicular stenosis, and chronic epiphora.

CT imaging is recommended in the setting of any trauma concerning for orbital injury. Penetrating or projectile injuries that suggest injury to deeper orbital structures or an intraorbital foreign body warrant further imaging. Significant blunt trauma or signs of orbital fractures such as step-offs along the orbital rim or orbital rim tenderness also require imaging to rule out orbital or facial fractures that may require surgical repair. Facial fractures can also predispose a patient to epiphora from nasolacrimal duct obstruction [6].

If tetanus vaccination occurred more than 10 years prior to the trauma, an intramuscular toxoid booster should be given [7]. Rabies vaccination may be pertinent in the case of an animal bite as well depending on the status of the animal. Though the face and ocular adnexa are well vascularized and unlikely to become infected after most traumas, antibiotic

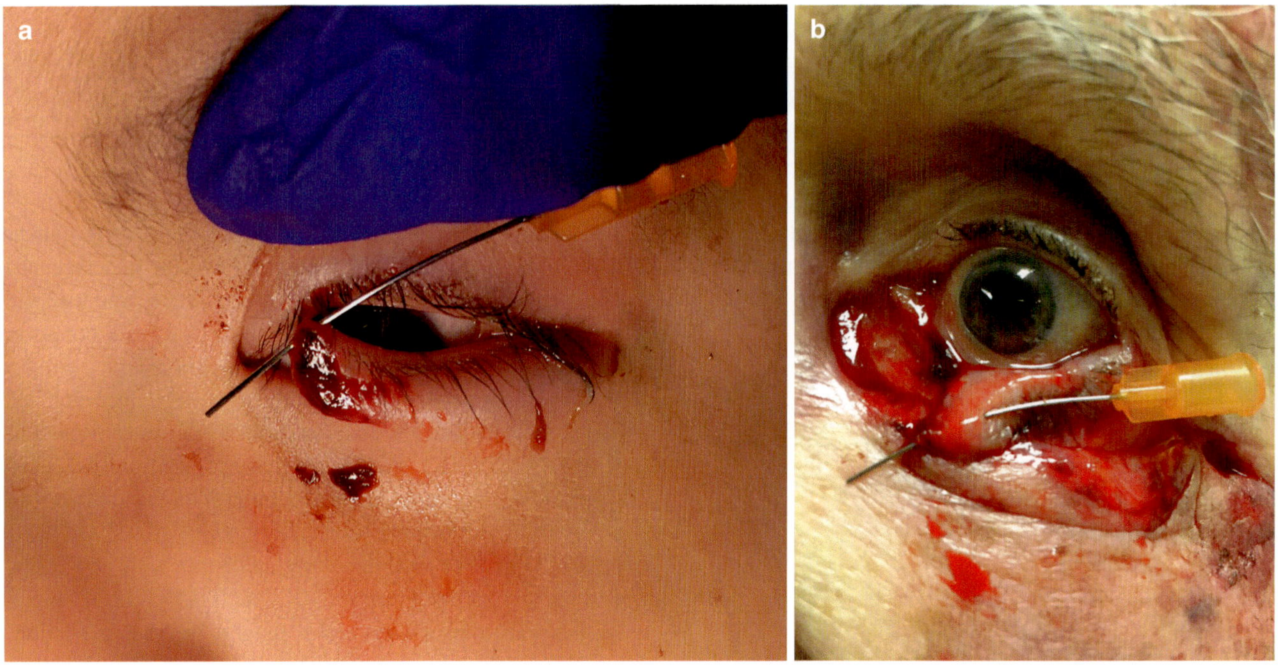

Fig. 56.2 Probing the lacrimal system. Demonstrated is a Bowman probe protruding through the proximal cut end of a lacerated inferior canaliculus in (**a**) a child and (**b**) an adult

prophylaxis with amoxicillin-clavulanate or similar coverage of gram-positives, gram-negatives, and atypicals are standard care after a penetrating animal bite [8]. Injuries involving "dirty" objects would also warrant antibiotic coverage.

Surgical Techniques

After thorough ophthalmic and trauma evaluations to rule out any more pressing comorbidities, surgical repair of the lacrimal system may commence. The goal of canalicular trauma repair is to reunite the two edges of the canaliculus in anatomic alignment and then repair the eyelid. Three different intubation techniques will be discussed below.

1. Repair using bicanalicular intubation with nasolacrimal duct intubation with Crawford tubes.
2. Repair using bicanalicular intubation with the pigtail probe.
3. Repair with a monocanalicular stent.

Classically, immediate repair is advocated, but multiple retrospective case series demonstrate non-inferior outcomes with repairs delayed up to 2 weeks [9]. If for some reason evaluation or repair must be delayed, adequate lubrication of the area with antibiotic ointment may prevent formation of scar tissue and premature closure of the severed canaliculi. Delayed closure can make finding the distal end of the canaliculus more challenging due to soft tissue contracture. As above, magnification and extra lighting may facilitate finding the distal cut canaliculus. Additionally, injecting the opposite, ipsilateral canalicular system with fluorescein (or other) dye may allow for regurgitation of irrigated fluid from the cut medial end, aiding its identification. Injection of air into the intact canaliculus while the traumatized area is submerged under saline and looking for bubbles exiting the severed medial end of the injured canaliculus is yet another method [10].

Choice of anesthesia may be physician preference or dependent on the age or demeanor of the patient. If intranasal tubes are placed, then general anesthesia is often preferred. If a simple repair is identified and a proximal monocanalicular stent will be placed, then the repair can be done under local anesthesia, with or without intravenous sedation. The use of magnification and a light source is often helpful for finding the distal end of the canaliculus, but this is based on physician preference.

Bicanalicular Intubation with Crawford Stent

Bicanalicular lacerations may be repaired using bicanalicular stents, which is considered the gold standard in stable stent placement. Available systems commonly used include Crawford stents (FCI Ophthalmics, Pembroke, MA) (Fig. 56.3a), as well as the Guboir (Fig. 56.3b) (Xomed Surgical Products Inc., Jacksonville, FL), Ritleng (FCI Ophthalmics, Pembroke, MA), O'Donoghue BD VisitecTM

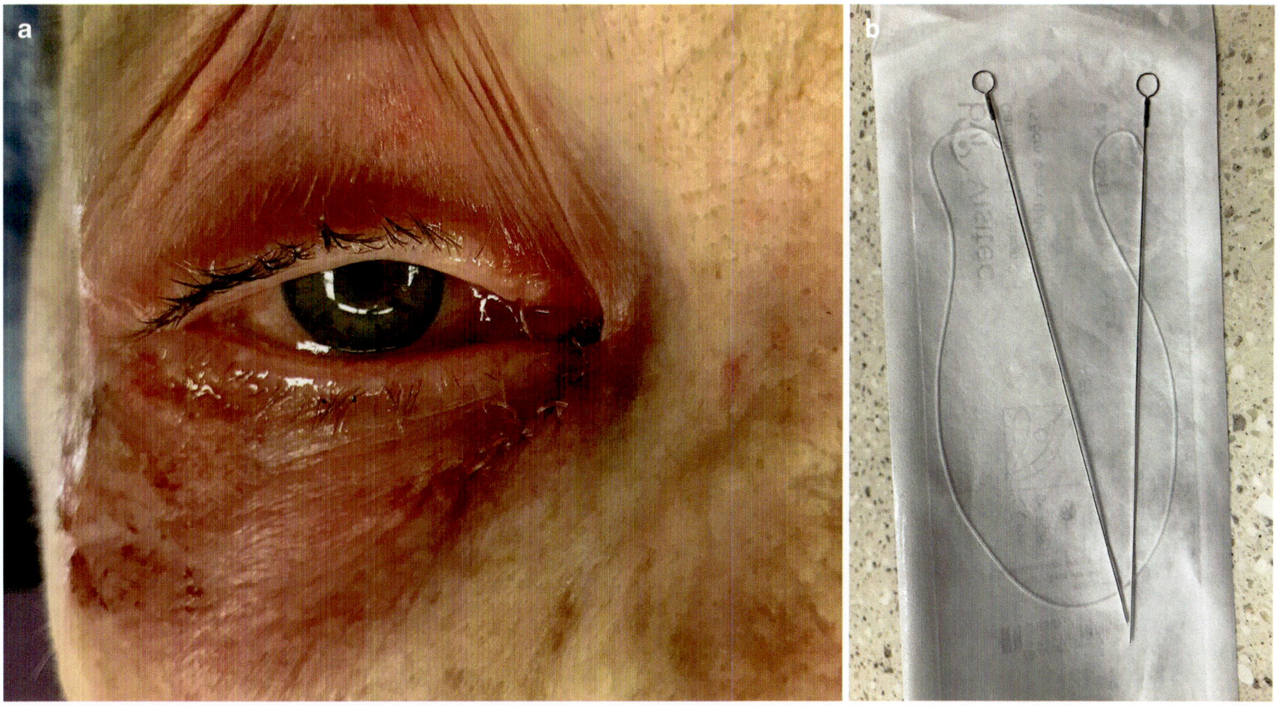

Fig. 56.3 Bicanalicular stenting. (**a**) Crawford bicanalicular intubation set in position after canalicular laceration repair. (**b**) The Guibor bicanalicular intubation system

DCR set (BD Visitec International Inc., Waltham, MA), and Bika stents (FCI Ophthalmics, Pembroke, MA).

The steps of canalicular laceration repair using the Crawford stents are listed below.

1. Identify the two ends of the cut canaliculus as above.
2. Pass the Crawford stent through the two ends of the canaliculus.
   (a) Pass the stent through the punctum first and out the first cut edge of the canaliculus. A dilator probe may be needed to enlarge the punctum in order to fit the stent.
   (b) Then pass the stent through the distal end of the cut canaliculus.
3. Using the lead wire with olive tip, pass the stent down the nasolacrimal duct and retrieve it in the nose using a Crawford hook. A nasal speculum or endoscope can be used to visualize the end of the Crawford tube if needed.
4. Pass the other end of the stent through the opposite canaliculus and retrieve it in the nose.
5. Suture the pericanalicular tissue around the stent and repair the eyelid laceration.
   (a) Suture the pericanalicular tissue together using two or three interrupted 7-0 polyglactin sutures to help approximate the two cut ends of the canaliculus.
   (b) Repair the eyelid margin defect and skin laceration in the usual technique for marginal eyelid laceration repairs.
   (c) If the eyelid has been avulsed, then a 4-0 or 5-0 polyglactin on a P-2 needle (or polyester or other) can be used to reinforce the medial canthal tendon before suturing the pericanalicular tissues. It is important to ensure that the medial eyelid has good apposition to the globe. A deeper medial bite than may be expected is necessary to ensure good apposition of the eyelid to the globe.
6. Remove the metal probes and tie the stent in the nose.
   (a) Be careful not to tie the knot too tight as it may put tension on the punctum and cause cheese-wiring of the punctum, which can impair function and may leave a scar. The authors prefer to tie a single square knot in the nose so the tubes can later be removed externally through the punctum.

The benefits of repair with bicanalicular silicone stents are several. Intubation of the distal system ensures the stents are in a correct passage if they are retrieved in the nose. Additionally, the bicanalicular and nasolacrimal duct placement may be less prone to dislodge. Furthermore, mono stents may be more prone to irritate the ocular surface owing to the phalange or "T" plate that rests at the eyelid margin. Downsides of the bicanalicular stents include that repair usually requires general anesthesia and retrieval of the tubes within the nose may be associated with a surgeon learning curve or may be difficult in some patients, i.e., in those with a narrow infra-turbinate fossa.

Pigtail Probing

For monocanalicular injuries, pigtail probing is an option for repair. In this technique, a curved metal instrument is passed through the uninvolved canaliculus, into the common canaliculus and into the distal cut end of the severed canaliculus. A suture and/or silicone stent is then passed through the punctum and lateral cut end of that traumatized canaliculus to connect both canaliculi.

The steps of canalicular laceration repair using the pigtail probe are listed below.

1. Pass the pigtail probe.
   (a) Enter the normal punctum and canaliculus and rotate the probe posterior to the MCT until the probe emerges from the cut end of the canaliculus on the opposite eyelid.
2. Thread a suture through the lower and upper canalicular system.
   (a) Thread a suture (6-0 Nylon or Prolene) through the eye of the pigtail probe.
   (b) Rotate the probe to pass the suture back through the canalicular system.
3. Thread stent back through canalicular system.
   (a) Thread approximately 25 mm of stent material back over the suture.
   (b) Rotate the suture to pass the stent through the canalicular system.
4. Suture the pericanalicular tissue as discussed above.
5. Tie the canalicular suture and allow the knot to retract into the stent so it does not irritate the ocular surface.
6. Repair the eyelid laceration.

The pigtail approach risks injuring the uninvolved canaliculus as well as creating a false passage when a common canaliculus is not present. However, some proponents argue that it allows for improved visualization of deep distal cut ends, especially in situations where the surgeon is struggling to find the distal end in an avulsed eyelid. If a closed system is not existent for air/fluid visualization, one may use cannulation of an intact canaliculus to laterally lift the lacrimal sac and facilitate direct visualization of the medial cut end [11].

Monocanalicular Repair

There are several options for monocanalicular stents. These include the Mono-Crawford monocanalicular stent (FCI Ophthalmics, Pembroke, MA) and the Mini Monoka monocanalicular stent (FCI Ophthalmics, Pembroke, MA). The Mono-Crawford stent is passed through the nasolacrimal duct and retrieved in the nose similar to the bicanalicular Crawford stent, and the stent usually requires general anesthesia. The Mini Monoka stent is best used for more proximal injuries. It is 30 mm long and has a punctal fixation device to keep it in place at the punctum.

The Mini Monoka monocanalicular stent is a popular in-office option for stenting simple monocanalicular traumas. In this technique, the stent is cut and inserted into the intact, dilated punctum of the lacerated canaliculus. A proximal phalanx sits in the punctum, fixing the stent into place, and the stent's distal end should rest in the lacrimal sac.

The main shortcoming of these monocanalicular stents is vulnerability to dislocation and requirement of good punctal integrity for their phalange to sit securely. They may be more challenging to use in avulsed eyelids as the stent has difficulty staying in position in the lacrimal system while the medial avulsed lid is repaired. Additionally, the phalange or T plate may irritate the ocular surface. Even in the context of monocanalicular trauma and in cases where the posterior medial canthal tendon is injured and unrepaired, bicanalicular stenting may allow for improved cosmetic and functional outcomes [12]. Therefore, the authors prefer to exercise the Mini Monoka option only in the case of necessity: i.e., due to lack of preoperative clearance for general anesthesia, other extenuating circumstances, or for exceedingly simple and proximal canalicular injuries.

Medial Canthal Tendon Injury

The medial canthal ligament is a fibrous tissue that anchors the medial tarsal plates to the medial bony orbital rim and serves as a structural support for the orbicularis oculi muscle. The anterior portion is attached firmly to the anterior lacrimal crest. The superior vertical portion is less securely attached along the frontal process of the maxilla and the frontal bone, and the third and weakest posterior portion attaches on the posterior lacrimal crest. The three insertions envelop the lacrimal sac [13]. Canalicular injuries are often due to trauma exerting lateral traction upon the medial eyelid, and 36% are reportedly associated with rupture of the weak posterior limb of the medial canthal tendon [14]. Recent evidence suggests that in the case of a ruptured posterior limb and intact anterior and superior MCT limbs, an intact Crawford stent is sufficient to prevent ectropion and to achieve tissue alignment, canalicular patency, and a good cosmetic outcome without the need for concomitant placement of a posterior lacrimal crest fixation suture [12].

In cases of anterior and posterior MCT avulsion, repair of the MCT with lacrimal crest fixation sutures may be undertaken to achieve adequate alignment and good apposition of the medial eyelids to the globe (Fig. 56.4). The MCT may be re-approximated by passing a 4-0 or 5-0 polyglactin suture, preferably on a P-2 needle, through the periosteum of the medial wall and then through the canthal tendon, superior and inferior to the canaliculi. Care must be taken to place a deep enough bite along the medial wall to ensure good placement of the medial canthus. If there is significant telecanthus from MCT injury, reconstructive options may include unilateral stainless steel fixation, transnasal wiring, osseous screw fixation with a bone anchor system (Mitek Products, Inc., Westwood, MA), microplate fixation, or intranasal wiring and button.

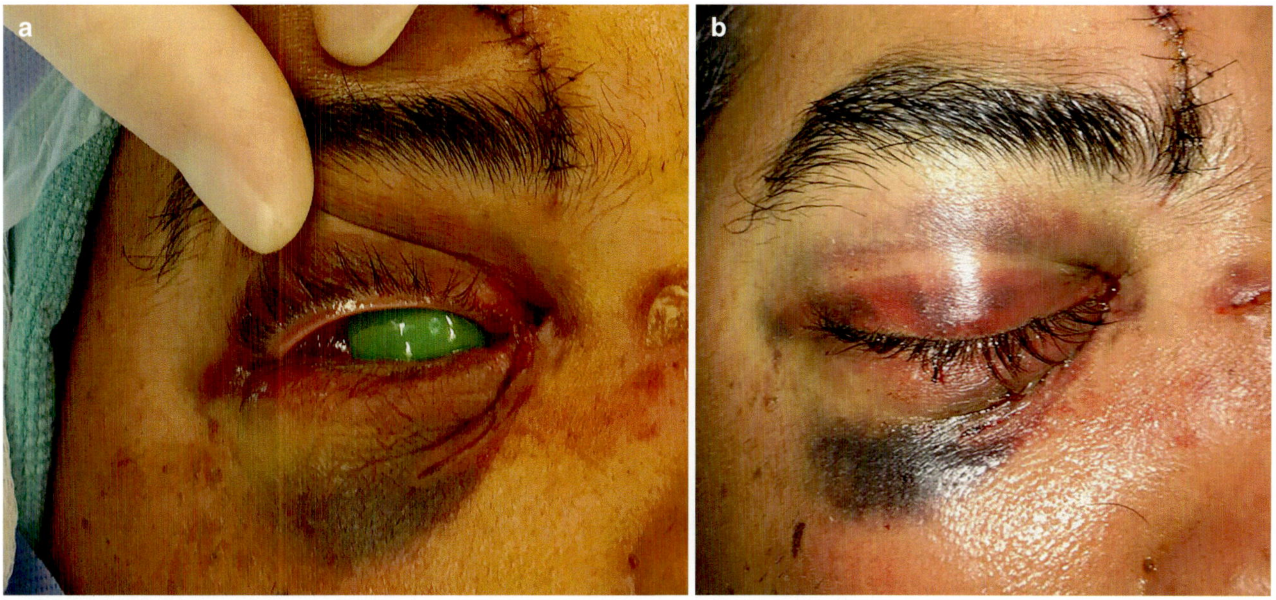

Fig. 56.4 Intubation in the context of medial canthal tendon injury. (**a**) Intraoperative photograph showing medial canthal laceration affecting both the upper and lower canaliculi. (**b**) Postoperative photograph after medial canthoplasty and bicanalicular intubation with a Crawford bicanalicular tube and orbital fracture repair showing a well-approximated medial canthus

Lacrimal Sac and Nasolacrimal Duct Injury

Simple lacrimal sac lacerations are usually repaired with direct closure. If concomitant canalicular injuries exist or if there is any concern, stenting as described above may be performed simultaneously.

Should there be irreparable injury to the NLD, or if fractures, scarring, or other related injuries preclude adequate repair of the lacrimal sac, a dacryocystorhinostomy (DCR) can be performed. The decision on primary versus secondary DCR is multifactorial, accounting for factors such as edema and comorbidities. If swelling is not significant, DCR may be performed alongside naso-orbito-ethmoid fracture repair.

Postoperative Recommendations and Management

Topical ophthalmic antibiotic ointment is applied to the area 2–3 times daily for approximately 5–7 days. Patients should be seen at 1 week postoperatively, and then stents are typically left in place for 6 weeks to 6 months. At this point, the stent is removed. A Crawford tube can be removed by cutting the tube between the upper and lower punctum and pulling the stent out from either punctum (if just one square knot in the nose was used). If the tube can be grasped from the nares, the tube can also be cut between the punctum and pulled out through the nose. Some prefer to remove through the nose and use endoscopic guidance in the office. The tube can be cut in between the punctum and the patient can blow their nose to remove the tube through the nose as well. If the tube becomes dislodged before the planned time for removal, it often needs to be removed. Alternatively, repositioning of the tube can be attempted. To remove a stent placed with a pigtail probe, rotate the suture to find the knot and cut the knot. Pull the knot and suture out together.

Complications

The most common complication of lacrimal system injury is the need for a repeat procedure due to persistent epiphora (*seen in 10–20% in most case series of canalicular repair*) [9]. Even adequate repair can be associated with strictures that cause insufficient tear drainage. These patients may require additional surgery, including a DCR or a conjunctivodacryocystorhinostomy with placement of a Jones tube. Other complications include premature extrusion of the lacrimal stent, cheese-wiring of the stent through the canaliculus, pyogenic granuloma formation, and epistaxis.

Conclusions

Lacrimal injuries are frequent. Lacerations most often affect canaliculi, but fractures may extend to the lacrimal sac or even impair the nasolacrimal duct. Chemical and thermal trauma are often isolated to the punctum and canaliculus. Early and astute treatment of patients with these injuries commonly allows for adequate tear drainage. Bearing in mind a patient's coexistent injuries is of vital importance for a surgeon when formulating a therapeutic plan. Patients should get a complete eye exam and ocular trauma should be ruled out prior to repair of a canalicular injury.

Disclosures Authors have no relevant financial disclosures.

References

1. Murchison AP, Bilyk JR. Pediatric canalicular lacerations: epidemiology and variables affecting repair success. J Pediatr Ophthalmol Strabismus. 2014;4:242–8. https://doi.org/10.3928/01913913-20140604-05.
2. Sadiq MA, Corkin F, Mangatos IS. Eyelid lacerations due to dog bite in children. J Pediatr Ophthalmol Strabismus. 2015;6:360–3. https://doi.org/10.3928/01913913-20150901-02.
3. White WL, Glover AT, Buckner AB, et al. Relative canalicular tear flow as assessed by dacryoscintigraphy. Ophthalmology. 1989;2:167–9.
4. Jones LT. An anatomical approach to problems of the eyelids and lacrimal apparatus. Arch Ophthalmol. 1961;66:111–24.
5. Lemke BN. Lacrimal anatomy. Adv Ophthalmic Plast Reconstr Surg. 1984;3:11–23.
6. Ali MJ, Gupta H, Honavar SG, et al. Acquired nasolacrimal duct obstructions secondary to naso-orbito-ethmoidal fractures: patterns and outcomes. Ophthal Plast Reconstr Surg. 2012;28:242–5. https://doi.org/10.1097/IOP.0b013e31823f3266.
7. Kaiser PK, Friedman NJ, Pineda R, editors. Eyelid Trauma. The Massachusetts eye and ear infirmary illustrated manual of ophthalmology. China: Elsevier Inc; 1998.
8. Chhabra S, Chhabra N, Gaba S. Maxillofacial injuries due to animal bites. J Maxillofac Oral Surg. 2015;2:142–53.
9. Chu YC, Wu SY, Tsai YJ, et al. Early versus late canalicular laceration repair outcomes. Am J Ophthalmol. 2017;182:155–9. https://doi.org/10.1016/j.ajo.2017.08.006.
10. Liu B, Li Y, Long C, et al. Novel air-injection technique to locate the medial cut end of lacerated canaliculus. Br J Ophthalmol. 2013;97:1508–9. https://doi.org/10.1136/bjophthalmol-2013-303822.
11. Cho SH, Hyun DW, Kang HJ, et al. A simple new method for identifying the proximal cut end in lower canalicular laceration. Korean J Ophthalmol. 2008;22:73–6. https://doi.org/10.3341/kjo.2008.22.2.73.
12. Tint NL, Alexander P, Cook AE, et al. Eyelid avulsion repair with bi-canalicular silicone stenting without medial canthal tendon reconstruction. Br J Ophthalmol. 2010;95:1389–92. https://doi.org/10.1136/bjo.2010.196246.
13. Rodriquez RL, Zide BM. Reconstruction of the medial canthus. Clin Plast Surg. 1988;15:255–62.
14. Dortzbach RK, Angrist RA. Silicone intubation for lacerated lacrimal canaliculi. Ophthalmic Surg. 1985;16:639–42.

Orbital Fractures

57

Adam J. Cohen

Evaluation

A baseline ocular examination should be performed with emphasis on intraocular pressure, pupil function, and the posterior segment to exclude compartment syndrome, traumatic optic neuropathy, and retinal breaks or detachments, respectively. Initial visual acuities can be unreliable depending on the extent of the injury, corneal pathology, and ocular adnexal edema.

If a compartment syndrome exists, immediate canthotomy and cantholysis is necessary to prevent compression optic neuropathy. Topical and oral antiglaucoma are indicated following cantholysis.

Traumatic optic neuropathy is seen in ~0.5–5% of orbital trauma patients [1]. If a traumatic optic neuropathy is suspected as evidenced by afferent pupil dysfunction and a normal appearing optic nerve head, high dose steroids may be started. No consensus exists on the efficacy of this treatment with regard to improvement of visual dysfunction.

Extraocular muscle dysfunction can be present secondary to several etiologies. Extraocular muscle entrapment is often thought of, but a neuropraxic injury may exist or myogenic etiology secondary to edema or hematoma of the muscles. Additionally, chemosis can restrict globe movement. Forced duction testing can be performed to exclude restriction but a false positive may occur secondary to muscle edema or hematoma. One study described approximately 80% of cases that present with extraocular muscle dysfunction resolve within a short period of time [2].

If a slit lamp examination is not possible, a pen light can be used to look for hyphema, flat anterior chamber, or iris irregularities.

If retinal pathology or a ruptured globe exists then these injuries supersede fracture repair.

A. J. Cohen (✉)
Eyelid & Facial Plastic and Reconstructive Surgery, Chicago and Glenview, IL, USA
e-mail: acohen@theartofeyes.com

Review of imaging is necessary for surgical decision making. A CT scan without contrast is the imaging modality of choice. Both coronal and axial images should be reviewed to thoroughly evaluate the orbit.

Orbital Fractures

Orbital Floor

By far the most common orbital fracture involves the floor with or without medial wall involvement.

Orbital fractures occur as result of increased intraorbital hydraulic pressure. The increased pressure travels in downward and medial directions, most commonly resulting in fractures of the posterior medial aspect of the orbital floor [3]. A less favorable theory supports a buckling of the orbit floor without displacement of the orbital floor.

In most instances orbital floor fractures do not repair. Operative inidcastions for non-urgent fractures that involve greater than 50% of the floor or greater than 1 cm^2, 2 mm or more of enophthalmos or hypoglobus (Fig. 57.1). Additionally, zygomaticomaxillary complex (ZMC) fractures, when poste-

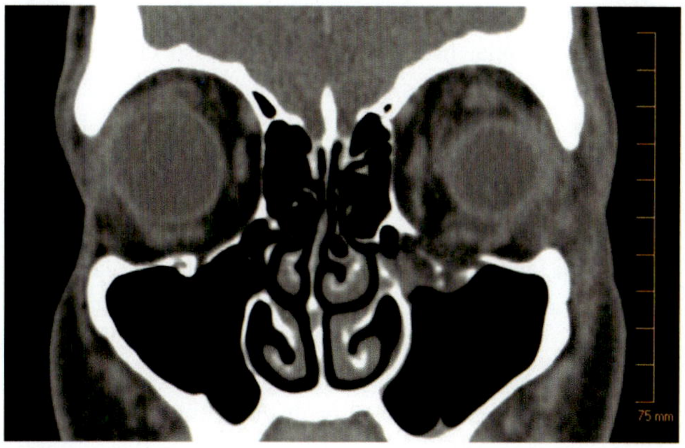

Fig. 57.1 Coronal CT scan with large right orbital floor fracture

A. J. Cohen, C. N. Burkat (eds.), *Oculofacial, Orbital, and Lacrimal Surgery*, https://doi.org/10.1007/978-3-030-14092-2_57

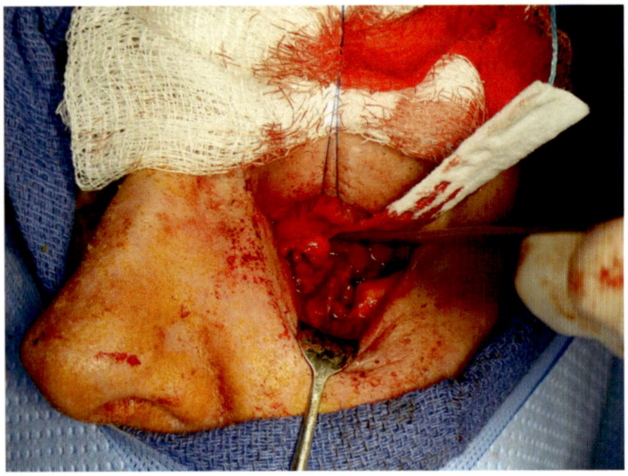

Fig. 57.2 Large left orbital floor fracture with significant rim involvement

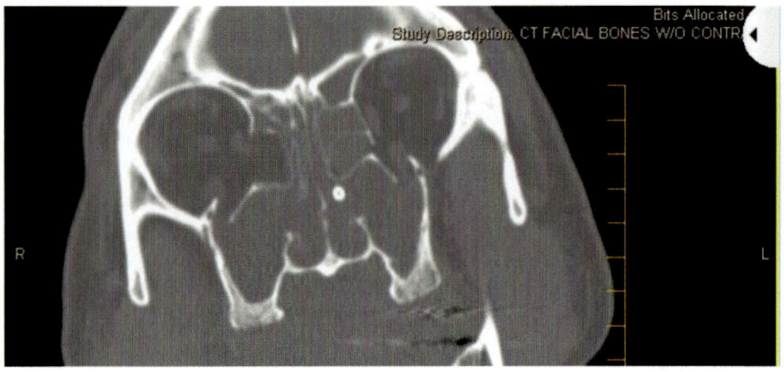

Fig. 57.3 Coronal CT scan with bilateral medial and orbital floor fractures

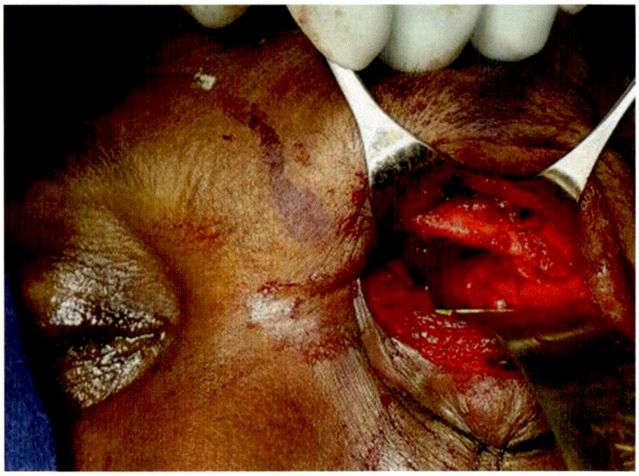

Fig. 57.4 Large left orbital roof fracture

riorly displaced, will cause the orbital floor to buckle posteriorly. When the ZMC is reduced into anatomic position, a significant orbital floor defect may be created, requiring surgical reconstruction. Surgical repair of the orbital floor is necessary in patients with 1 cm or more of posterior displacement [4]. Orbital exploration may also be considered whenever significant rotation of the ZMC segment is repaired to ensure that orbital contents were not incarcerated during the rotation. Additionally, involvement of orbital rim with a floor fracture usually warrants repair (Fig. 57.2).

Classically, 2 mm of enophthalmos, extraocular muscle entrapment, binocular diplopia within 30 ° of primary gaze, and a defect greater than 50% of the orbital floor are indications for repair. Infraorbital nerve dermatome paresthesia is never an indication for repair.

There is no consensus regarding timing of surgical repair of adult fractures, albeit most historical literature has been in favor of repair within 2 weeks of the injury. More recent studies, however, have demonstrated that delayed repair can allow for spontaneous healing, and have had similar postoperative outcomes if surgery is later indicated.

Pediatric orbital floor fractures warrant special consideration. A white-eyed blowout fracture can occur secondary to a greenstick fracture. The patient will have no significant findings on imaging, with little or no periocular ecchymosis and edema but will have binocular diplopia and extraocular muscle dysfunction. Patients can also experience nausea and vomiting, bradycardia, and syncope secondary to the oculocardiac reflex. Firriolo et al. found the presence of nausea and/or vomiting is related to tissue entrapment in pediatric patients with a sensitivity of 83.3% and a negative predictive value of 98.1% [5].

Medial wall fractures can result in medial rectus muscle entrapment, hemorrhage secondary anterior and/or posterior ethmoid artery laceration with compartment syndrome, and disruption of medial canthal tendon with secondary telecanthus. Nasolacrimal system damage may result with secondary epiphora. Lastly, pneumo-orbitalis rarely result in a compartment syndrome.

When both orbital floor and medial wall fractures exist (Fig. 57.3), repair is usually indicated secondary to enophthalmos that occurs because of disruption of bony support at the juncture of the medial wall and floor.

Orbital Roof Fractures

Orbital roof fractures warrant special consideration. Although most warrant observation, a percentage of can warrant repair (Fig. 57.4). If the roof fracture is full thickness, a cerebrospinal fluid leak may result, necessitating an intracranial approach to repair. In other instances enophthalmos or diplopia may result warranting repair via placement of an implant. In this situation an extremely thin, malleable implant is preferred given the curvature of the superior orbit with fixation with screws no more than 4 mm in length to reduce the chance of intracranial entry.

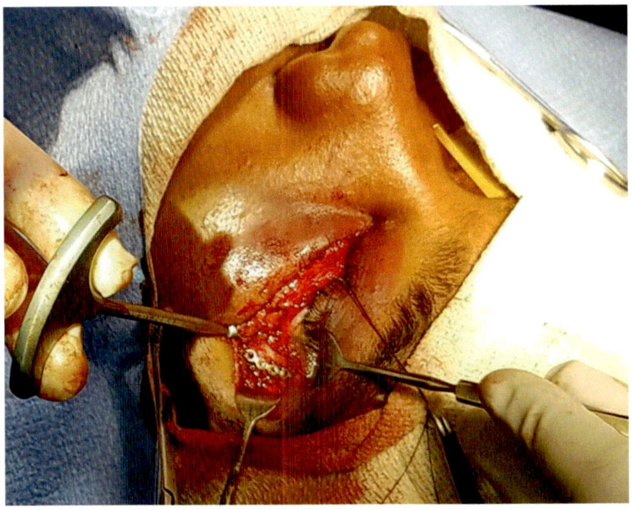

Fig. 57.5 Left lateral orbital rim fracture with fixation and zygoma fracture stabilized with Girard screw prior to fixation

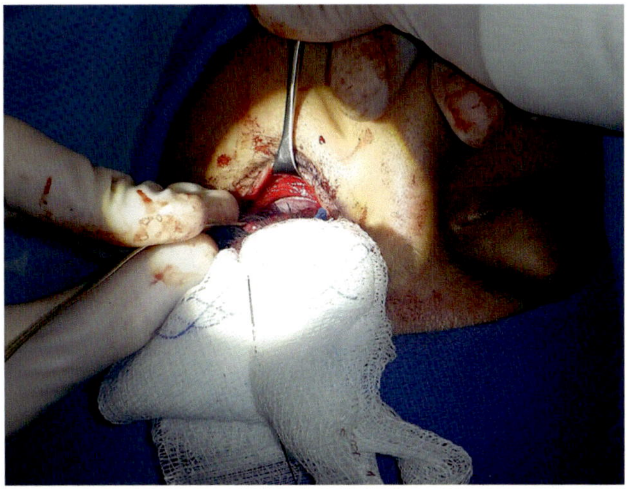

Fig. 57.6 Transconjunctival approach with lateral cantholysis with placement of implant for fracture repair

Orbital Lateral Wall and Rim Fractures

Most lateral wall fractures do not warrant repair. In certain instances lateral orbital rim fractures can occur most commonly at the frontozygomatic suture. If the fracture is displaced and associated with other orbital and malar fractures, repair is indicated. Repair of this fracture before other concomitant fractures will allow for stabilization and more efficacious repair of the remaining fractures (Fig. 57.5).

Surgical Repair

The approaches to repair of orbital fractures are similar between children and adults. The transconjunctival approach with or without lateral cantholysis is the favored approach of most surgeons because of its lower incidence of ectropion and reduced scarring (Fig. 57.6).

Isolated medial wall are amendable to an isolated transcaruncular approach or combined transconjunctival and transcaruncular approaches with concomitant floor fracture.

The lateral orbit and zygoma are easily accessible via a lateral canthotomy and cantholysis.

There are multiple autogenous, allograft, xenograft, and alloplastic reconstructive implants for orbital fracture repair. In general, autogenous grafts, including calvarium, iliac, rib, and cartilage (nasal septum, ear, rib), have the advantage of lower rates of infection and foreign body reaction, as well as less potential for fibrosis, migration, and extrusion than most alloplastic implants. However, when using autogenous grafts in children, extra consideration must be given to the effect this has on the skeleton at the donor site and the attendant growth disturbances that may ensue. Alloplastic implants decrease operative times, can be shaped and contoured readily, and provide both absorbable and nonabsorbable options.

Orbital fracture repair complications include infection, hemorrhage, extraocular muscle dysfunction, new or persistent diplopia, enopthalmos or exophthamos, infraorbital dysesthesia, implant extrusion or dislocation, symblepharon, and compressive optic neuropathy.

References

1. Steinsapir KD, Goldberg RA. Traumatic optic neuropathy. Surv Ophthalmol. 1994;38:487–518.
2. Back CPN, McLean NR, Anderson PJ, David DJ. The conservative management of facial fractures: indications and outcomes. J Plast Reconstr Aesthet Surg. 2007;60:146–51.
3. Patel S, Andrecovich C, Silverman M, Zhang L, Shkoukani M. Biomechanic factors associated with orbital floor fractures. JAMA Facial Plast Surg. 2017;19(4):298–302. 2153.
4. Tahernia A, Erdmann D, Follmar K, Mukundan S, Grimes J, Marcus JR. Clinical implications of orbital volume change in the management of isolated and zygomaticomaxillary complex-associated orbital floor injuries. Plast Reconstr Surg. 2009;123:968–75.
5. Firriolo JM, Ontiveros NC, Pike CM, et al. Pediatric orbital floor fractures: clinical and radiological predictors of tissue entrapment and the effect of operative timing on ocular outcomes. J Craniofac Surg. 2017;28(8):1966–71.

Midfacial Fractures

58

Hui Bae Harold Lee, Gregory G. Grecco, Meena Moorthy, and Kendall Burgett

Introduction

Hippocrates, born in 460 B.C., created, by way of closed reduction, techniques to repair fractures of the midface. His methods continued to be the standard of care until names like Lefort, Markowitz, Manson, Graefe, and Lang developed more modern models of internal and external fixation thousands of years later [1]. Certainly, the advent of radiographs, modern instrumentation, and hardware created advancement in standards and precision of care.

By definition, midfacial fractures involve anatomical structures between the frontal bone and the mandible. However, there is no hard delineation between nasal structures, the orbit, nor the naso/oropharynx within this region, but rather, each structure continues on to the next. As Albright stated, "there is no tenable basis for mapping geographic boundaries beyond which one discipline or the other must not step, for the very simple reason that injuries and disease processes do not recognize man-made stop signs" [2]. Thus, a multidisciplinary methodology is critical for optimal patient outcome and experience. However, for practical assessment of midfacial fracture management, anatomical landmarks can help the clinician survey and evaluate the facial trauma patient.

H. B. H. Lee (✉)
Department of Ophthalmology, St Vincent Hospital, Indianapolis, IN, USA

G. G. Grecco
Indiana University School of Medicine, Indianapolis, IN, USA
e-mail: ggrecco@iu.edu

M. Moorthy
Carmel, IN, USA
e-mail: mmoorthy@iu.edu

K. Burgett
Indiana University School of Medicine, Fishers, IN, USA
e-mail: kburgett@iu.edu

Anatomy

The midface is the central portion of the head and skull with the lower border of the frontal bones as its superior border and the floor of the maxilla as its inferior border. Commonly understood borders of the midface include its superior border (lateral, superior, and medial walls of the orbit along with the ethmoid structures), lateral border (the zygomatic bones), posterior border (the pterygoid process of the sphenoid), anterior border (frontal process of maxilla and nasal bones), and inferior border (palate) [3].

Classification

Markowitz and Manson's work reviewed CT patterns of midfacial fractures and categorized them into general classifications of Lefort type and nasoorbitoethmoid (NOE) fractures (Figs. 58.1 and 58.2) [5, 6]. These fractures involve mostly the central midface, but of course, have extension into the upper and lower face.

NOE fractures include traumatic injuries into the central pyramid of the face with involvement of the nose, orbit, ethmoids, the base of the frontal sinus, and the anterior cranial base (Fig. 58.3). The vertical medial buttresses that extend superiorly from the piriform aperture along with the frontal processes of the maxilla are primarily affected. In a Markowitz/Manson type 1 NOE fracture, there is a large fragmented segment where the medial canthal tendon is still attached to its insertions to the anterior and posterior lacrimal crests; often, minimal to no telecanthus is observed (see Fig. 58.4). In a Markowitz/Manson type 2 NOE fracture, there is more comminution, but the tendon is still attached. With a Markowitz/Manson type 3 NOE fracture, the comminution is typically greater, and the tendon is either detached or severed (see Fig. 58.5a). Because of the injury and displacement of the medial canthal tendon, telecanthus is classically seen with more severe NOE 2 and 3 fracture types.

A. J. Cohen, C. N. Burkat (eds.), *Oculofacial, Orbital, and Lacrimal Surgery*, https://doi.org/10.1007/978-3-030-14092-2_58

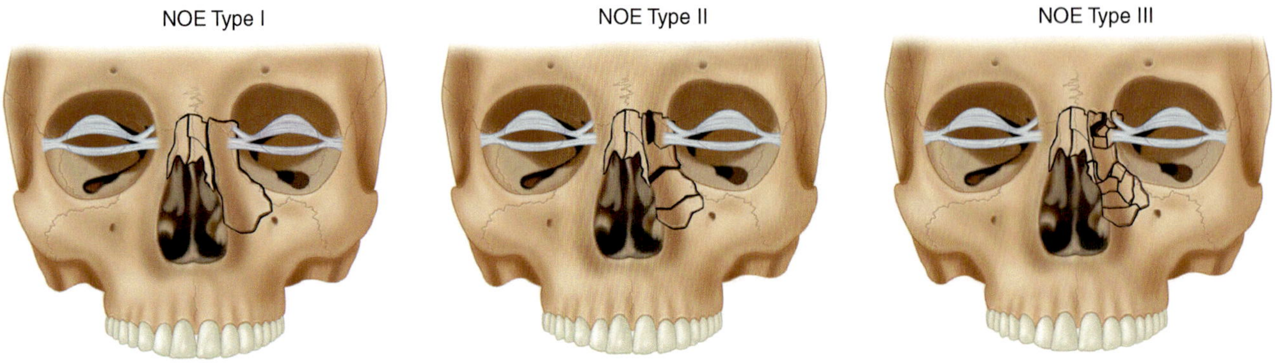

Fig. 58.1 Typing for Markowitz/Manson NOE fractures. Illustrations demonstrating the classical presentation for the three NOE-type fractures. While these illustrations depict involvement of the nasal bones in all three cases, nasal bone fractures per se are not required for NOE fractures [4]

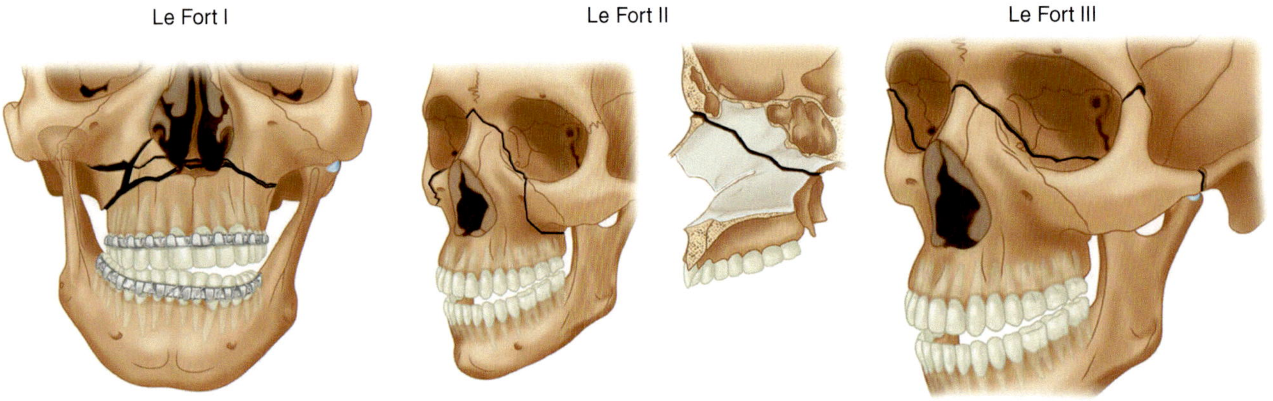

Fig. 58.2 Typing for Le Fort fractures. Illustrations demonstrating the classical presentation for the three Le Fort type fractures. Le Fort I fractures horizontally separate the palate and alveolar bone from the remainder of the face. In Le Fort II fractures, the nasal pyramid and palate are separated from the remainder of the face. Le Fort III fractures are craniofacial disjunction where the entire facial skeleton is fractured away from the skull base. All patterns can present as linear fractures or with communication [4]

An NOE fracture is not simply a nasal fracture combined with a medial wall fracture of the orbit. Classically, NOE fracture patterns are defined by telescoping of the nasal dorsum posteriorly. This usually results in fronto-nasal fractures as well as nasomaxillary components (see Fig. 58.5b).

Using cadaveric studies of traumatic injuries to the head and skull, the Frenchman, René Le Fort, developed categories of these classic fracture patterns. Lefort 1 fractures are primarily horizontal maxillary fractures that extend into the nasopharynx and involve the pterygoid plates. Lefort 2

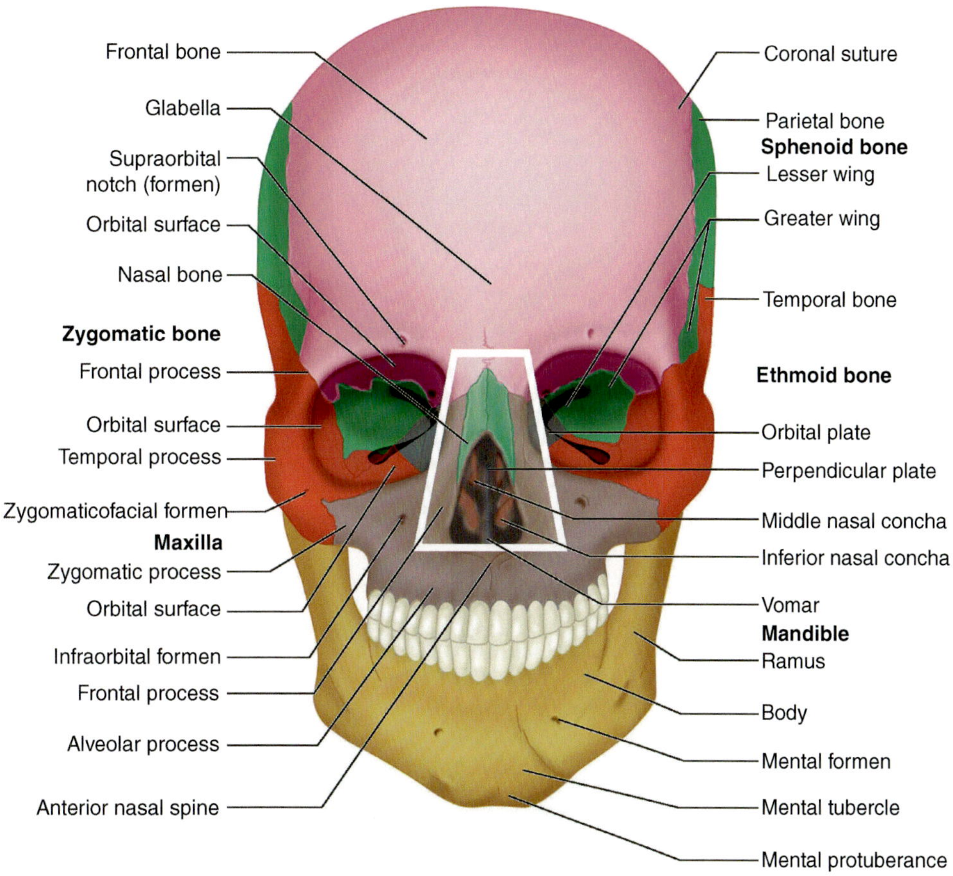

Fig. 58.3 Facial anatomy. Anatomic drawing demonstrating the bones of the skull and face. The concept of the central pyramid of the face is highlighted in orange [7]

fracture patterns involve the central pyramid of the face with extension from the zygomaticomaxillary complex to the inferior orbital rim, lacrimal bone/medial wall of the orbit, and into the nose (Fig. 58.6). Finally, Lefort 3 fractures are defined by a craniofacial disjunction that often involve the frontozygomatic suture line. These fractures extend into the lateral wall of the orbit and travel medially from the floor of the orbit up to the medial wall and nasal bones. The pterygoid plates are variably involved in both Lefort 2 and 3 fractures [8, 9].

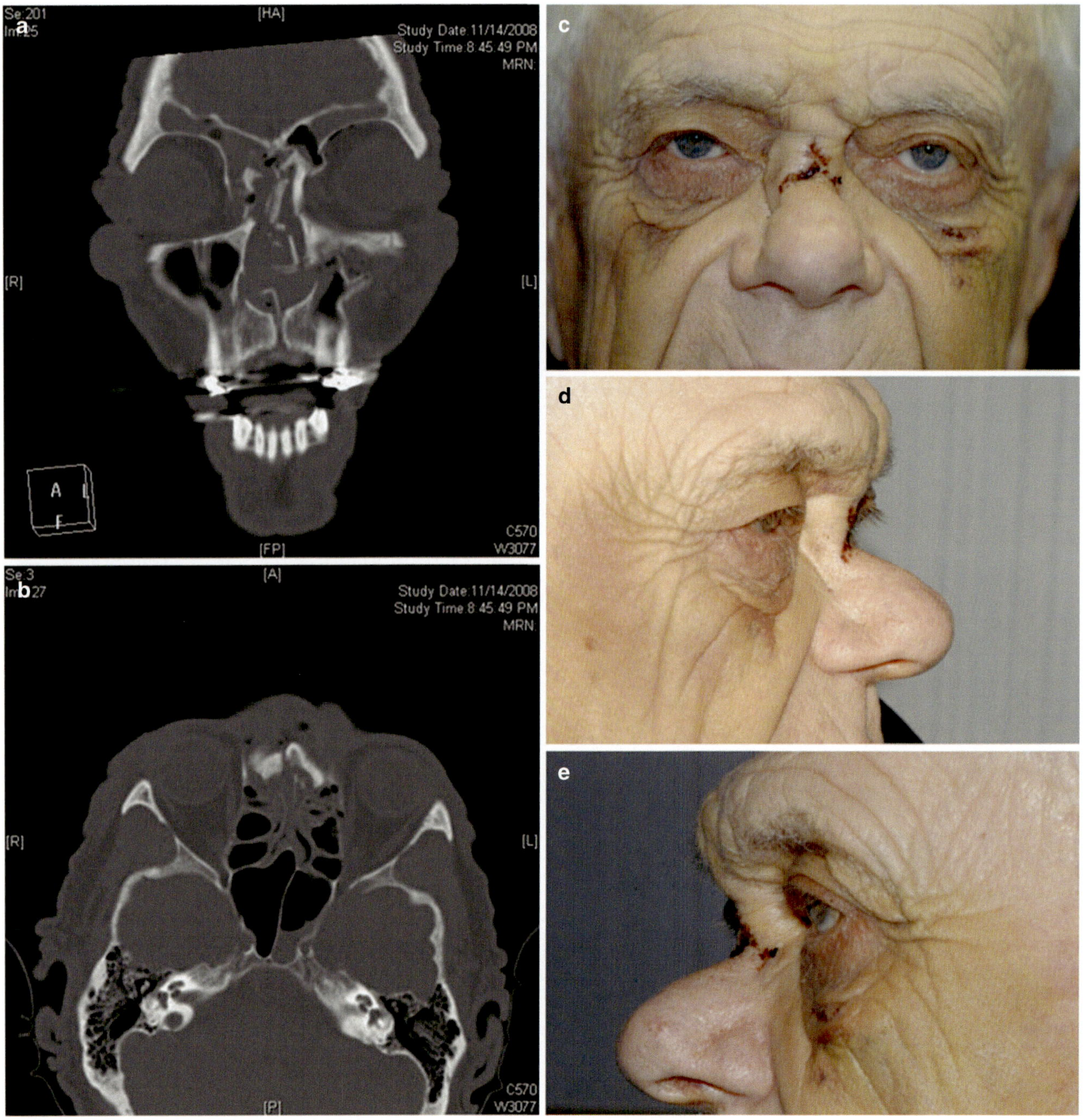

Fig. 58.4 Markowitz/Manson type I NOE fracture. Coronal (**a**) and axial (**b**) CT images show type I NOE fracture with involvement of the medial orbit and nose. Preoperative photos of the patient (**c**–**e**) demonstrate saddle-nose deformity without telecanthus

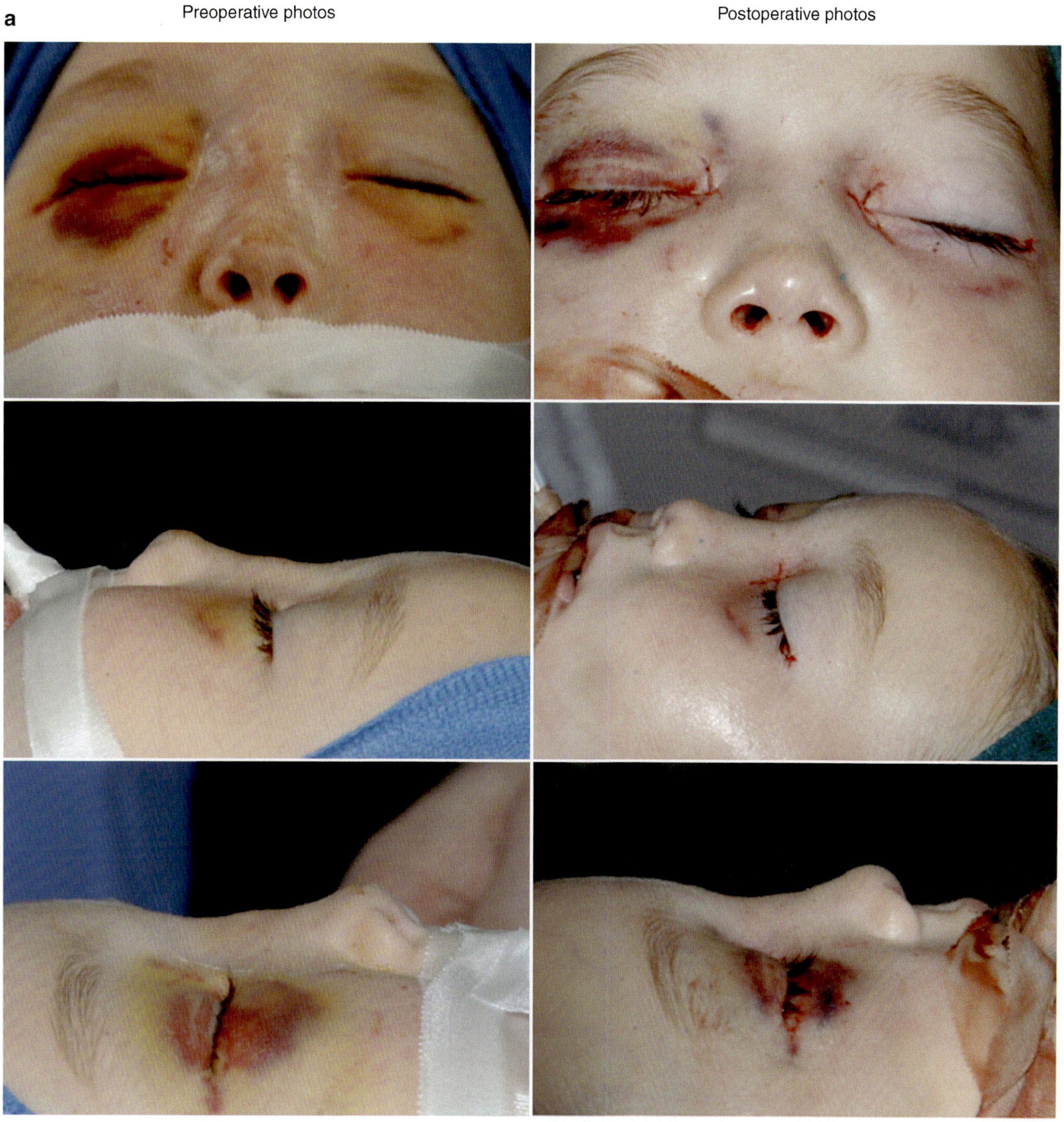

Fig. 58.5 Markowitz/Manson type III NOE fracture. (**a**) shows preoperative (*left*) and postoperative photos (*right*) for a Markowitz/Manson type III NOE fracture. Notice the traumatic telecanthus of the right eye. (**b**) Markowitz/Manson type III NOE fracture. CT images demonstrate posterior displacement of nasal pyramid with telescoping injury to medial orbital walls creating lateral displacement of the bony medial orbit

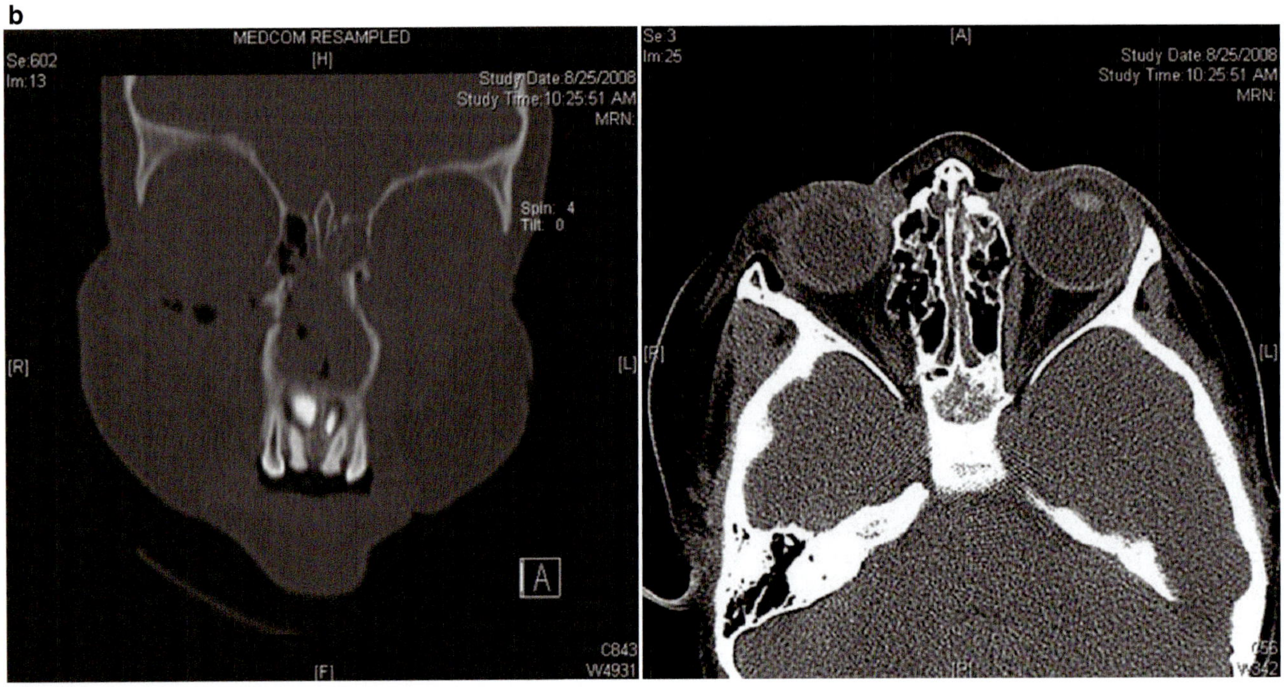

Fig. 58.5 (continued)

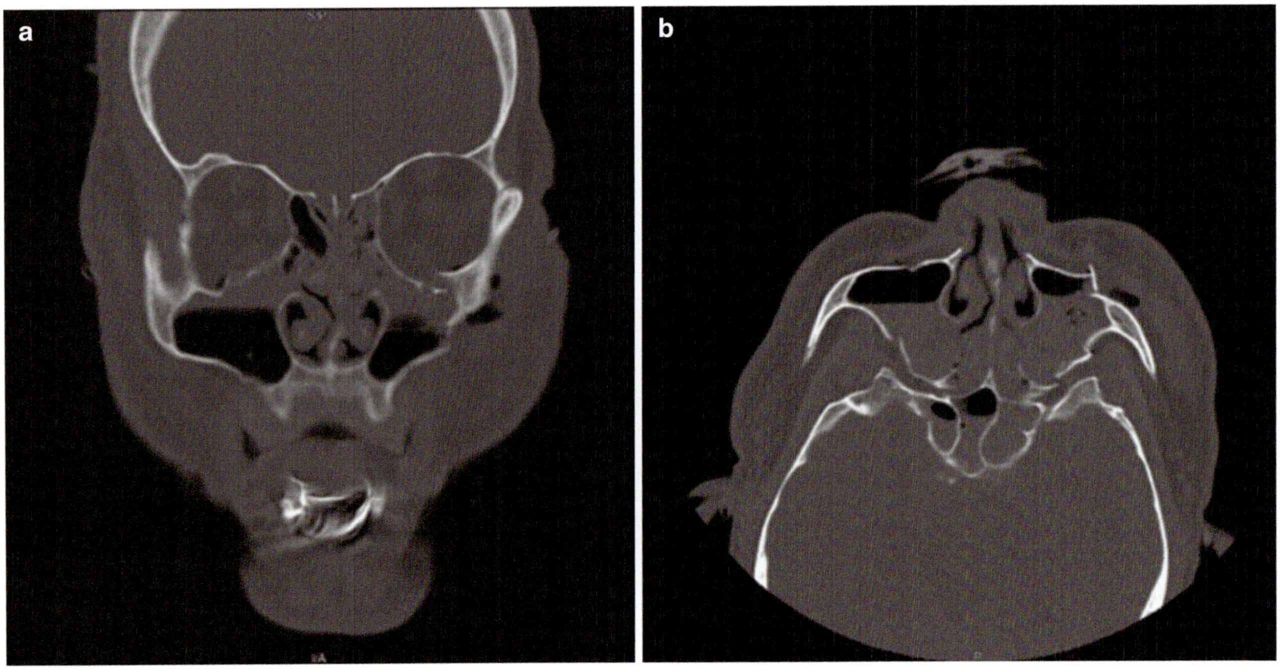

Fig. 58.6 Radiographic imaging of Lefort II fracture. Coronal (**a**) and axial (**b**) CT images show fractures of bilateral orbital floor fitting into fracture pattern of Lefort 2 fractures bilaterally with additional tripod fracture on left. Coronal (**c**) and axial (**d**) images after surgical reduction and fixation show proper anatomic alignment of orbital floors, malar eminences, zygomatic arches, and midface

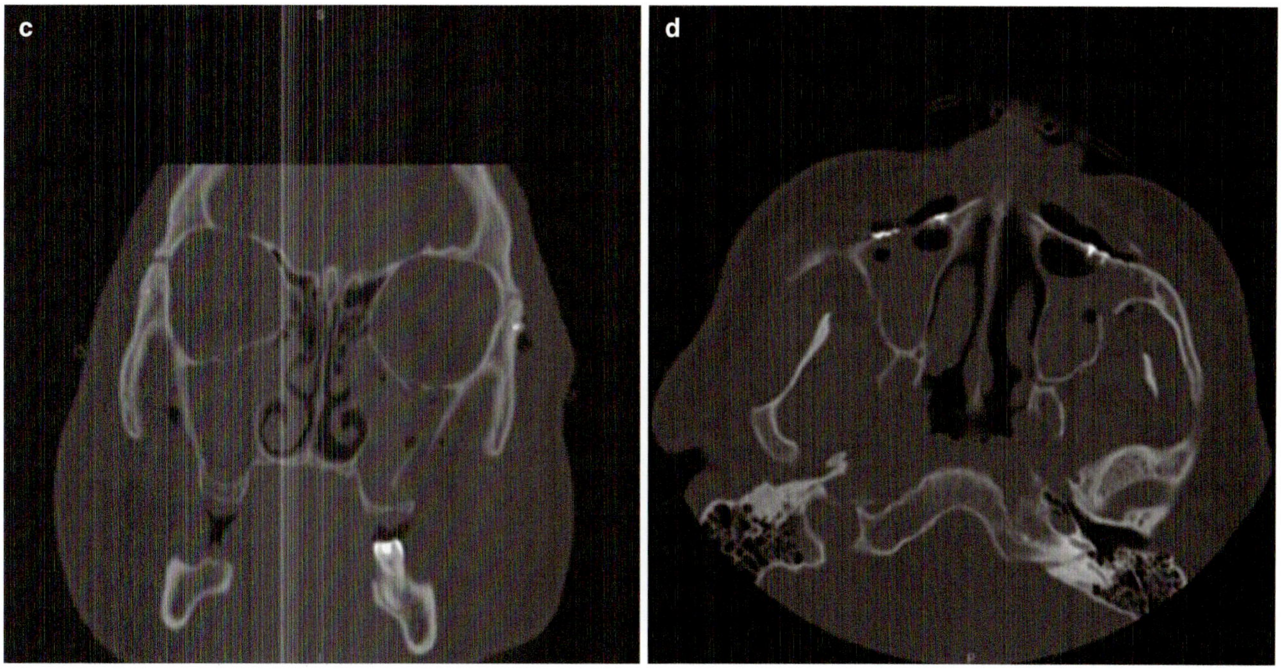

Fig. 58.6 (continued)

Epidemiology

In 1954, Bennett wrote an article concerning the rise of midfacial fractures in the "machine age" [3]. He reasoned the rise in high velocity facial injuries was secondary to increased motor vehicle use and subsequent collisions. Interestingly, in 2003, Maryam et al. found that the creation and use of seatbelts reduced the incidence of midfacial trauma [10].

When presenting to an emergency room setting, 37.5% of patients presenting with a facial injury have a fracture of their facial bones [11]. The large majority of patients with facial trauma are male (74.4–85%) [12, 13].

There is a wide range in the distribution of injury patterns and causes. Many different studies disagree largely on incidence of fracture patterns. Certainly, geographic locations combined with the development status of the study's country of origin play roles in evaluating the demographic of each study's analytic data. For example, one might expect zygomatic and orbital fractures to be more prevalent in assault- or sports-related injury. However, taken as a whole, data from previous studies appear to follow certain trends.

The most common modern causes of injury are motor vehicle collisions (12–71.3%), followed by assaults (9.5–61%), sports-related injuries (6–33%), and falls (3.3–36.7%) [11, 13–23]. The third decade of life is the age group most affected with craniofacial trauma with 28.3–39.2% occurring in 21–30-year-olds, followed by 19% in 31–40-year-olds and 4.6% in those younger than 10 years of age [12, 13, 24].

Interestingly, the greatest incidence (38%) of craniofacial trauma was observed in the late evening hours between 6 pm and 12 am with Saturdays being the day with the highest volume (44.7%) of injury. Tuesdays have the lowest incidence at 3.4% [13].

Craniofacial trauma affects portions of the face with different frequency. Although some reports vary widely, the highest frequency of injury appears to be the mandible and midface. The midface is involved in 25.3–71.5% of all facial fractures followed by the mandible 24.3–65% of the time [11, 12, 24].

Within the midface, the most common isolated fracture site is the zygoma (5.7–44%), followed by the nasal bone (7–37.7%), the orbit (7.6–21%), and maxilla (1.3–8.3%) [11, 12, 24].

Examination

Complex facial trauma often presents with concomitant traumatic injuries throughout other body systems. Any workup has to begin with initial emergency triage of vital organ systems. After the trauma team has stabilized the patient, the facial trauma service can evaluate the specifics within their field of expertise.

The patency of the airward is critical to the initial assessment of these complex fractures. Luckily, only 1.7% of facial trauma patients present with a compromised airway [25]. However, 34% of patients with Lefort type injuries need emergent airway establishment [26]. Emergency room evaluation may demonstrate poor airflow and even oxygen desaturation with straining. Edema, hemorrhage, tongue base prolapse, and collapse of midfacial structures with telescoping of the nose and maxilla can result in compromise of routes of intubation [27]. If traditional orotracheal intubation is not possible, options include nasal intubation or initiating surgical routes of securing the airway. If there are skull base injuries, intracranial penetration is a clear concern with this technique. Cricothyroidotomies or urgent tracheostomies can be performed in the emergency setting and even in preparation for maxillomandibular fixation with Lefort and mandible fractures.

All non-emergent airway decisions should consider fracture patterns and preparation for surgical manipulation. For example, nasotracheal intubation would make reduction of a NOE fracture quite difficult. Always consider alternative routes of intubation whenever maxillomandibular fixation is required. Because patients with maxillofacial trauma can be more likely to have cervical spine injuries, the state of the spine must be considered in all airway decisions on initial assessment and with operative planning [28]. Consultation with our otolaryngology and oral surgery colleagues may assist in planning, particularly with newer techniques of submental intubation [29–31].

Next, any frank hemorrhaging either from a direct laceration of blunt force (e.g., retrobulbar hemorrhage) must be addressed. Certainly, the circulatory system in general must be evaluated for other injuries that are life threatening. But, hemorrhages even within the head and neck can create complications that need to be addressed rapidly. Concerns for an orbital compartment syndrome should necessitate emergent canthotomy and cantholysis. Many techniques have been described to decompress the orbit in the setting of a retrobulbar hemorrhage, a true orbital emergency [32, 33]. Emergent eyelid release can and should be performed by the emergency room physician upon evaluation. We advocate a full thickness lid laceration to both upper and lower eyelids as proximal to the lateral canthus as possible as the simplest technique to manage retrobulbar hemorrhages. This technique has been shown to be as therapeutic as traditional canthotomy and cantholysis procedures, which many non-ophthalmic physicians are not as comfortable with [34].

Specific to the face, a screening nervous system examination must be performed looking at the cranial nerves within the field of injury. Olfactory nerve (cranial nerve I) injury may occur with neurotrauma from either direct nerve injury or transmission of shearing forces from blunt trauma. Vision and the range of ocular motility should be addressed looking for injuries to cranial nerves II, III, IV, and VI. We find that reduction of extraocular motility is the worst prognostic indicator of severe retrobulbar hemorrhage due to apical compression. Certain skull base, temporal bone, and zygomatic fractures along with lacerations along the course of the facial nerve may also result in facial paresis. Lacerations lateral to the lateral canthus should always raise suspicion of facial nerve injury. Notation of V2 hyposthesia should be made along with any other sensory issues including difficulty with smelling or hearing.

Once emergent airway, bleeding and neurologic deficits have been managed. A complete ophthalmic examination should be performed. Ophthalmic injuries of any kind are seen in 67–90% of midfacial fractures [35–37]. Ophthalmic complications related to facial trauma include ruptured globes, traumatic optic neuropathy, retrobulbar hemorrhages, retinal detachments, dislocated lenses, ocular restriction, and damage to the nasolacrimal system. Injuries sustained around the medial canthus raise suspicion for nasolacrimal duct damage as well as medial canthal tendon displacement. Decreased sensation in the distribution of the infraorbital nerve is common in patients with orbital floor fractures and should be documented on the initial examination. A trained ophthalmic surgeon should be involved in the care of all midfacial fractures and needs to be consulted on the initial examination whenever possible.

The ocular examination should include measurements of visual acuities, pupillary reflexes, motility, and intraocular pressure. A severe decrease in vision may suggest optic neuropathy from either direct or indirect injury to the nerve. The examiner must be skilled in evaluating the slightest pupillary abnormality including a relative afferent pupillary defect. A thorough extraocular motility examination should precede qualitative questioning of subjective diplopia when possible. Next, anterior segment examinations with a portable slit lamp or penlight should highlight important globe injuries. Fluorescein staining can help evaluate for both corneal abrasions and anterior globe lacerations. If extensive subconjunctival hemorrhage or hyphema, or distored pupil, is noted, there should be a high suspicion for a ruptured globe. The repair of a ruptured globe takes surgical precedence to the repair of associated facial and orbital injuries. Finally, a detailed posterior segment examination should begin to look for injuries including commotio retinae, retinal tears/detachments, vitreous hemorrhages, and optic nerve pathology.

Radiology

Standard imaging of facial fractures include computed tomography (CT) scans for most settings involving facial trauma. After stabilization of the airway and circulatory status, the patient is sent for imaging usually in an emergency department setting.

Conventional radiography generates single plane two-dimensional (2D) images. With the advent of multiplane two-dimensional and three-dimensional (3D) imaging techniques of CT and magnetic resonance imaging (MRI), massive improvements in diagnosis and surgical planning have been obtained. Kim et al. found a sensitivity of 85.7% for the detection of orbital floor fractures using CT imaging [38]. In other studies, up to 7.14% of all facial fractures are missed clinically but observed radiographically [12]. Contrarily, 6.37% of fractures were suspected clinically but not confirmed radiographically [12].

Foreign bodies within the head neck area present unique difficulties in surgical management and complications. In typical CT images, many types of wood in different hydrated states can be indiscernible in the black background of orbital fat. Because wood has absorption coefficients ranging from −999 to +54 HU, even large pieces of wood can be missed (standard CT scans are performed at a window width of 200–350 HU) [39]. The scale of CT imaging should be increased to at least 1000 Hounsfield units (HU) to increase the background signal of the orbital fat. Typically, "bone windows" settings (width, 4000 HU) can help discern vegetative foreign bodies of the face far greater than soft tissue windows.

MRI has its function in the acute setting of trauma as well. If unable to visualize nonmetallic foreign bodies using the techniques of CT, especially vegetative, MRI can be useful. Within the orbit, using T1-weighted images, intraorbital wooden foreign bodies appear hypointense compared to the hyperintense orbital fat [39]. Custer et al. studied wooden matter in environments consistent with orbital tissue [40]. He found that T1-weighted images created superior imaging quality and required less scanning time, particularly with small vegetative matter [40]. Additionally, T2-weighted images with fat suppression can help detect posttraumatic lesions associated with either direct or indirect traumatic optic neuropathy [41].

More recently, three-dimensional (3D) CT imaging has gained popularity within the facial trauma community. This modality may help define spatial relationships in the setting of midfacial trauma. Remmler et al. found that combining 2D and 3D techniques helped the diagnostic yield specifically in nasoorbitoethmoid fractures [42]. Although traditional CT techniques had higher sensitivity in evaluating medial wall orbit fractures, the addition of 3D techniques improved diagnosis of medial buttress displacement when reviewing intraoperative evaluation [42].

Surgical Management

Surgical management of midfacial fractures relies on an experienced surgeon with a detailed understanding of the facial anatomy. Surgical approaches include common anatomical dissections that the oculofacial plastic surgeon is not only comfortable with, but also include incisions that he is quite familiar with. Medial incisions include transcutaneous incisions that are identical to those used in dacryocystorhinostomy and medial wall decompressions (Fig. 58.7) [43, 44]. Approaches to the midface involve classic transconjunctival incisions that can be extended superiorly to meet the lateral wall of the orbit [45]. The gingival incisions that are commonly made in subperiosteal midface lifts are also essential for approaching the midface particularly in Lefort and zygomaticomaxillary complex (ZMC) fractures [46]. Coronal incisions are rarely necessary except for depressed frontal fractures or segmented zygomatic fractures [47–49].

The key to repairing these complex fractures starts with opening and accessing the central midface. Commonly, fractures are repaired with an outside-in technique. In this flawed

Medial orbitotomy incisions

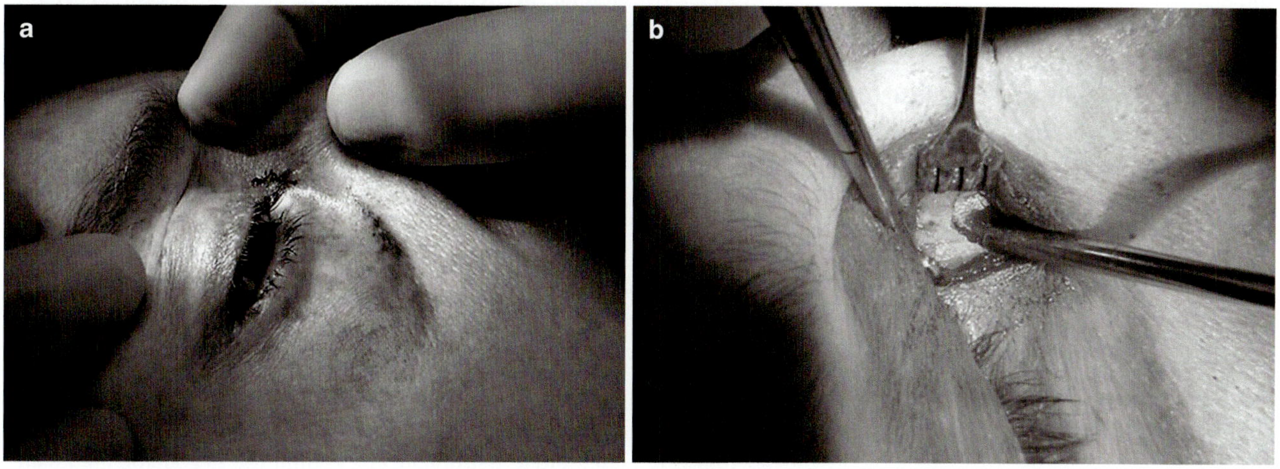

Fig. 58.7 Medial orbitotomy incisions. Medial orbitotomy incision is marked preparing for incision (**a**) creating easy and visible subperiosteal access to nasal bones and medial orbit (**b**) useful in the surgical management of midfacial fractures. This transcutaneous incision is identical to incisions used in dacryocystorhinostomy and medial wall decompression. (Source: Nunery and Tao [43])

An analogy for the orbito-centric approach

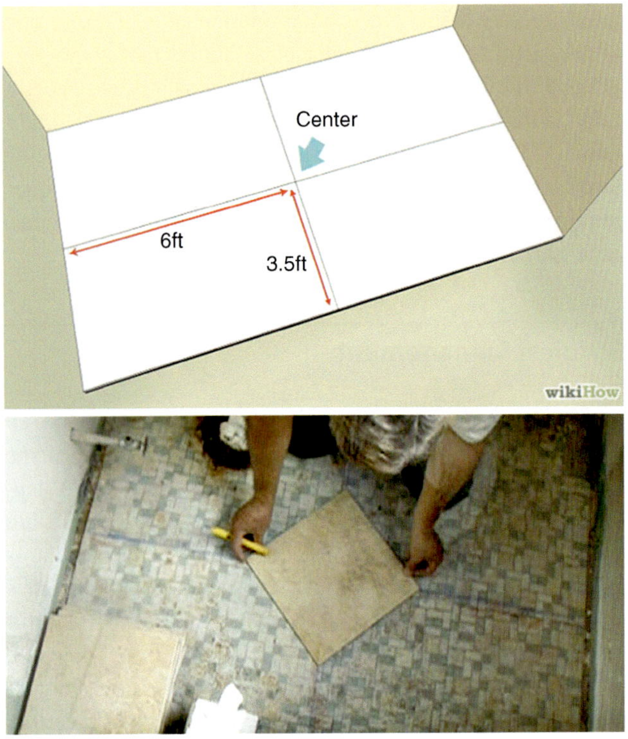

Fig. 58.8 Paradigm of the orbito-centric approach. Fracture repairs should be approached using an "inside-out" technique, rather than "outside-in." This is analogous to constructing a tile floor, in which starting in the center of the room and working peripherally yields the best results

approach, the lateral walls of the orbits are initially plated at the frontozygomatic fracture line followed by maxillomandibular reduction and fixation. At times, closed reduction of the nasal bones with splinting follows. Often, the critical portions of the central pyramid of the face are left unreduced and disregarded.

Our paradigm is to shift the mode of fracture repair from "outside-in" to "inside-out," similar in principle to preparing a bathroom floor for tiling (Fig. 58.8). One always starts at the center of the room and move to the periphery. Any imperfections or misalignments can be corrected and modified in the periphery. The critical portions that need to be exact and aligned are taken as priority. Otherwise, if one started from the periphery of the floor and moved in, he would compromise the perfection and symmetry of the central portion of the floor.

Linz studied the tracking of an observer's eyes when looking at children with synostosis [50]. He found that the observer would turn their gaze directly toward the child's eyes initially and focus their attention to the asymmetry related to the periocular area. Within cosmetic practices, most of the injectable agents (neurotoxic agents and fillers) are focused on the central midfacial pyramid. The highest concentration of these therapeutic agents involve the forehead, eyelid, and nasolabial folds. Trends suggest an increased volume of injections occurring in the midface area [51]. Biometric facial recognition software used by a variety of digital applications from facial identification to security issues utilize points within this central midfacial pyramid. The critical points of recognition involve computer algorithms using fiducial points such as eyes, nose, and mouth and their geometric relations [52]. There are modern day applications currently used in some smartphone devices for security access and even digital communication.

What these studies concerning facial recognition inform us is that the central midface holds the points which identify an individual as himself. These points and their geometric patterns must be aligned properly after a significant traumatic displacement to allow restoration of facial identity. The midface is not the location to compromise and sacrifice excellence but the arena to attempt perfection.

We then focus on the critical aspects of midfacial reduction and fixation. This starts with the medial canthal tendons and their three-dimensional location to the nasal bones, naso-frontal suture line, and frontal plane of the face. This critical alignment is where most commonly poor patient outcomes start. We advocate internal fixation of the nasal fragments whenever possible (Fig. 58.9). In cases of projectile injuries (e.g., missile injuries like gunshot wounds or explosions), this is not always possible, and closed reduction techniques like transnasal wiring are necessary. However, in blunt trauma, there is rarely a need to perform transnasal wiring as the medial canthal tendon tends to follow the lacrimal crest fixation. If the frontal process of the maxilla along with the anterior and posterior lacrimal crest is aligned, the medial canthal tendon will follow. Open reduction and fixation is achieved by transcutaneous medial canthal incision just anterior to the medial canthal tendon. This incision is much more posterior to a classic Lynch incision, which would create unsatisfactory anterior nasal incisions. This transcutaneous anterior incision allows full access to the nasal dorsum, naso-frontal suture line, lacrimal crest, and posterior medial wall of the orbit; all of which are points necessary in both NOE and Lefort 2 and 3 type fractures.

Many techniques can be used to manipulate the fragments into position. For zygomaticomaxillary complex fractures and Lefort fractures, the authors prefer using either a Boise elevator or Kocher forcep behind the arch to rotate the zygoma into position. Typically, the zygomatic fractures are rotated externally and posteriorly facilitated by positioning a large blunt instrument just behind the zygomatic arch using the Keen technique. By placing your opposite hand on the frontal bone, the surgeon can rotate the arch internally and

Intraoperative repair

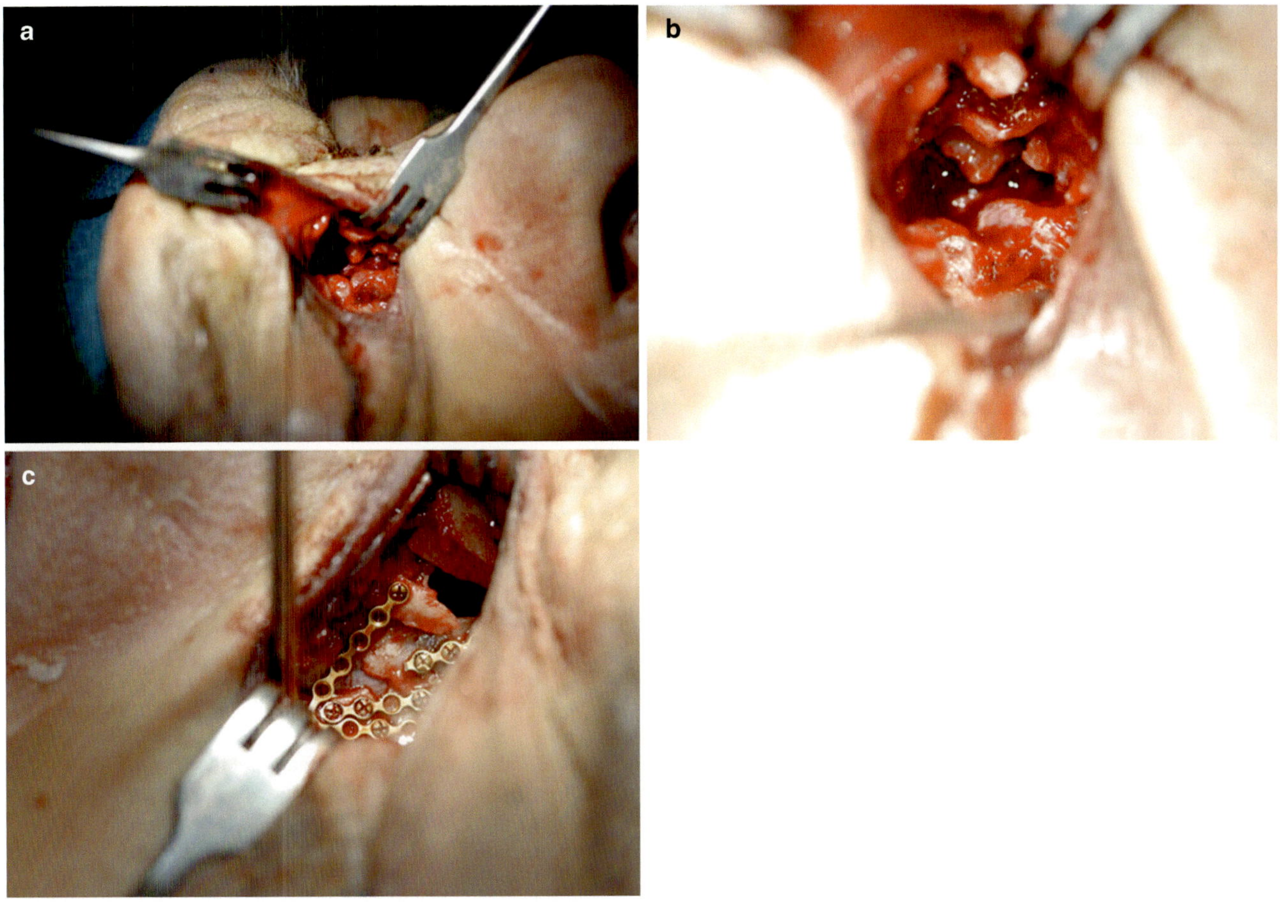

Fig. 58.9 Midfacial reduction and fixation—Intraoperative repair. Intraoperative photographs show severe disruption of nasal bones and anterior lacrimal crest (**a**, **b**). Reduction and fixation of multiple fragments (**c**) is typically possible even in severe fractures. Internal fixation of nasal fragments is encouraged whenever possible, as most poor outcomes are due to lack of critical alignment

anteriorly (AO Foundation Website reference). A Carroll-Girard screw can also be helpful to manipulate larger fragments, but the authors find it often unnecessary with the use of large blunt instruments.

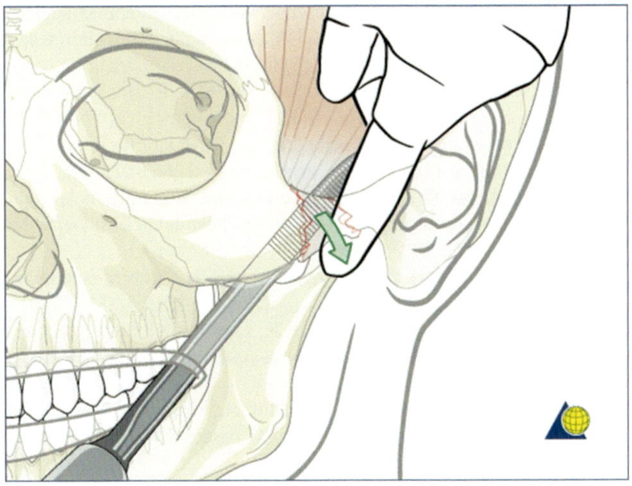

Any thin profile titanium screw is appropriate for internal fixation of buttress fractures. However, the authors advocate nonporous implants for use within the internal orbit. Implant material such as a nonporous, nylon sheet creates flexibility and margins when operating within the confines of orbital trauma. Fibrosis, scarring and adherence of orbital fat, ligaments and muscle to titanium and porous implants have been discussed broadly [53]. Nonporous implants (e.g., Supramid, Suprafoil) to repair internal orbital walls provide a cost efficient, safe, and forgiving material that is ideal in the environment of a dynamic orbit. Most repairs for internal orbital fractures should be focused on separating spaces (e.g., the orbit from the maxilla or ethmoid). Compartmentalization and nonadherence should be the priority of the implant choice. Supportive qualities such as found in larger thickness implants or titanium is not necessary as the anatomic walls of the internal orbit are thin and not structural. The surgeon should account for these factors when choosing the best option for orbital wall reduction. The ideal orbital implant should be nonadherent, widely available, and cost-efficient.

These qualities are found in nylon sheet implants such as Supramid, typically in a 0.35–0.4 mm thickness. Larger thickness sheets are also available, as well as porous implants embedded with titanium.

Complications

Midfacial fractures are commonly associated with ocular and supporting visual structure complications. These complications are well documented and range in severity dependent on fracture subtype, etiology of the fracture, and individual patient characteristics. A 2-year prospective study of 363 patients with midfacial fractures reported 90% of patients with midfacial fractures will likely experience some form of ocular injury; however, 63% of those ocular injuries were transient or minor injuries (e.g., subconjunctival hemorrhage/chemosis or eyelid swelling/bruising), 16% were moderate complications (e.g., enophthalmos, macular edema, or eyelid laceration), and the remaining were severe complications (gross proptosis, vitreous hemorrhage, retinal detachments, or traumatic optic neuropathy) [35]. Decreased visual acuity is the most common clinical finding occurring in nearly 70% of patients with midfacial fractures [35]. Other more frequently reported and characterized complications of midfacial fractures include diplopia, enophthalmos, convergence insufficiency and/or failure of accommodation, and optic neuropathy. Diplopia is a common ocular complication of midfacial fractures but varies significantly between fracture subtype (1% for middle third fractures and up to 86% of blow-out fractures) [35]. Blow-out fractures of the orbit are the most likely midfacial fracture to result in diplopia (36–86%) usually in association with road traffic accidents [35]. Diplopia as a result of midfacial trauma is regularly attributed to impairment of eye movement due to edema, hematoma, or injury to extraocular muscles or their nerve supply [35]. Following diplopia, enophthalmos reportedly occurs in 8% of patients after a midfacial fracture, most frequently in males who have experienced a blow-out fracture of the orbit during a road traffic accident or assault [35]. Weakness in accommodation and convergence results from varying etiologies, but the greatest contributing risk factor in midfacial fractures is associated head trauma [35]. Vision is lost in 1.6–5% of patients with midfacial fractures; the loss of vision is primarily attributed to permanent or temporary damage to the optic nerve in the region of the optic canal typically as a result of high velocity impact and strong force such as a midfacial fracture seen in road traffic accidents [54].

Following the surgical repair of midfacial fractures, complications may also arise. Inappropriate implant placement and errant surgical dissection can result in cicatrized eyelids, lower eyelid retraction or entropion, enophthalmos, and postoperative diplopia even in patients who had normal ductions postinjury. Orbital adherence syndrome can result from repairs of the orbit with titanium or porous implant material [53]. Reports have demonstrated that the titanium implant material can produce a fibrogenic response leading to restrictive diplopia and/or eyelid retraction [53]. However, removal of titanium hardware can improve diplopia if replaced with nylon foil implants [53]. Late implant complications can also occur, including implant migration, capsular hemorrhage, and implant infection. Non-ocular complications include anosmia, infraorbital nerve paresthesia, facial nerve injury, septal deviation, cerebrospinal fluid leak, malocclusion, trismus, and facial deformity [55]. Complications of repairs appear to be related to the location of the fracture such that the more superior the fracture the higher the rate of complications [55].

References

1. Gahhos F, Ariyan S. Facial fractures: hippocratic management. Head Neck Surg. 1984;6(6):1007–13.
2. Albright CR, McFarland PH Jr. Management of midfacial fractures. Oral Surg Oral Med Oral Pathol. 1972;34(6):858–79.
3. Bennett T. Midfacial fractures. South Med J. 1956;49(11):1252–7.
4. Cornelius CP, Gellrich N, Hillerup S, Kusumoto K, Schubert W, Fusetti S. AO Surgery Reference. 2013. Available from: https://www2.aofoundation.org/wps/portal/surgery.
5. Kelly KJ, Manson PN, Vander Kolk CA, Markowitz BL, Dunham CM, Rumley TO, Crawley WA. Sequencing LeFort fracture treatment (organization of treatment for a panfacial fracture). J Craniofac Surg. 1990;1(4):168–78.
6. Markowitz BL, Manson PN. Panfacial fractures: organization of treatment. Clin Plast Surg. 1989;16(1):105–14.
7. Jahan-Parwar B, Blackwell K. Facial bone anatomy. eMedicine. 2007; https://emedicine.medscape.com/article/835401-overview.
8. Tessier P. The classic reprint. Experimental study of fractures of the upper jaw. I and II. René Le Fort, M.D. Plast Reconstr Surg. 1972;50(5):497–506.
9. Patterson R. The Le Fort fractures: René Le Fort and his work in anatomical pathology. Can J Surg. 1991;34(2):183–4.
10. Maryam A, Saud AA, Hassan EA. Effects of seat belts on incidence, aetiology, and severity of maxillofacial injuries in eastern province, Saudi Arabia: a four year prospective study. J Pak Dent Assoc. 2003;12:170–5.
11. Gassner R, Tuli T, Hachl O, Rudisch A, Ulmer H. Craniomaxillofacial trauma: a 10 year review of 9543 cases with 21067 injuries. J Craniomaxillofac Surg. 2003;31(1):51–61.
12. Kumar R, Ahmed SS, Hashmi GS, Ansari MK, Rahman SA. Meta analysis of etiology and its clinical and radiological correlation in cases of Craniomaxillofacial trauma. J Maxillofac Oral Surg. 2016;15(3):336–44. https://doi.org/10.1007/s12663-015-0862-6.
13. Kapoor P, Kalra N. A retrospective analysis of maxillofacial injuries in patients reporting to a tertiary care hospital in East Delhi. Int J Crit Illn Inj Sci. 2012;2(1):6–10.
14. Lee JH, Cho BK, Park WJ. A 4 year retrospective study of facial fractures in Jeju, Korea. J Craniomaxillofac Surg. 2010;38(3):192–6.
15. Kamulegeya A, Lakor F, Kabenge K. Oral maxillofacial fractures seen at a Ugandan tertiary hospital: a six-month prospective study. Clinics. 2009;64(9):843–8.
16. Bakardjiev A, Pechalova P. Maxillofacial fractures in southern Bulgaria: retrospective study of 1706 cases. J Craniomaxillofac Surg. 2007;35(3):147–15021.

17. Maliska MC, Lima Junior SM, Gil JN. Analysis of 185 maxillofacial fractures in the state of Santa Catarina, Brazil. Braz Oral Res. 2009;23(3):268–74.
18. Brasileiro BF, Passeri LA. Epidemiological analysis of maxillofacial fractures in Brazil: a 5-year prospective study. Oral Surg Oral Med Oral Pathol Oral Radiol Endod. 2006;102:28–34.
19. Fasola AO, Nyako EA, Obiechina AE, Arotiba JT. Trends in the characteristics of maxillofacial fractures in Nigeria. J Oral Maxillofac Surg. 2003;61(10):1140–3.
20. Erol B, Tanrikulu R, Gorgun B. Maxillofacial fractures. Analysis of demographic distribution and treatment in 2901 patients (25-year experience). J Craniomaxillofac Surg. 2004;32(5):308–13.
21. Olasoji HO, Tahir A, Arotiba GT. Changing picture of facial fractures in northern Nigeria. Br J Oral Maxillofac Surg. 2002;40(2):140–3.
22. Hussain K, Wijetunge DB, Grubnic S, Jackson IT. A comprehensive analysis of craniofacial trauma. J Trauma. 1994;36:34–47.
23. Iida S, Kogo M, Sugiura T, Mima T, Matsuya T. Retrospective analysis of 1502 patients with facial fractures. Int J Oral Maxillofac Surg. 2001;30:286–90.
24. Hwang K, You SH. Analysis of facial bone fractures: an 11-year study of 2094 patients. Indian J Plast Surg. 2010;43:42–8.
25. Tung TC, Tseng WS, Chen CT, et al. Acute life-threatening injuries in facial fracture patients: a review of 1,025 patients. J Trauma. 2000;49:420–4.
26. Ng M, Saadat D, Sinha UK. Managing the emergency airway in Le Fort fractures. J Craniomaxillofac Trauma. 1998;4:38–43.
27. Kellman RM, Losquadro WD. Comprehensive airway management of patients with maxillofacial trauma. Craniomaxillofac Trauma Reconstr. 2008;1(1):39–47. https://doi.org/10.1055/s-0028-1098962.
28. Hackl W, Hausberger K, Sailer R, et al. Prevalence of cervical spine injuries in patients with facial trauma. Oral Surg Oral Med Oral Pathol Oral Radiol Endod. 2001;92:370–6.
29. Gordon NC, Tolstunov L. Submental approach to oroendotracheal intubation in patients with midfacial fractures. Oral Surg Oral Med Oral Pathol Oral Radiol Endod. 1995;79(3):269–72.
30. de Melo WM, Brêda MA Jr, Pereira-Santos D, Pereira CC, Sonoda CK, Araújo MM. Submental endotracheal intubation: a valuable resource for the management of panfacial fractures. J Craniofac Surg. 2012;23(6):1851–3. https://doi.org/10.1097/SCS.0b013e31826b8345.
31. Caron G, Paquin R, Lessard MR, Trépanier CA, Landry PE. Submental endotracheal intubation: an alternative to tracheotomy in patients with midfacial and panfacial fractures. J Trauma. 2000;48(2):235–40.
32. Oester AE Jr, Fowler BT, Fleming JC. Inferior orbital septum release compared with lateral canthotomy and cantholysis in the management of orbital compartment syndrome. Ophthal Plast Reconstr Surg. 2012;28(1):40–3. https://doi.org/10.1097/IOP.0b013e31823646f3.
33. Ballard SR, Enzenauer RW, O'Donnell T, Fleming JC, Risk G, Waite AN. Emergency lateral canthotomy and cantholysis: a simple procedure to preserve vision from sight threatening orbital hemorrhage. J Spec Oper Med. 2009;9(3):26–32.
34. Fu R, Lee HBH: Marvin H. Quickert thesis award candidate presentation. Orbital compartment syndrome: Effects of a full-thickness eyelid incision compared to the lateral canthotomy and cantholysis. 48th annual scientific symposium of the American Society of Ophthalmic Plastic and Reconstructive Surgery (ASOPRS). 2017. New Orleans.
35. al-Qurainy IA, Stassen LF, Dutton GN, Moos KF, el-Attar A. The characteristics of midfacial fractures and the association with ocular injury: a prospective study. Br J Oral Maxillofac Surg. 1991;29(5):291–301.
36. Holt JE, Holt GR, Blodgett JM. Ocular injuries sustained during blunt facial trauma. Ophthalmology. 1983;90(1):14–8.
37. Holt GR, Holt JE. Incidence of eye injuries in facial fractures: an analysis of 727 cases. Otolaryngol Head Neck Surg. 1983;91(3):276–9.
38. Kim SH, Ahn KJ, Lee JM, Choi KH, Han SH. The usefulness of orbital lines in detecting blow-out fracture on plain radiography. Br J Radiol. 2000;73(876):1265–9. https://doi.org/10.1259/bjr.73.876.11205669.
39. Glatt HJ, Custer PL, Barrett L, Sartor K. Magnetic resonance imaging and computed tomography in a model of wooden foreign bodies in the orbit. Ophthal Plast Reconstr Surg. 1990;6(2):108–14.
40. Custer PL, Lind A, Trinkaus KM. Complications of supramid orbital implants. Ophthal Plast Reconstr Surg. 2003;19:62–7. Wladis EJ: Are post-operative oral antibiotics required after orbital floor fracture repair? Orbit 2013;32(1):30–2.
41. Kubal WS. Imaging of orbital trauma. Radiographics. 2008;28(6):1729–39. https://doi.org/10.1148/rg.286085523.
42. Remmler D, Denny A, Gosain A, Subichin S. Role of three-dimensional computed tomography in the assessment of naso-orbitoethmoidal fractures. Ann Plast Surg. 2000;44(5):553–62. discussion 562–3.
43. Nunery WR, Tao JP. Medial canthal open nasal fracture repair. Ophthal Plast Reconstr Surg. 2008;24(4):276–9. https://doi.org/10.1097/IOP.0b013e318177f87c.
44. Timoney PJ, Sokol JA, Hauck MJ, Lee HB, Nunery WR. Transcutaneous medial canthal tendon incision to the medial orbit. Ophthal Plast Reconstr Surg. 2012;28(2):140–4. https://doi.org/10.1097/IOP.0b013e318248e62c.
45. Nunery WR. Lateral canthal approach to repair of trimalar fractures of the zygoma. Ophthal Plast Reconstr Surg. 1985;1(3):175–83.
46. Sullivan SA, Dailey RA. Endoscopic subperiosteal midface lift: surgical technique with indications and outcomes. Ophthal Plast Reconstr Surg. 2002;18(5):319–30.
47. Yanan W, Yanli H, Dilxat D, Weilong L, Hui L, Yi W, Lei L. Complications of supratemporalis approach with scalp coronal incision for orbital-zygomatic fracture. Hua Xi Kou Qiang Yi Xue Za Zhi. 2017;35(1):73–6.
48. Fattahi T, Salman S. An aesthetic approach in the repair of anterior frontal sinus fractures. Int J Oral Maxillofac Surg. 2016;45(9):1104–7.
49. Shetty SK, Saikrishna D, Kumaran S. A study on coronal incision for treating zygomatic complex fractures. J Maxillofac Oral Surg. 2009;8(2):160–3.
50. Linz C, Gerdes AB, Meyer-Marcotty P, Müller-Richter U, Böhm H, Ernestus RI, Kübler A, Alpers GW, Schweitzer T. Perception of children's faces with unilateral coronal synostosis—an eye-tracking investigation. Childs Nerv Syst. 2016;32(1):135–41. https://doi.org/10.1007/s00381-015-2798-z. Epub 2015 Aug 1.
51. Lee SK, Kim HS. Recent trend in the choice of fillers and injection techniques in Asia: a questionnaire study based on expert opinion. J Drugs Dermatol. 2014;13(1):24–31.
52. Bronstein AM, Bronstein MM, Kimmel R. Expression-invariant representations of faces. IEEE Trans Image Process. 2007;16(1):188–97.
53. Lee HB, Nunery WR. Orbital adherence syndrome secondary to titanium implant material. Ophthal Plast Reconstr Surg. 2009;25(1):33–6. https://doi.org/10.1097/IOP.0b013e3181929b6e.
54. Kallela I, Hyrkäs T, Paukku P, Iizuka T, Lindqvist C. Blindness after maxillofacial blunt trauma. Evaluation of candidates for optic nerve decompression surgery. J Craniomaxillofac Surg. 1994;22(4):220–5.
55. Haug RH, Prather J, Bradrick JP, Indresano AT. The morbidity associated with fifty maxillary fractures treated by closed reduction. Oral Surg Oral Med Oral Pathol. 1992;73(6):659–63.

Part V

Socket

Evisceration and Enucleation

59

Akshay Gopinathan Nair, Shubhra Goel,
and Cat Nguyen Burkat

Introduction

Evisceration and enucleation of the eye are commonly performed procedures in ophthalmic practice. Enucleation is the removal of the globe from the orbit that involves the separation of the globe from the extraocular muscles and the optic nerve [1]. It is possibly one of the oldest historical procedures in ophthalmic practice [2]. Evisceration is the removal of the contents of the globe, while retaining the sclera within the socket with the muscles undisturbed. Both of these procedures have special indications, although there exists some overlap. An ideal evisceration or enucleation surgery should result in adequate volume replacement in the form of an orbital implant; adequate surface area of the socket that should be lined with conjunctiva or any other mucus membrane; fornices that are deep enough to hold a prosthesis in place; good eyelid tone to retain the prosthesis within the fornices; and finally, acceptable aesthetic outcome of the prosthesis in terms of external appearance and transmitted motility. This chapter will review the indications, surgical techniques, and some common complications.

A. G. Nair
Ophthalmic Plastic Surgery and Ocular Oncology Services, Advanced Eye Hospital and Institute, Navi Mumbai, India

Ophthalmic Plastic Surgery and Ocular Oncology Services, Aditya Jyot Eye Hospital, Mumbai, India

S. Goel (✉)
Ophthalmic Facial Plastic and Cosmetic Surgery, Apollo Hospitals, Hyderabad, India

C. N. Burkat
Department of Ophthalmology and Visual Sciences, University of Wisconsin-Madison, Madison, WI, USA
e-mail: cburkat@wisc.edu

Enucleation

There are many factors that must be considered before advising enucleation to any patient: the psychological condition of the patient, the visual potential of the eye, cosmetic concerns of the patient, and the potential for suboptimal outcomes or complications [1]. The most common indication for enucleation is the presence of an intraocular malignancy. Other indications are painful blind eye, prevention of sympathetic ophthalmia, phthisis bulbi, neovascular glaucoma, and endophthalmitis (Table 59.1). Other less common indications include microphthalmia in children to stimulate the bony growth in an attempt to improve overall orbital and facial symmetry [3]. Another less common indication for primary enucleation is severe trauma leading to complete disruption of the ocular anatomy. In many such cases, ophthalmologists tend to primarily repair the globe first, regardless of the extent of damage. Primary enucleation in the setting of severe trauma may also alleviate concern that surgery to repair the globe may contribute to the potential risk of sympathetic ophthalmia in the fellow eye. However, the extremely low incidence of sympathetic ophthalmia, tests for early diagnosis, and improved medication have made this "prophylactic enucleation" somewhat controversial and debatable [4].

Table 59.1 Table listing the common indications and contraindications for enucleation and evisceration

	Enucleation	Evisceration
Intraocular malignancy	Indication	Absolute contraindication
Painful blind eye	Indication	Indication
Endophthalmitis	Indication	Indication
Penetrating trauma	Indication	Relative contraindication
Small phthisical eye	Indication (preferred)	Indication
Panophthalmitis	Contraindication	Indication

A. J. Cohen, C. N. Burkat (eds.), *Oculofacial, Orbital, and Lacrimal Surgery*, https://doi.org/10.1007/978-3-030-14092-2_59

The preferred anesthesia for enucleation surgery is general anesthesia. This helps allay patient anxiety and offers pain control and hypotension—both of which are important in enucleation. Preoperatively, if the media is opaque and limits view of the posterior pole, ocular imaging (ultrasonography or computed tomography (CT) scan) should be performed.

Intraoperatively, it is most important to confirm with the surgical staff that the correct eye is marked for surgery. An eyelid speculum can be placed to provide exposure of the operative field. Using Westcott scissors, a 360 ° circumcorneal peritomy is performed, taking care to incise close to the limbus in order to preserve maximum conjunctiva. The steps of the myoconjunctival technique are illustrated in (Figs. 59.1, 59.2, 59.3, and 59.4) [5]:

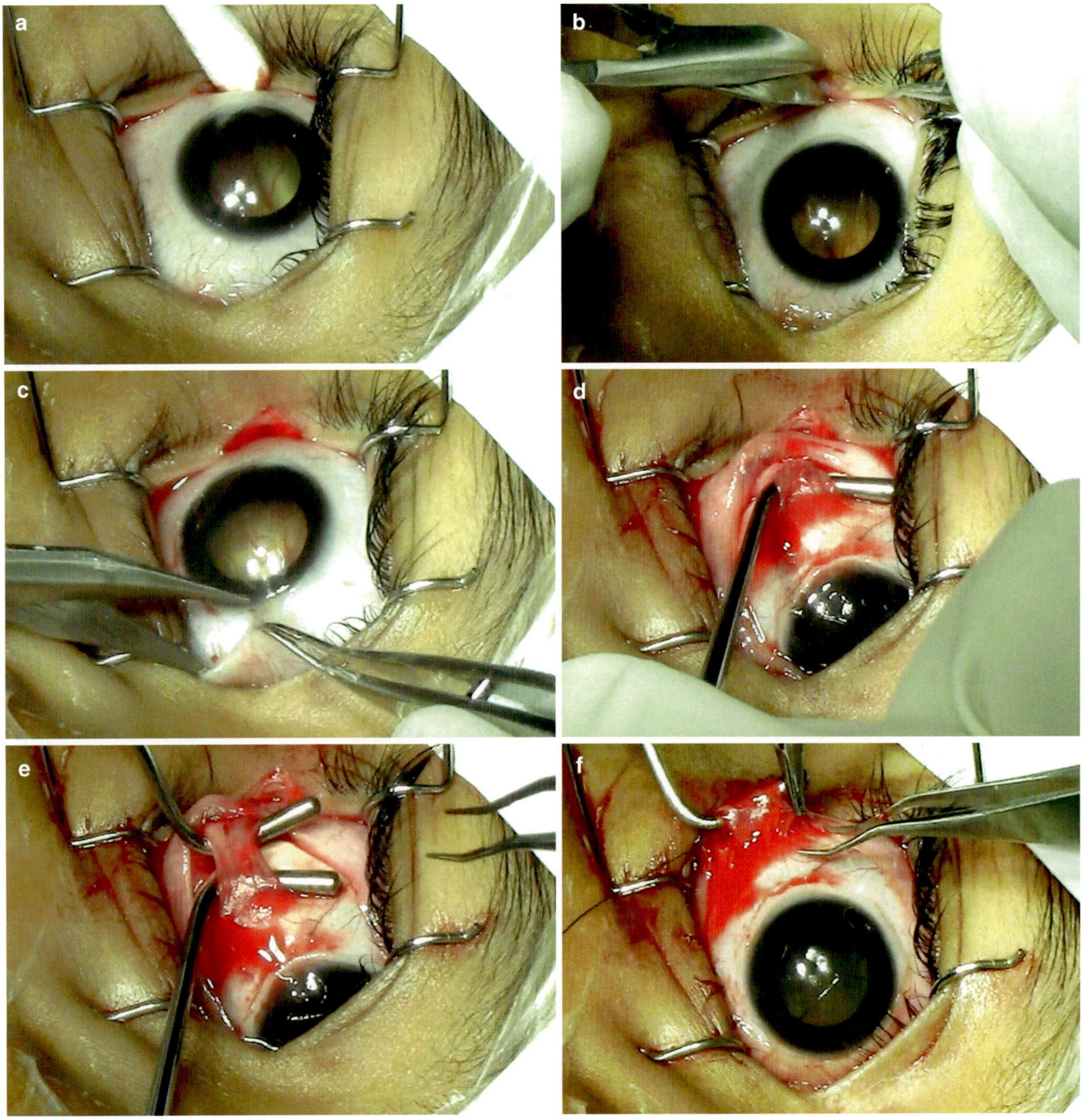

Fig. 59.1 Enucleation, surgical steps. A thorough examination of the eye is performed to confirm the correct operative eye (**a**). A lateral canthotomy can facilitate exposure and globe removal in some cases (**b**). Careful 360 ° peritomy is performed, preserving conjunctiva (**c**). The extraocular muscles are hooked (**d**) and isolated (**e**) and an optional traction suture can be placed with 6-0 silk close to the muscle insertion (**f**). The lateral rectus is isolated here

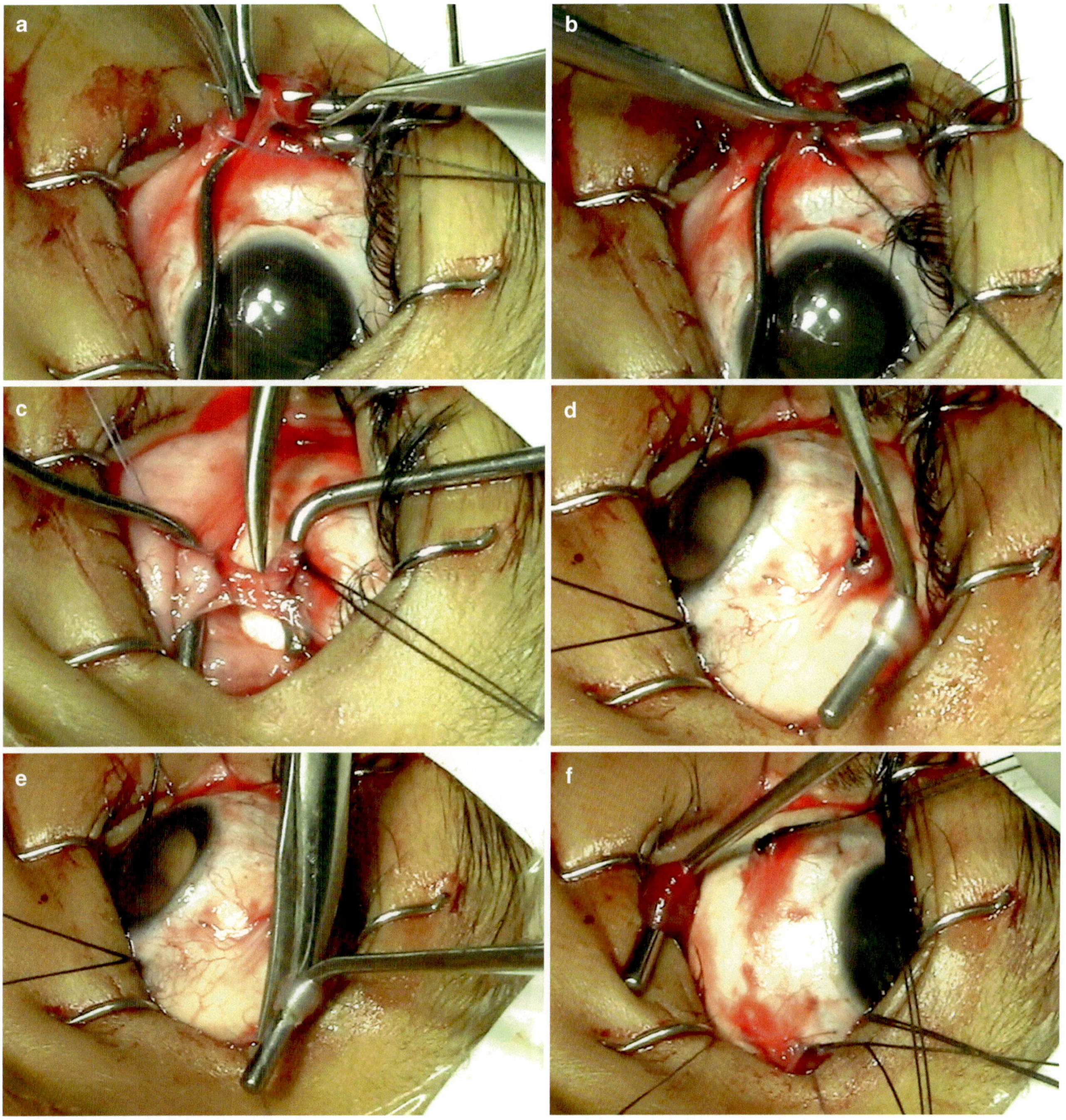

Fig. 59.2 Enucleation, extraocular muscle release. A double-armed 6-0 Vicryl suture is placed several millimeters distal to the initial traction suture (**a**), and the muscle is transected between the two sutures (**b**). Shown here is the lateral rectus muscle (**c**). After all recti have been cut, the superior oblique is hooked (**d**) and released without a suture (**e**). The inferior rectus is also isolated (**f**) and cut

- After limbal peritomy, subconjunctival dissection is performed in the quadrants between the rectus muscles and extended peripherally to separate Tenon's capsule from the sclera.
- Each of the four rectus muscles are hooked, and a 4-0 silk traction suture passed through the muscles, close to the insertion onto the globe. Several millimeters away, the muscle is secured with double-armed 6-0 polyglactin (Vicryl) sutures or other absorbable suture. Many surgeons prefer not to place traction sutures.
- The muscle is transected between the two sutures, leaving the traction suture on the muscle stump attached to the globe and the polyglactin (Vicryl) suture attached to the freed muscle. If no traction sutures are used, the muscle is typically cut at its scleral insertion. Leaving a small stump of muscle at the scleral insertion, however,

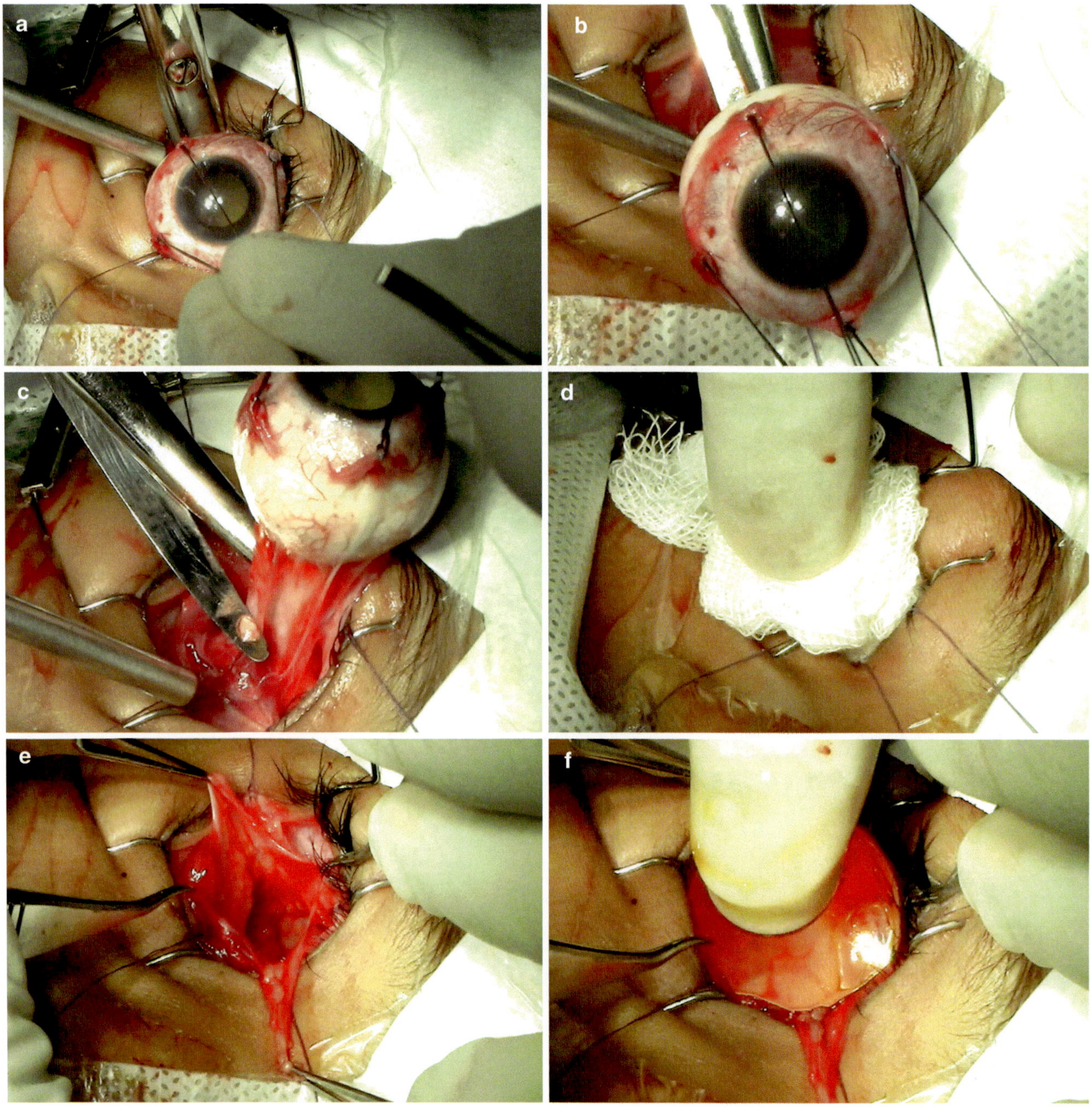

Fig. 59.3 Enucleation, removing the globe. Pulling up on the four silk traction sutures (**a**) provides upward traction to make the optic nerve taut. After strumming to feel the optic nerve; a slightly curved scissor is used to cut the optic nerve (**b**). After severing the optic nerve, the other posterior fibrous attachments are also cut (**c**). A gauze pack is used to stop bleeding (**d**) for several minutes with pressure. The intraconal space behind posterior Tenon's fascia is identified (**e**), and the implant is placed within (**f**)

can sometimes be useful to grasp the globe when transecting the nerve later.

- The superior and inferior oblique muscles are hooked and cut without tagging.
- Although not typically necessary, a lateral canthotomy may be performed to allow the globe to gently prolapse out of the socket.
- The optic nerve is then released from the posterior globe. A temporal approach with a curved or straight enucleation scissors, or a nasal approach using curved enucleation scissors are common techniques, depending on surgeon preference.
- Forward anterior traction by pulling the traction sutures with the non-dominant hand help makes the optic nerve taut. An enucleation spoon is preferred by some surgeons to provide traction and protect the posterior globe.
- The taut nerve can be strummed with closed scissor blades to assess the position and length of the optic nerve.

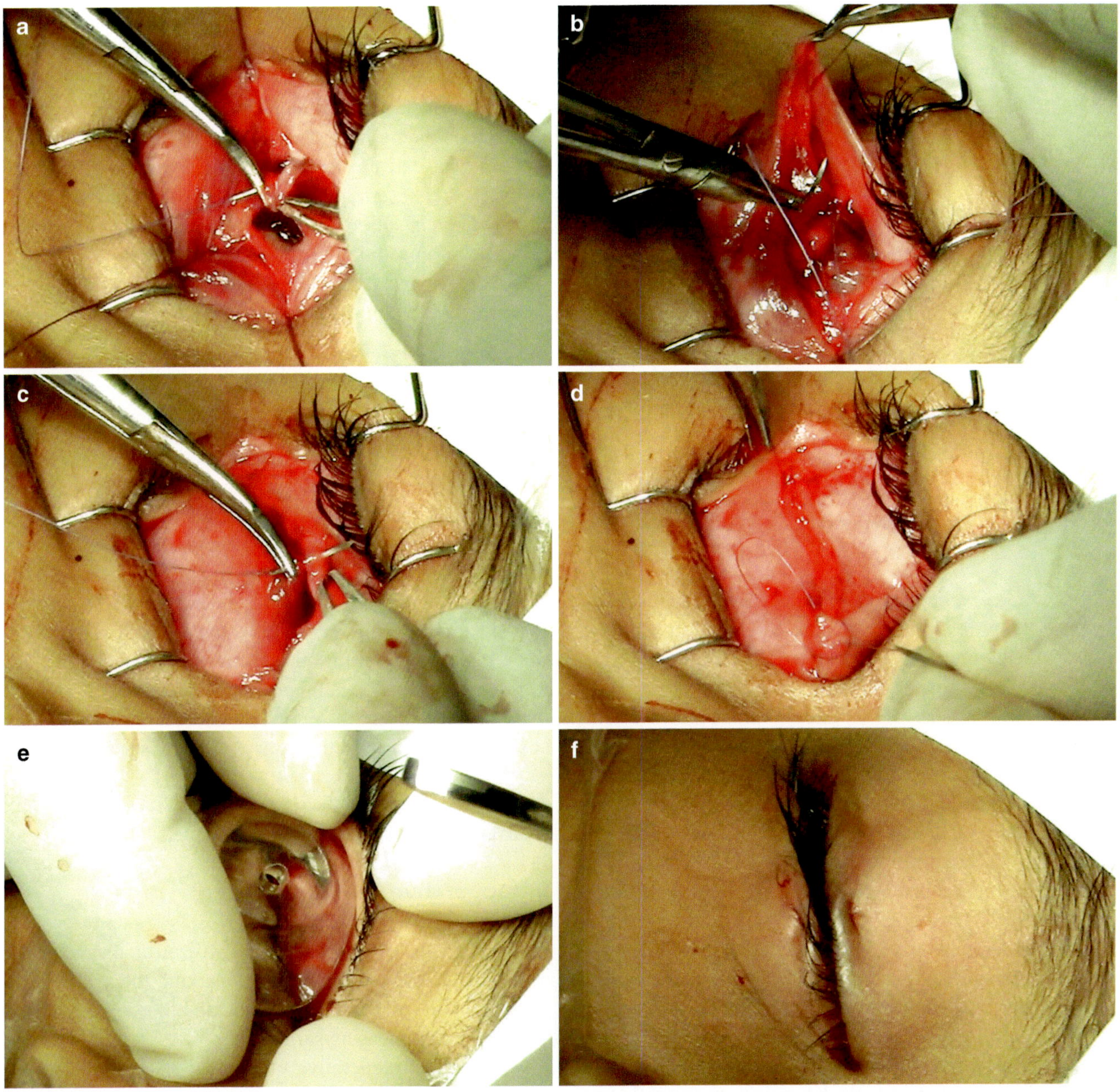

Fig. 59.4 Enucleation, surgical closure. The posterior Tenon's fascia is closed with interrupted absorbable sutures (**a**). The extraocular muscles are attached to the fornix by passing the double-armed Vicryl sutures out through the space between Tenon's and conjunctiva (**b**). The anterior Tenon's layer is closed with buried sutures (**c**). The conjunctiva is closed in a continuous fashion (**d**). A conformer is placed (**e**), followed by a temporary suture tarsorrhaphy (**f**)

- Severing the optic nerve is a critical step. One study reported that longer optic nerve segments were obtained at enucleation with mildly curved scissor blades from both temporal and nasal surgical approaches, but strongly curved scissors produced smaller specimens [6]. This is particularly important when enucleating eyes with intraocular malignancies, especially retinoblastoma. Obtaining a long optic nerve segment, such as 10 mm, allows pathology to evaluate whether the entire tumor has been removed since retinoblastoma commonly spreads via extension into the optic nerve (Fig. 59.5) [6].
- The tips of the scissors should be used to cut the nerve, in order to avoid transecting the muscles in the posterior orbit adjacent to the nerve. Once the tips are straddling the optic nerve, the tips should be tipped back towards the back of the orbit to avoid shortening the nerve segment as a result of the curved blades.

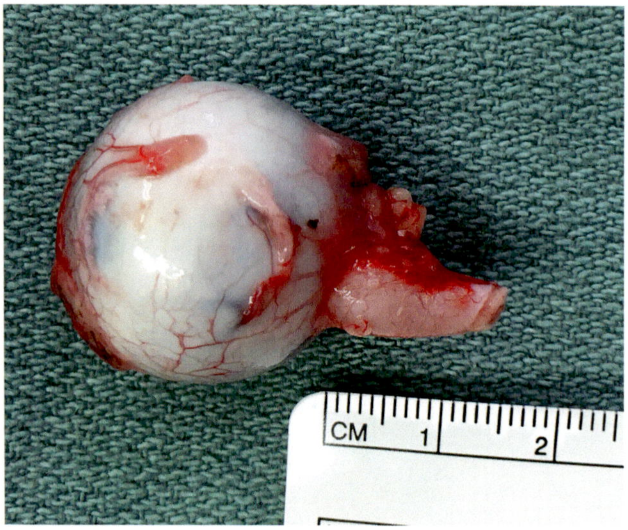

Fig. 59.5 Enucleation that includes a long segment of optic nerve is critical in cases of intraocular malignancy

- Once the nerve is cut, the globe is released and scissors are used to divide the remaining soft tissue attachments from the globe.
- The globe is placed in formalin for histopathology.
- Hemostasis is achieved by posterior orbital pressure using gauze for several minutes. Some surgeons will use bipolar cautery or hemostats to clamp the optic nerve prior to transection, to minimize bleeding. However, in cases of intraocular malignancy with concern for metastasis through the optic nerve, these techniques may limit the pathological specimen due to thermal or crush artifact of the nerve.
- An appropriately sized orbital implant is selected, typically a sphere, and placed within the muscle cone. This space can be identified by the presence of orbital fat and is posterior to Tenon's capsule. Ideally, an implant that is at least 20 mm in size should be placed to minimize postoperative superior sulcus deformity or anophthalmic socket syndrome from volume loss. Intraoperative implant sizers can help to determine the size selected, and often 20 mm implants can be placed even in children to facilitate stimulation of normal orbitofacial growth.
- The Tenon's capsule is closed in two distinct layers over the anterior implant using 4-0 or 5-0 absorbable polyglactin buried sutures.
- In the myoconjunctival technique, the previously secured rectus muscle edges are passed through the overlying conjunctiva and tied. The distance between the edge of the conjunctiva and the site of passing these sutures is approximately the same distance between the limbus and the insertions of the respective recti. Thus, the recti are attached "myoconjunctivally" to fornices on all four sides.
- The conjunctiva is closed in a continuous running or running locking fashion using absorbable sutures, such as 5-0 or 6-0 plain gut.
- A conformer is placed along with antibiotic ointment to maintain the fornices. This generic conformer is replaced with a custom prosthesis typically 2 months postoperatively after ensuring the socket has healed completely.
- A temporary suture tarsorrhaphy can be placed to provide pressure (in addition to an external gauze pressure patch) after surgery and is usually removed at the 1-week follow-up visit.

In addition to the myoconjunctival technique described here, other preferred enucleation techniques include suturing the muscles directly on the anterior face of the implant approximately 5–10 mm apart, or the imbrication technique, where the superior rectus is imbricated (overlapped and sutured) with the inferior rectus, and similarly, the medial rectus is imbricated with lateral rectus. In the integrated implant technique, where a porous implant is used, the muscles are directly sutured to the anterior implant surface, scleral cap, or the mesh used to wrap the implant. Although some surgeons prefer to suture the muscles in position close to former anatomic location, there are no studies to support that implant motility is improved over suturing the muscles close to one another on the anterior implant surface.

Complications of Enucleation

Intraoperative Complications

Enucleating the wrong eye is a grave error that must be avoided by clear communication, marking the eye prior to incision by the performing surgeon, and thorough examination before commencing surgery [1].

Common intraoperative complications include orbital hemorrhage and loss of muscle (slipped muscle). With the authorization of the treating cardiologist or primary care physician, patients should discontinue anticoagulant medications at least a week before surgery to minimize the risk of uncontrolled bleeding and postoperative hemorrhage.

In most cases of intraoperative bleeding, prolonged pressure using gauze will stop bleeding. Other options include injecting local anesthetic with epinephrine before cutting the optic nerve, or clamping a hemostat forceps around the nerve for a minute prior to transection [7]. In rare cases, orbital exploration may be required to identify the bleeding vessel and coagulate it with bipolar cautery. The use of gelfoam is also helpful in stopping such bleeds. The loss of a muscle can be prevented by tagging of the muscle prior to releasing it from the scleral insertion. However, the muscle can often be identified in the posterior orbit; following the muscular sheath can help locate the muscle if needed.

Postoperative Complications

Normal postoperative healing includes eyelid and socket edema, ecchymosis, and chemosis. Early postoperative complications may include hemorrhage, significant conjunctival prolapse, chemosis, and rarely infection. Conjunctival prolapse that falls over the lower eyelid margin or limits eyelid closure can usually be avoided by placing a suture tarsorrhaphy at the time of surgery.

Dehiscence of the wound with exposure of the implant, or even extrusion, can rarely occur, especially in the setting of a sudden orbital hemorrhage due to anticoagulants or Valsalva (Fig. 59.6). Meticulous layered tissue closure often minimizes this complication, as well as the tarsorrhaphy that provides pressure and prevents forward extrusion. Placing the appropriate size implant during surgery also needs to balance the need to replace orbital volume while avoiding too large an implant that increases the risk of dehiscence and exposure. Implant exposure and extrusion can be early or late complications, and have systemic factors as well.

The most common late complication following enucleation is post-enucleation socket syndrome (PESS). This term encompasses multiple clinical manifestations such as upper eyelid ptosis, enophthalmos, superior sulcus deformity, shallow anterior fornix, atrophy of orbital tissue, and entropion or ectropion of the lower lid. Enophthalmos occurs due to inadequate orbital volume replacement and can manifest as the surgical eye looking "sunken" or the contralateral eye appearing proptotic. A superior sulcus deformity is also primarily a sequelae of orbital volume deficit and loss of tone of the orbital tissues. It appears as a deep, darkly shadowed, groove or space between the upper eyelid and orbital rim, further exacerbating the appearance of enophthalmos and ptosis [1]. When multiple aspects of PESS are present, the orbital aperture size appears diminished, resulting in facial asymmetry and a less aesthetically acceptable outcome. In mild cases, the ocular prosthesis can be enlarged or the superior aspect modified such that more volume is incorporated and the superior ledge lifts the ptotic eyelid further.

Lower eyelid malposition can occur due to uncorrected eyelid laxity, or as a result of a heavy ocular prosthesis that creates mechanical ectropion. The fornix may be further obliterated with inferior fornix fat prolapse (Fig. 59.7), and in combination with ectropion, will result in the prosthesis sliding out of the socket. Lower eyelid malposition can be corrected using the normal techniques described in a separate chapter of this text.

Evisceration

Evisceration of the eye refers to removal of the intraocular contents, leaving the external shell, the sclera, intact. Typically, an implant is placed within the scleral shell with layered closure over it. An evisceration can also be performed comfortably under local anesthesia (peribulbar). While multiple variations in surgical technique exist, the primary steps remain the same (Figs. 59.8 and 59.9).

- As is the case in enucleation, it is important to recheck and confirm the correct eye to be operated upon before placing the speculum.
- A 360 ° peritomy is performed with Westcott scissors—a subconjunctival injection of anesthetic with epinephrine creates hydrodissection to facilitate easy peritomy. It is important to preserve as much conjunctiva as possible by incising the conjunctiva close to the limbus.

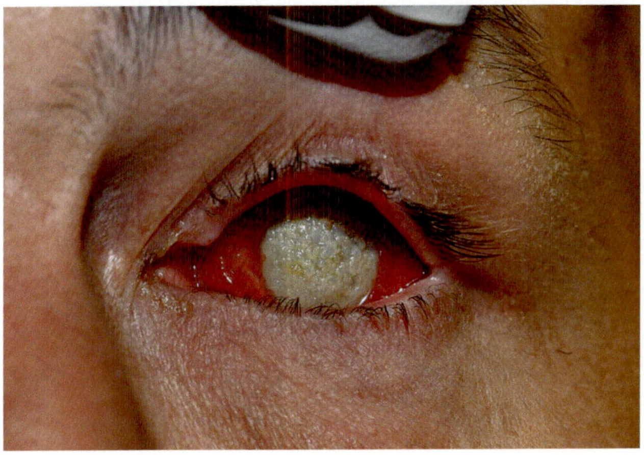

Fig. 59.6 Large exposure of a porous implant. Primary tissue closure over the implant is not possible with this size defect

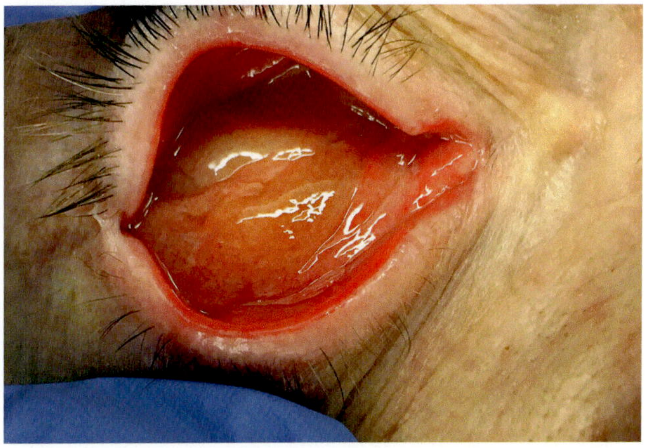

Fig. 59.7 The inferior fornix may be shallowed or obliterated with socket fat prolapse that may affect the ability to retain an ocular prosthesis, particularly when in combination with lower eyelid laxity

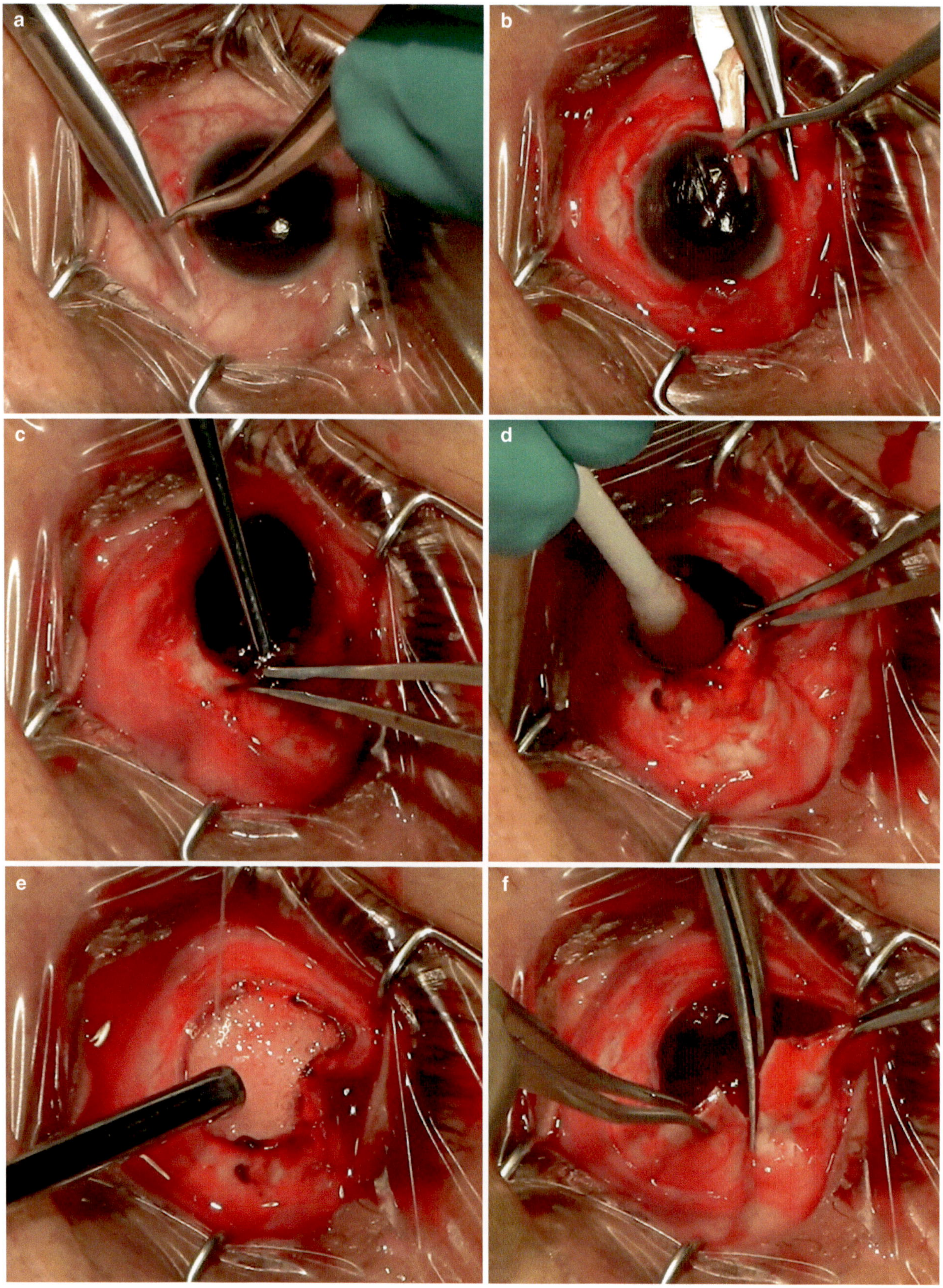

Fig. 59.8 Evisceration surgical steps. A 360 ° peritomy (**a**) is followed by removal of the corneal button (**b**). Dissection and complete removal of the intraocular contents (**c**) is followed by using absolute dehydrated alcohol to clean inside the scleral shell to denature residual uveal tissue (**d**). A thorough saline wash is essential as any residual alcohol can lead to severe postoperative inflammation (**e**). In this figure, scleral petals are fashioned by performing vertically linear cuts between each of the rectus muscles (**f**)

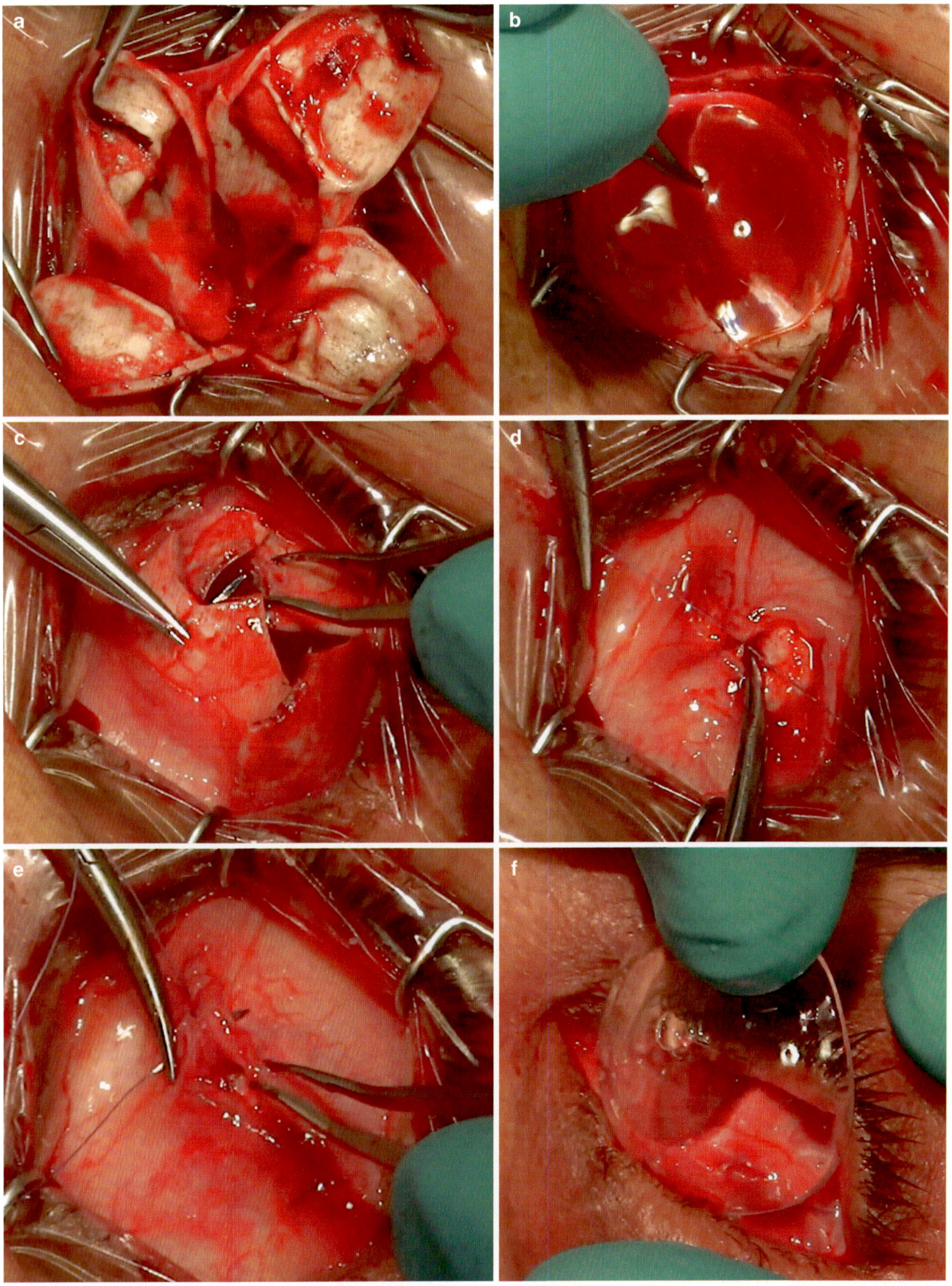

Fig. 59.9 Evisceration, four-petal technique. The scleral incisions extend posteriorly to the optic nerve attachment (**a**), and a circular posterior sclerotomy is incised around the optic nerve head. The implant is placed within the four petals (**b**) and the petals are overlapped and sutured to each other over the implant to provide maximum coverage (**c**). The Tenon's fascia is closed with absorbable sutures (**d**), followed by closure of the conjunctiva (**e**). A conformer is placed to maintain the fornices for a future prosthesis (**f**)

- A full-thickness limbal incision is made with an 11 or 15 scalpel blade while holding the adjacent sclera for countertraction.
- The entire corneal button is cut out with scissors. Some surgeons may leave the corneal button on, although most will remove the cornea which is often diseased or unhealthy (Fig. 59.8).
- Intraocular contents are then removed with the aid of an evisceration spoon, Freer periosteal elevator, or a scoop which is a round, flat curette. The instrument needs to be able to create a cleavage plane between the choroid and the sclera. Meticulous removal of all uveal tissue is essential—theoretically, this step decreases the potential risk of sympathetic ophthalmia [8].
- After removal of all uveal tissue, the inside surface of the scleral shell is vigorously cleaned with multiple cotton tip applicators dipped in absolute dehydrated alcohol. This causes denaturation of any residual uveal protein that might otherwise incite inflammation or present as the antigenic stimulus for sympathetic ophthalmia. Care should be taken to avoid dripping alcohol on the conjunctiva or socket tissues.
- The surgical field must then be thoroughly irrigated with saline to remove any residual alcohol that can cause postoperative inflammation.
- Two anterior scleral Burow's triangles are excised, 180 ° apart and between the rectus insertions, that will later facilitate suture of the sclera over the implant without a standing defect (dog ear).
- The orbital sphere implant is placed in the socket, either within the retained scleral shell, or placed behind the sclera. Whereas placement inside the sclera is simpler and requires less dissection, this can limit the size of implant that can be placed, particularly if the globe was phthisical or compressed by scleral bands or glaucoma implants (Fig. 59.10). One of the surgeons prefers using a modification of the transcleral technique originally described by Long et al. [9]. This technique requires opening the posterior sclera with a long linear incision that extends forward to just short of the anterior scleral edge. Through this incision, the optic nerve is then cauterized or clamped, and transected to release the posterior sclera. A large implant can then be easily placed through this posterior sclerotomy into the retrobulbar intraconal space—even in severely phthisical globes, a 20–23 mm implant can be placed as opposed to a smaller implant that would result in PESS. The freed posterior sclera is then pulled forward over the implant and essentially folded into itself to rest just under the anterior scleral edges. The other benefit of this technique is the double layer of sclera sutured over the implant that further minimizes the risk of implant exposure and extrusion.

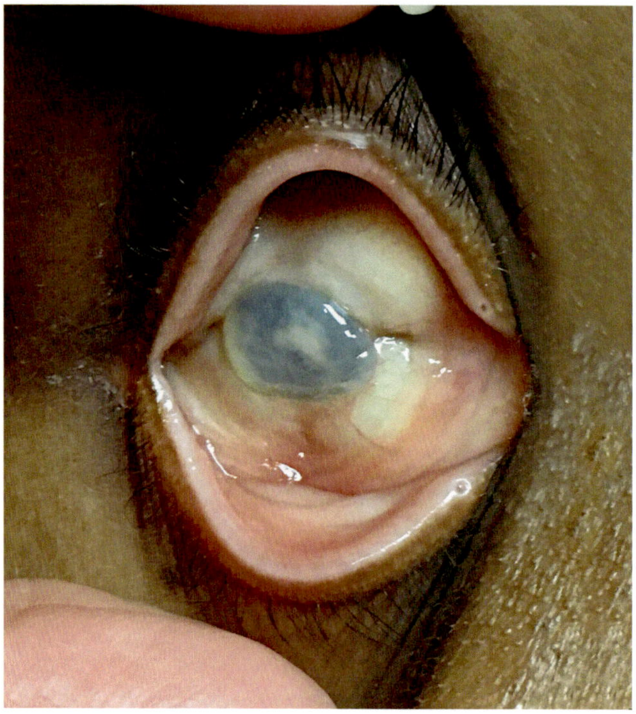

Fig. 59.10 Significant phthisis of the globe can limit the size orbital implant that can be placed within the scleral shell. The transcleral modification or other posterior sclerotomy techniques are indicated

- If placement inside the scleral shell is preferred, multiple sclerotomy techniques have been described to allow larger implants. One technique is to fashion four petals by creating linear sclerotomies in between the four rectus muscles [10]. The incisions extend from the scleral rim and run posteriorly to the optic nerve head insertion (Fig. 59.9). A circular posterior sclerotomy is performed around the optic nerve head to detach the nerve from the scleral petals, each of which is attached to a rectus muscle. The implant of choice is placed within the scleral petals. Layered closure is performed with overlap of the anterior edges of the petals.
- Tenon's fascia and conjunctiva are closed in layers with nonabsorbable sutures, as described for enucleation.
- A conformer lubricated with antibiotic ointment is placed, as well as a temporary tarsorrhaphy and/or pressure patch.
- Retrobulbar injection of bupivacaine after enucleation or evisceration can provide several hours of postoperative analgesia, if desired.
- A customized ocular prosthesis is placed after 4–8 weeks, depending on socket healing and the preference of the ocularist.

Of note, there are many different techniques for creating sclerotomies and scleral relaxing incisions to accommodate larger implants. Lee and colleagues advocated the creation of scleral windows posterior to each of the rectus muscle insertion [11]. Jordan and Anderson described a technique that involved disinsertion of the optic nerve and the creation of small radial sclerotomies [12]. Another technique called the "scleral quadrisection" has also been described by Yang et al. [13]. Massry and Hold have described obliquely splitting the scleral cavity into two sections, and releasing the flaps from their optic nerve attachments [14]. Some of the authors prefer the four-petal technique, described by Sales-Sanz and Sanz-Lopez, which created four complete sclerotomies from limbus to the optic nerve, with optic nerve disinsertion. These four petals, attached to a rectus muscle each, are then brought anteriorly to cover the implant [10]. Georgescu described a technique that was useful for phthisis bulbi and microphthalmos. In this technique, a 5-mm wedge of sclera was excised nasally and temporally and a 360 ° equatorial scleral incision was made, dividing the scleral into anterior and posterior halves [15].

Kaltreider and Lucarelli proposed an algorithm for selecting an implant size for patients undergoing enucleation, evisceration, and secondary implantation. Axial length of the contralateral eye was measured, and then 2 mm subtracted from it (to account for the scleral shell) to give the implant diameter. However, for evisceration and hyperopia, only 1 mm was subtracted. They found this formula allowed for 100% replacement of the volume removed and left space for a prosthesis of approximately 1.5–2.5 mm. It also minimized clinically unacceptable superior sulcus deformity and enophthalmos in most patients [16]. However, this algorithm results in additional costs for obtaining axial length measurements, and is not routinely used. Alternatively, sizers can be used intraoperatively to help in determining the ideal implant size that maximizes volume without creating tension on the wound.

Historically, the literature has suggested that evisceration was indicated for severe penetrating ocular trauma, despite the possibility of sympathetic ophthalmia. In such cases, the rationale behind evisceration was that removal of the eye (or its contents) prior to sensitization could be preventive. More recent studies have suggested that in severe ocular trauma with extensive disruption of the globe, it may not be feasible to reliably remove all uveal tissue in an evisceration. Therefore, enucleation may theoretically minimize the risk of sympathetic ophthalmia better [8].

An absolute contraindication for evisceration is suspected intraocular malignancy [17]. Otherwise, evisceration has traditionally been the procedure of choice for infections such as endophthalmitis, and enucleation is required for intraocular malignancies. For other indications such as a disfigured or painful blind eye, phthisis bulbi, or end-stage glaucoma, surgeons show varying preferences with no clear benefit between the two surgeries.

Orbital Implants

At the time of evisceration and enucleation, it is important to place an orbital implant in suitable cases. Although the primary function of implants is to replace lost orbital volume, they also have roles in promoting orbitofacial growth (especially in children), preventing socket contraction, and helping in motility of the final prosthesis. There are many different types of implants and multiple classification systems. Implants can be classified by shape, size, material, integration, and other means. An important and basic simplification is the division of implants into two groups: porous (bio-integrated) and nonporous or inert (non-integrated). The choice of implant type, and the different advantages and disadvantages of each, is covered in detail in a separate chapter.

Non-integrated implants typically do not have any provisions for attachment of the extraocular muscles or to the ocular prosthesis. They also do not allow for ingrowth of fibrovascular tissue. Resultant ocular motility using inert orbital implants is, therefore, the movement transmitted from the nonporous implant through the surface tension in the interface between the conjunctiva and the posterior surface of the ocular prosthesis, as well as movement of the fornices.

In order to allow for better prosthesis motility, these implants can be wrapped in any of a number of materials, such as donor sclera, bovine pericardium, processed human pericardium, polytetrafluoroethylene (e-PTFE), polyglactin mesh, among others [18]. The extraocular materials can then be secured to the wrapping material. However, non-integrated implants do not attach or directly interact with the prosthesis. Commonly used non-integrated, nonporous implants are polymethylmethacrylate (PMMA), silicone, glass, rubber, steel, gold, silver, and acrylic [19].

In contrast, porous implants allow for fibrovascular ingrowth throughout the implant, which may theoretically improve motility and/or decrease the risk of implant extrusion. The insertion of pegs that are directly connected to the posterior prosthesis can also be performed at 6–8 months after the initial surgery, once the implant is completely vascularized. Directly integrating the implant to the prosthesis through an externalized coupling mechanism would ideally provide the highest degree of prosthesis motility. However, pegged implants have been associated with increased risk of delayed implant infection, implant exposure, infection, and need for socket revision; thus, have largely fallen out of popularity.

Attachment of the extraocular muscles to the implant or its wrapping material is believed to improve implant motility and reduce the risk of implant migration. The amount of movement transmitted from the implant to the prosthesis determines the degree of final prosthetic motility.

Another category of implants includes the quasi-integrated implants, such as the Allen and the Iowa implants. These implants have irregularly shaped surfaces that create an indirect coupling mechanism between the implant and prosthesis. This is believed to impart a higher degree of movement to the prosthesis, without the risks associated with drilling a peg directly into the implant.

Porous orbital implants are manufactured from different materials including natural and synthetic sources. These materials are namely hydroxyapatite, aluminum oxide, and polyethylene. Hydroxyapatite is formed from a salt of calcium phosphate that is present in the mineralized portion of human bone and is reported to be nontoxic, nonallergenic, and biocompatible [1, 20]. While hydroxyapatite implants are typically spherical in shape and commercially available in many sizes, aluminum oxide and porous polyethylene implants are available in different shapes and sizes. Porous implants were historically thought to offer better implant movement than non-integrated implants due to direct muscle attachment to the implant, although this remains controversial [21].

Ceramic implants have gained some recent popularity primarily due to a highly interconnected pore network which allows them to act as a passive framework for host fibrovascular ingrowth. This fibrovascular integration with orbital tissue offers, at least theoretically, low complication rates with pegging while increasing motility of the prosthesis. The vascularization of porous implants was also thought to reduce the incidence of implant migration, exposure, and extrusion [22]. Furthermore, vascularization of a porous implant was believed to increase the success rate of surgical repair by conjunctival closure or patch grafting in cases of implant exposure [1, 23]. In contrast, some studies have demonstrated that porous implants were found to have higher exposure rates overall when compared to smoother synthetic implants [24].

Many factors are implicated in the development of implant exposure, such as postoperative infection, poor wound healing, or ill-fitting prostheses. Very small or tight prostheses can lead to development of pressure points between the implant and prosthesis, that over time, can result in a defect in the intervening conjunctiva and subsequent exposure/extrusion. Exposed implants can also be a nidus for further infection. In some cases, small defects over porous implants may close spontaneously or heal with simple closure of the conjunctiva and Tenon's layer. Most exposures require additional procedures such as scleral or mucous membrane patch grafts to promote conjunctival healing. Other materials that have been used to cover an exposed implant include hard palate mucosa, dermis fat graft (DFG), buccal mucosa, temporalis fascia, or amniotic membrane. The use of autologous serum drops to promote epithelial healing following surgery to cover the defect has also been reported [25]. If the exposure is large and the conjunctival surface area is limited, attempts to close the tissues over the implant will likely fail. Additionally, the implant needs to be removed if infected. In these cases, dermis fat grafts can provide excellent volume to the orbit, in addition to the dermal side contributing surface area to the conjunctiva to avoid fornix shortening and socket contracture.

Placement of an implant in an enucleation or evisceration being performed for fulminant infection is a controversial question. Conventional teaching states that in the presence of infection, the placement of a foreign body implant may hamper wound healing, delay infection clearance, and risk implant exposure and extrusion. However, many recent studies have reported the contrary, stating that evisceration with primary porous implant placement can be a viable treatment option for patients with endophthalmitis. Very few postoperative complications of implant exposure and infection were reported [26]. Tripathy and Rath reported that evisceration with primary placement of nonporous silicone implants in fulminant endophthalmitis/panophthalmitis provided good postoperative cosmetic outcome at an economical cost [27].

In summary, enucleation and evisceration surgeries may both be indicated in cases of painful blind eyes, but enucleation remains the procedure of choice when surgery is being performed on eyes with intraocular tumors. Whenever possible, adequate volume replacement with implants or dermis fat grafts should be done to reduce the potential for clinically apparent volume deficit within the anophthalmic socket. Conformers should be placed following surgery, to optimize the fornices prior to fitting of the final custom prosthesis. Factors, such as variations in surgical technique and the implant material and shape, are largely dependent on surgeon preferences.

Financial Disclosures None of the authors have any financial interests to disclose.

References

1. Moshfeghi DM, Moshfeghi AA, Finger PT. Enucleation. Surv Ophthalmol. 2000;44(4):277–301.
2. Beard CH. Enucleation. In: Ophthalmic surgery. Philadelphia: P. Blakiston's Son & Co; 1910. p. 457–77.
3. Nunery WR, Chen WP. Enucleation and evisceration. In: Bosniak S, editor. Principles and practice of ophthalmic plastic and reconstructive surgery, vol. 2. Philadelphia: W.B. Saunders Company; 1996. p. 1035–46.
4. Galor A, Davis JL, Flynn HW Jr, Feuer WJ, Dubovy SR, Setlur V, Kesen MR, Goldstein DA, Tessler HH, Ganelis IB, Jabs DA, Thorne JE. Sympathetic ophthalmia: incidence of ocular complications and vision loss in the sympathizing eye. Am J Ophthalmol. 2009;148(5):704–710.e2.

5. Shome D, Honavar SG, Raizada K, Raizada D. Implant and prosthesis movement after enucleation: a randomized controlled trial. Ophthalmology. 2010;117(8):1638–44.
6. Coats DK, Paysse EA, Chu Y. Obtaining maximal optic nerve length during Enucleation procedure. Arch Ophthalmol. 2000;118(1):70–3.
7. Stone W. Complications of evisceration and enucleation. In: Fasanella RM, editor. Management of complications in eye surgery. Philadelphia: W.B. Saunders; 1957. p. 278–317.
8. Phan LT, Hwang TN, McCulley TJ. Evisceration in the modern age. Middle East Afr J Ophthalmol. 2012;19(1):24–33.
9. Long JA, Tann TM, Girkin CA. Evisceration: a new technique of transcleral implant placement. Ophthal Plast Reconstr Surg. 2000;16:3225.
10. Sales-Sanz M, Sanz-Lopez A. Four-petal evisceration: a new technique. Ophthal Plast Reconstr Surg. 2007;23:389–92.
11. Lee SY, Kwon OW, Hong YJ, Kim HB, Kim SJ. Modification of the scleral openings to reduce tissue breakdown and exposure after hydroxyapatite implantations. Ophthalmologica. 1995;209:319–22.
12. Jordan DR, Anderson RL. The universal implant for evisceration surgery. Ophthal Plast Reconstr Surg. 1997;13:1–7.
13. Yang JG, Khwarg SI, Wee WR, Kim DM, Lee JH. Hydroxyapatite implantation with scleral quadrisection after evisceration. Ophthal Surg Lasers. 1997;28:915–9.
14. Massry GG, Holds JB. Evisceration with scleral modification. Ophthal Plast Recosntr Surg. 2001;17:42–7.
15. Georgescu D, Vagefi MR, Yang CC, McCann J, Anderson RL. Evisceration with equatorial sclerotomy for phthisis bulbi and microphthalmos. Ophthal Plast Reconstr Surg. 2010;3:165–7.
16. Kaltreider SA, Lucarelli MJ. A simple algorithm for selection of implant size for enucleation and evisceration: a prospective study. Ophthalmic Plast Reconstr Surg. 2002;18(5):336–41.
17. Manschot WA, van Peperzeel HA. Choroidal melanoma. Enucleation or observation? A new approach. Arch Ophthalmol. 1980;98:71–7.
18. Klapper SR, Jordan DR, Punja K, Brownstein S, Gilberg SM, Mawn LA, Grahovac SZ. Hydroxyapatite implant wrapping materials: analysis of fibrovascular ingrowth in an animal model. Ophthalmic Plast Reconstr Surg. 2000;16(4):278–85.
19. Beard C. Remarks on historical and newer approaches to orbital implants. Ophthalmic Plast Reconstr Surg. 1995;11:89–90.
20. Perry AC. Integrated orbital implants. Adv Ophthalmic Plast Reconstr Surg. 1990;8:75–81.
21. Shields CL, Shields JA, De Potter P, Singh AD. Problems with the hydroxyapatite orbital implant: experience with 250 consecutive cases. Br J Ophthalmol. 1994;78:702–6.
22. Jordan DR, Chan S, Mawn L, et al. Complications associated with pegging hydroxyapatite orbital implants. Ophthalmology. 1999;106:505–12.
23. Shields C, Shields J, Eagle R Jr, De Potter P. Histopathologic evidence of fibrovascular ingrowth four weeks after placement of the hydroxyapatite orbital implant. Am J Ophthalmol. 1991;111:363–6.
24. Custer PL, Kennedy RH, Woog JJ, et al. Orbital implants in enucleation surgery: a report by the American Academy of ophthalmology. Ophthalmology. 2003;110:2054–61.
25. Kamal S, Kumar S, Goel R. Autologous serum for anterior tissue necrosis after porous orbital implant. Middle East Afr J Ophthalmol. 2014;21(2):193–5.
26. Park YG, Paik JS, Yang SW. The results of evisceration with primary porous implant placement in patients with endophthalmitis. Korean J Ophthalmol. 2010;24(5):279–83.
27. Tripathy D, Rath S. Evisceration with primary orbital implant in fulminant Endophthalmitis/Panophthalmitis. Orbit. 2015;34(5):279–83.

Orbital Exenteration

60

Leon Rafailov, Roger E. Turbin, and Paul D. Langer

Background

Orbital exenteration, first described by George Bartisch in 1583 [1], is a surgery in which the globe and the surrounding orbital contents are surgically removed. Over the years, this surgery has evolved to allow varying degrees of tissue excision, with modern techniques permitting more conservative surgical approaches to spare tissue removal when possible and more extensive exenterations involving removal of orbital bone when necessary. Despite the progress in technique, orbital exenteration remains a surgery of last resort after all medical and other therapeutic options have been exhausted.

The indications for exenteration vary, but the surgery is performed most commonly to remove a malignant neoplasm; less frequently, exenteration is required to treat a benign neoplasm, an infection, or an inflammatory process. The great majority of neoplasms requiring exenteration are locally advanced skin cancers including basal cell carcinoma, sebaceous cell carcinoma, and squamous cell carcinoma, as well as melanomas of the conjunctiva and choroid with orbital invasion [2]. Exenteration may also be necessary for primary orbital tumors (such as sarcomas or lacrimal gland carcinomas) and for orbital extension of a sinus or intracranial malignancy. Locally advanced basal cell and squamous cell carcinomas remain the most common indications for surgery [3, 4], though newer chemotherapeutic agents such as hedgehog inhibitors may ultimately reduce the number of exenterations due to these skin cancers [5]. Exenteration to eradicate infection is reserved for cases of life-threatening disease and/or highly ischemic processes (e.g., mucormycosis and necrotizing fasciitis) that are poorly responsive to medical therapy and require debridement of widespread devascularized tissue [6–9]. Other much less common indications for exenteration include a blind painful orbit that may result from nonmalignant processes or infiltrative inflammatory diseases (such as extensive, uncontrolled sclerosing pseudotumor) and disfiguring neoplasms (such as massive lymphangiomas or neurofibromas), in which the disfigurement is so severe that an exenteration prosthetic provides the only cosmetically preferable alternative to the disease [10].

Patient Preparation

A generous amount of time should be spent counseling the patient and family members regarding the extensive nature of the surgery and the need for diligent postoperative care. It is important for patients to realize that while the surgery is disfiguring, there is potential for acceptable cosmetic rehabilitation. Determining whether a patient wants to wear a prosthesis may influence the technique used for reconstruction. In many cases, patients may elect to simply wear an eye patch despite reconstructive efforts to improve appearance [11].

The preoperative physical examination should include palpation of regional lymph nodes and testing of facial sensation, specifically to assess the function of the frontal and infraorbital nerves. In cases where patients have been referred from outside hospitals, it is prudent to obtain the original histopathology slides to confirm the diagnosis. The extent of disease and the possibility of metastatic spread must be determined prior to surgery, in many cases warranting positron emission tomography (PET) scanning and collaboration with an oncologist. The future need for radiation therapy should be determined if possible prior to surgery, as this factor may influence the technique chosen for reconstruction.

Orbital exenteration may be broadly divided into four techniques: standard or total exenteration, eyelid-sparing orbital exenteration, anterior or subtotal orbital exenteration, and extended exenteration.

L. Rafailov · R. E. Turbin · P. D. Langer (✉)
Institute of Ophthalmology and Visual Science, Rutgers New Jersey Medical School, Newark, NJ, USA
e-mail: planger@njms.rutgers.edu

A. J. Cohen, C. N. Burkat (eds.), *Oculofacial, Orbital, and Lacrimal Surgery*, https://doi.org/10.1007/978-3-030-14092-2_60

Standard or Total Exenteration

For all exenteration techniques, general anesthesia is highly preferred, although local anesthesia with sedation has been described [4]. The skin above the orbital rim is marked with a marking pen to outline the planned incision (Fig. 60.1a). If a neoplasm extends beyond the rim, a wider excision may be necessary. Lidocaine with epinephrine is then infiltrated into the skin at the level outside the rim. The upper and lower eyelid margins are secured with 4-0 silk sutures to allow for manipulation and traction during dissection. Then, using either a scalpel or a needle-tipped electrocautery device, the skin and subcutaneous tissue is incised and dissection carried down to the periosteum of the orbital rim for 360 °. The periosteum is incised with electrocautery, and further dissection is carried out in the subperiosteal plane parallel to the walls of the orbit (Fig. 60.1b–c).

The contents of the orbit can then be freed from the orbital walls using blunt dissection down to the orbital apex using a combination of electrocautery and a Freer periosteal elevator. Resistance to blunt dissection may be met when encountering the trochlea, the lateral orbital tubercle, the origin of the inferior oblique, and the insertions of the medial and lateral canthal tendons (Fig. 60.2a–d). The lacrimal sac can be severed at the point where it connects to the common canaliculus, or alternatively, at the point where the sac enters the bony nasolacrimal duct. Electrocautery can be used for hemostasis, especially to cauterize perforating vessels of the bony walls, specifically attending to the anterior and posterior ethmoidal arteries that penetrate the medial wall, and the zygomaticofacial and zygomaticotemporal arteries that emanate from the lateral wall. As the inferior and medial walls of the orbit are very thin, care must be taken not to apply excessive pressure that might create a bony dehiscence and increase the chances of a postoperative sino-orbital fistula.

The supraorbital nerve is generally sacrificed, leading to facial numbness in the V_1 dermatome. The infraorbital nerve can be preserved if not affected by malignancy by dissecting the orbital tissue off the surface of the nerve posteriorly. Both of these nerves and the bony orbital walls may be more reliably protected if using a supraperiosteal approach, which may be indicated with low-malignancy tumors.

Once the orbital contents are freed along the walls of the orbit, and the neurovascular bundles of the superior and inferior orbital fissures are cut, enucleation scissors are placed at the orbital apex and the remaining tissue severed (Figs. 60.1d and 60.2c–d). In some cases, a clamp can be placed around the tissue at the apex of the orbit (similar to the technique sometimes employed in enucleation) and the tissue cut anterior to the clamp. A snare, large Mayo scissors, or electrocautery may also be used in place of enucleation scissors.

In certain cases, when the tumor is believed to be of lower malignant potential, the deeper portions of the orbit can be spared for a subtotal exenteration. This technique uses the same steps as outlined above but the posterior orbital tissue is severed a few centimeters anterior to the apex at the discretion of the surgeon, creating a shallower orbital space that provides a better platform for granulation; however, the residual apical tissue may become a source of frequent bleeding if not cauterized aggressively. In an anterior exenteration, usually performed for untreatable conjunctival malignancies, the resection plane for the removal of the affected tissue lies just posterior to the sclera, often in conjunction with an eyelid-sparing technique (see below).

Once the tissue is removed from the orbit (Fig. 60.3), tamponade is achieved with cotton or gauze packing, which may be soaked with epinephrine, thrombin, or cold saline. Following a period of at least 5 min of pressure-based hemostasis, the packing is removed, and the remaining tissue and large vessels are cauterized.

Eyelid-Sparing Exenteration

Orbital exenteration with eyelid sparing has been introduced as an exenteration technique aimed at reducing the amount of skin removed and therefore improving reconstruction and rehabilitation [12]. This technique is reserved for tumors that do not involve the eyelid skin and most often arise within the orbit or conjunctiva; it can be used with a total exenteration or in an anterior exenteration. The technique differs from the standard technique in that the initial marking for the skin incisions is just outside the eyelid margin beyond the eyelash line. The anterior and posterior lamellae are then separated, and dissection is carried out in a plane parallel to the skin, posterior to the orbicularis oculi muscle, and anterior to the orbital septum, until the orbital rim is reached in all directions (Fig. 60.4). From that point forward, the technique is similar to that of the standard exenteration with the exception that the upper and lower eyelid skin can be approximated at the end of the surgery and sutured at the apex. If an anterior exenteration is performed (e.g., for a conjunctival malignancy), the posterior plane of tissue excision is directly behind the sclera. Upon closing, if there is space remaining between the two skin flaps, that area may be allowed to spontaneously granulate or be covered with a split-thickness skin graft. The preserved orbicularis provides an excellent blood supply to the bed of the orbit and the overlying skin allowing for quick healing (Figs. 60.5a–d and 60.6).

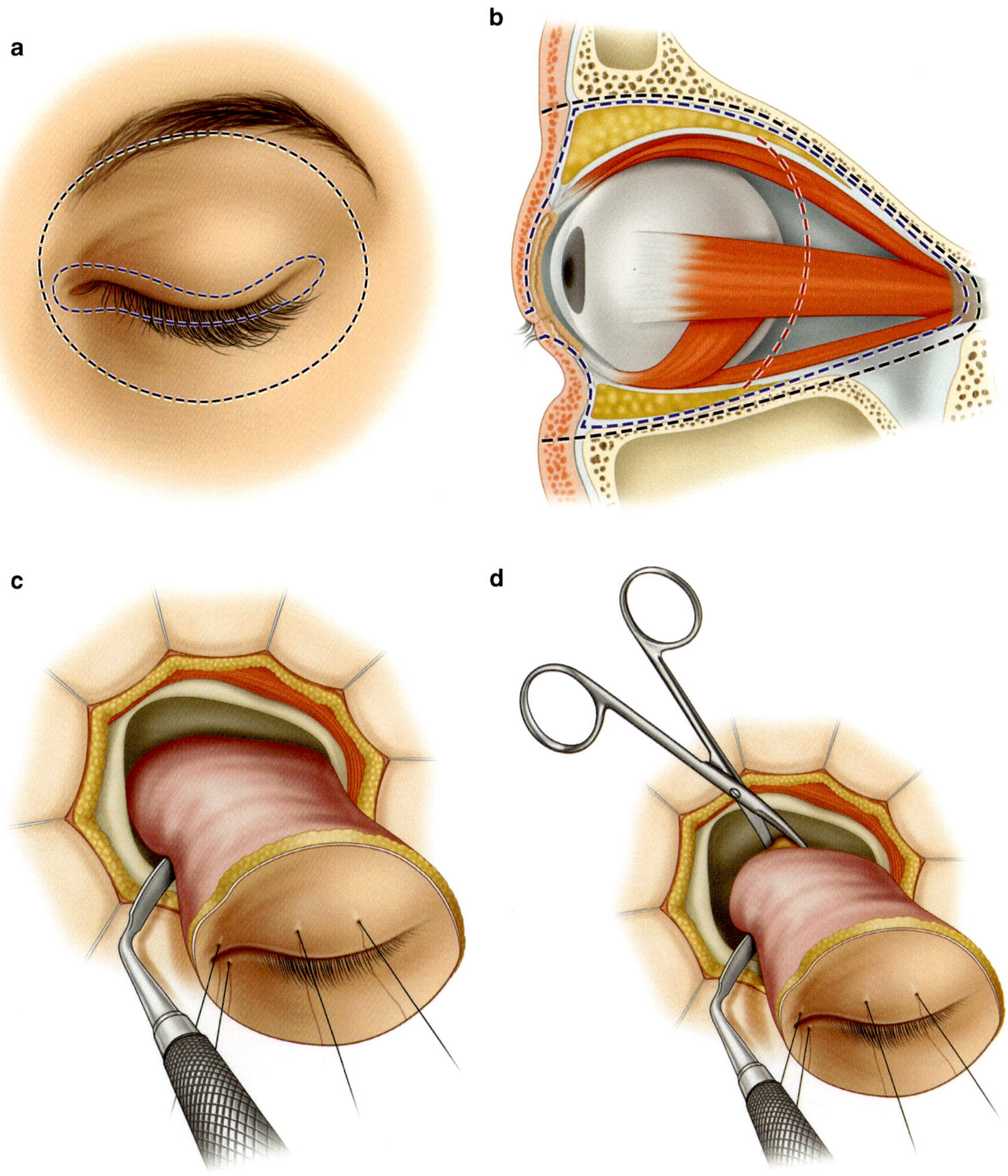

Fig. 60.1 (**a**) Incision lines for standard exenteration (black dotted line) and eyelid sparing exenetration (blue dotted line). (**b**) Sagittal view of incisions and dissection planes for standard exenteration (black dotted line) and eyelid sparing exenteration (blue dotted line). Either approach can be used when performing an anterior exenteration, in which the contents of the orbit are severed just behind the sclera (red dotted line). (**c**) With the aid of Sewall retractors, and using using 4-0 silk sutures for traction, the orbital contents are dissected from the bony orbital walls for 360 degrees down to the apex. (**d**) The tissues at the orbital apex are cut with a Mayo scissors

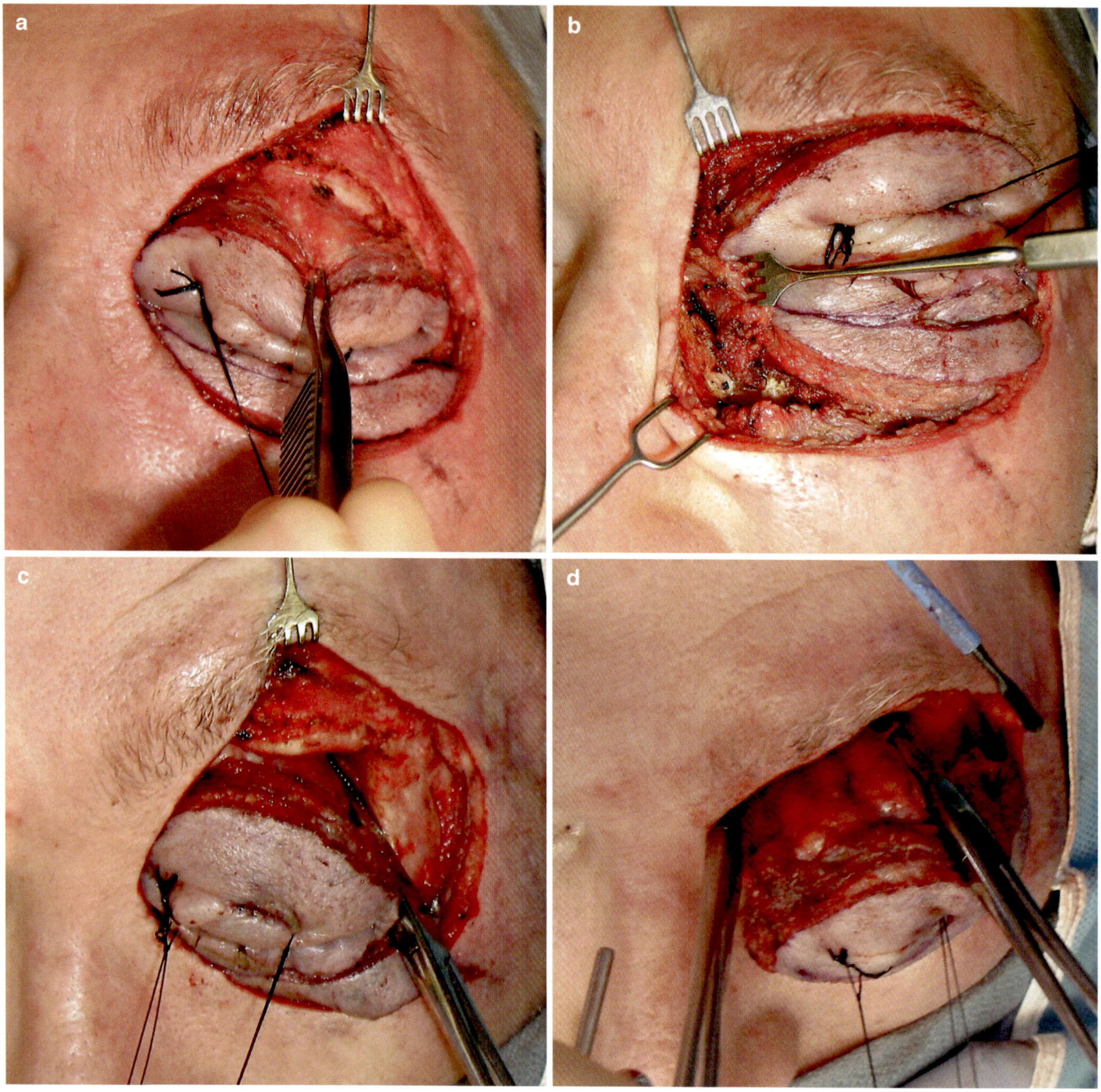

Fig. 60.2 (**a**) Dissection is carried down to the periosteum of the orbital rim for 360 °; (**b**) the medial canthal tendon and lacrimal sac are incised along the medial orbit; (**c**) a clamp can be placed around the tissue at the orbital apex; (**d**) enucleation scissors are used to sever the optic nerve, muscles, and tissues at the posterior orbit. (Photos courtesy of Cat N Burkat, MD FACS)

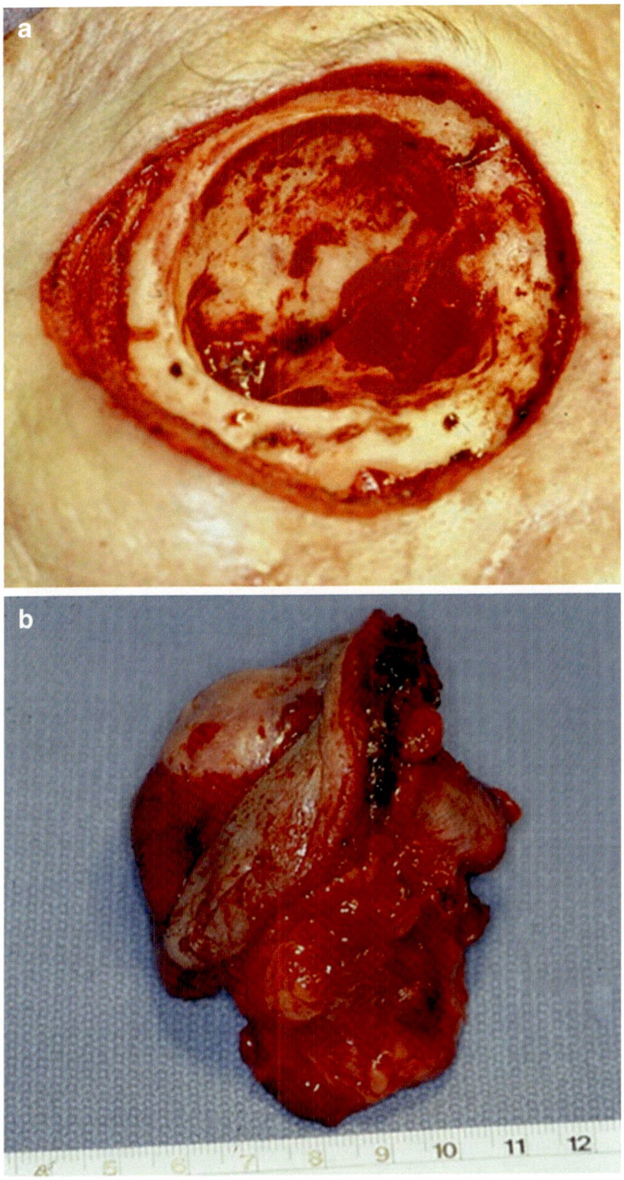

Fig. 60.3 (**a**) Bony walls of the orbit exposed after total exenteration. (**b**) Total exenteration specimen

Super-Exenteration or Extended Exenteration

For tumors invading the bones of the orbit or involving the lacrimal gland, an extended exenteration involving removal of orbital bone and periorbital tissue may be necessary. Often

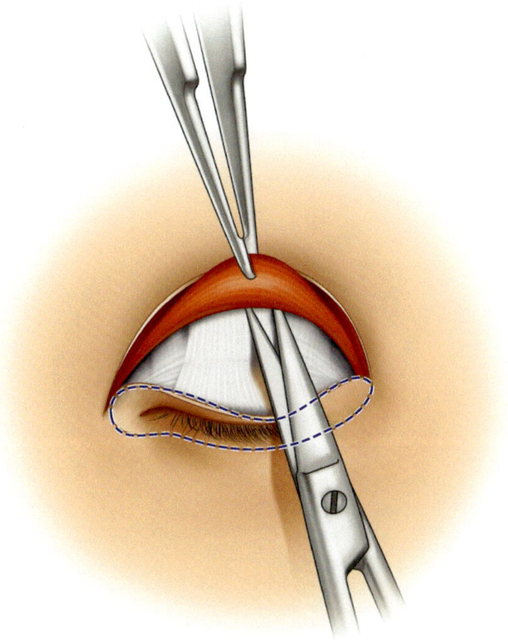

Fig. 60.4 In an eyelid sparing exenteration, a continuous incision is made extending a few millimeters above the upper eyelashes and a few millimeters below the lower eyelashes. A dissection plane (depicted) is then created between the orbicularis muscle and the septum that extends to the orbital rim for 360 degrees

this approach requires a team-based approach in collaboration with colleagues from otolaryngology, neurosurgery, and/or plastic surgery. The techniques for extended exenteration are highly variable and depend largely on the location and type of tumor.

Reconstruction

Reconstruction of the socket is usually performed by lining the socket with a free flap, a regional flap, a split-thickness skin graft, or an artificial dermal graft. Alternatively, the orbit is allowed to epithelialize over time by secondary granulation [13]. Deciding which reconstructive technique to use will require knowledge of the patient's cosmetic goals, sup-

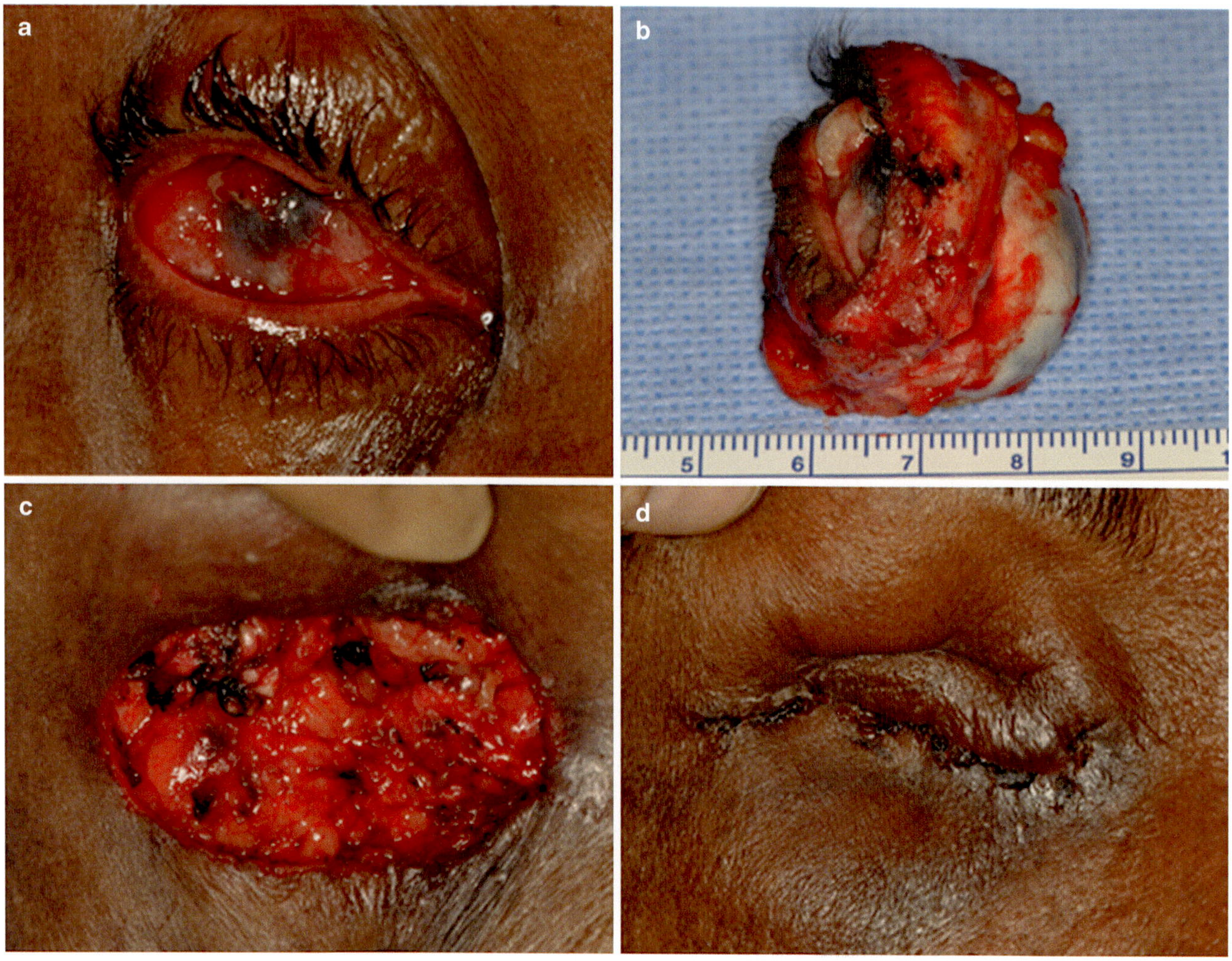

Fig. 60.5 Eyelid-sparing anterior exenteration. (**a**) Clinical photograph showing mucoepidermoid carcinoma involving the cornea and conjunctiva. (**b**) Specimen of anterior exenteration with eyelid-sparing technique. (**c**) Intraoperative photograph demonstrating remaining orbital tissue after anterior exenteration. (**d**) Wound healing and full coverage of the shallow base of the orbit on the ninth postoperative day

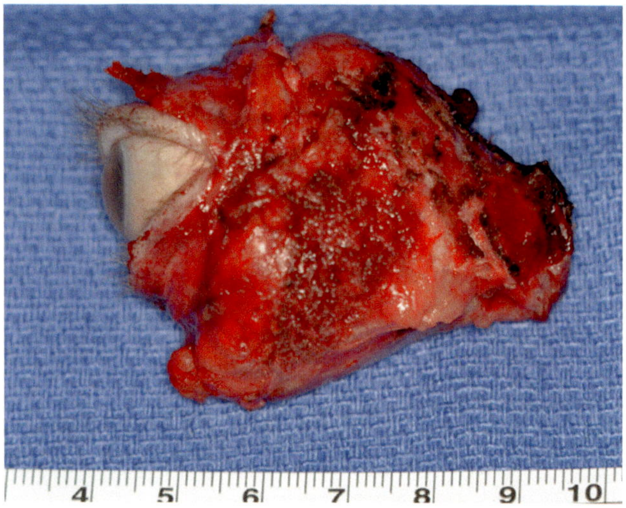

Fig. 60.6 Total exenteration specimen using the eyelid-sparing technique

port system, future plans for prosthetic fitting, and the need for further treatment through radiation.

Spontaneous granulation is the simplest reconstructive technique after uncomplicated exenteration, but it requires additional time and effort in the postoperative period, including frequent dressing changes and office or home debridement for several months [14, 15]. When relying on spontaneous granulation for healing, a gauze covered in antibiotic ointment or a petrolatum gauze is pressure-packed into the orbit at the conclusion of surgery and removed in 5–7 days. The packing is replaced and removed every few days or weekly until the granulation process has completely epithelialized the orbital cavity. In addition to saving time in the operating room and reducing operative morbidity, secondary granulation allows for early detection of recurrent tumor, as the overlying skin tends to be thin. Patients in whom the orbit is allowed to passively granulate must have a dependable support system to allow

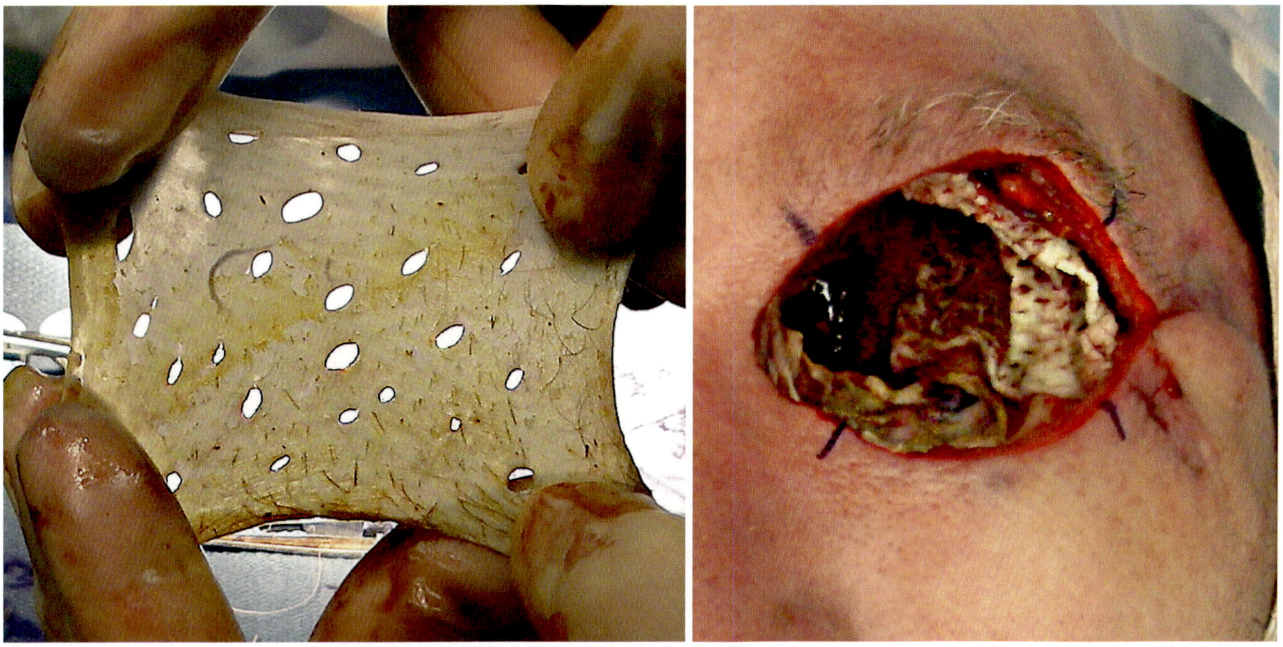

Fig. 60.7 Intraoperative photograph of a meshed split-thickness skin graft being trimmed for the socket. (Photo courtesy of Cat N Burkat, MD FACS)

assistance with dressing changes and wound maintenance, which requires socket cleaning every few days with hydrogen peroxide and cotton-tipped applicators when the dressing is changed.

A split-thickness skin graft may be used to line the socket to accelerate the granulation process, but it requires increased operative time and adds donor site morbidity. Typically, a split-thickness graft is harvested from the thigh and then meshed (in a 1:1.5 or 1:2 ratio) and placed directly over the walls of the exenterated orbit. The meshed skin is then adjusted to the specifications of the wound, trimmed, and sutured to the healthy surrounding skin (Fig. 60.7). The wound is then tightly packed with Xeroform gauze (or other petrolatum gauze) to allow reliable apposition of the graft to the underlying bone and/or soft tissue. Cleaning and wound care are similar to the spontaneous granulation technique but may be performed with less frequency. Complete epithelialization will usually occur earlier in the postoperative course (4–6 weeks) when compared to spontaneous granulation (10–14 weeks).

More recently, an artificial dermal substitute, Integra™ bilayer matrix wound dressing (Integra LifeSciences Holding Corporation, Plainsboro, New Jersey), has been successfully used in place of a skin graft following exenteration. This wound dressing consists of cross-linked bovine tendon collagen and glycosaminoglycan that serve as a dermal substitute, covered with a thin silicone layer to control moisture loss. The dressing promotes a faster and more reliable level of epithelialization compared to spontaneous granulation with the added benefit of less onerous postoperative care [16]. After exenteration, this dermal matrix may be applied to the inner bony walls (or residual soft tissue) of the orbit and sutured with nylon or Prolene sutures to the surrounding skin (Fig. 60.8). Care should be taken to trim and position the matrix flat on the bone, rather than folding into ridges or having overlap of the matrix. The matrix is then covered with antibiotic ointment, and dressing is packed into the wound, insuring tight apposition to the

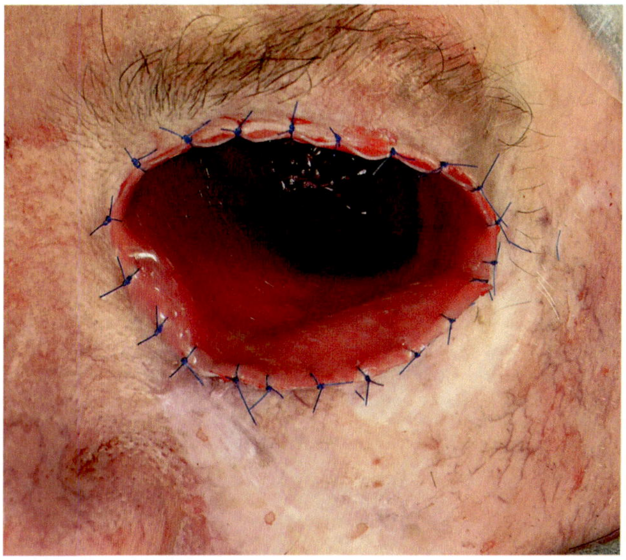

Fig. 60.8 Integra™ bilayer matrix wound matrix placed flat on the bone and sutured to the skin edges. (Photo courtesy of Cat N Burkat, MD FACS)

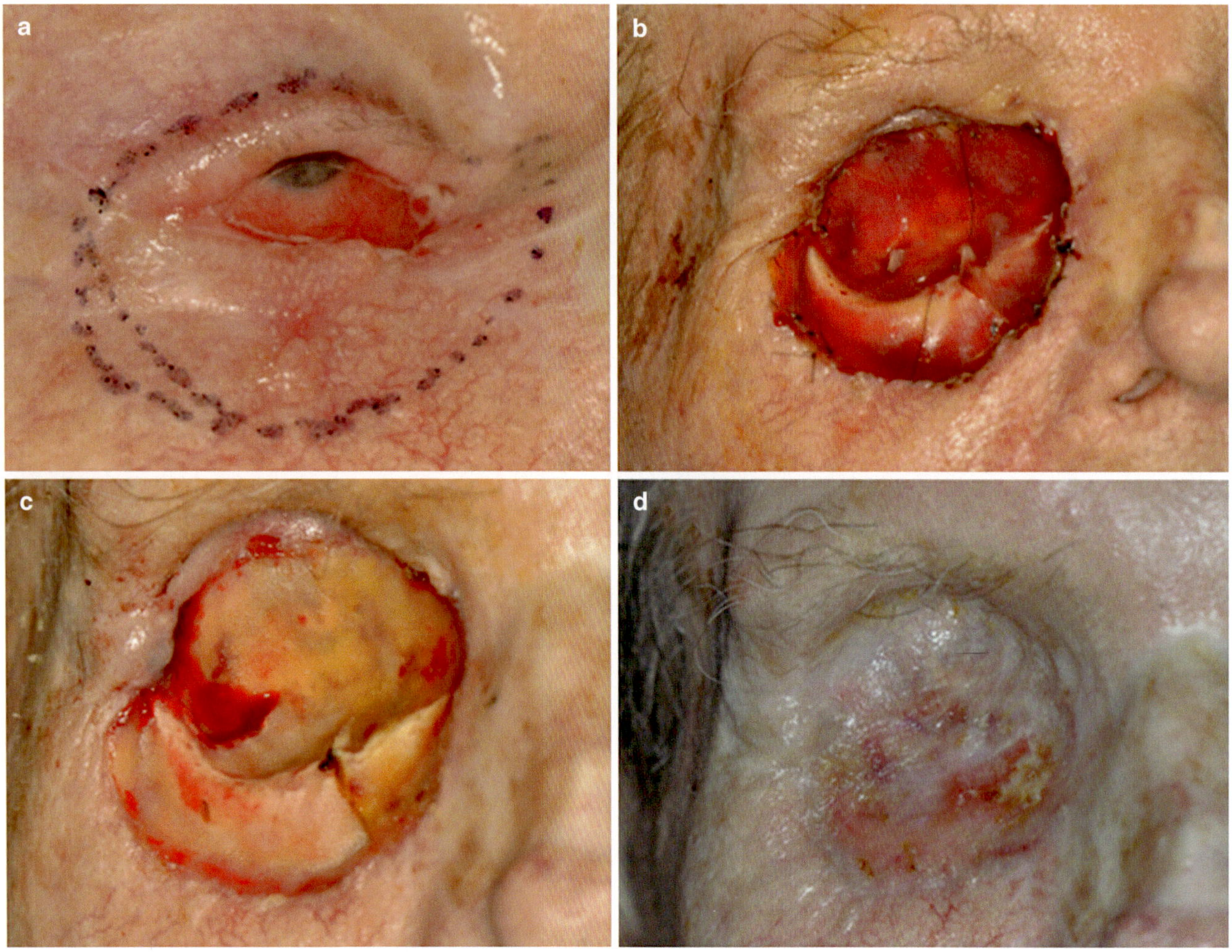

Fig. 60.9 Clinical photographs demonstrating the use of Integra™ bilayer matrix wound dressing within a 3-month postoperative period. (**a**) Squamous cell carcinoma of the right lower eyelid and anterior orbit (dissection was carried out at the outer dotted line; inner dotted line marks the palpable tumor edge). (**b**) 1 week following exenteration, an intact Integra™ bilayer covers the orbit as well as the exposed inferior orbital rim. (**c**) 4 weeks following exenteration, the silicone layer is removed, revealing the healthy neodermis. (**d**) Appearance of the orbit after successful epithelialization, with minimal postoperative management following use of the graft. (Courtesy of https://www.tandfonline.com. From Rafailov et al. [16]. Permission granted in writing by Taylor and Francis, Inc.)

orbital walls. The sutures and the superficial silicone layer are then removed in the office 3–4 weeks after surgery, when the silicone layer is crinkled and detaching itself. Once the silicone layer is removed, the underlying pinkish "neodermis" can then rapidly epithelialize (Figs. 60.9 and 60.10). In all cases where dermal or artificial dermal grafts are used, meticulous hemostasis is necessary to prevent postoperative bleeding beneath the graft that would jeopardize the graft's survivability.

Free flaps and regional flaps involve significant second site morbidity. They are commonly used only in cases where the defect is large, the patient is expected to undergo radiation, and when a prosthesis is not expected to be used postoperatively [17]. Such flaps are typically reserved for defects following extended exenterations when the walls of the orbit are removed. One of the most commonly employed regional flaps is the temporalis muscle flap, which requires splitting the anterior half of the temporalis muscle and rotating it either under or over the lateral orbital rim to blanket the socket [18]. Muscle flaps are often covered with split-thickness skin grafts. These flaps should be used with caution as they may mask recurrence of underlying neoplasm. Periodic surveillance MRIs may be required in the years following their placement.

Special considerations must be made for children who undergo exenteration. Because the orbital bones grow in proportion to intraorbital volume and pressure, children often experience growth retardation of the orbital wall and facial bones following exenteration. In order to prevent permanent asymmetry, children often require a combination of dermis fat grafts and porous implants to replace the lost orbital volume.

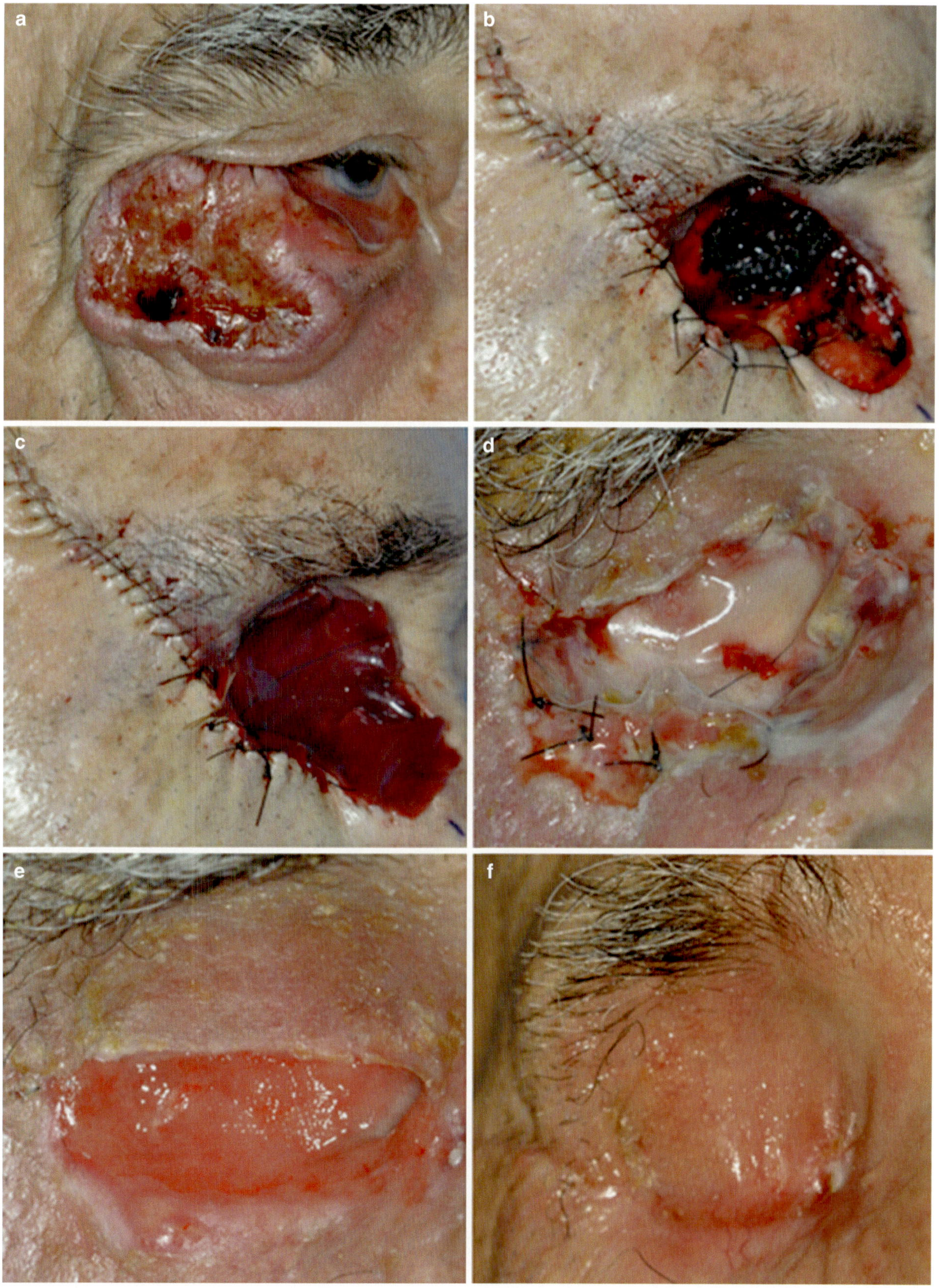

Fig. 60.10 Clinical images demonstrating Integra™ bilayer matrix wound dressing within a 3-month postoperative period. (**a**) A 69-year-old man with squamous cell carcinoma of the right lower eyelid and orbit. (**b**) Total exenteration with a large lateral defect closed with an advancement flap. (**c**) Intraoperative photograph following placement of the graft. (**d**) Orbit 4 weeks after exenteration, immediately prior to removal of silicone layer. (**e**) Orbit 4 weeks after silicone removal, healthy dermis present. (**f**) 3 months after exenteration with epithelialization complete. (Courtesy of: https://www.tandfonline.com. From: Rafailov et al. [16]. Permission granted in writing by Taylor and Francis, Inc.)

Table 60.1 Combined incidence of most frequent complications of orbital exenteration

	Fistula	Infection	Cerebrospinal fluid leak	Hemorrhage	Failed skin graft	Chronic discharge	Nonhealing ulcer
Bartley et al. [6] (1967–1986)	17/100	3/100	3/100	2/100			
Goldberg et al. [14] (1983–1999)	5/25					2/25	
Ben Simon et al. [16] (1999–2003)	2/34	1/34					1/34
Taylor et al. [19] (1993–2004)	7/14	6/14		1/14			
Rahman et al. [7] (1991–2004)	15/64		1/64		7/64	1/64	
Ali et al. [20] (1999–2012)	9/119	5/119					
Nagendran et al. [4] (2003–2013)	2/25		1/25		3/25		
Zhang et al. [5] (2005–2015)	4/102	1/102		1/102			1/102
Combined recorded complications (1967–2015)	61/483 (12.6%)	16/369 (4.3%)	5/189 (2.6%)	4/216 (1.9%)	10/89 (11.2%)	3/89 (3.4%)	2/136 (1.5%)

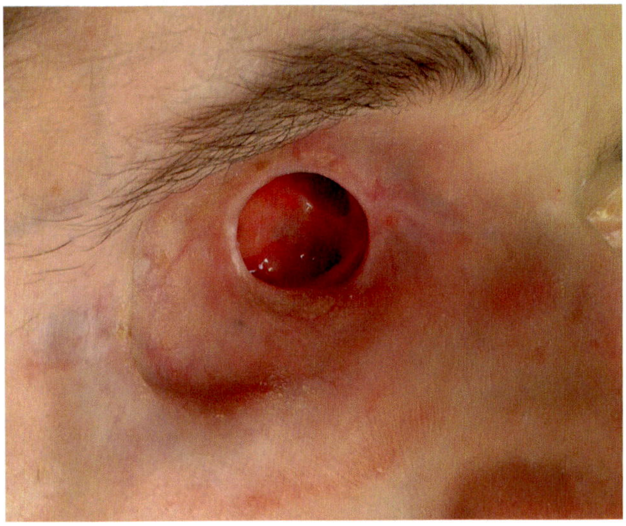

Fig. 60.11 A chronic sino-orbital fistula in an exenterated socket can create challenges for the prosthesis. (Photo courtesy of Cat N Burkat, MD FACS)

Complications of Exenteration

Complications from exenteration typically occur from iatrogenic trauma to the surrounding walls of the orbit during surgery, or in relation to problems with wound healing or infection (Table 60.1). Fractures of the medial or inferior walls may lead to a sino-orbital fistula, which may impede healing and can be difficult to treat (Fig. 60.11). Care must be taken to apply the minimum amount of pressure against the walls during dissection to prevent this complication. An opening into the sinus would obviously not allow for the placement of a skin graft over the fistula. Fracture of the superior wall may result in leakage of cerebrospinal fluid and in some cases may result in infection of the central nervous system. These fractures can be covered with bone wax if small and may require assistance from a neurosurgeon to close. Postoperative infections, most often from *Staphylococcus aureus*, can occur especially in the setting of delayed wound healing [19]. If radiation is required in the immediate postoperative period, wound healing may be delayed, especially when the socket is allowed to spontaneously granulate. In these cases, many surgeons advocate the use of thicker myocutaneous flaps, such as free flaps or regional flaps, as they provide a more durable protection of the socket through the radiation treatment than split-thickness skin grafts or spontaneous granulation [11]. Most complications of exenteration surgery can be avoided by careful dissection at the time of exenteration as well as by employing a tailored approach to reconstruction aimed to fit both the needs of the patient and the expected postoperative care.

Declaration of Interest The authors report no conflicts of interest. The authors alone are responsible for the content and writing of the paper.

References

1. Bartisch G. Ophthalmodoulcia. Dresden. 1583;3:208.
2. Nassab RS, Thomas SS, Murray D. Orbital exenteration for advanced periorbital skin cancers: 20 years experience. J Plast Reconstr Aesthet Surg. 2007;60(10):1103–9.
3. Bartley GB, Garrity JA, Waller RR, et al. Orbital exenteration at the Mayo Clinic. 1967–1986. Ophthalmology. 1989;96(4):468–73.
4. Rahman I, Cook AE, Leatherbarrow B. Orbital exenteration: a 13 year Manchester experience. Br J Ophthalmol. 2005;89(10):1335–40.
5. Sekulic A, Migden MR, Oro AE, et al. Efficacy and safety of vismodegib in advanced basal-cell carcinoma. N Engl J Med. 2012;366(23):2171–9.
6. Hargrove RN, Wesley RE, Klippenstein KA, et al. Indications for orbital exenteration in mucormycosis. Ophthal Plast Reconstr Surg. 2006;22(4):286–91.
7. Pelton RW, Peterson EA, Patel BC, Davis K. Successful treatment of rhino-orbital mucormycosis without exenteration: the use of multiple treatment modalities. Ophthal Plast Reconstr Surg. 2001;17(1):62–6.

8. Athavale DD, Jones R, O'Donnell BA, et al. Non-exenteration management of sino-orbital fungal disease. Ophthal Plast Reconstr Surg. 2017;33(6):426–9.
9. Shield DR, Servat J, Paul S, et al. Periocular necrotizing fasciitis causing blindness. JAMA Ophthalmol. 2013;131(9):1225–7.
10. Goldberg RA, Kim JW, Shorr N. Orbital exenteration: results of an individualized approach. Ophthal Plast Reconstr Surg. 2003;19:229–36.
11. Ben Simon GJ, Schwarcz RM, Douglas R, et al. Orbital exenteration: one size does not fit all. Am J Ophthalmol. 2005;139(1):11–7.
12. Shields JA, Shields CL, Suvarnamani C, et al. Orbital exenteration with eyelid sparing: indications, technique, and results. Ophthalmic Surg. 1991;22(5):292–7.
13. Mohr C, Esser J. Orbital exenteration: surgical and reconstructive strategies. Graefes Arch Clin Exp Ophthalmol. 1997;235:288–95.
14. Putterman AM. Orbital exenteration with spontaneous granulation. Arch Ophthalmol. 1986;104(1):139–40.
15. Lowry JC, Bartley GB, Garrity JA. The role of second-intention healing in periocular reconstruction. Ophthal Plast Reconstr Surg. 1997;13(3):174–88.
16. Rafailov L, Turbin RE, Langer PD. Use of bilayer matrix wound dressing in the exenterated socket. Orbit. 2017;36(6):397–400.
17. Hanasono MM, Lee JC, Yang JS, et al. An algorithmic approach to reconstructive surgery and prosthetic rehabilitation after orbital exenteration. Plast Reconstr Surg. 2009;123(1):98–105.
18. Naquin HA. Orbital reconstruction utilizing temporalis muscle. Am J Ophthalmol. 1956;41(3):519–21.
19. Taylor A, Roberts F, Kemp EG. Orbital exenteration – a retrospective study over an 11 year period analyzing all cases from a single unit. Orbit. 2006;25(3):185–93.
20. Ali MJ, Pujari A, Dave TV, et al. Clinicopathological profile of orbital exenteration: 14 years of experince from a tertiary eye care center in South India. Int Ophthalmol. 2016;36(2):253–8.

Orbital Implants: Classification and Outcomes

61

Sarah W. DeParis and Nicholas Mahoney

After the eye is removed in enucleation and evisceration surgery, an orbital implant is typically placed to restore lost volume to the orbit. This allows for support for an ocular prosthesis and provides structure for the periorbital tissue and eyelids [1, 2]. The ideal implant would be low cost, biocompatible, nondegradable, and easy to implant [1, 2]. A variety of materials have been used as orbital implants and meet these criteria to varying degrees; however, no implant has been made that is completely free of complications after placement. Postoperative problems and complications that occur include:

- Migration: movement within the orbit from the original placement location
- Exposure: erosion of the overlying tissue with uncovering of the implanted material (Fig. 61.1)
- Extrusion: severe exposure with potentially complete prolapse of the implant from the eye socket (Fig. 61.2)
- Infection: bacterial or fungal infiltration into implant materials, encapsulated implant space, or the orbital tissues (Fig. 61.3)
- Postenucleation socket syndrome: complex deformity of the orbital tissues arising from a combination of inadequate volume replacement, orbital atrophy, and rotation of the soft tissues

There are many factors used to classify implants, and all are considered in the selection of an orbital implant for a given case. Most surgeons get comfortable with a particular implant formulation, but availability might change, new materials might become available, or a postoperative complication from a different surgeon might need to be managed.

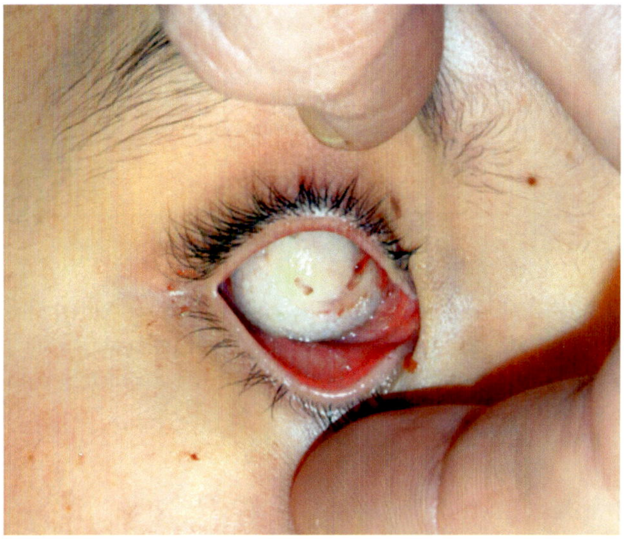

Fig. 61.1 Exposure without infection of a porous polyethylene implant

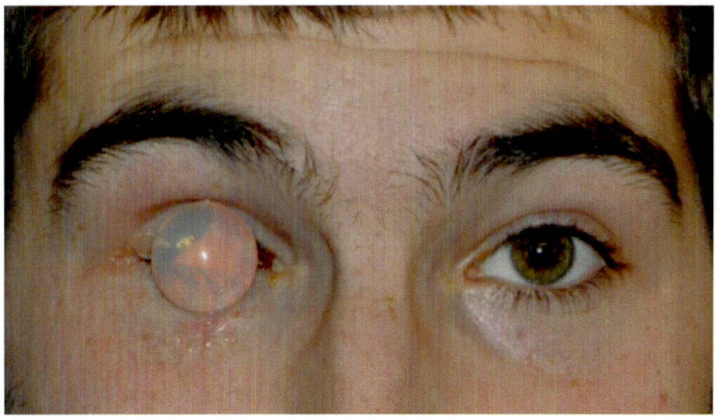

Fig. 61.2 Complete extrusion of a silicone implant placed after enucleation; the implant is still attached by polyester sutures to the extraocular muscles

In addition, various procedures and materials might suit a particular patient better. It is important to be familiar with the various implant compositions, shapes, and sizes available as well as the surgical techniques needed for proper placement.

S. W. DeParis
Department of Oculoplastic Surgery, Wilmer Eye Institute/Johns Hopkins Hospital, Baltimore, MD, USA

N. Mahoney (✉)
Department of Ophthalmology, Johns Hopkins Hospital, Baltimore, MD, USA
e-mail: nick.mahoney@jhmi.edu

A. J. Cohen, C. N. Burkat (eds.), *Oculofacial, Orbital, and Lacrimal Surgery*, https://doi.org/10.1007/978-3-030-14092-2_61

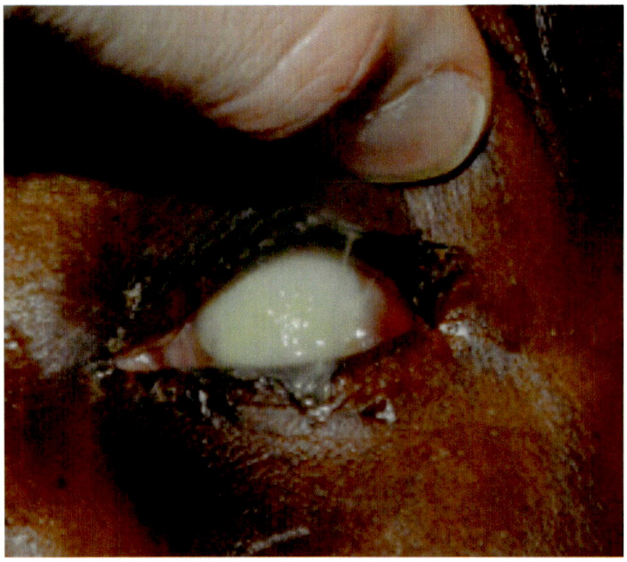

Fig. 61.3 Exposure and infection of hydroxyapatite implant

Orbital Implant Selection

Orbital implants can be broadly categorized by the type of material. In addition, implant shape and modifications such as integration, coatings, and nonuniform variations in design can also be discussed.

Implant Materials

The main distinguishing characteristic between materials available is the presence or absence of pores. A survey review of almost 2000 enucleations by Su and Yen reported around 20% use of nonporous materials and 72% of porous materials and 8% reliance on autologous dermis-fat grafting [3]. Great variability between surgical techniques in eye removal, implant placement, and tissue closure make comparison of exposure rates between implant material types difficult [4]. There is not a consensus from the multitude of studies looking at exposure rates, with a wide range of complication rates reported for both porous and nonporous implants [1, 2]. A 2018 meta-analysis by Wladis et al. of 25 studies and another by Schellini et al. in 2016 of 35 series both concur that both porous and nonporous materials are well-tolerated and likely comparable [5, 6]. Porous materials might be less prone to infection, migration, and extrusion with a range of exposures reported to be most typically between 0% and 9%, while nonporous materials are less expensive and have an extrusion rate of 0–7% [5, 6].

Nonporous Implants

Smooth, nonporous materials used to construct implants include glass, acrylic, polymethyl methacrylate (PMMA), and silicone. In general, they are low cost, inert, and well-tolerated, inciting minimal inflammatory response. Without pores in the material, these implants do not allow fibrovascular ingrowth and are not bio-integrated into the anophthalmic socket. Rather a pseudo-capsule of fibrosis tissue develops at the interface between the material and the orbital tissues [1, 2]. They have the benefit of relative ease of removal following placement, for example, in children who may require replacement with a larger implant later in life. However, they have greater rates of implant migration and extrusion than bio-integrated implants [1].

Glass implants were developed by Mules in 1885. These initial implants were brittle and had a high rate of extrusion [2]. Silicone implants have been used for over 50 years. They are flexible, have relatively low cost, and are easy to handle. The extraocular muscles can be sutured directly to the implant, allowing for improved motility. However, these implants are also prone to migration and extrusion. Acrylic or polymethyl methacrylate (PMMA) implants were first described in 1976 [2]. Similar to silicone implants, they offer ease of handling and removal but are prone to migration and extrusion. Silicone and acrylic orbital implants are currently commercially available from several manufacturers.

Porous Implants

Porous implants were first introduced in the 1980s and contain a network of interconnected pores. These pores provide channels for fibrovascular tissue ingrowth into the implant. This serves to anchor the implant within the orbit thereby decreasing implant migration and extrusion. This tissue and vascular ingrowth also results in bio-integration which can reduce infection rates and allow for healing and maintenance of overlying tissue breakdown [2]. Most notably, a peg can be placed through the anterior tissues into the implant to allow coupling of the implant to a prosthetic for enhancement of motility (Fig. 61.4). Though there is also a theoretical

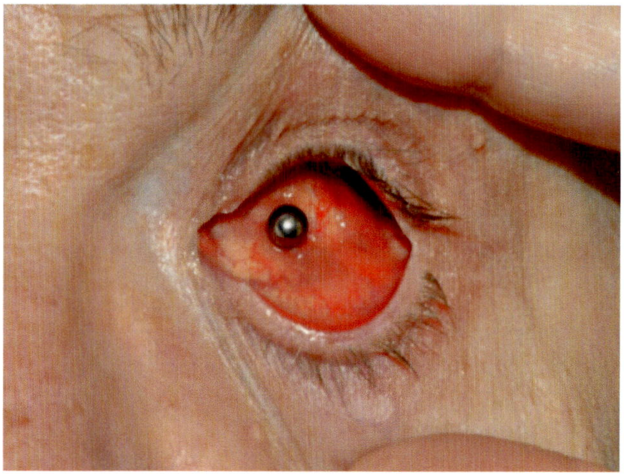

Fig. 61.4 Well-placed and well-tolerated motility peg

benefit of improved motility due to fibrovascular ingrowth alone, current literature has not found a clear benefit of porous implants for motility if a peg system is not placed [7, 8]. In addition, the more abrasive surface of porous implants may lead to mechanical breakdown of the anterior covering tissues resulting in exposure of the implant [4]. A meta-analysis by Custer and Trinkaus of 49 series of eye removal patients (both enucleation and evisceration) suggested an aggregate 4.9% exposure rate for coralline hydroxyapatite implants compared to 8.1% for porous polyethylene [9].

Hydroxyapatite

Hydroxyapatite (HA) has long been used in orthopedic surgery and dentistry for bone repair. This material was first used for orbital implants in the 1980s. It has the benefit of good biocompatibility and allows for rapid fibrovascular ingrowth. This ceramic material is brittle, prohibiting suturing of extraocular muscles directly to the implant without a wrapping material being placed. It has the downside of a more abrasive surface, which in the absence of wrapping could lead to thinning of the overlying Tenon's capsule and conjunctiva and greater difficulty of insertion due to tissue drag on the rough surface [1]. In general, wrapping of the implant is recommended for hydroxyapatite implants for these reasons.

Coralline HA implants were first developed in the mid-1980s and are derived from reef-building coral [1, 10]. They consist of calcium phosphate, a substance that occurs naturally in the human body [10]. The Bio-Eye (Bio-Eye Orbital Implants) is a coralline HA implant that was FDA approved in 1989 and is currently commercially available. A polymer-coated version is also available, and Shields et al. reported a low exposure rate of 2% with this implant in 126 enucleations [11].

There are several alternatives to coralline HA implants that have been developed and have similar benefits and complications. Synthetic HA implants such as the FCI3 implant (FCI Ophthalmics) are generally less expensive than their coralline counterparts and allow for easier drilling for peg placement, if desired [2]. Bovine HA implants such as the Molteno M-Sphere (Molteno Ophthalmic Limited) are composed of deproteinized cancellous bone from bovine fibula. These implants are less dense than coralline HA but are more fragile [1].

Porous Polyethylene

Porous polyethylene (PP) is a high-density hydrocarbon created via polymerization of ethylene under high pressure and temperature [12, 13]. It has been used for reconstruction of the bone and soft tissue in other fields for over 50 years and was developed in the 1980s as an orbital implant. The Medpor (Stryker Surgical) implant was first introduced in 1988. In PP implants, vascular ingrowth occurs slightly slower than HA over a 5–12-week period, but the final extent of vascularization is similar between the two materials [2, 14]. It is thought to be less inflammatory than HA [15, 16] and has a smoother surface making it easier to place within the orbit and allowing it to be used without wrapping. The PP material allows for direct suturing of the extraocular muscles to the implant, if desired, and some models come with pre-drilled holes for muscle attachment [12, 4]. In addition, newer iterations such as the SST-EZ implants (Stryker) have a cap anteriorly with smaller porosity to create a less abrasive surface, which may lead to a lower rate of exposure than other unwrapped PP implants as well as tunnels to allow muscle attachment (Figs. 61.5 and 61.6) [4]. Mahoney et al. reviewed 119 patients with such implants placed and reported an exposure rate of 3.5% [4].

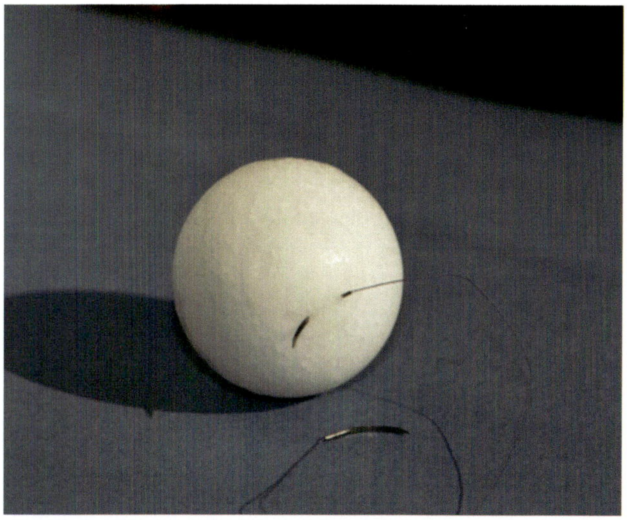

Fig. 61.5 Porous polyethylene implant with large pores diffusely and small pore anterior plate with tunnels for extraocular muscle attachment

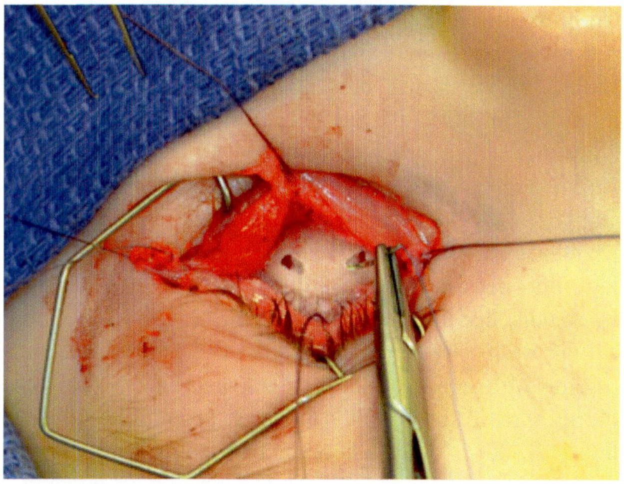

Fig. 61.6 Intraoperative photograph demonstrating porous implant placement during surgery with muscle attachment

Aluminum Oxide

Aluminum oxide or alumina porous orbital implants are the most recently introduced material for porous implants. This material is strong, resistant to wear, and highly biocompatible. They are also generally less expensive than HA implants. The bioceramic orbital implant (FCI Ophthalmic) was FDA approved in 2000. This type of implant has similar complications as HA implants due to an abrasive surface (need for wrapping). However, further study of this type of implant is needed [2]. A retrospective study of 419 patients by Jordan et al. showed an exposure rate of 9.1%, which is comparable to other porous implants [17].

Other Implant Materials

A number of other implant materials have been more recently developed. Polytetrafluoroethylene or Gore-Tex implants were studied in rabbits in the late 1990s but were found to be highly inflammatory, and further studies were largely abandoned [2]. Bioglass is thought to promote greater vascularization, and a PP/bioglass hybrid implant has been developed (Medpor Plus Sphere, Porex Surgical) [18]. However, a polyethylene/bioglass composite implant was studied in rabbits and showed no difference in fibrovascular ingrowth compared to PP [19]. Further studies of these orbital implants are needed to determine their safety and usefulness.

Material	Estimated cost ($)	Pore size (μm)
Coralline hydroxyapatite	600	300–700
Synthetic hydroxyapatite	450	300–500
Bovine hydroxyapatite	550	400–700
Porous polyethylene	500	100–1000
Aluminum oxide	450	500
Silicone sphere	30	–

Implant Shape Modifications

Quasi-integrated implants have an irregularly shaped anterior surface to allow a lock and key fit with the posterior surface of the ocular prosthesis, allowing for improved motility. This was first introduced in 1946 by Cutler. The Allen implant was developed in the 1940s and consisted of a PMMA implant connected by a peg to the patient's prosthesis. This was later redesigned as the Iowa acrylic implant, which had four mounds on the anterior surface corresponding with depressions on the posterior prosthesis surface. This was modified as the universal implant in the 1980s, an acrylic implant with lower-profile rounded mounds to reduce friction and exposure. Overall, these implants have higher rates of exposure, extrusion, and pain due to pinching of conjunctiva and Tenon's capsule between the implant and the prosthesis [20, 2]. The most recently developed quasi-integrated implant is the Medpor Quad-Motility PP implant [21]; however, this implant is no longer commercially available.

Implant Size

Regardless of the type or material chosen, the selected orbital implant should adequately replace the orbital volume lost with eye removal. This volume loss is often stated to be approximately 7 mL, based on the volume of an adult eye with a 24 mm axial length (volume = $4/3\pi r^3$) [22]. Many patients ultimately develop the so-called postenucleation socket syndrome secondary to inadequate orbital volume with enophthalmos, ptosis, deepened superior sulcus, or lower eyelid retraction [23, 24]. This presentation is a result of low orbital volume and also rotation of the orbital tissues inward and downward with preservation of suspensory ligaments such as Whitnall's. Attempts to improve cosmesis by having the ocularist enlarge the prosthetic volume and provide a superior bump may result in further weighing down of a loose lower eyelid and frank prosthetic prolapse. To prevent this, some have advocated for measurement of the volume of the enucleated eye using water displacement [22]. Unfortunately, some degree of volume loss from atrophy and prior medical care is likely to occur. In general, as large of an implant as can be safely placed without excessive tension in the surgical closure should be selected. Selection of an implant that is too large with undue tension on the wound may increase risk of implant exposure. Although it is tempting to place an implant deep in the orbit to allow maximum coverage, an anteriorly placed implant will likely have better cosmesis and motility. Ultimately, prosthetic support to the implant with a peg or postoperative volume augmentation may be needed.

Other Considerations in Implant Selection

Motility, Pegs, and Magnetic Coupling

Motility of the ocular prosthesis occurs due to surface tension between the conjunctival surface and the prosthetic and due to movement of the fornices. Several surgical factors may affect motility outcomes. Attachment of the extraocular muscles either directly to the implant, through predrilled tunnels, or to the wrapping material may facilitate improved motility. There was thought to be a theoretical advantage to porous implants for motility due to fibrovascular ingrowth. However, studies have not shown a clear motility advantage with porous implants if pegging is not performed [8, 7].

Pegging of an implant refers to placement of a peg into a drilled location in porous orbital implants, which is then coupled to the ocular prosthesis and improves motility, particularly in horizontal excursions [10]. MRI can be used to confirm that vascularization of the implant has occurred prior to peg placement, which is typically performed as a secondary procedure approximately 6 months after implant placement [25]. Primary peg placement at the time of eye

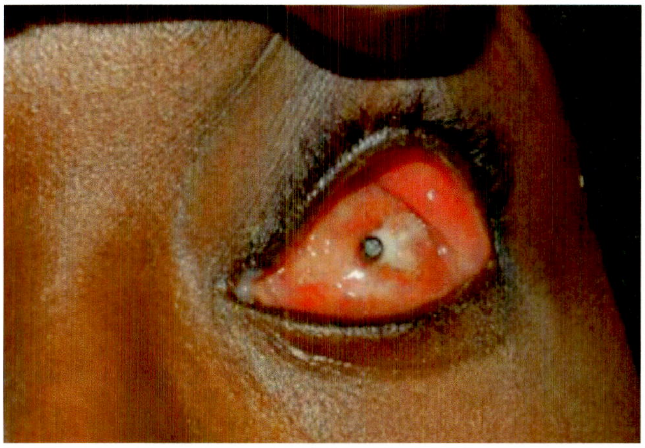

Fig. 61.7 Exposure next to a titanium motility peg. Patient desired to keep the peg for motility and to prevent lower eyelid retraction and/or prosthetic prolapse from her shallow orbit. Defect was closed by advancing conjunctiva in a bipedicle flap from the lateral aspect and the mucous membrane grafting to the donor site

removal surgery has also been described [26]. Complications can occur more frequently with peg placement, with some studies reporting a complication rate as high as 45% [27]. These can include peg extrusion, conjunctivitis and chronic discharge, an audible "click" noise with eye movements, and postoperative pain (Fig. 61.7). Titanium pegging systems show a lower rate of complications than sleeved PMMA and sleeved polycarbonate [28].

Pegging improves motility, particularly with large amplitude movements [25] and horizontal excursions [10]. However, as discussed previously, pegging has fallen out of favor due to a higher complication rate and need for a second surgical procedure in most cases [27, 2]. As discussed above, quasi-integrated implants should improve motility, though no direct comparison has been made between these and porous implants. One study showed no significant difference in motility between the Allen quasi-integrated implant and sclera-wrapped acrylic implant [29].

Magnetic implants were introduced in the mid-twentieth century and have a magnet embedded in the anterior surface of the implant which can couple with the patient's prosthesis to improve motility. Unfortunately, these implants had a high rate of extrusion, likely due to compression of conjunctiva and Tenon's capsule causing tissue breakdown. This occurred despite vaulting of the prosthetic. Motility was also felt to be less coupled than with traditional pegs [30]. In addition, the magnet is prone to rust, and MRI was prohibited in patients with these implants, and this implant type is no longer widely used [2].

Patient Characteristics

Individual patient characteristics may influence implant selection. For example, patients with a history of prior radiation or chemotherapy may have a greater risk of implant exposure or extrusion. In these patients, primary dermal fat graft placement may be considered. Patient age must also be considered. For example, pediatric patients may need later implant removal and replacement with one of a larger size, so some surgeons select nonporous implants in these instances to facilitate later ease of removal. Primary dermal fat grafting has also been used in the pediatric population as the graft will grow in size along with the patient [31].

Surgical Technique

Various small and large adjustments to technique may affect the outcome after implant placement. Higher rates of exposure with porous implants following evisceration surgery as compared to enucleation had been suggested, but other studies have shown similar exposure rates [12]. Surgeons have explored closing rectus and even oblique muscles together over implants and modifications to layered closure in enucleation. Similarly, surgeons have suggested placing implants posterior to the entire scleral shell for evisceration. Generally, the type of eye removal surgery should be selected based on the appropriate indications and contraindications, and surgeons should be comfortable with both techniques.

To improve motility, suturing of extraocular muscles to the implant may be a useful technique in enucleation surgery, which may result in less excursion compared to evisceration. This may be done directly to the implant in the case of nonporous implants, through predrilled tunnels in implants such as the SST-EZ or in prefabricated locations in coating such as the Bio-Eye, or to the wrapping material if one is used, such as with HA implants.

Wrapping of implants provides an extra barrier between the implant and the orbital tissues. Several different types of materials have been used for wrapping, including autogenous fascia and sclera, cadaveric sclera and fascia lata, bovine pericardium, acellular dermis, and synthetic materials such as polyglactin mesh. Autogenous fascia may be harvested from fascia lata, temporalis, rectus abdominus sheath, or the posterior auricular muscle complex [2]. Wrapping has several advantages, particularly with HA implants, including allowing precise attachment of the extraocular muscles to the implant and facilitating insertion by reducing tissue drag [2, 12]. The role of wrapping in implant exposure is controversial, as wrapping could reduce exposure by providing an extra barrier, but for the same reason may reduce vascularization which could increase exposure [1]. One study showed a greater rate of exposure for unwrapped PP and HA implants [14], but others have low exposure rates with unwrapped porous implants [12, 4]. There are several disadvantages to wrapping, including extra cost and operating time, slower vascularization of the implant, donor site morbidity if autologous tissue is used, or theoretical risk of disease transmission if non-autologous tissue is used [1]. Cutting windows in the wrapping material can increase the rate and extent of vascularization.

Outcomes

Complications

Exposure of the implant occurs secondary to tissue breakdown over its anterior surface. In extreme cases, the implant may become completely extruded from the orbit. Risk factors for exposure that have been proposed are prior history of extensive trauma, prior radiation or chemotherapy, poor wound closure, and infection [1]. Rates of exposure are greater for porous implants, but rates vary widely from 2% to 21% depending on the study, which may be due to wide variations in surgical technique [12]. Some studies have suggested greater exposure rates with porous implants in evisceration as compared to enucleation, but others have found no difference [12]. Wrapping of implants may reduce exposure, particularly with HA, though this has been debated [2]. Exposure rates for wrapped and unwrapped PP have been shown to be similar [12].

Conversely, complete implant extrusion is more common with nonporous implants. This may be due to the lack of vascularization anchoring the implant to the socket. In these implants, exposures generally will not resolve without surgical treatment [25]. Postoperative infection of orbital implants may also occur. Infection rates are thought to be lower with porous implants due to their robust vascular supply. There has been some controversy over whether an implant should be placed at the time of surgery in the setting of an active infection such as endophthalmitis, with some surgeons opting to perform a second procedure for secondary implant placement in these instances. However, primary implant placement in the setting of endophthalmitis has also been described [32].

Small exposures in porous implants may heal spontaneously with conservative treatment such as lubrication, topical antibiotics, prosthetic holiday, or prosthetic vaulting [1]. Exposures of any implant type that are small and recent may be closed primarily or with conjunctival advancement (Fig. 61.8). More chronic exposures often result in contraction of the conjunctiva, and advancement, especially when the tissues are adherent to the porous materials, can be difficult. Patch grafting with banked sclera or pericardium can provide an extra barrier to recurrence. If a porous implant has been colonized or infected, the implant can either be exchanged or burred until a level of high vascularity is noted and then either replaced or patched with dermis-fat graft (Fig. 61.9).

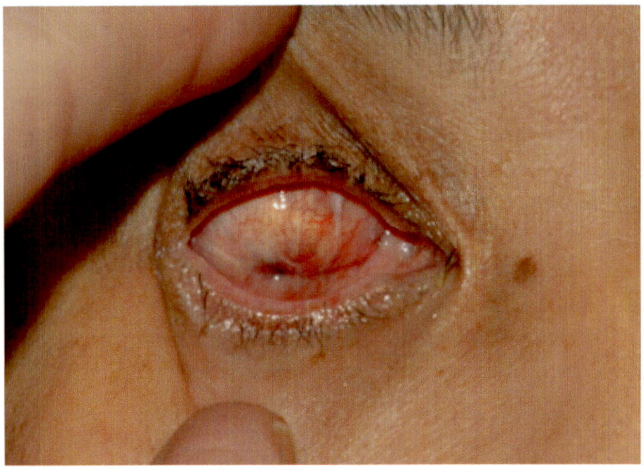

Fig. 61.8 Limited area of conjunctival dehiscence and exposure that might heal on its own

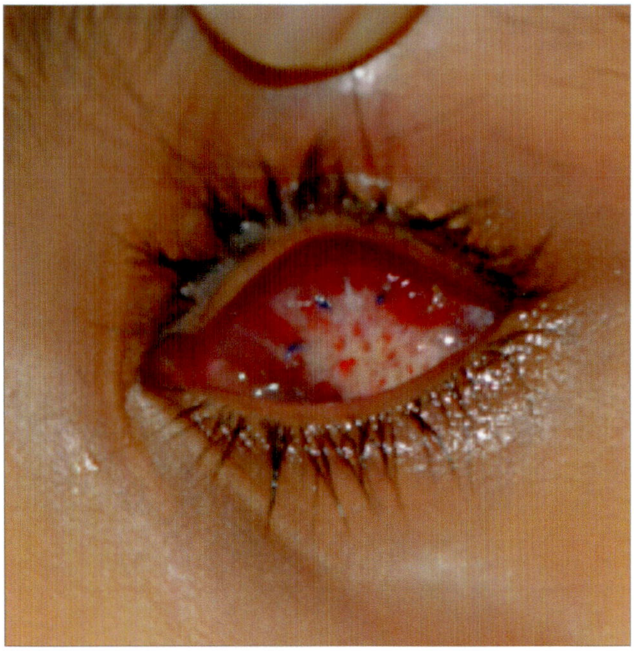

Fig. 61.9 One-week postoperative photograph demonstrating coverage of an exposed hydroxyapatite orbital implant placed during evisceration with a dermis-fat graft. The dermis is left uncovered, and nearby conjunctiva will epithelialize the dermal button and increase the conjunctival surface area

References

1. Chalasani R, Poole-Warren L, Conway RM, Ben-Nissan B. Porous orbital implants in enucleation: a systematic review. Surv Ophthalmol. 2007;52(2):145–55.
2. Baino F, Perero S, Ferraris S, et al. Biomaterials for orbital implants and ocular prostheses: overview and future prospects. Acta Biomater. 2014;10(3):1064–87.
3. Su GW, Yen MT. Current trends in managing the anophthalmic socket after primary nucleation and evisceration. Ophthal Plast Reconstr Surg. 2004;20(4):274–80.
4. Mahoney NR, Grant MP, Iliff NT, Merbs SL. Exposure rate of smooth surface tunnel porous polyethylene implants after enucleation. Ophthal Plast Reconstr Surg. 2014;30(6):492–8.
5. Wladis EJ, Aakalu VK, Sobel RK, Yen MT, Bilyk JR, Mawn LA. Orbital implants in enucleation surgery: a report by the American Academy of ophthalmology. Ophthalmology. 2018;125(2):311–7.
6. Schellini S, Jorge E, Sousa R, Burroughs J, El-Dib R. Porous and nonporous orbital implants for treating the anophthalmic socket: a meta-analysis of case series studies. Orbit. 2016;35(2):78–86.

7. Custer PL, Trinkaus KM, Fornoff J. Comparative motility of hydroxyapatite and alloplastic enucleation implants. Ophthalmology. 1999;106(3):513–6.
8. Colen TP, Paridaens DA, Lemij HG, Mourits MP, van Den Bosch WA. Comparison of artificial eye amplitudes with acrylic and hydroxyapatite spherical enucleation implants. Ophthalmology. 2000;107(10):1889–94.
9. Custer PL, Trinkaus KM. Porous implant exposure: incidence, management, and morbidity. Ophthal Plast Reconstr Surg. 2007;23(1):1–7.
10. Guillinta P, Vasani SN, Granet DB, Kikkawa DO. Prosthetic motility in pegged versus unpegged integrated porous orbital implants. Ophthal Plast Reconstr Surg. 2003;19(2):119–22.
11. Shields CL, Uysal Y, Marr BP, et al. Experience with the polymer-coated hydroxyapatite implant after enucleation in 126 patients. Ophthalmology. 2007;114(2):367–73.
12. Blaydon SM, Shepler TR, Neuhaus RW, White WL, Shore JW. The porous polyethylene (Medpor) spherical orbital implant: a retrospective study of 136 cases. Ophthal Plast Reconstr Surg. 2003;19(5):364–71.
13. Karesh JW, Dresner SC. High-density porous polyethylene (Medpor) as a successful anophthalmic socket implant. Ophthalmology. 1994;101(10):1688–95; discussion 1695–1686.
14. Rubin PA, Popham JK, Bilyk JR, Shore JW. Comparison of fibrovascular ingrowth into hydroxyapatite and porous polyethylene orbital implants. Ophthal Plast Reconstr Surg. 1994;10(2):96–103.
15. Jordan DR, Brownstein S, Dorey M, Yuen VH, Gilberg S. Fibrovascularization of porous polyethylene (Medpor) orbital implant in a rabbit model. Ophthal Plast Reconstr Surg. 2004;20(2):136–43.
16. Goldberg RA, Dresner SC, Braslow RA, Kossovsky N, Legmann A. Animal model of porous polyethylene orbital implants. Ophthal Plast Reconstr Surg. 1994;10(2):104–9.
17. Jordan DR, Klapper SR, Gilberg SM, Dutton JJ, Wong A, Mawn L. The bioceramic implant: evaluation of implant exposures in 419 implants. Ophthal Plast Reconstr Surg. 2010;26(2):80–2.
18. Ma X, Schou KR, Maloney-Schou M, Harwin FM, Ng JD. The porous polyethylene/bioglass spherical orbital implant: a retrospective study of 170 cases. Ophthal Plast Reconstr Surg. 2011;27(1):21–7.
19. Choi HY, Lee JE, Park HJ, Oum BS. Effect of synthetic bone glass particulate on the fibrovascularization of porous polyethylene orbital implants. Ophthal Plast Reconstr Surg. 2006;22(2):121–5.
20. Nunery WR, Cepela MA, Heinz GW, Zale D, Martin RT. Extrusion rate of silicone spherical anophthalmic socket implants. Ophthal Plast Reconstr Surg. 1993;9(2):90–5.
21. Anderson RL, Yen MT, Lucci LM, Caruso RT. The quasi-integrated porous polyethylene orbital implant. Ophthal Plast Reconstr Surg. 2002;18(1):50–5.
22. Thaller VT. Enucleation volume measurement. Ophthal Plast Reconstr Surg. 1997;13(1):18–20.
23. Tyers AG, Collin JR. Orbital implants and post enucleation socket syndrome. Trans Ophthalmol Soc U K. 1982;102(Pt 1):90–2.
24. Smit TJ, Koornneef L, Zonneveld FW, Groet E, Otto AJ. Computed tomography in the assessment of the postenucleation socket syndrome. Ophthalmology. 1990;97(10):1347–51.
25. Custer PL, Kennedy RH, Woog JJ, Kaltreider SA, Meyer DR. Orbital implants in enucleation surgery: a report by the American Academy of ophthalmology. Ophthalmology. 2003;110(10):2054–61.
26. Tawfik HA, Dutton JJ. Primary peg placement in evisceration with the spherical porous polyethylene orbital implant. Ophthalmology. 2004;111(7):1401–6.
27. Edelstein C, Shields CL, De Potter P, Shields JA. Complications of motility peg placement for the hydroxyapatite orbital implant. Ophthalmology. 1997;104(10):1616–21.
28. Yoon JS, Lew H, Kim SJ, Lee SY. Exposure rate of hydroxyapatite orbital implants a 15-year experience of 802 cases. Ophthalmology. 2008;115(3):566–572 e562.
29. Smit TJ, Koornneef L, Groet E, Zonneveld FW, Otto AJ. Prosthesis motility with and without intraorbital implants in the anophthalmic socket. Br J Ophthalmol. 1991;75(11):667–70.
30. Kawai S, Suzuki T, Kawai K. Mobility of hydroxyapatite orbital implant covered with autologous sclera. Jpn J Ophthalmol. 2000;44(1):68–74.
31. Heher KL, Katowitz JA, Low JE. Unilateral dermis-fat graft implantation in the pediatric orbit. Ophthal Plast Reconstr Surg. 1998;14(2):81–8.
32. Dresner SC, Karesh JW. Primary implant placement with evisceration in patients with endophthalmitis. Ophthalmology. 2000;107(9):1661–4; discussion 1664–1665.

Evaluation of the Anophthalmic Socket

62

David R. Jordan and Stephen R. Klapper

Introduction

Loss of an eye to tumor, trauma, or end-stage ocular disease can be devastating. The loss of binocular visual function with reduced peripheral visual field and loss of depth perception may result in difficulties with activities of daily living and have various vocational restrictions [1–6]. Individuals may experience a sense of facial disfigurement and poor self-esteem as a result of the "lost body part" [3–6]. Because eye contact is such an essential part of human interaction, it is extremely important for the patient with an artificial eye to maintain a natural, normal-appearing prosthetic eye (Fig. 62.1a, b).

Characteristics of the ideal anophthalmic socket include [7]:

1. A centrally placed, well-covered, buried implant of adequate volume, fabricated from a bioinert material that transmits motility from the implant to the overlying prosthesis
2. A socket lined with healthy conjunctiva and fornices deep enough to retain a prosthesis and to permit horizontal and vertical excursion of an artificial eye
3. Normal eyelid and eyelash position, appearance, and tone
4. A supratarsal eyelid fold that is symmetric with that of the contralateral eyelid
5. A comfortable ocular prosthesis that looks similar to the sighted, contralateral globe and in the same horizontal plane

The authors of this study do not have a commercial or proprietary interest in any of the products reviewed in this manuscript.

D. R. Jordan (✉)
Department of Ophthalmology, University of Ottawa Eye Institute, Ottawa, ON, Canada

S. R. Klapper
Department of Ophthalmology, Klapper Eyelid and Facial Plastic Surgery, Indiana University School of Medicine, Carmel, IN, USA
e-mail: steve@klapperplasticsurgery.com

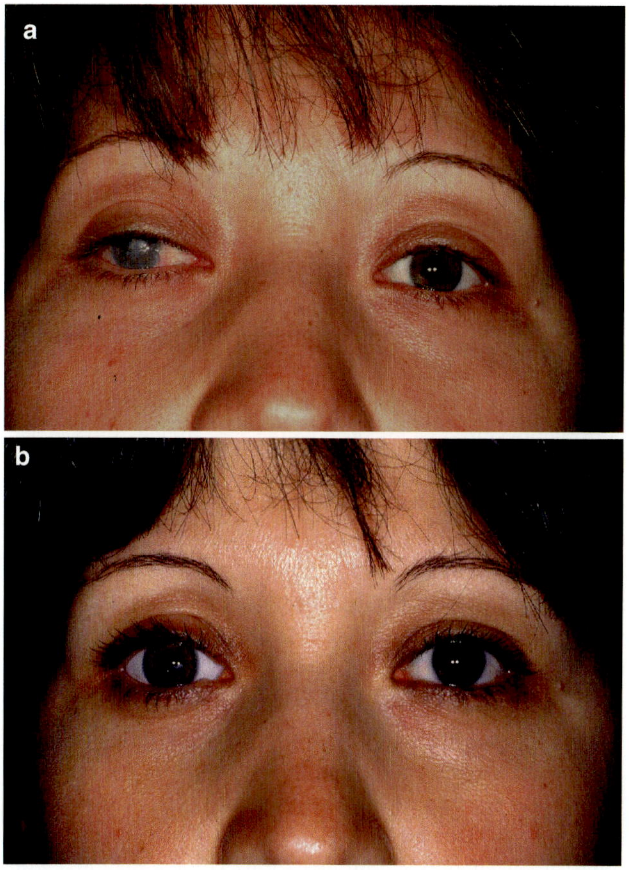

Fig. 62.1 (**a**) A 28-year-old female pre-evisceration surgery with a blind disfigured right eye. (**b**) Six months post-evisceration surgery with a porous orbital implant (hydroxyapatite) and a custom fit prosthetic eye

Close collaboration between the ophthalmologist and the ocularist is essential in order to obtain the best functional and cosmetic results with an ocular prosthesis and reduce the frequency of secondary orbital procedures. Excellent cosmetic results and long-term control of socket problems are the ideal but difficult to achieve in all cases. Secondary procedures can be helpful but at times may be emotionally unsatisfactory for

A. J. Cohen, C. N. Burkat (eds.), *Oculofacial, Orbital, and Lacrimal Surgery*, https://doi.org/10.1007/978-3-030-14092-2_62

both the patient and surgeon. Currently, no surgical procedure satisfies all the above requirements. Over the past two decades, there have been numerous developments and refinements in anophthalmic socket surgery with respect to implant material and design, implant wrapping, implant-prosthesis coupling, and socket volume considerations. Successful anophthalmic surgery is achieved when the anophthalmic patient obtains a painless, non-inflamed eye socket with adequate volume restoration and an artificial eye that looks and moves almost as naturally as a normal eye. Yearly follow-up examinations with the ocularist for prosthesis polishing and implant fit evaluation, as well as with the ophthalmologist to examine any socket issues that are more easily addressed when identified at an early stage (e.g., implant exposure), are important. This chapter will focus on the assessment of the anophthalmic socket and some of the common problems and complications that occur.

Assessment of the Anophthalmic Socket, Problems, and Complications

Anatomical Changes

In addition to the absence of the globe, the anophthalmic socket has other anatomic differences from a normal orbit. Postoperative socket changes begin a complex sequence of interrelationships that affects both the appearance of the socket and the function of the socket with a prosthesis. Progressive intraorbital volume loss after an enucleation/evisceration procedure with time results in rotary displacement of the orbital contents from the superior to the posterior and from the posterior to the inferior orbit [8, 9]. There is retraction of the superior rectus/levator muscle complex, a downward and forward redistribution of the orbital fat, and an upward movement of the distal end of the inferior rectus muscle resulting in a shallow inferior fornix and potential tilting of the prosthesis. The superior sulcus may deepen and upper eyelid ptosis may develop (Fig. 62.2a–d). Progressive lower eyelid laxity of senescence may be aggravated by the weight of an artificial eye. Loss of lower eyelid support and inferior fornix volume may make fitting and wearing of the custom prosthesis more difficult. Insufficient volume replacement, rotational socket changes, and tissue laxity associated with aging results in the "post-enucleation socket syndrome" or "anophthalmic socket syndrome" (deep superior sulcus, upper eyelid ptosis, an enophthalmic appearance, lower eyelid malposition) and may require a larger than desirable prosthesis [10–14].

As with other microsurgical ophthalmic procedures, enucleation and evisceration should be performed meticulously to attain the best functional and cosmetic result and to avoid deformities that may compound the patient's already challenging situation. Proper implant volume at the time of enucleation or evisceration may be determined either preoperatively or intraoperatively (enucleation cases) from the axial length of the eye or by determining the volume of fluid the enucleated eye displaces in a graduated cylinder [12–14]. Approximately 70–80% of the volume of an individual's normal globe ideally should be replaced with an orbital implant [12, 14]. This generally allows for a prosthetic volume that is 2.0–2.5 mL [11]. While the upper limit of prosthetic volume is around 4.0 mL, larger prostheses often result in progressive lower lid laxity and malposition due to the weight of the prostheses on the eyelid and the projection of the anterior surface of the artificial eye. Larger prostheses may also have limited socket excursion [12]. The preoperative or intraoperative calculated implant size is often greater than 22 mm [12–14]. Unfortunately, implants larger than 22 mm may have a higher exposure rate and if too large will hinder fitting of an acceptable custom prosthesis [12, 14]. In most adults we typically use 20–22 mm spherical implants following enucleation and 18–20 mm implants in evisceration procedures. Individualization of the implant size is important in optimizing orbital volume replacement and in achieving the best possible aesthetic result [11–14].

Fabrication, Care, and Maintenance of the Artificial Eye

Following enucleation, evisceration, or secondary implantation surgery, an acrylic (polymethylmethacrylate) conformer is placed in the conjunctival fornices to maintain the conjunctival space during the early postoperative healing phase. An anophthalmic socket without a conformer may be at risk for contraction, potentially compromising placement of an adequately sized prosthesis. The conformer is replaced with a custom-made ocular prosthesis typically fashioned in 4–8 weeks following enucleation, evisceration, or secondary implant surgery. Prefabricated or "stock eyes" (still used in underdeveloped countries) are unsatisfactory as they are generally not cosmetically optimal, limit motility, may trap secretions between the socket and prosthesis, and may not position well in the socket resulting in rotation and excursion. The ideal prosthetic eye is custom fit to the dimensions of the conjunctival fornices of each individual patient using the "modified impression technique" [15].

The time required for an individual patient to get used to the prosthetic eye is variable [16]. Some will be accustomed to it in a matter of hours, others may require days and a few never adjust comfortably. Ideally the prosthetic eye is left in the socket unless being professionally cleaned or adjusted. If the artificial eye is left out while sleeping or for more prolonged periods, it should be stored in soft contact lens saline solution. If the prosthesis is allowed to remain dry, the painted layers may separate and degrade.

Pine et al. have recently proposed a three-phase model that describes the response of the socket microenvironment

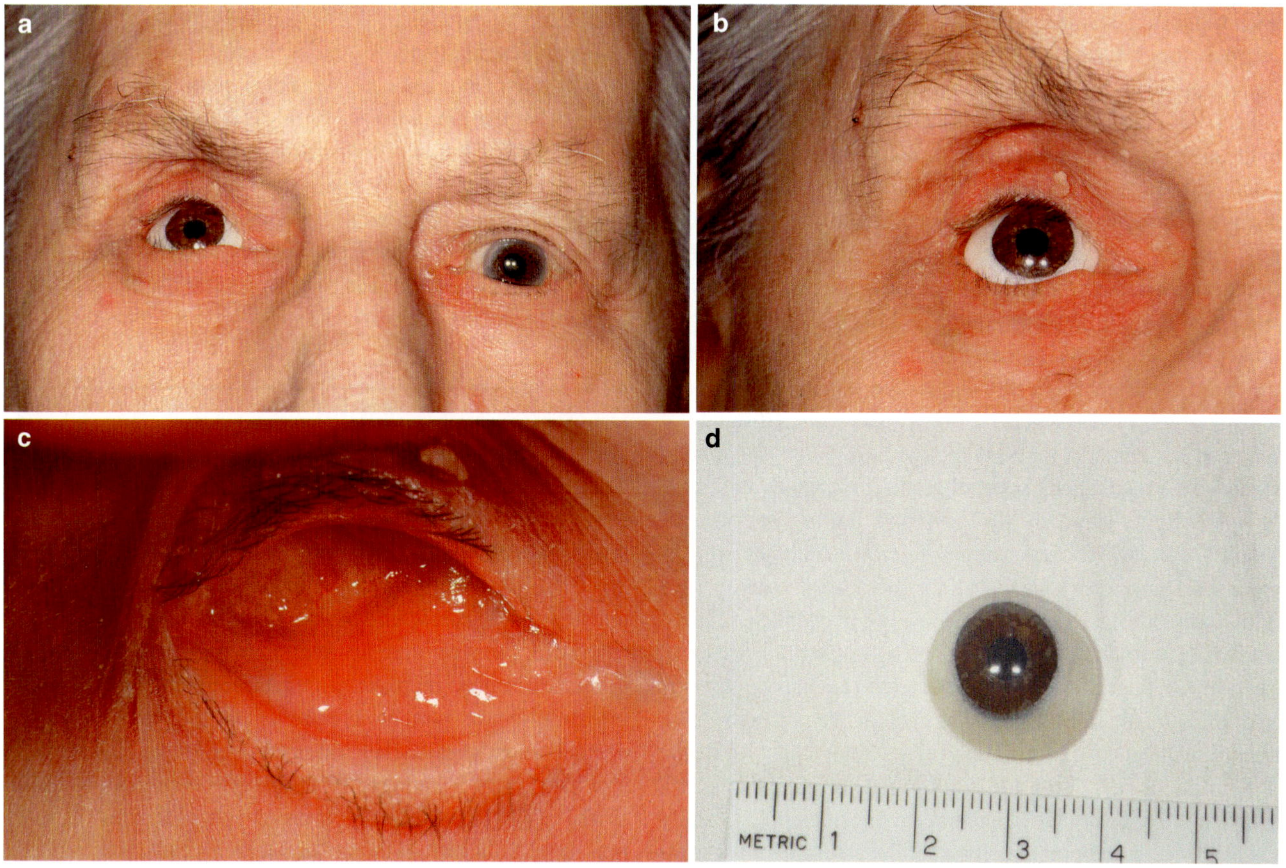

Fig. 62.2 (**a**) An 80-year-old female presented with difficulty wearing her prosthetic right eye. Following enucleation without an orbital implant 50 years earlier she was fit with a "stock eye" from a sample display. The right socket is enophthalmic with a deep superior sulcus as a result of volume loss (post-enucleation socket syndrome). (**b**) The superior edge of the prosthesis is tilted posteriorly, and the inferior edge has migrated anteriorly and pushing against the lower lid as a result of the rotary migration of the orbital tissues. The lower lid fornix is not well-formed and the eyelashes are vertical in position. (**c**) The superior and inferior fornices are shortened and the inferior fornix shows a bulge as a result of the inferior rectus/inferior oblique muscles rotating forward. (**d**) The stock eye was small and cracked, had lost its luster, and did not fit the socket well. It had not been changed or polished in 50 years. A new custom fit prosthesis made her more comfortable and allowed the artificial eye to stay in place. She remained enophthalmic

to prosthetic eye wear [17–21]. The phases include an *initial phase* of wear of a new (or recently polished) prosthesis when homeostasis is being established (or re-established) within the socket (conjunctival mucous coating of the prosthesis and tear balance); a second period *equilibrium phase* when beneficial surface deposits that facilitate wettability of the prosthesis build up on the prosthesis and wear is comfortable; and a third period or *breakdown phase* where there is an increasing likelihood of irritation from continued wear. The proposed model also provides a rationale for prosthesis cleaning to help manage non-specific mucoid discharge [17].

The initial period of wear when physiological homeostasis is being established within the socket is approximately a month [17]. The length of time beyond this homeostatic phase when the microenvironment starts to break down varies between individuals but is several months (e.g., 6–12 months) in duration. Artificial eye patients usually know as the artificial eye starts to have increased discharge and some irritation [17]. Frequent removal and manipulation of the artificial eye (e.g., daily or weekly) never allows the artificial eye socket microenvironment to get into the homeostatic (comfortable) phase. As a result, discharge is often more of a problem [17]. Frequent removal of the artificial eye also roughens the fine polished surface of the prosthesis and may lead to microtrauma of the conjunctiva with resultant socket irritation and discharge. If the prosthetic eye has to be removed by the patient (to remove lashes trapped behind it or other foreign bodies), proper cleaning and handling of the prosthetic eye is important. Cleaning (by the patient) approximately every 6–9 months is also suggested as prosthetic deposits accumulate continuously and after 6 months of wear may be thick enough to irritate the conjunctiva and cause discharge [17–19]. The ideal cleaning regime for most individuals will also be influenced by medical conditions (e.g., allergies), the wearing environment (e.g., dust, dirt, wind), and the standard surface finish of the prosthesis [17]. Although numerous cleaning techniques have been suggested over the years [16, 22–26] (many of which are contradictory), Pine et al. have recently reported that simply wiping all surfaces of the artificial eye under cool tap water with a wet paper towel is simple and works extremely well to clean the surface deposits that build up on the artificial eye over time [17–19]. This can easily be done by the patient in any environment should he/she have to remove the prosthetic eye. Dry paper towel or tissue (e.g., Kleenex) is ineffective in removing deposits and may wear away the highly polished surface of the prosthesis creating a rougher surface with a dull appearance. Similarly, solvents such as alcohol will damage the acrylic surface. The prosthetic eye patient should also return to their ocularist at least yearly to have the artificial eye assessed for damage, reassess fit, and have it "professionally cleaned and repolished to optical grade contact lens standard" [17–19]. Repolishing by the ocularists buffing instruments thoroughly removes deposits and microscratches as well as provides a smoother surface that not only looks better but also allows smoother movement of the eyelids over the prosthesis, decreasing conjunctival irritation and associated mucous production. Gradual changes to the eye socket such as fat atrophy and laxity of the upper and lower eyelids may cause rotation or malposition of the prosthetic eye. Minor changes in the shape or thickness of the artificial eye may provide the patient with a more comfortable fit and improve cosmesis [17]. Yearly checkups with an ophthalmologist allow assessment for post-enucleation socket syndrome or other complications (e.g., implant exposure) that are easier to repair if identified early.

Socket Dryness

Tear production gradually decreases over time in the anophthalmic socket [27–29], leading to burning and irritation within the socket in some individuals. Mucous secretion from the conjunctival goblet cells may increase as a compensatory mechanism and not uncommonly is interpreted as an infection by the patient. Artificial tears or gel applied throughout the day are very helpful. If tear supplements do not relieve dry eye symptoms, a drop of "light" mineral oil (a laxative purchased at any pharmacy) can be used on the artificial eye surface to allow the eyelids to glide smoothly over the prosthesis. Topical silicone oil (e.g., Sil-Ophtho – Stony Brook, Inc., Davenport, Iowa) may also be used and is often available through ocularists' offices.

Discharge and Irritation

Mucoid discharge with prosthetic eye wear often develops to some degree with time and can be a distressing condition that affects the quality of life of people who have lost an eye [17–20, 25, 26]. With an alteration in tear production post-enucleation/evisceration and the presence of a foreign body (the artificial eye), mucous secretion from the conjunctival goblet cells may increase which is often interpreted as an infection by the patient. Frequent handling may retard the normal prosthesis-socket microenvironment development and also result in damage to the highly polished prosthetic surface [17, 18]. Similarly, a prosthesis older than 5 years may develop an irregular surface leading to further mucous production. A poorly fit prosthetic eye may also have a sizeable dead space between the posterior surface of the prosthesis and the conjunctiva where mucoid debris (i.e., stagnant tears, dust particles, eyelashes) often accumulates giving the patient the impression they have a socket infection (Figs. 62.3a, b and 62.4a–e) [30–32].

When assessing the prosthetic eye patient with discharge, it is important for the physician to determine the age of the prosthesis and the patient's routine of prosthetic hygiene.

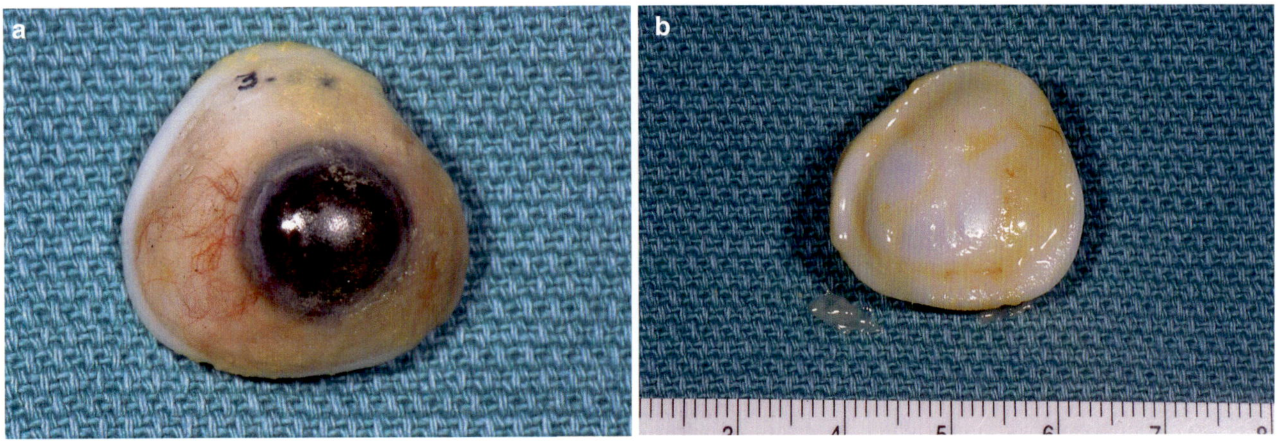

Fig. 62.3 (**a**, **b**) A 65-year-old male presented with socket discharge. He was wearing a 25-year-old prosthesis that hadn't been cleaned, polished, or adjusted since it was made. The prosthesis has multiple surface scratches and nicks. It has lost its luster and is discolored. In some areas the acrylic resin used to make the eye was breaking down. The discharge buildup is obvious (**b**)

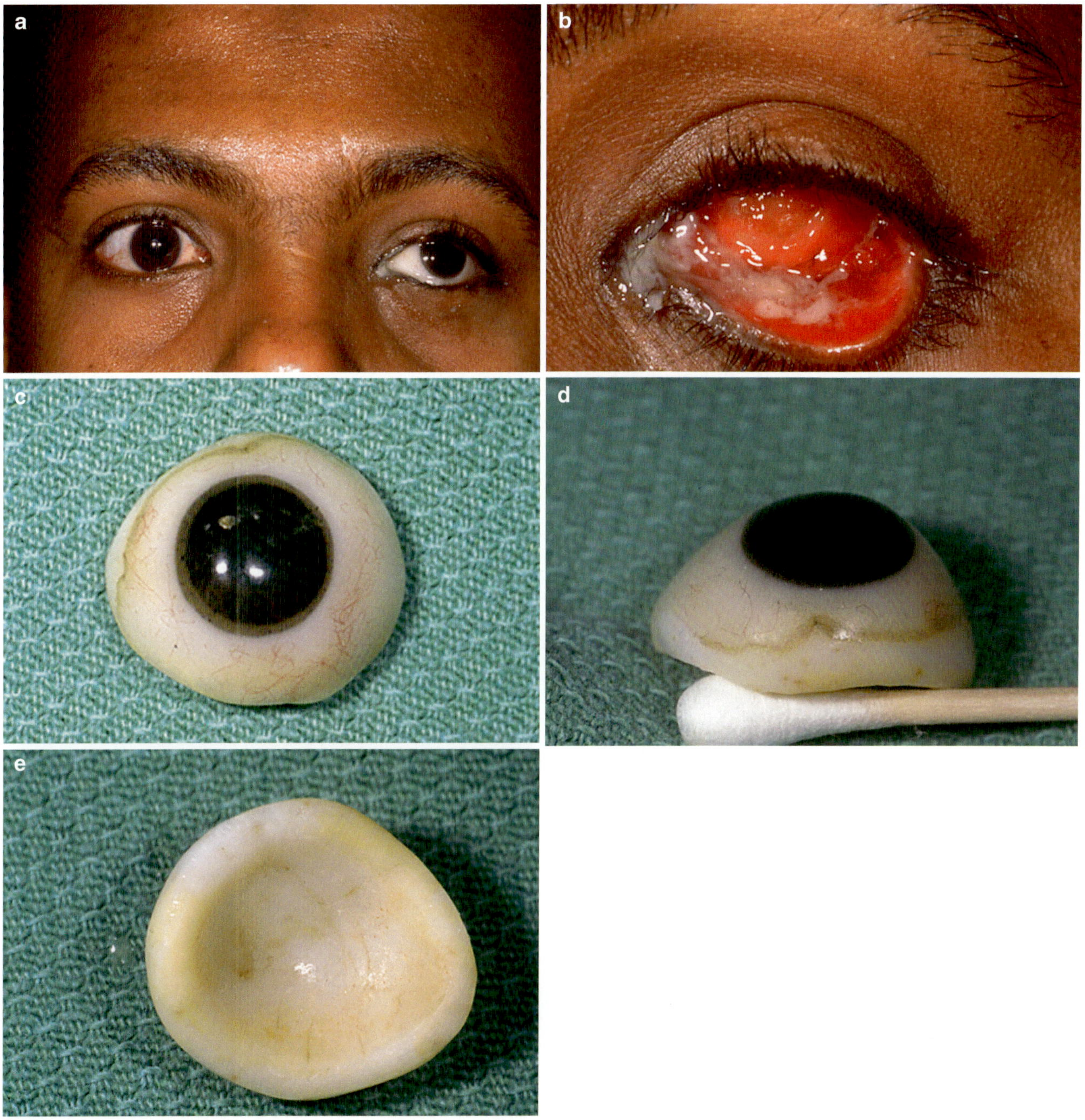

Fig. 62.4 (**a**) A 30-year-old male complaining of excessive discharge, burning, and irritation. The artificial eye was a "staock eye" and did not fit well since he acquired it 8 years earlier. He removed it frequently throughout the day to remove the discharge that accumulated behind the prosthesis. There was no improvement with a variety of antibiotic eye drops. (**b**) Discharge is seen in the inferior fornix as well as a great deal of conjunctival inflammation. (**c**) The artificial eye has lost its luster and is discolored around the edges. (**d**) The acrylic resin is breaking down along the edges of the prosthesis. (**e**) The posterior edge of the prosthetic eye was extremely rough and responsible for most of the conjunctival irritation and mucous production. The dead space posterior to the artificial eye accumulated the discharge which then migrated anteriorly to sit on the anterior surface of the artificial eye. The patient was sent for a custom-made prosthetic eye and placed on antibiotic-steroid drops. Within 2 weeks he was remarkably improved and more comfortable. The discharge had improved by 95%

Minimizing handling of the prosthesis should be encouraged. Prosthesis irregularities (e.g., nicks, scratches) and poor surface quality (loss of luster) are usually obvious at the slit lamp or when the prosthesis is taken out to assess the eye socket (Figs. 62.3a and 62.4c–e). Lubrication of the prosthesis should be evaluated as socket dryness with burning is not uncommon and artificial tears, gels, or other lubricants can be suggested. The patient should be asked when they were last in to see their ocularist. The ocularist will also evaluate the surface of the prosthesis for nicks and scratches as well as assess the fit of the artificial eye, being sure it is the appropriate size and there is no dead space between the prosthesis and orbital implant where mucous and other debris can accumulate. Most patients require annual polishing of the prosthesis but some sockets require semiannual polishing of the artificial eye to smooth the surface and remove the protein deposits. The average life of an artificial eye is typically 5–7 years but varies from socket to socket and is impacted by the daily, monthly, and annual hygiene administered. If discharge is still a problem after assessment by the ophthalmologist and ocularist, then treatment with a mild corticosteroid drop (i.e., FML) or a combined antibiotic-steroid drop (e.g., tobramycin- dexamethasone) once or twice daily often diminishes the discharge.

When more excessive discharge is present, a conjunctival infection (viral or bacterial) should be considered. Usually there are accompanying signs of acute or chronic conjunctivitis including edematous eyelids, conjunctival chemosis, hyperemia, and mucopurulent discharge in the conjunctival fornices (Fig. 62.5a, b). Conjunctival cultures are helpful in guiding appropriate antibiotic treatment.

There is also a subset of anophthalmic patients that have an exceptionally deep superior fornix, chronic conjunctival discharge, and ptosis [32]. The deep fornix and low-grade conjunctival inflammation lead to buildup of protein exudate that becomes colonized by bacteria leading to recurrent discharge [31, 32]. Rose described this “giant fornix syndrome” and suggested a cycle of progressively worsening symptoms not uncommonly treated with frequent topical antibiotics and/or systemic antibiotics [31, 32]. Jones et al. proposed eliminating the potential space harboring the chronic mucopurulent coagulum by shortening the fornix and concomitantly repairing the ptosis through a posterior surgical approach [32]. The superior conjunctivoplasty-Mullerectomy procedure resulted in significant improvement in their patients’ chronic socket discharge [32].

A pyogenic granuloma may also be the cause of recurrent socket discharge. Intermittent bleeding is often reported, and the vascular lesions are typically present along the conjunctival closure site or around an implant peg (Fig. 62.6). Pyogenic granulomas are a sign of local irritation or micro-

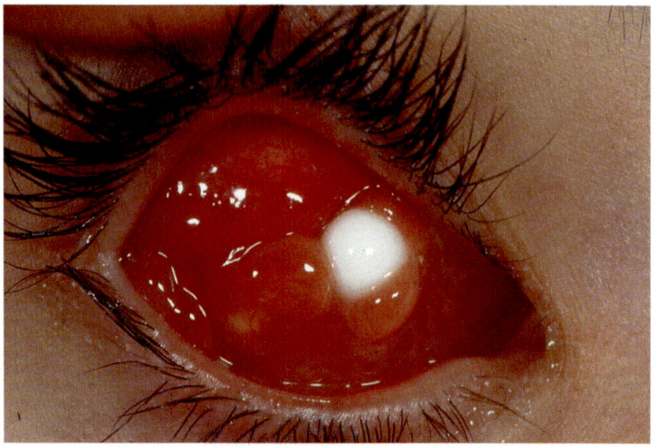

Fig. 62.6 Pyogenic granulomas are seen surrounding a polycarbonate peg

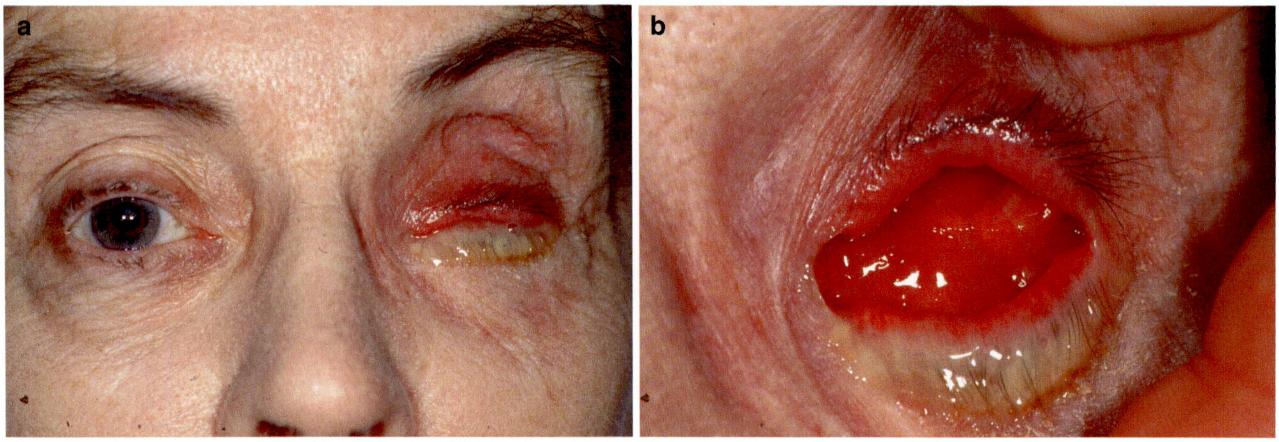

Fig. 62.5 (**a**) An 80-year-old female 6 weeks post-enucleation with a hydroxyapatite implant presented with recurrent discharge, recurrent pyogenic granulomas, socket tenderness, and no response to topical or oral antibiotics. An implant infection was suspected. (**b**) The conjunctiva was very inflamed with a large recurrent pyogenic granuloma laterally over the implant surface was present. Discharge was also seen along the lower lid margin. The porous implant was removed and grew Staphylococcus aureus on culture. She remained well with a comfortable socket following a secondary orbital implant (polymethylmethacrylate)

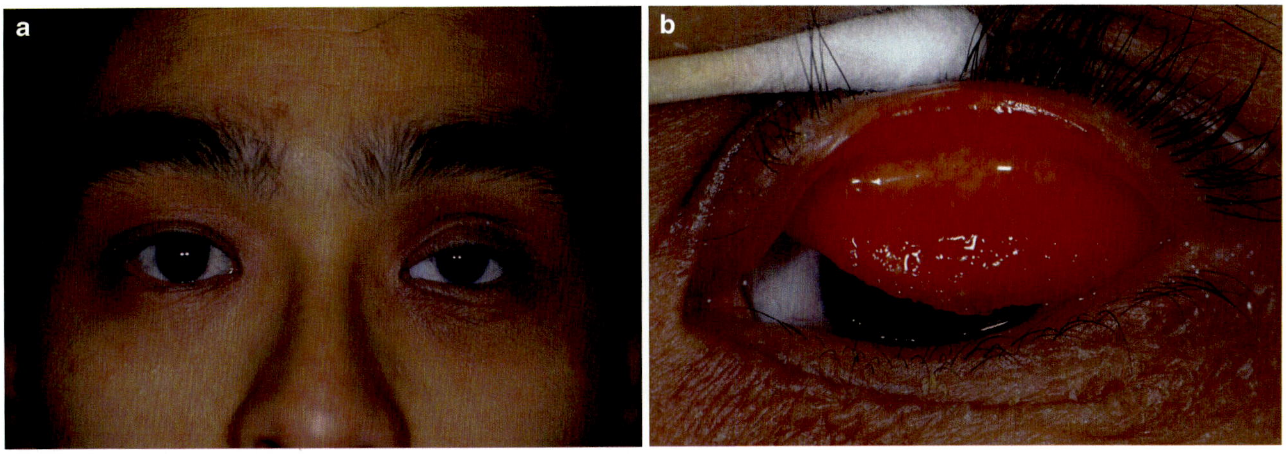

Fig. 62.7 (a) A 30-year-old man with a 5-year history of wearing an artificial eye presented with recurrent discharge and a left upper lid ptosis. (b) When the eyelid is flipped, giant cobblestones typical of giant papillary conjunctivitis were seen over the tarsal plate surface

trauma and may also indicate underlying implant exposure and/or infection [32, 33].

Recurrent and chronic socket discharge is also a distinguishing feature of giant papillary conjunctivitis or "GPC" [34, 35]. The etiology of GPC is not fully understood but is believed to be an immunologic reaction to an antigen present on the surface of the prosthesis. Giant papillae (>1 mm) on the tarsal conjunctiva of the upper eyelid is the hallmark of GPC (Fig. 62.7a, b). In severe cases, GPC may significantly limit the amount of time the patient can wear the prosthesis. Treatment can be difficult and may involve corticosteroid eye drops in conjunction with allergy drops. Topical cyclosporine eye drops or tacrolimus 0.03% ointment may also be helpful [36, 37]. In recalcitrant cases, carbon dioxide laser or cryoablation of the giant papillae can be attempted. Rarely, a prosthesis made of a different material (e.g., glass) may be considered.

Lagophthalmos with Exposure of the Prosthesis Surface

Some individuals with nocturnal lagophthalmos may develop unsightly dried matter on the anterior surface of the prosthesis that adheres the lid margin and/or lashes to the anterior surface of the prosthesis. As the eyelid attempts to open upon awakening, it is pulled away from the prosthesis surface causing discomfort and irritation. Sometimes the debris can be cleaned without removing the prosthesis by rinsing the surface of the prosthetic eye with a soft contact lens irrigating solution, or several drops of an artificial tear drop. If this is not successful, the artificial eye should be removed, and wiping the debris off the artificial eye under cool tap water with a wet paper towel works well. Light mineral oil or a lubricating eye ointment (e.g., lacrilube) should be used at bedtime on the anterior surface of the prosthesis if debris build up and eyelid sticking is a chronic problem.

Table 62.1 Causes of socket pain

Eyelid malpositions
Entropion, ectropion, incomplete eyelid closure
Conjunctival problems
Pyogenic granulomas, conjunctival inclusion cysts, giant papillary conjunctivitis, neoplasia (squamous cell)
Prosthesis issues
Poor fit, prosthetic surface breakdown, nicks, scratches, deposits, allergic reaction to the ocular prosthesis
Implant problems
Infection, inflammation, migration, exposure
Socket problems
Recurrent or new malignancy, amputation neuroma, trochleitis, scleritis (post-evisceration cases), socket contraction
Lacrimal gland
Dry socket
Referred pain from adjacent areas
Skull base/sinus/sphenoid wing tumors, postherpetic neuralgia
Others
Complex regional pain syndrome, phantom eye pain, drug-seeking behavior, factitious

Socket Pain

Pain and discomfort in the anophthalmic socket are uncommon but may range from the trivial to a more severe degree that affects daily life [2, 34, 39–46]. A wide variety of problems can cause socket pain and discomfort, most of which can be diagnosed through a careful history and clinical examination of the prosthesis and eye socket (Table 62.1). Prosthetic care and handling should be assessed as well as the fit of the artificial eye. The socket implant should be evaluated for signs of migration and the conjunctiva for signs of inflammation, infection or implant exposure. Migration of the implant may alter the fit of the prosthesis creating pressure on the tissue between the implant and prosthesis. Trochlear irritation/inflammation secondary to the prosthetic edge hitting the trochlear area on a recurrent basis is also a consideration [40]. Palpation of the trochlea recreates the discomfort experienced by the patient. If an evisceration was performed, recurrent scleritis and postherpetic neuralgia are rare causes of recurrent socket pain to consider. Patients with healthy-appearing sockets may be challenging, and more rare etiologies (e.g., phantom eye pain, drug-seeking behavior, secondary gain, factitious) should be considered [2, 34, 46]. Persistent socket pain warrants cranial neuroimaging (computerized tomography, magnetic resonance imaging) with attention to the orbit, paranasal sinus, and brainstem to rule out an amputation neuroma, sinus infection or mass, or an intraorbital or central nervous system abnormality [2].

Anterior Orbital Cysts

The development of a subconjunctival/anterior orbital cyst is occasionally seen and may be responsible for socket discomfort (aching, pressure sensation) as well as problems with the fit of a patient's prosthetic eye (Fig. 62.8) [47, 48]. These cysts arise from buried conjunctival epithelium that becomes incarcerated during wound closure. Management options include complete surgical excision of the cyst, marsupialization, absolute alcohol injection, and more recently trichloroacetic acid (TCA) injection [49–54]. Simple aspiration is inadequate treatment as it will only deflate the cyst for a few days.

Eyelid Malpositions

Lower eyelid laxity is a common problem that occurs with time in many artificial eye patients, and results from the aging eyelid supporting the weight of the prosthesis as well as tissue changes associated with removal of the eye (anophthalmic socket syndrome) [8, 9]. Lower eyelid laxity can be corrected with a tarsal strip-type procedure [55–57]. These procedures

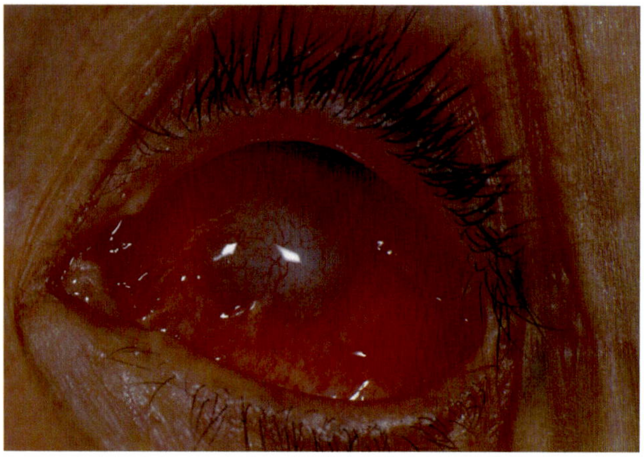

Fig. 62.8 A subconjunctival cyst is visible centrally. The patient presented with a pressure sensation in the socket

create a horizontal tightening, maintain the natural contour of the lower lid and lateral canthus, and provide improved support for the prosthesis without sacrificing the conjunctiva or inferior fornix. Some patients will also develop an inadequate inferior fornix secondary to anterior migration of inferior orbital fat and thinning or disruption of the suspensory ligament of the inferior fornix, resulting in anterior rotation of the lower edge of the prosthesis [58–60]. The fornix can be reconstructed with suture fixation of the conjunctiva to the orbital rim periosteum in some [60, 61]. In those patients with inferior eyelid retraction and/or vertically directed eye lashes with eyelid margin entropion associated with lower fornix contraction, eyelid rotational sutures or a marginal tarsotomy-type procedure may be required [61–65]. More advanced cases may require posterior lamellar lengthening with a spacer graft (e.g., mucous membrane, auricular or nasal cartilage, hard palate mucosa, acellular dermis) (Fig. 62.9a–d) [58–60].

Ectropion of the lower eyelid is frequently associated with significant lower eyelid laxity. This may initially present as an aesthetic issue but eventually leads to difficulties with prosthesis retention. A tarsal strip-type procedure and occasionally a posterior lamellar spacer graft may be required [55–58]. Occasionally there is a deficiency of anterior lamella (i.e., skin) requiring a skin graft or preferably a skin-muscle transposition pedicle flap from the upper eyelid to the lower eyelid.

Upper eyelid ptosis may result from inadequate implant size, migration of the orbital implant, a poorly fit prosthesis, laxity of the fibrous connective tissue framework in the superior orbit (including Whitnall's ligament) with rotation of the orbital tissues posteriorly and inferiorly (post-enucleation socket syndrome), trauma from the original injury/surgery, or senile dehiscence of the levator aponeurosis [66–68]. The mechanisms producing anophthalmic ptosis are multifactorial and should be assessed carefully before surgical repair to achieve optimal aesthetic results. Ocular prosthesis augmentation (artificial eye with a superior extension or flange) is a conservative non-surgical method to correct mild anophthalmic ptosis. Levator-Müller muscle involutional changes may be corrected with either an anterior or posterior approach (Fig. 62.10a, b) [68]. A superior conjunctivoplasty-Mullerectomy has been beneficial in those with an exceptionally deep superior fornix, ptosis, and chronic discharge (giant fornix syndrome) [31, 32]. Some anophthalmic patients with ptosis will require more than one surgical procedure to restore symmetry (Fig. 62.11a, b).

Deep Superior Sulcus and Enophthalmos

The socket soft tissue and volume changes that occur following enucleation or evisceration surgery causing upper eyelid ptosis and lower eyelid malposition also contribute to deepening of the superior sulcus [8, 9]. Inadequate volume replacement (too small an implant or no implant) at the time of the enucleation or evisceration procedure and postsurgical

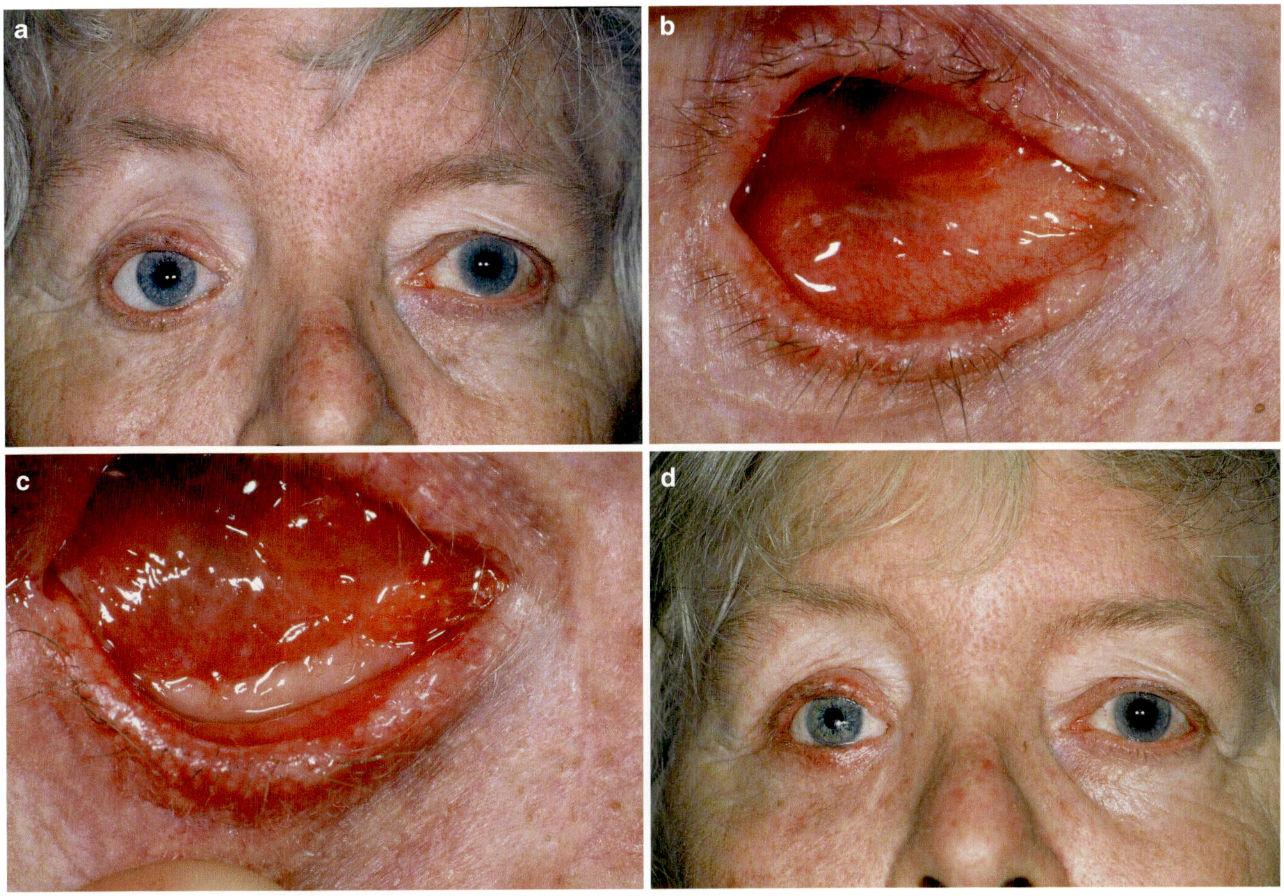

Fig. 62.9 (**a**, **b**) A 64-year-old female was seen with a retracted right lower eyelid as a result of inferior fornix shortening. (**c**) A hard palate graft was placed along the lower edge of tarsus and sutured in place. (**d**) Three months post-surgery, the right lower eyelid is in a more normal position

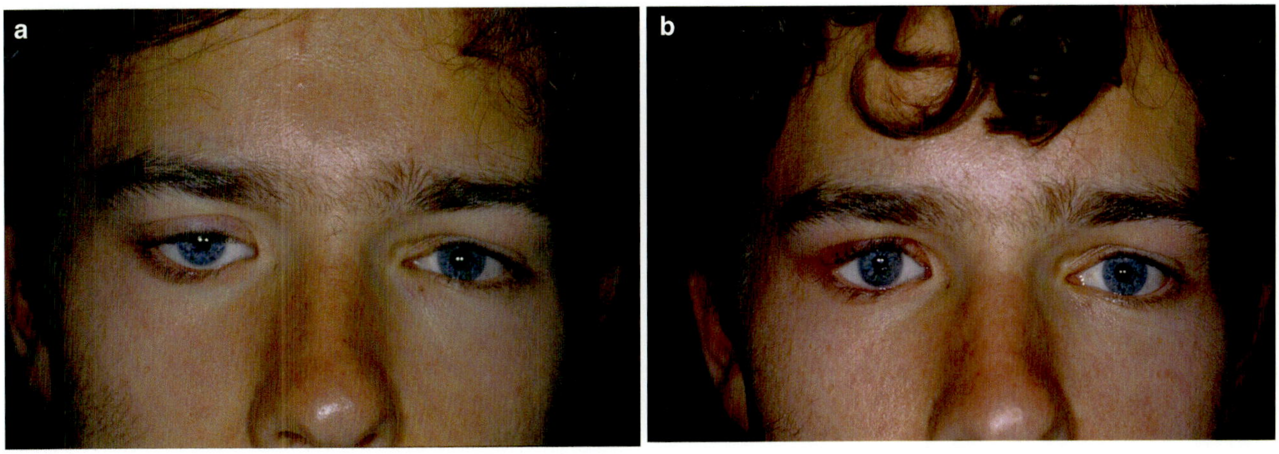

Fig. 62.10 (**a**) A 20-year-old male is seen with a right upper eyelid ptosis. The socket volume was fine. (**b**) Three months following an anterior approach levator advancement procedure, there is much better lid symmetry

orbital fat atrophy are other important factors in the development of a deep superior sulcus [8, 9, 11–14].

Conservative management of a superior sulcus deformity includes camouflage with lightly tinted spectacles or a weak plus lens (+1 to +2) that adds some magnification and helps make a narrow palpebral fissure appear larger. Alterations in the prosthesis can provide additional eyelid support and volume and help improve eyelid position and fullness. Surgical options include correcting any bone defects from old orbital fractures, adding additional socket volume (e.g., orbital floor

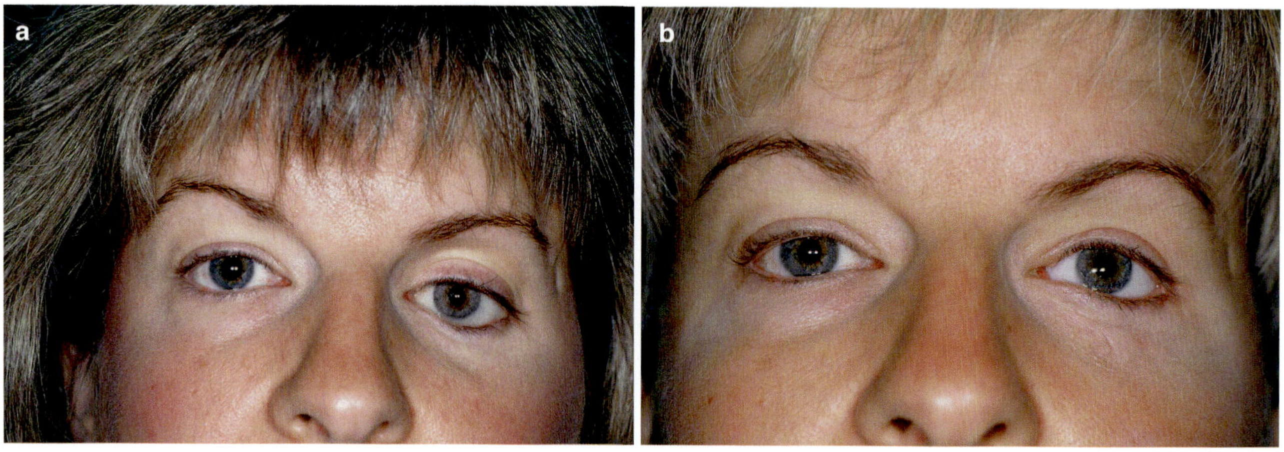

Fig. 62.11 (**a**) A 35-year-old female was seen for assessment of enophthalmos, left lower lid retraction and left upper eyelid ptosis. An orbital floor implant was put in place first (see Fig. 62.12a) followed in 3 months by a hard palate graft to the left inferior fornix, followed in 23 months by an anterior approach levator advancement procedure. (**b**) Four months following her last surgery and an adjustment to her artificial eye, she was happy with the symmetry between the two sides

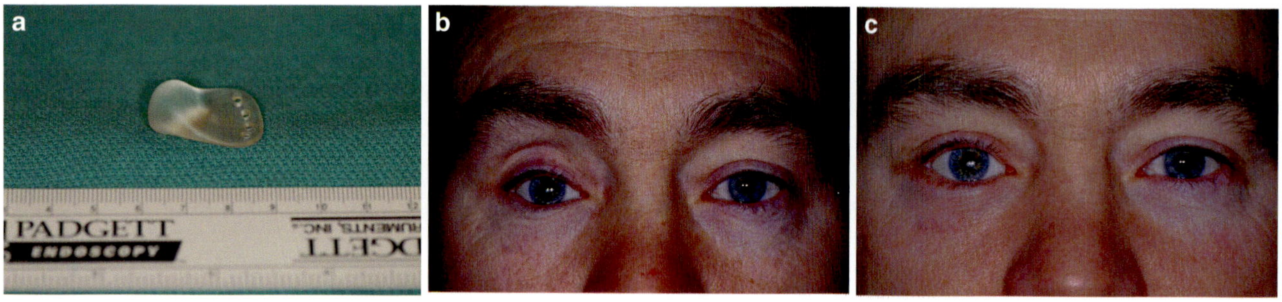

Fig. 62.12 (**a**) A subperiosteal floor implant ("Coderre implant," Oculoplastik[R], Inc., Montreal, Quebec). (**b**) A 35-year-old male presented 1 year post-evisceration with a deep superior sulcus on the right side. (**c**) Three months post-orbital floor implant, there was excellent superior sulcus symmetry

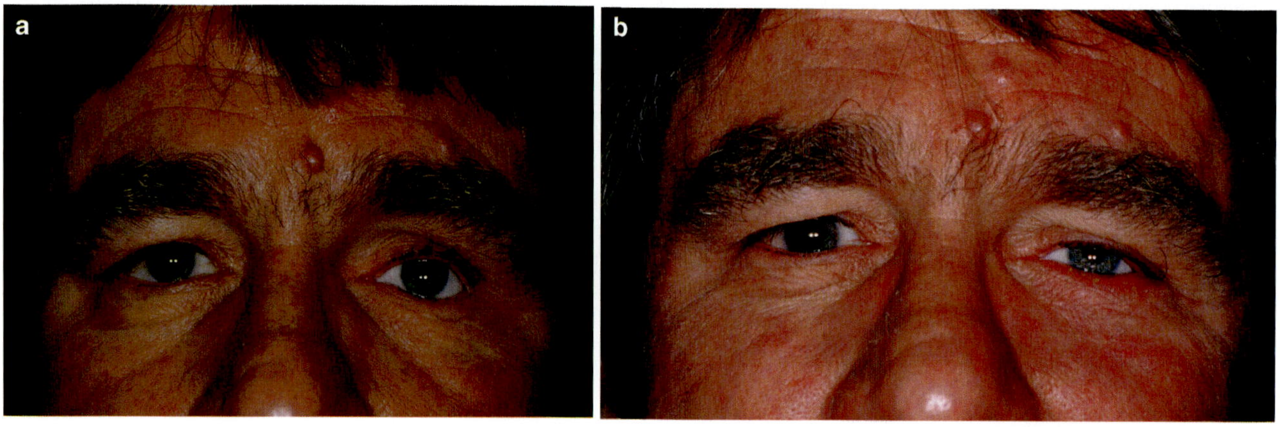

Fig. 62.13 (**a**) A 49-year-old male presented 3 years post-enucleation with a deep superior sulcus on the left side. (**b**) Three months post-orbital floor implant, there is excellent superior sulcus symmetry

implant; Fig. 62.12a), and superior sulcus tissue grafting (dermis fat grafting or acellular human dermis graft) (AlloDerm®, Lifecell Inc., Woodlands, Texas, USA, or DermaMatrix, Synthes, West Chester, PA, USA) [69–71]. Acrylic floor implants (polymethylmethacrylate) are commonly utilized for orbital volume augmentation (Figs. 62.12a–c and 62.13a, b), but other materials have been utilized including bone grafts, silicone beads, hydroxyapatite, silicone, teflon, supramid sheets, dermis fat, as well as a variety of injectable products such as autogenous fat, injectable hydroxylapatite (Radiesse), cross-linked collagen, silicone oil, self-inflating hydrogel pellet expanders, and hard tissue replacement polymer [72–76]. Soft tissue and dermal fillers (e.g., hyaluronic acid derived products) are another alternative to correct superior sulcus volume loss [38, 77].

Secondary Orbital Implantation

Enophthalmos may occur from fat atrophy secondary to orbital soft tissue changes post-enucleation/evisceration, inadequate implant volume replacement, or implant extrusion. Insertion of a secondary intraconal orbital implant is a consideration to correct the enophthalmos and superior sulcus depression (Fig. 62.14a, b). Secondary orbital implantation may also be indicated to improve prosthesis motility or for implant exposure or migration that has resulted in prosthetic fitting difficulties [78–83].

Secondary orbital implant surgery is often more complicated than enucleation or evisceration principally due to the disruption of anatomic planes, with disorganization and rearrangement of the orbital tissues. In addition, varying degrees of scarring are present throughout the orbital tissue as a result of the initial trauma or primary anophthalmic socket procedure. A variety of techniques for secondary orbital implantation have been described [78–82]. While secondary orbital implantation can be carried out without attempting to identify the rectus muscles, localization of the rectus muscles will typically help reposition the implant in a more anatomically correct position and improve socket motility [82].

Implant Migration

Implant migration may occur with long-standing orbital implants (e.g., nonporous alloplastic) as a result of the progressive orbital soft tissue changes that occur with time in the anophthalmic socket [8, 9]. Muscle imbrication over the anterior surface of a nonporous implant, a common practice many years ago, was formerly a predisposing factor to implant migration [83]. The overlapping muscles predisposed the orbital implant to an "up and out" or "down and in" migration over time. The increased use of porous orbital implants and improved surgical techniques have contributed to a significant decline in the incidence of implant migration. A migrated implant may lead to poor motility and an uncomfortable, poorly positioned prosthesis. Refitting the sockets with a new prosthesis may help socket motility and comfort. Alternatively, a secondary implant centrally positioned within the muscle cone and with reattachment of the rectus muscles may be required [78–82].

Implant Exposure and Extrusion

Implant exposure may occur with any type of implant days to years following anophthalmic surgery and may lead to implant infection, extrusion, or explantation (Fig. 62.15a, b, c). It was anticipated that porous orbital implants would have a lower incidence of implant exposure than traditional nonporous implants because of their associated fibrovascular ingrowth. However, complications gradually came to light with their widespread use over the past 25 years, and implant exposure is the complication discussed most often with reported implant exposure rates ranging from 0% to 50% [39, 40, 44, 84–111]. Implant exposure problems continue to deter some surgeons from using HA implants.

Factors predisposing to implant exposure include closing the wound under tension, poor wound closure techniques, infection, mechanical or inflammatory irritation from the spiculated surface of the porous implant, and/or delayed ingrowth of fibrovascular tissue with subsequent tissue breakdown [107]. It is believed that appropriate implant placement and proper tissue closure are of primary importance in helping to prevent porous implant exposure [46, 96, 107, 111–113].

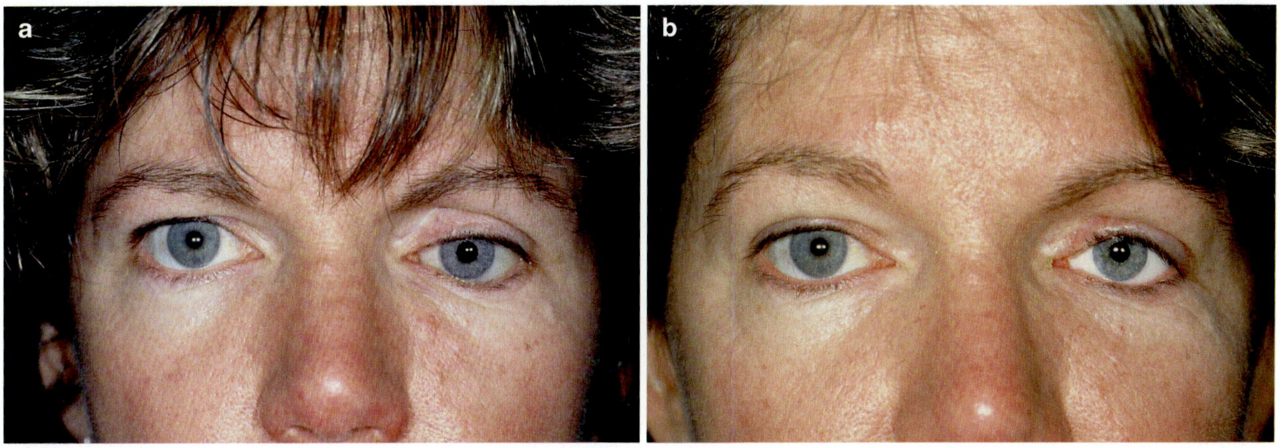

Fig. 62.14 (**a**) A 40-year-old female was seen with ptosis and enophthalmos of the left socket. As her orbital implant was put in as a child and was rather small, it was elected to put a larger implant in place as a first step to restore socket volume (16 mm implant removed, 20 mm implant inserted) followed by an anterior approach levator advancement ptosis correction 3 months later. (**b**) Six months post-surgery there was much more symmetry present between the two sides

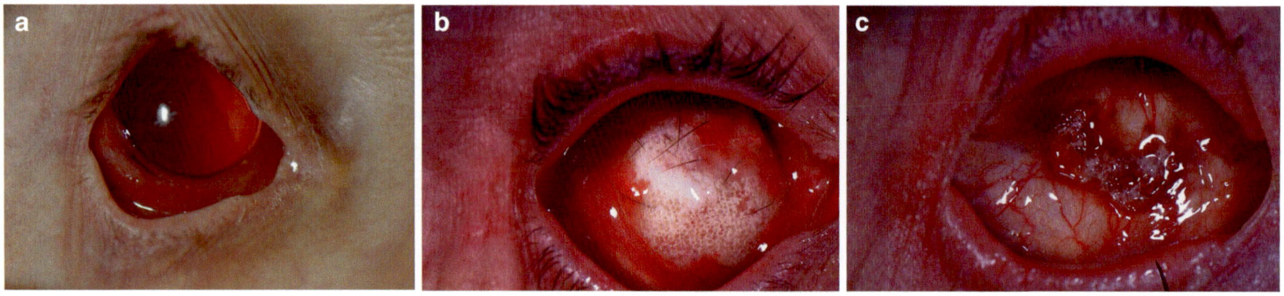

Fig. 62.15 (**a**) Exposed polymethylmethacrylate spherical implant. (**b**) Exposed aluminum oxide orbital implant 3 years post-enucleation surgery. (**c**) Exposed aluminum oxide orbital implant 5 year following evisceration surgery

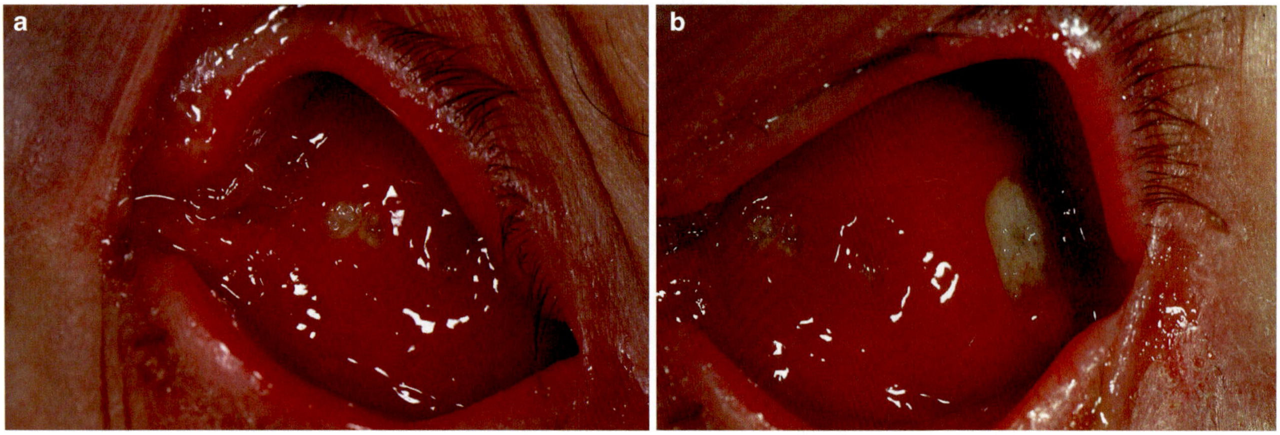

Fig. 62.16 (**a**) Left socket of a 40-year-old man post-enucleation with a porous polyethylene spherical implant. He was experiencing recurrent discharge, bloody secretions and discomfort when touching the implant. The porous polyethylene implant can be seen through the inflamed conjunctiva. Implant infection was suspected. (**b**) Another view of the same socket with at least 2 areas of exposed implant visible. The implant was removed and grew pseudomonas

A variety of techniques are available to manage implant exposure. For nonporous implants, implant removal and secondary implantation are usually required [82]. For porous implants management may include wound reclosure early on postsurgery (first few weeks) with or without a patch graft (e.g., sclera, temporalis fascia), vaulting of the prosthesis, and watchful waiting [113]. Persistent and/or large implant exposures may require additional surgery. A variety of graft and flap techniques have been advocated to repair implant exposure including Tenon's flaps, bipedicle conjunctival flaps, tarsoconjunctival pedicle flaps, scleral patch grafts, temporalis fascia or fascia lata grafts, hard palate mucosa or dermis fat grafts as well as other techniques [114–119].

Implant Infection

Infection of porous implants is a rare complication that may be difficult to control without implant removal [34, 120–124]. Factors predisposing to infection include early conjunctival dehiscence with implant exposure, poor or delayed vascular ingrowth secondary to chronic illness (e.g., diabetes, vasculopathy), chemotherapy, radiation therapy, prior socket reconstruction, or delayed fibrovascular ingrowth within a host scleral shell with no portals for vascular ingrowth [34]. Initial symptoms and signs are not always indicative of implant infection. Recurrent discharge, for example, may indicate implant infection but is also a common problem for some artificial eye patients without an infectious process. The constellation of socket findings including persistent mucopurulent discharge despite antibiotic coverage, recurrent pyogenic granuloma (indicative of implant exposure), and socket discomfort (aggravated by touching the implant) should raise one's suspicion for an implant infection (Fig. 62.16a, b) [120, 121]. Implant infection typically requires implant explantation with the risk of rectus or levator or oculomotor nerve injury as well as other socket tissue damage that may limit subsequent reconstructive options [120–124].

Pegging Problems and Complications

One of the main advantages of porous orbital implants (e.g., hydroxyapatite, aluminum oxide, porous polyethylene) is the ability to directly integrate them with an overlying artificial eye through a pegging system (Fig. 62.17). By coupling the orbital implant to the artificial eye via a peg, a wider range of prosthetic eye movements (as well as the fine darting eye movements seen during conversational speech) is possible. More dynamic artificial eye movement imparts a more life-like quality to the prosthetic eye. Infrared oculography has demonstrated objective and significant improvement in horizontal gaze after motility peg placement [125]. Despite the improved motility, many surgeons and patients still elect to avoid peg placement due to the satisfactory results without pegging and the possibility of post-pegging complications [126–136].

Potential problems and complications associated with pegging include increased discharge, recurrent pyogenic granulomas, implant exposure around the peg, implant infection, tissue overgrowth, peg dislocation, clicking noises, and various fitting problems (Fig. 62.18a–d) [126–136]. Refitting the prosthesis, scleral patch grafting, peg removal, and at times implant removal may be required [126].

Although pegging has declined dramatically over the past decade, a precise and meticulous technique under local anesthesia with or without intravenous sedation in the appropriately

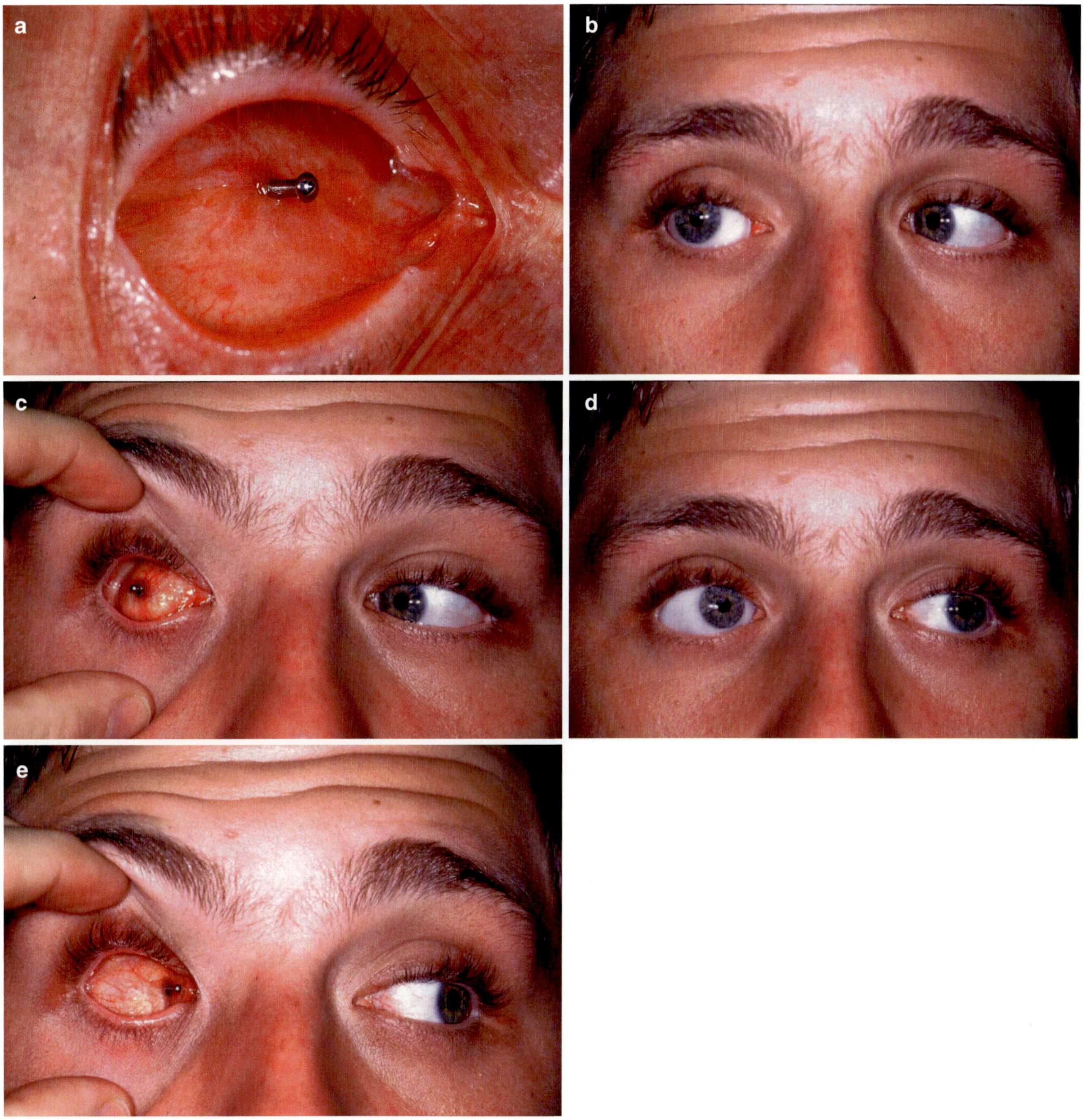

Fig. 62.17 (**a**) A well-positioned titanium peg with quiet conjunctiva surrounding is illustrated. (**b**) Post-evisceration patient with an aluminum oxide porous orbital implant looking to his right with excellent excursion in abduction. (**c**) The underlying titanium peg has also moved into abduction, explaining the excellent movement of the overlying prosthetic eye. (**d**) Patient looking to his left. (**e**) The underlying titanium peg has moved into adduction

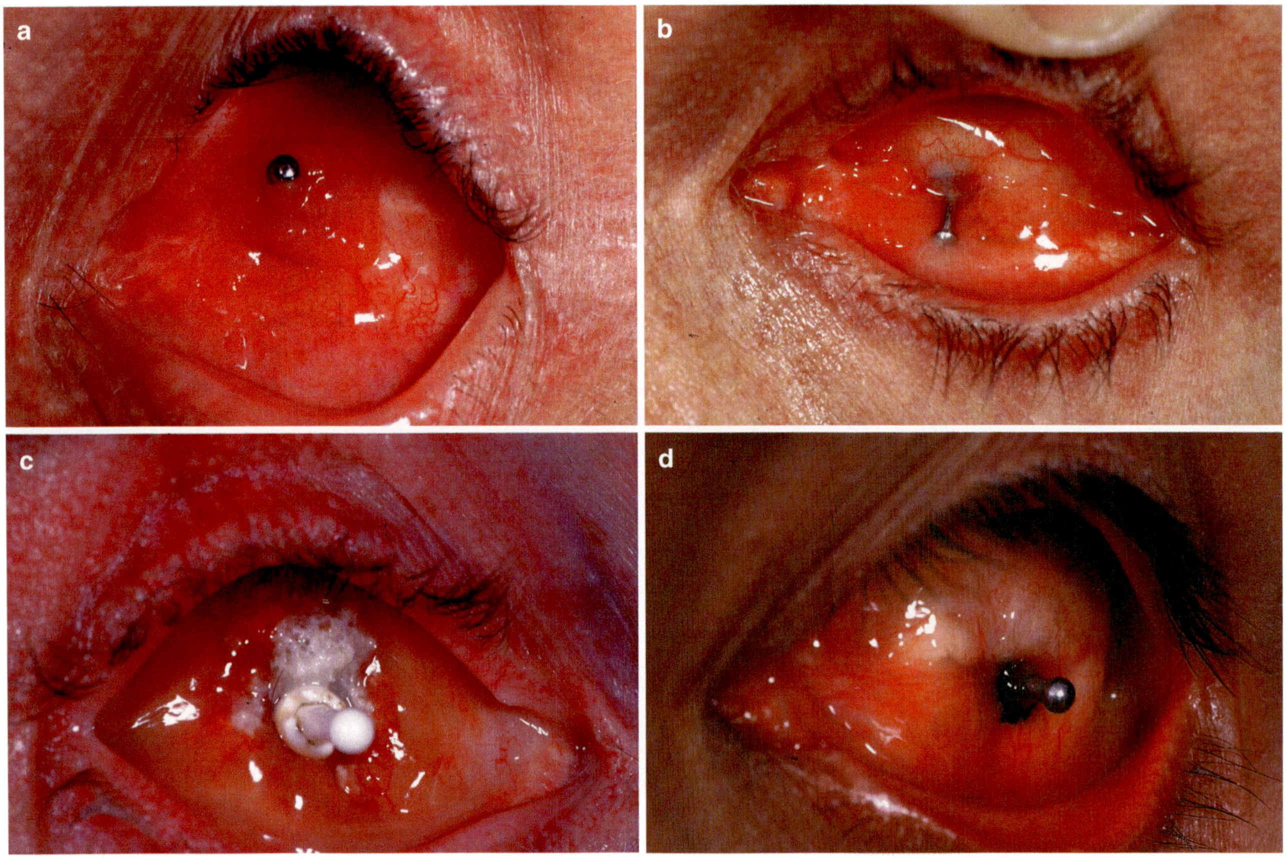

Fig. 62.18 (**a**) A large pyogenic granuloma surrounding a titanium peg. The patient was experiencing recurrent mucoid discharge. (**b**) The severe angulation downward of this peg made it very difficult to couple the overlying prosthetic eye with the peg. (**c**) Exposure of the peg sleeve and adjacent aluminum oxide orbital implant. (**d**) Accumulation of a black deposit that has leached away from the titanium peg is seen in the conjunctiva surrounding the peg

selected patient can be a successful outpatient procedure [134, 135]. It is important to be selective in deciding which patients are candidates for a peg system. Proper care of the artificial eye and regular follow-up visits with the ocularist and ophthalmic plastic surgeon are important to help ensure minimal problems with the peg system. If the patient is unlikely, unable, or unwilling to have adequate postoperative care, then pegging should be avoided. Children under 15 years of age, the elderly (those over 75 years of age approximately), or individuals of any age with a chronic illness or vasculopathy (e.g., a collagen vascular disease, sarcoidosis, diabetes mellitus, immunosuppressive therapy, prior orbital radiation therapy, etc.) should not be considered for pegging in the author's opinion [135].

Acquired Socket Contracture

Acquired socket contracture results from shrinkage and shortening of part or all of the orbital tissues in the anophthalmic orbit, resulting in conjunctival fornices that are inadequate to allow retention of a prosthesis [137, 138]. Socket contracture may occur as a result of several processes including scar tissue associated with the initial injury, poor surgical techniques during previous surgeries (e.g., excessive destruction of conjunctiva, traumatic dissection/cauterization within the socket), multiple socket operations (poor vascular supply), prior ischemic ocular disease, alkali/acid burns, cicatrizing conjunctival diseases, radiation therapy (plaque or external beam), chronic socket inflammation, infection, not wearing a conformer or prosthesis, and a poorly fitting prosthesis (Fig. 62.19a–c).

The goal of treatment in socket contracture is to identify and correct the underlying cause(s) (if possible), allow the patient to comfortably wear a prosthesis and achieve the best motility and cosmesis possible. In advanced cases of socket contracture, success may be limited to the ability of the patient to wear a prosthesis, with motility of the prosthesis and symmetry to the contralateral side secondary considerations. No single surgical technique exists for the treatment of the contracted socket, particularly in advanced cases. The management of each case must be individualized to correct the specific problem of the affected socket [139–157]. It is also important to remember that each surgical procedure may cause more tissue trauma to the socket, with disruption of the already compromised vasculature, resulting in further contracture of the socket (Fig. 62.20a–e).

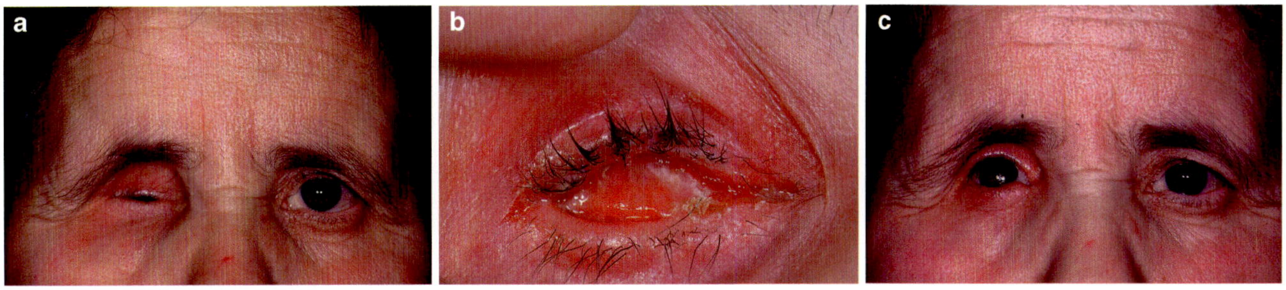

Fig. 62.19 (**a**) A 75-year-old female stopped wearing her artificial eye several years earlier and presented with a desire to have it refit. The right upper lid appears ptotic. (**b**) Close-up socket view illustrates almost complete loss of the superior and inferior fornix. (**c**) Following a mucous membrane graft to the upper and lower fornix, the patient was able to wear her prosthetic eye

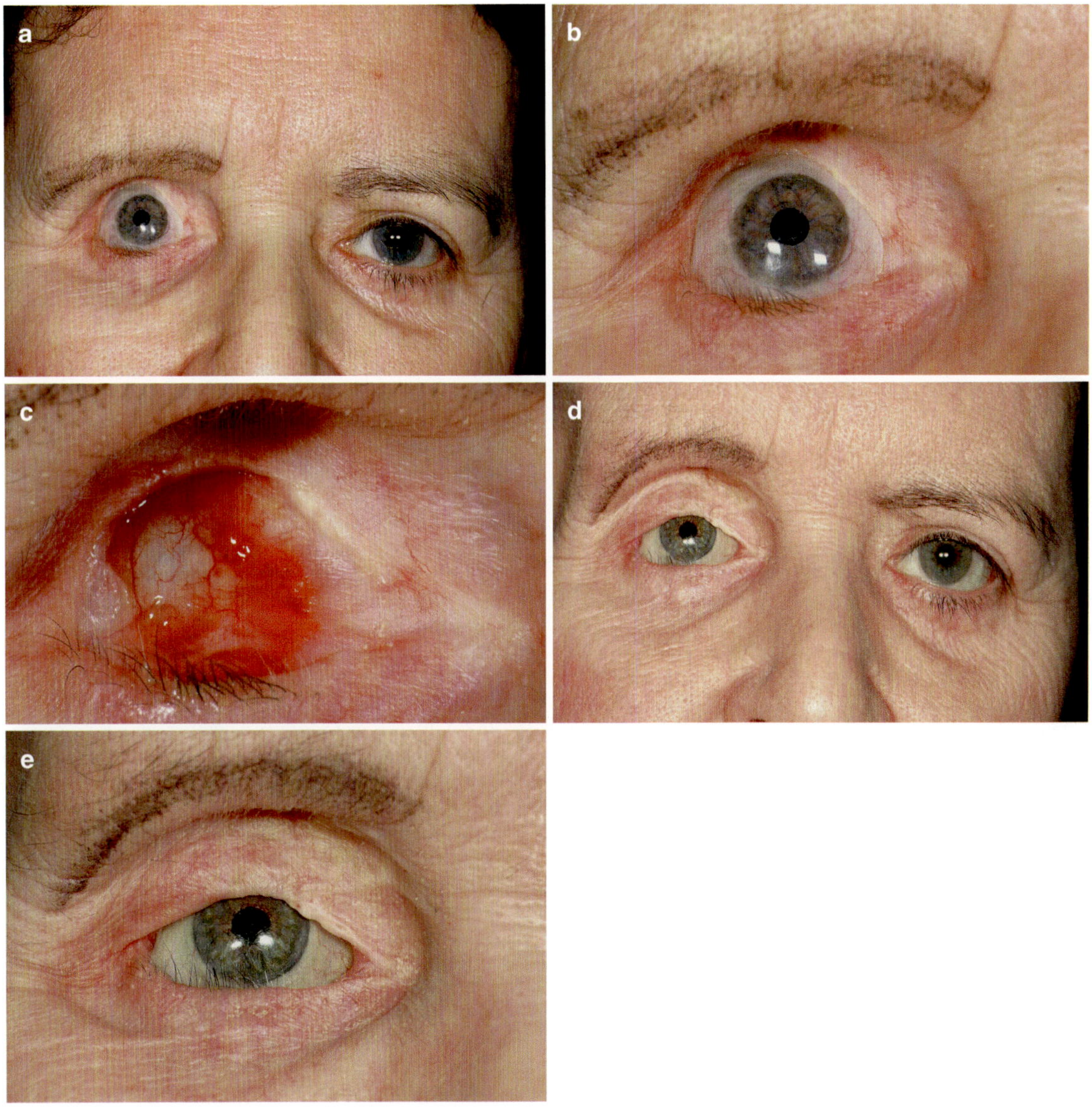

Fig. 62.20 (**a**) A 66-year-old female with an inability to wear her prosthetic eye comfortably. Following resection of a basal cell carcinoma from the right upper eyelid with postoperative radiation, the right cornea developed severe exposure then perforation. The right eye required enucleation. (**b**) There is enophthalmos with partial loss of the right upper eyelid margin and atrophic adjacent skin from the radiation treatment. (**c**) There was also severe deficiency of the superior fornix on the right. (**d, e**) Following multiple surgeries the patient was able to comfortably wear an artificial eye. She initially had a temporalis muscle transfer into the eye socket via a small bone tunnel in the lateral orbital wall for revascularization of the orbital tissues. A split thickness mucous membrane graft was carried out as a second procedure to recreate the superior fornix. A skin graft from the supraclavicular area was done during a third operation. Twelve weeks following the last surgery, the patient is seen wearing her prosthetic eye. It was comfortable and no longer fell out

Summary

Loss of an eye following trauma, malignant tumors, or severe ocular disease is a devastating circumstance. Since eye contact is an essential part of human interaction, it is extremely important for the anophthalmic patient to maintain a natural, normal-appearing prosthetic eye. In the past few decades, there have been numerous developments and refinements in anophthalmic socket surgery with respect to implant material and design, implant-prosthesis coupling, and socket volume consideration. Anophthalmic socket surgery is no longer simply about replacing a diseased eye with a basic orbital implant. Ophthalmic surgeons working closely with ocularists must be focused on restoring a natural appearance to the patient's prosthesis with comfort, some motility, appropriate orbital volume, and eyelids that look symmetrical, so they can blend into the society with a near-normal appearance. Although evisceration surgery has recently increased in popularity and is favored by many surgeons because of the simplicity of the technique, less disruption to the socket anatomy, and excellent cosmetic results, enucleation is still required in patients with known or potentially occult ocular malignancies as well as blind, painful, and/or unsightly eyes with opaque media and unknown or unclear past ocular histories [158].

References

1. Coday MP, Warner MA, Jarling KU, Rubin PAD. Acquired monocular vision, functional consequences form the patients perspective. Ophthalmic Plast Reconstr Surg. 2002;18:55–63.
2. Bohman E, Roed Rassmussen ML, Dafgard KE. Pain and discomfort in the anophthalmic socket. Curr Opin Ophthalmol. 2014;25:455–60.
3. Rasmussen ML, Ekholm O, Prause JU, Toft PB. Quality of life of eye amputated patients. Acta Ophthalmol. 2012;90:435–40.
4. Ahn JM, Lee SY, Yoon JS. Health related quality of life and emotional status of anophthalmic patients in Korea. Am J Ophthalmol. 2010;149:1005–11.
5. Masdottir S, Sahlin S. Patient satisfaction and results after evisceration with a split-sclera technique. Orbit. 2007;26:241–7.
6. McBain HB, Ezra DG, Rose GE, Newman SP. The psychological impact of living with an ocular prosthesis. Orbit. 2014;33:33–9.
7. Gougelmann HP. The evolution of the ocular motility implant. Int Ophthalmol Clin. 1970;10(4):689–711.
8. Smit TJ, Koornneef L, Zonnereld FW, Groet E, Otto AJ. Computed tomography in the assessment of the postenucleation socket syndrome. Ophthalmology. 1990;97:137–40.
9. Smit TJ, Koornneef L, Zonnereld FW, Groet E, Otto AJ. Primary and secondary implants in the anophthalmic orbit: preoperative and postoperative computed tomographic appearance. Opthalmology. 1991;98(1):106–10.
10. Soll DB. The anophthalmic socket. Ophthalmology. 1982; 89:407–23.
11. Kaltreider SA. The ideal ocular prostheses. Analysis of prosthetic volume. Ophthalmic Plast Reconstr Surg. 2000;16(5):388–92.
12. Kaltreider SA, Lucarelli MJ. A simple algorithm for selection of implant size for enucleation and evisceration. Ophthalmic Plast Reconstr Surg. 2002;18:336–41.
13. Custer PL, Trinkaus KM. Volumetric determination of enucleation Implant size. Am J Ophthalmol. 1999;128:489–94.
14. Thaller VT. Enucleation volume measurement. Ophthalmic Plast Reconstr Surg. 1997;13:18–20.
15. Allen L. Modified impression fitting. Int Ophthalmol Clin. 1970;10:747–62.
16. Parr GR, Goldman BM, Rahn AO. Post insertion care of the ocular prosthesis. J Pros Dentistry. 1983;49(2):220–4.
17. Pine KR, Sloan BH, Jacobs RJ. A proposed model of the response of the anophthalmic socket to prosthetic eye wear and its application to the management of mucoid discharge. Med Hypothesis. 2013;81:300–5.
18. Pine KR, Sloan B, Stewart J, Jacobs RJ. The response of the anophthalmic socket to prosthetic eye wear. Clin Exp Optom. 2013;96:338–93.
19. Pine KR, Sloan B, Jacobs RJ. Deposit build up on prosthetic eyes and implications for conjunctival inflammation and mucoid discharge. Clin Ophthalmol. 2012;12(6):1755–62.
20. Pine KR, Sloan B, Stewart J, Jacobs RJ. A surgery of prosthetic eye wearers to investigate mucoid discharge. Clin Ophthalmol. 2012;1(6):707–13.
21. Pine KR, Sloan B, Jacobs RJ. The development of measurement tools for prosthetic eye research. Clin Exp Optom. 2013;96:32–8.
22. Osborn KL, Hottler D. A survey of recommendations on the care of ocular prostheses. Optometry. 2010;81:142–5.
23. Trawnik WR. Care of the ocular prostheses. Adv Ophthalmic Plast Reconstr Surg. 1990;8:146–8.
24. Fett DR, Scott R, Putterman AM. Evaluation of lubricants for prosthetic eye wearers. Ophthalmic Plast Reconstr Surg. 1986;2(1):29–31.
25. LeGrand JA. Chronic exudate: an unnecessary evil. J of Ophthal prosthetics. 1999;4(1):757–9.
26. Jones CA, Collin JRO. A classification and review of the causes of discharging sockets. Trans Ophthalmol UK. 1983;103:351–3.
27. Larned DC. Lacrimal mechanics in the enucleated state. Ophthalmic Plast Reconstr Surg. 1992;8:202–7.
28. Allen L, Kolder HE, Bulgarelli EM, Bulgarelli DM. Artificial eyes and tear measurements. Ophthalmology. 1980;87:155–7.
29. Kim SE, Yoon JS, Lee SY. Tear measurements in prosthetic eye users with Fourier-Domain optical coherence tomography. Am J Ophthalmol. 2010;149:602–7.
30. Vasquez RJ, Linberg JV. The anophthalmic socket and prosthetic eye: a clinical and bacteriologic study. Ophthalmic Plast Reconstr Surg. 1989;5:277–80.
31. Rose GE. The giant fornix syndrome: an unrecognized cause of chronic, relapsing, grossly purulent conjunctivitis. Ophthalmology. 2004;111:1539–45.
32. Jones DF, Lyle CE, Fleming JC. Superior conjunctivoplasty-Mullerectomy for correction of chronic discharge and concurrent ptosis in anophthalmic socket with enlarged superior fornix. Ophthalmic Plast Reconstr Surg. 2010;26:172–5.
33. Jordan DR, Brownstein S, Lee-Wing M, Ashenhurst M. Pyogenic granulomas following oculoplastic procedures: an imbalance in angiogenesis regulation. Can J Ophthalmol. 2001;36(5):260–8.
34. Jordan DR, Brownstein S, Dorey MW. Clinicopathologic analysis of 15 explanted hydroxyapatite implants. Ophthalmic Plast Reconstr Surg. 2004;20(4):285–90.
35. Chang WJ, Tse DT, Rosa RH, Huang A, et al. Conjunctival cytologic features of giant papillary conjunctivitis associated with ocular prostheses. Ophthalmic Plast Reconstr Surg. 2005;21(1):39–45.
36. Scrinivasan OD, Jakobiec FA, Iwamoto T, DeVoe G. Giant papillary conjunctivitis with ocular prostheses. Arch Ophthalmol. 1979;97:892–5.
37. Kymionis GD, Goldman D, Ide T, Yoo SH. Tacrolimus ointment 0.03% in the eye for treatment of giant papillary conjunctivitis. Cornea. 2008;27:228–9.

38. Attas-Fox L, Barkena Y, Iskhakov V, Rayvich S. Topical tacrolimus 0.03% ointment for intractable allergic conjunctivitis: an open-label pilot study. Curr Eye Res. 2008;33:545–9.
39. Remulla HD, Rubin PAD, Shore JW, Sutula FC, Townsend DJ, Woog JJ, Jahrling KV. Complications of porous spherical orbital implants. Ophthalmology. 1995;102:586–93.
40. Jordan DR, Bawazeer A. Experience with 120 synthetic hydroxyapatite implants (FCI_3). Ophthalmic Plast Reconstr Surg. 2001;17:184–90.
41. Glaft HJ, Googe PB, Powers T, Apple DJ. Anophthalmic socket pain. Am J Ophthalmol. 1993;116:357–62.
42. Rasmussen ML, Prause JU, Toft PB. Phantom pain after eye amputation. Acta Ophthalmol. 2011;89:10–6.
43. Gerding H, Vo O, Husstedt IW, Evers S, Soros P. Phantom pain after enucleation. Ophthalmology. 2003;100:943–9.
44. Jordan DR. Anophthalmic orbital implants. Ophthal Clin NA. 2000;13(4):587–608.
45. Massary GC, Holds JB. Coralline hydroxyapatite spheres as secondary orbital implants in anophthalmos. Ophthalmology. 1995;102:161–6.
46. Jordan DR, Nerad J, Tse DT. An unusual case of orbital cellulitis. Can J Ophthalmol. 1990;25(4):210–2.
47. McCarthy RW, Beyer CK, Dallow RL, Burke JF, Lessell S. Conjunctival cysts of the orbit following enucleation. Ophthalmology. 1981;88(1):30–5.
48. Owji N, Aslani A. Conjunctival cysts of the orbit after enucleation: the use of trichloroacetic acid. Ophthalmic Plast Reconstr Surg. 2005;21(4):264–6.
49. Sanchez EM, Formento NA, Peres-Lopez M, Jimenez AA. Role of trichloroacetic acid in treating posterior conjunctival cyst in anophthalmic socket. Orbit. 2009;28:101–3.
50. Hornblass A, Bosniak S. Orbital cyst following enucleation: the use of absolute alcohol. Ophthalmic Surg. 1981;12:123–6.
51. Smit TJ, Koorneef L, Zonneveld FW. Conjunctival cysts in anophthalmic orbits. Br J Ophthalmol. 1991;75:342–3.
52. Goldstein MH, Soparkar CNS, Kersten RC, Orcutt JC, Patrinely JR, Holds J. Conjunctival cysts of the orbit. Ophthalmology. 1998;105(11):2056–60.
53. Hanig CJ, Hornblass A. Treatment of postenucleation orbital cysts. Ann Ophthalmol. 1986;18:191–3.
54. Juneman A, Holbach LM. Epithelial giant inclusion cyst 50 years after enucleation without orbital implant. Klin Monatsbl Augenheilkd. 1998;212:127–8.
55. Anderson RL. The tarsal strip procedure for correction of eyelid laxity and canthal malposition in the anophthalmic socket. Ophthalmology. 1981;88:895–903.
56. Anderson RL, Gordy DD. The Tarsal strip procedure. Arch Ophthalmol. 1979;97(11):2192–6.
57. Jordan DR, Anderson RL. The lateral tarsal strip revisited: the enhanced tarsal strip. Arch Ophthalmol. 1989;107(4):604–6.
58. Smith RJ, Malet T. Auricular cartilage grafting to correct lower conjunctival fornix retraction and eyelid malposition in anophthalmic patients. Ophthalmic Plast Reconstr Surg. 2008;24(1):13–8.
59. Ma'luf RN. Correction of the inadequate lower fornix in the anophthalmic socket. Br J Ophthalmol. 1999;83:881–2.
60. Neuhaus RW, Hawes MJ. Inadequate inferior cul-de-sac in the anophthalmic socket. Ophthalmology. 1992;99:153–7.
61. Rougraff PM, Tse DT, Johnson TE, Feuer W. Involutional entropion repair with fornix sutures and lateral tarsal strip. Ophthalmic Plast Reconstr Surg. 2001;17(4):281–7.
62. Ho SF, Pherwani A, Elsssherbiny SM, Reuser T. Lateral tarsal strip and quickert sutures for lower eyelid entropion. Ophthalmic Plast Reconstr Surg. 2005;21(5):345–8.
63. Kersten RC, Kleiner FP, Kulwin DR. Tarsotomy for the treatment of cicatricial entropion with trichiasis. Arch Ophthalmol. 1992;110:714–7.
64. Weis FA. Surgical treatment of entropion. J Int Coll Surg. 1954;21:758–60.
65. Allen LH. Four-snip procedure for involutional lower lid entropion: modification of Quickert and Jones Procedures. Can J Ophthalmol. 1991;26(3):139–43.
66. Kaltreider S, Shields MD, Heipperd SC, Patrie J. Anophthalmic ptosis: investigation of the mechanisms and statistical analysis. Ophthalmic Plast Reconstr Surg. 2003;19(6):421–8.
67. Vistnes LM. Mechanism of upper eyelid ptosis in the anophthalmic orbit. Plast Reconstr Surg. 1976;58:539–45.
68. Karesh JW, Putterman AM, Fett DR. Conjunctival-Muellers muscle excision to correct anophthalmic ptosis. Ophthalmology. 1986;93:1068–71.
69. Lee EW, Berbos Z, Zaldivar RA, Lee MS, Harrison AR. Use of a Dermatrix graft in Oculoplastic Surgery. Ophthalmic Plast Reconstr Surg. 2010;26(3):153–4.
70. Rubin PA, Fay AM, Remulla HD, Maus M. Ophthalmic plastic applications of acellular dermal allografts. Ophthalmology. 1999;106:2091–7.
71. Shorr N, Perry JD, Glodberg RA, et al. The safety and applications of acellular human dermal allograft in ophthalmic plastic and reconstructive surgery. Ophthalmic Plast Reconstr Surg. 2000;16:223–30.
72. Vagefi MR, McMullan TFW, Burroughs JR, White GW, McCann JD, Anderson RL. Injectable calcium hydroxylapatite for orbital volume augmentation. Arch Facial Plast Surg. 2007;9(6):439–42.
73. Cahill KV, Burns JA. Volume augmentation of the anophthalmic orbit with cross-linked collagen (Zyplast). Arch Ophthalmol. 1989;107(11):1684–6.
74. Hunter PD, Baker SS. The treatment of enophthalmos by orbital injection of fat autograft. Arch Otolaryngol Head Neck Surg. 1994;120(8):835–9.
75. Huang ZL, Ma L. Restoration of enophthalmos in anophthalmic socket by HTR polymer. Ophthalmic Plast Reconstr Surg. 2005;21(4):318–21.
76. Tenag MA, Madura T, Yano K, Hosokawa K. Use of calcium phosphate cement paste in orbital volume augmentation. Plast Reconstr Surg. 2006;117(4):1186–93.
77. Morley AMS, Mehryar T, Malhorta R, Goldberg R. Use of Hyaluronic acid gel for upper eyelid filling and contouring. Ophthalmic Plast Reconstr Surg. 2009;25:440–4.
78. Smit TJ, Koornneef L, Mourits MP, et al. Primary versus secondary intraorbital implants. Ophthalmic Plast Reconstr Surg. 1991;6:115–8.
79. Georgiadis NS, Tezidou CD, Dimitriadis AS. Restoration of the anophthalmic socket with secondary implantation of a coralline hydroxyapatite sphere. Ophthalmic Surg Lasers. 1998;29:808–14.
80. Frueh BR, Kelker GV. Baseball implant, a method of secondary insertion of an intraorbital implant. Arch Ophthalmol. 1976;94:429–30.
81. Massry GG, Holds JB. Coralline hydroxyapatite spheres as secondary orbital implants in anophthalmos. Ophthalmology. 1995;102:161–6.
82. Jordan DR. Localization of Extraocular muscles during secondary orbital implantation surgery. The tunnel technique: experience with 100 patients. Ophthalmology. 2004;111:1048–54.
83. Allen L. The argument against imbrication the rectus muscles over spherical orbital implants after enucleation. Ophthalmology. 1983;90:1116–20.
84. Perry AC. Advances in enucleation. Ophthalmic Plast Reconstr Surg. 1991;4:173–82.
85. Dutton JJ. Coralline hydroxyapatite as an ocular implant. Ophthalmology. 1991;98:370–7.
86. Sheilds CL, Sheilds JA, Potter D, et al. Lack of complications of the hydroxyapatite orbital implant in 250 consecutive cases. Trans Am Ophthalmol Soc. 1993;91:177–89.

87. Sheilds CL, Sheilds JA, De Potter P, et al. Problems with the hydroxyapatite orbital implant: experience with 250 consecutive cases. Br J Ophthalmol. 1994;78:702–6.
88. Nunery WR, Heinz GW, Bonnin JM, Martin RT, Cepela MA. Exposure rate of hydroxyapatite spheres in the anophthalmic socket: histopathologic correlation and comparison with silicone sphere implants. Ophthalmic Plast Reconstr Surg. 1993;9:96–104.
89. Goldberg RA, Holds JB, Ebrahimpour J. Exposed hydroxyapatite orbital implants: report of six cases. Ophthalmology. 1992;99:831–6.
90. Kim YD, Goldberg RA, Shorr N, Steinsapir KD. Management of exposed hydroxyapatite orbital implants. Ophthalmology. 1994;101:1709–15.
91. Oestreicher JH, Liu E, Berkowitz M. Complications of hydroxyapatite orbital implants: a review of 100 consecutive cases and a comparison of Dexon mesh (polyglycolic acid) with scleral wrapping. Ophthalmology. 1997;104:324–9.
92. Jordan DR, Brownstein S, Jolly SS. Abscessed hydroxyapatite orbital implants: a report of two cases. Ophthalmology. 1996;103:1784–7.
93. Yoon JS, Lew H, Kim SJ, et al. Exposure rate of hydroxyapatite orbital implants. Ophthalmology. 2008;115:566–72.
94. Shoamanesh A, Pang N, Oestreicher JH. Complications of orbital implants: a review of 542 patients who have undergone orbital implantation and 275 subsequent peg placements. Orbit. 2007;25:173–82.
95. Custer PL, Trinkaus KM. Porous implant exposure: incidence, management, and morbidity. Ophthalmic Plast Reconstr Surg. 2007;23:1–7.
96. Jordan DR, Klapper SR, Gilberg SM. The use of vicryl mesh in 200 porous orbital implants. Ophthalmic Plast Reconstr Surg. 2003;19:53–61.
97. Wang JK, Liao SL, Lai PC, et al. Prevention of exposure of porous orbital implants following enucleation. Am J Ophthalmol. 2007;143:61–7.
98. Blaydon SM, Shepler TR, Neuhaus RW, White WL, Shore JW. The porous polyethylene (Medpor) spherical orbital implant: a retrospective study of 136 cases. Ophthalmic Plast Reconstr Surg. 2003;19:364–74.
99. Karesh JW, Dresner SC. High density porous polyethylene (Medpor) as a successful anophthalmic implant. Ophthalmology. 1994;101:1688–96.
100. Ma Y, Schou KR, Maloney-Schou M, Harwin FM, Ng J. The porous polyethylene/Bioglass spherical orbital implant: a retrospective study of 170 cases. Ophthalmic Plast Reconstr Surg. 2011;27:21–7.
101. Mahoney NR, Grant MP, Illiff NT, Merbs SL. Exposure rate of smooth surface tunnel porous polyethylene implants after enucleation. Ophthalmic Plast Reconstr Surg. 2014;30:492–8.
102. Jordan DR, Munro SM, Brownstein S, Gilberg SM, Grahovac SZ. A synthetic hydroxyapatite implant: the so-called counterfeit implant. Ophthalmic Plast Reconstr Surg. 1998;14(4):244–9.
103. Jordan DR, Mawn L, Brownstein S, McEachren TM, Gilberg SM, Hill V, Grahovac SZ, Adenis JP. The bioceramic orbital implant: a new generation of porous implants. Ophthalmic Plast Reconstr Surg. 2000;16:347–55.
104. Jordan DR, Gilberg S, Mawn LA. The bioceramic orbital implant: experience with 107 implants. Ophthalmic Plast Reconstr Surg. 2003;19:128–35.
105. Alwitry A, West S, King J, Foss AJ, Abercrombie LC. Long term follow-up of porous polyethylene spherical implants after enucleation and evisceration. Ophthalmic Plast Reconstr Surg. 2007;23:11–5.
106. Ahmed Sadiq S, Mengher LS, Downes R. Integrated orbital implants – a comparison of hydroxyapatite and porous polyethylene implants. Orbit. 2008;27:37–40.
107. Jordan DR, Klapper SK, Gilberg SM, Dutton JJ, Wong A, Mawn L. The bioceramic implant: evaluation of implant exposures in 419 implants Ophthalmic. Plast Reconstr Surg. 2010;26: 80–2.
108. Wang JK, Lai PC, Liao SL. Late exposure of the bioceramic orbital implant. Am J Ophthalmol. 2009;147:162–70.
109. Karslioglu SK, Buttanri IB, Fazil K, Serin D, Akbaba M. Long-term outcomes of pegged and unpegged bioceramic orbital implants. Ophthalmic Plast Reconstr Surg. 2012;28:264–7.
110. Jordan DR, Gilberg SM, Bawazeer A. The coralline hydroxyapatite orbital implant (Bio-Eye™): experience with 170 Patients. Ophthalmic Plast Reconstr Surg. 2004;20(1):69–71.
111. Jordan DR, Klapper SR. Anophthalmic orbital implants: current concepts and controversies. Compr Ophthalmol. 2005;6(6):287–96.
112. Jordan DR. Problems after evisceration surgery with porous orbital implants: experience with 86 patients. Ophthalmic Plast Reconstr Surg. 2004;20(5):374–80.
113. Pelletier C, Gilberg D, Jordan DR. Use of temporalis fascia for management of exposed hydroxyapatite implants. Ophthalmic Plast Reconstr Surg. 1998;14(3):198–203.
114. Buettner H, Bartley GB. Tissue breakdown and exposure associated with orbital hydroxyapatite implants. Am J Ophthalmol. 1992;113:669–73.
115. El-Sharhed FS, Sherief MM, Ali AT. Management of tissue breakdown and exposure associated with orbital hydroxyapatite implants. Ophthalmic Plast Reconstr Surg. 1995;11:91–4.
116. Neuhaus RW, Shorr N. Use of temporalis fascia and muscle as an auto graft. Arch Ophthalmol. 1983;101:262–4.
117. Oestreicher JH. Treatment of exposed coral implants after failed scleral patch graft. Ophthalmic Plast Reconstr Surg. 1994;10(2):110–3.
118. Wiggs EO, Becker BB. Extrusion of enucleation implants: treatment with secondary implants and autogenous temporalis fascia or fascia lata patch grafts. Ophthalmic Surg. 1992;23: 472–6.
119. Soporkar CNS, Patrinely JR. Tarsal patch flap for orbital implant exposure. Ophthalmic Plast Reconstr Surg. 1998;6:391–7.
120. Jordan DR, Brownstein S, Joly SS. Abscessed hydroxyapatite orbital implants: a report of 2 cases. Ophthalmology. 1996;103:1784–7.
121. Jordan DR, Klapper SR, Mawn L, et al. Abscess formation within a synthetic hydroxyapatite implant. Can J Opthalmol. 1998;33:329–32.
122. Ainbinder DJ, Haik BG, Tallado M. Hydroxyapatite orbital implants abscess: histopathologic consideration of an infected implant following evisceration. Ophthalmic Plast Reconstr Surg. 1994;10:267–70.
123. Jordan DR, Brownstein S, Rawlings N, Robinson J. An infected porous polyethylene orbital implant. Ophthalmic Plast Reconstr Surg. 2007;23(5):413–5.
124. Jordan DR, Brownstein S, Robinson J. An infected Aluminum oxide orbital implant. Ophthalmic Plast Reconstr Surg. 2006;22(1):66–7.
125. Guillinta P, Vasani SN, Granet DB, Kikkawa DO. Prosthetic motility in pegged versus unpegged integrated porous orbital implants. Ophthalmic Plast Reconstr Surg. 2003;19:119–22.
126. Jordan DR, Chan S, Mawn L, Gilberg S, Dean T, Brownstein S, Hill VE. Complications associated with pegging hydroxyapatite orbital implants. Ophthalmology. 1999;106:505–12.
127. Fahim DK, Frueh BR, Musch DC, Nelson CC. Complications of pegged and non-pegged hydroxyapatite orbital implants. Ophthalmic Plast Reconstr Surg. 2007;23:206–10.
128. Jordan DR, Chan S, Mawn L, Gilberg SM, Brownstein S, Hill V. Complications associated with pegging hydroxyapatite orbital implants. Ophthalmology. 1999;106:505–12.

129. Edelstein C, Shields CL, DePotter P, Shields JA. Complications of motility peg placement for the hydroxyapatite orbital implant. Ophthalmology. 1997;104:1616–21.
130. Lin CJ, Lio SL, Jou JR, Kao SC, Hou PK, Chen MS. Complications of motility peg placement for porous hydroxyapatite orbital implants. Br J Ophthalmol. 2002;86:394–6.
131. Jordan DR. Spontaneous loosening of hydroxyapatite peg sleeves. Ophthalmology. 2001;108:2041–4.
132. Cheng MS, Lio SL, Lin L. Late porous polyethylene implant exposure after motility coupling post placement. Am J Ophthalmol. 2004;138:420–4.
133. Lee SY, Jang JW, Lew H, Kim SJ, Kim HY. Complications in motility peg placement for hydroxyapatite orbital implants in anophthalmic socket. Jpn J Ophthalmol. 2002;46:103–7.
134. Jordan DR, Klapper SR. A new titanium peg system for hydroxyapatite orbital implants. Ophthalmic Plast Reconstr Surg. 2000;16:380–7.
135. Johnson RLC, Ramstead CL, Nathoo N. Periocular mass lesions secondary to dermatologic fillers: report of 3 cases. Ophthalmic Plast Reconstr Surg. 2011;27:74–5.
136. Yazici B, Akova B, Sanli O. Complications of primary placement of motility post in porous polyethylene implants during enucleation. Am J Ophthalmol. 2007;143:828–4.
137. Krishna G. Contracted sockets (etiology and types). Indian J Ophthalmol. 1980;28:117–20.
138. Tawfik HA, Raslan AO, Talib N. Surgical management of acquired socket contracture. Curr Opin Ophthalmol. 2009;20:406–11.
139. Klein M, Manneking H, Bier J. Reconstruction of the contracted ocular socket with free full-thickness mucosa graft. Int J Oral Maxillofac Surg. 1993;29:96–8.
140. Molgat YM, Hurwitz JJ, Webb MC. Buccal mucous membrane-fat graft in the management of the contracted socket. Ophthalmic Plast Reconstr Surg. 1993;9:267–72.
141. Massry GG, Hornblass A, Rubin P, Holds JB. Tarsal switch procedure for the surgical rehabilitation of the eyelid and socket deficiencies of the anophthalmic socket. Ophthalmic Plast Reconstr Surg. 1999;15:333–40.
142. Holck DE, Foster JA, Dutton JJ, Dillon HD. Hard palate mucosal grafts in the treatment of the contracted socket. Ophthalmic Plast Reconstr Surg. 1999;15:202–9.
143. Lee AC, Fedorovich I, Heinz GW, Kikkawa DO. Socket reconstruction with combined mucous membrane and hard palate mucous grafts. Ophthalmic Surg Lasers. 2002;33:463–8.
144. Karesh JW, Putterman AM. Reconstruction of the partially contracted ocular socket or fornix. Arch Ophthalmol. 1988;106:552–6.
145. Klein M, Menneking H, Bier J. Reconstruction of the contracted ocular socket with free full thickness mucous membrane graft. Int J Oral Maxillofac Surg. 2000;29:96–8.
146. Betharia SM, Patil ND. Dermis fat grafting in contracted sockets. Indian J Ophthalmol. 1988;36:110–2.
147. Lee YH, Kim HC, Lee JS, Park WJ. Surgical reconstruction of the contracted orbit. Plast Reconstr Surg. 1999;4:1129–36.
148. Suh IS, Yang YM, Oh SJ. Conjunctival cul-de-sac reconstruction with radial forearm free flap in anophthalmic orbit syndrome. Plast Reconstr Surg. 2001;107:914–9.
149. Aihara M, Sakai S, Matsuzaki K, Ishida H. Eye socket reconstruction with free flaps in patients who have had postoperative radiotherapy. J Craniomaxillofac Surg. 1998;26:301–5.
150. Anita NH, Arora S. Malignant contracture of the eye socket. Plast Reconstr Surg. 1984;74:292–4.
151. Tahara S, Susuki T. Eye socket reconstruction with free radial forearm flap. Ann Plast Surg. 1989;23:112–6.
152. Sterker I, Frerich B. Secondary reconstruction of the eye socket with a free radial forearm flap. Ophthalmology. 2007;104:978–82.
153. Li D, Jie Y, Liu H, Liu J, Zhu Z, Mao C. Reconstruction of anophthalmic orbits and contracted eye sockets with microvascular radial forearm free flaps. Ophthal Plast Reconstr Surg. 2008;24:94–7.
154. Soutar DS, Scheker LR, Tanner NS. The radial forearm flap: a versatile method for intra-oral reconstruction. Br J Plast Surg. 1983;36:1–8.
155. Bajaj MS, Pushker N, Kumar KS, Chandra M, Ghose S. Evaluation of amniotic membrane grafting in the reconstruction of contracted socket. Ophthal Plast Reconstr Surg. 2006;22(2):116–20.
156. Poonyathalang A, Preechawat P, Pomsathit J, Mahaisaviriya P. Reconstruction of contracted eye socket with amniotic membrane graft. Ophthalmic Plast Reconstr Surg. 2005;21:359–62.
157. Putterman AM, Karesh JW. A surgical technique for the successful and stable reconstruction of the totally contracted ocular socket. Ophthalmic Surg. 1988;19(3):193–201.
158. Timothy NH, Feilich DE, Linberg JV. Perspective: evisceration versus enucleation, the ocularists standpoint. Ophthal Plast Reconstr Surg. 2003;19(6):417–20.

Surgical Management of the Contracted Socket

63

A. K. Grover, Amrita Sawhney, and Shaloo Bageja

An *acceptable anophthalmic socket*, both functionally and aesthetically, is one which has a centrally placed implant, adequate epithelial lining of conjunctiva, and eyelids of normal length and tone.

Contracted socket, or socket contracture, is defined as the shrinkage and shortening of all or a part of orbital tissues causing a decrease in depth of the fornices and orbital volume, leading to the inability to retain an ocular prosthesis [1, 2]. It can either be due to soft tissue or bony contraction.

The management of anophthalmic sockets has been highly challenging and requires a close collaboration between the ophthalmologist and the ocularist to obtain best functional and cosmetic results. A successfully rehabilitated anophthalmic socket must support a prosthetic device that would simulate the normal fellow eye.

An Ideal Anophthalmic Socket (Fig. 63.1a, b)
- Centrally placed implant of adequate volume
- A socket lined with healthy conjunctival epithelium
- Adequately deep inferior and superior fornices to retain the prosthesis
- Optimal implant-prosthesis coupling to ensure motility of the artificial eye
- Normal position and adequate tone of eyelids
- Well-fitted prosthesis that looks similar to the contralateral eye

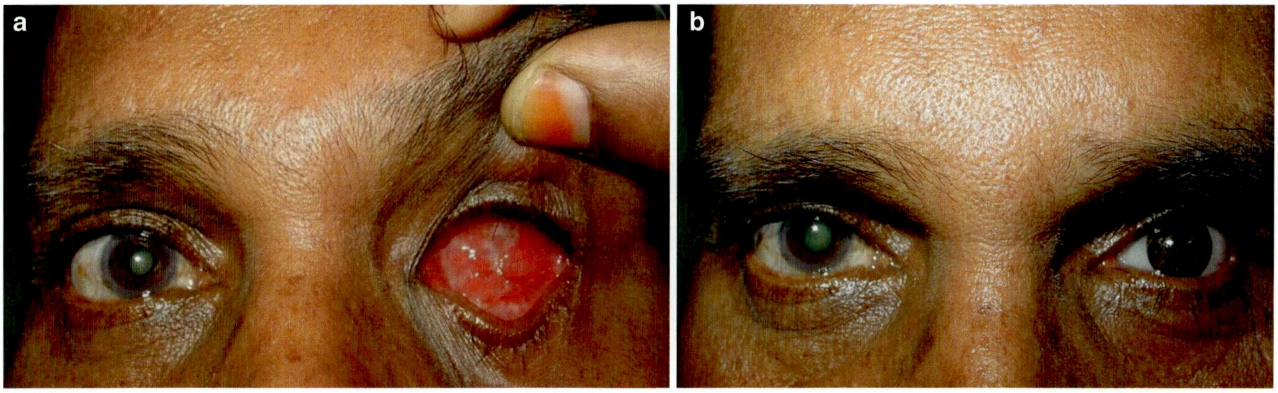

Fig. 63.1 (**a**) A healthy anophthalmic socket. (**b**) A well-fitted prosthesis, left side

A. K. Grover (✉)
Sir Ganga Ram Hospital, New Delhi, India

A. Sawhney
Associate Consultant, Ophthalmology, New Delhi, India

S. Bageja
Senior Consultant, Ophthalmology, New Delhi, India

A. J. Cohen, C. N. Burkat (eds.), *Oculofacial, Orbital, and Lacrimal Surgery*, https://doi.org/10.1007/978-3-030-14092-2_63

Causes of Contracted Socket

Socket contracture can either be congenital or acquired. Congenital variants include congenital anophthalmos, cystic ocular remnants, or microphthalmos.

Acquired socket contracture can occur as a result of extensive dissection of orbital tissues during enucleation or evisceration, improper suturing of conjunctiva and Tenon's capsule, multiple socket surgeries, implant exposure or migration, incorrect conformer size, or ill-fitting prosthesis. Other acquired causes leading to contracted socket include radiation therapy, trauma which includes acid or alkali burns or extensive lacerations of eyelid and orbital tissues, cicatricial conjunctival diseases, and implant or socket infection [3].

Causes of Contracted Socket

1. *Congenital causes*
   - Congenital anophthalmos
   - Cystic ocular remnants
   - Microphthalmos
2. *Acquired causes*
   (a) *Surgery-related causes*
   - Enucleation/evisceration with extensive dissection of orbital tissues
   - Conjunctiva and Tenon's capsule not preserved or sutured properly
   - Multiple socket surgeries

   (b) *Implant-, conformer-, and prosthesis-related causes*
   - Implant exposure/migration
   - Delay in wearing conformer
   - Conformer of incorrect size
   - Prosthesis non-compliance
   - Ill-fitting prosthesis

   (c) *Etiology-related causes*
   - Radiation therapy – poorly vascularized socket
   - Trauma – acid/alkali burns/extensive lacerations of eyelid and orbital tissues
   - Cicatricial conjunctival diseases
   - Implant/socket infection
   - Exposure/extrusion of orbital implant

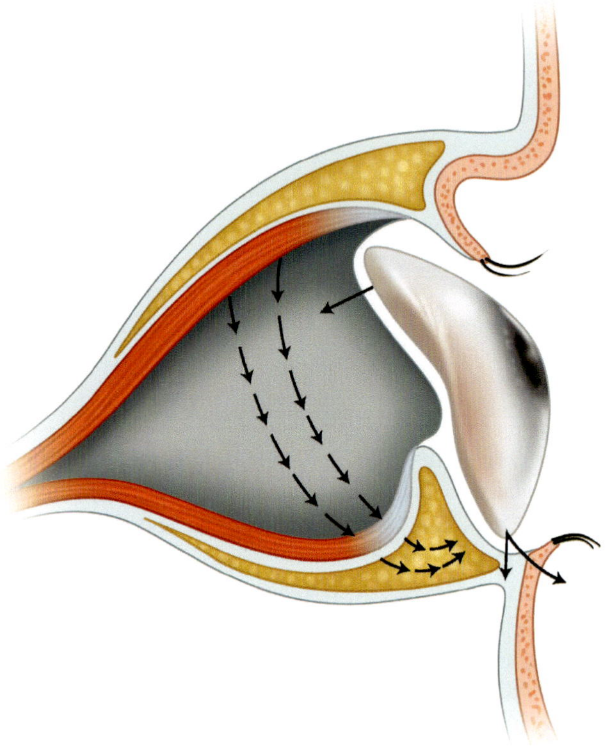

Fig. 63.2 Diagrammatic representation of prosthesis tilt in a contracted socket

Radiographic studies have reported the following changes in the anophthalmic socket after simple uncomplicated enucleation:

1. Redistribution of intraorbital fat downward and forward.
2. Inferior displacement of the superior rectus-levator complex that leads to the hollow and sunken appearance of the post-enucleation superior eyelid sulcus (also known as superior sulcus deformity).
3. Inferior fornix and distal inferior rectus (near the orbital rim) are elevated.

The effect of volume loss following enucleation is a rotation of intraorbital contents. A prosthesis with a large superior modification is then required to replace the residual volume loss and elevate the ptotic eyelid. Despite this compensatory shape, the superior prosthesis tends to shift back, such that it causes depression in the superior sulcus, and pushes against the lower eyelid inferiorly.

The above changes in the anophthalmic socket lead to the recognized "post-enucleation socket syndrome," which is characterized by the following findings:

- Deepening of the upper eyelid sulcus (superior sulcus deformity)
- Upper eyelid ptosis (with upper eyelid dysfunction/lagophthalmos)
- Lower eyelid laxity and ectropion

Pathogenesis of Contracted Socket and the Post-enucleation Socket Syndrome (Fig. 63.2)

Simple enucleation without placement of an implant leads to contraction of extraocular muscles resulting in retraction and collapse of Tenon's capsule, eventually leading to disfiguring upper eyelid entropion.

Over time, the lower eyelid progressively stretches due to prosthesis tilt and leads to a combination of involutional and mechanical ectropion. This eyelid malposition further reduces the inferior fornix. Attempting to enlarge the prosthesis size to maintain retention would, in turn, worsen the ectropion [4]. Ideally, adequate orbital volume replacement by placing an appropriately sized implant at the time of primary surgery can prevent this cascade of events.

Prevention

Surgical orbital procedures, such as enucleation and evisceration, should be performed meticulously to attain best cosmetic and functional results. Minimal forniceal dissection with preservation of as much conjunctiva as possible, limited cauterization of tissues, and layer-by-layer closure of Tenon's capsule and conjunctiva without any tension are critical steps during surgery that minimize the risk of postoperative socket contracture. Layered closure over the implant is performed preferably in different directions, with vertical conjunctival closure potentially allowing for better inferior and superior fornices, as tension is not placed on the fornices.

Placing an appropriately sized orbital implant is a primary factor in reducing the risk of post-enucleation socket syndrome from volume loss after enucleation or evisceration. The average volume of the globe is 7.2 ml, and the combined volume of the implant and prosthesis should equal the volume of the removed globe. The average volume of a prosthesis is 2.5 ml; thus the implant needs to equal almost two thirds of the volume of the globe. Increasing the volume of the prosthesis may result in mechanical ectropion of the lower eyelid from the heavier weight.

On average, the adult socket can accommodate an orbital implant of 20–22 mm in diameter. Orbital sizers placed during surgery, or measuring the contralateral globe axial length preoperatively, can help guide the implant size to select. Placing an excessively large implant carries increased risk of dehiscence, implant extrusion, and difficulty in fitting of the ocular prosthesis. On the other hand, placing a small implant of less than 20 mm will result in more noticeable post-enucleation socket syndrome. In the setting of a phthisical globe, various surgical techniques such as transecting the optic nerve, or placing radial or circumferential posterior scleral cuts, can create space behind or within the scleral cavity for accommodation of a larger implant.

As the overall implant diameter is less than the globe, this typically leads to an alteration in functional length of the levator-superior rectus complex, thereby decreasing levator function and resulting in ptosis. Adding to the superior margin of the prosthesis helps restore the functional length of the levator muscle.

Aesthetically, the goal is to also restore a natural appearance and movement to the prosthetic eye. In the routine enucleation technique, the extraocular muscles are sutured to each other or close to each other on the anterior implant surface. It has been hypothesized that muscle contraction is compromised by unduly stretching the muscle beyond its original length, thus reducing motility. The myoconjunctival approach to enucleation has been suggested to improve prosthesis motility as extraocular muscles are sutured to the implant in normal anatomic positions and then sutured to the fornices.

Routine follow-up examinations of the socket and prosthesis with the ophthalmologist and ocularist, respectively, can help identify and address socket issues at an early stage.

Management of Contracted Socket

The primary aim of management is to create a socket that will allow for proper fitting of a prosthesis, in order to achieve an acceptable cosmetic appearance. Before starting definitive treatment, it is important to classify socket contracture and eliminate any precipitating factors.

Classifications of Contracted Socket

According to the Gopal Krishna classification [5], soft tissue socket contraction is graded from grade 0 to 5:

- **Grade-0:** Socket is lined with healthy conjunctiva and has deep and well-formed fornices.
- **Grade 1:** Shallow or shelving/shortening of the lower fornix
- **Grade 2:** Loss of upper and lower fornices
- **Grade 3:** Loss of upper, lower, medial and lateral fornices
- **Grade 4:** Loss of all fornices and reduction of palpebral aperture in horizontal and vertical dimensions
- **Grade 5:** Recurrence of socket contracture despite repeated reconstruction attempts

Other simpler classifications described mild, moderate, and severe degrees of socket contracture [3]:

- **Mild:** Only one fornix is involved (usually lower fornix) + shortening of posterior lamellae of the eyelids
- **Moderate:** Both superior + inferior fornices are involved (decrease in area)
- **Severe:** All fornices are involved + phimosis of palpebral aperture (loss of area + volume)
- **Malignant:** Severe loss of area, volume, with associated bony contracture [6]

Another accepted classification of socket contracture was described by Tawfik et al. [7]:

- **Grade 1:** Minimal or no actual contracture of socket. Patient complains of inability to retain the prosthesis mainly due to horizontal eyelid laxity with subsequent prolapse of the inferior fornix.
- **Grade 2:** Mild contracture of the inferior or superior fornix. Patient has difficulty with the prosthesis or may complain of rolling-in of the upper and lower eyelid margins.
- **Grade 3**: Scarring is more advanced making it impossible to wear the prosthesis. Cicatrization involves the entire upper and lower fornices.
- **Grade 4:** Severe phimosis of the palpebral fissure both vertically and horizontally. Recurrent cases of contracted socket and irradiated sockets are included in grade 4 disease.

Ideally, an updated classification may be necessary that encompasses all the factors such as socket moisture, eyelid malposition, previous surgeries, radiation exposure, and bony contracture.

History and Examination

A thorough history and clinical examination should be obtained when evaluating a patient with a contracted socket, as these will guide the treatment plan. A detailed history should include all previous ocular surgeries, specific technique used, muscle attachment, type of implant placed, and complications during or after surgery. The time interval between the procedure and onset of fibrosis will reveal an acute or chronic nature of the disease. History of ocular malignancy, trauma, or congenital malformations is also necessary.

The clinical evaluation of the socket should be performed with and without the prosthesis, and should include the periorbital external examination as well as the slit-lamp examination. Photographic documentation is mandatory.

1. Volume assessment: The socket volume is assessed by measuring the relative depth of the socket compared to the fellow eye. Superior sulcus deformity is a sign of volume loss (Fig. 63.3).
2. Depth: A shallow/shortened inferior fornix leads to poor fitting of the prosthesis (Fig. 63.4 b, c).
3. Surface area: Surface area of the socket and depth of the fornices are noted. It is important to assess the fornices and the socket lining. Fibrous bands and symblepharon (Fig. 63.5), granulomas (Fig. 63.6), implant exposure (Fig. 63.7), implant extrusion (Fig. 63.7b), or chronic inflammation or infection should be documented appropriately.
4. Moisture: It should be noted whether the socket is dry or wet.

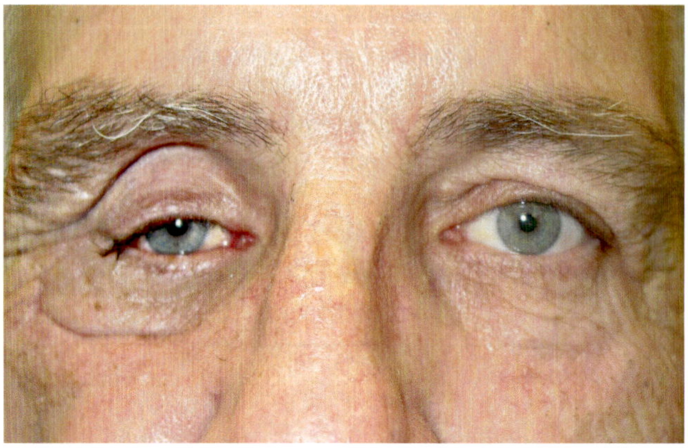

Fig. 63.3 Right superior sulcus deformity showing a deep hollowed sulcus, as well as ptosis of the upper eyelid. (Image courtesy of Cat Nguyen Burkat, MD FACS)

5. Palpation: Palpation of the socket assesses for the presence and position of the implant. An inferiorly displaced implant can often obliterate the inferior fornix.
6. Eyelids: Examination of the eyelids may demonstrate excessive eyelid or canthal tendon laxity that should be addressed.
7. Motility: Other features that should be assessed are the extraocular movements (Fig. 63.8) and tone of the orbicularis muscle.
8. A computed tomographic scan (CT scan) may be necessary to assess for orbital cavity size (which may be hypoplastic in congenital anophthalmos), bony contracture, and associated orbital fractures which may be contributing to a sunken appearance (cases with previous trauma) and to ascertain the presence, size, and position of an orbital implant (Fig. 63.9).

Management of the Contracted Socket

The management of the contracted socket is highly challenging, and varies depending on congenital or acquired etiologies, degree of contracture, and the periorbital deformities associated with it.

Congenital Contracted Socket

Socket contracture can either be due to congenital anophthalmos, where the optic vesicle fails to develop, or due to congenital microphthalmos, where remnants of vestigial eye tissue are present.

Congenital microphthalmos is more common and can be further categorized into pure microphthalmos, in which the eye appears normal but axial length is decreased, and complex microphthalmos, in which the globe is abnormal.

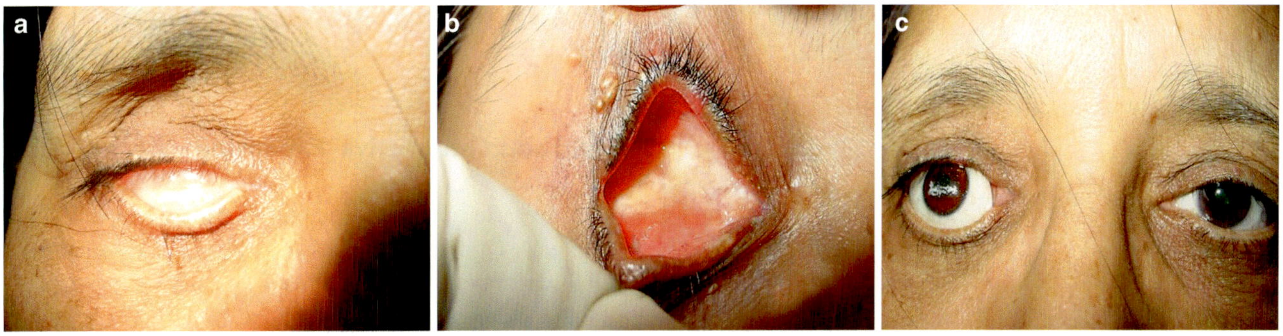

Fig. 63.4 (**a**) Inferior fornix shelving with socket tissue prolapse limits the ability to retain a prosthesis. (**b**) Inferior fornix shortening. Pinch test of the patient shows that the surface is adequate, but depth of fornix is inadequate to hold the prosthesis. (**c**) Poor stability of prosthesis and inferior scleral show, suggesting lower eyelid laxity

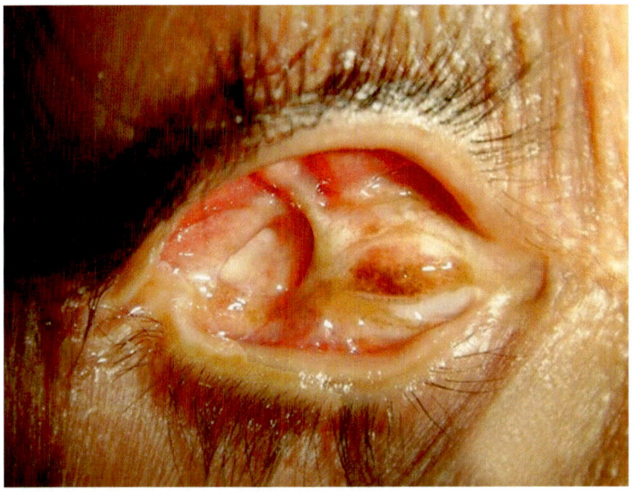

Fig. 63.5 Fibrous bands and symblepharon in the socket

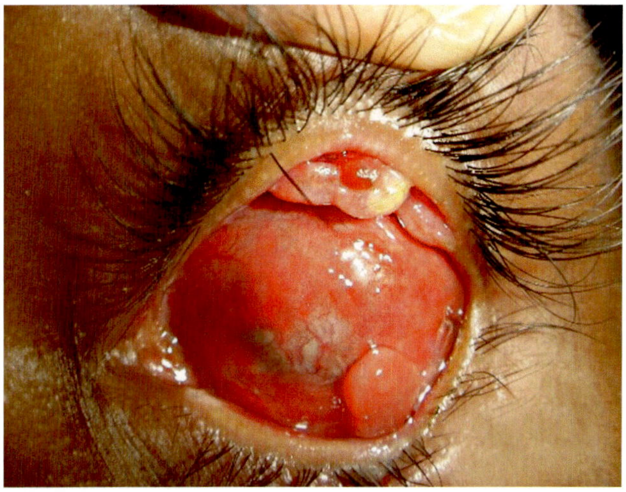

Fig. 63.6 Multiple granuloma formation in the socket may be secondary to poor tissue closure technique, poor prosthesis fit with chronic surface irritation, or other inflammatory etiology

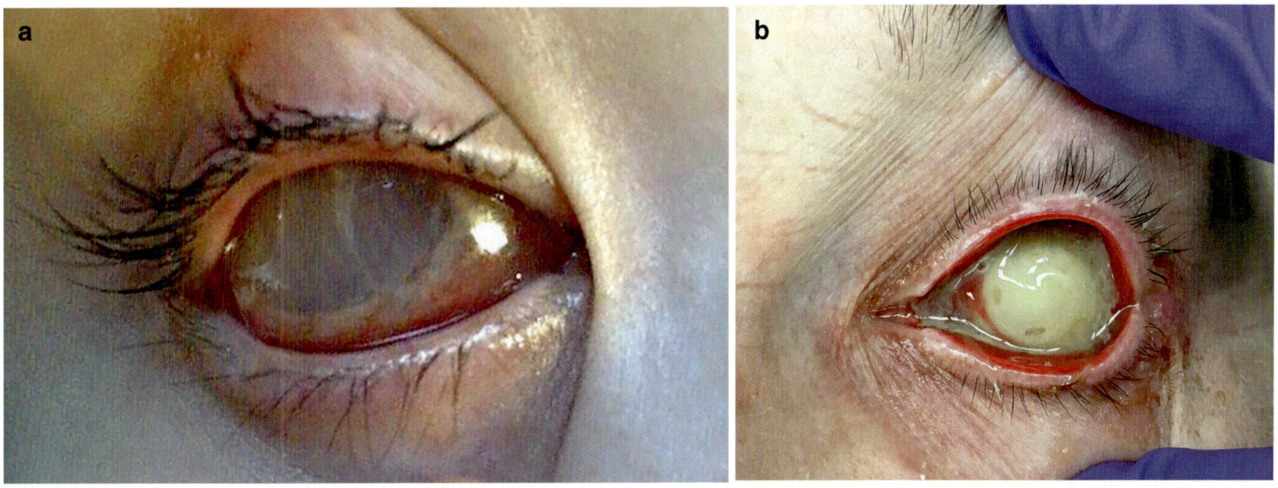

Fig. 63.7 (**a**) Large exposure of a nonporous silicone implant. (Image courtesy of Cat Nguyen Burkat, MD FACS). (**b**) Extensive extrusion of a porous polyethylene implant. (Image courtesy of Cat Nguyen Burkat, MD FACS)

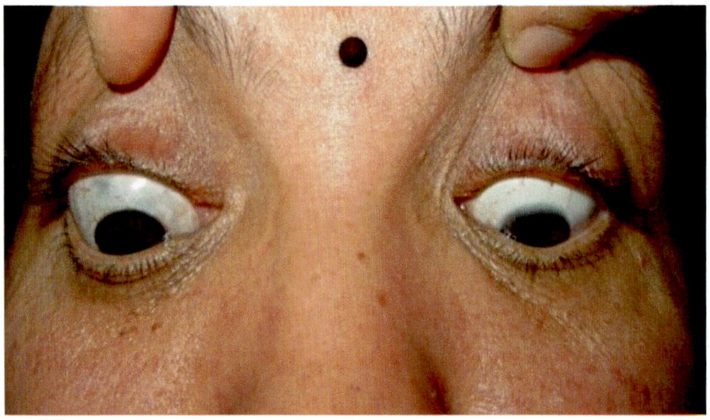

Fig. 63.8 Transmission of motility from implant to overlying prosthesis

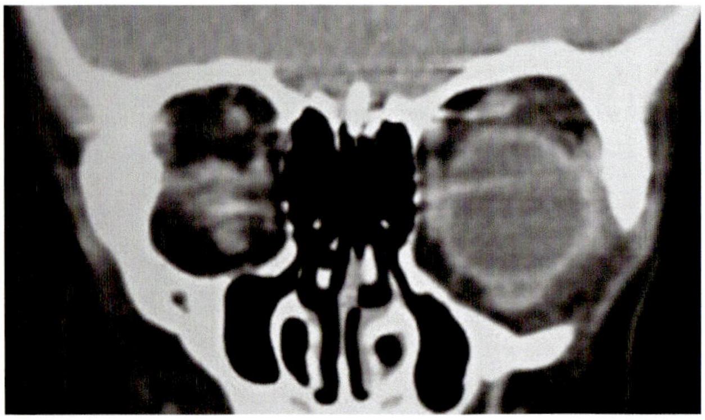

Fig. 63.9 CT scan, coronal view, demonstrates right orbital bony hypoplasia due to congenital anophthalmos

In both anophthalmos and microphthalmos, there is shortening of the vertical and horizontal dimensions of eyelids leading to phimosis, blepharoptosis due to the absence of levator muscle, shortened conjunctival fornices with deficiency of palpebral and bulbar conjunctiva, hypoplasia of the bony orbit, and facial asymmetry due to reduction in soft tissue volume [8].

Treatment

A complete history and systemic examination must be carried out to rule out associated anomalies. Visual acuity assessment with visual evoked potential (VEP) and early refraction should be considered in microphthalmic eyes to determine maximum visual potential of the eye. Ocular examination of both eyes including ultrasonography and electroretinogram (ERG) will guide the management plan.

When treating a congenital contracted socket, it is necessary to consider both soft tissue and bony hypoplasia. Treatment should commence as early as possible as early intervention will help stimulate the growth of the orbital bones and the periocular and midfacial tissues.

The steps of reconstruction are:

(a) Expansion of horizontal and vertical eyelid apertures.
(b) Recreation of fornices.
(c) Expansion of bony orbit.
(d) Replacement of volume.

Eyelid and Conjunctival Expansion

There are various methods used for the purpose of soft tissue eyelid and conjunctival expansion, with the gold standard of serial conformers ideally initiated as early as possible to maximize outcomes.

Conformers

Anophthalmia or microphthalmia with or without orbital cyst can be treated with increasingly larger conformers alone. Once the socket has developed sufficiently with serial conformers, the cyst can be removed, if indicated, with or without removal of the ocular remnant. Often, the globe and cyst can be left intact as they provide necessary orbital volume for socket growth. Volume replacement can later be performed with free dermis fat graft [9]. Other options for soft tissue expansion include:

- Expanding *hydrogel conformers* can also stimulate socket expansion, particularly for expanding the palpebral fissures. The socket expanders are small when dry, ranging from 6 to 9 mm in diameter, for easy insertion. Due to high hydrophilic properties, they expand to 11, 14, and 18 mm when fully hydrated, which typically takes 2–4 weeks. If necessary, the hydrogel conformer can then be replaced with a larger expanding conformer for additional results (Fig. 63.10a–d). Other authors have used 2-octyl cyanoacrylate glue to adhere the eyelid margins together in a temporary tarsorrhaphy over the conformer in order to minimize surgery with anesthesia for a young patient.
- *Dumbbell-shaped or champagne glass configuration acrylic conformers* [10]
- These conformers help expand soft tissues and encourage bony growth by transmitting pressure to the socket by application of tape over its external component. The conformer size requires changing every week for several months initially, and then every 6–8 weeks.
- *Custom scleral shell*
- Custom scleral shells can be useful in cases of microphthalmic eyes to promote orbital growth. Custom clear shells can be made for mild to moderate microphthalmia with positive response to visual evoked potential testing, in order to allow the eye to achieve its maximum visual potential. The custom prosthesis can be painted for optimal cosmetic appearance [11].

In general, it is preferable to preserve the microphthalmic eye even if there is no vision as the globe volume provides stimulus for eyelid and orbital growth, which may potentially

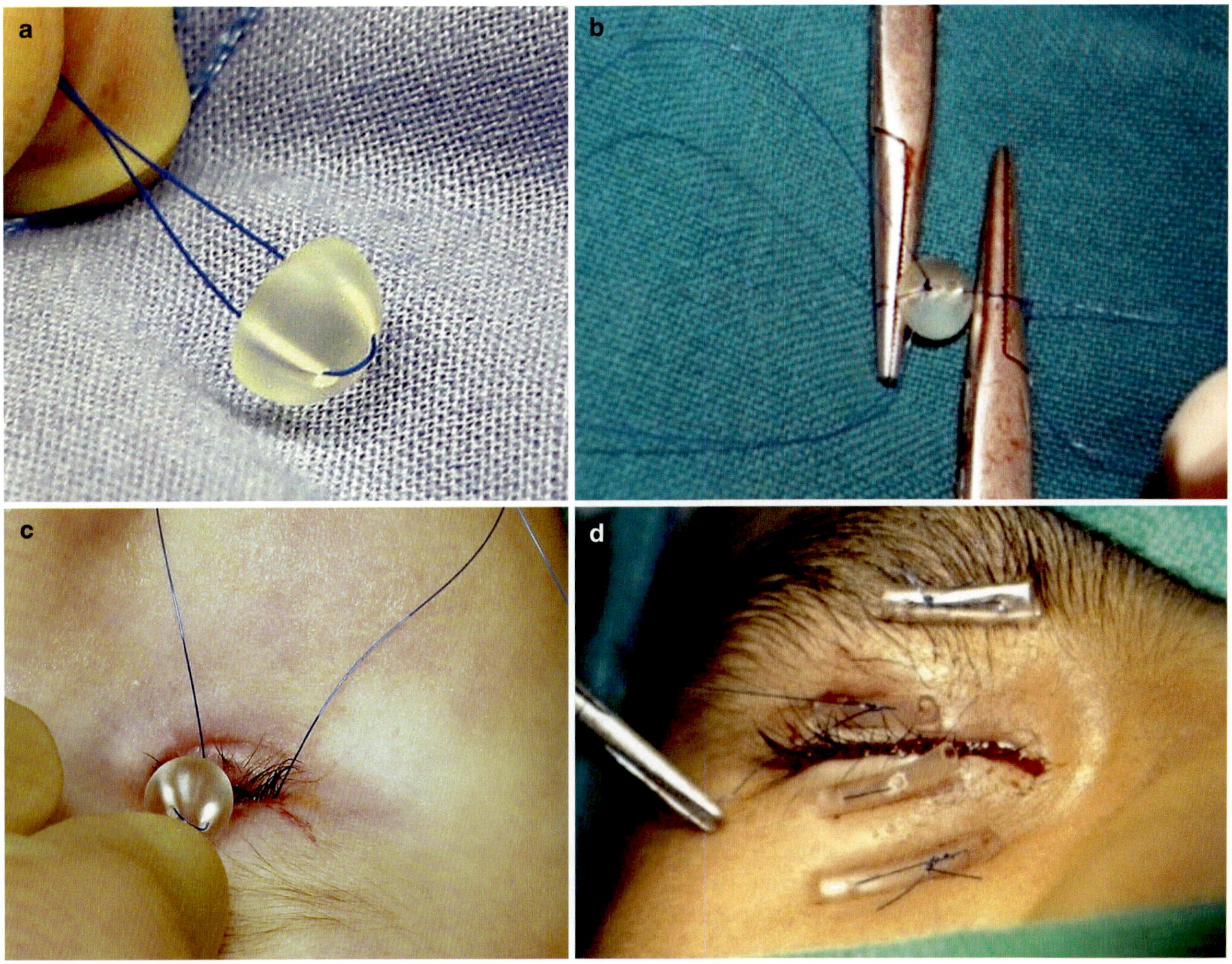

Fig. 63.10 (**a**) A hydrogel socket hemisphere expander. (Image courtesy of Cat Nguyen Burkat, MD FACS). (**b**) A Prolene suture is passed through the conformer leaving enough laxity in the sutures to allow for expansion of the conformer. (**c**) The hydrogel expander is being sutured to the socket with sutures passed from deep in the fornices to exit on the eyelid. (Image courtesy of Cat Nguyen Burkat, MD FACS). (**d**) The Prolene sutures are tied over bolsters on the eyelid

delay the need for early surgical intervention. If maximal expansion has been achieved with serial conformers and above options, then surgical lengthening of the fornices and posterior lamella may be required with mucous membrane grafting.

Orbital Expansion

The most common methods described for expansion of the orbit include:

- Intraorbital implantation of non-expanding orbital implants
- Balloon expanders
- Dermis fat grafts
- Hydrogel expanders
- Integrated orbital tissue expander
- 3D osteotomies for small bony sockets

Orbital Implants (Non-expanding)

Traditionally, static orbital implants were used but had limited results as smaller implants failed to expand the orbit adequately and larger implants carried a high risk of extrusion [12]. A range of sizes and materials of implants have been used with varying success. These are discussed in more detail in a separate chapter.

Balloon (Inflatable Soft Tissue) Expanders

These expanders are typically implanted through an orbitotomy or bicoronal approach, with the balloon inflated with monthly injections of saline through an external inflation port. The ideal expander diameter is 22 mm, and the target inflation period ranges from 20 to 36 weeks. This technique has the advantage of predictable orbital and soft tissue growth [13]. Complications include implant extrusion, tissue ischemia or pressure necrosis, infection, need for multiple injections, inflation pressure spikes, lack of control over direction of expansion, and conformer displacement due to forward protrusion of the expander [14].

Dermis Fat Grafts

These grafts are another form of dynamic orbital expanders, as they exert enough pressure and volume to expand the socket soft tissue and orbit. The dermis fat graft (DFG) is harvested from areas of abundant subcutaneous fat, such as the abdomen, buttocks, inner thigh, and removed as an ellipse or circular button measuring 20 mm in diameter. The epidermis is removed using scissors or a blade until the pinpoint reticular dermis layer is encountered. A wide button of underlying fat is then excised with the attached dermis. The contracted socket is incised horizontally and the fibrosis released to allow the conjunctiva and Tenon's layer to recess into the fornix. The DFG is then placed within the socket cavity and the conjunctival edges sutured to the DFG border. Over the next several weeks, the conjunctival epithelium migrates over the graft and expands the surface area. Thus, the DFG provides both orbital volume and surface area to the contracted or deficient conjunctival layer. This subsequently allows the conjunctival layer to recess without tension, thus creating improved fornices for prosthesis stability. The main disadvantage of this technique is the unpredictable fat absorption resulting in superior sulcus deformity, more commonly seen in adults. Studies have demonstrated that young children treated with DFG may have hypertrophy of the fat, to the extent that later debulking of the graft fat is necessary [15]. Since it is anticipated that a portion of the transplanted DFG will absorb, the DFG can be oversized slightly for placement into the socket deficit. However, an overly large DFG can also cause tissue compression of the fat, resulting in more rapid necrosis and fat atrophy. Placement of DFG for orbital volume can be performed concurrently with serial conformers for eyelid expansion.

Hydrogel Expanders

Hydrogels are hydrophilic polymers that expand up to 6–12 times their original volume, and thus the orbital tissues, by osmotically imbibing tissue fluid. Hydrogel expanders can be molded into desired shapes and their expansion can be precisely controlled. They are self-inflating without injection ports and therefore have less complications related to inflation, such as sudden pressure necrosis. These characteristics render them suitable for reconstruction in congenital anophthalmos [16].

Three types of hydrogel implants are available: (1) hemisphere self-expanding conformers for conjunctival fornix expansion as discussed earlier, (2) orbital sphere implants to expand the bony orbit, and (3) pellet expanders for microphthalmic eyes [17].

The conjunctival conformer is placed into the fornices and secured with tissue glue or sutures with bolsters. Gradual expansion is achieved to its maximum within 2–3 weeks and then it can be replaced with a larger hydrogel hemisphere conformer or a conventional prosthesis.

Orbital expanders can be spherical or pellet-shaped depending on the absence or presence of a microphthalmic eye, respectively. These are placed either through a small conjunctival incision, lateral soft tissue incision, or inserted intraorbitally using a customized trocar.

The limitations of hydrogel expanders include anterior orbital migration, hemorrhage, and the inability to maintain continued pressure on the orbit after expansion. In hypoplastic orbits with anophthalmia, the limited orbital space on neuroimaging may indicate placement of the smallest hydrogel sphere. Once maximum expansion is achieved, however, it can be exchanged with subsequently larger hydrogel spheres in order to further stimulate orbital and soft tissue expansion.

Integrated Orbital Tissue Expander (OTE)

This consists of a flexible expander anchored to the lateral orbital wall by a titanium plate. As the expander is fixed to the orbital wall, it has the advantage of sustained and unidirectional expansion. A 1 cc syringe with a 30 gauge needle is used to expand the OTE via an injection port to apply increasing pressure to the orbit. These expanders can therefore be inflated and deflated, as needed, without additional surgeries. In addition to the expansion of the bony orbit, the OTE can induce growth of the associated frontal, maxillary, and zygomatic bones. Growth of these facial bones results in improved eyebrow position, cheek fullness, and forward projection of the lateral canthal angle, further improving facial symmetry. Overall, integrated orbital tissue expanders have been demonstrated to be safe and effective in managing the anophthalmic socket with good long-term outcomes.

Complications include difficulty in locating the injection port, displacement of the titanium plate, tissue necrosis around the plate, and spontaneous deflation of the expander [18].

3D Osteotomies for Small Bony Sockets

C- and U-shaped osteotomies (Fig. 63.11) can be created to expand the roof, lateral wall, and orbital floor. The osteotomy segments are advanced forward and away from the center of the orbital cavity. The orbital floor and rim are placed at a higher level compared to the normal side to provide better support to the prosthesis. Bone grafts are used to fill the defect [19].

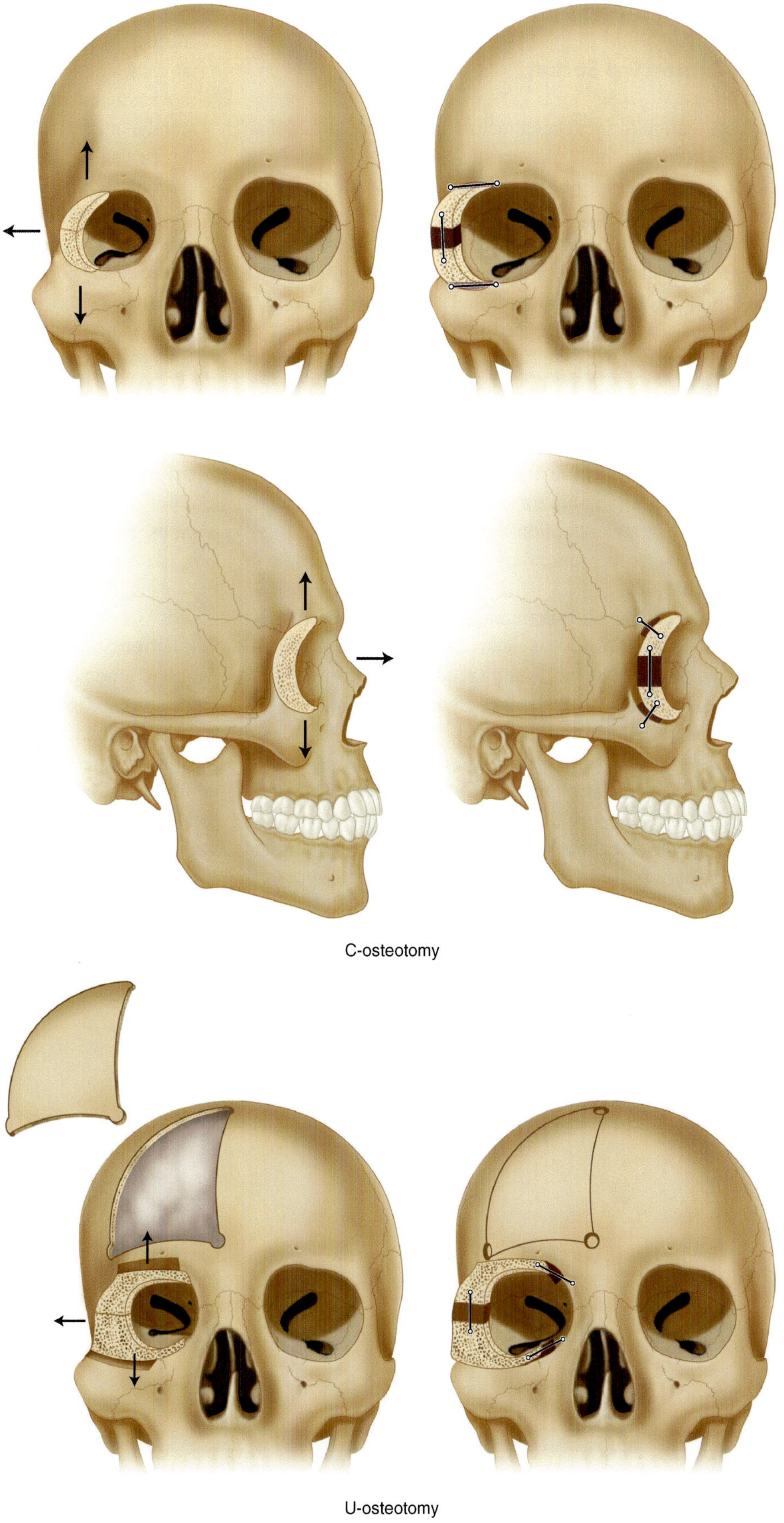

Fig. 63.11 Diagrammatic representation of C-shaped and U-shaped osteotomies. Interpositional bone grafts are demonstrated as shadowed segments along the lateral wall

Acquired Contracted Socket

Mild Contracted Socket

Patients with mild socket contracture usually complain of an inability to retain the ocular prosthesis, such as a history of the prosthesis falling out when bending forward or during coughing or sneezing. Often the underlying cause is lower eyelid laxity with minimal shortening of the inferior fornix [20]. Treatment depends on the adequacy of the inferior fornix. Preoperative examination should also include evaluation of the socket without the prosthesis as an oversized or migrated implant may be seen to be the cause of fornix shallowing.

1. With adequate fornix presenting as lower eyelid entropion or laxity: Cicatricial shortening of the posterior eyelid lamella can result in entropion but with adequate fornices. Treatment options include:
   - Transverse blepharotomy with marginal rotation of eyelid.
   - Horizontal eyelid shortening if eyelid laxity coexists.
   - In recurrent or severe cicatricial cases, lengthening of the posterior eyelid lamella requires a free graft interposed inferior to the tarsus (tarsus, hard palate, ear cartilage, acellular dermix matrix).
2. With shallowing/shortening of fornix (usually inferior): Closed method fornix repair may be considered for mild contracture (Fig. 63.12a, b).
   Procedure: After local infiltration, several double-armed sutures are passed through the inferior fornix and periosteum away from the globe, to exit through the lower eyelid skin. Each suture arm is passed through a silicone or rubber bolster and tied. A clear conformer is placed to further ensure that the inferior fornix is appropriately stretched and deepened toward the orbital rim. The sutures are removed after 2–3 weeks, at which point a prosthesis can be attempted if the fornix is improved. Suture fornix repair can be combined with a lateral canthal tightening procedure if horizontal laxity is present [21].
3. With shallowing of fornix and fat prolapse: An open method for fornix repair may be preferred [22].
   Procedure: Fornix reconstruction requires conjunctival incision, complete release of fibrosis by dissection under the conjunctiva to the orbital rim, horizontal tightening, and posterior lamellar lengthening with either tarsal substitutes or buccal mucous membrane grafts (Fig. 63.13a–f).

Moderate and Severe Contracted Socket

Various graft options can be utilized for socket reconstruction, with preferences depending on whether the socket is dry or moist.

Treatment of a Moist Socket

Mucous membrane grafts (partial-thickness or full-thickness) are the gold standard treatment for a moist contracted socket and provide repair in a single stage [23, 24]. Partial-thickness mucous membrane grafts are more susceptible to shrinkage and contracture compared to full-thickness grafts. Donor site complications for full-thickness grafts are minimal. However, mucous membrane grafts lack rigidity and are therefore best for establishing the inferior fornix. They are less ideal for replacing eyelid posterior lamella, for which firmer substitutes are indi-

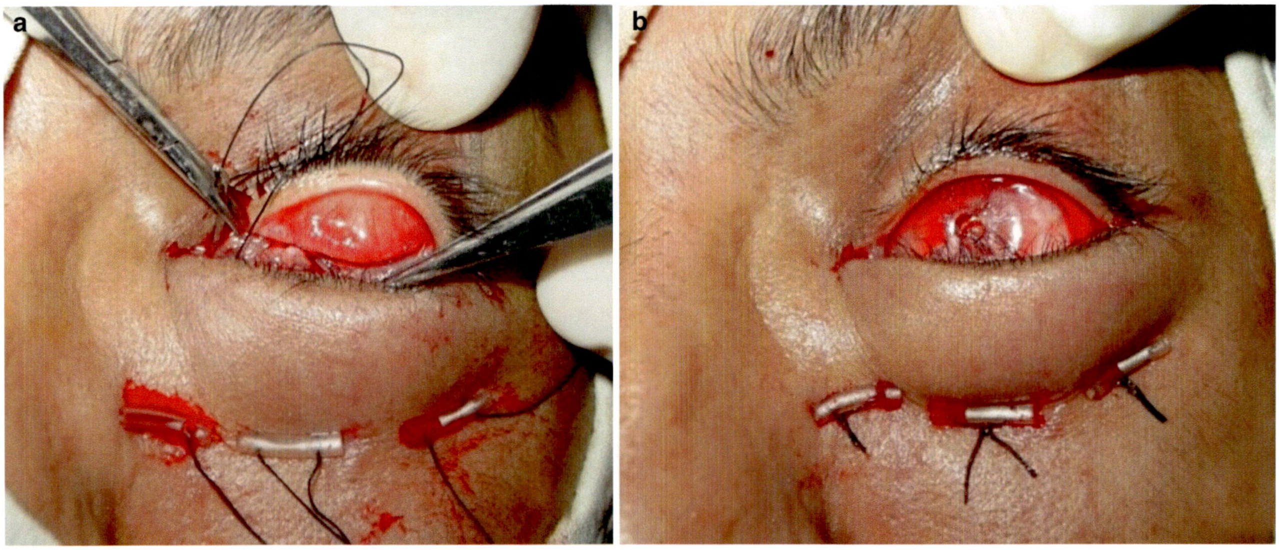

Fig. 63.12 (**a**) Sutures are passed deep through the inferior fornix and periosteum at the orbital rim, brought out through skin, and passed through bolsters. (**b**) The sutures are tied over the bolsters and removed after several weeks

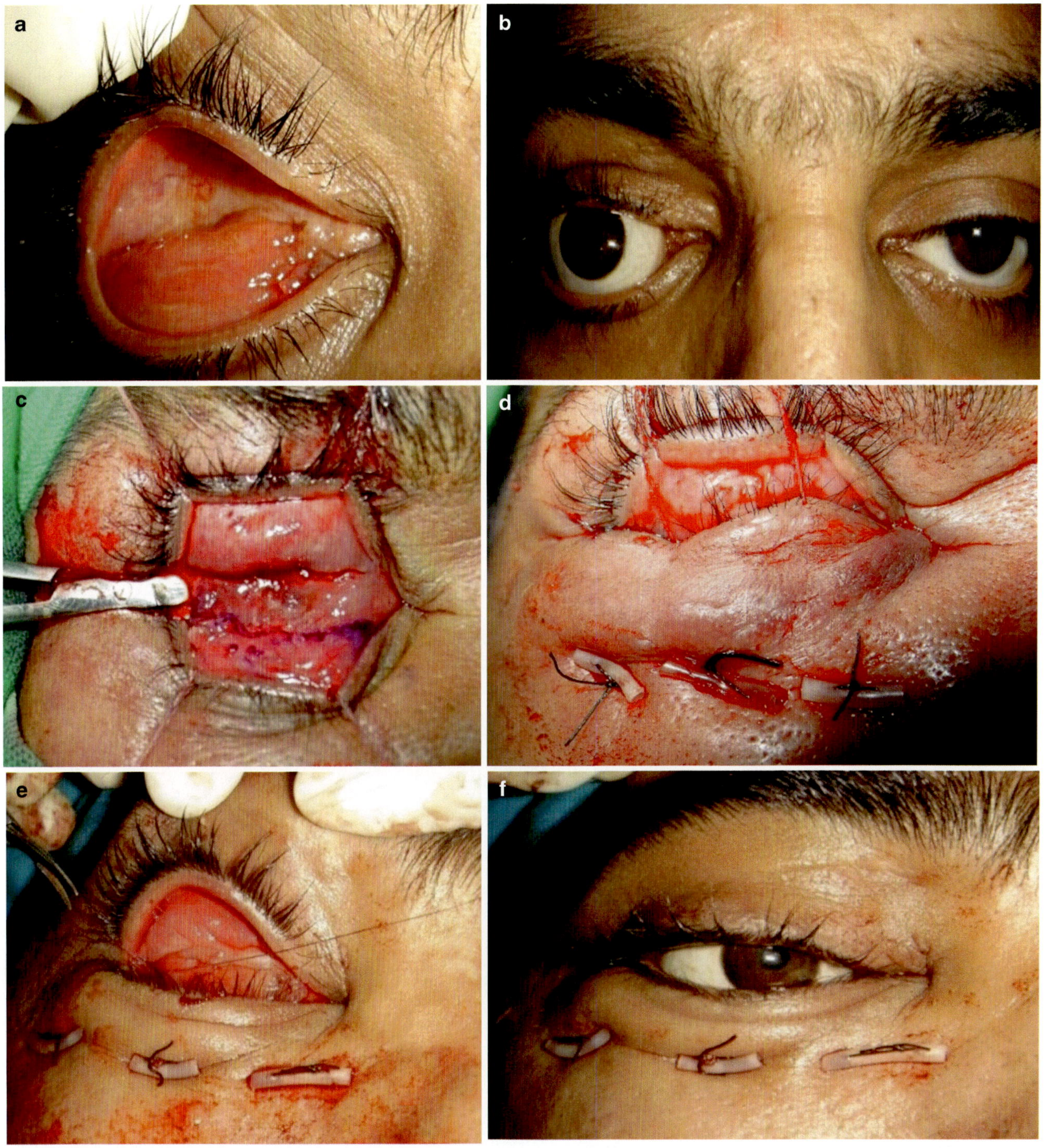

Fig. 63.13 (**a**) Preoperative image showing a shelved inferior fornix with fat prolapse. (**b**) Preoperative image demonstrates a poor fitting ocular prosthesis with upward rotation and lower eyelid laxity. (**c**) Conjunctival undermining to the orbital rim through a small temporal vertical incision. (**d**) Fornix-deepening sutures are passed through the conjunctival fornix at a position determined by placing an appropriate-sized conformer in the socket. The sutures are externalized and tied over bolsters. (**e**) Lateral canthal tendon tightening is performed. (**f**) Prosthesis is in optimal position at the end of the procedure

cated, such as tarsal autografts, hard palate, ear or nasal cartilage.

A full-thickness mucous membrane graft can be obtained from:

- Oral buccal mucosa of the inner cheek and lips (optimal choice)
- Hard or soft palate
- Skin of the labia and rectum

Harvesting of Buccal Mucous Membrane Graft (Fig. 63.14a, b)

The site of harvest is marked with a marking pen on the inner mouth or lower lip mucosa. The area is infiltrated with 2% lidocaine with epinephrine to decrease bleeding and also to facilitate removal of mucosa. Although mucous membrane grafting was first described from the lower lip, the cheek became more popular as it minimized the risk of scarring of the frenulum and subsequent lip deviation or retraction. However, grafts from the oral mucosa may be relatively contraindicated in patients who:

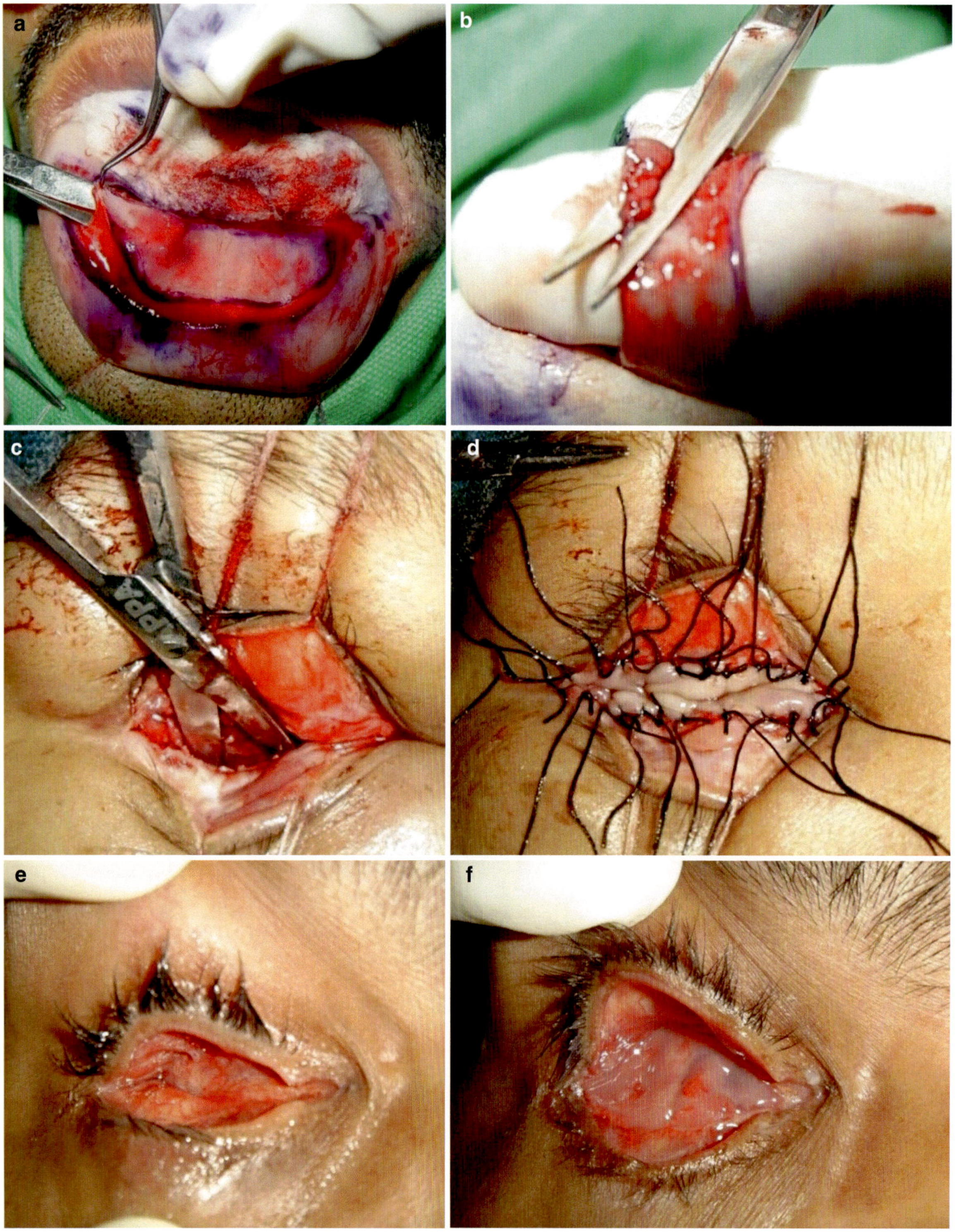

Fig. 63.14 (**a**) Harvesting of buccal mucosal graft from inside the lower lip. (**b**) Submucosal tissue is trimmed from the posterior aspect of the graft. (**c**) Dissection is performed in the inferior fornix to release the scar tissue. (**d**) The harvested mucous membrane graft is trimmed and sutured to the host bed with absorbable polyglactin or chromic gut sutures. (**e**) Preoperative photo of a right contracted socket with shortened fornices. (**f**) Postoperative photo demonstrates adequate surface and improvement in fornix depth

- Chew tobacco
- Chew betel nuts or other areca nut products (pan masala, gutka, mainpuri)
- Have a current infectious disease of the mouth (candida, lichen, varicella-virus, herpes virus)

Marking in the cheek should take care to avoid iatrogenic injury to the salivary duct (Stensen duct) near the upper second molar. If the Stensen duct cannot be clearly identified, placing several drops of lemon juice to the tongue can stimulate secretion from the parotid gland. A mouth retractor can also be helpful in providing adequate exposure. A #15 Bard-Parker blade is used to incise the mucosa, and the full-thickness graft is removed using blunt and cutting dissection in the submucosal plane with blunt-tipped scissors. A graft measuring approximately 25% larger than the anticipated defect (to allow for subsequent contracture with healing) is procured and the submucosal tissue trimmed from the posterior graft. Cautery should be minimized to avoid scarring of the lip. Although vascular mucosal healing is rapid, the graft site can be closed with running, or running locking, 5-0 absorbable suture (such as mild chromic or plain gut) to facilitate patient comfort. The graft can be placed on a wet saline gauze until used later in the procedure.

Preparation of Recipient Site (Fig. 63.14c, d)
The socket is first infiltrated with 2% lidocaine with epinephrine.

The conjunctiva is incised horizontally several millimeters below the tarsus to avoid the vascular arcade, and careful dissection is performed to release the conjunctiva from underlying cicatrix and fibrotic tissue. Subconjunctival dissection is carried out to the eyelid margin and inferiorly toward the orbital rim, until the lower eyelid is freely mobile superiorly. This results in a posterior eyelid and fornix tissue deficit. The harvested mucous membrane graft is placed into position with the mucosal side facing the ocular surface, and sutured to the recipient fornix and palpebral conjunctiva with 6-0 polyglactin or gut interrupted sutures. The graft should be slightly oversized in order to allow for postoperative contraction.

Quilting sutures are applied to the center of the graft for better apposition of the graft to the recipient bed to minimize dead space and promote vascularization of the graft [25]. Fornix reformation sutures are passed through the graft at the desired site of the deepened superior and/or inferior fornix, to exit through the skin and tightened over bolsters. A conformer is inserted to be left until the graft is healed (approximately 3 weeks). Postoperative antibiotic and lubricating drops are prescribed, betadine mouth washes for 5 days, and instructions for a soft and non-spicy diet.

Hard palate grafts (HPG) can also be used for socket reconstruction, particularly when the lower eyelid requires more support and elevation. These grafts not only have a mucosal layer to line the posterior eyelid but also a fibrous collagen matrix that provides rigidity to minimize eyelid retraction [26]. They can be easily harvested and undergo minimal graft shrinkage.

Amniotic membrane grafts (AMG) can be useful in mild to moderate contracted sockets, and are antifibrotic and anti-inflammatory. These grafts act as a substrate to provide growth factors along with basement membrane over which the normal conjunctival epithelial cells can migrate and differentiate. However, they cannot be used in cases of severely contracted sockets if there is a lack of normal conjunctival epithelial cells. In contrast, mucous membrane grafts are a substitute graft (replacement graft) and can still be beneficial in the absence of normal conjunctival cells [27].

Dermis Fat Graft
A dermis fat graft is an optimal autologous implant to correct both surface and volume deficits in a contracted socket. It is readily available, inexpensive, and has negligible allergic risks. Dermis fat grafts consist of the de-epithelialized dermis layer that is attached to and supplies nutrients to the adjacent subcutaneous fat tissue.

Harvesting of Dermis Fat Graft (Fig. 63.15a, b, c)
The preferred site of harvest is often the upper outer quadrant of the gluteal region, although dermis fat grafts can be harvested from other areas with abundant subcutaneous fat, such as the buttocks, lower abdomen, and inner thigh. The advantage of the outer gluteal site is that it is non-weight-bearing, and there is no risk of sciatic nerve damage. The graft is harvested from an area approximately 5 cm below the midpoint of the line that joins the anterior iliac crest and ischial tuberosity. A circle with a diameter of 20–25 mm is marked on the skin. The circle can also be converted to an ellipse in preparation to avoid standing defects (dog ears) upon closure. The epidermis is carefully shaved superficially with a #15 blade scalpel until fine pinpoint bleeding is visible, which represents the reticular dermis. The incision should not extend further into dermis to avoid compromising the graft viability. A deep incision is then made perpendicular to the surface, through the dermis and into subcutaneous fat, taking care to avoid narrowing the deep base of the fat plug. The depth of the fat plug should be at least 20–30 mm. The dermis fat graft is typically oversized approximately

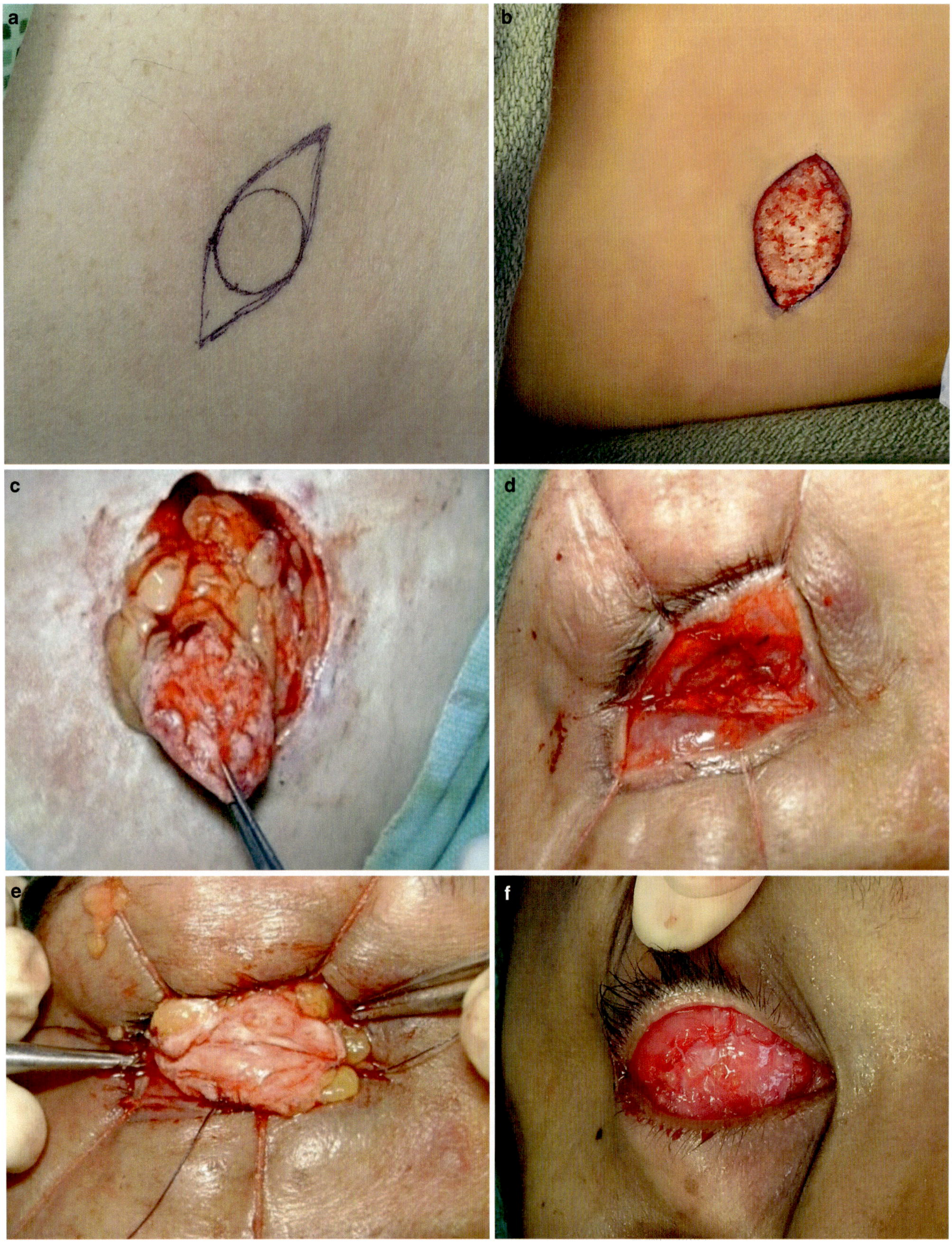

Fig. 63.15 (**a**) A 25 mm diameter circle is marked on the skin of the gluteal region. (Image courtesy of Cat Nguyen Burkat, MD FACS). (**b**) Epidermis is incised superficially until minute pinpoint bleeding is visible. (Image courtesy of Cat Nguyen Burkat, MD FACS). (**c**) The harvested dermis fat graft is 20–30 mm in depth. (**d**) Subconjunctival dissection is performed to prepare the host bed. (**e**) The dermis fat graft is transferred to the orbital recipient site. (**f**) The dermis fat graft completely sutured into the socket without excessive tension. (Image courtesy of Cat Nguyen Burkat, MD FACS)

15–20% in anticipation of fat atrophy, although it is difficult to predict the degree of atrophy. The donor site is closed with buried interrupted 3-0 or 4-0 absorbable sutures placed through fat and subcutaneous tissue, followed by skin closure.

Preparation of Recipient Site (Fig. 63.15d, e, f)

The recipient site is prepared by performing a conjunctival incision from the caruncle horizontally through the center to the lateral canthus and subconjunctival dissection performed to release all cicatrix and create a host cavity in the anophthalmic socket. The dermis fat graft is transferred into the recipient site without creating excessive pressure. At times, gentle pressure may be necessary to keep the fat within the orbit. The graft is expected to balloon outward initially until it is sutured into place; however, forcing overly abundant fat tissue into the socket could create pressure to the fat and result in more rapid fat atrophy. The fat base is placed deep in the orbit, and the dermal side faces the conjunctiva. The margin of the conjunctiva is reapproximated to the edge of the dermis with multiple 6-0 polyglactin interrupted and running sutures. A conformer is inserted over the dermis fat graft to maintain the fornices, and a pressure patch is placed for 2–3 days. Abundant literature exists that demonstrates good cosmetic and functional results in contracted sockets revised with dermis fat grafts. As dermis is included, good vascularity of the fat allows for minimal contracture and atrophy. As also mentioned previously, these grafts have the particular benefit of augmenting orbital volume as well as providing conjunctival surface area to a contracted socket.

Complications of Dermis Fat Grafts

1. Significant atrophy of graft.
2. Necrosis of graft due to infection.
3. Pressure necrosis of graft.
4. Loss of transplant due to postoperative hemorrhage.
5. Donor site wound dehiscence or infection.
6. Scar formation and deformity.

Treatment of Dry and Grossly Contracted Socket

Split-thickness skin grafting is used in these cases and may be combined with pressure molding and external wiring.

Harvesting of Graft (Fig. 63.16a, b)

The sites most commonly used are the inner aspect of the thigh or upper arm. A dermatome is helpful to obtain the appropriate split-thickness skin graft.

Preparation of Recipient Site (Fig. 63.16c–f)

The recipient site is prepared by performing a conjunctival incision from the caruncle horizontally through the center to the lateral canthus and subconjunctival dissection is performed to the superior and inferior fornices. The split-thickness skin graft is transferred to the socket, and sutured to the host bed with an overlapping suturing technique. Fornix-forming sutures are passed and tied over external skin bolsters. A pressure dressing is placed for 3–4 days after surgery.

Optical Methods for Cosmesis

1. Spectacle prosthesis
2. Tinted lenses
3. Convex lenses to magnify microphthalmic socket
4. Concave lenses to minimize buphthalmic socket

Management of Recalcitrant Cases

Dortzbach and Callahan have advocated exenteration of the eyelid and residual socket material to create a cavity into which a prosthesis is fitted [28]. An osseointegrated orbitofacial prosthesis can also be considered that provides excellent retention via magnets, as well as good aesthetic symmetry [29].

Prosthesis Fitting

The ocular prosthesis is an important option for restoration of facial symmetry and aesthetics. The ocular prosthesis can be either a stock or custom-made prosthesis. Although more affordable, a stock ocular prosthesis does not optimally match the fellow eye as it is produced in bulk and not individualized. Some patients, however, may opt to wear a stock prosthesis until the socket is healed and a custom-fit prosthesis can be made.

A custom ocular prosthesis is typically created over 1–2 days with a patient in the office to precisely match the iris color, sclera, arcus, and blood vessel pattern [30]. Patients typically are seen by the ocularist every 6–12 months for polishing and fitting adjustments of the prosthesis. Any history of discomfort, pain, redness, bleeding, or discharge from the eye should be referred back to the ophthalmologist [31]. More details regarding ocular prostheses are covered in a separate chapter.

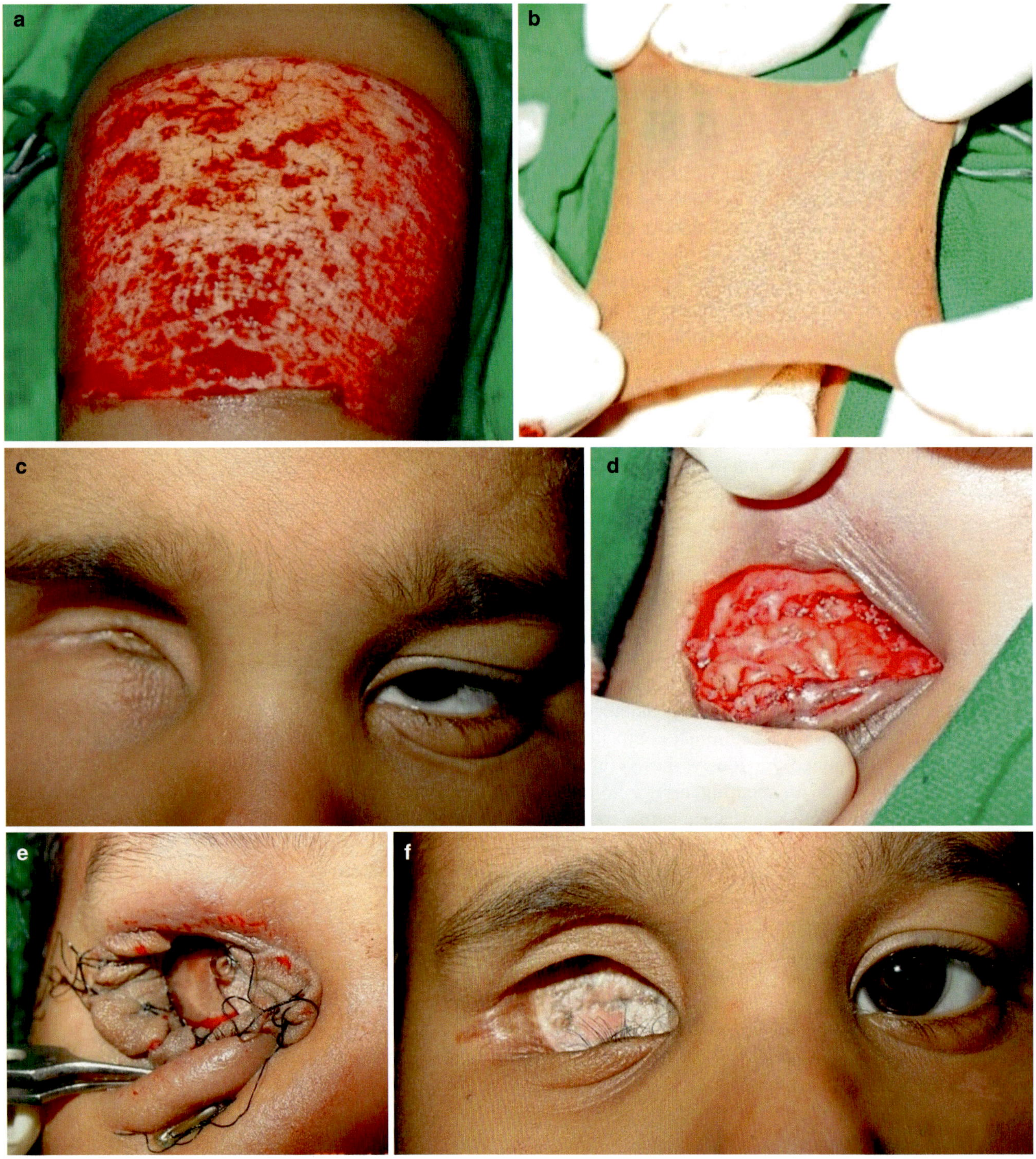

Fig. 63.16 (**a**) Split-thickness skin graft is harvested from the inner aspect of the thigh. (**b**) Harvested split-thickness graft is demonstrated. (**c**) Grossly contracted socket. (**d**) Conjunctival incision and dissection to create the recipient bed. (**e**) Split-thickness skin graft is sutured to the host bed. (**f**) The postoperative image demonstrates improved volume and surface area of the socket after split-thickness skin grafting

Conclusion

Patients with a contracted socket can be managed with gratifying outcomes by appropriate evaluation and choice of surgical procedure. Although these can be extremely challenging for both the surgeon and patient, the sockets with mild contracture or with minimal posterior laminar shortening can often have good functional results, with the main goals of creating a socket that can retain a prosthesis and, ultimately, improving facial symmetry. Cases with severe socket contracture can be more difficult and patients should be informed prior to surgery about the higher risk of persistent contracture, recurrence, or need for additional procedures.

References

1. Nesi FA, Lisman RD, Levine MR. Evaluation and current concepts in the management of anophthalmic socket. In: Smith's ophthalmic plastic and reconstructive surgery. 2nd ed. St. Louis: Mosby; 1998. p. 1079–124.
2. Kim CY, Woo YJ, Lee SY, Yoon JS. Postoperative outcomes of anophthalmic socket reconstruction using an autologous buccal mucosal graft. J Craniofac Surg. 2014;25(4):1171–4.
3. Schaefer D. Evaluation and management of the anophthalmic socket and socket contracture. In: Nesi F, Lisman RD, Levine MR, editors. Smith's ophthalmic plastic and reconstructive surgery. 2nd ed. St. Louis: Mosby; 1997. p. 115–1120.
4. Smith TJ, Koornneef L, Zonnereld FW, Groet E, Otto AJ. Computed tomography in the assessment of the postenucleation socket syndrome. Ophthalmology. 1990;97:1347–51.
5. Krishna G. Contracted sockets-I (Aetiology and types). Indian J Ophthalmol. 1980;28:117–20.
6. Vistnes L. The eye socket. In: Repair and reconstruction in the orbital region. 3rd ed. London: Churchill Livingstone; 1991. p. 335.
7. Tawfik HA, Raslan AO, Talib NL. Curr Opin Ophthalmol. 2009;20:406–11. Wolters Kluwer Health I Lippincott Williams & Wilkins, 1040–8738.
8. Yago K, Furuta M. Orbital growth after unilateral enucleation in infancy without orbital implant. Jpn J Ophthalmol. 2001;45(6):648–52.
9. Wiwatwongwana D, Rootman J. Bilateral microphthalmos with cyst with free fat graft. Ophthal Plast Reconstr Surg. 2009;25(3):241–3.
10. Gundlach KKH, Gutoff RF, Hingst VHM, et al. Expansion of the socket and orbit for congenital clinical anophthalmia. Plast Reconstr Surg. 2005;116:1214–22.
11. Ragge NK, Subak-Sharpe ID, Collin JRO. A practical guide to the management of anophthalmia and microphthalmia. Eye (Lond). 2007;21:1290–300.
12. Mazzoli R, Raymond WR, Ainbinder DJ, Hansen EA. Use of self-expanding, hydrophilic expanders (hydrogel) in the reconstruction of congenital clinical anophthalmos. Curr Opin Ophthalmol. 2004;15:426–31.
13. Gossman M, Mohay J, Roberts DM. Expansion of the human microphthalmic orbit. Ophthalmology. 1999;106:2005–9.
14. Drennan M. Balloon expansion therapy in clinical anophthalmos. J Ophthalmic Prosthet. 2002;5:9–15.
15. Mitchell KT, Hollsten DA, White WL, et al. The autogenous dermis fat orbital implant in children. JAAPOS. 2001;5:367–9.
16. Ronert MA, Hofheinz H, Manassa E, Asgarouladi H, Olbrish RR. The beginning of a new era in tissue expansion: self-sealing osmotix expander- four year clinical experience. Plast Reconstr Surg. 2004;114:1025–31.
17. Schittkowski MP, Guthoff RF. Injectable self-inflating hydrogel pellet expanders for the treatment of orbital volume deficiency in congenital microphthalmos: preliminary results with a new therapeutic approach. Br J Ophthalmol. 2006;90:1173–7.
18. Tse DT, Abdulhafez M, Orozco MA. Evaluation of an integrated orbital tissue expander in congenital anophthalmos: report of preliminary clinical experience. Am J Ophthalmol. 2011;15(3):470–82.
19. Zhang R. Reconstruction of the anophthalmic orbit by orbital osteotomy and free flap transfer. J Plast Reconstr Aesthet Surg. 2007;60:232–40.
20. Krastinova D, Mihaylova M, Martin B. Surgical management of the anophthalmic orbit, part 2: post tumoral. Plast Reconstr Surg. 2001;108:827–36.
21. Ma'Luf RN. Correction of the inadequate lower fornix in the anophthalmic socket. Br J Ophthalmol. 1999;83(7):881–2.
22. Neuhaus RW, Hawes MJ. Inadequate inferior cul-de-sac in the anophthalmic socket. Ophthalmology. 1992;99(1):153–7.
23. Bowen Jones EJ, Nunes E. The outcome of oral mucosal grafts to the orbit: a three-and -a-half-year study. Br J Plast Surg. 2002;55:102–4.
24. Tawfik HA, Raslan AO, Talib N. Surgical management of acquired socket contracture. Curr Opin Ophthalmol. 2009;20:406–11.
25. Naugle TC, Lee WW, Couvillion S. Use of quilting sutures in ophthalmic plastic surgery. Ophthal Plast Reconstr Surg. 2004;20:237–9.
26. Siegel RJ. Palatal grafts for eyelid reconstruction. Plast Reconstr Surg. 1985;76:411–4.
27. Bajaj MS, Pushker N, Kumar KS, Chandra M, Ghose S. Evaluation of amniotic membrane grafting in the reconstruction of contracted socket. Ophthal Plast Reconstr Surg. 2006;22(2):116–20.
28. Dortzbach RK, Callahan A. Advances in socket reconstruction. Am J Ophthalmol. 1970;70:800–13.
29. Wei LA, Brown JJ, Hosek DK, Burkat CN. Osseointegrated implants for orbito-facial prostheses: preoperative planning tips and intraoperative pearls. Orbit. 2016;35(2):55–61. Epub 2016 Jan 28.
30. Mishra SK, Chowdhary R. Reproduction of custom made eye prosthesis maneuver- a case report. J Dent Oral Hyg. 2009;1:59–63.
31. Cafiero-Chin M, Marques C, Danz HJ. Ocular prosthesis: indications to management. Can J Optom. 2015;77:24–32.

64 Management of Clinical Anophthalmos in Children

Iris Lee, John D. Ng, Kevin R. Schou, Maureen Maloney-Schou, and Katherine Schou

Introduction

True anophthalmos is defined as the absence of the embryologic formation of an optic vesicle. It lies on a spectrum of disease that depends on the timing and extent of interruption of eye development, and includes microphthalmos, or an underdeveloped, disorganized small eye. Anophthalmos is divided into three categories based on embryologic development. In primary anophthalmos the optic vesicle fails to develop, whereas in secondary anophthalmos, there is failure of development of the entire anterior neural tube. Consecutive or degenerative anophthalmos occurs when the optic vesicle degenerates, and may be difficult to distinguish from severe microphthalmos [1]. Primary and secondary anophthalmos tend to occur with insults in the first 4 weeks of gestation, whereas degenerative anophthalmos occurs between weeks 4–8 [2]. Clinical anophthalmos includes both anophthalmos and severe microphthalmos, where vestigial tissue may only be identified histologically or with imaging.

Worldwide, these two conditions are responsible for 15–20% of blindness and severe visual impairment in children [3, 4]. During childhood, growth of the globe provides important stimulus for development of the surrounding bone and tissue. The lack of this interplay makes the management of the anophthalmic socket in these children a constantly evolving process requiring a multidisciplinary management strategy.

Incidence

The incidence of microphthalmos and anophthalmos has been studied in several cohorts and ranges from 1 to 3/10,000 births [3, 4]. Regional variations in incidence have been observed with a rate of 30/100,000 births in Scotland from 1981 to 1996 [5] to 0.18 /10,000 among live and still births in California from 1989 to 1997 [6]. Rates in Thailand (7.7%) and Sri Lanka (7.1%) were the highest among 26 countries in a survey by Hornby et al. conducted between 1990 and 1998. Among children 3–15 years in schools for the blind and community-based rehabilitation, 10.7% had microphthalmos, and 2.3% had anophthalmos [4].

Etiology

A variety of specific genetic loci with different inheritance patterns have linked with anophthalmos. SOX2 is one of the most common monogenic causes of major ocular malformations, causing 15–40% of bilateral anophthalmia and severe microphthalmia [7, 8]. Most mutations in a German cohort were observed to be sporadic [9], although an autosomal dominant pattern has also been observed [8]. Located at locus 3q26.3-q27, it is important during early development for cell differentiation and early organogenesis, including the nervous system [10]. It binds a variety of protein products from genes that have also been associated with anophthalmia including PAX6.

Genes involved in the development of eye substructures [5] also contribute to the development of clinical anophthalmos. PAX6, which was one of the earliest genes found to have an association with anophthalmos and microphthalmos [8], is involved in the development of the lens placode [10].

I. Lee
Casey Eye Institute, Oregon Health & Science University, Portland, OR, USA

J. D. Ng (✉)
Departments of Ophthalmology and Otolaryngology/Head & Neck Surgery, Casey Eye Institute, Oregon Health & Science University, Portland, OR, USA
e-mail: ngj@ohsu.edu

K. R. Schou · M. Maloney-Schou
Maloney's Custom Ocular Prosthetics Inc, Lake Oswego, OR, USA
e-mail: kevin@Ocularconcepts.com

K. Schou
Lake Oswego, OR, USA

A. J. Cohen, C. N. Burkat (eds.), *Oculofacial, Orbital, and Lacrimal Surgery*, https://doi.org/10.1007/978-3-030-14092-2_64

CHX10, OTX2, and RAX are involved in retinal expression [5]. PAX6 and CHX10 are both inherited in a dominant fashion, whereas OTX2 and RAX are inherited in an autosomal recessive pattern [10].

Mutations in genes involved vitamin A processing and delivery have also been observed in anophthalmic children. STRA6 is involved in transmembrane transport of retinol and RARB is involved in downstream signaling after activation by retinol A [11]. ALDH1A3 is involved in retinoic acid synthesis [12, 13]. RBP4 has also been recently characterized as a transport protein that delivers retinol from the liver to the placenta and eye [14].

Nongenetic factors include gestational infections and environmental factors. Toxoplasmosis, rubella, cytomegalovirus, and influenza during pregnancy can all cause microphthalmia. Environmental factors include vitamin A deficiency, x-ray exposure during pregnancy, solvent abuse, and thalidomide.

Importance of Treating Anophthalmia

Studies in the 1960s and 1970s on both animal and humans skulls estimated the impact of anophthalmos on bony orbit formation. In anophthalmic cat skulls, not only was the orbit smaller, but the quality of the bone was affected. Importantly, placement of an orbital implant can reduce the severity of some of these changes [15, 16] (Figs. 64.1, 64.2, and 64.3).

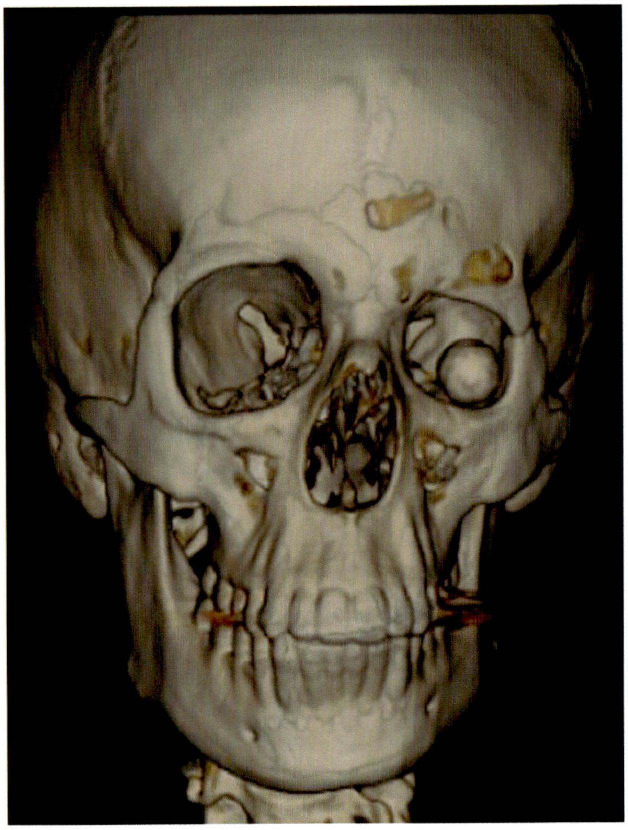

Fig. 64.1 3D reconstruction of computed tomography imaging from a patient with hypoplastic left orbit

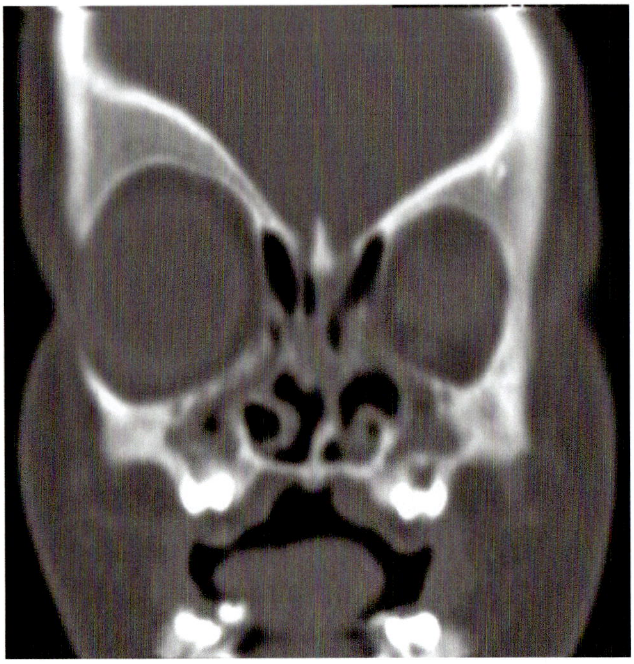

Fig. 64.2 Coronal computed tomography image from a patient with hypoplastic left orbit

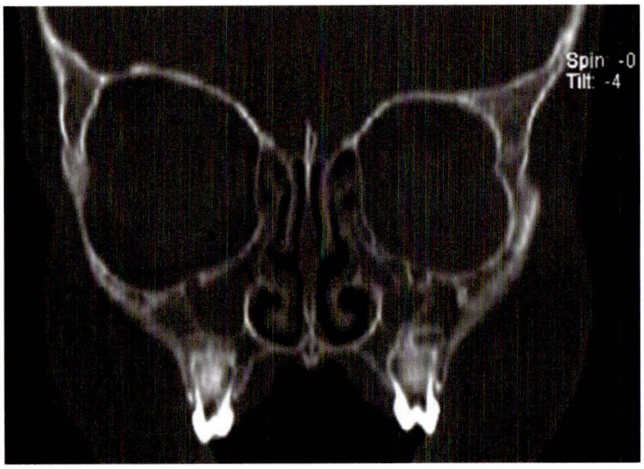

Fig. 64.3 Coronal computed tomography image of a patient who has responded well to orbital expansion. There been some inferolateral migration of the implant and bone remodeling around the implant

As the orbit makes up the central one third of the face, severe hypoplasia results in adjacent underdevelopment of the ipsilateral face, especially the cheek and brow areas. The amount of hemifacial hypoplasia varies and may occur not only due to orbital hypoplasia but concomitant developmental anomalies. In such cases, the hemifacial asymmetry tends to be more pronounced. Without adequate expansion of the orbit, brow hypoplasia and associated ptosis are inevitable [17, 18]. The issue of ptosis can be compounded by poor levator function. The superior rectus and levator palpebrae superioris may be present on imaging but hypoplastic and less likely to function well [19].

Beyond surgical management, management of psychosocial issues is an important aspect of treating anophthalmos. The birth of any child is a significant event for parents and family with its own set of stressors. The birth of a child with anophthalmia brings its own set of challenges. As with many chronic diseases, treatment of the child requires both counseling and involvement of the parents. The ophthalmologist, ocularist, and pediatrician must work in tandem with the parents from early in the child's clinical course to produce good cosmetic and positive psychosocial outcomes, which are inevitably entwined.

Initial Presentation

Prenatal Diagnostics

As mentioned previously, anophthalmia and microphthalmia can be caused by a variety of gene mutations. Chorionic villous sampling can be conducted at 10–12 weeks for karyotyping and more detailed genetic analysis. SOX2 mutations have been detected prenatally using fluorescence in situ hybridization [20]. However, the variety of genetic causes for clinical anophthalmia limits the sensitivity of this testing for detecting all cases of clinical anophthalmia. The genetic cause for anophthalmia, microphthalmia, and coloboma is determined postnatally in fewer than 50% of patients [13]. Furthermore, many of these genes have variable penetrance [5].

Prenatal imaging with ultrasound and MRI has been used to demonstrate anophthalmia [17, 21]. These malformations in utero can be detected with ultrasound as early as the late first to early second trimesters. Described by Jeanty et al. in 1982, in utero assessment of anophthalmia involves measurement in an axial plane where the eyes were of the largest possible diameter [22]. Ultrasound at this point is also useful to determine other comorbidities as described below.

Assessment in the Perinatal Period

Ultrasound is not only important prenatally, but also in the perinatal period. After birth, when clinical anophthalmia may be first noticed despite prenatal imaging [23], ultrasound may show a spectrum of phenotypes from complete absence of tissue to the presence of ocular remnant or cyst. Associated findings include variable neural and surrounding tissue as well as reduced orbital dimensions [24]. Imaging can also be used to distinguish clinical anophthalmos from cryptophthalmos, cyclopia/synophthalmia, and congenital cystic eye.

An important component of the perinatal assessment includes the evaluation for associated developmental abnormalities, both in the other eye in cases of unilateral anophthalmos and systemically. Findings in the fellow eye can include coloboma, sclerocornea, optic nerve hypoplasia, retinal dystrophy, or cataract [25, 26]. These abnormalities can occur in 25–47.4% of fellow eyes in unilateral anophthalmos, resulting in rates of legal blindness of 12.5–34.2% [25].

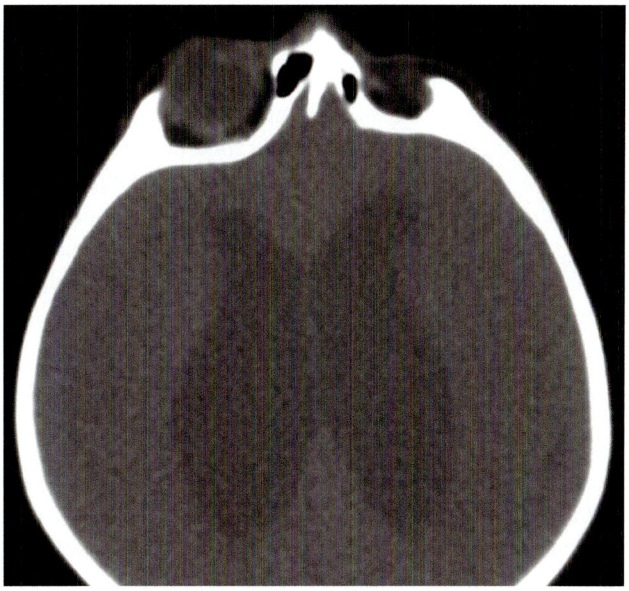

Fig. 64.4 Computed tomography imaging of the brain showing enlargement of the lateral ventricles

The laterality of the anophthalmia might also hold predictive value for expected types of developmental anomalies. In their cohort of children with bilateral anophthalmos, Albernaz noted a higher rate of malformations associated with maldevelopment of forebrain structures. These include dysgenesis or complete absence of the corpus callosum and absence of the optic chiasm. In addition to findings in the fellow eye as discussed above, unilateral anophthalmos seemed to be associated with first and second branchial arch defects [24]. In total, estimates of the rate of associated systemic abnormalities range from 33% to 73% [27–29] and can be described in syndromic conditions including trisomy 13, Lenz syndrome, Goldenhar-Gorlin Syndrome, and Waardenburg syndrome. SOX2 is associated with male genital tract anomalies, myopathy, spastic diplegia, seizures, hippocampal malformation, pituitary hypoplasia, and corpus callosum hypoplasia or agenesis [30]. Major organ systems that tend to be involved include the brain (Fig. 64.4), musculoskeletal system, and face. The heart and kidney may also be involved. A combination of magnetic resonance imaging, computed tomography, and ultrasound can be used to diagnose these changes.

Initial Management of Clinical Anophthalmos

Initial Exam

Cases of anophthalmos should be referred to an ophthalmologist soon after birth. The initial ophthalmic examination should include an exam under anesthesia at which time cycloplegic refraction, dilated fundus exam, and intraocular pressure check can be performed. Visual evoked potential may be carried out for those infants determined to have microphthalmos since the presence of vision impacts the treatment strategy, a topic that is beyond the scope of this discussion. External lid measurements and imaging for orbital dimensions are useful for informing decisions about initial interventions. Management of the anophthalmic socket involves addressing microorbitism, conjunctival sac atresia, and short, phimotic lids [31].

Anatomical Considerations

Treatment of anophthalmos is a dynamic process as the bones and soft tissue mature in children. CT studies of orbit volume in infants showed that the orbital size changes the most rapidly in the first 2 years of age, and reaches 77–96% of adult mean values by 5–8 years [15, 32]. Aspects of bony orbit development to consider include orbital volume and orbital rim dimensions (orbital entrance and projection of the superior, lateral, and inferior orbital rims), which impact the size of orbital expanders that can be used.

Development of the eyelids and socket space are intimately related, and often addressed first in the management of anophthalmos because they control access to the more posterior orbital space. Conformers used to expand these areas of the face must exert a balance of anterior, posterior, and radial pressure [33]. Measurements pertaining to the eyelid and socket space include the horizontal palpebral fissure, vertical palpebral fissure, and forniceal depth. Adequate development of both these structures is important for conformer or prosthesis retention as well as improved cosmetic result.

Occasionally, microphthalmia or anophthalmia with cyst is found on imaging. On physical exam, these may present as a bulge, often in the lower eyelid, with a bluish hue. These cysts are usually left in place to contribute to orbital growth. Indications for removal include asymmetric growth (either too large or small compared with the other side, especially if protruding through the palpebral fissure in the cases of large cysts) and pain [5, 34].

Initial Strategies (Conjunctival Expansion)

Early expansion of the conjunctival sac with acrylic conformers (Figs. 64.5 and 64.6) is essential for creating a stable environment for future prosthesis placement. It also helps to expand the orbital rim [31, 35], which is important for maximizing the size of the orbital expander that can be used [16]. Before treatment can begin for patients with anophthalmos, a discussion between the ophthalmologist and the ocularist is strongly recommended. A plan of sizes, designs, and goals to be achieved should be discussed. The ocularist should be present for the examination of the sockets and impression at the earliest exam under anesthesia in order to begin expansion therapy as soon as possible. The younger the patient, the more frequent return appointments to the ocularist should be made; one to 2 weeks on average for the first 8 months of life. This time frame should be tailored to each individual patient, dependent on growth factors.

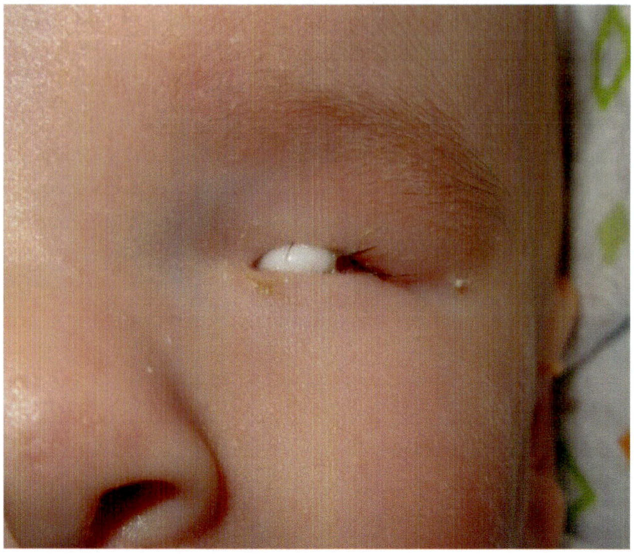

Fig. 64.5 Child with acrylic conformer in place

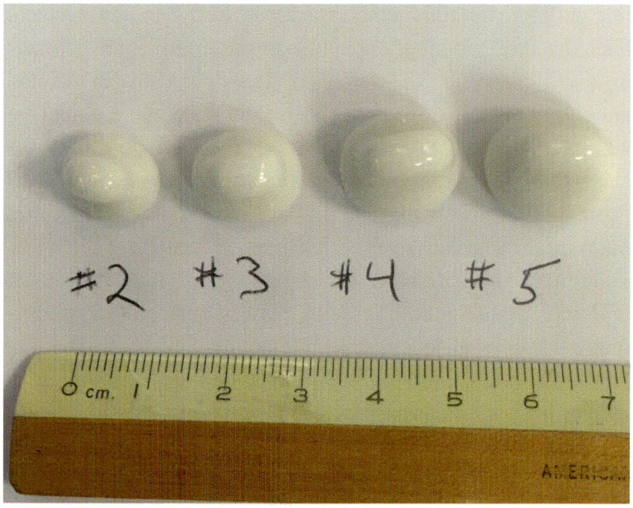

Fig. 64.6 Examples of acrylic conformers of various sizes

Conformers that are too large in a socket can have adverse effects—the rapidity of expansion must be balanced against excessive stretch, which may cause contraction [36]. A conformer that fills the socket with slight stretching and periodical enlargements will enlarge the socket faster, and with fewer complications. Adding to the periphery at one appointment and to the anterior-posterior diameter at the next appointment has shown to be a successful treatment plan. If the patient has a small palpebral fissure, a bar can be constructed to just protrude past the lid margins for stabilization and stretching of the palpebral fissure.

In eyes where the anophthalmic socket is extremely constricted or where the fornices are not well developed, expanding hydrophilic socket implants can be good alternative to acrylic conformers [36, 37]. Blepharophimosis, for example, presents with contracted and small lids and reduced conjunctival surface and can be challenging for initial acrylic conformer placement. Hydrogel expanders consist of a copolymer of methylmethacrylate and vinyl pyrrolidone, and are available for both the conjunctival pocket and the orbit. Hydrogel expanders in the conjunctival space expand to their full size (determined by the swelling capacity of the material) within weeks in older series [37] and 2 days in a more recent series [36]. In their patients, Gundlach and Schittkowski found that a hydrogel conformer could be replaced with an acrylic counterpart or prosthesis in 2 and 2.8 months, respectively [35, 36]. Complications of hydrogel implants include degradation of the implant, causing irritation. Most other early complications resulted from wrong implant size (too small or too large) resulting in expander loss. As mentioned above, loss of conjunctival expanders result in regression of expansion results if not rapidly replaced.

Conformers can also cause a variety of eyelid pathologies that impact management of anophthalmos. The weight of the conformer can cause both mechanical ectropion, found more commonly in the lower lid, and entropion. Entropion can also be caused if excessive stretch has caused eyelid contractures, which may present with the patient's eyelashes plastered against the conformer. Lagophthalmos is almost universally present and is caused by a combination of conjunctival tissue insufficiency and the mechanical effects of the prosthesis. Lastly, retraction can also occur through both cicatricial and mechanical mechanisms. Insufficient orbital volume also contributes to upper lid retraction [38]. Correction of lid malposition in these children can be challenging because of a shortage of tissue, scarring, and unpredictable healing, requiring the use of hard palate and spacer grafts, tissue augmentation, or mechanical stretching of the lid (Figs. 64.7, 64.8, 64.9, 64.10, and 64.11). During the process of expansion, it is also important to remind parents of the importance of keeping conformers in place because regression occurs quickly [18, 35, 36].

Once the socket is deemed to have stretched as far as possible by the use of conformers, then the surgeon should place

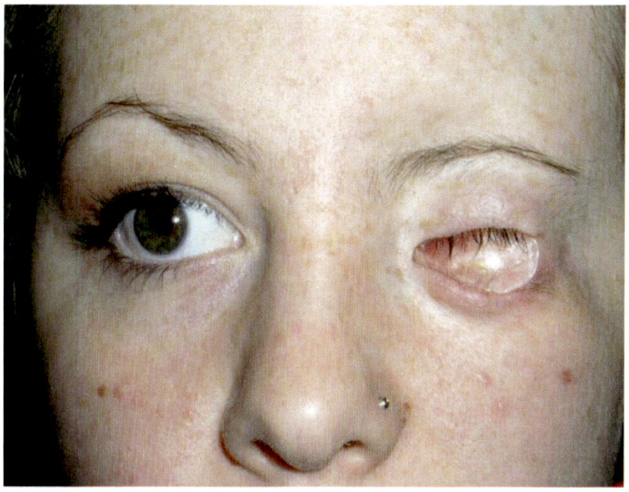

Fig. 64.7 Patient with inferior lid retraction, brow hypoplasia, reduced palpebral fissure

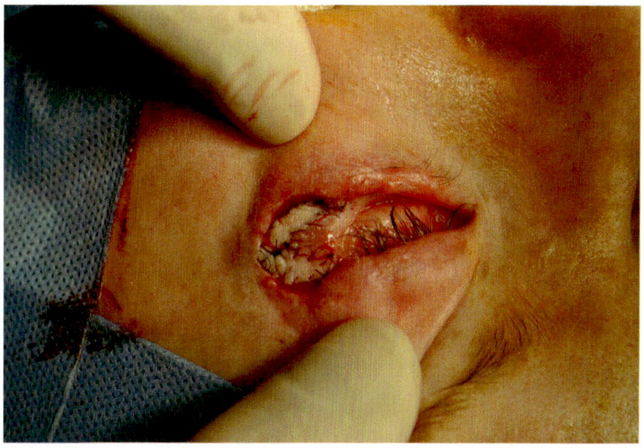

Fig. 64.8 Intraoperative photograph using graft to augment conjunctival space

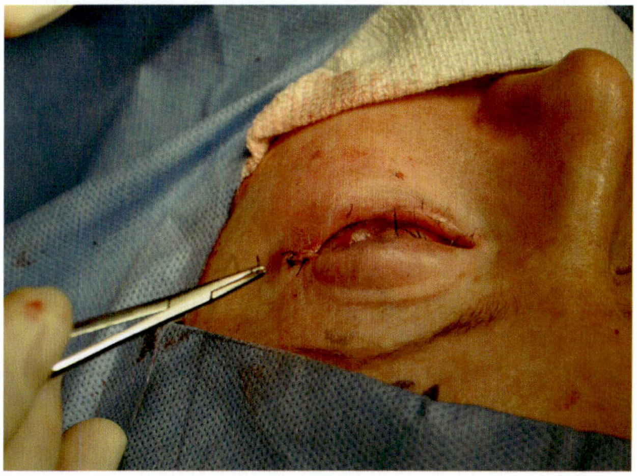

Fig. 64.9 Intraoperative photograph after expansion of conjunctival space

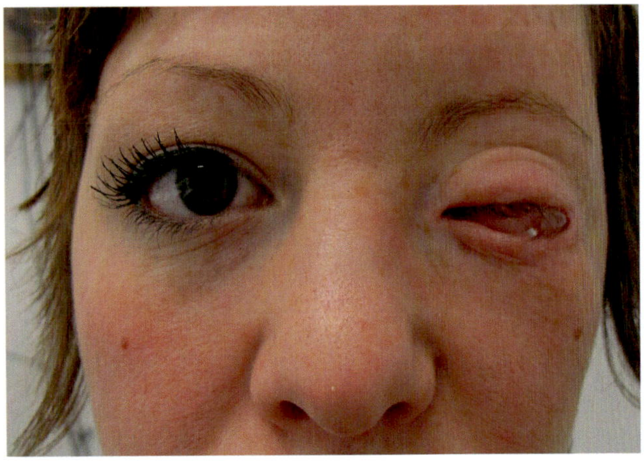

Fig. 64.10 Patient with expanded conjunctival space, improved forniceal contour

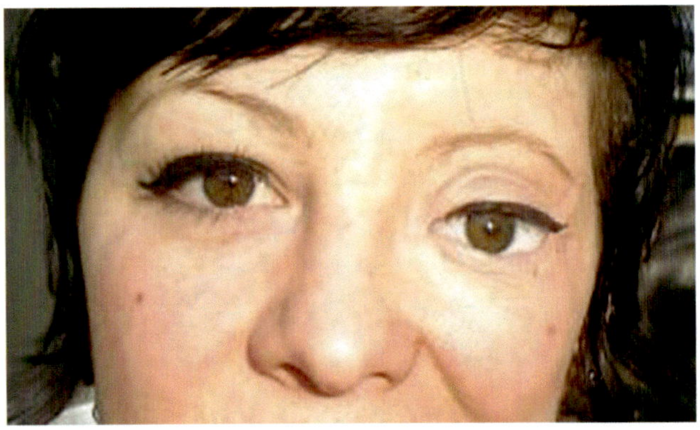

Fig. 64.11 Patient with conformer in place

a spherical implant or dermis fat graft as discussed in the next section. After an implant is placed, the ocularist can use a more conventional conformer shape.

Orbital Expansion

There are multiple options for augmentation of orbital volume once the orbital rim has expanded sufficiently. These historically included hard spherical implants, inflatable soft tissue expanders, dermis fat grafts, hydrogel expanders, and integrated orbital tissue expanders. Today, spherical implants, hydrogel expanders, and dermis fat grafts are the most widely used. Several surgical approaches for both primary placement and exchange are available and include entry through upper or lower lid creases [36], the lateral canthus [19], or the conjunctiva [37]. Our preference is the lateral approach (Figs. 64.12 and 64.13) in order to reduce the risk of extrusion. Using this technique, the implant is placed in the orbit through a path along the periosteum of the lateral wall, preventing lateral

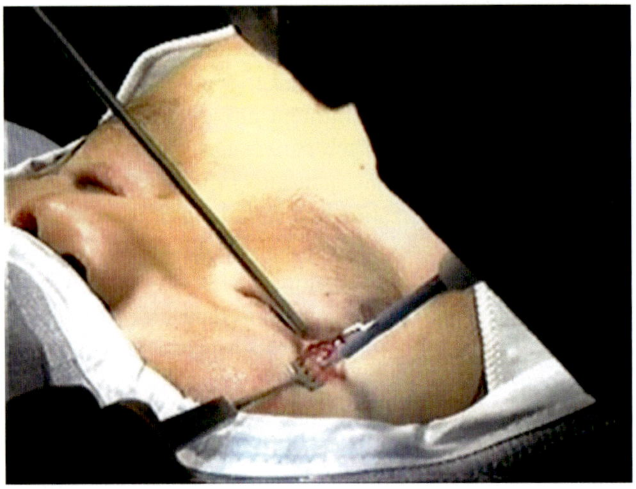

Fig. 64.12 Infant with acrylic conformer in place

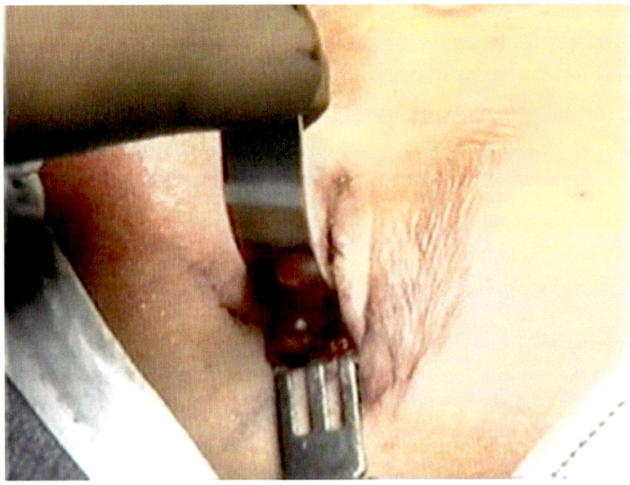

Fig. 64.13 Lateral approach for placement of orbital expanders

extrusion. In contrast, both the conjunctival or upper lid crease approaches can result in extrusion back through the path created by a more direct surgical approach, especially with the rapid expansion that can occur with hydrogels.

When deciding on the size of an orbital expander, a balance must be struck between fitting an expander that is too large, and risking extrusion, versus an expander that is not large enough, yielding suboptimal results. The static nature of silicone spheres can exacerbate the problem of adequate sizing, especially if orbital rim dimensions limit the size of the sphere. Hydrogel orbital expanders were initially described in 1999 along with their conformer counterparts [37]. The properties of hydrogels were discussed previously with hydrogel conformers. The benefit of hydrogel expanders is twofold—that they can fit in through a small incision, and because they can be fragmented, they can be removed

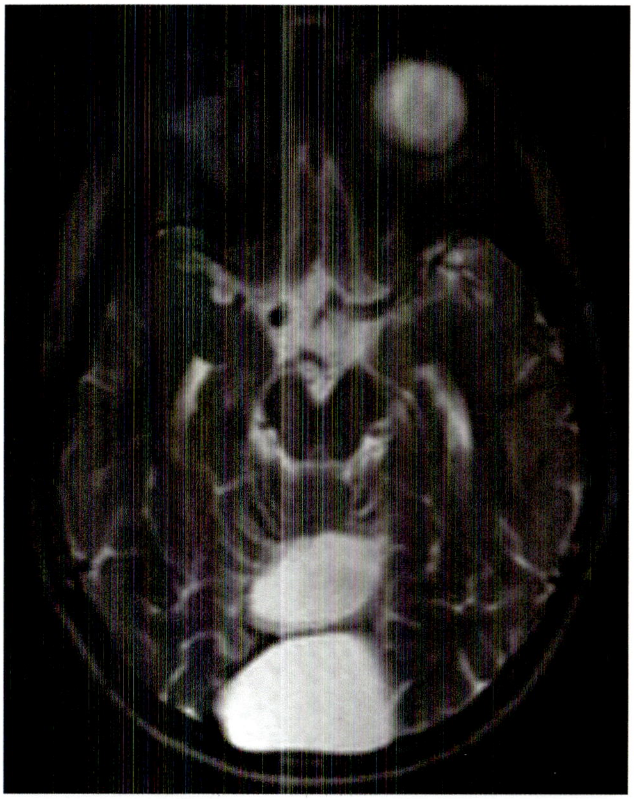

Fig. 64.14 Magnetic resonance imaging of dermis fat graft in the right orbit

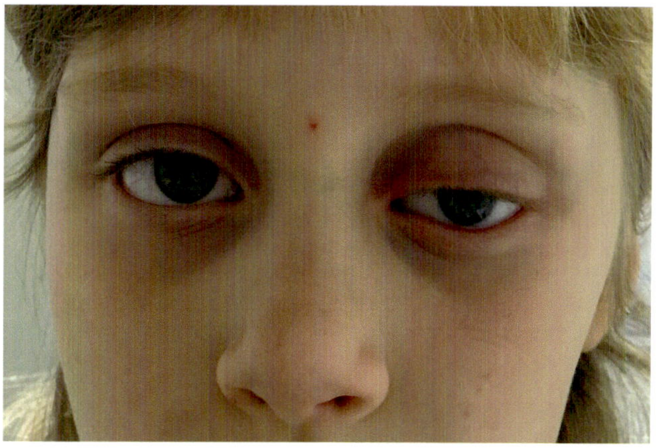

Fig. 64.15 Patient with dermis fat graft

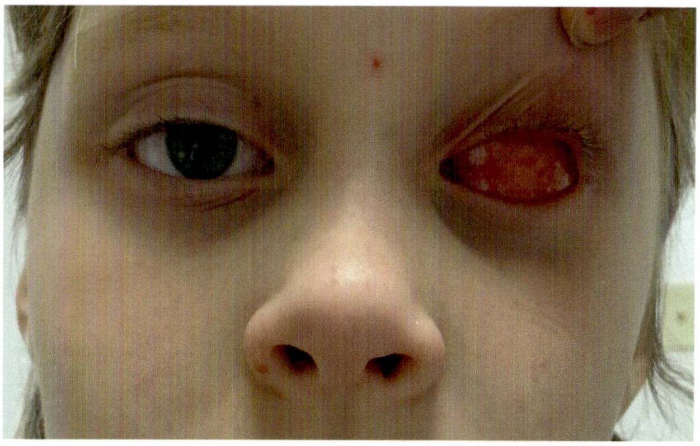

Fig. 64.16 Patient with dermis fat graft with conformer in place

during exchange through a similarly small incision [36]. Although also available, biointegratable implants are more difficult to exchange. Also, higher rates of extrusion were observed by Li et al. [39].

Dermis fat grafts offer another option for orbital expansion in the pediatric population (Figs. 64.14, 64.15, and 64.16), especially when implanted at less than three to 4 years of age [19, 40]. The benefit of this type of graft is that it grows with the patient, continuing to provide stimulus for orbital expansion. However, fat grafts can prove challenging when trying to fit a pediatric patient with a prosthesis due to this growth. Fat grafts can also be an unstable foundation for prosthesis, contributing to spinning, ptosis, and conformer loss due to rapid growth.

In our experience, dermis fat grafts placed in the orbits of children with clinical anophthalmos have less of an issue of fat overgrowth than those placed in the orbits of children who undergo enucleation. However, it is not uncommon for several debulking surgical procedures to be required over a period of several years. Frequent surgical procedures can prove emotionally detrimental for the patient and their families. When considering a dermis fat graft, great care and extensive communication regarding expected compliance between the surgeon, ocularist, and family will likely provide the best result.

Besides the issue of debulking, there are a variety of other complications that are common to all implants. Early issues include pain, both from surgery and pressure from implant. Hemorrhage and infection as also possible. Delayed complications include exposure and extrusion of the implant with orbital implants tending to migrate inferolaterally [41] (Fig. 64.3).

Continuing Management

Both silicone sphere and hydrogel implants require exchange, either with another implant or with a dermis fat graft. The process of anterior expansion with conformers will continue, usually with a step down in size of the conformer in size due to partial obliteration of the socket volume from the deeper orbital space occupying implants. The process of improving cosmetic and psychosocial outcomes for these children is necessarily individualized and dynamic. However, with compliant parents and child, and close communication with the family, ophthalmologist, and ocularist, good outcomes can be achieved.

References

1. Vachha BA, Robson CD. Imaging of pediatric orbital diseases. Neuroimaging Clin N Am. 2015;25(3):477–501.
2. Albernaz VS, Castillo M, Hudgins PA, Mukherji SK. Imaging findings in patients with clinical anophthalmos. Am J Neuroradiol. 1997;18(3):555–61.
3. Dolk H, Busby A, Armstrong BG, Walls PH. Geographical variation in anophthalmia and microphthalmia in England, 1988–94. BMJ. 1998;317(7163):905–9.
4. Hornby SJ, Gilbert CE, Rahi JK, Sil AK, Xiao Y, Dandona L, et al. Regional variation in blindness in children due to microphthalmos, anophthalmos and coloboma. Ophthalmic Epidemiol. 2000;7(2):127–38.
5. Verma AS, Fitzpatrick DR. Anophthalmia and microphthalmia. Orphanet J Rare Dis. 2007;2:47.
6. Shaw GM, Carmichael SL, Yang W, Harris JA, Finnell RH, Lammer EJ. Epidemiologic characteristics of anophthalmia and bilateral microphthalmia among 2.5 million births in California, 1989–1997. Am J Med Genet A. 2005;137(1):36–40.
7. Williamson KA, FitzPatrick DR. The genetic architecture of microphthalmia, anophthalmia and coloboma. Eur J Med Genet. 2014;57(8):369–80.
8. Fitzpatrick DR, van Heyningen V. Developmental eye disorders. Curr Opin Genet Dev. 2005;15(3):348–53.
9. Gerth-Kahlert C, Williamson K, Ansari M, Rainger JK, Hingst V, Zimmermann T, et al. Clinical and mutation analysis of 51 probands with anophthalmia and/or severe microphthalmia from a single center. Mol Genet Genomic Med. 2013;1(1):15–31.
10. Bardakjian TM, Schneider A. The genetics of anophthalmia and microphthalmia. Curr Opin Ophthalmol. 2011;22(5):309–13.
11. Srour M, Chitayat D, Caron V, Chassaing N, Bitoun P, Patry L, et al. Recessive and dominant mutations in retinoic acid receptor beta in cases with microphthalmia and diaphragmatic hernia. Am J Hum Genet. 2013;93(4):765–72.
12. Fares-Taie L, Gerber S, Chassaing N, Clayton-Smith J, Hanein S, Silva E, et al. ALDH1A3 mutations cause recessive anophthalmia and microphthalmia. Am J Hum Genet. 2013;92(2):265–70.
13. Yahyavi M, Abouzeid H, Gawdat G, de Preux AS, Xiao T, Bardakjian T, et al. ALDH1A3 loss of function causes bilateral anophthalmia/microphthalmia and hypoplasia of the optic nerve and optic chiasm. Hum Mol Genet. 2013;22(16):3250–8.
14. Chou CM, Nelson C, Tarle SA, Pribila JT, Bardakjian T, Woods S, et al. Biochemical basis for dominant inheritance, variable penetrance, and maternal effects in RBP4 congenital eye disease. Cell. 2015;161(3):634–46.
15. Kennedy RE. Growth retardation and volume determinations of the anophthalmic orbit. Am J Ophthalmol. 1973;76(2):294–302.
16. Tucker SM, Sapp N, Collin R. Orbital expansion of the congenitally anophthalmic socket. Br J Ophthalmol. 1995;79(7):667–71.
17. Chen CP, Wang KG, Huang JK, Chang TY, Lin YH, Chin DT, et al. Prenatal diagnosis of otocephaly with microphthalmia/anophthalmia using ultrasound and magnetic resonance imaging. Ultrasound Obstet Gynecol. 2003;22(2):214–5.
18. Quaranta-Leoni FM. Congenital anophthalmia: current concepts in management. Curr Opin Ophthalmol. 2011;22(5):380–4.
19. Jordan DRKS. Evaluation and management of the anophthalmic socket and socket reconstruction. In: Black EHNF, Calvano CJ, Gladstone GJ, Levin MR, editors. Smith and Nesi's ophthalmic plastic and reconstructive surgery. New York: Springer; 2012. p. 1131–73.
20. Guichet A, Triau S, Lepinard C, Esculapavit C, Biquard F, Descamps P, et al. Prenatal diagnosis of primary anophthalmia with a 3q27 interstitial deletion involving SOX2. Prenat Diagn. 2004;24(10):828–32.
21. Mashiach R, Vardimon D, Kaplan B, Shalev J, Meizner I. Early sonographic detection of recurrent fetal eye anomalies. Ultrasound Obstet Gynecol. 2004;24(6):640–3.
22. Jeanty P, Dramaix-Wilmet M, Van Gansbeke D, Van Regemorter N, Rodesch F. Fetal ocular biometry by ultrasound. Radiology. 1982;143(2):513–6.
23. Blazer S, Zimmer EZ, Mezer E, Bronshtein M. Early and late onset fetal microphthalmia. Am J Obstet Gynecol. 2006;194(5): 1354–9.
24. Albernaz VS, Castillo M, Hudgins PA, Mukherji SK. Imaging findings in patients with clinical anophthalmos. AJNR Am J Neuroradiol. 1997;18(3):555–61.
25. Schittkowski MP, Guthoff RF. Systemic and ophthalmological anomalies in congenital anophthalmic or microphthalmic patients. Br J Ophthalmol. 2010;94(4):487–93.
26. Ragge NK, Subak-Sharpe ID, Collin JR. A practical guide to the management of anophthalmia and microphthalmia. Eye. 2007;21(10):1290–300.
27. Morrison D, FitzPatrick D, Hanson I, Williamson K, van Heyningen V, Fleck B, et al. National study of microphthalmia, anophthalmia, and coloboma (MAC) in Scotland: investigation of genetic aetiology. J Med Genet. 2002;39(1):16–22.
28. Skalicky SE, White AJ, Grigg JR, Martin F, Smith J, Jones M, et al. Microphthalmia, anophthalmia, and coloboma and associated ocular and systemic features: understanding the spectrum. JAMA Ophthalmol. 2013;131(12):1517–24.
29. Tucker S, Jones B, Collin R. Systemic anomalies in 77 patients with congenital anophthalmos or microphthalmos. Eye. 1996;10. (Pt 3:310–4.
30. Fantes J, Ragge NK, Lynch SA, McGill NI, Collin JR, Howard-Peebles PN, et al. Mutations in SOX2 cause anophthalmia. Nat Genet. 2003;33(4):461–3.
31. Krastinova D, Kelly MB, Mihaylova M. Surgical management of the anophthalmic orbit, part 1: congenital. Plast Reconstr Surg. 2001;108(4):817–26.
32. Bentley RP, Sgouros S, Natarajan K, Dover MS, Hockley AD. Normal changes in orbital volume during childhood. J Neurosurg. 2002;96(4):742–6.
33. Mazzoli RA, Raymond WR, Ainbinder DJ, Hansen EA. Use of self-expanding, hydrophilic osmotic expanders (hydrogel) in the reconstruction of congenital clinical anophthalmos. Curr Opin Ophthalmol. 2004;15(5):426–31.
34. McLean CJ, Ragge NK, Jones RB, Collin JR. The management of orbital cysts associated with congenital microphthalmos and anophthalmos. Br J Ophthalmol. 2003;87(7):860–3.
35. Gundlach KK, Guthoff RF, Hingst VH, Schittkowski MP, Bier UC. Expansion of the socket and orbit for congenital clinical anophthalmia. Plast Reconstr Surg. 2005;116(5):1214–22.
36. Schittkowski MP, Katowitz JA, Gundlach KKH, Guthoff RF. Self-inflating hydrogel expanders for the treatment of congenital anophthalmos. In: Guthoff RF, Katowitz JA, editors. Oculoplastics and orbit, Essentials in ophthalmology. Berlin: Springer Berlin Heidelberg; 2006. p. 205–21.
37. Wiese KG, Vogel M, Guthoff R, Gundlach KK. Treatment of congenital anophthalmos with self-inflating polymer expanders: a new method. J Craniomaxillofac Surg. 1999;27(2):72–6.
38. Shams PN, Selva D. Upper eyelid retraction in the anophthalmic socket: review and survey of the Australian and New Zealand Society of ophthalmic plastic surgeons (ANZSOPS). Ophthal Plast Reconstr Surg. 2014;30(4):309–12.
39. Li T, Shen J, Duffy MT. Exposure rates of wrapped and unwrapped orbital implants following enucleation. Ophthal Plast Reconstr Surg. 2001;17(6):431–5.
40. Heher KL, Katowitz JA, Low JE. Unilateral dermis-fat graft implantation in the pediatric orbit. Ophthal Plast Reconstr Surg. 1998;14(2):81–8.
41. Tao JP, LeBoyer RM, Hetzler K, Ng JD, Nunery WR. Inferolateral migration of hydrogel orbital implants in microphthalmia. Ophthal Plast Reconstr Surg. 2010;26(1):14–7.

Ocular and Scleral Shell Prostheses

65

James Johnston

Introduction

Ocular prostheses are utilized for the anatomical and cosmetic rehabilitation of patients who have undergone enucleation or evisceration surgery, or in cases of trauma or disease of the globe which result in blind, unsightly, and sometimes uncomfortable eyes that may not require further surgical intervention.

The two main different types of ocular prostheses that are utilized, as well as pediatric applications of prosthetic therapy, will be discussed. Although fabrication and fitting of artificial eyes following enucleation or evisceration and scleral shell ocular prostheses fitted over an existing blind globe are, indeed, quite similar, there are some significant differences that warrant separate consideration.

Overview of Ocularistry

Custom-fitted prosthetic eyes were first developed in Germany during the mid- to late nineteenth century. These artificial eyes were empirically fitted and fabricated of hand-blown, thin-walled, cryolite glass and were fitted by skilled glass craftsman specifically to the patients' anophthalmic sockets. Due to the fragility of these hollow glass eyes and the domestic scarcity of the raw materials needed for their fabrication during the mid-1940s, plastic prosthetic eyes became the standard in the United States. Current technology in ocularistry involves the use of polymethylmethacrylate acrylic (PMMA) which is also utilized in dentistry for the manufacture of dental implants and materials. The transition to this more moldable, adjustable acrylic material allowed for an accuracy of fitting not previously possible, ultimately leading to the ability to fit prosthetic devices over blind eyes, often obviating the need for surgical removal or alteration of many non-painful, non-sighted eyes.

Prosthetic specialists in artificial eyes, called ocularists, are trained in carefully fitting these acrylic prostheses by utilizing direct, physical impressions of the eye socket, as well as techniques of empirical shaping. Most artificial eyes are still hand-painted on site by the ocularist to best match the patient's companion eye, but there are some ocularists who now utilize pre-colored, digitized, and printed iris images that can be laminated within the completed prostheses. Evaluation and fitting of prosthetic eyes by an ocularist are directly based on referral from an ophthalmologist or oculoplastic surgeon.

Ocularistry, as a craft, involves very specific artistic and technical abilities. It also requires a thorough understanding of orbital anatomy and function, as well as specific skills directing patient management of prosthetic issues and clinical communication with the referring ophthalmologist and/or oculoplastic surgeon.

Post-enucleation and Post-evisceration Prostheses

The post-enucleated or post-eviscerated socket is usually ready to begin prosthetic rehabilitation with the ocularist at 2–6 weeks after surgery depending upon several factors including healing of implant closure, removal of tarsorrhaphy (if placed), residual edema, patient sensitivity, and motivation. In most cases, a generic post-surgical conformer is placed by the surgeon in the operating room in order to protect the suture line from the blinking of lids, as well as to maintain the conjunctival fornix, for this period prior to the ocularist visit.

The initial patient visit with the ocularist will usually entail the fitting of a custom shaped temporary prosthesis, designed to gently encourage deepening of the superior and inferior fornix, and provide quicker cosmetic benefit for the

J. Johnston (✉)
Ocularists Limited, Des Plaines, IL, USA
e-mail: midwestop@comcast.net

A. J. Cohen, C. N. Burkat (eds.), *Oculofacial, Orbital, and Lacrimal Surgery*, https://doi.org/10.1007/978-3-030-14092-2_65

patient following surgery. An impression, or final fitting of the prosthesis, at this early stage will not generally be an accurate representation of the completely healed socket and can even create tangential stress to the suture line, thus risking wound dehiscence and implant exposure. The fitting and wearing of a temporary prosthesis earlier, however, allows for the patient's cosmetic concerns to be more easily managed during the healing phase. This initial temporary prosthesis is generally worn for 2–6 weeks while the socket and chemosis heal. In cases of shortened or contracted fornices, deeper than usual superior sulcus depression, cicatricial adhesions, or blepharoptosis due to residual lid edema, the socket may require additional temporary prostheses of gradually larger sizes to better develop the socket prior to the fitting, fabrication, and delivery of the final prosthesis. Those with ptosis or superior sulcus volume loss may sometimes benefit from modification of the prosthesis to enlarge the superior portion to elevate the eyelid.

Once the socket and eyelids are adequately healed and developed, the final prosthesis is fabricated, painted, and delivered. The process of fabricating the final prosthesis may take anywhere from 1 day to several weeks depending upon the particular clinical setting and ocularist preference. The patient will then follow up with the ocularist several times during the first year to ensure that any socket changes are coordinated with appropriate adjustments to the prosthesis. The goal of the final prosthesis should be that it fits well in the socket, is comfortable, and requires minimal maintenance by the patient. Any remaining deficiencies such as continuing blepharoptosis, inferior displacement of the orbital contents, floppy eyelid syndrome, ectropion or entropion, can be referred back to the surgeon for consultation and appropriate surgical correction.

Patient Care of Prosthetic Eyes Following Enucleation and Evisceration

The ocular prosthesis should be removed by the patient for cleaning approximately once every month to once every 6 months, depending upon factors such as mucus discharge, dryness, and overall patient sensitivity. A daily rinse with saline solution, eye wash, or distilled water is sometimes recommended to reduce and control any mucus discharge. Over-the-counter lubricating drops are recommended for the management of dryness, as needed. The patient should be instructed to avoid using harsh chemicals or alcohol wipes to clean the prosthesis.

Daily removal of the ocular prosthesis is generally not encouraged, as mechanical irritation from frequent tissue manipulation and the possibility of introducing infective organisms can actually lead to an increase in mucus secretion and conjunctival inflammation or infection. In addition, frequent removal can predispose to eyelid laxity, resulting in upper eyelid ptosis or lower eyelid ectropion or canthal angle dystopia.

An ocular prosthesis should be professionally cleaned and polished by the ocularist every 6–12 months, adjusted as needed for socket changes, and replaced approximately every 5–7 years, on average.

Scleral Shell Ocular Prostheses for Phthisical Eyes

Scleral shell ocular prostheses are artificial eye prostheses that are designed to be worn over blind, but unsightly eyes that do not require further surgical intervention (Figs. 65.1 and 65.2). While there is tremendous cosmetic potential and benefit to the patient wearing a scleral shell over a blind disfigured eye, real consideration must be given to the increased comfort a properly fitted scleral shell can provide when fitted to a phthisical, hypotonic, or otherwise disfigured globe. Fitting a scleral shell over such a blind eye can often obviate the need for enucleation, evisceration, or eyelid correction

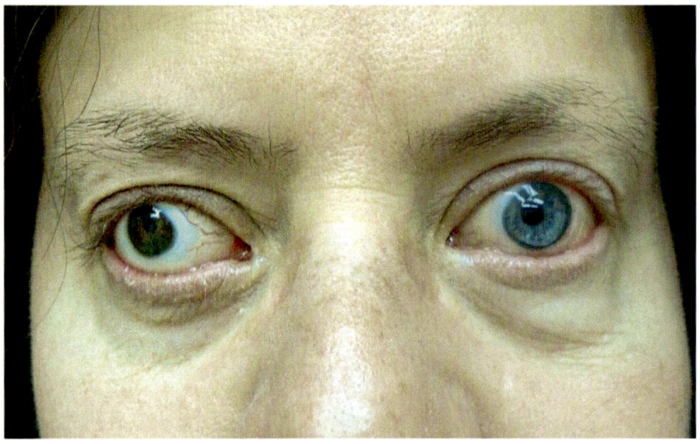

Fig. 65.1 Patient with a blind, phthisical right eye who may benefit from a scleral shell prosthesis

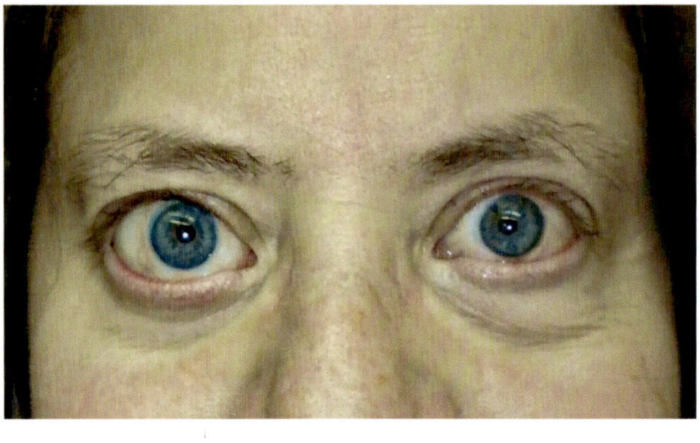

Fig. 65.2 Scleral shell in place over the phthisical right globe

surgeries by ameliorating superficial irritations that can be a problem with these blind and disfigured globes.

A scleral shell prosthesis is almost always fitted following a careful alginate or polyvinyl siloxane impression mold of the blind eye, in the ocularist clinic. Proper clearance of the cornea is critical in cases where a clear, "live" cornea is present. Unlike the fitting of a contact lens, a prosthetic shell directly contacts only the scleral portion of the globe and has a central vaulting designed to create a tear chamber in the interface between the anterior cornea and posterior surface of the scleral shell. This vaulting or doming above the cornea, along with a properly placed anterior/posterior fenestration through the shell, ensures proper tear and oxygen exchange to the cornea. This configuration provides a stable, comfortable habitat for any sensitive corneal tissue, not unlike a well-fitted bandage contact lens.

To ensure proper fitting of the scleral shell prosthesis, the ocularist will first fabricate a transparent scleral shell from the direct impression of the globe, in order to accurately visualize this tear chamber through the shell, as well as delineate any pressure points that may need to be identified for adjustment prior to proceeding to the opaque, painted scleral shell prosthesis. Once it is apparent that the clear shell is properly mating with the blind globe, the opaque scleral shell is fabricated and the colors are matched to the companion eye, similar to a full ocular prosthesis after enucleation. The patient is followed by both the ocularist and ophthalmologist on a regular schedule.

Patient Care of Scleral Shell Ocular Prostheses

Unlike a standard prosthesis, the scleral shell should generally be treated as a hard contact lens; it should be removed at night, handled carefully by the patient to avoid scratches or contamination, and placed in fresh sterile saline or contact lens solution when not being worn.

A scleral shell prosthesis should be polished every 6–12 months by the ocularist, adjusted as needed for anatomical changes and patient comfort. On average, a well-fitting scleral shell prosthesis would be expected to last approximately 5–7 years before replacement is required.

Pediatric Considerations Regarding Ocular Prostheses

Due to congenital conditions such as microphthalmia, retinoblastoma, congenital glaucoma, and cataracts, in addition to severe ocular traumas, prosthetic therapy is often utilized to achieve positive functional and cosmetic outcomes in children. The utilization of custom temporary prosthetic conformers is of prime importance to expand the ocular and orbital tissues with increasingly larger volume replacements. It is widely acknowledged that the orbital contents play a large role in stimulating bony growth of the orbit and midface, during the first 5–8 years of life. In recent years, there has been some surgical advancement with expandable, implantable devices to stimulate the orbital growth; but prosthetic therapy is still required, with or without these newer expandable implants, for maximal volume and lifelong optimal results. The earlier the prosthetic therapy is instituted, the greater the window for increasing facial symmetry for the child.

Infants that are born with congenital microphthalmia or anophthalmia should ideally be seen by the ocularist within the first weeks of life for the initial temporary prosthesis. Generally, these first temporaries are fabricated of clear acrylic to allow for visual evaluation, while in place, of the socket soft tissues. However, some ocularists will utilize solid white custom conformers, and some add small pegs on the anterior surface that extend between the eyelids to help the family manipulate the conformers more easily. Patient and family cooperation is essential, as the child needs to be seen regularly on a 4-week to several month schedule to expand the size of the temporary conformers. Some young children need to be seen even more frequently initially if the eyelid tissues are expanding well and the conformer becomes loose and falls out. If the conformer is too loose, it is not stimulating tissue and bony growth with enough volume replacement. Also, if the conformer falls out for a long period of time without replacement, the socket tissues may contract and negate all progress. The parents do not generally remove the conformer, but instead clean the prosthesis externally with saline or eye rinse. Again, lubricating drops or ointments are utilized as needed for dryness. In cases of trauma requiring enucleation or surgical reorganization of ocular tissue, a similar course is followed. The serial conformers are utilized for 2–3 years, or until the trajectory of soft tissue expansion plateaus, at which point, surgical options may be indicated. If surgery is deferred or the family is satisfied with the conformers, the child can wear a painted prosthesis that has been fabricated to match the companion eye. The conformers, in general, are required to expand the eyelids and fornices, which are crucial to having the ability to wear a custom ocular prosthesis in the future. They also expand the periorbital tissues to improve facial symmetry, which can be documented by measuring the horizontal palpebral fissure from the medial to lateral canthal angle to follow progress. Although studies have demonstrated that conformers can also stimulate moderate growth in an anterior-posterior direction, often the bony orbit will require additional treatments, such as hydrogel orbital implants, dermis fat grafts, or static sphere orbital implants.

Care of the ocular prosthesis follows a schedule similar to the adult care described earlier, with the exception that a pediatric prosthesis is not expected to last more than 3 years, on average, due to anatomical changes of the socket tissues or microphthalmic globe due to normal growth.

Conclusions

When working with patients with anophthalmia (congenital or acquired), microphthalmia, or those with phthisical globes, ocular prostheses should be considered necessary in order to facilitate both healthy tissue function and optimal cosmesis. A good working relationship between the patient, ophthalmologist, and ocularist is necessary for success. Although every individual requiring an ocular or scleral shell prosthesis poses a unique set of clinical challenges, maintaining communication across disciplines ensures the most fulfilling outcomes for our patients.

Oculofacial Prosthetic Rehabilitation and Osseointegrated Implants

66

Julie Jordan Brown, Megan Spindel Thomas, and Cat Nguyen Burkat

Introduction

Acquired orbital defects resulting from trauma, exenteration, or other extensive orbitofacial surgery can be severely disfiguring [1]. Patients with orbital defects must not only adapt to the functional disability of monocular vision but also the emotional distress that accompanies altered self-perception and social interaction. Our eyes are described as the psychological center of the face, crucial to interpersonal communication and expression of emotion [2]. It follows that timely reconstruction of acquired orbital defects following extensive surgery or traumatic injury is crucial to the patient's ability to function optimally in society [3].

Surgical reconstruction of extensive orbital defects may be technically impossible or hold poor potential for a satisfactory result. Rehabilitation of large orbital and facial defects requires a combination of surgical reconstruction and prosthetic rehabilitation. Facial appearance is central to human identity and normal function; therefore, restoration of natural appearance is fundamental to oculofacial prosthetics. Anaplastology is a basic prerequisite for rehabilitation of patients with extensive orbital defects, providing a prosthetic substitute for lost anatomy that looks normal, both topographically and optically, and has borders that become part of the natural movements of the adjacent periorbital and facial tissue [4]. Considerable skill and experience are required to create an oculofacial prosthesis that meets the criteria for successful prosthetic rehabilitation. Careful planning and performance of surgical procedures can facilitate prosthetic design and retention. This requires collaboration between the oculoplastic surgeon and the anaplastologist as well as other members of the treatment team.

J. J. Brown · M. S. Thomas
Anaplastology, Medical Art Resources, Inc, Milwaukee, WI, USA
e-mail: info@medicalartresources.com; mthomas@medicalartresources.com

C. N. Burkat (✉)
Department of Ophthalmology and Visual Sciences, University of Wisconsin-Madison, Madison, WI, USA
e-mail: cburkat@wisc.edu

Patient Referral for Prosthetic Rehabilitation

Clinical anaplastology is a systematic approach that provides patients with prosthetic rehabilitation designed and fabricated to normalize the appearance of parts of the face and body impacted by congenital malformation, traumatic injury, disease, or excisional surgery for tumors. Clinical anaplastologists are health-care specialists educated and trained in the provision and management of prostheses that may include custom-made facial, ocular, and/or somatic prostheses based on a physician's referral and clinical assessment [5]. A comprehensive background that includes an academic foundation in art and the basic medical sciences is required. Artistic skills and sensibilities are necessary, first to perceive the form, texture, and colors present and then to replicate what is seen [4]. Additionally, technical instruction regarding materials and fabrication technique, patient management coursework, and clinical experience are necessary to develop the professional skills required of an anaplastologist. Educational paths are varied among anaplastologists, but most are highly skilled medical illustrators, maxillofacial prosthodontists, or maxillofacial prosthetic technicians with specialization in facial prosthetics. Certified clinical anaplastologists (CCA) have met minimal, continuing competency, ethical, and professional standards set forth by the Board for Certification in Clinical Anaplastology (BCCA). Oculoplastic or facial reconstructive surgeons should establish a working relationship with a clinical anaplastologist prior to patient referral.

When an orbital exenteration is planned, the patient should be referred to the anaplastologist prior to surgery. Most patients are not familiar with prosthetic treatment of extensive facial defects and may have misconceptions about

A. J. Cohen, C. N. Burkat (eds.), *Oculofacial, Orbital, and Lacrimal Surgery*, https://doi.org/10.1007/978-3-030-14092-2_66

what is possible. The patient may anticipate that the oculofacial prosthesis will be surgically attached and never need to be removed. The anaplastologist can begin to establish realistic expectations, but must do this carefully and with compassion in order to avoid increasing the anxiety or emotional distress the patient and family are already experiencing.

A presurgical appointment is helpful to provide the patient with information and demonstrate examples of results that can typically be expected. It allows the patients to anticipate the appearance of the defect and begin to envision to what extent a prosthesis will restore their appearance. Benefits and limitations are discussed as well as methods of retention. The anaplastologist may take photos, facial molds, or a 3-D scan. This office visit can help reduce the anxiety a patient might experience prior to a surgical procedure that will result in a significant facial defect. If placement of osseointegrated craniofacial implants is possible at the time of excisional surgery, planning for implant location can be initiated in collaboration with the surgeon. In the meantime, the surgeon can discuss the exenteration procedure with the patient to help prepare the patient for his or her postsurgical appearance and healing period.

Treatment Options

Oculofacial prostheses are superficial removable synthetic substitutes for lost normal anatomy and must be custom designed and fabricated for each individual. The extent of tissue loss dictates the type of oculofacial prosthesis, but all encompass a custom ocular prosthesis. Oculofacial prostheses, also known as epitheses or camouflage prostheses, include upper eyelid, lower eyelid, orbital, upper facial, and hemifacial prostheses.

An upper or lower eyelid prosthesis is appropriate for patients who have suffered traumatic injury or when the eyelid has retracted over time due to radiation therapy. When an in-dwelling ocular prosthesis alone does not successfully normalize appearance (Fig. 66.1a, b), an eyelid prosthesis can be designed to restore a more symmetrical gaze and fill in distracting concavities (Fig. 66.2a–c).

An orbital prosthesis restores both eyelids and the bony and soft tissue of the orbit. It may also include the eyebrow (Fig. 66.3a, b). When tissue loss is more extensive and the defect encompasses the orbit plus significant adjacent facial structures such as the soft tissue of the cheek or forehead, the prosthesis is classified as an upper facial prosthesis.

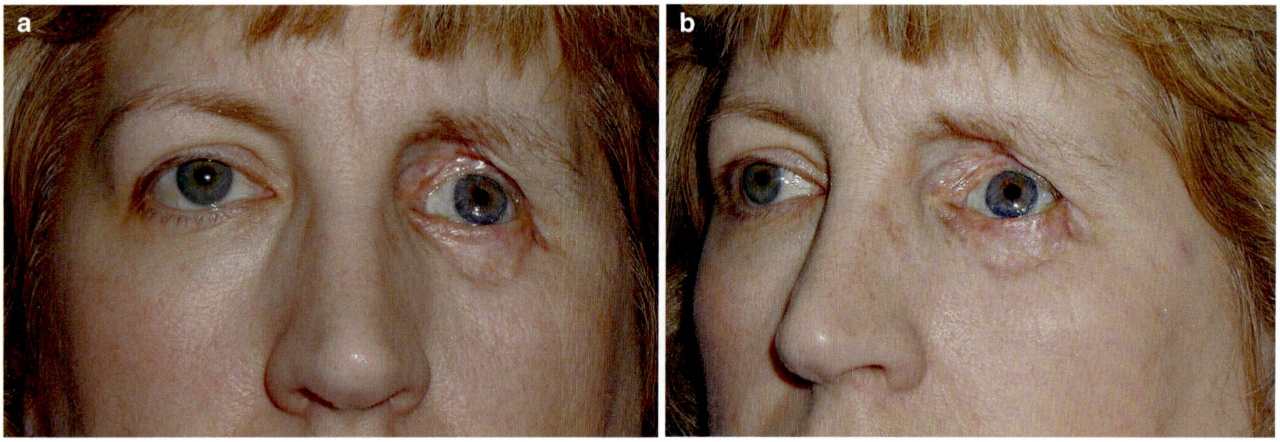

Fig. 66.1 (**a**, **b**) An ocular prosthesis alone does not restore this patient's retracted upper eyelid resulting from childhood irradiation (**a**). The ocular gaze is negatively impacted by the retracted eyelid (**b**)

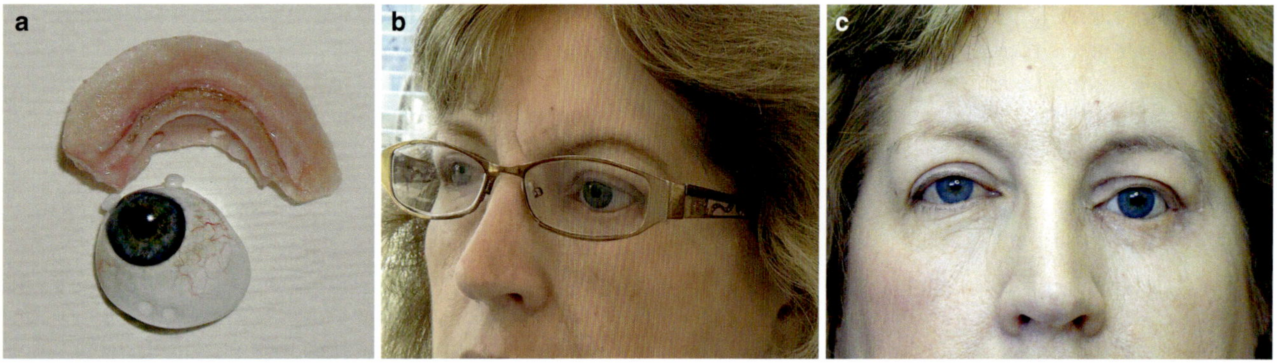

Fig. 66.2 (**a**–**c**) An *upper eyelid prosthesis* that keys onto the ocular component (**a**) restores the deficient upper eyelid and creates a more symmetrical gaze (**b** and **c**)

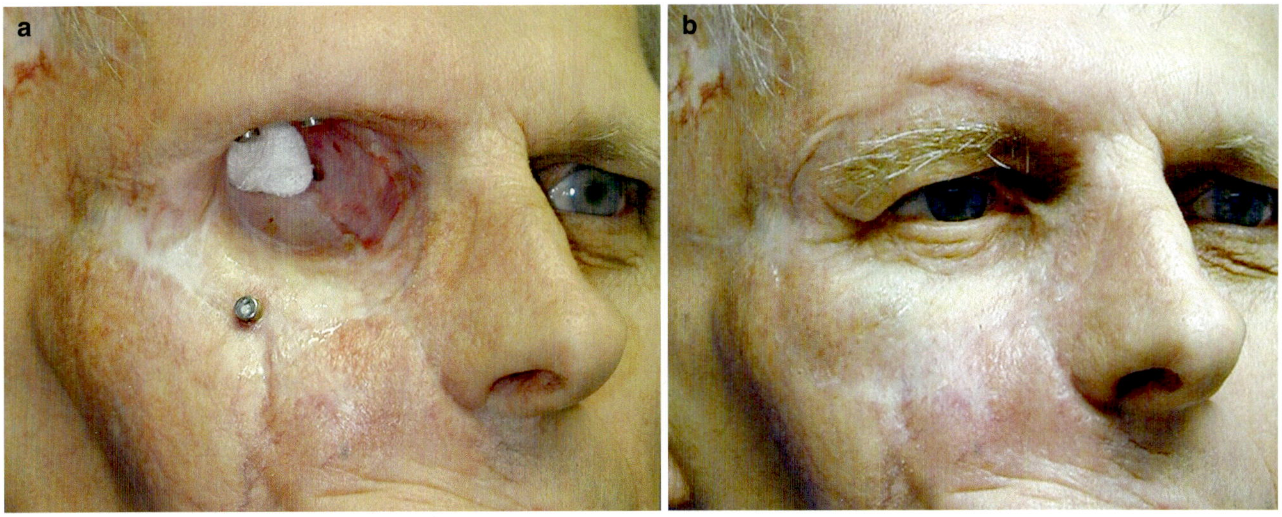

Fig. 66.3 (**a**, **b**) An *implant-retained orbital prosthesis* (**a**) restores both eyelids and the bony and soft tissue of the orbit, and may include the eyebrow (**b**)

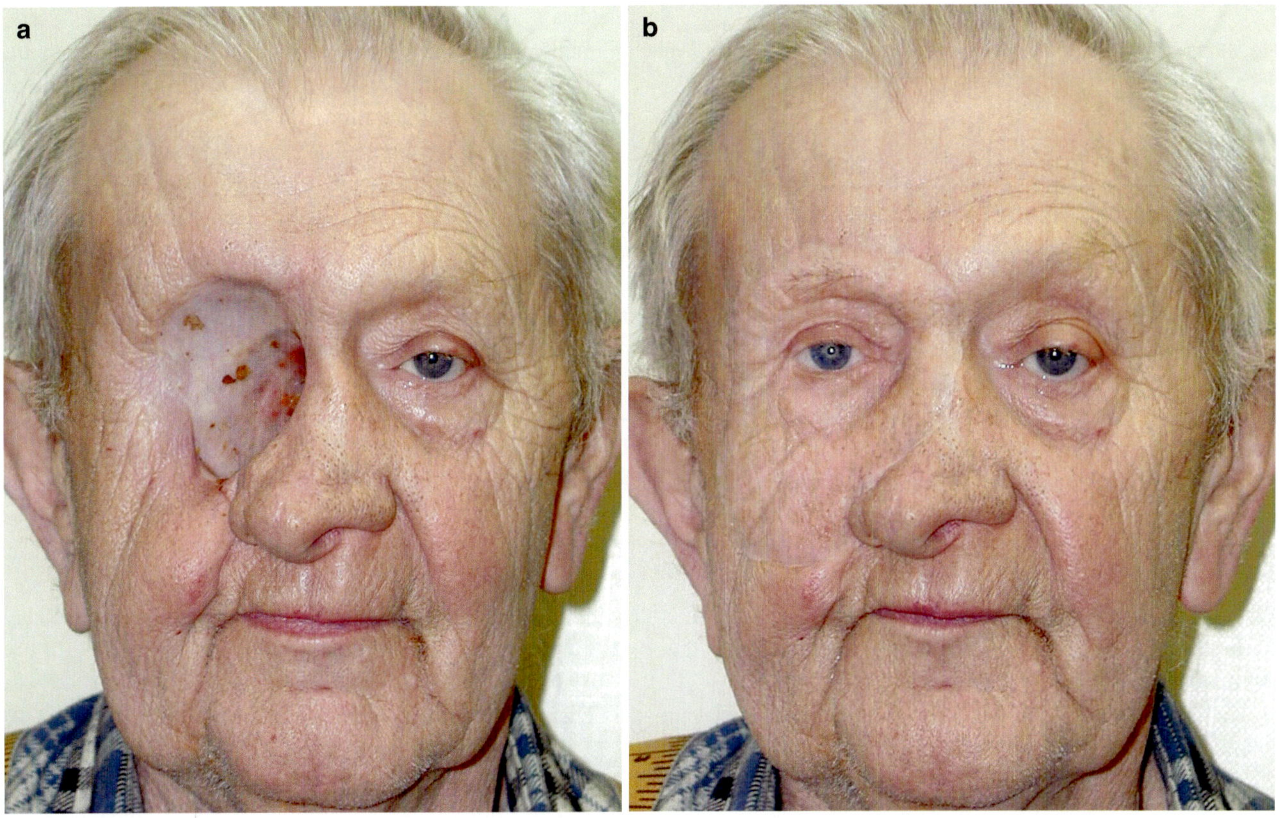

Fig. 66.4 (**a**, **b**) A *hemifacial prosthesis* is more extensive and restores part of the nose in addition to other adjacent structures

A hemifacial prosthesis is more extensive and restores part of the nose in addition to the orbit plus significant adjacent facial tissues (Fig. 66.4a, b).

Some patients with an orbital defect may prefer an eye patch or eyeglass shield instead of an oculofacial prosthesis. Unfortunately, commercially available eye patches are often inadequate in shape and size to cover extensive orbital defects and may interfere with eyeglasses. Patients should be aware that eye patches can be custom-made in the size/shape desired without a stiff substructure so that the defect is covered and eyeglasses can be worn comfortably (Fig. 66.5). Patients may also elect to "go natural" without an eye patch or bandage.

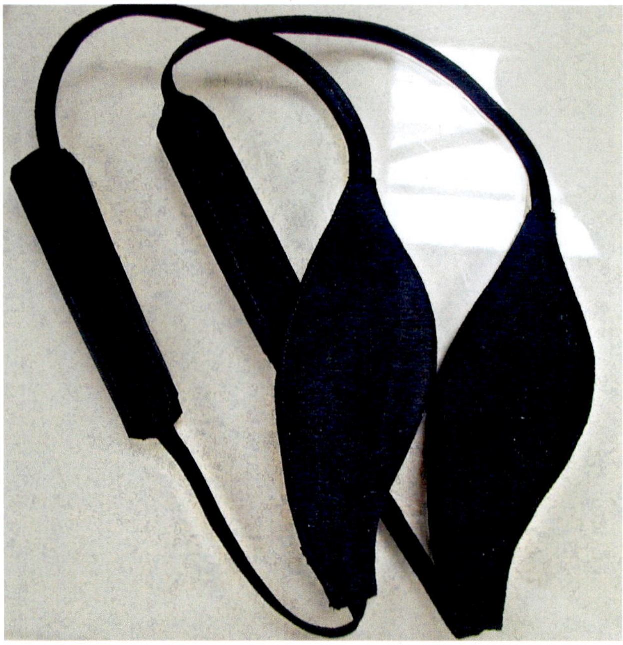

Fig. 66.5 Custom-made eye patches that are flexible and fitted to the individual defect may be preferable to patients as an alternative to a prosthesis or off-the-shelf patch

Benefits and Limitations of Prosthetic Rehabilitation

The goal of prosthetic rehabilitation is to restore lost anatomical form and appearance, social confidence, and quality of life. The prosthesis may also support eyeglasses and protect sensitive tissue and fistulas into the sinuses or the oral cavity. Many patients with a facial disfigurement express the desire to continue their life without a focus on the cause of the disfigurement—the traumatic accident or life-threatening disease. Eye patches and bandages seem to invite questions and comments that the individual may prefer to avoid. Without prosthetic rehabilitation, an extensive orbital defect becomes public evidence of a personal medical history that the patient may prefer to keep private.

Natural human eye movement sends a constant stream of messages; thus as an artificial substitute for complex living anatomy, an oculofacial prosthesis has significant limitations [2]. Oculofacial prostheses lack the complex animation of the living eye: blink, directional gaze, facial expression, as well as dilation and constriction of the pupil. Although there are fabrication techniques that provide some simulation of movement and pupil dilation, the lack of animation remains a disappointment to clinicians and patients. There is ongoing research with the intent to create an orbital prosthesis that can blink in synchrony with the intact eye using electromyographic signals of the orbicularis oculi muscle [6, 7]. It is likely that virtual reality could play a future role in the simulation of movement in oculofacial prostheses.

Synthetic substitutes for living tissue are limiting. Silicone does not have the self-cleansing, replicating, and repair properties of the skin. It is subject to abrasion, tearing, yellowing, and the discoloration caused by absorption of environmental contaminants, such as smoke and body excretions. As a result, silicone prostheses need periodic replacement to maintain hygiene and aesthetics [4]. Removal is necessary on a daily basis for cleaning of the prosthesis and underlying skin. This is a disappointment to patients who may anticipate permanent placement and minimal maintenance of a prosthetic device.

The useful life of a facial prosthesis ranges from 1 to 3 years. Factors influencing durability include the method of retention, environmental exposure, hygiene, and patient care, as well as the design of the prosthesis. Tobacco use and prolonged exposure to ultraviolet light adversely affect the color stability of a prosthesis. Nicotine stains prosthetic materials and exposure to ultraviolet light bleaches some pigments within the prosthesis [8]. Limitations of prosthetic rehabilitation should be fully disclosed so that the patient develops realistic expectations.

Stable and reliable retention is problematic in some cases due to soft tissue movement, such as around the cheek and forehead. In these situations, even a well-designed and properly fitted prosthesis may gap or dislodge with extreme changes in facial expression. Patients may be able to minimize the conspicuousness of these troublesome areas with carefully selected eyeglass frames.

Criteria for a Successful Oculofacial Prosthesis

The desired goal of any camouflage prosthesis is to assist in restoring optimal function and normalizing appearance. Clinical anaplastologists use the following criteria to evaluate a prosthetic device:

- The prosthesis is inconspicuous (Fig. 66.6a, b).
  - The sculptural form creates a natural symmetrical appearance.
  - The color and texture simulate a lifelike appearance.
  - Edges are thin and conform to facial movement.
- The prosthesis is secure and comfortable.
- The prosthesis is designed and fabricated to minimize health and safety risks to the patient.
- The prosthesis can be applied and removed with relative ease.
- The prosthesis is designed for durability.
- The prosthesis uses appropriate cosmetic or health grade materials [5].

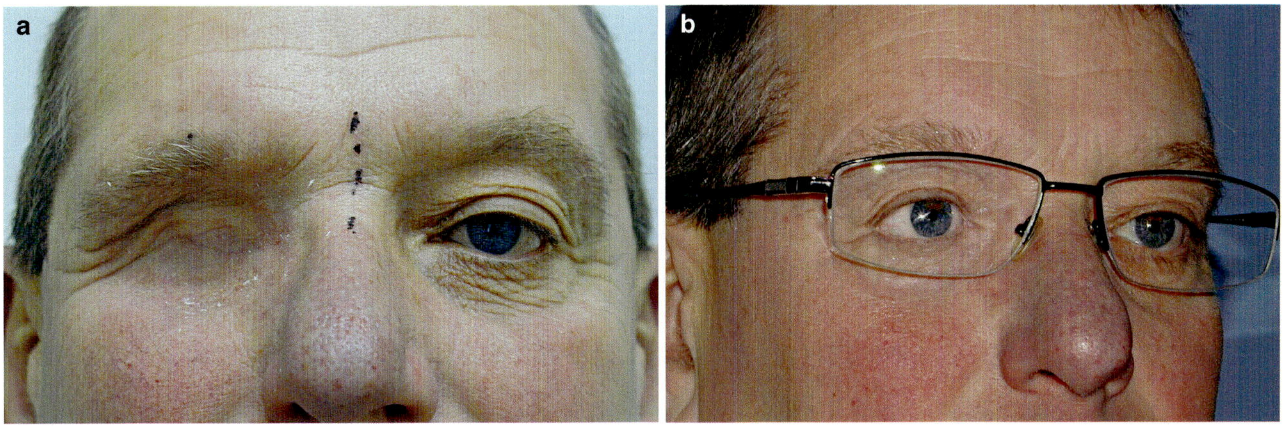

Fig. 66.6 A successful prosthesis on the right is inconspicuous, especially with concurrent use of eyeglasses (**a**, **b**)

Prosthetic Materials and Methods of Retention

Ongoing improvement in materials and techniques available to anaplastologists has resulted in prostheses that can closely simulate missing anatomy [4]. Silicone elastomers are the material of choice because they are durable, translucent, and biocompatible, are available with varying properties, and can easily be pigmented to match the patient's skin [9]. Silicone is often used in combination with methyl methacrylate and light-cure dental acrylic. Medical and health grade materials are selected and used in combination to replicate the texture and elasticity of the lost anatomy as closely as possible. For example, a high tear strength silicone may be used at the edges in combination with a lower durometer silicone to replicate the eyelids (Fig. 66.7). The ocular component is fabricated from laminar layers of silicone or methyl methacrylate plastic.

The most beautiful and lifelike prosthesis is useless to the patient, however, if it cannot be reliably positioned and retained [4]. Each patient is evaluated to determine the best method of retaining his or her prosthesis comfortably and securely. Retention of oculofacial prostheses can be achieved using the following methods:

- Anatomical retention (to existing anatomical structures such as undercut areas in the orbital cavity)
- Mechanical anchorage (attachment to eyeglass frames or to an intraoral prosthesis)
- Adhesive retention
- Surgically placed osseointegrated titanium implants [10]

Anatomical retention is possible when the contour of the orbital defect provides undercuts, such as behind the supraorbital rim. The undercut areas can be gently engaged by the prosthesis to provide reliable retention. The benefits to the patient in terms of ease of use outweigh the technical challenges that anatomical retention presents to the anaplastologist [11]. Filling the defect with a solid mass should be avoided, as this will likely cause too much friction and lead to skin breakdown. The part of the prosthesis that engages the socket should be relatively thin-walled and flexible (Fig. 66.8a–c).

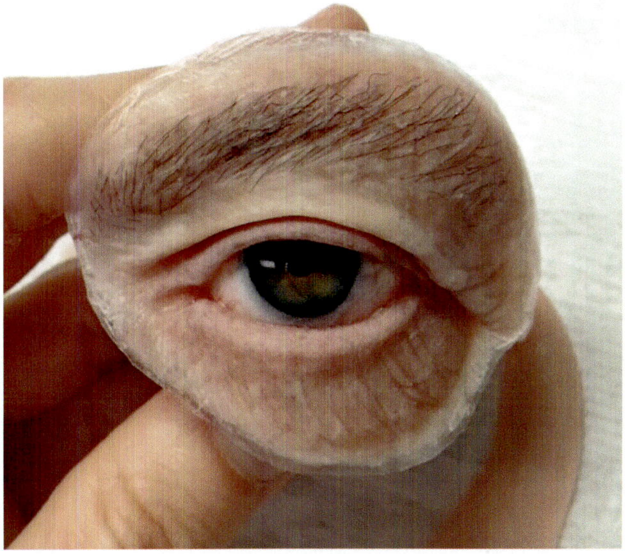

Fig. 66.7 High tear strength silicone is used at the edges in combination with lower durometer silicone for the eyelids

Mechanical anchorage to eyeglasses is considered a last resort because it is difficult to avoid gapping at the margins of the prosthesis when eyeglasses slip out of place. However, it is an option for patients who may not be a candidate for osseointegrated implants and are unable to manage skin adhesives. In the case of extensive facial defects with communication between the orbital cavity and the oral cavity, the oculofacial prosthesis may be coupled to an intraoral appliance or obturator (Fig. 66.9a, b) [9].

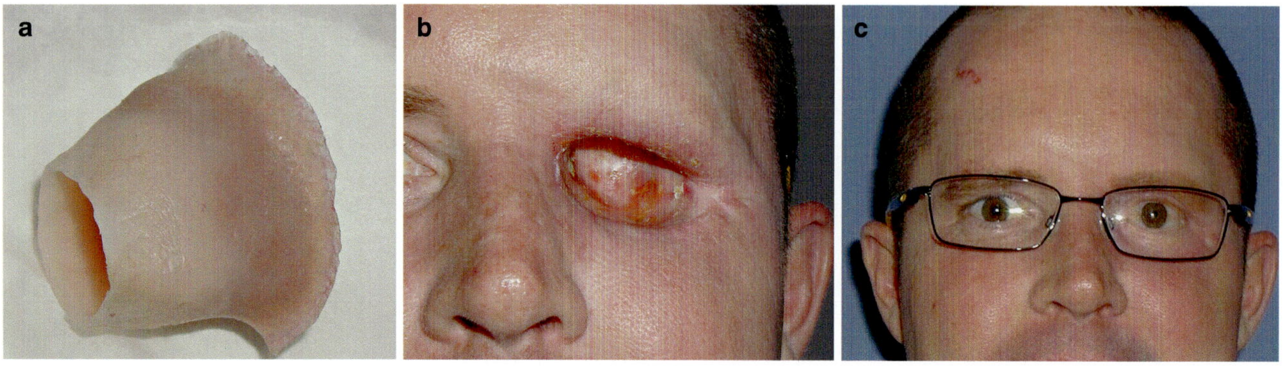

Fig. 66.8 (**a**–**c**) Intaglio view (**a**) of an *anatomically retained orbital prosthesis* that engages undercuts in the orbit (**b** and **c**). The prosthesis should be thin-walled and flexible to prevent skin breakdown

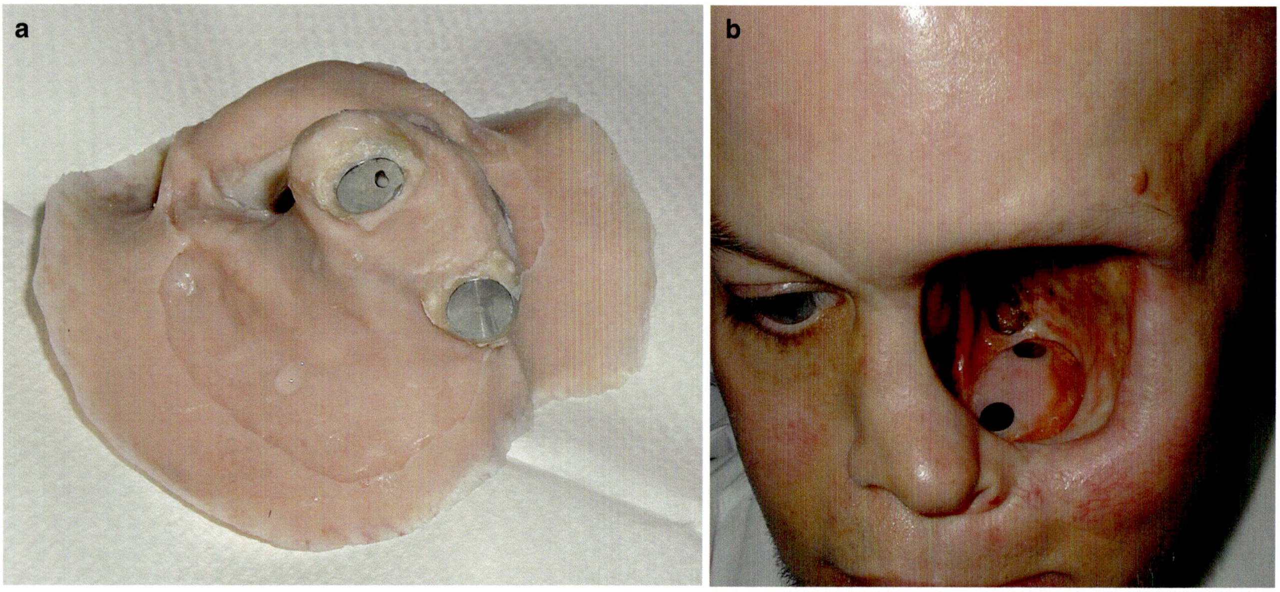

Fig. 66.9 (**a**, **b**) The intaglio surface of a *mechanically retained prosthesis* that attaches with magnets (**a**) to the patient's intraoral obturator (**b**)

Skin adhesive retention can be used successfully, although there are disadvantages associated with skin adhesives in terms of handling products and cleaning the prosthesis. Good dexterity and adequate vision are necessary to manage skin adhesive retention unless a supportive caregiver can assist with application and removal. There are a variety of products available, from liquid adhesives to biface tape (Fig. 66.10). Skin preparation products and mild adhesive removers reduce skin problems when used as instructed [9]. Products must be carefully chosen by the anaplastologist for the individual patient and instructions given for their use. Even with correct application, skin adhesives can be problematic for orbital defects due to soft tissue movement of the eyebrow and cheek with subsequent dermatitis (Fig. 66.11a). In addition, compromised

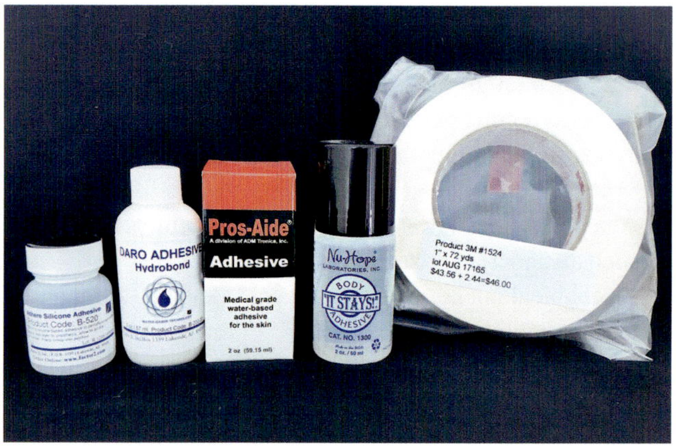

Fig. 66.10 Skin adhesive products range from gentle, water-based formulas to high-strength solvent-based products to biface tape

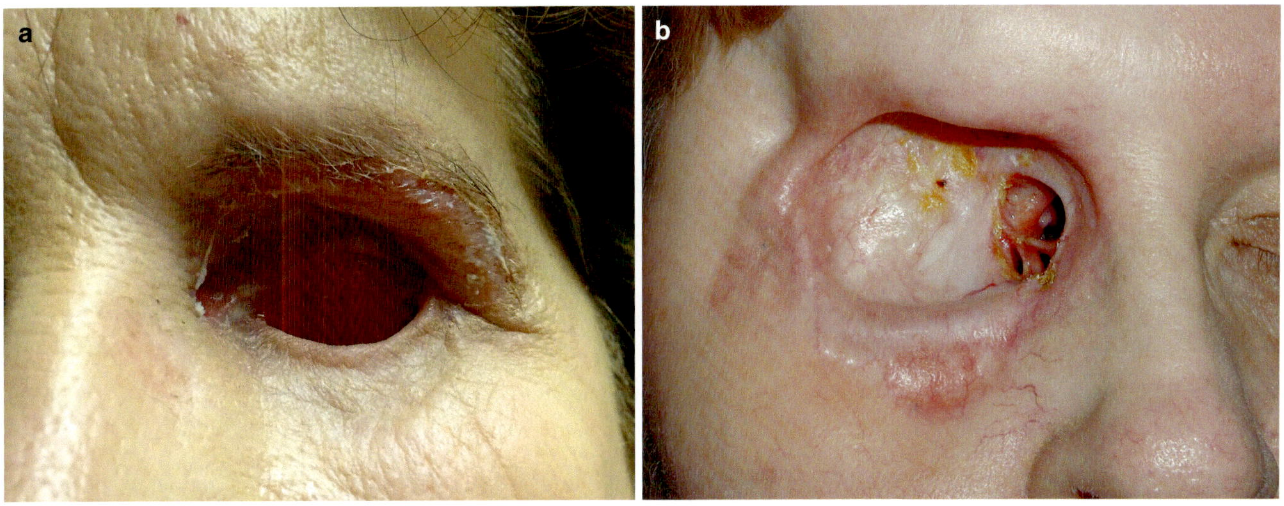

Fig. 66.11 (**a**, **b**) Periorbital contact dermatitis related to long-term daily skin adhesive use in irradiated socket

tissue lining of the orbital defect is often fragile and sensitive, particularly when the orbit has been irradiated (Fig. 66.11b).

Osseointegrated titanium implants are screw-shaped fixtures surgically placed into the bone, allowed to heal, and subsequently activated with skin penetrating abutments to which the prosthesis attaches [12, 13]. Per-Ingvar Brånemark coined the term "osseointegration" in 1977 to describe "a direct structural and functional connection between ordered, living bone and the surface of a load-carrying implant" [14]. The principle of osseointegration or bone anchorage has had long-term successful application to anchor dental prostheses, which prompted development of components for extraoral prosthetic attachment [4]. Bone anchorage of oculofacial prostheses has the following advantages over other forms of retention that contribute to improved quality of life:

- Secure and reliable retention
- Improved comfort due to minimal skin contact
- Stability less affected by physical activity, climate, and facial expression
- Consistent location of the prosthesis at every application, which can be challenging for patients with reduced vision
- Elimination of adhesive products which can be tedious or cause dermatitis
- Ease of use and improved patient confidence
- Reduced skin friction resulting in less skin irritation
- Improved longevity of thin, transparent edges of the silicone prosthesis [10, 15]

Disadvantages of osseointegrated implants for retention include:

- Surgical procedure(s) with associated risks
- Daily hygiene of abutment/skin interface
- Risk of minor skin complications
- Patient acceptance of skin penetrating abutments and attachment hardware
- Possible implant failure

For osseointegrated implants to be successful, there must be bone of adequate volume, thickness, and density to allow their proper placement, i.e., a sufficient number of implants of adequate length and properly distributed with due regard to their alignment [4]. It follows that surgical placement of craniofacial implants requires preoperative treatment planning with the anaplastologist, who can provide a surgical template to guide implant placement [16]. Oculofacial implants are increasingly used to improve aesthetic results, ease of use for the patient, security and stability of the prosthesis, as well as extending the useful life of the prosthesis (Fig. 66.12a–c) [17].

Surgical Preparation of the Defect

Preservation or surgical reconstruction of anatomic landmarks in a symmetrical position will enhance the aesthetic outcome possible. Displacement of the eyebrow should be avoided if possible (Fig. 66.13). In the orbital and periorbital regions, primary wound closure may result in distortion of adjacent facial features and negatively impact the prosthetic result. Lining the defect with a thin skin graft allows more immediate fitting of the prosthesis and creates a more desirable surface for placement of the prosthesis than allowing the defect to granulate [18].

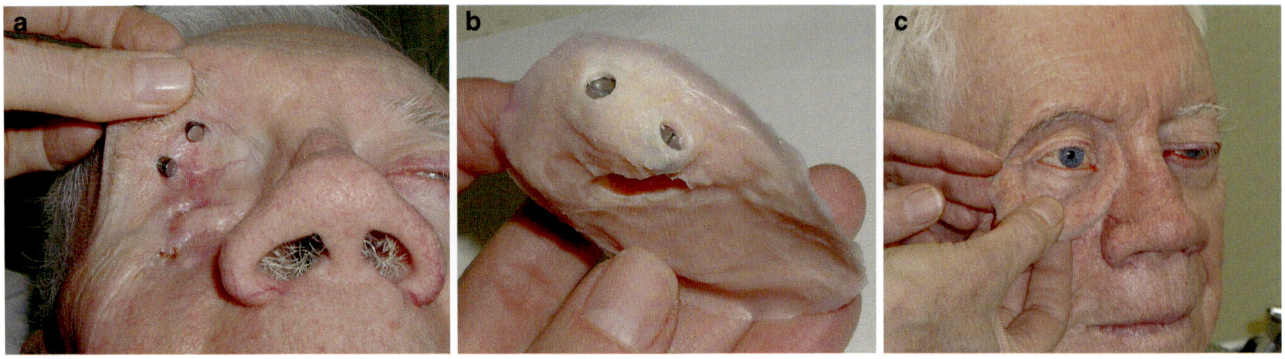

Fig. 66.12 (a–c) This implant-retained oculofacial prosthesis attaches with magnets to two osseointegrated fixtures

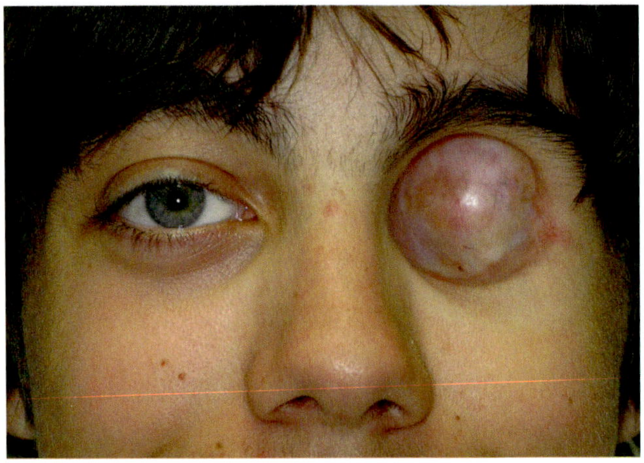

Fig. 66.13 The preservation of anatomical landmarks in a symmetrical position and a closed, skin-lined orbit is ideal for prosthetic restoration

Successful prosthetic restoration of extensive orbital defects, such as following exenteration, is dependent on adequate orbital depth and space nasally to allow symmetrical placement of the ocular component that is embedded within the facial prosthesis. Reconstructive efforts focus on achieving a durable lining of the orbital cavity that protects the sinonasal and cranial cavities while accommodating a prosthesis if desired [19]. When the eyelid skin and orbicularis muscles are not involved by tumor or trauma, the anterior lamella of the eyelid can be spared and used for coverage of the orbital defect [20–22]. The simplest treatment of healing by secondary intention and granulation has disadvantages associated with a lengthy healing process of several months and daily wound care, as well as potentially suboptimal prosthetic outcomes [20]. When completely healed by secondary intention, the orbital cavity often becomes slightly shallower, especially if an alloplastic mesh has been used. A meshed or unmeshed split-thickness skin graft, or full-thickness graft, can be used to line the orbital cavity to accelerate wound healing [20]. The thinness of the graft provides a deep cavity that is conducive to prosthetic design and retention and an excellent site for percutaneous abutments associated with osseointegrated implants. These methods are usually successful when there is no history of prior radiation or postoperative radiation and also allow easy inspection for local tumor recurrence [20].

For patients with prior radiation or subsequent planned radiation therapy, a more durable, well-vascularized lining of the orbital cavity with soft tissue is necessary to avoid bone exposure and osteoradionecrosis [20]. The most commonly used pedicled flaps are the temporalis muscle flap and temporoparietal fascial flap. The relatively thin temporalis muscle flap may preserve reasonable space for an adhesive-retained or implant-retained orbital prosthesis, but results in a depression at the donor site that may be undesirable [23]. Donor site deformity is reduced with the use of a temporoparietal fascial flap covered by a full or split-thickness skin graft. However, the reach of these local pedicled flaps is limited and in some cases does not extend enough for complete coverage of the defect. A bulky free-flap reconstruction or transposed forehead tissue flap may eliminate oculofacial prosthetic rehabilitation as a treatment option if the orbital cavity becomes too shallow or even nonexistent (Fig. 66.14) [18].

An extended orbital exenteration that involves removal of orbital bony walls, as well as other structures such as the sinuses, may result in a structural and soft tissue cavity that is too extensive to be covered with local or regional flaps [20]. In some cases, a total maxillectomy or suprastructure maxillectomy is combined with orbital exenteration (orbitomaxillectomy), with the reconstructive priority shifting away from prosthetic rehabilitation and instead focused on closure of the nasal cavity [20].

Complications following exenteration include fistulae, tissue necrosis, exposed bone, and infection; therefore, it is critical that the healing process and contracture of surrounding tissue is complete before definitive prosthetic rehabilitation begins [24]. When adjuvant radiation therapy is indicated, prosthetic rehabilitation should be delayed until edema has resolved.

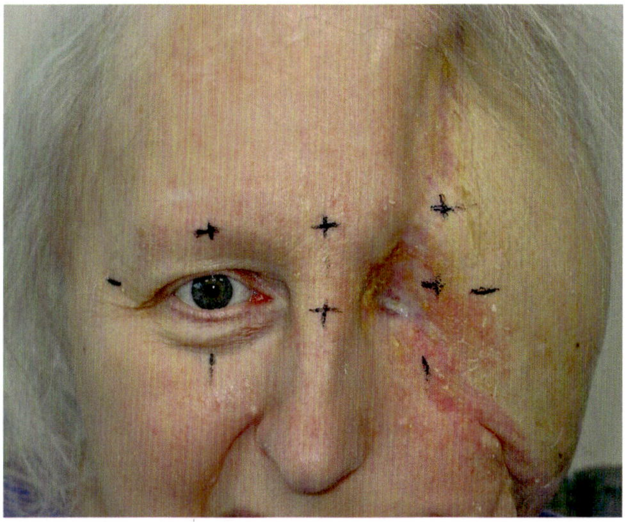

Fig. 66.14 A bulky free-flap reconstruction may create a shallow orbital cavity that cannot accommodate a symmetrically placed ocular or orbital prosthesis

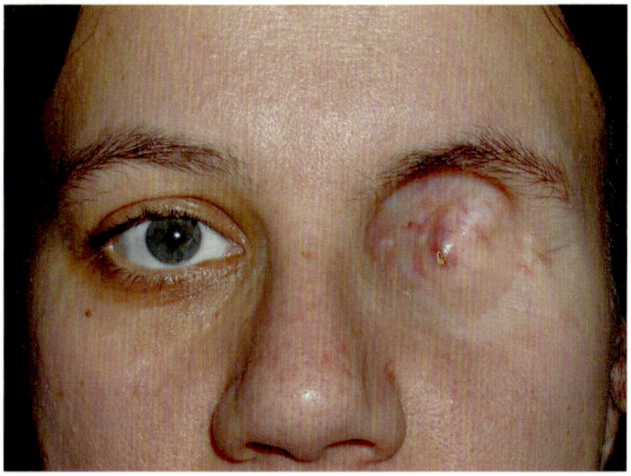

Fig. 66.15 The ideal orbital cavity is lined with thin skin and allows adequate depth for accurate placement of the ocular

Oculoplastic surgeons can optimize the prosthetic outcome by creating a defect site that allows the anaplastologist to design an aesthetic and stable prosthesis. The retention strategy dictates the preferred attributes of the defect site; in particular, if the patient prefers an osseointegrated prosthetic option, the surgeon should attempt to line the orbital cavity with thin tissue to allow for the deepest orbital space to house the integrated orbital and ocular prostheses, and to keep the tissues extremely thin in the desired location of future planned titanium implants (Fig. 66.15). This further reinforces the importance of preoperative consultation and communication between the surgeon, clinical anaplastologist, ocularist, and other members of the multidisciplinary team.

Osseointegrated Implants for Attachment of Oculofacial Prostheses

"Osseointegration is a process whereby clinically asymptomatic rigid fixation of alloplastic materials is achieved, and maintained, in bone during functional loading" [25]. Albrektsson et al. named the following important factors that contribute to long-term stability of the implant:

- Biocompatibility of the material
- Implant design and length
- Implant surface
- Condition of the recipient
- Surgical technique
- Type and period of the functional loading [26]

Implant systems relevant to bone-anchored oculofacial prostheses are classified as either solitary implants or grouped implants. Solitary implants are based on the dental application of the classic Brånemark system, which uses a series of solitary screw implants that rely on osseointegration with percutaneous abutments arising from each implant.

Grouped implants refer to grid and plate systems, which are secured by several smaller bone screws with percutaneous abutments arising from any location along the grid [10]. Examples of extraoral/craniofacial systems with solitary implants currently include the Brånemark System marketed by Cochlear Americas under the brand name Vistafix in the United States and Nobel Biocare in European and other markets and the International Team for Implantology (ITI) marketed by the Straumann company, Panthera Dental, and Southern Implants [10].

Extraoral systems with grouped implants are useful when viable bone is not sufficient in the desired locations. Forces are distributed across the plate or grid with several titanium bone screws. Grouped systems rely on osteosynthesis for high stability [10]. The Epitec System (Leibinger company) and the Epiplating System by Medicon are examples of grouped implant systems.

The basic principles of surgical technique are centered on minimizing surgical trauma to the bone that could limit implant osseointegration [4]. The following points are of importance:

- Use of a new and sharp drill/cutting burr
- Low drill speed (1500–2000 rpm)
- Extensive cooling–continuous irrigation [10, 27]
- Specific torque control

Self-tapping titanium screws are available for all established systems, which require special instrumentation. For solitary implant systems, the surgeon palpates the base of

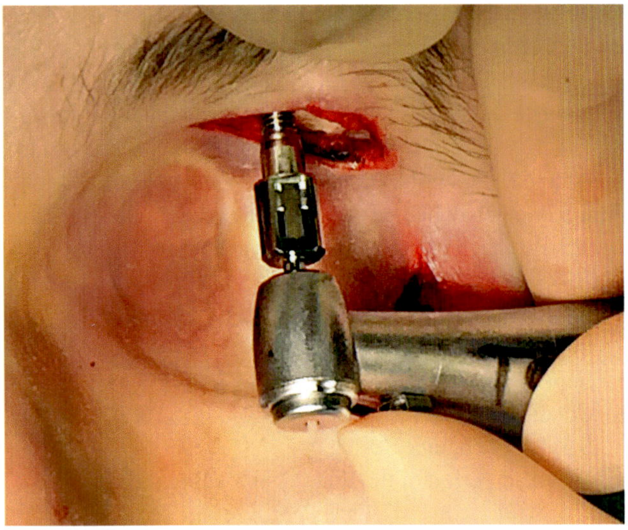

Fig. 66.16 The handpiece is used to place the oculofacial implant with appropriate torque. Excess torque or drilling speed compromises the osseointegration

the implant site repeatedly for bone presence with a dissector and performs visual inspection. In order to avoid contamination, titanium fixtures should only be handled with titanium instruments. With torque control, the titanium fixture is screwed in mechanically with torque specific to type of fixture (Fig. 66.16). The use of 4 mm long fixtures is preferred. There should be at least 10 mm between implants/abutments. In most orbital cases, the implant fixtures are capped with a cover screw, and the implant is allowed to heal before the fixtures are activated with a skin-penetrating abutment.

Skin thinning of the peri-abutment subcutaneous tissue is recommended to establish and maintain reaction-free skin penetration. The skin around the abutment should be hairless and subcutaneous tissue removed to minimize skin mobility in relation to the abutment (Fig. 66.17). The periosteum must remain intact to maintain the blood supply required for healing [27].

The osseointegration period for solitary implants is a minimum of 12 weeks and possibly longer depending on the thickness and quality of the bone encountered at stage one. The poorer the bone quality, the longer the time between stages one and two [27]. For patients who have undergone irradiation, a two-stage procedure with a 4- to 6-month interval between implant placement and abutment connection is recommended.

For grouped implant systems, the instrumentation is consistent with those commonly used in osteosynthesis with the addition of a few special instruments. The implants are inserted subperiosteally and are adapted to follow the contour of the bone as closely as possible in order to avoid stressing the hardware and the bone. Holes are drilled for the

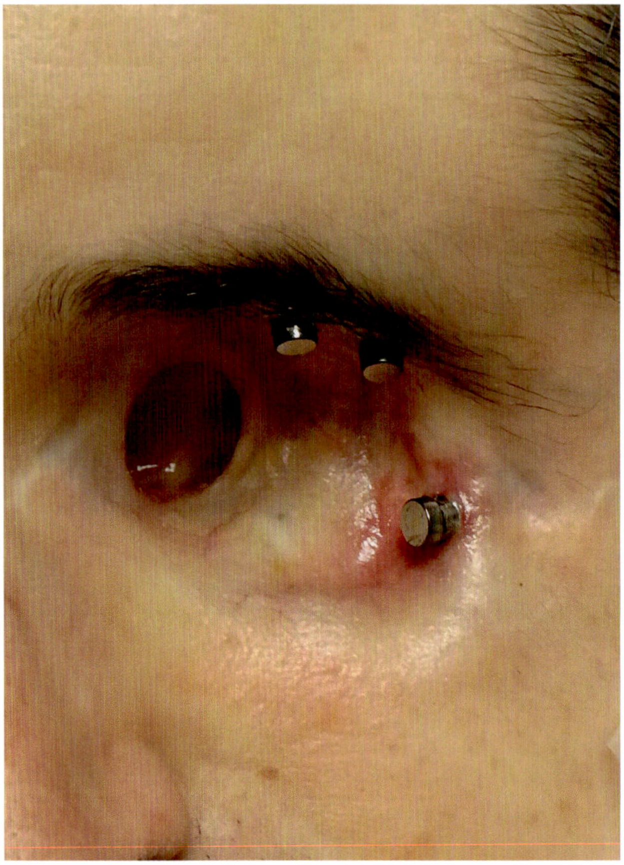

Fig. 66.17 Ideal peri-abutment tissue is thin, immobile, and hair-free

self-tapping titanium bone screws using a spiral drill (1.6 mm diameter). A minimum of three screws should be used for stability with care being taken not to overtighten the screws. Percutaneous abutments are attached to bone screws through tapped holes in the plate. Soft tissue management is still important, but soft tissue reduction is more conservative than with the Brånemark technique. Grouped implant systems require a minimum 2- to 3-month healing period for integration [10].

Resonance frequency analysis (RFA) is an option that can supply clinically relevant information about the state of the implant to bone interface at any stage of the treatment or follow up examination. The measurement is performed with a small SmartPeg, which acts as a transducer attached to the implant or abutment [27]. Studies indicate that implants with high and increasing implant stability quotient (ISQ) values are successfully integrated [28]. Future developments for implant attachment are likely to involve attachment without skin penetration. This is routinely used for bone anchored hearing devices in the form of magnets. Currently the size of the magnets would preclude use in the orbit. Disadvantages include skin thinning and breakdown over the magnet and less reliable retention [29].

Contraindications and Complications for Osseointegrated Implants

Patient-specific factors that affect implant survival include high-dose radiation therapy, chemotherapy, prolonged time between radiation and implant placement, age, osteoporosis, smoking, and concurrent disease [1, 30, 31]. Adjunctive use of hyperbaric oxygen therapy may reduce the risk of osteoradionecrosis and subsequent implant loss in patients who have had radiation [31]. Absolute contraindications with regard to implantation are severe psychiatric disorders and cachexia. Poor hygiene, drug or alcohol addiction, and minor psychiatric disorders are relative contraindications and should be individually assessed [10].

Postoperative complications should also be discussed with the patient preoperatively and may include paresthesia, cellulitis, or peri-implant soft tissue inflammation and bone infection leading to osteoradionecrosis and implant loss [27, 32]. The most common complications are adverse skin reactions arising at the sites of skin penetration. In contrast to gingival penetration associated with intraoral implants in which saliva provides continual cleansing of the abutment region, skin penetration stimulates an inflammatory response. Skin thinning and personal hygiene are important factors in reducing inflammation. Chronic persistent skin problems can be due to loose fixtures or abutments and can be avoided by properly checking the torque on components [14]. A classification of skin reactions was developed by Holgers et al.: 0 = no reaction, 1 = reddish, 2 = red and moist, 3 = granulation tissue, and 4 = skin infection to such a degree that the abutment has to be removed [33]. Appropriate antimicrobial and anti-inflammatory treatment can be prescribed as needed. Skin conditions such as acne vulgaris and seborrheic eczema can cause local problems and can be managed with local cleaning and appropriate medications. Patients with diabetes mellitus are more likely to experience peri-abutment skin necrosis. Keloid formation can be treated with local compression or local excision combined with steroid injection [14, 27].

Patients should be cautioned about removing the prosthesis and external components prior to MRI procedures. This will eliminate the risk of implant loss and minimize artifacts. The intraosseous implants and abutments are not ferromagnetic and will not cause any problems during MRI (up to 3 T) [34, 35]. If the patient already has implants and is scheduled for radiation therapy of the implant area, the skin-penetrating abutments should be removed and a cover screw placed on the implant. Osseointegrated implants can be left in place under the intact skin [27].

Traumatic implant loss is rare with orbital implants since the abutments are tucked into the orbital cavity under the supraorbital rim and thus not easily dislodged during sporting activities.

Preoperative Planning and Surgical Pearls for Osseointegrated Implants

If osseointegrated implants are the selected method of retention, then surgical planning for implant position is initiated. Position of the implants should be selected in collaboration with the anaplastologist for the best aesthetic and functional outcome. Preoperative planning and proper patient selection is key. Planning should consist of three main issues: (1) careful clinical exam of the orbital deformity by the surgeon and anaplastologist with particular attention paid to soft tissue mobility and thickness, (2) orbital CT scan, and (3) analysis of socket topography to ensure adequate depth and space for all the implant and ocular components of the prosthesis to avoid an aesthetic compromise in the final prosthesis [1]. The anaplastologist may initiate planning using traditional techniques such as facial molds and resulting positive model, photographs, and sculpture of an initial prototype. Three-dimensional computer imaging, virtual surgical planning, and 3-D printing can also be applied to the precise and proper placement of implants in viable bone and are well described by others [36, 37]. Intraoperative stereotactic image guidance has also been described to aid in proper positioning of implants, particularly in thinner, poor quality bone [38].

If traditional methods are used, the preliminary sculpture is developed and implant locations selected for optimal retention and to accommodate the ocular and prosthetic attachment components [1]. Radio-opaque CT spots are affixed to the patient's skin in the desired locations just prior to an orbital CT. This allows a direct transfer of the ideal locations that are marked on the patient model. The surgeon and anaplastologist review the orbital CT for bone volume and density, keeping in mind soft tissue movement. Ideally, locations are selected where orbital rim bone demonstrates adequate thickness to solidly house an implant and away from proximity to the cranial cavity, sinuses, or lacrimal fossa. In general, the medial orbital wall tends to be less optimal for implant placement.

The number of implants is dependent on the extent and contour of the defect. Smaller orbital defects may only allow sufficient space for two fixtures, while an extensive upper facial or hemifacial prosthesis may require four or even five implants for secure retention. Ideally, for an oculofacial prosthesis following exenteration, a tripod configuration is optimal with one implant in the central superior orbital rim (lateral to the frontal sinus), one at the superolateral frontal bone (above or below the frontozygomatic suture), and a lateral or inferolateral implant in the zygomatic bone. This third implant affords the prosthesis slightly more stability and retention. When possible, superior and lateral or superior and inferior implants are desired for stable attachment due to different vectors. A typical configuration for implants is shown in Fig. 66.18. Locations and angles are adjusted based on analysis of the CT scan, also making sure to space the implants sufficiently apart so that the intervening bone is not weakened or would limit osseointegration. The surgeon may elect to place an additional implant with a cover screw as a sleeper implant if osseointegration is in question [27]. In addition, the abutments that are later placed through the skin are wider, and thus require additional space to avoid contact. On average, this requires that the implant fixtures be placed a minimum of 10 mm apart. Incorporation of the ocular component (made by the ocularist or anaplastologist) in the correct location in three-dimensional space is central to the anaplastologist's recommendation for implant location. The implant site locations must be selected with this is mind, with the implant sites placed in a way as to avoid compromising the expected placement of the ocular component.

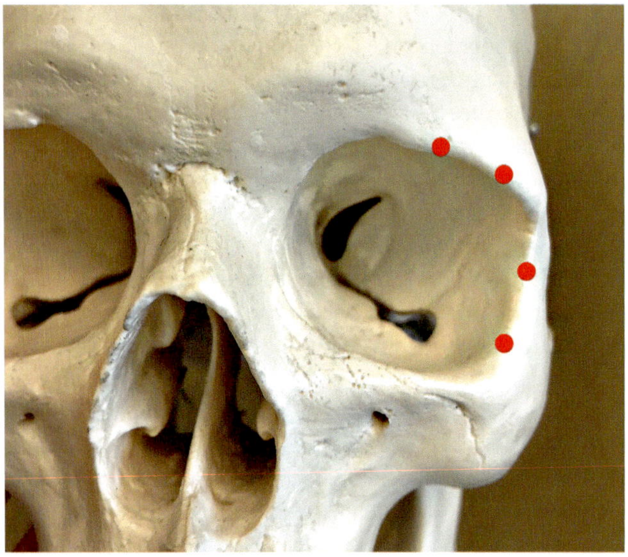

Fig. 66.18 Optimal implant locations include the central superior orbital rim, superolateral frontal bone, and lateral or inferolateral zygomatic bone. Two implants may suffice for a smaller prosthesis, while up to five may be necessary for a more extensive prosthesis

Similarly, the depth of the socket cavity must be evaluated as a very shallow orbit limits the ability to house all the titanium implants, ocular and facial components, and corresponding magnets and abutments. If necessary, the surgeon should plan to deepen the socket if possible, and thin the soft tissue so that only very thin skin is overlying the bone where the implants are placed. Otherwise, thick tissue can easily cover over the implant and abutment, leading to implant loss (Fig. 66.19a, b). Likewise, placement of an implant in an area of very mobile tissue such as the eyebrow is suboptimal as the tissue can move and cover over the implant or lead to friction. Although longer skin-penetrating abutments are available, they will subsequently take up more space in the final oculofacial prosthesis, and potentially compromise the outcome. If eyelashes and eyelids are present, a permanent tarsorrhaphy can be placed to minimize dead space and chronic discharge and to limit movement of tissues under the prosthesis that could affect the magnetic attachment. The desired implant positions are then recorded for fabrication of a surgical template (Fig. 66.20a, b) [39].

The angle of the implant is as important as the location in order to avoid compromise in the aesthetic outcome. Unfortunately implant system instrumentation is not designed for the orbital cavity which makes optimal angulation of the implants challenging for the surgeon (Fig. 66.21). The goal is to insert the implants with a low angle profile,

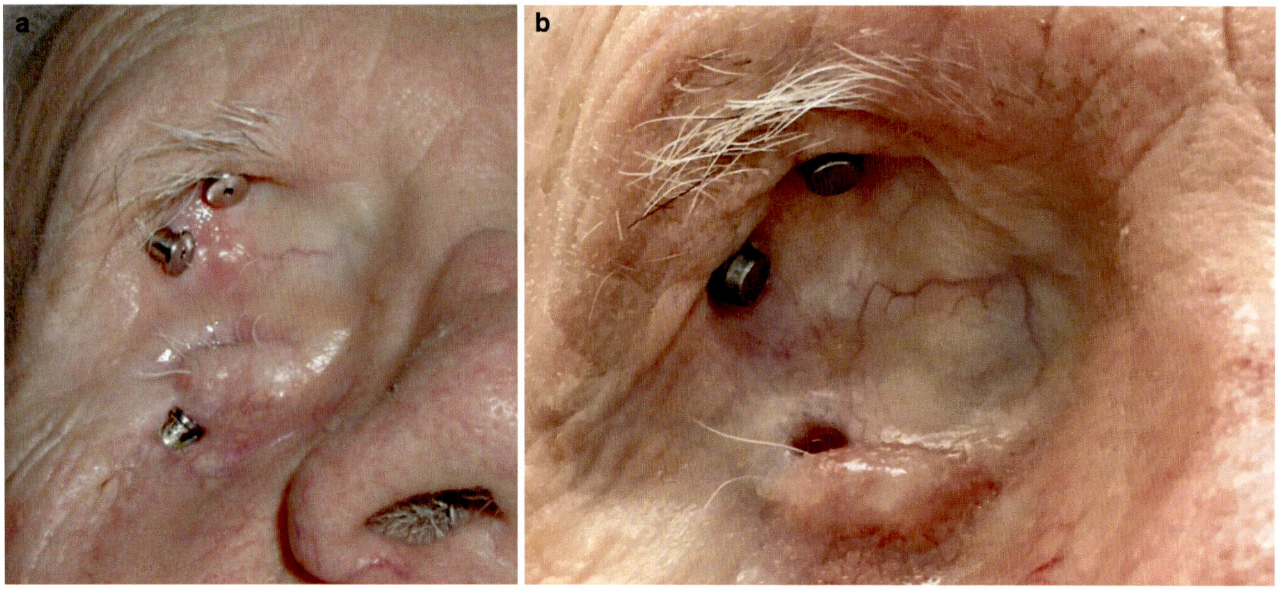

Fig. 66.19 (**a**, **b**) Thick, mobile cheek and socket tissue ultimately buried the inferior abutment (**a**), leading to its removal (**b**)

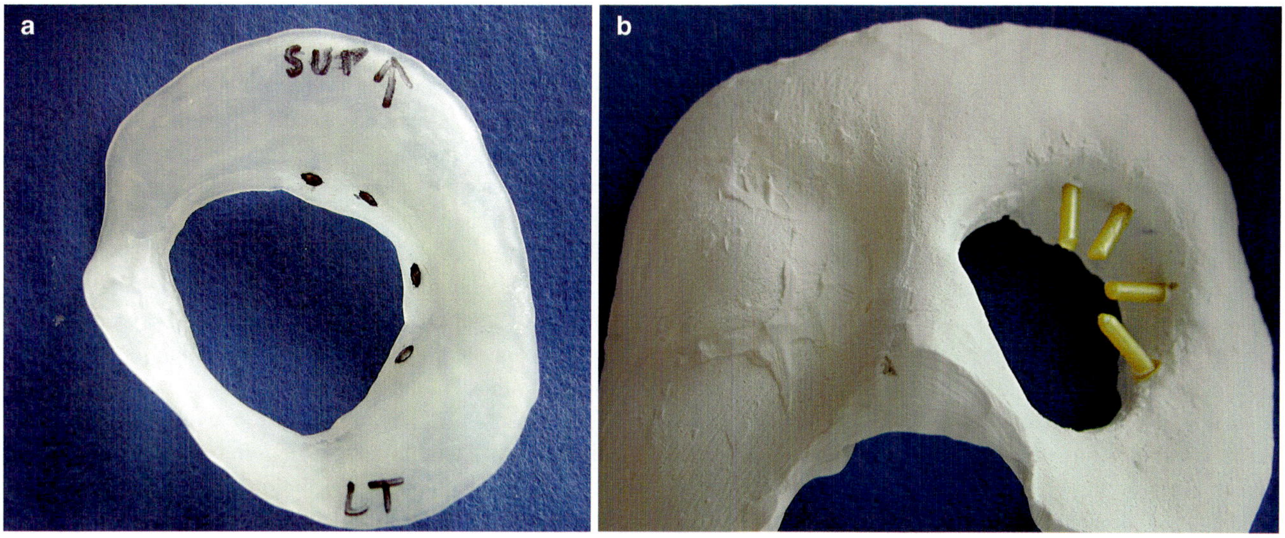

Fig. 66.20 (**a, b**) A surgical template indicates optimal implant location (**a**), and a positive model of the patient demonstrates the desired implant angle (**b**)

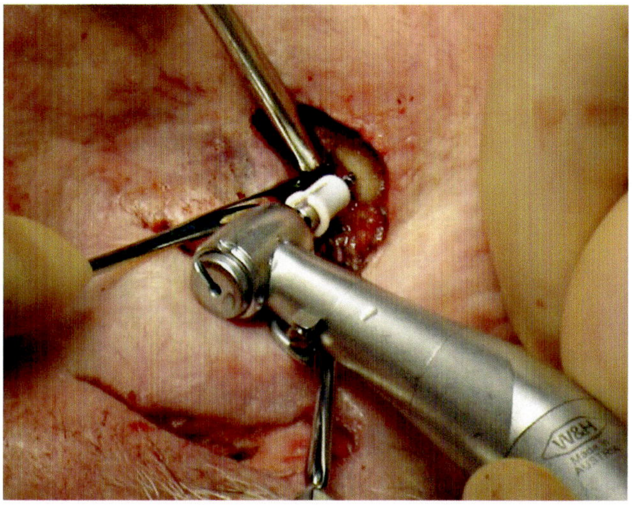

Fig. 66.21 Implant system instrumentation that is not designed for the orbital cavity makes optimal angulation of the implants challenging for the surgeon. Subsequent generation instruments have been made for easier use in the orbital cavity

tucked inside the orbital rim, so that the corresponding magnets and components can be optimally hidden within the prosthesis. If the angulation is sharper and pointing more anteriorly from the socket (which is naturally easier to place due to the tight orbital space and nose), the oculofacial prosthesis may potentially be much thicker and extend further forward than the contralateral face in order to cover the components. In contrast, placing the implants too flat behind the orbital rim may possibly make it more difficult for the patient to attach the prosthesis to the magnets. During surgery a model of the patient that demonstrates the desired angle of the implants is a useful reference (Fig. 66.20b). If computer-aided design is used, a 3-D model of the patient's partial skull can be printed as a reference for orientation of the surgical guide [37].

Magnet components have improved significantly in the past decade in terms of their strength and size. These improvements have reduced the use of complex bar splints, which are difficult for the patient to clean [15]. The surgical template or guide must be accurate and able to withstand sterilization. The template can be custom-made by the anaplastologist from rigid acrylic or flexible silicone as long as it is extensive enough to orient with confidence onto the orbital defect. Bone level guides are well described by Huang et al. and can be 3-D printed based on CT data [37].

During surgery, the smallest punch biopsy that can be used is best for creating the opening for drilling. This is typically a 4 mm punch size. Alternatively, a blade can be used to minimally open skin at the marked implant sites. As mentioned previously, the best sites for implant placement that will minimize implant loss are in areas of very thin and nonmobile tissue (Fig. 66.22). Thicker tissues surrounding the implants risk coverage of the implants and difficulty accessing the magnets. When drilling the implants into the bone, it is critical to use only the speed recommended, as faster speeds generate more heat and temperature rise and thus risk osseous damage that could affect the healing and osseointegration of implants. Although healing abutments can be placed at the primary surgery, this is often tedious for the patient to place compression wraps around the abutments on a routine basis to keep the surrounding tissue compressed to avoid covering the abutments. Therefore, it is often easier to close the skin over the implant fixture with a healing cap, which allows the patient to wear their current prosthesis in the interim healing period, and to later perform a second stage to open skin and place the final abutments in the implants after allowing appropriate time for osseointegration.

Process for Design and Fabrication of the Oculofacial Prosthesis

Correct and thorough assessment of the needs and priorities of each individual patient will contribute to the success of the prosthesis in terms of design, retention strategy, and patient acceptance [15]. A high level of compassion and empathy from the anaplastologist helps the patient express concerns and desires regarding prosthetic reconstruction of the orbital defect. Overcoming these obstacles is crucial for the patient and engaged caregivers in terms of hygiene of the defect and being able to apply and remove a prosthesis.

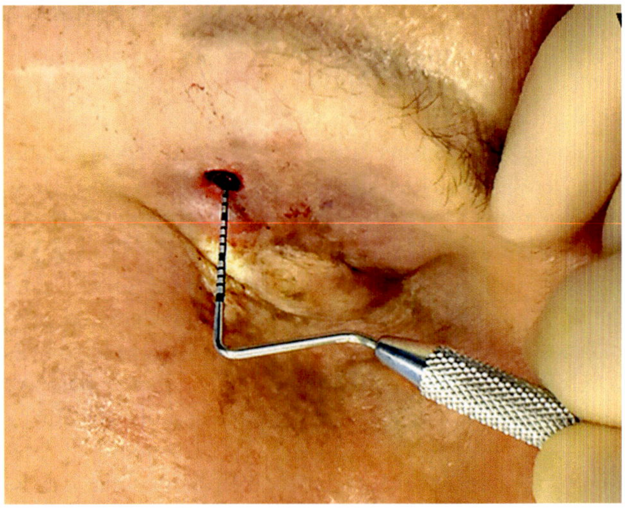

Fig. 66.22 After a biopsy punch is used to create the site of skin penetration, a dental perio probe can be used to measure skin thickness, which guides the selection of the implant to be placed. An implant that extends too far out from the skin will require more space within the prosthesis

Once a treatment plan and retention strategy has been developed, work can begin on the ocular component of the prosthesis. Ocular fabrication can be done while the orbital cavity is healing, which can encourage the patient by seeing some progress. The ocular should be custom-made so that every detail is tailored to match the individual. The correct anterior curvature of the eye is critical to the success of the sculpture of the eyelids. The iris size, pupil size, scleral tinting, and veining must be individualized for a convincing symmetrical match to the companion eye. The ocular prosthesis becomes the centerpiece around which the rest of the orbital prosthesis is created (Fig. 66.23a–c) [21].

The process of fabricating a custom eyelid, orbital, upper facial, or hemifacial prosthesis requires a minimum of four office visits by the patient. Appointments with the anaplastologist can be scheduled weekly or at the convenience of the patient. Because some patients travel a considerable distance to the anaplastologist's office, consolidated appointments may be arranged so that a prosthesis can be created over a 5-day period. The process should not take months to complete unless this is the patient's preference.

When the orbital defect is sufficiently healed, the anaplastologist needs to develop a replica of the defect area and the contralateral orbital region. A data acquisition appointment involves a facial moulage, 3-D facial scans, and/or photographs to facilitate sculpture of a prototype for the prosthesis. All of these processes are painless and efficient ways to collect the data necessary to begin sculpting the eyelids and surrounding tissue.

Locating the ocular prosthesis within the defect in the correct symmetrical position in all three dimensions is crucial to development of a convincing sculpture. Although the prototype is typically sculpted by hand in clay or wax (Fig. 66.24), a virtual prototype can also be created using computer-aided design and relevant software [40, 41].

At a subsequent appointment, the prototype is tried on the patient and input is solicited regarding comfort, contours, and appearance. Soft tissue movement and fit are analyzed and the prototype is modified until an appropri-

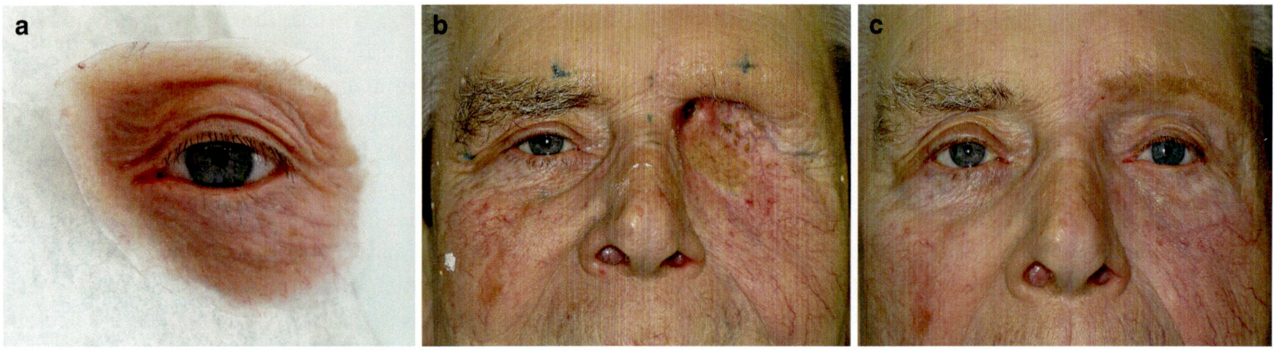

Fig. 66.23 (**a**–**c**) The ocular should be custom-made so that every detail is tailored to create a convincing symmetrical match

ate shape and fit is achieved. At this appointment, five or more individualized color formulae are developed to replicate subtle variations in the patient's complexion such as the caruncle, shadows and highlights, freckling, and capillaries (Fig. 66.25).

The anaplastologist spends considerable time in the lab finalizing the sculpture – recreating every skin fold, wrinkle, and textural detail. This can be done using traditional sculpting techniques or digital technologies [41]. Regardless of the methods used to produce the final sculpture, the anaplastologist must possess a mastery of the skills necessary to achieve a convincing likeness of the lost anatomy.

Considerable attention must also be devoted to design of the fitting or intaglio surface of the prosthesis. The intaglio surface must be as carefully designed as the external surface. It should be smooth and easy to clean – designed to minimize skin friction. When the treatment plan includes attachment to osseointegrated implants, the intaglio surface is commonly hollowed out so that the prosthesis only makes contact at the periphery (Fig. 66.26a, b). A substructure is designed to encase components of retention, such as magnets, to facilitate secure attachment.

Upon completion of the prototype, a durable mold is fabricated which provides for reproduction of the prosthesis in the selected materials. Mold fabrication can be achieved

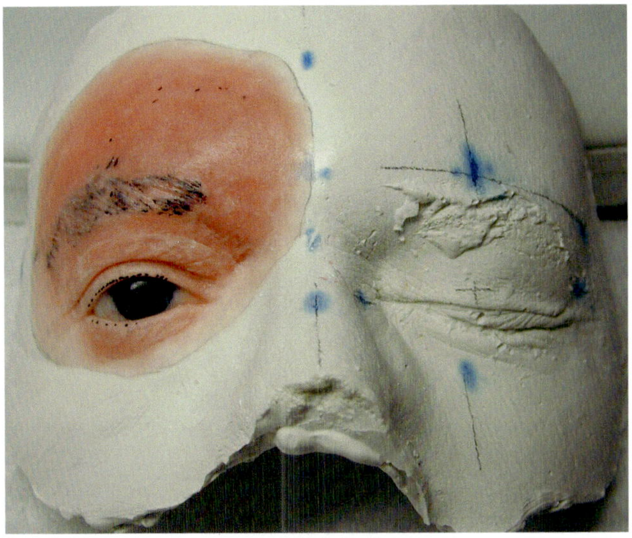

Fig. 66.24 Hand-sculpted wax prototype on patient cast

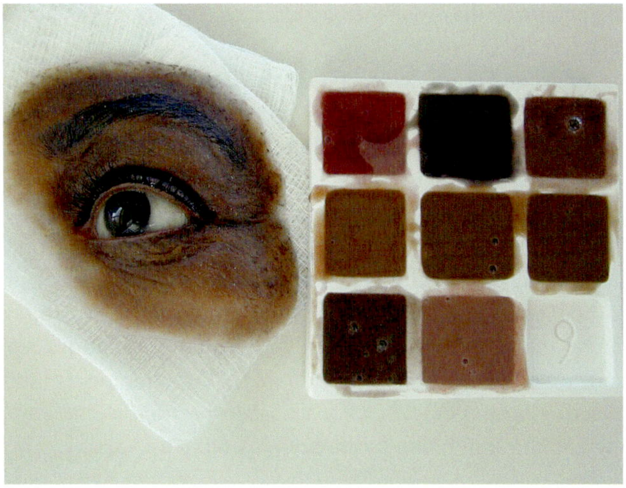

Fig. 66.25 Individualized color formulae are developed to replicate each patient's complexion

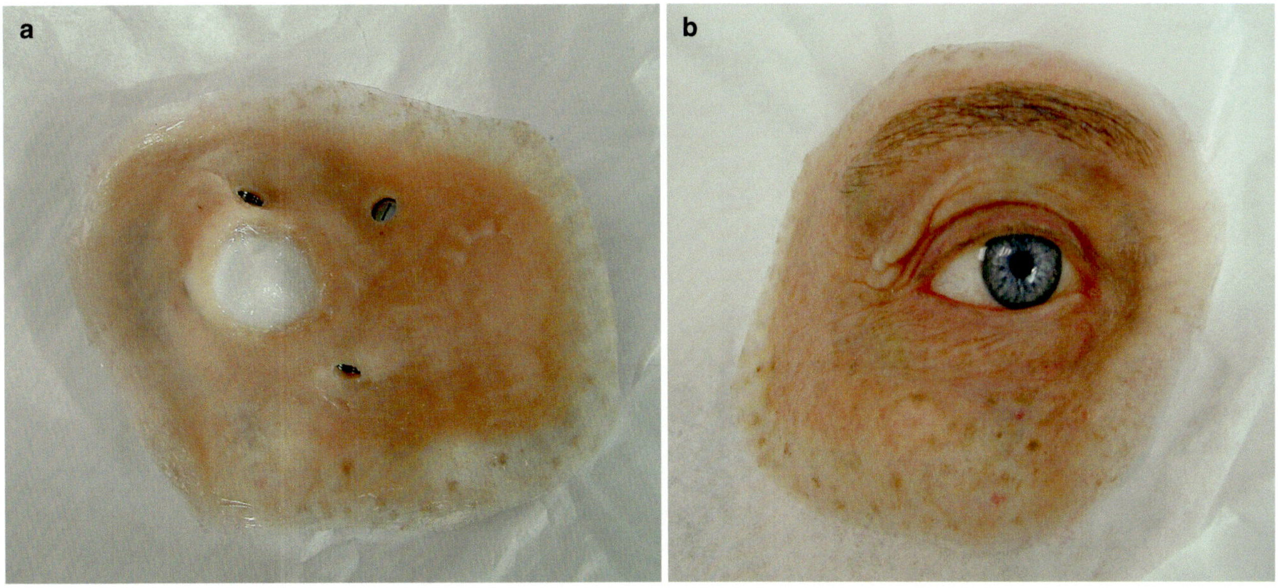

Fig. 66.26 (**a**, **b**) The intaglio surface (**a**) of this implant-retained hemifacial prosthesis (**b**) has been hollowed out so that the prosthesis only makes contact at the periphery

using standard mold making techniques or digital technology [41]. The mold should be designed to produce thin marginal edges and to be durable for repeated castings.

When the mold is complete pigmented silicone is painted onto its surface to imitate the anatomical layers that comprise the details of the patient's complexion. The ocular component is duplicated and becomes a third piece of the mold. Brow hairs can be laminated into the intrinsic coloration for a realistic appearance and durability (Fig. 66.27a, b). The mold is closed and allowed to cure, usually with heat. The patient returns for his/her delivery appointment and the prosthesis is tried on the patient – necessary adjustments are made and final color detail added extrinsically. Hair may be individually inserted simulating the eyebrow and eyelashes to enhance the realistic appearance of the prosthesis (Fig. 66.28).

Wear and care instructions are demonstrated for the patient and provided in writing, as the delivery appointment can be overwhelming for patients. The prosthesis can be worn for all normal daily activities, but adhesive retention can be challenging for swimming and some impact sports. The prosthesis should be removed for sleeping. Good hygiene of the prosthesis and the underlying skin is critical to maintaining normal usage of the prosthesis. The orbital cavity should be gently cleaned with a mild pH neutral soap and water or a sensitive skin baby wipe. Wipes are useful for cleaning orbital defects since visual inspection is challenging and the skin lining of the cavity is often thin and fragile. When implants are involved, the area around the abutments is best cleaned during or after bathing as the soap and water will soften any debris or crusting around the abutments.

The prosthesis should be cleaned each time it is removed with clear dish soap and water or isopropyl alcohol. However care should be taken not to soak the ocular component in alcohol. The prosthesis should be thoroughly dried and stored in a safe place at night. Semiannual or annual office

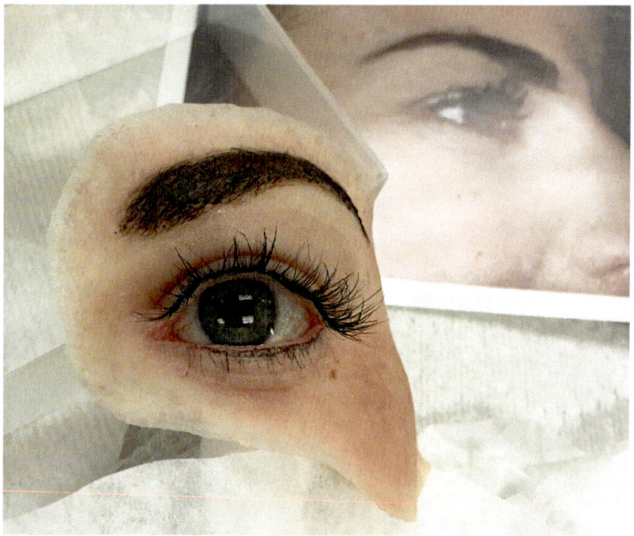

Fig. 66.28 Hair may be individually inserted into the prosthesis to simulate eyebrows and eyelashes

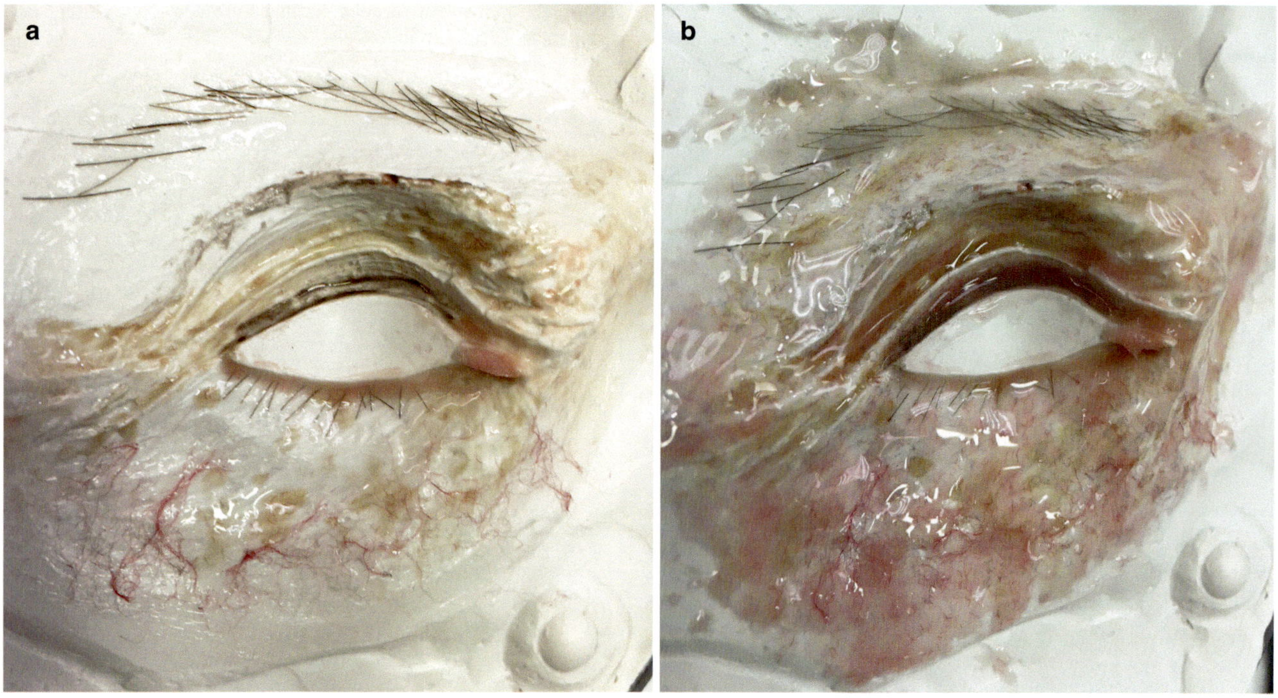

Fig. 66.27 (**a**, **b**) Progression of pigmented silicone being layered into the mold to replicate human skin. In addition to silicone, thread and hair may be laminated into the mold to mimic blood vessels, eyebrows, and eyelashes

visits may extend the life of the prosthesis by providing an opportunity for the anaplastologist to thoroughly clean the prosthesis, refresh eyelashes and brow hair, and touch up coloration. It is typical for color to fade over time, especially red pigments, and for the silicone to gradually yellow as it absorbs skin secretions [8].

Oculofacial prostheses have a useful life of 1–3 years. When the appearance of the prosthesis has degraded and can no longer be restored, the prosthesis should be replaced. If the prosthesis still fits properly, a replacement can be fabricated from the durable mold archived by the anaplastologist in a single appointment. If patient contours and fit have changed, then the fabrication process must be repeated to adapt to anatomical changes.

Conclusion

There is a lifetime relationship forged between the patient living with an orbitofacial defect and the anaplastologist. However, the anaplastologist is just one member of a larger team of medical professionals. Cross-disciplinary communication is crucial to oculofacial prosthetic rehabilitation, and the participation of an anaplastologist in the presurgical selection of optimum position and direction of anchoring elements is essential to the final outcome [4]. Patient acceptance of prosthetic substitution for an anatomical feature so fundamental to expression of emotion, self-perception, and social interaction depends on compassionate and ongoing communication.

References

1. Wei LA, Brown JJ, Hosek DK, Burkat CN. Osseointegrated implants for orbito-facial prostheses: preoperative planning tips and intraoperative pearls. Orbit. 2016; https://doi.org/10.3109/01676830.2015.1099699.
2. McNeill D. The face. New York: Little, Brown and Company; 1998.
3. Macgregor FC. Some psycho-social problems associated with facial deformities. Am Sociol Rev. 1951;16:629–38.
4. Brånemark PI, De Oliveira MF, editors. Craniofacial prostheses: anaplastology and osseointegration. Chicago: Quintessence Books; 1997.
5. Brown JJ, Duncan G. Anaplastology clinical practice standards: American Anaplastology Association; 2006.
6. Akamatsu T, Kawashima N, Tsunekuni T, Imagawa K, Miyasaka M. A blinking periorbital prosthesis using surface electromyographic signals of the orbicularis oculi muscle. Eur J Plast Surg. 2015;38(5):371–6.
7. Altman SM, Broderick CG, Caffrey E, Rond DS, inventors; Altman SM, Broderick CG, Caffrey E, Rond DS, assignees. Blink actuation mechanism for a prosthetic eye. United States patent US 9161833B1. 2013.
8. Visser A, Raghoebar GM, van Oort RP, Vissink A. Fate of implant-retained craniofacial prostheses: life span and aftercare. Int J Oral Maxillofac Implants. 2008;23(1):89–98.
9. McKinstry RE. Fundamentals of facial prosthetics. Arlington: ABI Professional Publications; 1995.
10. Federspil P. Implant-retained craniofacial prostheses for facial defects. GMS Curr Top Otorhinolaryngol Head Neck Surg. 2009;8(3):97–104
11. Brown JJ. Aesthetic maxillofacial prosthetic rehabilitation. In: Snow SN, Mikhail GR, editors. Mohs micrographic surgery. Madison, WI: The University of Wisconsin Press; 2004. p. 233–8.
12. Toljanic JA, Eckert SE, Roumanas E, Beumer J, Huryn JM, Zlotolow IM, et al. Osseointegrated craniofacial implants in the rehabilitation of orbital defects: an update of a retrospective experience in the United States. J Prosthet Dent. 2005;94(2):177–82.
13. Parel SM, Brånemark PI, Tjellström A, Gion G. Osseointegration in maxillofacial prosthetics. Part II: extraoral applications. J Prosthet Dent. 1986;55(5):600–6.
14. Granström G. Invited review craniofacial osseointegration. Oral Dis. 2007;13:261–9.
15. Thomas K. The art of clinical anaplastology. Great Britain: 4Edge Limited; 2006.
16. Asher ES, Evans JH, Wright RF, Wazen JJ. Fabrication and use of a surgical template for placing implants to retain an auricular prosthesis. J Prosthet Dent. 1999;81:228–33.
17. Wilkes GH, Wolfaardt JF. Craniofacial osseointegrated prosthetic reconstruction. In: Habal MB, editor. Advances in plastic and reconstructive surgery, vol. 15. St Louis: CV Mosby, Inc; 1998. p. 51–90.
18. Davis BK, Roumanis ED, Nishimura RD. Prosthetic-surgical collaborations in the rehabilitation of patients with head and neck defects. Otolaryngol Clin of North Am NA. 1997;30:631–45.
19. Hanasono MM, Lee JC, Yang JS, Skoracki RJ, Reece GP, Esmaeli B. An algorithmic approach to reconstructive surgery and prosthetic rehabilitation after orbital exenteration. Plast Reconstr Surg. 2009;123(1):98–105.
20. Hanasono MM. Reconstructive surgery for head and neck cancer patients. Adv Med. 2014; https://doi.org/10.1155/2014/795483.
21. Pine KR, Sloan BH, Jacobs RJ. Clinical ocular prosthetics. Cham: Springer; 2015.
22. Rahman I, Cook AE, Leatherbarrow B. Orbital exenteration: a 13 year Manchester experience. Br J Ophthalmol. 2005;89(10):1335–40.
23. Hanasono MM, Utley DS, Goode RL. The temporalis muscle flap for reconstruction after head and neck oncologic surgery. Laryngoscope. 2001;110(10):1719–25.
24. Tyers AG. Orbital exenteration for invasive skin tumours. Eye. 2006;20:1165–70.
25. Zarb GA, Albrektsson T. Osseointegration – a requiem for the periodontal ligament? Int J Periodontics Restorative Dent. 1991;11:88–91.
26. Albrektsson T, Brånemark PI, Hansson HA, Lindström J, Hallen O, Ohman A. Osseointegrated implants in the treatment of edentulous jaw. Experience from a 10-year period. Scand J Plast Reconstr Surg. 1977;11:1–175.
27. Vistafix. Treatment and surgery guide. Göthenburg: Vistafix; 2012.
28. Sennerby L, Meredith N. Implant stability measurements using resonance frequency analysis: biologic and biomechanical aspects and clinical implications. Periodontology. 2000;47:51–66.
29. Reinfeldt S, Hakansson B, Taghavi H, Eeg-Olofsson M. New developments in bone-conduction hearing implants: a review. Med Devices (Auckl). 2015;8:79–93.
30. Granström G, Tjellström A, Albrektsson T. Postimplantation irradiation for head and neck cancer treatment. Int J Oral Maxillofac Implants. 1993;8(4):1–6. (WAS 27).
31. Granström G, Bergström K, Tjellström A, Brånemark PI. A detailed analysis of Titanium implants lost in irradiated tissues. Int J Oral Maxillofac Implants. 1994;9:653–662. (WAS 28).
32. Curi MM, Oliveira MF, Molina G, Cardoso CL, de Oliveira LG, Brånemark PI, et al. Extraoral implants in the rehabilita-

tion of craniofacial defects: implant and prosthesis survival rates and peri-implant soft tissue evaluation. J Oral Maxillofac Surg. 2012;70(7):1551–7.

33. Holgers KM, Tjellström A, Bjursten LM, Erlandsson BE. Soft tissue reactions around percutaneous imlants: a clinical study on skin-penetrating titanium implants used for bone-anchored auricular prostheses. Int J Maxillofac Implants. 1987;2:35–9.
34. Fritsch MH, Naumann IC, Mosier KM. Baha devices and magnetic resonance imaging scanners. Otol Neurotol. 2008;29(8):1095–9.
35. Arndt S, Kromeier J, Berlis A, Maier W, Laszig R, Aschendorff A. Imaging procedures after bone anchored hearing aid implantation. Laryngoscope. 2007;117(10):1815–8.
36. Bedrossian E, Brånemark PI. Systematic treatment planning protocol for patients with maxillofacial defects: avoiding living a life of seclusion and depression. Atlas Oral Maxilofac Surg Clin North Am. 2012;20(1):135–58.
37. Huang YH, Seelaus R, Zhao L, Patel PK, Cohen M. Virtual surgical planning and 3D printing in prosthetic orbital reconstruction with percutaneous implants: a technical case report. Int Med Case Rep J. 2016;9:341–5.
38. Meltzer N, Garcia J, Byrne P, Boahene D. Image-guided titanium implantation for craniofacial prosthetics. JAMA Fac Plast Surg. 2009;11(1):58–61.
39. Reisberg D, Habakuk S. Use of a surgical positioner for bone-anchored facial prostheses. Int J Oral Maxillofac Implants. 1997;12:376–9.
40. Salazar-Gamarra R, Seelaus R, Lopes da Silva JV, Moreira da Silva A, Dib LL. Monoscopic photogrammetry to obtain 3D models by a mobile device: a method for making facial prostheses. J Otolaryngol Head Neck Surg. 2016;45:33.
41. Perry R. The development of an orbital prosthesis workflow using advanced digital technologies [thesis]. Baltimore: Johns Hopkins University; 2015. https://jscholarship.library.jhu.edu/handle/1774.2/39443

Index

A. J. Cohen, C. N. Burkat (eds.), *Oculofacial, Orbital, and Lacrimal Surgery*, https://doi.org/10.1007/978-3-030-14092-2

M

T

GPSR Compliance

The European Union's (EU) General Product Safety Regulation (GPSR) is a set of rules that requires consumer products to be safe and our obligations to ensure this.

If you have any concerns about our products, you can contact us on ProductSafety@springernature.com

In case Publisher is established outside the EU, the EU authorized representative is:

Springer Nature Customer Service Center GmbH
Europaplatz 3
69115 Heidelberg, Germany

Batch number: 10756636

Printed by Printforce, the Netherlands